ASH-SAP: American Society of Hematology Self-Assessment Program

ASH®-SAP
American Society of Hematology Self-Assessment Program

FOURTH EDITION

Editors

Stephanie A. Gregory, MD   Keith R. McCrae, MD

Chapter Authors

Donald M. Arnold, MD
Alan B. Cantor, MD, PHD
David C. Dale, MD
Georgette A. Dent, MD
Charles S. Eby, MD
Amy E. Geddis, MD, PHD
Irene M. Ghobrial, MD
Victor R. Gordeuk, MD
Timothy A. Graubert, MD
Stephanie A. Gregory, MD
Janna M. Journeycake, MD
Marc J. Kahn, MD
Neil E. Kay, MD
Ginna G. Laport, MD
Jacob P. Laubach, MD

Hillard M. Lazarus, MD, FACP
Cindy A. Leissinger, MD
Ross L. Levine, MD
Daniel C. Link, MD
Gary H. Lyman, MD, MPH
Alice D. Ma, MD
Jaroslaw P. Maciejewski, MD, PHD, FACP
Keith R. McCrae, MD
Bruno C. Medeiros, MD
Martha P. Mims, MD, PHD
Stephan Moll, MD
Vicki A. Morrison, MD
Charles H. Packman, MD
Josef T. Prchal, MD

Ching-Hon Pui, MD
Karen Quillen, MD, MPH
Charles T. Quinn, MD, MS
A. Koneti Rao, MD
Paul G. Richardson, MD
Gail J. Roboz, MD
Michal G. Rose, MD
Kerry J. Savage, MD, BSC, MSC
Amy D. Shapiro, MD
Don L. Siegel, MD, PHD, BSC
David P. Steensma, MD
Wendy Stock, MD
Lillian Sung, MD, PHD
Geoffrey L. Uy, MD
Guy Young, MD

© The American Society of Hematology

Published by

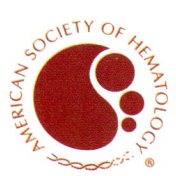

© 2010 The American Society of Hematology. All rights reserved. No parts of this publication may be reproduced, stored in a retrieval system, or transmitted in any form or by any means, electronic or mechanical, including photocopy, without prior consent of the American Society of Hematology.

American Society of Hematology
2021 L Street, NW, Suite 900
Washington, DC 20036
202-776-0544

ASH Customer Service Toll-Free (within U.S. only)
866-828-1231

First edition 2003
Second edition 2005
Third edition 2007
Fourth edition 2010

ISBN-13: 978-0-9828435-0-5

ISBN-10: 0-9828435-0-X

Set in 10/13pt Minion by Cadmus Communications.
Printed and bound by Cadmus Communications, Easton, PA.

Cover image copyright American Society of Hematology.
Blood image courtesy of Jing Huang and J. Evan Sadler, MD, Howard Hughes Medical Institute, Chevy Chase, MD.

Contents

Authors, ix
Acknowledgments, xi
Preface, xii
CME information, xiii
Disclosures, xiv
Claiming CME and ABIM credit, xx

Chapter 1: Molecular basis of hematology

Basic concepts, 1
Analytic techniques, 6
Clinical applications of DNA technology in hematology, 13
Glossary, 20
Bibliography, 23

Chapter 2: Consultative hematology

The role and effectiveness of the consultant, 27
Consultation for surgery and invasive procedures, 27
Intensive care unit, 35
Consultation for hematologic complications of solid organ transplantation, 40
Pregnancy, 42
Selected outpatient hematology topics, 52
Consultation in pediatric patients, 57
Bibliography, 64

Chapter 3: Hematopoietic growth factors

Myeloid growth factors, 75
Erythroid growth factors, 81
Platelet growth factors, 86
Other HGFs, 88
Bibliography, 88

Chapter 4: Iron metabolism, iron overload, and the porphyrias

Regulation of iron homeostasis, 93
Hereditary hemochromatosis and other iron overload syndromes, 96
The porphyrias, 101
Bibliography, 107

Chapter 5: Acquired underproduction anemias

Underproduction anemias resulting from nutritional deficiencies, 110
Megaloblastic anemias, 115
Underproduction anemias resulting from organ dysfunction, 121
Marrow failure states leading to underproduction anemias, 125
Anemia secondary to marrow infiltration or abnormalities in the marrow microenvironment, 127
Complex/multifactorial anemias, 128
Bibliography, 130

Chapter 6: Hemolytic anemias

Overview, 133
Hemolysis due to intrinsic abnormalities of the RBC, 134
Hemolysis due to extrinsic abnormalities of the RBC, 160
Bibliography, 175

Chapter 7: Thrombosis and thrombophilia

Pathophysiology of thrombosis, 179
Thrombophilias, 180
Antithrombotic drugs, 195
Venous thromboembolism, 202
Arterial thromboembolism, 210
Acknowledgment, 212
Bibliography, 212

Chapter 8: Bleeding disorders

Overview of hemostasis, 217
Approach to the patient with excessive bleeding, 219
Disorders of primary hemostasis, 220
Disorders of secondary hemostasis, 227
Disorders of fibrinolysis, 236
Bibliography, 238

Chapter 9: Disorders of platelet number and function

Platelet biology: structure and function, 241
Regulation of platelet number, 243
Immune causes of thrombocytopenia, 243
Nonimmune causes of thrombocytopenia, 250
Disorders of platelet function, 254
Bibliography, 260

Chapter 10: Laboratory hematology

General concepts, 263
Terminology, 263
Specific laboratory tests, 263
Bibliography, 288

Chapter 11: Transfusion medicine

Red blood cell transfusion, 291
Platelet transfusion, 297
Granulocyte transfusion, 303
Transfusion of plasma products, 304
Pretransfusion testing, 306
Apheresis, 308
Transfusion support in special clinical settings, 312
Transfusion risks, 321
Bibliography, 327

Chapter 12: Cellular basis of hematopoiesis and stem cell transplantation

Introduction and historical perspective, 331
Hematopoietic stem cell concepts, 331
Ontogeny of hematopoiesis, 334
Stem cell enrichment strategies, 335
Transplantation for specific diseases, 354
Late effects and long-term follow-up after transplantation, 365
Summary, 367
Bibliography, 367

Chapter 13: Myeloid disorders

Granulocytes: neutrophils, eosinophils, and basophils, 373
Monocytes and tissue histiocytes, 375
Dendritic cells, 376
Neutrophilia, 376
Neutropenia, 378
Disorders of neutrophil function, 385
Monocytosis, 388
Monocytopenia, 388
Disorders of histiocytes and DCs, 388
Lysosomal storage diseases, 392
Bibliography, 394

Chapter 14: Myeloproliferative neoplasms

Epidemiology, 398
Chronic myelogenous leukemia, *BCR-ABL1* positive, 398
Chronic neutrophilic leukemia, 406
Systemic mastocytosis, 407
Myeloid (and lymphoid) neoplasms associated with eosinophilia and abnormalities of *PDGFRA*, *PDGFRB*, or *FGFR1*, 410
Chronic eosinophilic leukemia, not otherwise specified, 413
Polycythemia vera, 414
Essential thrombocythemia, 425
Primary myelofibrosis, 431
Myeloproliferative neoplasm, unclassifiable, 437
Bibliography, 437

Chapter 15: Marrow failure syndromes

Congenital bone marrow failure syndromes, 443
Acquired bone marrow failure conditions, 450
Bibliography, 472

Chapter 16: Acute myeloid leukemia

Definition and epidemiology, 475
Clinical manifestations, 475
Subtype classification, 476
Prognostic factors, 477
Treatment, 479
Monitoring residual disease, 480
AML relapse, 480
Older patients with AML, 481
Acute promyelocytic leukemia (APL), 481
Pediatric AML, including Down syndrome, 483
Bibliography, 483

Chapter 17: Acute lymphoblastic leukemia and lymphoblastic lymphoma

Classification and diagnosis of ALL, 489
Immunophenotyping, 489
Cytogenetics, 490
Molecular genetics, 491
Prognostic factors, 492
Treatment of ALL, 493
Lymphoblastic lymphoma, 503
Late complications of therapy, 504
Bibliography, 504

Chapter 18: Lymphomas

Overview of lymphocyte development, 511
Non-Hodgkin lymphomas, 516
Immunodeficiency-associated lymphoproliferative disorders, 539
Hodgkin lymphoma, 541
Acknowledgment, 547
Bibliography, 548

Chapter 19: Chronic lymphocytic leukemia

Chronic lymphocytic leukemia, 555
Diagnosis, 557
Clinical and laboratory features, 559
Staging, 560
Prognostic factors, 560
Therapy, 564
Approach to newly diagnosed patients with high-risk disease, 569
Complications of CLL, 571
Quality-of-life issues, 572
Other indolent cell leukemias, 573
The future, 574
Bibliography, 574

Chapter 20: Plasma cell dyscrasias

Plasma cell development, 581
Etiology and incidence, 582
Molecular pathogenesis, 583
Plasmacytoma, 597
Other plasma cell disorders, 597
Acknowledgment, 599
Bibliography, 599

Index, 605

Authors

Donald M. Arnold, MD
Assistant Professor of Medicine
McMaster University
Hamilton, Ontario, Canada

Alan B. Cantor, MD, PHD
Assistant Professor of Pediatrics
Children's Hospital Boston Hospital
Division of Hematology/Oncology
Boston, MA

David C. Dale, MD
Professor of Medicine
Department of Medicine
University of Washington
Seattle, WA

Georgette A. Dent, MD
Associate Professor of Pathology and Laboratory Medicine
Associate Dean for Student Affairs
University of North Carolina School of Medicine
Chapel Hill, NC

Charles S. Eby, MD
Associate Professor of Medicine
Department of Pathology and Immunology
Laboratory and Genomic Medicine Division
Washington University School of Medicine
Saint Louis, MO

Amy E. Geddis, MD, PHD
Associate Professor of Pediatrics
University of California, San Diego
San Diego, CA

Irene M. Ghobrial, MD
Instructor of Medicine
Dana-Farber Cancer Institute
Boston, MA

Victor R. Gordeuk, MD
Director, Center for Sickle Cell Disease
Director, Division of Hematology and Oncology
Professor of Medicine, College of Medicine
Howard University
Washington, DC

Timothy A. Graubert, MD
Associate Professor of Medicine
Oncology Division, Stem Cell Biology Section
Washington University
Saint Louis, MO

Stephanie A. Gregory, MD
The Elodia Kehm Professor of Medicine
Director, Section of Hematology
Rush Medical College/Rush University Medicine Center
Chicago, IL

Janna M. Journeycake, MD
Associate Professor of Medicine
Department of Pediatrics
University of Texas Southwestern Medical Center at Dallas
Dallas, TX

Marc J. Kahn, MD
Professor of Medicine
Section of Hematology/Medical Oncology
Associate Dean for Admissions and Student Affairs
Tulane University School of Medicine
New Orleans, LA

Neil E. Kay, MD
Professor of Medicine
Mayo Clinic
Rochester, MN

Ginna G. Laport, MD
Associate Professor of Medicine
Division of Bone and Marrow Transplantation
Stanford University Medicine Center
Stanford, CA

Jacob P. Laubach, MD
Instructor in Medicine
Harvard Medical School
Dana-Farber Cancer Institute
Cambridge, MA

Hillard M. Lazarus, MD, FACP
Professor of Medicine
University Hospitals Case Medical Center
Cleveland, OH

Cindy A. Leissinger, MD
Professor of Medicine, Pediatrics, and Pathology
Chief, Section of Hematology and Medical Oncology
Director, Louisiana Comprehensive Hemophilia Center
Tulane University School of Medicine
New Orleans, LA

Ross L. Levine, MD
Geoffrey Beene Junior Faculty Chair
Human Oncology and Pathogenesis Program
Memorial Sloan-Kettering Cancer Center
New York, NY

Daniel C. Link, MD
Professor of Medicine
Oncology Division
Washington University Medicine School
Saint Louis, MO

Gary H. Lyman, MD, MPH
Professor of Medicine
Department of Medicine
Duke Comprehensive Cancer Center
Durham, NC

Alice D. Ma, MD
  Associate Professor of Medicine
    Division of Hematology and Oncology
  University of North Carolina, Chapel Hill
  Chapel Hill, NC

Jaroslaw P. Maciejewski, MD, PHD, FACP
  Chair, Department of Translational Hematology and Oncology
    Research
  Cleveland Clinic
  Cleveland, OH

Keith R. McCrae, MD
  Professor of Molecular Medicine
  Cleveland Clinic Lerner College of Medicine,
    and Taussig Cancer Institute
  Cleveland, OH

Bruno C. Medeiros, MD
  Assistant Professor of Medicine
  Stanford Comprehensive Cancer Center
  Stanford, CA

Martha P. Mims, MD, PHD
  Associate Professor of Medicine, Hematology/Oncology
  Baylor College of Medicine
  Houston, TX

Stephan Moll, MD
  Associate Professor of Medicine
  Division of Hematology and Oncology
  Department of Medicine
  University of North Carolina School of Medicine
  Chapel Hill, NC

Vicki A. Morrison, MD
  Associate Professor of Medicine
  Sections of Hematology/Oncology and Infectious Disease
  VA Medical Center
  Minneapolis, MN

Charles H. Packman, MD
  Chief, Hematology-Oncology Division
  Carolinas Medical Center
  Charlotte, NC

Josef T. Prchal, MD
  Professor of Internal Medicine
  Hematology Division
  University of Utah
  Salt Lake City, UT

Ching-Hon Pui, MD
  Chair, Department of Oncology
  St. Jude Children's Research Hospital
  Memphis, TN

Karen Quillen, MD, MPH
  Associate Professor of Pathology and Laboratory
    Medicine and of Medicine
  Boston Medical Center
  Boston, MA

Charles T. Quinn, MD, MS
  Director, Hematology Clinical and Translational Research
  Associate Professor of Clinical Pediatrics
  Cincinnati Children's Hospital Medicine Center
  Cincinnati, OH

A. Koneti Rao, MD
  Director, Sol Sherry Thrombosis Research Center
  Section Chief, Hematology
  Temple University School of Medicine
  Philadelphia, PA

Paul G. Richardson, MD
  Clinical Director, Jerome Lipper Center for Multiple Myeloma
  Associate Professor of Medicine
  Dana-Farber Cancer Institute
  Boston, MA

Gail J. Roboz, MD
  Associate Professor of Medicine
  Director, Leukemia Program
  Weill Medical College, Cornell University
  New York, NY

Michal G. Rose, MD
  Director, West Haven VA Cancer Center
  Associate Professor of Medicine
  Yale Medical School
  West Haven, CT

Kerry J. Savage, MD, BSC, MSC
  Assistant Professor
  British Columbia Cancer Agency
  Vancouver, British Columbia, Canada

Amy D. Shapiro, MD
  Medical Director
  Indianapolis Hemophilia and Thrombosis Center
  Indianapolis, IN

Don L. Siegel, MD, PHD, BSC
  Professor of Pathology and Laboratory Medicine
  University of Pennsylvania Medicine Center
  Philadelphia, PA

David P. Steensma, MD
  Associate Professor of Medicine
  Hematological Malignancies
  Dana-Farber Cancer Institute
  Boston, MA

Wendy Stock, MD
  Professor of Medicine
  Department of Medicine
  University of Chicago
  Section Hematology/Oncology
  Chicago, IL

Lillian Sung, MD, PHD
  Assistant Professor of Pediatrics
  Department of Pediatrics, Division of Hematology/Oncology
  The Hospital for Sick Children
  Toronto, Ontario, Canada

Geoffrey L. Uy, MD
  Assistant Professor of Medicine
  Division of Oncology
  Washington University
  School of Medicine
  Saint Louis, MO

Guy Young, MD
  Associate Professor of Pediatrics
  Director, Hemostasis/Thrombosis Program
  Children's Hospital Los Angeles
  Los Angeles, CA

Acknowledgments

The editors and authors of this fourth edition of the *American Society of Hematology Self-Assessment Program* (*ASH-SAP*) would like to acknowledge the efforts of the authors of the third edition, published by the American Society of Hematology. Content from selected chapters in the third edition formed the foundation of certain chapters or sections in the fourth edition of the *ASH-SAP*, and we are grateful to the following authors for the use of this content:

Thomas C. Abshire, MD
Kenneth C. Anderson, MD
George R. Buchanan, MD
Alan B. Cantor, MD, PHD
Mark A. Crowther, MD, MSC, FRCPC
Henry C. Fung MD, FRCPE
Francis J. Giles, MD
Jay H. Herman, MD
Teru Hideshima, MD, PHD
Meghan A. Higman, MD, PHD
Sima Jeha, MD
Thomas R. Klumpp, MD, FACP
Michael Linenberger, MD
Dana C. Matthews, MD

Robert E. Richard, MD, PHD
Nita L. Seibel, MD
Jamile M. Shammo, MD, FASCP
Kevin Shannon, MD
Akiko Shimamura, MD, PHD
Jamie E. Siegel, MD
Lewis R. Silverman, MD
F. Marc Stewart, MD
Mark M. Udden, MD
Koen van Besien, MD
Parameswaran Venugopal, MD
Ted Wun, MD, FACP
Marc S. Zumberg, MD

ASH would also like to thank the following individuals for their assistance in reviewing the *ASH-SAP* and/or providing other services contributing to the product:

Tahamtan Ahmadi, MD, PHD
Kenneth A. Bauer, MD
Nancy Berliner, MD
Hal E. Broxmeyer, PHD
Linda J. Burns, MD
Nicholas Burwick, MD
Douglas B. Cines, MD
Joseph M. Connors, MD
Rupali Das, MSC, PHD
Sherine F. Elsawa, PHD
Patrick F. Fogarty, MD

David Garcia, MD
Richard M. Kaufman, MD
Kevin Kuo, MD
John Lazarchick, MD
Jacob M. Rowe, MD
J. Evan Sadler, MD, PHD
Mikkael A. Sekeres, MD
Leslie E. Silberstein, MD
Lawrence A. Solberg, Jr., MD, PHD
Ramon V. Tiu, MD
James W. Vardiman, MD

Preface

This fourth edition of the *American Society of Hematology Self-Assessment Program* (*ASH-SAP*) serves as a resource for fellows in training, both as a review and as a resource to prepare for subspecialty board certification. It is also intended for the practicing hematologist as an update in the discipline that also provides continuing medical education credit and points toward American Board of Internal Medicine (ABIM) Maintenance of Certification. ABIM awarded ASH the ability to provide 70 points toward Maintenance of Certification as a result of the merit of the *ASH-SAP* case-based multiple-choice questions as well as the thoroughness of *ASH-SAP* as a complete hematology educational resource.

ASH-SAP provides material that is up to date, concise, and presented in an easy-to-read format. As with other editions, the material in the fourth edition has been extensively peer reviewed by selected external reviewers, authors of *ASH-SAP* chapters, the ASH Committee on Educational Affairs, and members of the ASH Trainee Council.

The fourth edition of *ASH-SAP* encompasses pediatric and adult hematology, including benign disorders, malignant disorders, stem cell transplantation, laboratory hematology, and transfusion medicine. Each chapter has been updated from the previous edition(s), and the multiple-choice questions are new. Moreover, five new chapters that focus on areas of rapid change and significant importance have been added to this current edition. A major goal of *ASH-SAP* is to provide challenging and informative multiple-choice questions for hematologists studying for certification or recertification exams. It has been said that the teacher's job is to make the act of decision making so difficult that the student can escape only by learning. Toward that end, the multiple-choice questions are challenging and designed to enforce an educational concept that is expanded upon in the critique.

In addition to updated text, the fourth edition has several other new elements:

- A new chapter on plasma cell dyscrasias
- A new chapter on thrombosis and thrombophilia
- A new chapter on disorders of platelet number and function
- A new chapter on bleeding disorders
- A new chapter of chronic lymphocytic leukemia and related disorders
- All new case-based multiple-choice questions with critiques
- Many new authors who are authorities in the topics they address
- New and updated clinical vignettes
- Updated links to other online resources including PubMed articles, articles in *Blood*, ASH Image Bank case studies and image sets, and *Hematology*, the ASH Education Program Book

As with the previous edition of *ASH-SAP*, the fourth edition builds on the contributions of authors of the first, second, and third editions, whom we would like to thank and acknowledge. We would also like to thank the current chapter authors, ASH Executive Committee, ASH Trainee Council, ASH Education Committee, and ASH leadership for their valuable input and insight. We are again indebted to Mr. Charles Rossi, Consulting Editor. His expert consultative review of each multiple-choice question provided assurance of outstanding educational value and consistency. Ms. Helena Mickle very ably served as Managing Editor, organizing and coordinating all aspects of development and production. We also wish to acknowledge Cadmus Communications Corp., especially Ms. Eve Malakoff-Klein, for assistance in the production of the printed books. Ms. Polly Siegel at HighWire Press was instrumental in producing the electronic component.

We hope that you find the fourth edition of *ASH-SAP* to be as valuable a resource as its previous editions, and we welcome your feedback concerning ways that we can continue to improve the usefulness and quality of *ASH-SAP*. Comments and/or recommendations can be forwarded to the ASH Education & Training Department at *cme@hematology.org*.

Stephanie A. Gregory, MD
Rush Medical College/Rush University Medical Center

Keith R. McCrae, MD
Cleveland Clinic Lerner College of Medicine,
and Taussig Cancer Institute

CME information

Two versions of this self-assessment are available: one is the standard version for *AMA Category 1 PRA Credit*™, and one awards lifelong learning points toward the American Board of Internal Medicine (ABIM) Maintenance of Certification program in addition to CME credits. The standard version includes a printed syllabus divided into chapters dedicated to specific topical areas in hematology, as well as a self-assessment exam book that includes case-based, multiple-choice questions and critiques. A Web-based multimedia component reflects the same information contained in the printed text and adds the platform for the online exam. For the *ASH-SAP* with Maintenance of Certification module, the printed question book is withheld, but access to the online hematology text and the online exam is included.

Accreditation

The American Society of Hematology (ASH) is accredited by the Accreditation Council for Continuing Medical Education to sponsor CME for physicians. ASH designates the standard version of this educational activity for a maximum of 50 *AMA PRA Category 1 Credits*™. Physicians should only claim credit commensurate with the extent of their participation in the activity. Physicians who participate in this CME activity but are not licensed in the United States are also eligible for *AMA PRA Category 1 Credits*™.

ASH designates the *ASH-SAP* with Maintenance of Certification module educational activity for a maximum of 50 *AMA PRA Category 1 Credits*™. Physicians should only claim credit commensurate with the extent of their participation in the activity.

Target audience

ASH-SAP is a high-quality educational product offering up-to-date information in the field of hematology for hematologists, medical oncologists, internists, pediatricians, and hematology-oncology fellows and trainees.

Educational objectives

The self-assessment's goals are:
1. to provide timely clinical updates on new developments in hematology
2. to help practicing physicians prepare for recertification
3. to serve as a tool for board review

Date of release:
July 2010

Online access expires/last date for users to claim CME credit for this edition:

July 2013

Disclosures

As a provider accredited by the Accreditation Council for Continuing Medical Education (ACCME), the American Society of Hematology must ensure balance, independence, objectivity, and scientific rigor in all of the educational activities it sponsors. All authors are expected to disclose any financial relationships with any proprietary entity producing health care goods or services that have occurred within 12 months from the start of or during the production of the work and that are relevant to the author's content. If an author has such a financial interest, then s/he must disclose the name of the commercial interest and nature of the relationship (e.g., consultant, grantee, etc.). If the author has no such financial relationship, s/he must declare that s/he has nothing to disclose. The intent of this disclosure is not to prevent an author with a significant financial or other relationship from making a presentation, but rather to provide readers with information on which they can make their own judgments. It remains for the audience to determine whether the author's interests or relationships may influence the work with regard to exposition or conclusion.

	Employ	Consultancy	Equity	Research funding	Honoraria	Patents, royalties	Speakers' bureau	Membership on board of directors or advisory committee	Other (specify)
Donald M. Arnold, MD		Amgen Canada		Hoffman-La Roche	CME lectures at McMaster University, funded by unrestricted educational grant from GlaxoSmithKline				
Alan B. Cantor, MD, PHD									
David C. Dale, MD		Amgen, Biota, Regeneron, Schering-Plough, Tarix, Telik		Amgen, Genzyme, Merck, Schering-Plough, Telik, Barth Foundation, National Institutes of Health, University of Washington	Amgen, Biota, Caremark, Cellerant, Regeneron, Schering-Plough, Tarix, Telik, BCDecker, Wolters Kluwer Health (Lippincott Williams & Wilkins), American College of Physicians, US Department of Health and Human Services	Book chapters and editing for Wolters Kluwer Health (Lippincott Williams & Wilkins)	Amgen	Cellerant (Scientific Advisory Board), Schering-Plough (Data Safety Monitoring Board)	
Georgette A. Dent, MD									
Charles S. Eby, MD		Barr Pharmaceuticals		Osmetech, Beckman-Coulter, Stago Diagnostica	Genome Quebec				
Amy E. Geddis, MD, PHD				Amgen				Amgen	
Irene M. Ghobrial, MD				Millennium	Millennium, Celgene		Millennium, Celgene, Novartis	Millennium, Celgene, Novartis	
Victor R. Gordeuk, MD		Merck, Amgen, Ikaria		Merck, TRF Pharma, Biomarin			Novartis		
Timothy A. Graubert, MD									
Stephanie A. Gregory, MD		Amgen, Genentech		Amgen, Boehringer Ingelheim, Celgene, CTI, Genentech, GenMab, GlaxoSmithKline, Gloucester Pharmaceuticals, Millennium, NCIC CTG, Rigel Pharmaceuticals			Genentech, GlaxoSmithKline, Millennium		

(Continued)

	Employ	Consultancy	Equity	Research funding	Honoraria	Patents, royalties	Speakers' bureau	Membership on board of directors or advisory committee	Other (specify)
Janna M. Journeycake, MD					Baxter Healthcare			Physicians Advisory Council of Baxter Healthcare	Grant support: NIH K23 Career Development Award
Marc J. Kahn, MD									
Neil E. Kay, MD		Cephalon		Celgene, Genentech, Polyphenon E International, Hospira				Genentech, Biogen Idec	
Ginna G. Laport, MD					Genzyme				
Jacob P. Laubach, MD								Novartis	
Hillard M. Lazarus, MD, FACP					Genentech/Biogen IDEC		Genentech/Biogen IDEC		
Cindy A. Leissinger, MD									
Ross L. Levine, MD		Novartis, Cephalon, TargeGen (all on one-time basis)			Novartis, Cephalon (paid talks)				
Daniel C. Link, MD									
Gary H. Lyman, MD, MPH				Amgen			Amgen		
Alice D. Ma, MD									
Jaroslaw P. Maciejewski, MD, PHD, FACP									
Keith R. McCrae, MD		GlaxoSmithKline			GlaxoSmithKline				
Bruno C. Medeiros, MD		Millennium, Antisoma		Genentech			Celgene, Novartis		

Martha P. Mims, MD, PHD	Amgen, Genentech, Imclone, Roche, IDEC		Grant support: CDC grant
Stephan Moll, MD	Bayer, Roche Diagnostics, International Technidyne Corp., Lundbeck, GTC Biotherapeutics, Talecris, Ortho McNeil-Janssen Pharmaceuticals	International Technidyne Corp.	Lundbeck, Talecris
Vicki A. Morrison, MD			Merck, Pfizer, Genentech, Celgene, Amgen	Merck, Celgene
Charles H. Packman, MD			
Josef T. Prchal, MD			
Ching-Hon Pui, MD		EUSA Pharma, Sanofi-Aventis	
Karen Quillen, MD, MPH			
Charles T. Quinn, MD, MS			
A. Koneti Rao, MD			
Paul G. Richardson, MD			Celgene, Millennium, Johnson & Johnson	Celgene, Millennium, Johnson & Johnson
Gail J. Roboz, MD		Celgene, Eisai, Genzyme, Novartis, Cephalon	
Michal G. Rose, MD			

(Continued)

	Employ	Consultancy	Equity	Research funding	Honoraria	Patents, royalties	Speakers' bureau	Membership on board of directors or advisory committee	Other (specify)
Kerry J. Savage, MD, BSC, MSC					Roche, Eli Lilly				
Amy D. Shapiro, MD		Baxter BioScience, Inspiration Biopharmaceuticals, Syntonix					Baxter BioScience, Novo Nordisk	Baxter BioScience, Novo Nordisk, Bayer Healthcare, Inspiration Biopharmaceuticals, Catalyst Biosciences, American Thrombosis and Hemostasis Network, National Hemophilia Foundation	Clinical research protocols: Baxter BioScience, Novo Nordisk, Bayer Healthcare Pharmaceuticals, Wyeth Pharmaceuticals, Inspiration Biopharmaceuticals; NIH/NHLBI: Clinical Trial Review Board, Data Safety Management Board
Don L. Siegel, MD, PHD, BSC									
David P. Steensma, MD				Amgen, Johnson & Johnson, Novartis					
Wendy Stock, MD		Hana Biosciences		Enzon	Enzon				
Lillian Sung, MD, PHD									
Geoffrey L. Uy, MD		Genzyme		Genzyme, Novartis Oncology	Novartis Oncology		Genzyme		
Guy Young, MD		Novo Nordisk, Baxter, Bayer			Novo Nordisk, Baxter, Bayer			Novo Nordisk, Baxter, Bayer	

In compliance with ACCME policy, the American Society of Hematology also requires all authors to disclose any discussion of off-label drug use.

Dr. Arnold will discuss rituximab for ITP.

Dr. Ghobrial will discuss bortezomib in Waldenström macroglobulinemia and use of lenalidomide in upfront therapy for myeloma.

Dr. Gregory will discuss rituximab maintenance after rituximab chemotherapy in lymphoma, radioimmunotherapy for consolidation therapy after chemotherapy for initial treatment of lymphoma, bortezomib and combinations in Waldenström macroglobulinemia, rituximab in hairy cell leukemia, R-CHOP in localized DLBCL, and thalidomide in mantle cell lymphoma.

Dr. Journeycake will discuss anticoagulant agents in children.

Dr. Kay will discuss pentostatin and lenalidomide for CLL.

Dr. Maciejewski will discuss off-label use of cyclosporine A, prednisone, and danazol.

Dr. Moll will discuss new oral anticoagulants rivaroxaban, apixaban, and dabigatran.

Dr. Quillen will discuss use of recombinant factor VII in refractory bleeding.

Dr. Rao will discuss DDVAP for treatment of platelet disorders.

Dr. Richardson will discuss upfront use of lenalidomide.

Dr. Savage will discuss rituximab maintenance after rituximab chemotherapy in lymphoma, radioimmunotherapy for consolidation therapy after chemotherapy for initial treatment of lymphoma, bortezomib and combinations in Waldenström macroglobulinemia, rituximab in hairy cell leukemia, R-CHOP in localized DLBCL, and thalidomide in mantle cell lymphoma.

Dr. Shapiro will discuss rFVIIa as high-dose therapy and for rare disorders.

Dr. Siegel will discuss use of recombinant factor VIIa for bleeding.

Dr. Young will discuss rFVIIa (Novoseven) for management of bleeding in hemophilia at doses and regimens that are not approved and for other off-label indications and prothrombin complex concentrates (various brand names) for treatment of warfarin overdose, vitamin K deficiency, and liver disease.

Claiming CME and ABIM credit

Scores of 80% or better on the self-assessment exams are eligible to claim credit for the activity. On **July 31, 2013**, on-line access expires; this is also the last date for users to claim credit for this edition. The remainder of this section details the types of credit available for completing this activity. For questions about credit, please contact the ASH Education & Training Department at *cme@hematology.org* or call toll-free 866-828-1231 (within United States only).

Category 1 CME Credits
Two versions of this self-assessment are available, and each version is designated for a maximum of 50 *AMA PRA Category 1 Credits*™. Physicians should only claim credit commensurate with the extent of their participation in the activity.

Standard Version
In order to receive *AMA PRA Category 1 Credits*™ for participation in this activity, you must first complete the self-assessment test. To receive 50 Category 1 CME Credits for the standard version, go to *www.ash-sap.org* to complete the exam for the standard version. The test can be taken all at once, or parts of it can be completed at the end of each chapter and saved until the entire program is completed.

ASH-SAP with Maintenance of Certification Module
In order to receive 50 *AMA PRA Category 1 Credits*™ for participation in the *ASH-SAP* with American Board of Internal Medicine (ABIM) Maintenance of Certification (MOC) Module version, you must first complete the ABIM-MOC self-assessment test online at *www.ash-sap.org*. The test can be taken all at once, or parts of it can be completed at the end of each chapter and saved until the entire program is completed.

ABIM Maintenance of Certification points
You may only receive lifelong learning points toward the ABIM Maintenance of Certification program if you are using the *ASH-SAP with ABIM Maintenance of Certification Module* version of this activity, and you must complete this exam **online** at *www.ash-sap.org*. You must also be currently enrolled in the ABIM Maintenance of Certification program to earn these points.

Please refer to the *ASH-SAP* website at *www.ash-sap.org* for further information about the number of lifelong learning points to be awarded and how these points are processed.

CHAPTER 01

Molecular basis of hematology

Martha P. Mims, Timothy A. Graubert, and Josef T. Prchal

Basic concepts, 1
Analytic techniques, 6
Clinical applications of DNA technology in hematology, 13
Glossary, 20
Bibliography, 23

Basic concepts

Advances in recombinant DNA technology over the past 25 years have substantially altered our view of biologic processes and have immediate relevance to our understanding of both normal hematopoietic cell function and hematologic pathology. A complete review of molecular genetics is beyond the scope of this text, but the following is intended as a brief review of the concepts of the molecular biology of the gene, an introduction to epigenetics and genomics, an outline of noncoding RNAs, and an explanation of the terminology necessary for understanding the role of molecular biology in breakthrough discoveries. Emerging diagnostic and therapeutic approaches in hematology and an outline of gene therapy approaches will be reviewed. The promise of inducible pluripotent stem cells (iPSCs) will be introduced. The concepts outlined in the following sections are also illustrated in Figure 1-1; in addition, bolded terms in the text are summarized in a glossary at the end of the chapter. Several examples of how these concepts and techniques are applied in clinical practice are included.

Anatomy of the gene
Structure of DNA

DNA is a complex, double-stranded molecule composed of **nucleotides**. Each nucleotide consists of a **purine** (adenine or guanosine) or **pyrimidine** (thymine or cytosine) base attached to a deoxyribose sugar residue. Each strand of DNA is a succession of nucleotides linked through phosphodiester bonds between the 5′ position of the deoxyribose of one nucleotide and the 3′ position of the sugar moiety of the adjacent nucleotide. The 2 strands are connected through hydrogen bonds between paired purine–pyrimidine nucleotides. Hydrogen bonding can occur only between strict pairs of purines and pyrimidines; that is, adenine must be paired with thymine (A-T) and guanosine must be paired with cytosine (G-C). This is known as Watson–Crick base pairing. Consequently, the 2 strands of DNA are said to be **complementary**, in that the sequence of one strand determines the sequence of the other through the demands of strict base pairing. The 2 strands are joined in an antiparallel manner so that the 5′ end of one strand is joined with the 3′ end of the complementary strand. The strand containing the codons for amino acid sequences is designated as the sense strand, whereas the opposite strand that is transcribed into messenger RNA (mRNA) is referred to as the antisense strand.

Structure of the gene

DNA dictates the biologic functions of the organism by the flow of genetic information from DNA to RNA to protein. The functional genetic unit responsible for the production of a given protein, including the elements that control the timing and the level of its expression, is termed a **gene**. The gene contains several critical components that determine both the amino acid structure of the protein it encodes and the mechanisms by which the production of that protein may be controlled. The **coding sequence**, which dictates protein sequence, is contained within **exons**; these stretches of DNA may be interrupted by intervening **noncoding sequences**, or **introns**. In addition, there are **flanking sequences** in the 5′ and 3′ ends of the coding sequences that often contain

---

Conflict-of-interest disclosure: *Dr. Mims:* equity: Amgen, IDEC; research funding: Genentech, Imclone, Roche, Novartis. *Dr. Graubert* declares no competing financial interest. *Dr. Prchal* declares no competing financial interest.

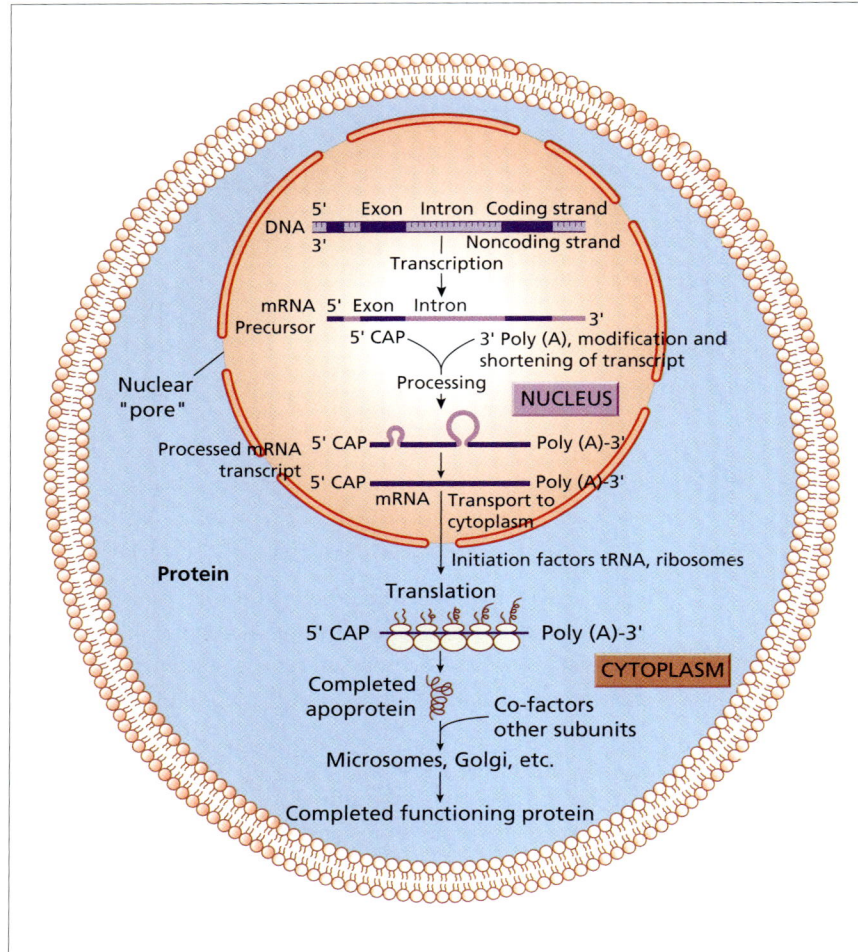

Figure 1-1 Flow of genetic information from DNA to RNA protein. DNA is shown as a double-stranded array of alternating introns and exons. Transcription, posttranscriptional processing by splicing, polyadenylation, and capping are described in the text. The mature transcript passes from the nucleus to the cytoplasm, where it is translated and posttranslationally modified to form a mature protein. Reproduced with modifications with permission from Benz EJ Jr. Anatomy and physiology of the gene. In: Hoffman R, Benz EJ Jr, Shattil SJ, Furie B, Cohen HJ, eds. *Hematology: Basic Principles and Practice.* New York, NY: Churchill Livingstone; 1991.

important regulatory elements that control the expression of the gene.

Genes are arrayed in a linear fashion along **chromosomes**, which are long DNA structures complexed with protein. Within chromosomes, DNA is bound in **chromatin**, a complex of DNA with histone and nonhistone proteins that "shield" the DNA from the proteins that activate gene expression. For a gene to be expressed, this tight complex must be unwound and made more accessible to regulatory proteins. Both histone deacetylation and methylation contribute to repression of gene expression. Generally, histone deacetylases maintain chromatin in the repressed state. In addition to being complexed with protein, the DNA of inactive genes is modified by the addition of methyl groups to cytosine residues. **Methylation** is generally a marker of an inactive gene, and changes in gene expression can often be correlated with characteristic changes in the degree of methylation of the 5′ regulatory sequences of the gene. Methylation and other DNA changes separate from the nucleotide sequence may be modulated by nutrition or drugs and may also be heritable. These changes constitute **epigenetic** control of gene expression.

Epigenetics
DNA methylation

Epigenetic modulation of gene expression was first recognized in studies of glucose-6-phosphate dehydrogenase (G6PD), a protein encoded by an X-linked gene. Ernest Beutler deduced the principle of random embryonic X chromosome inactivation from studies of G6PD deficiency. His observations and the studies of Mary Lyon and Susumu Ohno on the mechanism of dosage compensation in mammals led to the understanding of X chromosome inactivation in females. This was the first example of stochastic epigenetic silencing in humans, demonstrating that human females are mosaics of activity of X chromosome–encoded genes. Using this principle in tumor tissue derived from females led to the strongest evidence that neoplastic diseases are, for the most part, clonal. Indeed, these studies, performed 40 years ago, predicted the importance of epigenetics years before most of the scientific community fully understood it. X chromosome inactivation is largely modulated by a differential methylation of DNA and histone sequences.

Monozygotic twins accumulate different methylation patterns in the DNA sequences of their somatic cells as they age, increasing phenotypic differences. Lifestyle disparities, especially smoking, result in even greater differences in their DNA methylation patterns. Thus despite having identical DNA sequences, twins become increasingly dissimilar due to epigenetic changes that result in different expression of their identically inherited genes. Epigenetic DNA modulation changes gene activity; thus in one form of hereditary colorectal cancer, methylation of the promoter region of the *MLH1* gene, whose protein product repairs damaged DNA, results in colon cancer.

Mendelian genetics is based on the principle that the phenotype is the same whether an allele is inherited from the mother or the father, but this does not always hold true. Some human genes are transcriptionally active on only one copy of a chromosome such as the copy inherited from the father, whereas the other copy of the chromosome inherited from the mother is transcriptionally inactive. This mechanism of gene silencing is known as **imprinting**, and these transcriptionally silenced genes are said to be "imprinted." When genes are imprinted, they are usually heavily methylated in contrast to the nonimprinted copy of the allele, which is typically not methylated.

A classical example of imprinting is associated with deletion of approximately 4 megabases (Mb) on the long arm of chromosome 15. When this deletion is inherited from the father, the child manifests Prader-Willi syndrome, whose features include short stature, hypotonia, obesity, mild mental retardation, and hypogonadism. The same deletion, when inherited from the mother, causes Angelman syndrome, which is characterized by severe mental retardation, seizures, and an ataxic gait. The deletions that cause Prader-Willi and Angelman syndromes are indistinguishable at the DNA sequence level and affect the same group of genes. The causative gene of Angelman syndrome encodes a ligase essential for ubiquitin-mediated protein degradation during brain development. In brain tissue, this gene is active only on the chromosome copy inherited from the mother. Consequently, a maternally transmitted deletion removes the single active copy of this gene. Several genes in the critical region are associated with Prader-Willi syndrome, and they are transcribed only on the chromosome transmitted by the father. A paternally transmitted deletion removes the only active copies of these genes, producing the features of Prader-Willi syndrome.

Another mechanism of Prader-Willi syndrome is **uniparental disomy**. Uniparental disomy occurs when 2 copies of a chromosome, or part of a chromosome, are inherited from one parent but none are inherited from the other parent as a result of an error during meiosis. When 2 copies of the maternal chromosome 15 are inherited, Prader-Willi syndrome results because no active paternally transmitted genes are present. When this occurs during mitotic division of somatic cells, acquired uniparental disomy can contribute to cancer because of a reduction in tumor suppressor gene expression or an increase in oncogene expression. Acquired uniparental disomy is the mechanism by which the homozygous *JAK2* V617F mutation develops in polycythemia vera.

More recently, it has been described that epigenetic control of gene expression is determined by location of the gene in relationship to the nuclear core and nuclear pores and its association with lamina-associated proteins, lamins, which can affect the transcriptional activity of the affected gene(s) by their subnuclear localization.

Flow of genetic information
Transcription

RNAs are mostly single-stranded molecules that differ from DNA in 2 ways: by a sugar backbone composed of ribose rather than deoxyribose, and by containing the pyrimidine uracil rather than thymine. The first step in the expression of protein from a gene is the synthesis of a **premessenger RNA** (premRNA). The **transcription** of premRNA is directed by **RNA polymerase II**, which in conjunction with other proteins generates an RNA copy of the DNA sense strand. This transcribed mRNA is complementary to the DNA antisense strand. The premRNA contains the sequences of all of the gene's exons and introns. The introns are then removed by a complex process called mRNA **splicing**. This process involves the recognition of specific sequences on either side of the intron that allow its excision in a precise manner that maintains the exon sequence. The mRNA may then undergo modifications at the 5′ and 3′ ends (**capping** and **polyadenylation**, respectively). Although RNA splicing was thought to be nucleus specific, recently it has been shown to take place in the cytoplasm of platelets and neutrophils activated by external stimuli.

Splicing of mRNA is a critical step in gene expression with important implications for understanding hematologic disease. Splicing is controlled by the spliceosome, a large complex of proteins (50–100) and 5 small nuclear ribonuclear proteins (snRNPs). mRNA splicing is an important mechanism for generating diversity of the proteins produced by a single gene. Some genes exhibit **alternative splicing**, a process by which certain exons are included in or excluded from the mature mRNA, depending on which splice sequences are used in the excision process. For example, this is the means by which some erythroid-specific proteins of heme synthesis (aminolevulinic acid [ALA] synthase) and energy metabolism (pyruvate kinase) are generated, contrasting with the alternatively processed genes in liver and other tissues. This permits functional diversity of the products of the same gene and is one of several determinants of tissue specificity of cellular proteins. Mutations in the sequences of either introns or exons can derange the splicing process by either creating or destroying a splice site so that intron sequence is not removed or exon sequence is eliminated. If abnormal splicing results in a premature stop codon (nonsense mutation), then a surveillance pathway known as **nonsense-mediated decay (NMD)** may result in degradation of the abnormal mRNA. This mechanism generally applies to stop codon mutations in the first one third to one half of the mRNA and works to prevent synthesis of mutant peptides. When mutations occur in the last one third of the mRNA molecule, abnormal peptides may be produced.

Translation

The mature mRNA is transported from the nucleus to the cytoplasm, where it undergoes **translation** into protein. The mRNA is "read" in a linear fashion by **ribosomes**, structures composed of ribonucleoprotein that move along the mRNA and insert the appropriate amino acids, carried by **transfer RNAs (tRNAs)**, into the nascent protein. The amino acids are encoded by 3 base triplets called **codons**, the **genetic code**. The 4 bases can encode 64 possible codons; because there are only 20 amino acids used in protein sequences, more than one codon may encode the same amino acid. For this reason, the genetic code has been termed **degenerate**. However, although an amino acid may be encoded by more than one codon, any single codon encodes only one amino acid. The beginning of the coding sequence in mRNA is encoded by AUG codon that has a variable translation initiation activity determined by the neighboring nucleotide sequences (Kozak sequence); that modulates translation by eukaryotic ribosomes. The Kozak sequence is ACCATGG. In addition, there are 3 **termination codons** (UAA, UAG, and UGA) that mark the end of the protein sequence.

In the context of these facts, single base pair alterations in the coding sequence of genes may have a range of effects on the resultant protein. Because the genetic code is degenerate, some single base pair changes may not alter the amino acid sequence, or they may change the amino acid sequence in a manner that has no effect on the overall function of the protein; these will be phenotypically silent mutations. Sickle cell disease, however, is caused by a single base pair change (point mutation), resulting in an amino acid alteration that critically changes the chemical characteristics of the resultant globin molecule. Other mutations may change a codon to a termination codon, resulting in premature termination of the protein (nonsense mutation). Finally, single or multiple base pair insertions or deletions can disrupt the reading of the sequence of a gene's 3 base pairs (bp). These **frameshift mutations** render the gene incapable of encoding normal protein. These latter 2 abnormalities account for some β thalassemias and for polycythemia due to gain of function in the erythropoietin receptor. Clinically important mutations may occur in the noncoding region of genes, such as in the regulatory elements upstream of the initiation codon or within intronic splicing sites.

Control of gene expression

With the exception of lymphocytes (which undergo unique changes in the DNA encoding immunoglobulin and/or the T-cell receptor) and germ cells (which contain only half the DNA of somatic cells), each nucleated cell of an organism contains identical DNA. Consequently, biologic processes are critically dependent on **gene regulation**, the control of gene expression such that proteins are produced only at the appropriate time within the appropriate cells. Gene regulation is the result of a complex interplay of specific sequences within a gene locus, chromatin, and regulatory proteins (transcription factors) that interact with those sequences to increase or decrease the transcription from that gene.

DNA sequences that lie in proximity to and regulate the expression of genes, which encode protein, are termed *cis-acting regulatory elements*. Within the first 50 bases 5′ to the **structural gene** is a site for binding of RNA polymerase II for nearly all genes; this is called the **promoter** region. Other sequences that regulate the level of transcription of the gene are located at less predictable distances from the structural gene. Such sequences may increase (**enhancers**) or decrease (**silencers**) expression. A special type of enhancer is locus control region (LCR), which was first and best defined in the β-globin cluster of genes on chromosome 11. It is located approximately 50 kilobases (kb) upstream from the β globins gene, controls all genes in the β-globin locus, and also has a strong tissue-specific activity (erythroid specific).

Control of gene expression is exerted through the interaction of the *cis*-acting elements described previously with proteins that bind to those sequences. These nuclear DNA binding proteins are termed ***trans*-acting factors**, or **transcription factors**. Most of these proteins have a DNA binding domain that can bind directly to regulatory sequences within the gene locus; many of them contain common motifs, such as **zinc-fingers** or **leucine zippers**, which are shared by many transcription factors. In addition, they frequently have unique domains that allow them to interact with other transcription factors. Thus, a complex pattern is emerging whereby the expression of different transcription factors, which may interact both with one another and with specific regions of DNA to increase or decrease transcription, determines the unique tissue and stage-specific expression of the genes within a given cell.

Recently, the role of small interfering RNAs (**siRNAs**) and **microRNAs** in gene expression has also been recognized. It has been estimated that only approximately 1% of the genome encodes protein, but a much larger fraction is transcribed, most of which is noncoding. A portion of this noncoding RNA participates in the RNA interference pathway illustrated in Figure 1-2. Some portion of this RNA forms hairpin loops that are cleaved by the enzymes **Drosha** and **Dicer** into short 21- to 23-bp double-stranded RNAs. These short double-stranded RNAs contain both sense strands and antisense strands that correspond to coding sequences in mRNAs. These small microRNAs are then incorporated into a larger complex known as a **RISC** (RNA-induced silencing complex). The microRNA is then unwound in a strand-specific manner, and the single-stranded RNA locates mRNA targets by Watson–Crick base pairing. Gene silencing results from cleavage of the target mRNA (if there is complementarity at the scissile site) or translational inhibition (if there is a mismatch at the scissile site). This gene-silencing pathway is known as RNA interference. Recent studies suggest that as much as 20% of cellular RNA is regulated by RNA interference. These small RNAs play regulatory roles in development and differentiation, and they are also expressed in a tissue-specific manner. Several lines of evidence suggest that siRNAs may have a role in hematologic malignancies. In B-cell chronic lymphocytic leukemia, evaluation of common deletions at the 13q14 locus revealed deletion and down-regulation of 2 microRNA genes.

Genomics

The ability to analyze data obtained from the entire human genome (**genomics**) is changing biology, and many of these advances have been initiated with studies of hematologic disorders. Genomics is based on identification of human alleles and their variations recognizable by artificial oligonucleotides. These oligonucleotides match different alleles (DNA sequences at known chromosomal locations) in populations; most of these alleles are single nucleotide polymorphisms (**SNPs**). The investigations have been facilitated by the International Haplotype Map Project (HapMap), which was designed to identify a set of SNPs that provide maximum information about potential disease associations.

In 2001, a rough draft of the complete sequence of the human genome was published, followed by a more complete sequence in 2003. This gargantuan accomplishment has led to a number of realizations about the organization and structure of the human genome. One of the most important discoveries is the identification of single-base DNA differences (SNPs) that occur at more than 10 million positions in the human genome. The complete diploid sequences of individuals from several distinct populations have now been obtained, revealing that each individual

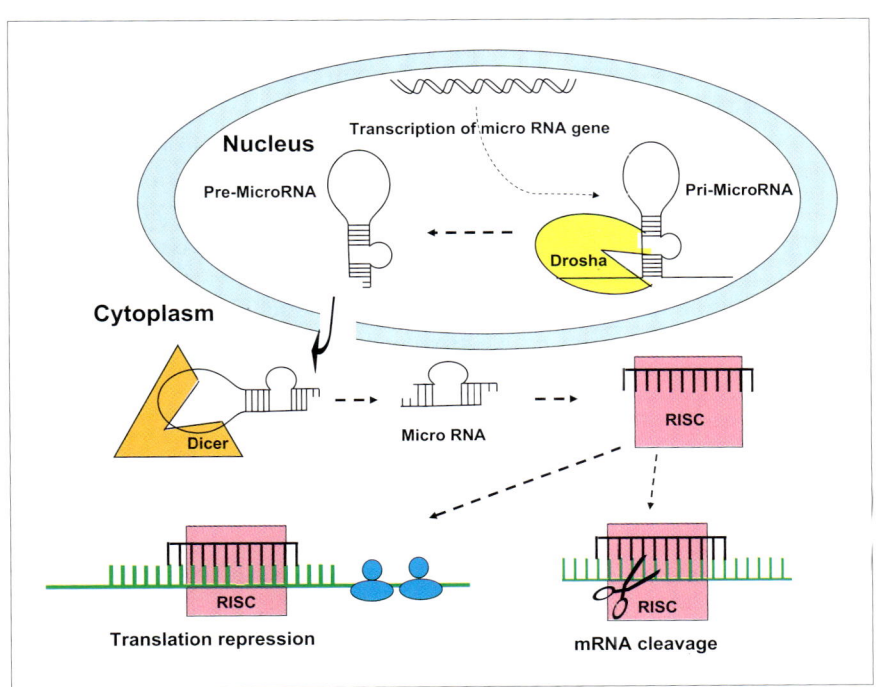

Figure 1-2 MicroRNA production. Production of microRNA begins with transcription of the microRNA gene to produce a stem-loop structure called a pri-microRNA. This molecule is processed by Drosha to produce the shorter pre-microRNA. The pre-microRNA is exported from the nucleus; the cytoplasmic Dicer enzyme cleaves the pre-microRNA to produce a double-stranded mature microRNA. The mature microRNA is transferred to RISC, where it is unwound by a helicase. Complementary base pairing between the microRNA and its target mRNA directs RISC to destroy the mRNA (if completely complementary) or halt translation (if a mismatch exists at the scissile site).

harbors approximately 3.5 million SNPs. In addition, study of the human sequence revealed that human recombination is concentrated into short hot spots that occur at intervals along the genome. **Alleles** (which are alternative forms of particular genes) located between these hot spots show strong statistical association known as **linkage disequilibrium**. The HapMap project was begun with the goal of mapping the structure of this allelic association across the genome. Over 3 million SNPs have been genotyped across the genomes of 270 people in 4 geographic populations in the first 2 phases of this project. Thus far, it appears that because of linkage disequilibrium, a select set of SNPs (called **tag SNPs**) reliably defines the DNA surrounding them, making it possible to locate relevant genes by comparing the haplotype patterns in different groups. This observation should not only permit mapping of disease-relevant genes by comparing the pattern of these tag SNPs in patients versus controls, but also provide further insight into how evolution has shaped the human genome. The catalog of naturally occurring human variants will be extended by the 1000 Genomes Project, which aims to uncover all common variants (ie, those with a frequency of at least 1%). In addition to SNPs, larger segments of DNA (ranging from 1 kb to >1 Mb) vary in copy number between individuals. These **copy number variants (CNVs)** contribute to phenotypic diversity and must be distinguished from somatically acquired copy number alterations that occur in hematologic malignancies.

Analytic techniques

Digestion and separation of nucleic acids

DNA may be cut, or digested, into predictable, small pieces using **restriction endonucleases**. Each of these bacterially derived enzymes recognizes a specific sequence of 4 to 8 bp in double-stranded DNA. These recognition sequences are usually palindromic (that is, they read the same sequence 5′ to 3′ on both strands). The DNA is cleaved by the enzyme on both strands at the site of the recognition sequence. After restriction endonuclease digestion, DNA fragments may be separated by size using agarose gel electrophoresis, with the smallest fragments running faster (closer to the bottom of the gel) and the largest fragments moving more slowly (closer to where the samples were loaded). DNA can be visualized in the gel by staining with ethidium bromide, a chemical that inserts itself between the DNA strands and fluoresces upon exposure to ultraviolet light. A desired fragment of DNA may be isolated and then purified from the gel. Some restriction enzymes generate overhanging single-stranded tails, known as "sticky ends." Complementary overhanging segments may be used to join, or ligate, pieces of DNA to one another (Figure 1-3). These methods form the backbone of recombinant DNA technology.

Hybridization techniques

DNA is chemically stable in the double-stranded form. This tendency of nucleic acids to assume a double-stranded structure is the basis for the technique of **nucleic acid hybridization**. If DNA is heated or chemically denatured, the hydrogen bonds are disrupted, and the 2 strands separate. If the denatured DNA is then placed at a lower temperature in the absence of denaturing chemicals, the single-stranded species will **reanneal**, or reassociate, in such a way that the complementary sequences are again matched and the hydrogen bonds reform. If the denatured DNA is incubated with radioisotope- or fluorogen-labeled, single-stranded complementary DNA or RNA, the radiolabeled species will **anneal** to the denatured, unlabeled strands. This hybridization process can be used to determine the presence and abundance of an identical DNA species. The technique of molecular hybridization is the basis for **Southern blotting** and many other molecular techniques.

To perform Southern blot analysis, DNA is isolated from peripheral blood, bone marrow, or tumor tissue. The total cellular DNA is then digested with specific restriction enzymes. This results in a wide range of fragments that may be separated by size using agarose gel electrophoresis. Because the DNA will be digested into thousands of fragments, genomic DNA will appear in the gel as a continuous smear. The DNA in the gel is denatured by exposure to alkaline buffer, and the resulting single-stranded species are transferred and fixed to a nitrocellulose or nylon membrane.

Detection of a specific gene fragment requires the use of a **probe**. A probe is a labeled, single-stranded fragment of DNA that is specific to the gene of interest. Probes can be produced from any portion of gene whose sequence is known or that has been previously isolated, such as globin, immunoglobulin heavy- and light-chain genes, the genes encoding the T-cell receptor loci, and the genes encoding the coagulation proteins such as factor VIII and von Willebrand factor. The denatured, labeled probe dissolved in hybridization solution is incubated with the denatured Southern blot membrane, which contains single-stranded DNA corresponding to the entire cellular DNA. By molecular hybridization, the probe will anneal to complementary sequences within the DNA fixed to the membrane. After the membrane is washed to remove excess unbound probe and probe that has stuck nonspecifically to areas of low-sequence homology, the membrane is exposed to radiographic film or a fluorescence detection system. The resultant autoradiogram will allow visualization of the DNA fragment or fragments that represent the gene of interest with a sequence complementary to the probe (Figure 1-4).

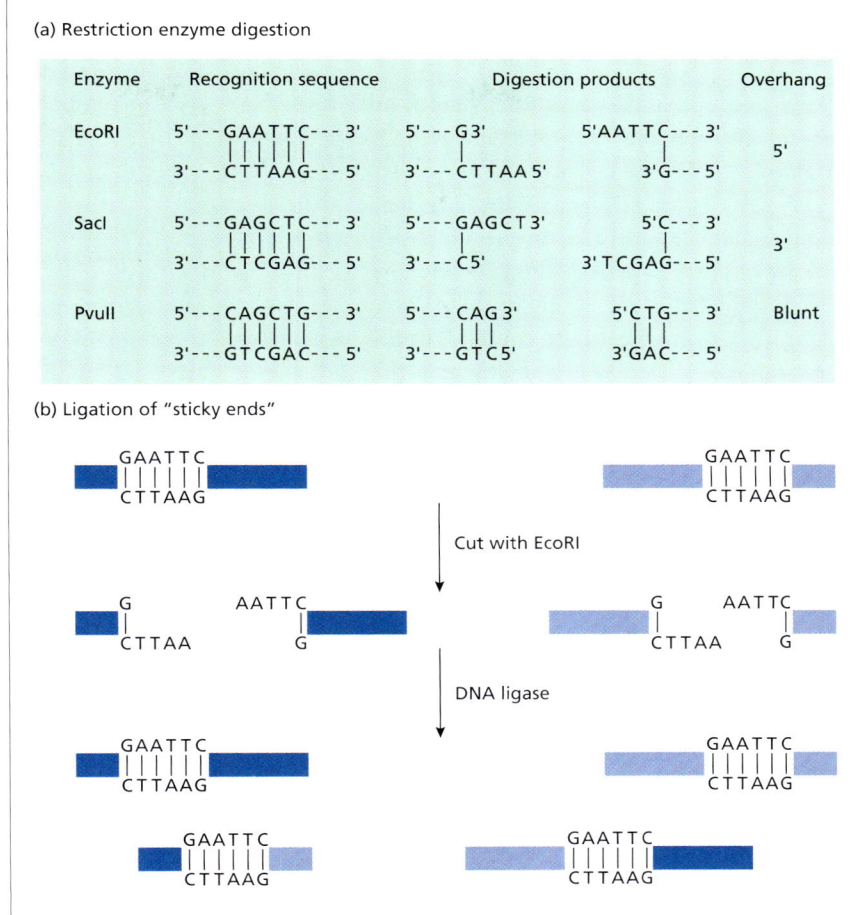

Figure 1-3 Restriction endonuclease digestion. (a) Diagram of typical restriction enzyme recognition sequences and the pattern of cleavage seen upon digestion with that enzyme. (b) Means by which restriction enzyme can be exploited to form recombinant proteins. Digestion of the 2 fragments with the enzyme *Eco*RI results in 4 fragments. Ligation with DNA ligase can regenerate the original fragments, but can also result in recombinant fragments in which the 5′ end of one fragment is ligated to the 3′ end of the second fragment. This recombinant DNA can then be used as a template for generation of recombinant protein in expression vectors.

Southern blotting may be used to determine whether a gene is present or absent, or grossly rearranged by deletion, insertion, or recombination.

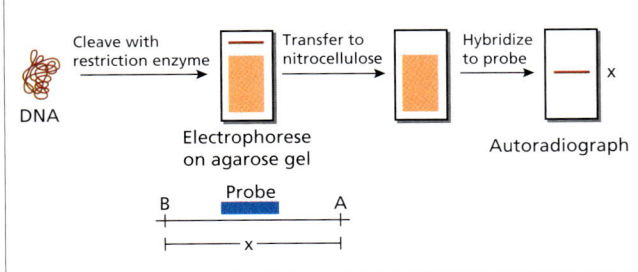

Figure 1-4 Southern blot analysis of DNA. DNA is cleaved with restriction endonuclease, electrophoresed through an agarose gel, and transferred to nitrocellulose. The probe, as illustrated at the bottom of the figure, lies on a piece of DNA of length x when DNA is digested with the enzyme. Hybridization of the probe to the blot, with appropriate washes and exposure to radiograph, shows a single band of length x on the autoradiogram.

Restriction fragment length polymorphism (RFLP) analysis is a Southern blot–based technique with many useful applications in hematology. Using this technique, inherited disease-associated alleles may be identified and traced by the presence of inherited mutations or variations in DNA sequence that create or abolish restriction sites. Rarely, a single-base, disease-causing DNA mutation will coincidentally fall within a recognition sequence for a restriction endonuclease. If a probe for the mutated fragment of DNA is hybridized to total cellular DNA digested with that enzyme, then the detected DNA fragment will be of different size. The β-globin point mutation resulting in hemoglobin S may be detected in this way. More commonly, genetic diseases are not the result of single base pair mutations that conveniently abolish or create restriction enzyme sites. However, a similar technique may be used to detect the presence of an RFLP that is linked to a disease locus within a family or group but does not directly detect the molecular abnormality responsible for the disease. This is because there are normal variations in DNA sequence among individuals that are inherited but silent in that they do not cause disease. These

polymorphisms are often located in intronic sequences or outside of but relatively close to the gene. They are "innocent bystanders" that serve simply to mark the DNA surrounding the gene in question. Because RFLPs are transmitted from parent to offspring, they are extremely useful in the diagnosis of many genetic diseases.

RFLP analysis has also been used to locate, or map, disease-associated genes within the genome by **linkage analysis**. Pieces of DNA have been cloned whose precise location in the genome is known. Many of these random pieces of DNA are useful because they contain readily identifiable polymorphisms. These RFLPs allow for the subsequent identification of genes close to them. Because the spontaneous mutation rate of the genome is high and relatively constant, the "genetic distance" can be measured by the frequency with which 2 pieces of DNA become separated as a result of recombination across chromosome pairs during meiosis. By analyzing a family pedigree for which 2 RFLPs are defined, the frequency with which the 2 RFLPs are transmitted from parent to offspring as a linked pair can be analyzed. If, for example, the RFLPs are from loci on 2 different chromosomes, assortment of the 2 will be random. If, however, they are from adjacent genes, they will almost always be transmitted together; the configuration of these close polymorphisms constitutes a gene haplotype. Linkage analysis has made the identification of the genes responsible for diseases possible without available information about what the genes encode. For example, the gene for hemochromatosis has long been known to be linked to the histocompatibility (human leukocyte antigen [HLA]) locus. The HLA haplotype can predict which members of an affected family will have the disease. The association between HLA and hemochromatosis stems from the fact that the HLA locus is close to the gene for hemochromatosis. By identifying RFLPs in the vicinity of the HLA locus and examining the neighboring DNA sequences, the gene for hemochromatosis was identified. Subsequent analysis of the sequence of that gene, its predicted protein product, and its mutation has provided important insights into the pathogenesis of hemochromatosis.

Hybridization techniques can also be applied to RNA. Although RNA is generally an unstable single-stranded species, it is stabilized when converted to the double-stranded form. Therefore, if placed under hybridization conditions, RNA will complex with complementary, single-stranded nucleic acid species in the same fashion as DNA. **Northern blotting** is analogous to Southern blotting but involves electrophoresis of RNA with subsequent transfer and hybridization to a probe. Whereas Southern blotting detects the presence of a gene or its integrity, Northern blot analysis detects the presence or absence of that gene's expression within a specific cell type.

Protein can be detected by the blotting technique referred to as **Western blotting**. Proteins are detected by specific antibodies directed against the protein of interest. A labeled anti-immunoglobulin antibody raised in another species can then be used to detect the specific antibody bound to the blot.

Cytogenetic techniques
Conventional cytogenetics

Uniform, nonrandom chromosomal abnormalities found in a malignant cellular population, termed **clonal** abnormalities, and inherited chromosomal abnormalities are detected by **cytogenetics**, or chromosomal analysis. Conventional cytogenetic techniques can detect numeric chromosomal abnormalities (too many or too few chromosomes), as well as deletion or translocation of relatively large chromosomal fragments among chromosomes. Certain chromosomal translocations are considered pathognomonic of specific diseases, such as the t(15;17) in acute promyelocytic leukemia (APL). Normally chromosomes cannot be seen with a light microscope, but during cell division, they become condensed and can be easily analyzed. To collect cells with their chromosomes in this condensed state, bone marrow or tumor tissue may be briefly maintained in culture and then exposed to a mitotic inhibitor, which blocks formation of the spindle and arrests cell division at the metaphase stage. Thus, cytogenetic studies require dividing cells.

Conventional cytogenetic studies have several limitations. First, these studies require active cell division, which may not be obtainable. Second, the technique is insensitive to submicroscopic abnormalities. Finally, because only a very small number of cells are analyzed, the technique is relatively insensitive for measurement of minimal residual disease burden.

Fluorescence in situ hybridization

Fluorescence in situ hybridization (FISH) studies complement conventional cytogenetic analysis by adding convenience, specificity, and sensitivity. This technique applies the principles of complementary DNA hybridization. A specific single-stranded DNA probe corresponding to a gene or chromosomal region of interest is labeled for fluorescent detection. One or more probes are then incubated with the fixed cellular sample and examined by a fluorescence microscope. FISH probes have been developed that are capable of identifying specific disease-defining translocations, such as the t(15;17) that characterizes APL. A probe corresponding to the *PML* gene on chromosome 15 is labeled with a fluorescent marker, such as rhodamine, which is red. Another fluorescent marker, such as fluorescein, which is green, is linked to a probe corresponding to the *RARα* gene on chromosome 17. When the t(15;17) chromosomal translocation is present, the 2 genes are juxtaposed, the 2 probes are in close proximity, and the fluorescent signals merge to generate a yellow signal. The specificity of FISH is highly dependent on the specificity of the probes that are used. Numeric abnormalities, such as monosomy and trisomy, may be identified using centromere-specific probes.

The major advantage of FISH is that it can analyze known cytogenetic abnormalities in nondividing cells (interphase nuclei); thus, peripheral blood slides can be directly processed. FISH studies are most useful when assessing for the presence of specific molecular abnormalities associated with a particular clinical syndrome or tumor type and are approximately one order of magnitude more sensitive than morphology and conventional cytogenetic studies in detecting residual disease. FISH panels are now available to detect recurrent genetic changes in leukemias, lymphomas, and multiple myeloma. These panels are particularly useful in predicting prognosis when conventional cytogenetic studies are normal.

Since their introduction nearly 30 years ago, FISH techniques have evolved rapidly for use in hematologic disorders. A number of improvements have been made in the probes themselves; for instance, probes can now be labeled with quantum dots, which are nano-sized fluorophores with extremely high fluorescence efficiency. Quantum dots have sharp emission spectra, making them useful in a wide range of bioimaging techniques including FISH. Another innovation is the use of probes such as peptide nucleic acids (PNAs), which are synthetic analogs of DNA in which the deoxyribose phosphate backbone is replaced by a noncharged peptide backbone. In the absence of charge repulsion, the uncharged PNA oligomers bind more tightly than DNA oligomers to their complementary DNA. Conversely, single-base mismatches affect PNA–DNA hybridization much more than DNA–DNA hybridization, giving PNA probes greater power to discriminate single-base sequence differences. Beyond technical improvements in FISH probes, more sensitive and specific FISH techniques have also evolved. For instance, double fusion FISH (D-FISH) uses differentially labeled large probes that each span one of the 2 **translocation breakpoints**. This allows simultaneous visualization of both fusion products and reduces false-negative results. Another technique known as split-signal FISH uses differentially labeled probes targeting the regions flanking the breakpoint. Thus in normal cells, the signals appear fused, but split upon translocation. This technique has been used to detect t(8;14) in Burkitt lymphoma and t(11;14) in mantle cell lymphoma. Labeling probes with unique combinations of fluorophores in multiplex FISH (M-FISH) has not only permitted simultaneous detection of every chromosome, but has also now been used to analyze specific chromosomal regions and can detect subtle rearrangements.

Comparative genomic hybridization

In **comparative genomic hybridization (CGH)**, DNA extracted from a test sample and from a normal control are differentially labeled and applied to target metaphase chromosomes to compete for complementary hybridization sites. The ratio of test to reference fluorescence along the chromosomes is quantified using digital image analysis. Gains and amplifications in the test DNA are identified as regions of increased fluorescence ratio, and losses are identified as areas of decreased ratio. In an even more sensitive technique known as array CGH, large numbers of mapped clones or oligonucleotides are spotted onto a glass slide or synthesized in situ and then hybridized to differentially labeled test and normal reference genomes. In array CGH, resolution of the analysis is restricted only by probe size and the density of probes on the array. These and other techniques permit high-resolution, genome-wide detection of genomic copy number changes. Careful analysis of AML genomes using these approaches has revealed few somatic copy number changes that are not detectable by routine cytogenetics. In contrast, ALL genomes are characterized by recurring copy number alterations, frequently involving loss of genes required for normal lymphoid development (eg, *PAX5*, *IKZF1*).

SNP chips

Currently, genomic techniques for studying human and other genomes depend on examining large quantities of data that require accurate processing, analysis, and interpretation. Thus, a new field of bioinformatics has emerged. Fluorescently labeled single-stranded DNA from a subject is hybridized with the oligonucleotides on the slide to determine, for a specific region in the genome, which DNA sequence undergoes complementary base pairing with that of the subject. The pattern of hybridization signals is analyzed by a computer, providing a detailed profile of genetic variation specific to an individual's DNA. With current technology, enough probes can be placed on a single **microarray** to analyze variation in 1 million SNPs in an individual, as well as copy number variations (SNP chips). SNP microarrays are now used routinely to perform genome-wide association studies, in which the frequencies of each SNP are compared in disease cases and unaffected controls. These SNP chips are also used to examine copy number variants, methylation patterns in an individual's genome, and genetic variation.

Sequence-based studies

A variety of novel high-throughput DNA sequencing technologies (collectively termed **Next-Gen sequencing**) have greatly accelerated the pace and lowered the cost of large-scale sequence production. At the core of each of these technologies is the capture of individual DNA fragments, which are then clonally amplified and sequenced by synthesis in multiple parallel reactions. Sequencing both ends of captured fragments ("paired-end reads") improves the efficiency of data production and allows for identification of insertions, deletions, and translocations. With these approaches, the search for inherited and somatic mutations associated with hematologic malignancies and congenital blood disorders has evolved from a candidate gene approach to whole chromosome, whole **exome**, and even whole genome analysis.

Polymerase chain reaction

The polymerase chain reaction (PCR) is a powerful technique for amplifying very small quantities of DNA of known sequence. Two oligonucleotide primers are required; one is complementary to a sequence on the 5′ strand of the DNA to be amplified, and the other is complementary to the 3′ strand. The DNA template is denatured at a high temperature; the temperature is then lowered for the primers to be annealed to the DNA. The DNA is then extended with a temperature-stable DNA polymerase (such as *Taq* polymerase), resulting in 2 identical copies of the original DNA from each piece of template DNA. The products are denatured, and the process is repeated. The primary product of this reaction is the fragment of DNA bounded by the 2 primers (Figure 1-5). Thus, a minute quantity of DNA may be

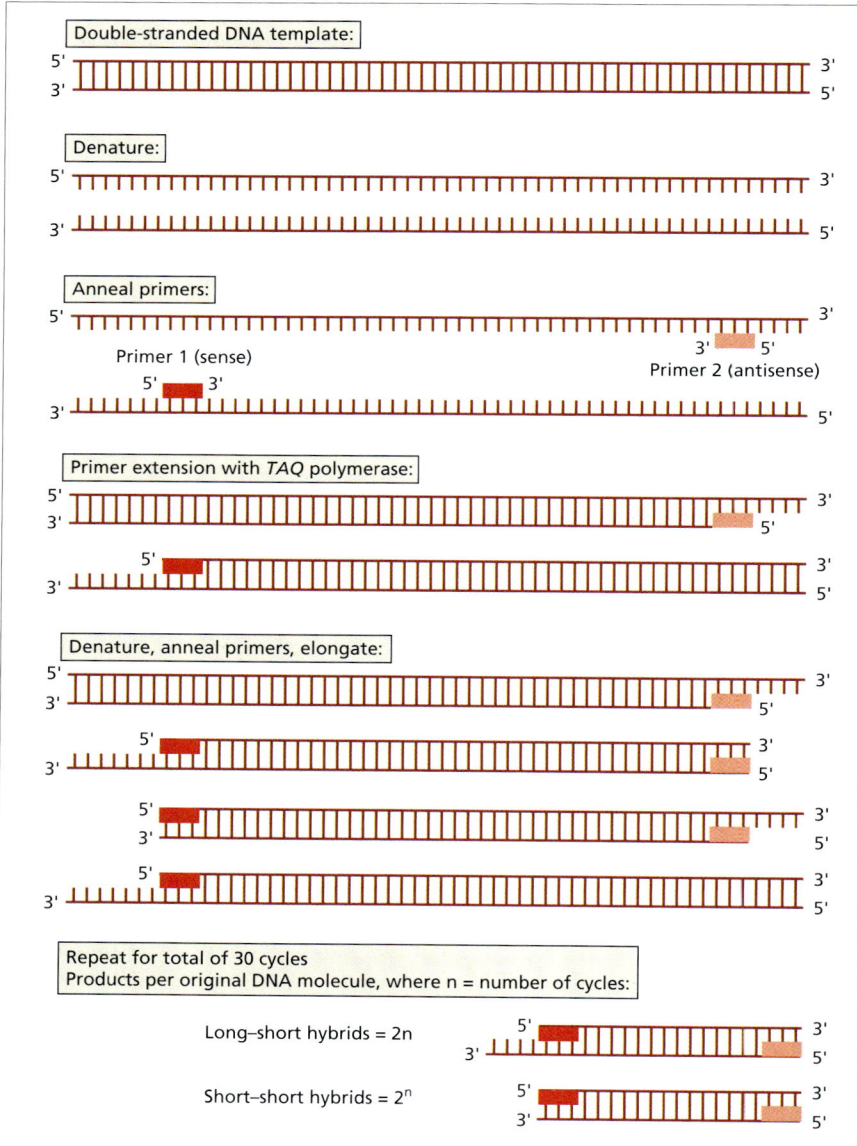

Figure 1-5 Polymerase chain reaction. The DNA template is denatured at high temperature and allowed to anneal to oligonucleotide primers flanking the DNA of interest. The temperature at which this annealing is performed is dependent on the characteristic melting temperature of the oligonucleotide primers. The temperature is then raised to 72°C to allow elongation of the primers using *Taq* DNA polymerase. This creates a DNA copy of the DNA extending from the specific oligonucleotide. The temperature is then raised to denature the products, and the process is repeated. Because the *Taq* polymerase is temperature stable, it withstands cycling without the addition of enzyme at each cycle. As the reaction proceeds, newly synthesized strands of DNA originating from the primer serve as templates for subsequent amplification. The result of this is the formation of a product that is bounded on both ends by the flanking oligonucleotides. As shown in the lower panel, the primary product of the PCR after multiple cycles is this fragment of DNA bounded by the 2 primers (short–short hybrid). Reproduced with permission from Berliner N. Use of molecular techniques in the analysis of hematologic disease. In: Hoffman R, Benz EJ Jr, Shattil SJ, Furie B, Cohen HJ, eds. *Hematology: Basic Principles and Practice*. New York, NY: Churchill Livingstone; 1991.

used to synthesize large quantities of a specific DNA sequence. This technique has superseded many blotting techniques for prenatal diagnosis and cancer diagnostics. Using multiple primer pairs in the same reaction, multiplex PCR can efficiently amplify several fragments simultaneously.

Reverse transcriptase PCR (RT-PCR) is a modification of the PCR technique that allows for the detection and amplification of expressed RNA transcripts. **Complementary DNA (cDNA)** is generated from RNA using reverse transcriptase, an enzyme that mediates the conversion of RNA to DNA. The resultant cDNA is then subjected to routine PCR amplification. Because cDNA is generated from processed mRNA transcripts, no intronic sequences are obtained. RNA is much less stable than DNA; thus, amplification of mRNA from tissue or blood requires careful preservation of source tissue or blood samples.

Quantitative PCR is another modification of the PCR technique. Various techniques have been developed that allow the number of target sequences present in a PCR reaction to be estimated by quantitation of the product in comparison to the product from a known concentration of template. An automated technology, **real-time PCR** has superseded other approaches. A fluorogenic tag is incorporated into an oligonucleotide that will anneal to the internal sequence of the *Taq* DNA polymerase-generated PCR product. This tag consists of a fluorescent "reporter" and a "silencing" quencher dye at opposite ends of the oligonucleotide. When annealed to the internal sequence of the PCR product, fluorescence from the reporter is quenched because the silencer lies within the same stretch of sequence. After completion of each cycle of PCR amplification, the reporter is not incorporated to the product but is cleaved by *Taq* DNA polymerase (because this enzyme also has exonuclease activity). This fluorogen tag is released, generating a fluorescent signal. Real-time PCR detects the number of cycles when amplification of product is exponential and expresses this as a ratio to standard housekeeping RNA such as ribosomal RNA or glyceraldehyde-3-phosphate dehydrogenase (GAPDH) mRNA. This number can be easily converted to the number of molecules of mRNA present in the tested sample. This is becoming the preferred technique for precise measurement of minimal residual disease.

The power of the PCR technique lies in its great sensitivity, which theoretically allows the detection of DNA from a single cell. This great sensitivity is, however, also its major weakness because small amounts of contaminating DNA or RNA from other sources can cause false-positive results. Clinical laboratories that use PCR for critical diagnostic tests require elaborate quality assurance protocols to prevent inappropriate diagnosis. Equally troublesome can be false-negative results that result from inappropriate primer design, degraded RNA, or inappropriate temperature parameters for the annealing of primers.

The amplified sequence of interest can then be rapidly evaluated for presence of mutation(s) by direct sequencing, restriction enzyme digestion (if a suitable enzyme that discriminates between mutant and wild-type alleles is available), allele-specific PCR (discussed later in this chapter), or other techniques.

DNA microarray technology: expression arrays

With the cloning of the human genome, it has become feasible to analyze the level of expression of thousands of genes simultaneously in a given cell or tissue. Microarray technology provides a more complete characterization of the gene expression patterns within the cells of interest, referred to as a **gene expression profile**. These studies have yielded an explosion of new data. This enormous wealth of data may be used to classify disease, predict response to therapy, and dissect pathways of disease pathogenesis. A major shortcoming of expression arrays is that defects not caused by loss or gain of gene transcripts, such as those from microRNA changes, or missense mutations are not detected by these analyses. There are 2 principle types of DNA microarray methods: oligonucleotide microarrays and cDNA microarrays. Both methods rely on the hybridization of fluorescently labeled mRNA from a cell population of interest to DNA probes fixed on a solid support. The oligonucleotide microarray is produced by the synthesis of gene-specific oligomers of approximately 25 bp in length immobilized on a glass surface. mRNA is extracted from samples, and double-stranded cDNA is synthesized from the RNA template. Then, biotinylated complementary RNA (cRNA) is generated from the cDNA template by in vitro transcription using biotin-labeled nucleotides. The biotinylated cRNA is fragmented and hybridized to the chip. Hybridization is then detected using a streptavidin-phycoerythrin stain, and the fluorescence intensity of each feature of the array is quantified using a confocal argon laser microarray scanner. cDNA arrays are generated by the robotic deposition of a panel of DNA fragments corresponding to genes onto a glass slide. In general, the cDNA fragments are 1000 to 10,000 bp in length. Unlike the oligonucleotide array, mRNA is extracted from both test and control samples and used as a template to generate cDNA containing fluorescently tagged nucleotides. Test and control samples tagged with different fluors then compete for hybridization to the specific probes on the array. Message abundance is measured as a ratio of the fluorescent intensity of one sample compared with a reference sample. It is advisable that any significant difference in mRNA expression in a tested sample be confirmed by real-time PCR.

Two main computational approaches have been used to analyze microarray data: unsupervised and supervised learning. Unsupervised learning methods cluster samples based on gene expression similarities without a priori knowledge of class labels. Hierarchical clustering and self-organizing maps are 2 commonly used algorithms of unsupervised learning. One potential application of unsupervised learning is for discovery of previously unrecognized disease subtypes. The strength of this method is that it provides an unbiased approach to identifying classes within a data set. A weakness is that these data sets are complex and the structure uncovered by clustering may not reflect the underlying biology of interest. The second computational approach, supervised learning, uses known class labels to create a model for class prediction. For example, a training data set is used to create an expression profile for tumor samples from patients with "cured" versus "relapsed" disease. These profiles are then applied to an independent data set to validate the ability to make the prognostic distinction. In either method, it is important to demonstrate statistical significance and assure that the tested sample is compared with the appropriate control.

The main limitation of microarray expression technology is that it analyzes only mRNA abundance. It does not reveal important translational and posttranslational modifications and protein–protein interactions. Some of these shortcomings are circumvented by microRNA and DNA methylation arrays. Purity of the cell population is also essential for these analyses, and one must assure that the control and analyzed cells are homogeneous, of same cell type, and of comparable differentiation.

Proteomics

Proteins are the effectors of most cellular functions. Genetic defects perturb normal cellular functions because they result in changes in the level or the function of the proteins they encode. Many proteins undergo extensive posttranslational modifications that influence their activity and function, including cleavage, chemical modification such as phosphorylation and glycosylation, and interaction with other proteins. These posttranslational events are not encoded by the genome and are not revealed by genomic analysis or gene expression profiling. Proteomics is the systematic study of the entire complement of proteins derived from a cell population.

Proteomic analysis relies on complex bioinformatic tools applied to mass spectroscopy data. In general, these techniques require some sort of separation of peptides, usually by liquid chromatography, followed by ionization of the sample and mass spectrometry. In matrix-associated laser desorption/ionization time of flight (MALDI-TOF) mass spectrometry, the time of flight of the ions is detected and used to calculate a mass-to-charge ratio. The spectrum of mass-to-charge ratios present within a sample reflects the protein constituents within the sample. Supervised or unsupervised learning approaches, as described previously, are then used to identify patterns within the data. More recently, protein microarrays have been developed. Analytical protein microarrays are composed of a high density of affinity reagents (antigens, antibodies, etc) that can be used to detect the presence of specific proteins in a mixture. Functional protein microarrays contain a large number of immobilized proteins; these chips can be used to examine protein–protein, protein–lipid, protein–nucleic acid, and enzyme–substrate interactions. Although all of these technologies hold enormous potential, clinical applications have yet to be realized.

Transgenic and knockout mice

Analysis of both inherited and acquired diseases by "reverse genetics" has resulted in the identification of many disease-related genes for which the function is unknown. Once a disease-related gene has been identified, either by linkage mapping (eg, the gene for cystic fibrosis) or by identifying rearranged genes (eg, the *bcr* gene at the breakpoint of the Philadelphia chromosome), the challenge lies in identifying the function of the protein encoded by that gene and characterizing how changes in the expression of that gene can contribute to the disease phenotype. Understanding of the role of these genes and their encoded proteins has been greatly aided by the development of techniques to alter or introduce these genes in mice using recombinant DNA technology.

Mice can be produced that express an exogenous gene and thereby provide an in vivo model of the gene's function. Linearized DNA is injected into a fertilized mouse oocyte pronucleus, and the oocyte is then reimplanted into a pseudopregnant mouse. The resultant **transgenic mice** can then be analyzed for the phenotype induced by the injected transgene. Placing the gene under the control of a strong **constitutive promoter**, which is active in all tissues, allows the assessment of the effect of widespread overexpression of the gene. Alternatively, placing the gene under a tissue-specific promoter will elucidate the function of that gene in an isolated tissue. A third approach is to use the control elements of the gene to drive expression of a gene that can be detected by chemical, immunologic, or functional means. For example, the promoter region of a gene can be joined to the β-galactosidase cDNA, and activity of the enzyme in various tissues in the resultant transgenic mouse can be assessed. Use of such a reporter gene will show the normal distribution and timing of expression of the gene from which the promoter elements are derived. These transgenic mice contain multiple copies of exogenous genes that have inserted randomly into the genome of the recipient and are thus not always properly regulated and are generally expressed in decreased amounts. In contrast, one can specifically alter any defined genetic locus in totipotent embryonic stem (ES) cells by targeted recombination between the locus and a plasmid carrying an altered version of that gene that abrogates the expression of a gene (a null mutation). If a plasmid contains that altered gene with enough flanking DNA identical to that of the normal gene locus, **homologous recombination** will occur at a very low rate; however, cells undergoing the desired recombination can be selected by a selection marker present in the plasmid, such as neomycin resistance gene. The altered ES cell is then introduced into the blastocyst of a developing embryo. The resultant animals will be **chimeric**, in that only some of the cells in the animal will contain the targeted gene. If the new gene becomes part of the germline, the siblings of the same litter can then be bred to yield mice homozygous for the null allele. Such **knockout mice** can illuminate the function of the targeted gene by the phenotype induced by the targeted gene's absence. Technology also exists to replace the mouse gene in ES cells by a desired gain-of-function mutated human gene.

Many genes of interest participate in pathways that are vital for viability or fertility; thus, full knockout mice cannot be generated. Conditional gene modification using Cre-*loxP* technology allows the gene of interest to be knocked out in specific tissues or at specific times. This is accomplished by inserting the altered gene with flanking DNA-containing *loxP* sites. If animals containing the *loxP* sites are then bred with a second strain of mice that expresses an enzyme called Cre recombinase, recombination will take place between the *loxP* sites, removing the desired portion of the gene and ligated flanking sequences. Further, if the Cre recombinase is expressed under the control of a tissue promoter or drug-specific (such as tetracycline) promoter, then tissue-specific and conditional knockout mice can be generated. The use of transgenic knockout and conditional knockout mice has been invaluable in elucidating the function of large numbers of genes implicated in the pathogenesis of both inherited and acquired diseases.

Transgenic technology is laborious, time consuming, and expensive. Some of these disadvantages are circumvented by using rapidly reproducing and inexpensive organisms such as zebrafish or even yeast. However, like transgenic mice, these models do not detect human-specific pathophysiology. Rapidly emerging technology using dedifferentiated somatic cells reprogrammed to become totipotent cells now appears feasible. These cells, called **induced pluripotent stem (iPS) cells**, are produced by reprogramming of adult somatic cells to become embryonic-like cells, which in turn can be further differentiated along specific lineages. In 2006, Yamanaka's group published a landmark paper demonstrating that mouse fibroblasts could be reprogrammed into ES cell–like cells by expression of only 4 transcription factors (Oct4, Sox2, Klf4, and c-Myc). Moreover, more recent studies showed that potentially oncogenic c-Myc is not required and that a combination of Oct4, Sox2, Nanog, and Lin28 is also successful for generation of iPS. The concrete demonstration that iPS cells may be used to treat disease was replacement of the sickle globin gene with a normal β-globin gene in mice. Corrected iPS cells from sickle mice were differentiated into hematopoietic progenitors in vitro, and these cells were transplanted into irradiated sickle mice recipients. Erythroid cells derived from these progenitors synthesized high levels of human hemoglobin A and corrected the sickle cell disease phenotype. These results pioneered a method for producing patient-specific, ES-like cells without the ethical concerns of using embryos. This approach holds promise for replacing retroviral and other vector-mediated gene transfer with potentially more efficient and safer strategies. At present, human iPS cells have already been differentiated into cardiovascular cells and hematopoietic stem cells. Reprogramming of somatic cells into pluripotent stem cells may soon replace ES cells as a potential source of tissue for clinical use.

Clinical applications of DNA technology in hematology

Molecular biology has revolutionized the understanding of molecular pathogenesis of disease in ways that have profoundly affected the diagnostic armamentarium of the hematologist. Several examples of how molecular studies are used for diagnosis and clinical decision making in hematology are described in this section.

Applications to germline (inherited) mutations

The diagnosis of hemoglobinopathies has been at the forefront of prenatal diagnosis by means of molecular biology. For diseases such as sickle cell anemia, where the affected gene is known at the level of DNA sequence, the digestion of genomic DNA with *Mst*II restriction enzyme results in a longer restriction fragment of a chromosome bearing the mutation (Figure 1-6). By using PCR, oligonucleotides flanking the β-globin gene are used to amplify the locus, and the amplified DNA can be analyzed by restriction enzyme digestion. This requires only minute quantities of DNA and can be performed in a matter of a few hours. With diseases such as hemophilia or von Willebrand disease, where the genes are sequenced but where the specific molecular defects are heterogeneous and largely undefined, RFLP analysis is usually used in linkage studies to identify affected individuals in families known to carry the disease. For example, in

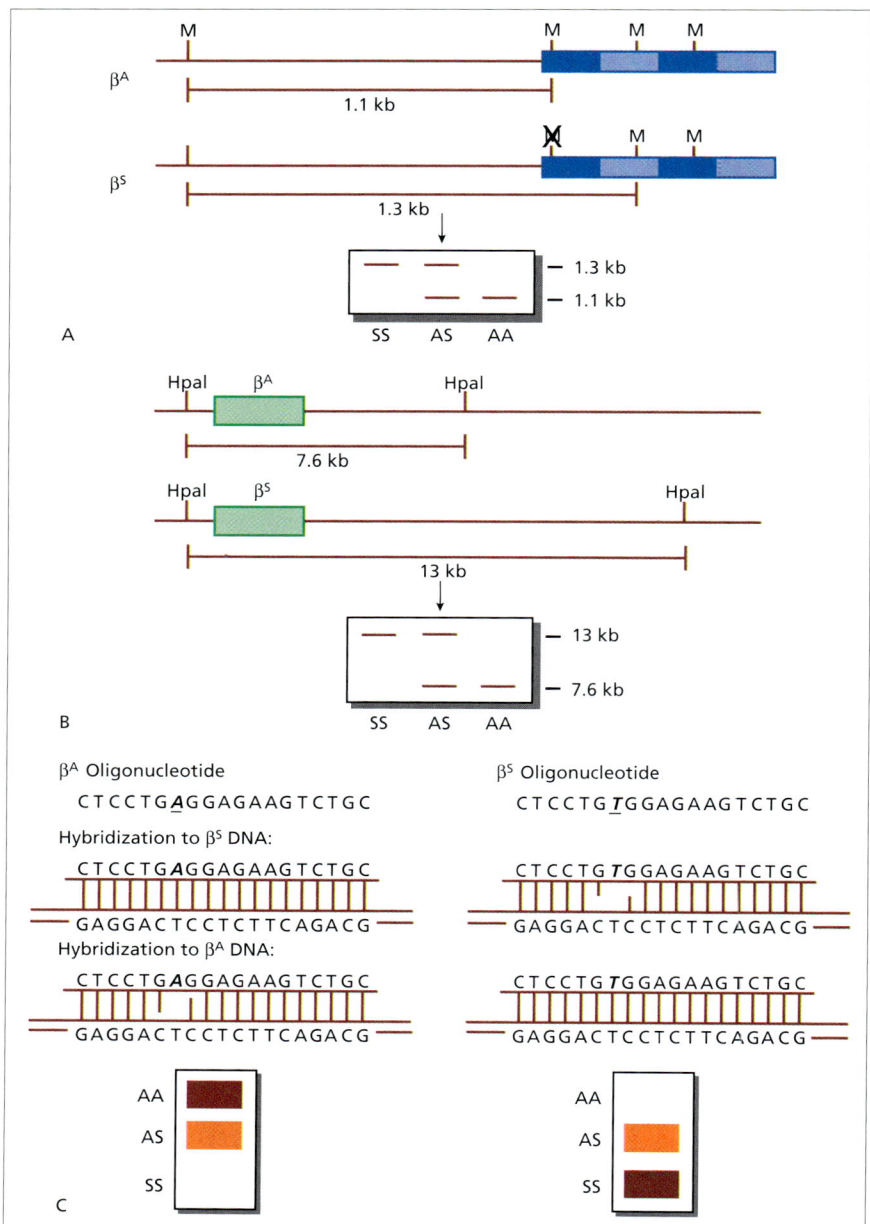

Figure 1-6 A, Polymorphism created by pathogenic point mutation. B, Flanking polymorphism associated with disease allele. C, Oligonucleotide hybridization.

hemophilia A, the disease-carrying X chromosome in an affected patient usually can be identified by an associated RFLP. Once the RFLP pattern of an affected patient is known, subsequent analysis of the RFLP pattern of parents and further offspring can predict whether future male offspring will inherit the disease. This allows identification of affected male and carrier female offspring.

Screening with oligonucleotides and PCR

Another approach is to detect the specific point mutation, such as those in the β-globin gene in sickle cell disease and β thalassemias, by hybridization techniques. Using stringent washing conditions permitting hybridization of the labeled single-stranded oligonucleotide that is perfectly complimentary to the mutation, single-base changes in DNA sequence can be detected (Figure 1-6B).

A more recent advance in the use of PCR has been to use real-time PCR technology for allele-specific determination. In these assays, a set of PCR primers flanking the polymorphism of interest is combined with 2 short oligonucleotides corresponding to the normal and the mutant SNPs and the patient's DNA. Each of the 2 oligonucleotides (corresponding to the alternative SNPs) is labeled with a fluorophore on one end and a quencher on the other end. During the PCR reactions, if the DNA polymerase enzyme encounters a fluorescently labeled oligonucleotide perfectly paired to its corresponding sequence, then the fluorophore will be cleaved off of the oligonucleotide, move away from the quencher, and generate fluorescence. If each oligonucleotide is labeled with a differently colored fluorophore, then after multiple rounds of PCR amplification, fluorescence can be analyzed and used to determine which alleles the patient carries. The advantages of this technology are its sensitivity, speed, accuracy, and the ability to evaluate samples from multiple patients in a single 96-well plate.

Applications to somatic (acquired) mutation

The power of molecular biology to provide important insights into the basic biology of disease is perhaps most dramatically shown by the evolving concepts of malignancy. The recognition of the role of oncogenes in the pathogenesis of neoplasia is primarily a result of an integration of observations of tumor virology and cytogenetics made possible by the techniques of molecular biology. The development of techniques for DNA transfer into tissue culture cells resulted in the observation that the transforming capability of many RNA tumor viruses, or **retroviruses**, was attributable to single genes. Southern blotting techniques identified these transforming genes, termed **oncogenes**, to be present in the normal genome of eukaryotic cells as "proto-oncogenes." Subsequently, blotting techniques revealed that these same genes were often involved and altered in characteristic chromosomal translocations that had already been established as pathognomonic markers of certain malignancies. Several examples of how molecular techniques have enhanced our understanding of the pathogenesis of hematologic malignancies, as well as their diagnosis and treatment, are provided in the following sections.

Gene rearrangement studies in lymphoproliferative disease: T-cell and B-cell mutations

Lymphocytes are one of the exceptions to the rule that DNA in all cells in an individual is identical. During the development of a mature lymphoid cell from an undifferentiated stem cell, somatic rearrangements of the immunoglobulin and T-cell receptor loci take place, resulting in an extensive repertoire of composite genes that creates immense immunoglobulin and T-cell diversity. These somatic rearrangements result in deletion of intervening DNA sequences in the vicinity of the immunoglobulin and T-cell receptor genes. These deletions can be detected by Southern blot analysis or PCR. The details of this process in lymphocyte ontogeny are further outlined in Chapter 18. Southern blot analysis showing clonal rearrangement of the immunoglobulin κ light chain is illustrated in Figure 1-7.

PCR-based approaches are now replacing Southern blotting in the diagnostic setting because they are more rapid, are less technically demanding, and require less DNA. The majority of the PCR-based techniques evaluate rearrangement of the immunoglobulin H locus in suspected B-cell neoplasms and the T-cell receptor γ locus in suspected T-cell disorders. Despite their power, molecular clonality studies should always be interpreted in the context of the clinical, morphologic, and immunophenotypic diagnosis. False-positive PCR results can occur in several circumstances; for example, when very small tissue samples are used, a few reactive T cells in the sample might result in the appearance of oligoclonal bands. Similarly in reactive lymph nodes from patients infected with Epstein-Barr virus (EBV) or cytomegalovirus (CMV), a restricted T-cell receptor repertoire may result in T-cell receptor gene oligoclonality. A similar oligoclonal pattern can be seen in patients recovering from stem cell transplantation.

Identification of cryptic translocation in pediatric acute lymphoblastic leukemia: prognostic significance

As many as 20% of children with pre–B-cell acute lymphoblastic leukemia (ALL) have a translocation that fuses the *AML1* gene on chromosome 8 with the *TEL* gene on chromosome 12 in the t(12;21) translocation. Both of these genes encode transcription factors that regulate hematopoietic differentiation. Although this translocation is common, it is rarely seen by standard cytogenetic techniques. However, it can be routinely identified with FISH or with RT-PCR using specific *TEL-AML1* probes. The identification of this translocation is important because it has been associated with a favorable outcome in pediatric ALL.

Nucleophosmin mutations in acute myeloid leukemia

Up to 25% of acute myeloid leukemia (AML) cases have no chromosomal abnormalities visible by conventional karyotyping. Nucleophosmin (NPM) is a nucleocytoplasmic shuttling protein involved in leukemia-associated chromosomal translocations and shows abnormal cytoplasmic expression in the leukemic cells of approximately 35% of primary AML in adults. Direct sequencing of the *NPM1* gene in genomic DNA from bone marrow mononuclear cells from adults with non-M3 AML demonstrated a mutation in exon 12 that correlated with the aberrant cytoplasmic NPM localization associated mainly with normal karyotype. *NPM1* mutations have also been found in 27.1% of children with AML and normal karyotype. Children and adults with *NPM1* gene mutations had good response to induction chemotherapy, and the mutation may represent a new target for monitoring minimal residual disease.

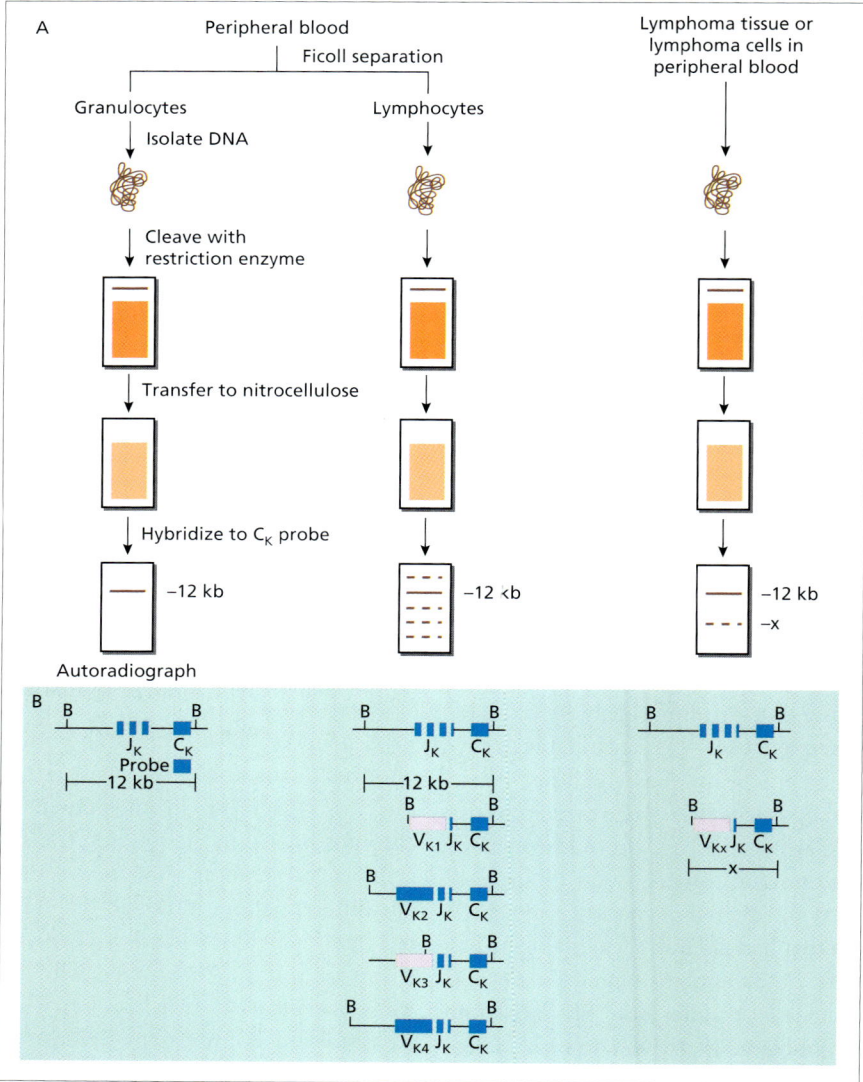

Figure 1-7 Southern blot analysis of κ light-chain rearrangement to establish clonality of populations of B lymphocytes. In A, the Southern technique and its predicted results in different cell populations are diagrammed; in B, the molecular configurations of the κ locus are outlined. In the leftmost panel, genomic DNA, as represented in peripheral blood granulocytes, is analyzed. Because all of these cells retain their immunoglobulin genes in the germline configuration, there is a single band on Southern blot analysis corresponding to germline κ locus. In the middle panel, polyclonal lymphocytes also show only a germline band on Southern analysis. However, as shown in B, this does not reflect the fact that the cells do not have rearrangement of the κ locus. It is instead a reflection of the fact that there are insufficient cells of any one clone to be detectable as a discrete band on Southern analysis. Because a significant fraction of the cells will retain one κ locus that is unrearranged, a germline band is detectable. (In normal peripheral lymphocytes, this band also partly reflects T cells, which of course do not rearrange their immunoglobulin gene loci.) The rightmost panel diagrams the Southern pattern produced by monoclonal tumor cells bearing a κ light chain. All of the cells of the population will have an identical rearrangement of the κ genes that will be apparent as a rearranged band on Southern blot analysis. The figure demonstrates the pattern of cells in which one κ locus has rearranged. If both chromosomes are rearranged, then there will be 2 rearranged bands and the germline band will no longer be present. Reproduced with permission, from Berliner N. Use of molecular techniques in the analysis of hematologic disease. In: Hoffman R, Benz EJ Jr, Shattil SJ, Furie B, Cohen HJ, eds. *Hematology: Basic Principles and Practice.* New York, NY: Churchill Livingstone; 1991.

Monitoring minimal residual disease in CML

The development of PCR has markedly increased the sensitivity of tests available for the monitoring of minimal residual disease. With the availability of real-time PCR, the relative abundance of the fusion transcript can now be monitored to assess trends of increase or decrease over time. Risk groups can now be stratified based on transcript quantity rather than simply presence or absence of transcript. The accuracy and reliability of real-time quantitative PCR as a measure of *bcr-abl* transcript level is dependent on the quality control procedures carried out by the laboratory. Normalization of the results to an appropriate control gene is required to compensate for variations in RNA quality and the efficiency of the **reverse transcriptase** reaction. *BCR* and *ABL* have been used as control genes, and both seem to be suitable because they are expressed at low level and have similar stability to *bcr-abl*. A major molecular response to imatinib has been defined as a 3-log reduction in *bcr-abl* transcripts (*bcr-abl*/reference gene) compared with a standardized baseline obtained from patients with untreated newly diagnosed CML. Unfortunately, not all laboratories have defined a baseline, and there is significant variation of baseline levels between laboratories. The use of standardized control samples that can be used to adjust results between laboratories should help harmonize results from various testing facilities.

Minimal residual disease detection in lymphoma

Immunoglobulin and T-cell receptor gene rearrangement studies allow the detection of residual disease in the blood and/or bone marrow of patients who have undergone treatment of a lymphoid malignancy. PCR-based techniques have greatly increased the sensitivity of such studies. Southern blot analysis can detect residual disease to the level of approximately 1 in 10^3 to 1 in 10^4 cells. PCR increases the sensitivity by at least one order of magnitude. However, because each gene rearrangement is unique, the PCR detection of gene rearrangements at this level of sensitivity is a labor-intensive undertaking. PCR of original tumor tissue is performed using primers based on consensus sequences shared by the variable and joining regions of the appropriate locus (immunoglobulin or T-cell receptor genes). The specific rearrangement must then be sequenced so that an oligonucleotide specific to the unique rearrangement in that patient's tumor can be synthesized. PCR can then be done using this **allele-specific oligonucleotide**, with adequate sensitivity to detect 1 in 10^5 cells. As such studies become increasingly available, they will play an important role in estimating prognosis and determining eligibility for autologous transplantation and other therapeutic modalities.

Expression profiling: applications to diagnosis and treatment

DNA microarray studies have yielded important new insights into leukemia pathogenesis and should facilitate the development of therapeutic interventions. Early studies demonstrated that the distinction between ALL and AML could be made with 100% accuracy on the basis of gene expression profiles alone. Later studies demonstrated that distinct molecular subtypes of ALL and AML could be discriminated based on expression profiling. For example, the application of DNA microarray technology to the evaluation of infant ALL with rearrangement of the *MLL* gene located at chromosome 11q23 suggested a molecular signature distinct from ALL and AML with molecular features of both. In addition, this work identified the *FLT-3* gene as one of the genes distinguishing infants with *MLL*-associated ALL from those with non–*MLL*-rearranged, pre–B-cell ALL. Microarray technology may also accurately delineate subtypes of a heterogeneous disorder, such as pediatric ALL. For example, hierarchical clustering has been used to distinguish pediatric ALL subtypes: *E2A-PBX*, *MLL*, T-ALL, hyperdiploid, *BCRABL*, and *TEL-AML1* (Figure 1-8).

Microarray studies are also facilitating the classification of lymphomas and outcome prediction for specific patient populations with this disease. For example, expression profiling was used to create a prediction model that identified 2 categories of patients with diffuse large B-cell lymphoma (DLBCL): good and poor prognosis. In addition, this study identified genes overexpressed in patients with poor prognosis. Two of these genes, *PDE4B* and *PKC*-β, may represent potential therapeutic targets.

Pharmacogenomics and treatment of ALL

Pharmacogenomics is the study of how an individual's genetic inheritance affects the body's response to drugs. The term comes from the words *pharmacology* and *genomics* and is thus the intersection of both disciplines. Germline SNPs and gene expression patterns in ALL cells have been linked to both the toxicity and the efficacy of chemotherapy. For instance, germline polymorphisms in the thiopurine methyltransferase gene result in loss of functional protein and predispose patients to severe hematologic toxicity unless the dose of mercaptopurine is reduced by 90% to 95%. ALL cells have been subjected to gene expression analysis and in vitro drug sensitivity to help identify patients at high risk of treatment failure so that therapy can be adjusted. These techniques hold promise for individualizing and optimizing treatments for many tumor types.

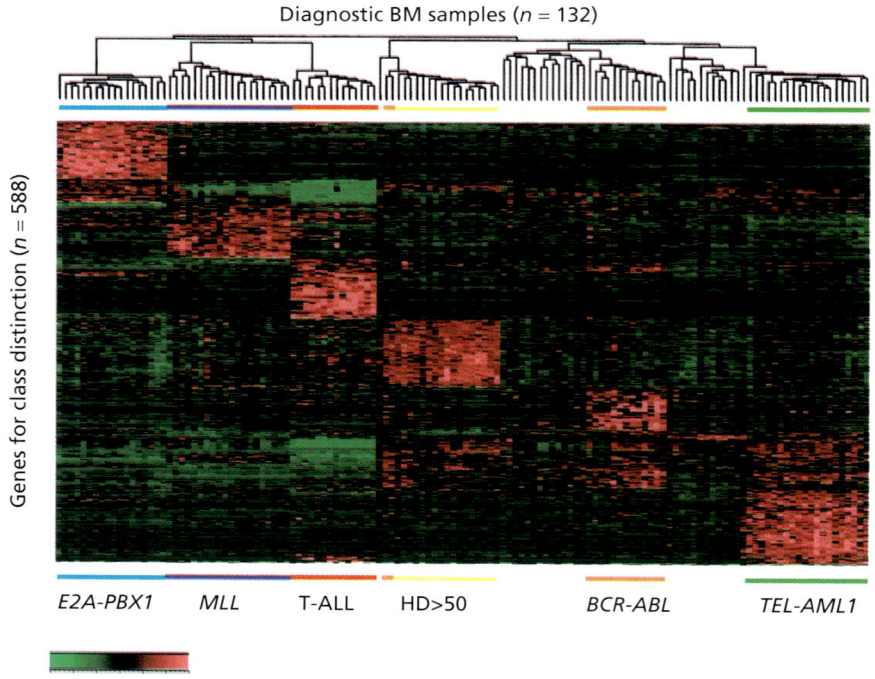

Figure 1-8 Expression profile of pediatric ALL diagnostic bone marrow blasts. In this figure, each column corresponds to a single leukemia sample, and each row represents the expression level of a probe set across the cases, with red representing expression above the mean and green representing expression below the mean. As shown, the pattern of expression of groups of either overexpressed or underexpressed genes distinguished among distinct ALL clinical and molecular phenotypes. Reproduced from Ross ME, Downing JR. Classification of pediatric acute lymphoblastic leukemia by gene expression profiling. *Blood*. 2003;102:2951–2959.

Applications to stem cell transplantation
HLA typing for stem cell transplantation

Molecular techniques have been important to the further understanding of the diversity of HLA genotypes. The serologic testing for HLA antigens often identifies broad groups of cross-reactive antigens. Because there is an increased incidence of severe graft-versus-host disease (GVHD) in patients who receive transplantations from serologically compatible but genotypically incompatible unrelated donors, it is important to identify the individual antigens within these cross-reactive groups. Genotypic HLA typing can be achieved by PCR amplification of the HLA locus followed by hybridization to specific oligonucleotides corresponding to the different alleles within a given cross-reactive group. Such genotyping is much more predictive of successful transplantation and the risk of GVHD than serologic study or the mixed lymphocyte assay (MLC), and it has supplanted these assays for the identification of optimal donors, especially unrelated donors. This is discussed in detail in Chapter 12.

Analysis of bone marrow engraftment

When donor and recipient are of opposite sex, the assessment of donor engraftment is based on conventional cytogenetics and is relatively straightforward. When donor and recipient are of the same sex, RFLP analysis of donor and recipient bone marrow allows the detection of polymorphic markers to distinguish DNA from the donor and recipient. After transplantation, RFLP analysis of recipient peripheral blood cells then can be used to document engraftment, chimerism, graft failure, and disease relapse. In most centers, PCR amplification and genotyping of short tandem repeat (STR) or variable number tandem repeat (VNTR) sequences that are polymorphic between donor and recipient pairs are now used to assess chimerism.

Applications to novel therapies
Antisense and RNA interference therapy

The recognition that abnormal expression of oncogene products plays a role in malignancy has led to the proposal that suppression of that expression might reverse the neoplastic phenotype. One way of blocking mRNA expression is through the use of **antisense oligonucleotides**. These are short pieces of single-stranded DNA or RNA, 17 to 20 bases long, called **oligonucleotides**, which are synthesized with a sequence complementary to the transcription or the translation initiation site in the mRNA. These short single-stranded species enter the cell freely, where they complex to the mRNA through the complementary sequence. Investigation of the mechanism of action of antisense oligonucleotides led to the discovery that naturally occurring double-stranded RNA molecules suppress gene expression better than antisense sequences and helped to unravel the mechanism of RNA interference. RNA interference has significant advantages over antisense therapy in that much lower concentrations are required. Numerous studies are under way in hematologic diseases; however, methods for delivery of siRNA are still far from perfect. In one study, adult stem cells from sickle cell patients were infected with a viral vector carrying a therapeutic γ-globin gene harboring an embedded siRNA precursor specific for $β^S$ globin. The newly formed red blood cells made normal hemoglobin and suppressed production of sickle β globin. In another study, a retroviral system for stable expression of siRNA directed to the unique fusion junction sequence of TEL-PDGFβR resulted in profound inhibition of TEL-PDGFβR expression and inhibited proliferation of TEL-PDGFβR–transformed cells. When applied to mice, this strategy slowed tumor development and death in mice injected with these cells compared with cells not containing the siRNA. Stable siRNA expression sensitized transformed cells to the PDGFβR inhibitor imatinib, suggesting that stable expression of siRNAs, which target oncogenic fusion genes, may potentiate the effects of conventional therapy for hematologic malignancies.

Gene therapy

The application of gene therapy to genetic hematologic disorders has long been an attractive concept. In most cases, this involves insertion of normal genes into autologous hematopoietic stem cells with subsequent transplantation back into the patient. Candidate hematologic diseases for such therapy include hemophilia, sickle cell disease, thalassemia, and severe combined immune deficiency syndrome (SCIDS). Rapid advances in technology for the separation of hematopoietic stem cells and techniques of gene transfer into those cells have advanced efforts toward this goal, and many clinical trials have begun. Although significant methodologic hurdles remain, research in this field continues to move forward. It should be recognized, however, that correction of diseases such as hemophilia, sickle cell disease, and thalassemia requires efficient gene transfer to a large number of hematopoietic stem cells with high levels of expression of the β-globin gene in erythroid precursors. Long-term repopulating stem cells have been relatively resistant to genetic modification; thus, many investigators have focused on gene therapy applications in which low levels of expression could restore patients to health.

A major impediment to successful gene therapy has been the lack of gene delivery systems that provide safe, efficient, and durable gene insertion and that can specifically target the cells of interest. Currently used approaches include retroviral vectors, adenoviral vectors, other viral vectors, and nonviral vectors. Features of each of these are outlined in Table 1-1.

RNA tumor viruses, or retroviruses, are unique in that their genetic information is contained in RNA rather than DNA. When the retrovirus infects a cell, its RNA is copied into DNA by the enzyme reverse transcriptase, and the cDNA then inserts into the host genome. In addition to the role that they play in human disease, retroviruses have become important as vectors for gene transfer. Retroviral vectors are constructed from retroviruses that are rendered unable to replicate because the genes (*gag*, *pol*, and *env*) necessary for reproduction of infectious viral particles are deleted. The desired gene is inserted into the retroviral genome, where the viral regulatory sequences direct high-level expression of the inserted gene. The recombinant retrovirus is then produced in a packaging cell line that contains the deleted genes necessary to make complete viral particles. The recombinant retrovirus then enters the target cell through a specific receptor, is reverse transcribed into DNA, and integrates randomly into the host genome. Vectors based on viruses of the Retroviridae family include those based on Oncovirinae (eg, Moloney murine leukemia viruses), Lentivirinae (eg, human immunodeficiency virus [HIV]-1), and Spumavirinae (eg, human foamy viruses).

Retroviral vectors have the major advantage of high transduction efficiency because they can stably transduce most target cells. However, their use has several limitations. They require the appropriate viral receptor for entry into the target cell, and this limits their host range. Perhaps more importantly, viral integration requires a proliferating target cell, and hematopoietic stem cells are generally noncycling.

Table 1-1 Methods of gene transfer for gene therapy.

Gene transfer method	Requires dividing cells	Insertion into host genome	Wide host range	Potential *in vivo* transfer	Stable expression
Retroviruses	Yes	Yes	No	No	Yes
Adenovirus	No	No	Yes	Yes	No
AAV	No	Yes	Yes	Yes	Yes
Lipofection	No	Probably not	Yes	Yes	No
CaPO4	No	Yes	Yes	No	Yes

AAV = adeno-associated virus

However, as shown in animal models, the HIV-based lentiviral vectors may be efficient for gene transfer into noncycling cells, such as hematopoietic stem cells. There is further evidence that cycling cells engraft less well than quiescent stem cells; therefore, induction of cycling to enhance transduction may impede successful transplantation of transduced cells. Third, the retroviral genome is subject to rearrangement and deletion, especially during purification and concentration of transducing viruses. The need for a packaging cell line to generate high-titer virus has also been associated with a low but measurable rate of transfer of replication competence to the recombinant virus. Finally, because the genes are inserted into the genome, there is a risk of insertional mutagenesis. Initially it was thought that this integration was random, but emerging evidence suggests that there is bias toward integration into actively transcribed genes in target cells with the potential that integration itself could alter the subsequent biologic properties of the target cell. Such a complication has been observed in 5 children who received retroviral-based gene therapy for treatment of X-linked SCIDS. Although the therapy was successful in 18 of 20 children who received it, 5 boys in 2 separate trials have developed T-cell leukemia. Interestingly, in children treated with gene therapy for SCIDS due to adenosine deaminase deficiency, no such event has developed. Investigators now believe that in X-linked SCIDS, activity of the newly expressed protein along with deregulated expression of proto-oncogenes cooperated to produce a lymphoproliferative disorder. Studies in monkeys suggest that such an observation may not be limited to X-linked SCIDS. Ingenious ideas to increase the safety of viral vectors in gene therapy include the use of vectors that are self-inactivating with better gene transfer and integration site choices, adding so-called insulator elements to the flanking regions of transgenes to prevent activation of nearby genes after integration, and the use of cellular promoters rather than viral promoters to obtain more physiologic regulation of gene expression.

Adenoviral vectors differ from retroviruses in several ways. They can infect nondividing cells, but they do not integrate into the host genome. Because infection with adenovirus results in lytic infections, adenoviral vectors must be rendered defective to prevent lytic infection. In infected, viable cells, the transduced DNA is not integrated but propagates within the cells. Adenoviral vectors have been used in human clinical trials, notably in gene therapy for cystic fibrosis. Results have indicated that the major problem with these vectors is their short-term efficacy secondary to rapid immune response to the infecting virus and toxicity secondary to acute inflammatory reactions. Other viral vectors include adeno-associated virus (AAV), herpesvirus, and RNA viruses. AAV is of interest for hematopoietic cell transfer because it does not require dividing cells for transduction. Interestingly, wild-type AAV integrates in a known preferred location on chromosome 19, decreasing the risk of random insertional mutagenesis. However, targeted integration may be less reliable with recombinant virus compared with wild-type virus. Preliminary clinical results, however, as in trials of gene therapy for hemophilia, have indicated that host immune response to the virus may result in inflammatory complications as well as destruction of transduced cells. Adenoviral vectors have proved useful, however, in the field of adoptive immunotherapy where immune cells can be transduced ex vivo and used to expand lymphoid populations specific for viruses such as CMV and EBV. These studies have also led to the development of successful tumor vaccines in which patients' own tumor cells are transduced with genes that enhance the immune response.

Nonviral gene transfer removes the risk of toxicity related to active viral infection secondary to contaminating packaging virus (with retroviral vectors) or reversion to competence for lytic infection (with adenoviral vectors). These methods introduce DNA into cells by complexing DNA to ligands for specific receptors or by physical methods such as lipofection (fusion of cells with liposomal vesicles) or direct injection of DNA but are much less efficient than viral transduction. Further study is needed to establish the durability of the expression of transgenes introduced by these methods.

A large number of clinical trials of gene therapy have been undertaken. They fall into 3 broad categories: (i) studies in which the transferred gene is a marker gene, which allows the documentation of successful gene transfer as well as insight into the natural history of disease (for example, to prove the origin of relapse in transplanted cells after autologous bone marrow transplantation); (ii) studies in which the transferred gene is inserted to correct an inherited genetic defect (for example, to introduce a normal adenosine deaminase [ADA] gene into T cells and stem cells to correct ADA-deficient SCIDS); and (iii) studies in which therapeutically active genes are introduced for the treatment of acquired disease (primarily as vaccines against tumors). Although some trials have been unsuccessful from a therapeutic standpoint, much has been learned, and there is continued optimism that gene therapy approaches will eventually be safe and effective.

Glossary

alleles Alternative forms of a particular gene.
allele-specific oligonucleotide Oligonucleotide whose sequence matches that of a specific polymorphic allele. Most commonly applies to oligonucleotides matching the sequence of unique immunoglobulin or T-cell receptor

gene rearrangements that are used for polymerase chain reaction (PCR) detection of minimal residual disease.

alternative splicing Selective inclusion or exclusion of certain exons in mature RNA by utilization of a varied combination of splicing signals.

anneal Association of separated DNA strands or DNA and RNA strands via complementary base pairing.

antisense oligonucleotides Oligonucleotides with a base sequence complementary to a stretch of DNA- or RNA-coding sequence.

capping Addition of the nucleotide 7-methylguanosine to the 5′ end of mRNA. This is a structure that appears to stabilize the mRNA.

chimeric Containing an alteration in only some of the cells of the animal.

chromatin Complex of genomic DNA with histone and nonhistone proteins.

chromosome Large linear DNA structures tightly complexed to nuclear proteins.

***cis*-acting regulatory elements** Sequences within a gene locus, but not within coding sequences, that are involved in regulating the expression of the gene by interaction with nuclear proteins.

clonal Arising from the proliferation of a single cell.

coding sequence Portion of the gene contained within exons that encodes for the amino acid sequence of the protein product.

codon The 3-nucleotide code that denotes a specific amino acid.

comparative genomic hybridization (CGH) A technique allowing detection of subtle chromosomal changes (deletions, amplifications, or inversions that are too small to be detected by conventional cytogenetics techniques).

complementary Sequence of the second strand of DNA that is determined by strict purine–pyrimidine base pairing (A-T; G-C).

complementary DNA (cDNA) Double-stranded DNA product from an RNA species. The first strand is synthesized by reverse transcriptase to make a DNA strand complementary to the mRNA. The second strand is synthesized by DNA polymerase to complement the first strand.

constitutive promoter A promoter that drives high-level expression in all tissues.

copy number variant (CNV) A segment of DNA at least 1 kb in length that varies in copy number between individuals.

cytogenetics Study of the chromosomal makeup of a cell.

degenerate Characteristic of the genetic code whereby more than one codon can encode the same amino acid.

Dicer A component of processing mechanism of formation of microRNA and siRNA.

Drosha A component of processing mechanism of formation of microRNA.

enhancer *cis*-Acting regulatory sequence within a gene locus that interacts with nuclear protein in such a way as to increase the expression of the gene.

epigenetics Changes in gene expression caused by mechanisms other than alteration of the underlying DNA sequence.

exome All protein coding portions of genes (exons) in the genome.

exon Portion of the structural gene that encodes for protein.

flanking sequences DNA lying 5′ and 3′ of a structural gene that frequently contain important regulatory elements.

fluorescence in situ hybridization (FISH) High-resolution mapping of genes by hybridization of chromosome spreads to biotin-labeled DNA probes and detection by fluorescent-tagged avidin.

frameshift mutation Mutation within the coding sequence of a gene that results from deletion or insertion of a nucleotide that disrupts the 3-base codon structure of the gene, completely altering the predicted amino acid sequence of the protein encoded by that gene.

gene Functional genetic unit responsible for the production of a given protein, including the elements that control the timing and the level of its expression.

gene expression profile Analysis of the global expression of a collection of cells using hybridization to microarrays.

gene regulation Process controlling the timing and level of expression of a gene.

genetic code System by which DNA encodes for specific protein through 3-nucleotide codons, each encoding a specific amino acid.

genomics The study of the entire DNA sequence of organisms and interactions between various genetic loci.

homologous recombination Alteration of genetic material by alignment of closely related sequences. In targeting genes by homologous recombination, plasmids that contain altered genes flanked by long stretches of DNA that match the endogenous gene are introduced into embryonic stem cells. A rare recombination event will cause the endogenous gene to be replaced by the mutated gene in the targeting plasmid. This is the means by which knockout mice are obtained.

imprinting Genetic process in which certain genes are expressed in a parent-of-origin–specific manner.

intron Intervening sequence of noncoding DNA that interrupts coding sequence contained in exons.

induced pluripotent stem (iPS) cells A type of pluripotent stem cell derived from a somatic cell, by inducing expression of 3 to 4 transcription factors.

knockout mouse Mouse in which one or both of the copies of a gene have been disrupted by a targeted mutation. Such mutations are achieved by homologous recombination using plasmids containing the mutated gene flanked by long stretches of the normal endogenous gene sequence.

leucine zipper Leucine-rich side chains shared by a group of transcription factors that allow protein–protein interactions.

linkage analysis Analysis of a gene locus by study of inheritance pattern of markers of nearby (linked) loci.

linkage disequilibrium Where alleles occur together more often than can be accounted for by chance, indicating that the 2 alleles are physically close on the DNA strand.

methylation DNA modification by addition of methyl groups to cytosine residues within genomic DNA. Hypermethylation is a characteristic of inactive DNA; reduction in methylation is associated with increased transcriptional activity.

microarray Glass slide or silicon chip on which cDNAs or oligonucleotides have been spotted to allow the simultaneous analysis of expression of hundreds to thousands of individual mRNAs. Hybridization of labeled cDNAs from a tissue of interest allows the generation of a gene expression profile.

microRNA Small RNA molecules encoded in the genomes of plants and animals. These highly conserved, approximately 21-mer RNAs regulate the expression of genes both by changing stability of mRNAs as well as by translational interference.

Next-Gen sequencing Massively parallel sequence production from single-molecule DNA templates.

noncoding sequences DNA sequences that do not directly encode for protein; these sequences lie within introns or in intragenic regions.

nonsense-mediated decay (NMD) Nonsense mutation (premature stop codon) of one allele of mRNA may result in degradation of the abnormal mRNA.

Northern blotting Analysis of RNA expression by gel electrophoresis, transfer to nitrocellulose or nylon filter, and hybridization to single-stranded probe.

nucleic acid hybridization Technique of nucleic acid analysis via association of complementary single-stranded species.

nucleotide Basic building block of nucleic acids, composed of a sugar moiety linked to a phosphate group and a purine or pyrimidine base.

oligonucleotide Short single-stranded DNA species, usually composed of 15 to 20 nucleotides.

oncogene Cellular gene involved with normal cellular growth and development, the altered expression of which has been implicated in the pathogenesis of the malignant phenotype.

polyadenylation Alteration of the 3′ end of mRNA by the addition of a string of adenosine nucleotides ("poly-A tail") that appear to protect the mRNA from premature degradation.

polymorphism In one popular concept, phenotypically silent mutation in DNA that is transmitted from parent to offspring; also used when a mutation in any gene exceeds an arbitrary threshold (eg, 5%) in any given population.

premessenger RNA Unprocessed primary RNA transcript from DNA, including all introns.

probe Fragment of DNA derived from a genetic locus that can be labeled, denatured, and used to analyze that gene.

promoter Region in the 5′ flanking region of a gene that is necessary for its expression; includes the binding site for RNA polymerase II.

purine Two of the bases found in DNA and RNA nucleotides: adenine and guanine.

pyrimidine Bases found in DNA and RNA nucleotides: cytosine and thymine in DNA; cytosine and uracil in RNA.

quantitative PCR PCR in which the product is quantitated in comparison to the PCR product resulting from a known quantity of template. This allows quantitation of the template in the reaction; it can, for example, allow an estimate of the degree of contamination with tumor cells in a cell population.

real-time PCR Automated technique for performing quantitative PCR using a fluorogenic reporter to detect levels of target sequences during early cycles of the PCR reaction.

reanneal Reassociation of 2 complementary single-stranded nucleic acid species.

restriction endonucleases Enzymes produced by bacteria that cleave double-stranded DNA at specific recognition sequences.

restriction fragment length polymorphism (RFLP) Polymorphism in which a silent mutation occurs within the recognition sequence for a restriction endonuclease. This results in an alteration in the size of the DNA fragment resulting from digestion of DNA from that DNA locus.

retrovirus RNA tumor virus.

reverse transcriptase Enzyme encoded by retroviruses that mediates conversion of its RNA genome to a DNA replica.

reverse transcriptase polymerase chain reaction (RT-PCR) Amplification of RNA sequences by conversion to cDNA by reverse transcriptase, followed by the polymerase chain reaction.

ribosome Ribonuclear protein complexes that bind to mRNA and mediate its translation into protein by "reading" the genetic code.

RISC RNA-induced silencing complex. A multiprotein complex that combines with microRNAs to target complementary mRNA for degradation or translation inhibition.

RNA polymerase II Enzyme-mediating transcription of most structural genes.

silencer *cis*-Acting regulatory sequence within a gene locus that interacts with nuclear protein in such a way as to decrease the expression of the gene.

siRNA Small interfering RNAs that act in concert with large multiprotein RISC complexes to cause cleavage of complementary mRNA or prevent its translation.

SNP Single nucleotide polymorphism. Naturally occurring inherited genetic variation between individuals at the level of single nucleotides (eg, C>T).

Southern blotting Analysis of DNA by gel electrophoresis, transfer to nitrocellulose or nylon filter, and hybridization to single-stranded probe.

splicing Process by which intron sequences are removed from premRNA.

structural gene Portion of a gene that is transcribed into mRNA.

tag SNP A single nucleotide polymorphism that is closely associated and inherited with nearby SNPs and can be used to define the DNA sequence in a small chromosomal region.

termination codon One of 3 codons that signal the termination of translation.

trans-acting factor Protein that interacts with *cis*-acting regulatory region within a gene locus to regulate transcription of that gene. Also called transcription factor.

transcription Process by which premRNA is formed from the DNA template.

transcription factor Protein that interacts with *cis*-acting regulatory region within a gene locus to regulate transcription of that gene. Also called *trans*-acting factor.

transfer RNA (tRNA) Small RNA molecules that bind to the ribosome and covalently bind specific amino acids, allowing translation of the genetic code into protein.

transgenic mouse A mouse that expresses an exogenous gene (transgene) introduced randomly into its genome. Linearized DNA is injected into the pronucleus of a fertilized oocyte, and the zygote is reimplanted. Resultant mice will carry the transgene in all cells.

translation Process by which protein is synthesized from an mRNA template.

translocation breakpoint Site of junction of 2 aberrantly juxtaposed (translocated) chromosomal fragments.

uniparental disomy Occurs when 2 copies of a chromosome, or part of a chromosome, are derived from one parent and no copies derive from the other parent. In a somatic cell, this can result in progeny with 2 copies of the wild-type allele or 2 copies of the mutant allele.

Western blotting Detection of specific proteins via binding of specific antibody to protein on a nitrocellulose or nylon membrane.

zinc-finger Structural feature shared by a group of transcription factors. Zinc-fingers are composed of a zinc atom associated with cysteine and histidine residues; the fingers appear to interact directly with DNA to affect transcription.

Bibliography

Basic concepts

Beutler E, Yeh M, Fairbanks VF. The normal human female as a mosaic of X-chromosome activity: Studies using the gene for G-6-PD deficiency as a marker. *Proc Natl Acad Sci USA*. 1962;48(1):9–16.

Lyon MF, Searle AG, Ford CE, Ohno S. A mouse translocation suppressing sex-linked variegation. *Cytogenetics*. 1964;3(15):306–323.

Epigenetics

Gruenbaum Y, Margalit A, Goldman RD, Shumaker DK, Wilson KL. The nuclear lamina comes of age. *Nat Rev Mol Cell Biol*. 2005;6:21–31. *A review describing what is known about the nuclear lamina and the role of lamin-dependent complexes in chromatin organization, gene regulation, and signal transduction.*

Lalande M, Calciano MA. Molecular epigenetics of Angelman syndrome. *Cell Mol Life Sci*. 2007;64:947–960. *A thorough description of what is known about imprinting and Angelman syndrome.*

Rice KL, Hormaeche I, Licht JD. Epigenetic regulation of normal and malignant hematopoiesis. *Oncogene*. 2007;26:6697–6714. *A nice review detailing the interaction between lineage-specific transcription factors and a series of epigenetic tags, including DNA methylation and covalent histone tail modifications, such as acetylation, methylation, phosphorylation, SUMOylation, and ubiquitylation.*

Sahoo T, del Gaudio D, German JR, et al. Prader-Willi phenotype caused by paternal deficiency for the HBII-85 C/D box small nucleolar RNA cluster. *Nat Genet*. 2008;40:719–721. *An elegant description of the specific genetic defect in Prader-Willi syndrome.*

RNA interference

Calin GA, Ferracin M, Cimmino A, et al. A microRNA signature associated with prognosis and progression in chronic lymphocytic leukemia. *N Engl J Med*. 2005;353:1793–1801. *A description of a unique microRNA signature is associated with prognostic factors and disease progression in chronic lymphocytic leukemia.*

Hammond SM. Dicing and slicing: the core machinery or the RNA interference pathway. *FEBS Lett.* 2005;579:5822–5829. *A review describing the discovery of the RNA interference pathway and discussion of future lines of work.*

Prchal JT. MicroRNAs: a new player in human malignancies? *Hematologist.* 2005;2:19. *A brief discussion of microRNAs.*

HapMap

Crawford DC, Nickerson DA. Definition and clinical importance of haplotypes. *Annu Rev Med.* 2005;56:303–320. *A review of the basic concepts of high-density genetic maps of SNPs and haplotypes and how they are typically generated and used in human genetic research.*

McVean G, Spencer CC, Chaix R. Perspectives on human genetic variation from the HapMap Project. *PLoS Genet.* 2005;1:413–418. *A review focusing on what the HapMap Project has taught us about the structure of human genetic variation and the fundamental molecular and evolutionary processes that shape it.*

The International HapMap Consortium. A second generation human haplotype map of over 3.1 million SNPs. *Nature.* 2007;449:851–861. *A description of the Phase II HapMap, which characterizes over 3.1 million human SNPs genotyped in 270 individuals from four geographically diverse populations.*

Molecular techniques

Botstein D, White RL, Skolnick M, et al. Construction of a genetic linkage map in man using restriction fragment length polymorphisms. *Am J Hum Genet.* 1980;32:314–331. *One of the first descriptions of the basis for the construction of a genetic linkage map of the human genome.*

McKusick VA. The morbid anatomy of the human genome: a review of gene mapping in clinical medicine. 4. *Medicine (Baltimore).* 1988;67:1–19. *An early and thorough review of the use of gene mapping to define the genetic origin of inherited disease.*

Minden MD, Messner HA, Belch A. Origin of leukemic relapse after bone marrow transplantation detected by restriction fragment length polymorphism. *J Clin Invest.* 1985;75:91–93. *A description of the use of restriction fragment length polymorphism analysis to determine the origin of recurrent leukemia cells in which no identifying chromosome was present.*

Southern EM. Detection of specific sequences among DNA fragments separated by gel electrophoresis. *J Mol Biol.* 1975;98:503–517. *The seminal paper describing the Southern blotting technique.*

Cytogenetics, FISH, and sequencing studies

Le Beau MM, Rowley JD. Chromosomal abnormalities in leukemia and lymphoma: clinical and biological significance. *Adv Hum Genet.* 1986;15:1–54. *An early review of the significance of chromosomal abnormalities in hematologic malignancies.*

Ley TJ, Mardis ER, Ding L, et al. DNA sequencing of a cytogenetically normal acute myeloid leukaemia genome. *Nature.* 2008;456:66–72. *This study establishes whole-genome sequencing as an unbiased method for discovering novel mutations associated with cancer.*

Ried T, Baldini A, Rand TC, et al. Simultaneous visualization of seven different DNA probes by in situ hybridization using combinatorial fluorescence and digital imaging microscopy. *Proc Natl Acad Sci USA.* 1992;89:1388–1392. *A description of the combinatorial labeling of probes to increase the number of target sequences that can be detected simultaneously by FISH.*

Volpi EV, Bridger JM. FISH glossary: an overview of the fluorescent in situ hybridization technique. *Biotechniques.* 2008;45:385–409. *A succinct review of the many FISH strategies available.*

Willman CL. Molecular evaluation of acute myeloid leukemia. *Semin Hematol.* 1999;36:390–400. *A review of the molecular genetic features of different forms of AML and automated molecular technologies for residual disease assessment.*

Polymerase chain reaction

Chebab FF, Kan YW. Detection of specific DNA sequences by fluorescence amplification: a color complementation assay. *Proc Natl Acad Sci USA.* 1989;86:9178–9182. *This paper describes the development of a color complementation assay that allows rapid screening of specific genomic DNA sequences. The technique is based on the simultaneous amplification of 2 or more DNA segments with fluorescent oligonucleotide primers such that the generation of a color, or combination of colors, can be visualized and used for diagnosis.*

Guo Z-M, Xu K, Yue Y, et al. Temporal control of Cre recombinase-mediated in vitro DNA recombination by Tet-on gene expression system. *Acta Biochim Biophys Sin.* 2005;37:133–138. *This paper describes the use of the Cre-loxP system to induce conditional knockout mice.*

Mullis K, Faloona F, Scharf S, et al. Specific enzymatic amplification of DNA in vitro: the polymerase chain reaction. *Cold Spring Harb Symp Quant Biol.* 1986;51:263–273. *One of the earliest descriptions of the polymerase chain reaction.*

Transgenic and knockout mouse models

Palmiter RD, Brinster RL. Germ-line transformation of mice. *Ann Rev Genet.* 1986;20:465–499. *A nice early review on the creation of transgenic mice.*

Sauer B. Inducible gene targeting in mice using the Cre/lox system. *Methods.* 1998;14:381–392. *A thorough review explaining the Cre-Lox system and its various uses.*

Thomas KR, Capecchi MR. Site directed mutagenesis by gene targeting in mouse embryo-derived stem cells. *Cell.* 1987;51:503–512. *Straightforward description of the creation of a transgenic mouse containing a mutation in the hypoxanthine phosphoribosyl transferase gene.*

Hemoglobinopathies

Boehm CD, Stylianos EA, Phillips JA, et al. Prenatal diagnosis using DNA polymorphisms: report on 95 pregnancies at risk for sickle cell disease or beta-thalassemia. *N Engl J Med.* 1983;308:1054–1058. *One of the earliest descriptions of the use of SNPs linked to a gene for diagnosis of disease.*

Hanna J, Wernig M, Markoulaki S, et al. Treatment of sickle cell anemia mouse model with iPS cells generated from autologous skin. *Science.* 2007;318(5858):1920–1923. *Using a humanized sickle cell anemia mouse model, these investigators showed that that mice can be "rescued" after transplantation with "corrected" hematopoietic progenitors obtained in vitro from autologous iPS cells.*

Lymphoproliferative disease

Arnold A, Cossman J, Bakhshi A, et al. Immunoglobulin-gene rearrangements as unique clonal markers in human lymphoid neoplasms. *N Engl J Med.* 1983;309:1593–1599. *An early study showing that the detection of immunoglobulin gene rearrangements by Southern blotting is a sensitive marker for clonality and B-cell lineage in lymphoid malignancies.*

Minden MD, Mak TW. The structure of the T cell antigen receptor genes in normal and malignant T cells. *Blood.* 1986;68:327–336. *A nice review describing rearrangements of the β chain of the T-cell antigen receptor and the use of these rearrangements to identify clonality in T-cell neoplasms.*

Cryptic translocations in leukemia

Maloney K, McGavran L, Murphy J, et al. TEL-AML1 fusion identifies a subset of children with standard risk acute lymphoblastic leukemia who have an excellent prognosis when treated with therapy that includes a single delayed intensification. *Leukemia.* 1999;13:1708–1712. *A beautiful example of how the presence of a molecular marker can be used to predict response to chemotherapy.*

Minimal residual disease monitoring

Cave H, van der Werff ten Bosch J, Suciu S, et al. Clinical significance of minimal residual disease in childhood acute lymphoblastic leukemia. European Organization for Research and Treatment of Cancer–Childhood Leukemia Cooperative Group. *N Engl J Med.* 1998;339:591–598. *One of the earliest studies demonstrating that detection of residual disease using a sensitive technique such as PCR is a strong predictor of ultimate outcome in acute lymphoblastic leukemia.*

Diverio D, Rossi V, Avvisati G, et al. Early detection of relapse by prospective reverse transcriptase polymerase chain reaction analysis of the PML-RARα fusion gene in patients with acute promyelocytic leukemia enrolled in the GIMEMA-AIEOP Multicenter AIDA trial. *Blood.* 1998;92:784–789. *A demonstration that conversion to PCR positivity for PML/RARα during remission from acute promyelocytic leukemia predicts subsequent hematologic relapse.*

Hughes T, Branford S. Molecular monitoring of BCR-ABL as a guide to clinical management in chronic myeloid leukaemia. *Blood Rev.* 2006;20(1):29–41. *A description of the use of real-time PCR to monitor BCR-ABL transcripts in chronic myeloid leukemia.*

Nucifora G, Larson RA, Rowley J. Persistence of the 8;21 translocation in patients with acute myeloid leukemia type M2 in long-term remission. *Blood.* 1993;82:712–715. *This article describes the interesting observation that detection of the 8;21 translocation in patients with AML M2 does not necessarily foretell relapse.*

Gene expression profiling

Alizadeh AA, Eisen MB, Davis RE, et al. Distinct types of diffuse large B-cell lymphoma identified by gene expression profiling. *Nature.* 2000;403:503–511. *One of the first papers to demonstrate diversity in gene expression among diffuse large B-cell lymphomas and the fact that gene expression reflects tumor proliferation rate, host response, and differentiation state of the tumor.*

Armstrong SA, Kung AL, Mabon ME, et al. Inhibition of FLT3 in MLL. Validation of a therapeutic target identified by gene expression based classification. *Cancer Cell.* 2003;3:173–183. *An elegant study demonstrating that identification of an overexpressed gene can be used to help direct therapy.*

Armstrong SA, Staunton JE, Silverman LB, et al. MLL translocations specify a distinct gene expression profile that distinguishes a unique leukemia. *Nat Genet.* 2002;30:41–47. *An interesting demonstration that a unique gene expression profile in patients with acute lymphoblastic leukemia predicts a chromosomal translocation.*

Shipp MA, Ross KN, Tamayo P, et al. Diffuse large B-cell lymphoma outcome prediction by gene-expression profiling and supervised machine learning. *Nat Med.* 2002;8:68–74. *A study demonstrating that gene expression in tumor samples from patients with diffuse large B-cell lymphoma can be used to predict the outcome after standard CHOP therapy.*

Yeoh EJ, Ross ME, Shurtleff SA, et al. Classification, subtype discovery, and prediction of outcome in pediatric acute lymphoblastic leukemia by gene expression profiling. *Cancer Cell.* 2002;1:133–143. *Further evidence that gene expression predicts important leukemia subtypes and therapeutic outcome.*

Pharmacogenomics

Cheok MH, Pottier N, Kager L, Evans WE. Pharmacogenetics in acute lymphoblastic leukemia. *Semin Hematol.* 2009;46:39–51. *A thorough description using ALL as an example of how pharmacogenetics can be used to tailor therapy to individual patients to optimize efficacy and safety through better understanding of human genome variability and its influence on drug response.*

Stem cell transplantation

Knowlton RG, Brown VA, Braman JC, et al. Use of highly polymorphic DNA probes for genotypic analysis following bone marrow transplantation. *Blood.* 1986;68:378–385.

DNA markers known as restriction fragment length polymorphisms are a sensitive and informative method of distinguishing patient and allogeneic donor cells after bone marrow transplantation.

Antisense and RNA interference therapy

Chen J, Wall NR, Kocher K, et al. Stable expression of small interfering RNA sensitizes TEL-PDGFbetaR to inhibition with imatinib or rapamycin. *J Clin Invest.* 2004;113:1784–1791. *A description of how siRNAs directed at a particular fusion transcript might be used therapeutically in combination with other targeted agents.*

Guinness ME, Kenney JL, Reiss M, et al. Bcl-2 antisense oligodeoxynucleotide therapy of Epstein-Barr virus-associated lymphoproliferative disease in severe combined immunodeficient mice. *Cancer Res.* 2000;60:5354–6358. *A mouse study demonstrating that oligonucleotides directed against the first 6 codons of Bcl-2 prevented development of fatal EBV-positive lymphoproliferative disease in immune-compromised animals.*

Samakoglu S, Lisowski L, Budak-Alpdogan T, et al. A genetic strategy to treat sickle cell anemia by coregulating globin transgene expression and RNA interference. *Nat Biotechnol.* 2006;24:89–94. *An ingenious strategy to "turn off" expression of the sickle β globin with RNA interference while simultaneously delivering a γ-globin gene.*

Gene therapy

Aiuti A, Cattaneo F, Galimberti S, et al. Gene therapy for immunodeficiency due to adenosine deaminase deficiency. *N Engl J Med.* 2009;360:447–458. *An extended follow-up report on 10 patients with SCID due to ADA deficiency.*

Cavazzana-Calvo M, Hacein-Bey S, de Saint Basile G, et al. Gene therapy of human severe combined immunodeficiency (SCID)-X1 disease. *Science.* 2000;288:669–672. *The fascinating description of immune reconstitution in 5 infants with X-linked SCID who underwent gene therapy.*

Hacein-Bey-Abina S, Von Kalle C, Schmidt M, et al. LMO2-associated clonal T cell proliferation in two patients after gene therapy for SCID-X1. *Science.* 2003;302:415–419. *A report of uncontrolled clonal proliferation of mature T cells in 2 patients with X-linked SCIDS treated with gene therapy.*

Kohn DB, Candotti F. Gene therapy fulfilling its promise. *N Engl J Med.* 2009;360:518–521. *An informative editorial describing the issues surrounding gene therapy for SCID.*

Mulligan RC. The basic science of gene therapy. *Science.* 1993;260:926–932. *An insightful description of the technical issues involved in gene therapy.*

Nienhuis AW. Development of gene therapy for blood disorders. *Blood.* 2008;111:4431–4444. *A comprehensive description of the use and potential for gene therapy in benign and malignant blood disorders.*

Nonsense-mediated decay

Amrani N, Sachs MS, Jacobson A. Early nonsense: mRNA decay solves a translational problem. *Nat Rev Mol Cell Biol.* 2006;7:415–425. *A review of the mechanisms of nonsense-mediated decay.*

Khajavi M, Inoue K, Lupski JR. Nonsense-mediated mRNA decay modulates clinical outcome of genetic disease. *Eur J Hum Genet.* 2006;14:1074–1081. *A review of the physiologic role of nonsense-mediated decay, its implications for human diseases, and its importance to an understanding of genotype–phenotype correlations in various genetic disorders.*

Sheth U, Parker R. Targeting of aberrant mRNAs to cytoplasmic processing bodies. *Cell.* 2006;125:1095–1109. *An insightful model for nonsense-mediated decay in which 2 successive steps distinguish normal and aberrant mRNAs.*

Proteomics

Service RF. Proteomics ponders prime time. *Science.* 2008;321:1758–1761 *An editorial review of the challenges facing proteomics.*

Unwin RD, Whetton AD. How will haematologists use proteomics? *Blood Rev.* 2007;21:315–326. *A complete discussion of the technologies available for the study of the proteome that offer realistic opportunities in hematology.*

CHAPTER 02

Consultative hematology

Marc J. Kahn, Amy E. Geddis, and Keith R. McCrae

The role and effectiveness of the consultant, 27	Intensive care unit, 35	Selected outpatient hematology topics, 52
Consultation for surgery and invasive procedures, 27	Consultation for hematologic complications of solid organ transplantation, 40	Consultation in pediatric patients, 57
	Pregnancy, 42	Bibliography, 64

The role and effectiveness of the consultant

A hematology consultant provides expert advice about the diagnosis and management of benign or malignant hematologic disorders to requesting physicians and other health care providers. A consultation request might involve an adult general medical patient, a child or adolescent, a pregnant woman, a perioperative patient, or an individual who is critically ill. Given the relatively low numbers of physicians specifically trained in hematology, in some situations, a hematologist may also be asked to render an opinion on patient management to another physician, perhaps from a distance, without having directly seen the patient; requests such as these should be considered carefully given that complete patient information may not be directly available. Other consultative responsibilities of the hematologist may include serving on committees that maintain a formulary, developing clinical practice guidelines, establishing policies and procedures for transfusion services, or monitoring quality and efficiency. In some cases, consultation for the federal government or pharmaceutical industry may also be requested. Although these latter roles will not be specifically addressed in this chapter, the data management, organizational, and communication skills that are critical for patient consultation are also useful when working within advisory groups.

A clinical hematologist must also understand the principles of effective consultation and the extreme importance of interphysician communication (Table 2-1). Consultants need to communicate effectively not only with other staff physicians and consultants, but also with house staff, fellows, students, and the patient and family. The value of group meetings to discuss complex patients should not be overestimated. A commitment to effective communication ensures maximal compliance with recommendations and the highest quality of multidisciplinary patient care.

Consultation for surgery and invasive procedures

Clinical case

You are consulted to help manage a 72-year-old man with a mechanical mitral valve who is scheduled to undergo extraction of his remaining 7 teeth. The patient is maintained on warfarin to keep his international normalized ratio (INR) between 2 and 3. The oral surgeon is concerned about the patient's bleeding risk but is reluctant to stop warfarin because of the patient's mechanical mitral valve. You estimate the patient to be at high risk for thromboembolism if warfarin is stopped. As such, you recommend continuing warfarin at the prescribed dose with the use of a mouthwash containing ε-aminocaproic acid to control local bleeding and reconsultation should this approach not be sufficient.

Preoperative assessment of bleeding risk

Avoiding hemorrhage is a prime concern during surgery, invasive procedures, and spinal anesthesia. The risk of hemorrhage is proportional to the extent of the intervention, the vascularity of the involved tissue, the potential for local fibrinolysis, the effects of pressure from a hematoma, the ability to achieve surgical hemostasis, and the possibility that elements of the procedure might induce a hemostatic defect, as with cardiopulmonary bypass. Additionally, considering

---

Conflict-of-interest disclosure: *Dr. Kahn* declares no competing financial interest. *Dr. Geddis*: research funding: Amgen; membership on board of directors or advisory committee: Amgen. *Dr. McCrae*: consultancy: GlaxoSmithKline; honoraria: GlaxoSmithKline.

Table 2-1 Principles of effective consultation and interphysician communication.

Principle	Comment
Determine the question that is being asked	The consultant must clearly understand the reason for the consultation
Establish the urgency of the consultation and respond in a timely manner	Urgent consultations must be seen as soon as possible (communicate any expected delays promptly); elective consultations should be seen within 24 hours
Gather primary data	Personally confirm the database; do not rely on secondhand information
Communicate as briefly as appropriate	Compliance is optimized when the consultant addresses specific questions with ≤5 succinct and relevant recommendations
Make specific recommendations	Identify major issues; limit the diagnostic recommendations to those most crucial; and provide specific drug doses, schedules, and treatment guidelines
Provide contingency plans	Briefly address alternative diagnoses; anticipate complications and questions
Understand the consultant's role	The attending physician has primary/ultimate responsibility; the consultant should not assume primary care or write orders without permission from the attending
Offer educational information	Provide relevant evidence-based literature and/or guidelines
Communicate recommendations directly to the requesting physician	Direct verbal contact (in person or by phone) optimizes compliance and minimizes confusion or error
Provide appropriate follow-up	Continue involvement and progress notes as indicated; officially sign-off the case or provide outpatient follow-up

Adapted from Goldman L, Lee T, Rudd P. Ten commandments for effective consultations. *Arch Intern Med.* 1983;143:1753–1755; and Sears CL, Charlson ME. The effectiveness of a consultation. Compliance with initial recommendations. *Am J Med.* 1983;74:870–876.

whether hemorrhage could lead to severe or permanent functional impairment (particularly within the central nervous system [CNS], spinal canal, or eye) is important in assessing the bleeding risk of a procedure.

The most important and relevant preoperative assessment necessary to determine the risk of bleeding is a detailed personal and family history. Abnormalities found on preoperative hemostatic testing and significant bleeding after the procedure are most strongly predicted by a personal history of abnormal bleeding; a history of family members with bleeding disorders; the use of antiplatelet, anticoagulant, or other medications that could affect hemostasis; a history of prior bleeding associated with hemostatic challenges; or a history of known medical comorbidities associated with a bleeding diathesis. By comparison, patients with no suspicious history and no obvious comorbidities rarely have abnormal screening tests, and abnormal hemostatic laboratory results in patients without a bleeding history generally do not correlate closely enough with outcome to modify treatment decisions. This applies to high-risk procedures, including liver biopsy, kidney biopsy, prostate surgery, coronary artery bypass surgery, tonsillectomy, and gynecologic surgery, where screening hemostatic test results have low sensitivity and poor positive predictive value.

Despite the lack of evidence to support laboratory screening in asymptomatic patients, a limited hemostatic evaluation remains standard practice for patients undergoing major surgery. These tests include the prothrombin time (PT), activated partial thromboplastin time (aPTT), and platelet count. Tests for platelet function, including the bleeding time and platelet function analyzer (PFA-100), do not predict the bleeding risk of invasive procedures and are not warranted in the absence of a history suggestive of a bleeding disorder. It is important to remember that most tests of coagulation and/or platelet function were not developed as screening tools for procedure-induced bleeding; thus, it is not surprising that they do not perform well in that setting. For example, a normal aPTT result might fail to identify a patient with mild von Willebrand disease (vWD), particularly if that patient's history was uninformative because he or she had never been subjected to a significant prior hemostatic stress. Alternatively, the aPTT may yield an abnormal result that is not associated with a bleeding diathesis, such as a deficiency of a contact factor protein or a lupus anticoagulant.

The hematologist is most often consulted about patients who have a suspicious history of bleeding, abnormal preprocedure hemostatic screening results, a preexisting characterized bleeding disorder, or exposure to drugs that affect hemostasis. The approach to a preoperative patient with either a suggestive history or abnormal screening tests should mimic the approach to the bleeding patient (see Chapter 8). This begins with completing the historical, clinical, and laboratory database and determining whether a suspected defect involves primary or secondary hemostasis.

The risks for patients with known hemostatic disorders must be determined based on the nature of the defect and the specific procedure that is planned. For high-risk procedures, preoperative factor replacement therapy is indicated to correct the PT/INR to ≤1.5, the aPTT to ≤1.5 times control (in the case of hemophilia, a factor level of 80%–100%), and the fibrinogen to ≥1 g/L. For low- to moderate-risk procedures, a PT/INR of ≤2 is usually adequate. Although randomized trials are lacking, patients with thrombocytopenia should achieve a platelet count of ≥50,000/μL before moderate- to high-risk procedures. However, a platelet count of ≥100,000/μL is desired before neurosurgical interventions or ophthalmologic procedures, where even limited bleeding may lead to catastrophic outcomes. Patients with immune thrombocytopenia often tolerate surgery well even with platelet counts <50,000/μL. Data to support the use of platelet transfusions in this setting are not available. Special considerations may be warranted for patients with severe liver disease, deficient factor production, delayed factor clearance, and accelerated fibrinolysis. Acquired platelet dysfunction may also contribute to a bleeding diathesis.

Patients with normal baseline hemostasis who are taking antiplatelet or anticoagulant drugs must be evaluated in the context of the indications for antithrombotic therapy and the bleeding risks associated with the specific procedure. For example, consumption of aspirin or clopidogrel within the week prior to coronary artery bypass graft surgery is associated with a significant increase in perioperative bleeding, transfusion requirements, and reoperation. These risks, however, must be counterbalanced against the improved graft outcomes in the presence of antiplatelet therapy, and some recommendations suggest that aspirin be continued up until the time of surgery, whereas clopidogrel should be discontinued at least 5 days and preferably 10 days prior to surgery. A similar approach applies to patients receiving abciximab or other specific inhibitors of platelet glycoprotein (GP) IIb/IIIa. However, because the GPIIb/IIIa antagonists have a short half-life, delaying surgery for 12 hours after stopping the drug may be a safe alternative approach.

Due to the specific nature of current recommendations and the particular clinical situation in question, we recommend review of the American College of Chest Physicians (ACCP) current guidelines concerning the perioperative management of antithrombotic and antiplatelet medications for complete evidenced-based guidelines (http://chestjournal.chestpubs.org). Aspirin can also be safely continued in outpatients undergoing cataract surgery, simple dental extractions, and certain dermatologic procedures. However, clopidogrel and dipyridamole are usually discontinued prior to invasive biopsies, arthroscopies, traumatic dental surgeries, and outpatient procedures that may be accompanied by a high risk of bleeding.

For patients on warfarin, management prior to and following invasive procedures should be guided by evidence-based recommendations for either temporary interruption or bridging anticoagulation (Table 2-2). Patients on low molecular weight heparin (LMWH) should stop therapy 24 hours before surgery or epidural anesthesia and not resume it until 24 hours after the procedure. Because dosage is difficult to calculate, protamine sulfate is not generally used to reverse LMWH. Unfractionated heparin (UFH) should be stopped 6 hours before surgery. If surgery must take place in <4 hours, UFH can be reversed with protamine sulfate. Although selective serotonin reuptake inhibitors

Table 2-2 Management of patients receiving bridging anticoagulation.

Clinical situation	Guidelines
Patients taking VKA prior to surgery	Use SC LMWH for bridging as an outpatient.
Patients receiving therapeutic-dose LMWH as bridge	Stop LMWH 24 hours prior to surgery. Give 50% of total dose as last dose, rather than 100%. For minor procedures, resume LMWH 24 hours after procedure. Delay LMWH for 48–72 hours for major procedures. Always consider bleeding risks prior to restarting anticoagulation.
Patients taking aspirin or clopidogrel prior to surgery	Stop 7–10 days prior to surgery. Can resume aspirin or clopidogrel 24 hours after surgery if adequate hemostasis.
Patients receiving aspirin or clopidogrel at high risk for cardiac events without stents	Continue aspirin up to and beyond time of surgery. Stop clopidogrel at least 5 days prior to surgery.
Patients with bare metal stents within 6 weeks of placement who require surgery	Continue aspirin and clopidogrel in perioperative period.
Patients with drug-eluting stent within 12 months of placement who require surgery	Continue aspirin and clopidogrel in perioperative period
Patient requiring minor dental procedures, dermatologic procedures, or cataract surgery who are taking VKAs, aspirin, or clopidogrel	Continue VKA and/or aspirin and coadminister oral prohemostatic agent. For patients taking clopidogrel, see clopidogrel recommendations above.

Adapted from Douketis JD, Berger PB, Dunn AS, et al. Perioperative management of antithrombotic therapy: American College of Chest Physicians Evidence-Based Clinical Practice Guidelines (8th Edition). Chest. 2008;133:299S–339S.

LMWH = low molecular weight heparin; SC = subcutaneously; VKA = vitamin K antagonists.

impair platelet function and may be associated with increased bleeding in patients undergoing surgery, there are no general guidelines that address their discontinuation in the preoperative patient, and thus, individuals on these agents must be considered on an individual basis.

Perioperative hemorrhage, hemostatic agents, and transfusion

Intraoperative hemorrhage

Intraoperative hemorrhage may be due to inadequate local hemostasis or a systemic coagulation defect. The consultant may be called to assist the surgeon in making a rapid decision regarding the possibility of a coagulation defect and advisability of reexploring the wound. A need for reexploration is most evident when the PT, aPTT, and platelet count are normal, although it is not uncommon to have surgical bleeding due to inadequate local hemostasis and abnormal coagulation parameters concurrently. Potential causes of intraoperative coagulopathy and generalized bleeding that must be considered include unrecognized preexisting defects such as factor XI deficiency or vWD, hypothermia, hyperfibrinolysis, drugs, uremia, disseminated intravascular coagulation (DIC), and postransfusion (dilutional) coagulopathy. Not to be overlooked is the increased risk of bleeding induced by common issues such as acid–base disturbances and surgery-induced hypothermia.

Excessive blood loss occurs in 6% to 25% of patients undergoing bypass surgery. This is mostly due to the effects of cardiopulmonary bypass on platelet function, but may also be due to the use of antiplatelet agents, heparin, or other anticoagulants. Liver transplantation also carries unique risks due to temporary cessation of coagulation factor synthesis and enhanced fibrinolysis. During reperfusion of the transplanted liver, tissue-type plasminogen activator (tPA) is released into the circulation, and proteolysis of vWF occurs. Factor replacement, antifibrinolytic therapy, and, in selected patients with active bleeding, recombinant factor VIIa (rFVIIa) are sometimes used on an empiric basis to control hemorrhage. Of note, 2 recent randomized, placebo-controlled trials showed that single- or multiple-dose prophylactic rFVIIa did not decrease the number of perioperative red blood cell transfusions required by patients undergoing orthotopic liver transplantation for end-stage liver disease. As an alternative to rFVIIa, fibrin sealant has been used on the liver surface intraoperatively to ensure adequate local hemostasis.

Hemostatic agents

Intraoperative hemorrhage can be prevented or controlled under certain circumstances by the use of hemostatic agents. Such agents include conjugated estrogens, desmopressin (DDAVP), lysine analogs, aprotinin, rFVIIa, and fibrin sealant. Oral or intravenous conjugated estrogens, given for 5 to 7 days preoperatively, may decrease platelet-related bleeding in patients with chronic renal failure. Acquired platelet dysfunction due to uremia, underlying vWD, or congenital platelet dysfunction may also improve after intravenous or intranasal administration of DDAVP. However, a recent meta-analysis of 17 randomized, double-blind, placebo-controlled trials showed no significant impact of DDAVP on transfusion requirements among patients undergoing cardiac bypass, whereas treated patients suffered a 2.4-fold increased incidence of perioperative myocardial infarction (MI).

The lysine analogs, ε-aminocaproic acid and tranexamic acid, inhibit plasminogen activation to plasmin, thus impairing lysis of fibrin clots. These agents are useful in coagulation factor–deficient hemorrhage involving mucous membranes, where local fibrinolysis adds to the hemostatic impairment (eg, dental procedures, epistaxis, menorrhagia). For many dental procedures specifically, ε-aminocaproic acid mouthwashes are effective at controlling local bleeding. Lysine analogs have also been shown to reduce postoperative bleeding after cardiac surgery, liver transplantation, and prostatectomy. A recent observational study of 4374 patients undergoing coronary revascularization surgery with cardiopulmonary bypass showed that ε-aminocaproic acid and tranexamic acid were effective in significantly reducing surgical blood loss, and neither agent was associated with an increased risk of thromboembolism or other complications. The efficacy and safety of ε-aminocaproic acid in this trial concurs with prior meta-analyses that revealed a 30% to 40% reduction in bleeding after cardiac surgery. Because tranexamic acid is no longer commercially available in the United States, ε-aminocaproic acid has become the hemostatic agent of choice for routine use in cardiac surgery with bypass.

Aprotinin is a bovine lung-derived serine protease inhibitor that inhibits plasmin and kallikrein and attenuates fibrinolysis. It has been used most extensively for prophylaxis of intraoperative and postoperative hemorrhage in patients undergoing coronary artery bypass graft surgery with cardiopulmonary bypass. This agent also reduces bleeding associated with liver transplantation, noncardiac thoracic surgeries, and orthopedic surgeries. Preclinical data and early clinical experience with aprotinin raised concerns about potential nephrotoxicity and intravascular thrombosis. In 2006, a large observational study revealed that aprotinin use in patients undergoing coronary revascularization and cardiopulmonary bypass was associated with a 1.5- to 2.5-fold increased risk of renal failure, MI, heart failure, stroke, and encephalopathy, compared with rates in control patients and those who received ε-aminocaproic acid or tranexamic acid. In addition, a propensity-score, case-control comparison of aprotinin and tranexamic acid in high transfusion risk cardiac surgery patients showed that aprotinin may be associated with worsening renal function among patients with preexisting renal dysfunction. In 2007, a US Food and Drug Administration (FDA) panel decided not to withdraw aprotinin from US markets but advocated restricting its usage to high-risk patients undergoing complex procedures. End-organ complications related to aprotinin are believed to be due to ischemic microthrombotic tissue injury, particularly in the renal microvasculature.

rFVIIa is approved for the treatment of bleeding in hemophilia A or B patients with acquired inhibitors. Off-label indications, however, account for the majority of rFVIIa usage in US academic medical centers. Most of these indications are for the prevention and treatment of bleeding associated with invasive procedures and surgeries in patients with hepatic or renal insufficiency and coagulopathy. Small nonrandomized studies have shown that rFVIIa can reduce bleeding and/or transfusion requirements in patients undergoing retropubic prostatectomy, noncoronary cardiac surgery with cardiopulmonary bypass, and orthotopic liver transplantation, although the benefit in these settings appears to be small. rFVIIa has also been used successfully in a small number of patients with profound thrombocytopenia and severe qualitative platelet defects.

A multicenter assessment of rFVIIa usage for all off-label indications revealed that a single dose can effectively correct the INR in >80% of cases (although the INR has not been proven to be a surrogate for hemostatic efficacy) and that hemostasis can be achieved in roughly 50% of bleeding patients within 6 hours of treatment. However, rebleeding and hemorrhagic deaths occur in roughly one fourth and one third of cases, respectively. Thromboembolism, line thrombosis, MI, ischemic stroke, and other potential rFVIIa-associated adverse events occurred in 9.8% of patients. A recent survey of the FDA's Adverse Event Reporting System (AERS) revealed that roughly two thirds of the thromboembolic events associated with rFVIIa occurred among patients receiving the drug for off-label indications. Arterial and venous events, which were equally prevalent, resulted in significant morbidity, and thromboembolic complications were the probable cause of death in roughly three fourths of the case fatalities. A prospective randomized trial that compared rFVIIa with placebo for nonsurgical intracranial hemorrhage observed a >3-fold incidence of serious thrombotic events (predominantly MI and cerebral infarction) among the predominantly elderly patients receiving rFVIIa (7% vs 2%, respectively; P = not significant), although this did not significantly alter long-term neurologic outcomes. Despite the lack of statistical significance in this trial, these observations compelled the FDA to issue a warning regarding off-label use of rFVIIa and thrombotic risk. A significant incidence of thrombosis has also been observed in patients who receive rFVIIa following trauma. At this point, well-designed, prospective, randomized trials are needed to accurately define the risk–benefit ratio and cost-effectiveness of this therapy. At present, for surgical patients who might potentially benefit from off-label use, the consultant must also consider patient age, history of atherosclerotic disease, other medical comorbidities, and concurrent medications that might contribute to a thromboembolic complication.

Fibrin sealant (eg, Tisseel, Hemaseel), also known as fibrin glue, is composed of purified, virally inactivated human fibrinogen and human thrombin. Fibrin sealant also contains aprotinin, which may be undesirable in certain settings (eg, middle ear surgery). Although randomized clinical trial data and evidence-based guidelines are lacking, fibrin sealant has proven to be effective in cardiac surgery, urologic procedures, orthopedic surgery, dental procedures, trauma, and neurosurgery, where it is used to seal dural leaks and repair otic ossicles and bony defects. It is useful for achieving local hemostasis in patients with factor VIII deficiency or congenital hemostatic defects.

Transfusion

The collection and transfusion of autologous blood in the perioperative setting was most popular and widespread in the early 1990s when concerns about the medical and legal risks of allogeneic transfusion were greatest. With the routine use of nucleic acid testing (NAT), a unit of homologous blood currently conveys a risk of <1 in 2,000,000 and perhaps <1 in 8,000,000 of transmitting human immunodeficiency virus (HIV) and hepatitis C, and this risk will be even smaller if individual donor NAT replaces minipool NAT methods. The risk of transmission of hepatitis B with serologic screening is currently 1 in 60,000 to 1 in 150,000, and this risk will also decrease substantially with future NAT. Although preoperative autologous blood donation (PABD) can eliminate the risks of transmitting these viral infections, autologous donors are still susceptible to other transfusion-related hazards, including complications from the donation itself. Autologous donors receive less homologous blood perioperatively, but they are more likely to be transfused with their own blood. They are therefore subject to clerical errors, bacterial contamination, and complications related to blood processing. Additional disadvantages of PABD include a higher likelihood of perioperative anemia (because of the autologous donation) and a 6 in 100,000 risk that the autologous collection will be associated with a severe adverse reaction requiring hospital admission, particularly if this is the donor's first experience. It is recommended that PABD not be used if the likelihood of perioperative transfusion is <10%.

Predetermined hemoglobin "triggers" should not be used in perioperative transfusion management. The decision to transfuse should be based on individualized assessment and evidence-based guidelines. A number of studies have demonstrated that inappropriate perioperative red blood cell and/or platelet transfusions correlate with increased risks of cardiac, renal, pulmonary, and infectious complications, in addition to a higher mortality. Controlled trials have shown no improvement in outcome from maintaining a critically ill patient's hemoglobin above an arbitrary value (see subsequent section on transfusion in the intensive care setting).

Postoperative bleeding

Surgical reexploration is urgently indicated when active bleeding of bright red blood is observed in a normothermic, nonacidotic postoperative patient with hemostatically adequate values of the PT, aPTT, and platelet count. In this case, a technical or vascular etiology of bleeding is most likely. However, a postoperative patient with persistent oozing or low-volume bleeding is more likely to have a mild, undiagnosed hemostatic defect, such as vWD, platelet dysfunction, or mild hemophilia, despite a normal aPTT. In such patients, measurement of the activities of vWF and factors VIII, IX, and XI is indicated. Men with mild factor XI deficiency and no history of pathologic bleeding may develop severe hemorrhage after dental extraction or prostate surgery. Isolated prolongation of the PT/INR suggests vitamin K deficiency, undiagnosed liver disease, or surreptitious warfarin ingestion. Multiple hemostatic abnormalities and thrombocytopenia should prompt consideration of DIC and/or dilutional coagulopathy due to hypertransfusion.

DDAVP, cryoprecipitate, factor concentrate, or recombinant factor VIII can be used to correct various degrees of factor VIII deficiency; although of these, cryoprecipitate is the only product that does not undergo viral inactivation. Fresh frozen plasma or, more commonly, factor IX–containing concentrates or recombinant factor IX are required to control bleeding in factor IX deficiency. Hemophilia or vWD-related mucous membrane bleeding may also improve with the use of ε-aminocaproic acid. Transfusion of plasma, cryoprecipitate, and/or platelets is indicated to correct the defects and stop the bleeding in patients with vitamin K deficiency, hypofibrinogenemia, and DIC. ε-Aminocaproic acid and, for highly selected patients, rFVIIa may be considered for persistent or uncontrolled bleeding.

Thromboprophylaxis and postoperative thrombosis
Prophylaxis for thromboembolism

Postoperative thromboembolism complicates a variety of procedures, particularly large joint surgery or joint replacement, thoracic or abdominal procedures lasting >30 minutes under general anesthesia, cancer surgery, major trauma, and spinal cord injury. The risks are increased in patients who are immobilized and those with active cancer, a past history of venous thromboembolism (VTE), thrombophilia, or recent VTE. Without postoperative anticoagulation, 50% of patients who have surgery within a month of a DVT will develop a recurrence, and 6% of those events will be fatal. Anticoagulation can reduce the risk of recurrence by 90%, but 3% of patients have severe postoperative hemorrhage (with the possibility of permanent disability), and 3% of these patients (0.09% overall) will die of bleeding.

The risk of VTE after surgery can be estimated based on the type of procedure, the age of the patient, and presence of additional medical comorbidities (Table 2-3). After the risk of perioperative VTE is determined, a prophylactic strategy can be recommended according to evidence-based guidelines. Prophylactic measures include combinations of lower extremity intermittent pneumatic compression devices or graduated compression stockings, along with chemical prophylaxis with UFH, LMWH, fondaparinux, and oral anticoagulation (Table 2-3).

The timing of the initiation of prophylaxis varies based on the procedure and regional practice patterns. For hip replacement surgery, fewer DVTs occur when LMWH is started between 2 and 6 hours postoperatively, compared with starting warfarin or LMWH 12 hours after surgery. For other procedures, the timing of initiation of prophylaxis does not significantly correlate with outcomes. In Europe, LMWH therapy is usually started at half doses 12 hours before surgery, whereas in the United States, it is common to start full doses (eg, 30 mg of enoxaparin every 12 hours) at 12 to 24 hours after surgery; the bleeding rates are low, 0.9% and 3.5%, respectively. Prophylactic warfarin begun just before or immediately after surgery is less commonly associated with hemorrhage into the replaced knee but is also less effective in preventing DVT. A meta-analysis showed that hip replacement under spinal anesthesia is less often followed by DVT than when it is performed under general anesthesia. Thromboprophylaxis is generally continued for at least 7 to 10 days postoperatively. Extended therapy, for up to 28 to 35 days, should be considered for hip replacement or hip fracture surgery, cancer surgery involving the chest or abdomen, or postoperative patients with spinal cord injury.

The pentasaccharide fondaparinux is an acceptable alternative to UFH or LMWH. Recent large randomized clinical

Table 2-3 VTE risk stratification for surgical patients and evidence-based guidelines for prophylactic anticoagulation.

Level of risk	Definition	VTE risk (%)	Recommended prophylaxis
Low risk	Minor surgery in patients <40 years old with no additional risk factors*	Calf DVT: 2	Early and aggressive ambulation
		Proximal DVT: 0.4	
		Clinical PE: 0.2	
		Fatal PE: <0.01	
Moderate risk	Minor surgery with additional risk factors* or	Calf DVT: 10–20	LDUH (every 12 hours) or LMWH, or GCS or IPC device (if bleeding risk)
	Surgery in patients 40–60 years old with no additional risk factors or	Proximal DVT: 2–4	
	Major surgery in patients <40 years old with no additional risk factors	Clinical PE: 1–2	
		Fatal PE: 0.1–0.4	
High risk	Surgery in patients >60 years old or	Calf DVT: 20–40	LDUH (every 8 hours) or LMWH or IPC device (if bleeding risk)
	Surgery in patients 40-60 years old with additional risk factors*	Proximal DVT: 4–8	
		Clinical PE: 2–4	
		Fatal PE: 0.4–1	
Highest risk	Major surgery in patients >40 years old with additional risk factors* or	Calf DVT: 40–80	LMWH or fondaparinux or oral anticoagulation (INR 2–3) or GCS/IPC device + LDUH (every 8 hours) or GCS/IPC device + LMWH
	Hip or knee arthroplasty or	Proximal DVT: 10–20	Consider extended prophylaxis (ie, >7–10 days) for cancer surgery, hip arthroplasty, hip fracture surgery, or spinal cord injury
	Hip fracture surgery or	Clinical PE: 4–10	
	Major trauma or	Fatal PE: 0.2–5	
	Spinal cord injury		

* Additional risk factors: prior VTE, obesity, heart failure, cancer, hypercoagulable state.
Adapted from Geerts WH, Bergqvist D, Pineo GF, et al. Prevention of venous thromboembolism: American College of Chest Physicians Evidence-Based Clinical Practice Guidelines (8th Edition). *Chest.* 2008;133(Suppl 3):381S–453S.
DVT = deep venous thrombosis; GCS = graduated compression stocking; INR = international normalized ratio; IPC = intermittent pneumatic compression; LDUH = low-dose unfractionated heparin; LMWH = low molecular weight heparin; PE = pulmonary embolism; VTE = venous thromboembolism.

trials have indicated that prophylactic fondaparinux (started 4–8 hours after surgery) is at least as effective as LMWH (ie, dalteparin or enoxaparin) for patients undergoing abdominal surgery and major orthopedic procedures (knee or hip arthroplasty or hip fracture surgery); initiation of fondaparinux ≥6 hours after surgery alleviates the slight increased bleeding risk associated with this agent. Similar to LMWH, extended-duration fondaparinux (for 19–23 days) after hip fracture surgery further reduces the risk of VTE (by 96%), compared with therapy for only 6 to 8 days, without a significant increase in bleeding.

Additional considerations for thromboprophylaxis in surgical patients include the potential need for dose adjustments or avoidance of LMWH and fondaparinux in patients with renal failure and measures to avoid perispinal hematoma in patients receiving neuraxial anesthesia/analgesia (Table 2-4). Oral factor X agents have shown promising results in phase III clinical prophylaxis trials and may present another option for thromboprophylaxis in the near future.

Treatment of postoperative deep vein thrombosis

When VTE occurs in a postoperative patient, the consultant may be asked for treatment recommendations. For most low-risk procedures, full anticoagulation can be safely initiated within 12 to 24 hours after surgery. The agent of choice in the immediate postoperative period is continuous-infusion UFH because of the short half-life and ability to reverse rapidly with protamine if bleeding develops. Relative contraindications to immediate postoperative anticoagulation include certain neurosurgical or ophthalmologic procedures in which bleeding would risk permanent disability or blindness. Absolute contraindications to anticoagulation in a patient with lower

Table 2-4 Recommendations to minimize the risk of perispinal hematoma in surgical patients undergoing neuraxial anesthesia/analgesia.

Avoid neuraxial anesthesia/analgesia in patients who have bleeding disorders

Avoid neuraxial anesthesia/analgesia in patients who have drug-related preoperative impairment of hemostasis

Delay catheter insertion/spinal needle for 8–12 hours after a subcutaneous dose of heparin or a twice-daily dose of LMWH

Delay catheter insertion/spinal needle for 18 hours after a once-a-day injection of LMWH

Delay anticoagulant prophylaxis if a hemorrhagic aspirate (ie, "bloody tap") is seen during initial insertion

Remove epidural catheter when the anticoagulant effect is at a minimum (ie, just before next scheduled dose)

Delay anticoagulant prophylaxis at least 2 hours after catheter is removed

With warfarin prophylaxis, continuous epidural analgesia should be limited to 1–2 days and the PT/INR should be <1.5 at the time of catheter removal

The safe use of fondaparinux prophylaxis with continuous epidural anesthesia is under investigation

Adapted from Horlocker TT, Wedel DJ, Benzon H, et al. Regional anesthesia in the anticoagulated patient: defining the risks (the second ASRA Consensus Conference on Neuraxial Anesthesia and Anticoagulation). *Reg Anesth Pain Med.* 2003;28:172–197; and Geerts WH, Bergqvist D, Pineo GF, et al. Prevention of venous thromboembolism: American College of Chest Physicians Evidence-Based Clinical Practice Guidelines (8th Edition). *Chest.* 2008;133(Suppl 3):381S–453S.

INR = international normalized ratio; LMWH = low molecular weight heparin; PT = prothrombin time.

---

extremity thrombosis may require that placement of a temporary or permanent inferior vena cava filter be considered.

In general, by the third postoperative day after uncomplicated surgery, the risks of anticoagulation are comparable to those in a nonsurgical patient. Initial therapy in such patients could include LMWH and warfarin as prescribed in standard doses for nonsurgical patients with DVT. The patient's prior experience with therapy for thrombosis may influence the recommendation.

Postphlebitic syndrome is a distressing and morbid condition. To prevent it, thrombolytic therapy may be considered for carefully selected postsurgical patients with massive iliofemoral DVT. It is worth noting that clinical trials of thrombolytic agents have shown marginal improvement in survival and long-term morbidity despite the immediate discernable benefits of thrombolysis. The use of elastic compression stockings (pressure of 30–40 mm Hg) for the first 2 years after a DVT has been shown to decrease the incidence and severity of postphlebitic syndrome. The duration of anticoagulation with warfarin after an uncomplicated postoperative VTE is usually 3 months; however, longer treatment may be indicated in the setting of certain hypercoagulable conditions, such as cancer or antiphospholipid antibody syndrome, a history of multiple thromboembolic episodes, or persistent venous obstruction with severe postphlebitic syndrome.

Excessive warfarin dosing

The management of patients treated with warfarin who have INR measurements outside of the therapeutic range depends on the presence and severity of bleeding in addition to the magnitude of the INR increase. Management recommendations for such patients are summarized in Table 2-5. For patients with INR measurements minimally outside of the therapeutic range who have no bleeding, no change in management may be necessary. For patients on warfarin with life-threatening bleeding, regardless of INR, immediate intervention is required as outlined in Table 2-5. To prevent excessive anticoagulation with warfarin, INR monitoring should be initiated after the initial 2 or 3 doses of warfarin have been administered. INR measurements should be repeated until a stable level is obtained. Patients on stable warfarin dosing should receive INR testing no less frequently than every 4 weeks. Care should be taken when giving warfarin to elderly patients, to patients who are malnourished or debilitated, and to patients with liver disease or on medications that affect warfarin metabolism, to ensure that overdosing does not occur.

Key points

- Preoperative hemostatic screening test abnormalities and postoperative bleeding risk are most strongly associated with a personal or family history of bleeding, the use of antiplatelet or anticoagulant agents, prior procedure-related bleeding, and known medical comorbidities associated with a bleeding diathesis.
- Intraoperative hemorrhage may be due to inadequate local/surgical hemostasis and/or a preexisting or acquired systemic coagulation defect.
- Coagulation tests and tests of primary hemostasis (bleeding time or PFA-100) are neither sensitive nor specific in predicting surgical bleeding.
- The risk of VTE after surgery and the appropriate anticoagulant prophylaxis strategy should be determined according to the type of procedure, the age of the patient, and presence of additional medical comorbidities.
- Management of acute VTE in a postoperative patient is similar to the approach in a nonsurgical patient, except that bleeding risks and contraindications to anticoagulation and thrombolysis must be carefully considered in the context of the procedure.
- Hemostatic agents such as conjugated estrogens, DDAVP, lysine analogs, aprotinin, rFVIIa, and fibrin sealant may be useful for selected surgical patients with an increased risk of bleeding; however, potential adverse effects and cost must also be considered.

Table 2-5 Abbreviated management recommendations of patients treated with warfarin who have INR measurements outside of the therapeutic range.

INR	Recommendation
Increased, but <5.0; no significant bleeding	Lower warfarin dose or omit 1 dose. Monitor more frequently and resume at adjusted dose when INR is therapeutic.
≥5.0 but <9.0; no significant bleeding	Omit next 1 or 2 warfarin doses. Monitor more frequently and resume at adjusted dose when INR is therapeutic. If patient is at increased risk of bleeding, 1 dose can be omitted and administer 1.0–2.5 mg oral vitamin K.
>9.0; no significant bleeding	Administer 2.5–5.0 mg oral vitamin K while holding warfarin. Monitor more frequently and administer additional vitamin K if necessary. May take 24–48 hours to reduce INR.
Serious bleeding at any elevation of INR	Hold warfarin and give 10 mg vitamin K by slow IV infusion. May supplement with fresh frozen plasma, prothrombin complex concentrates, or recombinant factor VIIa (rVIIa) depending on urgency of situation. Repeat vitamin K every 12 hours for persistent elevation of INR.
Elevated with life-threatening bleeding	Hold warfarin and give fresh frozen plasma, prothrombin complex concentrates, or rVIIa supplemented by vitamin K 10 mg via slow infusion. Repeat as necessary.

Adapted from Ansell J, Hirsch J, Hylek E, Jacobson A, Crowther M, Palareti G. Pharmacology and management of the vitamin K antagonists. *Chest*. 2008;133:161s–198s.

INR = international normalized ratio; IV = intravenous.

Intensive care unit

Anemia

Many patients hospitalized in intensive care units (ICUs) for acute medical illnesses have anemia at the time of admission, and most of those who do not will develop it. In a recent observational study, 37% of all patients admitted to ICUs received a mean of 4.8 units of packed red blood cells during their time in the ICU. The pathophysiology of anemia in acutely ill patients is multifactorial and, although acute in nature, largely resembles the anemia of chronic inflammation. Anemia in acutely ill patients is also exacerbated by bleeding and frequent phlebotomy; in one study, an average of 41 mL of blood per day was obtained from patients in the ICU for laboratory tests.

Over the last decade, considerable debate has centered on the role of transfusion in critically ill patients, largely based on the realization that transfusion may be associated with an increased risk of a number of adverse short- and long-term outcomes in addition to transmission of infectious disease. These include immunosuppression, renal failure, stroke, and perhaps even malignancy. Moreover, transfused blood may not impart the expected increase in oxygen delivery to tissues due to a number of alterations such as decreased levels of 2,3-diphosphoglycerate (and thus decreased oxygen unloading capacity), loss of nitric oxide activity, and proinflammatory effects. The landmark Transfusion Requirements in Critical Care (TRICC) trial examined the role of transfusion in 838 critically ill patients with hemoglobin values <9.0 g/dL, randomizing patients to a liberal transfusion strategy in which the hemoglobin was maintained at 10 to 12 g/dL or a restrictive group, in which the hemoglobin was maintained between 7 and 9.9 g/dL. In-hospital mortality was significantly lower in the restricted group, although no differences were observed in 30-day mortality. This study suggests that a restrictive transfusion policy is preferable in the majority of critically ill patients, and several subsequent studies have confirmed these initial observations. However, although recent surveys suggest that transfusion practices have changed toward a more restrictive approach, this has not been universal, with more liberal policies often being used in surgical ICUs, specific institutions, and by individual physicians. Moreover, controversy still exists as to the utility of red blood cell transfusion in specific patient populations, in particular those with acute ischemic cardiac disease. One study that reviewed outcomes of patients in a Medicare database who were hospitalized for acute MI identified improved outcomes in patients with hematocrit levels <33% who received red blood cell transfusion. However, several other studies, most of which have been retrospective, but including a subgroup analysis of patients from the TRICC study, have yielded different and conflicting outcomes, with either clear benefits of transfusion not observed or a trend toward improved outcomes with transfusion only in severely anemic individuals with a hematocrit <25% or hemoglobin <7.0 g/dL.

Due to the potentially adverse affects of transfusion on the outcomes of patients with critical illness, several studies have addressed the utility of recombinant erythropoietin in this setting. As with transfusion, these studies have yielded conflicting results, with some, but not all, demonstrating modest reductions in the need for red blood cell transfusion. Moreover, a recent randomized, placebo-controlled trial that did not demonstrate a reduction in transfusion requirements suggested that erythropoietin administration may lead to decreased mortality in patients with trauma, despite an increase in thrombotic events. A meta-analysis of 9 studies of erythropoietin use in critically ill patients suggested that erythropoietin use was associated with reduced transfusion requirements but no decrease in overall mortality. Thus, at the present time, erythropoietin cannot be universally recommended for treatment of anemia in critically ill patients, and additional studies are required.

Thrombocytopenia

Approximately 40% of patients in medical or surgical ICUs develop a platelet count <150,000/μL; 20% to 25% develop a platelet count <100,000/μL, and 12% to 15% develop severe thrombocytopenia, with a platelet count <50,000/μL. The development of thrombocytopenia in patients in the ICU is a strong independent predictor for ICU mortality. The spectrum of disorders that may cause thrombocytopenia in this setting is extensive. Some causes of thrombocytopenia are summarized in Table 2-6, several of which are described in detail in this section.

Evaluation of the patient with thrombocytopenia should include a detailed history, thorough physical examination, and close inspection of the peripheral blood film. A history of chronic or prior thrombocytopenia and the setting in which it occurred should be queried. Underlying marrow disease and preexisting morbidities that may induce chronic thrombocytopenia, such as liver disease, neoplasia, or immune thrombocytopenia (ITP), may be largely excluded by the documentation of normal hematologic parameters prior to the onset of the acute illness. Abnormalities on the peripheral blood film that may aid in reaching a diagnosis include: (i) platelet clumping when blood is collected in ethylenediaminetetraacetic acid–containing tubes, suggesting pseudothrombocytopenia; (ii) schistocytes, which may suggest an underlying thrombotic microangiopathy such as thrombotic thrombocytopenic purpura (TTP), the hemolytic uremic syndrome (HUS), or DIC; (iii) poikilocytes or nucleated red blood cells, which may reflect a myelophthisic

Table 2-6 Diagnosis of thrombocytopenia in the intensive care unit.

Diagnosis\finding	Clinical findings	Special	LDH	aPTT	aPL antibody	Platelet morphology	Red blood cell morphology
Pseudothrombocytopenia	None	Platelet count normal in citrate or heparin	Normal	Normal	Absent	Clumps	Normal
Drug-induced thrombocytopenia	None, bleeding/petechiae if severe	Higher incidence with certain drugs	Normal	Normal	Absent	Normal	Normal
ITP	None, bleeding/petechiae if severe	Often associated with prior history	Normal	Normal	Absent or present	Normal or mildly enlarged	Normal
Heparin-induced thrombocytopenia	May be associated with thrombosis	5–14 days after starting heparin, unless reexposure, may have DIC as well	Normal	Prolonged due to heparin	Absent	Normal	Normal
DIC	Underlying illness usually identifiable	Increased D-dimer or FDP, decreased fibrinogen (in some), mildly prolonged PT, may have microangiopathic hemolytic anemia	Normal or mild increase	Usually normal	Absent	Normal	Schistocytes in some
Catastrophic aPL syndrome	Infection, fever, at least 3 organs involved	Small vessel microthrombi	Normal or mildly increased	Normal or increased	Present	Normal	Normal
TTP-HUS	Thrombocytopenia and microangiopathic hemolytic anemia without other apparent cause; may also have renal dysfunction, neurologic changes, fever	Microangiopathic hemolytic anemia, ADAMTS <5% may help confirm diagnosis, but diagnosis is clinical	Increased	Normal	Absent	Normal or mildly enlarged	Schistocytes

aPL = antiphospholipid; aPTT = activated partial thromboplastin time; DIC = disseminated intravascular coagulation; FDP = fibrin degradation product; HUS = hemolytic uremic syndrome; ITP = idiopathic thrombocytopenic purpura; PT = prothrombin time; TTP = thrombotic thrombocytopenic purpura.

process; or (iv) abnormal leukocytes, which may suggest a hematologic malignancy or myelodysplasia or accompany a syndrome of congenital thrombocytopenia. Bone marrow aspiration and biopsy should be pursued when an underlying marrow disorder is suspected.

Drug-induced thrombocytopenia

Acutely ill patients are commonly treated with several drugs, many of which may be capable of inducing thrombocytopenia through a variety of mechanisms. A partial list of offending agents includes heparin, trimethoprim/sulfamethoxazole, β-lactam antibiotics, vancomycin, cephalothin, carbamazepine, hydrochlorothiazide, nonsteroidal anti-inflammatory drugs, phenytoin, procainamide, quinidine and quinine, rifampin, sulfasalazine, sulfonylureas, and valproic acid. Ticlopidine and, less commonly, clopidogrel are thienopyridine adenosine diphosphate receptor antagonists that may induce a TTP-HUS–like syndrome in which thrombocytopenia is accompanied by a microangiopathic hemolytic anemia. Thrombocytopenia may also develop in 0.5% to 1.0% of patients treated with the GPIIb/IIIa inhibitor abciximab, often within hours of the infusion, and less commonly with other GPIIb/IIIa inhibitors such as eptifibatide. Because thrombocytopenia due to these latter agents is accompanied by inhibition of platelet aggregation, a more aggressive platelet transfusion approach may be indicated for patients in whom the platelet count decreases to <20,000/μL.

An expanded list of drugs and the level of evidence for their association with thrombocytopenia are maintained at Platelets on the Web (http://www.ouhsc.edu/platelets/index.html). However, in theory, almost any drug may induce thrombocytopenia, and review of company files may be useful in the absence of published reports implicating specific drugs with thrombocytopenia.

The diagnosis of drug-induced thrombocytopenia is a diagnosis of exclusion and may be difficult in the complicated ICU patient with multiple potential reasons for thrombocytopenia. A clear understanding of the temporal relationship between the institution of the drug and the onset of thrombocytopenia is essential. The decision on whether to discontinue the administration of a potentially offending drug depends on the level of suspicion that this is the offending agent, the relative importance of that drug to the patient's treatment plan, and the feasibility of alternative management approaches. In some circumstances, measurement of drug-dependent antiplatelet antibodies may be useful, although management decisions will likely need to be made before the results of such assays become available. Following discontinuation of an offending drug, the time to resolution of thrombocytopenia depends on the rate of clearance of that drug and its metabolites from plasma or tissue and the mechanism by which thrombocytopenia is induced. However, most cases of drug-induced thrombocytopenia resolve within 7 to 10 days, although heparin-induced thrombocytopenia (HIT) may resolve more rapidly in many cases.

Heparin is a common cause of drug-induced, antibody-mediated thrombocytopenia and is commonly used in ICU patients. One to 2% of heparin-treated patients develop isolated thrombocytopenia (HIT), and in 25% to 50% of these individuals, HIT is accompanied by thrombosis (HITT). Some comments pertaining to HITT are of particular relevance in the ICU setting. First, because patients with HITT may be thrombocytopenic for a number of other reasons in addition to HITT, an acute decrease in the platelet count may not be routinely observed prior to HIT onset; thus, some patients with HITT in the ICU may present with only new thrombosis in the presence of preexisting thrombocytopenia. Second, it is important to recognize that immunologic tests for heparin-PF4 antibodies are common in some subgroups of patients, particularly in the post–cardiac bypass setting. However, although 50% or more of such patients may have positive enzyme-linked immunosorbent assay tests for heparin-PF4 antibodies and 10% to 15% may have positive tests for heparin-dependent platelet activation, clinical HITT is only thought to occur in 1% to 2% of postbypass patients. Third, despite the importance of vigilance for HITT in any clinical setting, recent studies suggest that HITT is a relatively uncommon cause of thrombocytopenia in acutely ill patients in the ICU setting. Fourth, although thrombosis in patients with HITT is most commonly venous, this ratio is reversed in patients who have undergone recent arterial vascular procedures. Finally, due to the frequent presence of renal and hepatic dysfunction in patients in the ICU, antithrombotic agents used for therapy of presumptive HITT should be initiated with extreme caution, and dosing should be increased slowly as needed to reach a therapeutic range. Recent studies, for example, suggest that a bolus of lepirudin should not be used to initiate therapy.

Infection and DIC

Sepsis is another common cause of thrombocytopenia in critically ill patients, often leading to the development of thrombocytopenia within the first 4 days of intensive care. In a recent review of 69 patients admitted to the ICU with septic shock, thrombocytopenia was present in 38 (55%), with 13 patients developing platelet counts <20,000/μL. Patients with thrombocytopenia had significantly higher values for serum creatinine, a lower Pao_2/Fio_2 ratio, and a higher Sequential Organ Failure Assessment score. The mechanisms of infection-induced thrombocytopenia include impaired platelet production, enhanced clearance of immunoglobulin-coated platelets, cytokine-driven hemophagocytosis of platelets in response to elevated levels of macrophage colony-stimulating factor, and infection of bone marrow stromal cells and megakaryocytes with viruses such as HIV or cytomegalovirus (CMV). Several uncommon infections may also be associated with severe thrombocytopenia. Hantavirus is a flu-like illness endemic in the western United States that is associated with rapid development of noncardiac pulmonary edema. Ehrlichiosis is a tick-borne infection that occurs in the southern and upper midwestern United States, associated with high fever, headache, myalgias, and CNS symptoms. Meningococcemia with superimposed DIC and Rocky Mountain spotted fever with vasculitis are other causes of severe thrombocytopenia. Management of infection-induced thrombocytopenia consists of treating the underlying infection and administering platelet transfusions as needed (see discussion below of platelet transfusions in patients with DIC).

DIC is another cause of thrombocytopenia in the ICU that may result from a number of causes including amniotic fluid embolism, malignancy, and trauma, among others. Although commonly associated with hemorrhage, DIC may occasionally lead to thrombotic phenomena, in particular peripheral ischemic manifestations. A scoring system that establishes a uniform platform for the diagnosis of overt and nonovert DIC has been developed by the International Society for Thrombosis and Hemostasis; scoring for overt DIC is based on the presence or absence of an appropriate underlying disorder, thrombocytopenia, elevated fibrin-related markers (eg, fibrin degradation products, D-dimer), a prolonged PT, and a decreased fibrinogen level. In some cases, all of these criteria may not be present; for example, fibrinogen is an acute-phase reactant and may be elevated in patients with acute or chronic inflammation. Thus, significant reductions from the baseline fibrinogen level in such individuals caused by DIC may not result in hypofibrinogenemia as defined by standard laboratory ranges.

Guidelines for the management of DIC have recently been published by the British Committee for Standards in Hematology and highlight the importance of treating the underlying condition that precipitated the syndrome. Therapy with blood components must be individualized based on the patient's clinical condition. The use of platelet transfusions in thrombocytopenic patients with DIC should be based on the presence of bleeding rather than an absolute platelet count. For example, it is recommended that platelet transfusion should be considered for patients with bleeding or at high bleeding risk and with a platelet count <50,000/μL. Similarly, treatment of a prolonged PT is recommended only for patients who are bleeding or require an invasive procedure. Cryoprecipitate or fibrinogen concentrates may be used for patients with severe hypofibrinogenemia (fibrinogen <100 g/dL) that persists after plasma therapy. The use of low doses of heparin should be considered for patients with significant thrombotic manifestations, and activated protein C has been shown to enhance survival in a subgroup of patients with DIC with severe sepsis accompanied by an Acute Physiology and Chronic Evaluation (APACHE) score of ≥25 and/or dysfunction of 2 or more organs.

Massive transfusion-induced thrombocytopenia

Transfusion of >15 to 20 units of packed red blood cells after posttraumatic and surgical hemorrhage may lead to a dilutional thrombocytopenia that can be accompanied by hypothermia, platelet dysfunction, and a dilutional coagulopathy. Hypofibrinogenemia is also common in this setting. Therapy includes transfusion of plasma, platelets, and if needed, cryoprecipitate or fibrinogen concentrates.

Thrombotic thrombocytopenic purpura and hemolytic uremic syndrome

Due to the importance of prompt recognition and therapy of TTP and HUS, initial management is customarily undertaken in the ICU. TTP and HUS are thrombotic microangiopathies that share the central processes of microangiopathic hemolytic anemia and thrombocytopenia. Each of these disorders may be accompanied by other clinical manifestations, including neurologic abnormalities, renal dysfunction, and fever. In current practice, however, the presence of microangiopathic hemolytic anemia and thrombocytopenia without another apparent cause are considered sufficient criteria for institution of treatment. In general, patients with TTP have a higher incidence of neurologic manifestations, whereas those with HUS have a greater frequency and extent of renal involvement. The presence of severely decreased activity of the von Willebrand factor (vWF)-cleaving protease, ADAMTS13, is common in TTP but not HUS. However, the clinical manifestations of these disorders overlap extensively, and they are considered by some as a single disorder (TTP-HUS). Attempting to differentiate classic adult TTP from HUS may be useful in guiding therapy, although when this cannot be definitively accomplished, a trial of plasma-based therapy should be initiated.

There are 2 major variants of HUS. The most common follows enteric infection with verotoxin-producing *Escherichia coli* (VTEC). Infection is followed by abdominal pain and bloody diarrhea. Up to 20% of patients with bloody diarrhea progress to HUS and acute renal failure within the next 5 to 6 days. This variant of HUS is most common in children, often occurs in epidemics, and is generally self-limited, although affected patients may require extensive support including dialysis, and the long-term prognosis in terms of renal function is not as favorable as once believed. Plasma exchange has not been shown to improve the outcomes of patients with this variant. The second variant of HUS is referred to as *atypical*, *sporadic*, or *D(−) HUS* and is most common in adults in the postpartum period. This variant is associated with loss of function mutations in several complement regulatory proteins including factor H, factor I, thrombomodulin, and membrane complement protein (CD46); deletion of factor H–related molecules 1 and 3 has also been described, as have gain of function mutations in complement factors B and C3.

The thrombotic microangiopathies that complicate stem cell transplantation, chemotherapy, cyclosporine, and clopidogrel therapy generally present with clinical manifestations similar to those seen in atypical HUS, with a preponderance of renal insufficiency, although the importance of genetic contributions to these disorders is uncertain. New classification schemes that incorporate the rapid increases in understanding of the molecular pathogenesis of these disorders are emerging.

The pathogenesis of TTP involves deficiency of the vWF-cleaving protease, ADAMTS13. Deficiency of the protease leads to increased levels of ultra-large vWF multimers (ULvWF) that promote the agglutination of platelets in the microvasculature and induce microvascular thrombosis. ADAMTS13 deficiency most commonly results from neutralizing antibodies against the protease, although a minority of anti-ADAMTS13 antibodies are nonneutralizing and enhance protease clearance. A congenital variant of TTP, the Upshaw-Schulman syndrome, results from inherited deficiency of the ADAMTS13 but, in some cases, may not present until adulthood.

Management of TTP in the acute care setting should be focused on rapid institution of daily plasma exchange with 1.0 to 1.5 plasma volumes. The utility of corticosteroids in acute TTP remains controversial, although given the immune nature of the disorder, corticosteroids are generally used. It is essential that therapy be initiated rapidly based on a clinical diagnosis because TTP is associated with a 90% fatality rate if untreated but an 85% remission rate following plasma exchange. Although documentation of a severely reduced ADAMTS13 level (<5%) in the appropriate clinical setting is useful for confirmation, awaiting such measurements should not be allowed to delay institution of therapy. Therapy should also not be withheld in a patient with a clinical diagnosis of TTP in whom the ADAMTS13 level is not severely reduced. For patients with refractory disease, rituximab has been used successfully in some individuals. Immunosuppression with rituximab and use of mycophenolate mofetil or splenectomy have also shown promise in reducing the relapse rate of TTP, which is approximately 30% within the first 12 months after an initial remission.

Catastrophic antiphospholipid antibody syndrome

The catastrophic antiphospholipid antibody syndrome is a rare but serious complication that may occur in patients with antiphospholipid antibodies (APLAs). This disorder is characterized by (i) evidence of involvement of 3 or more organs, systems, and/or tissues; (ii) development of manifestations simultaneously or in <1 week; (iii) confirmation by histopathology of small vessel occlusion in at least one organ or tissue; and (iv) laboratory confirmation of the presence of APLAs (lupus anticoagulants and/or anticardiolipin antibody and/or anti-β_2GPI antibodies). A registry containing clinical, laboratory, and therapeutic data on reported cases of the catastrophic antiphospholipid antibody syndrome is maintained at the European Forum on Antiphospholipid Antibodies Web site (http://www.med.ub.es/MIMMUN/FORUM/CAPS.HTM).

Infection is the most commonly identified precipitant of the catastrophic antiphospholipid antibody syndrome, but other triggers such as trauma, withdrawal of anticoagulation, and neoplasia have also been described. However, approximately 40% of patients with catastrophic antiphospholipid antibody syndrome have no obvious underlying cause. Although affecting <1% of antiphospholipid antibody syndrome patients, mortality may be as high as 50%.

Due to the rarity of catastrophic antiphospholipid antibody syndrome, recommendations for therapy are largely anecdotal, and no formal trials have been conducted. However, anticoagulation and high-dose corticosteroids form the mainstay of treatment, and additional benefit may be provided by plasma exchange and/or intravenous immunoglobulin (IVIg). The efficacy of these latter 2 approaches has neither been directly compared nor proven.

> **Key points**
>
> - Anemia develops in most patients treated in the intensive care setting. In these patients, a conservative transfusion strategy aimed at maintaining the hemoglobin between 7 and 9.9 g/dL is associated with fewer complications and potentially reduced mortality compared with a more liberal transfusion strategy.
> - Recombinant erythropoietin may be able to reduce the incidence of transfusion in patients in the ICU, although this has not been observed in all studies. One study suggested that erythropoietin may be associated with decreased mortality in trauma patients, although these observations require more rigorous study.
> - Thrombocytopenia in ICU patients is often multifactorial and may result from drugs, infection, or other causes. A history of a normal platelet count prior to the onset of acute illness generally suggests that the cause of thrombocytopenia is related to the acute illness or other intervention.
> - The diagnosis of HIT remains primarily clinical, and laboratory testing should be regarded as confirmatory. In patients in whom HIT is suspected with moderate to high preclinical probability, heparin should be discontinued and alternative anticoagulation initiated even in the absence of thrombosis.
> - First-line therapy for TTP/HUS remains plasma exchange. Emerging evidence suggests that rituximab may be beneficial in refractory cases, as well as in reducing relapse rates, although a prospective randomized study evaluating its utility has yet to be performed.

Consultation for hematologic complications of solid organ transplantation

> **Clinical case**
>
> You are asked to see a 33-year-old woman 48 hours after orthotopic liver transplantation for primary biliary cirrhosis. Postoperatively, she has been having hemolysis due to antibodies directed against the A antigen. The patient is A positive and received a liver from an O-positive donor. The blood bank is having difficulty cross-matching the patient with O-positive blood. You determine that she most likely has hemolysis from passenger lymphocytes in the donor liver that are making antibodies to both the A and B antigen. You recommend transfusing compatible cells when needed and suggest that the syndrome should to be short-lived. You also suggest plasma exchange as an alternative if the hemolysis becomes brisk.

Transfusion support

A consultant hematologist may be asked to assist with transfusion management in a patient undergoing solid organ transplantation. Of all solid organ transplantations, transfusion management is most challenging for patients undergoing liver transplantation due to the underlying coagulopathy that develops in these patients. The typical liver transplantation is associated with transfusion of 10 to 22 units of packed cells. This amount is decreased significantly when a Cell Saver (Haemonetics, Braintree, MA) is used. In addition to red blood cells, liver transplantation is associated with a large requirement for transfused plasma and platelets, although because of the concern for thrombosis, platelets have recently been used more sparingly. Heart-lung and heart transplantations also require transfusion support, whereas kidney and kidney-pancreas transplantations can often be performed without blood product support. Transfusion therapy for solid organ transplantation carries the potential risks of infection, human leukocyte antigen (HLA) alloimmunization, and rarely transfusion-associated graft-versus-host disease (GVHD).

In the past, pretransplantation transfusion was used as a form of immunomodulation to minimize the possibility of solid organ rejection. Recent randomized studies have shown, however, that pretransplantation transfusion does not improve renal graft survival and modern immunosuppressives are more effective at preventing graft rejection. Exposure to allogeneic lymphocytes can induce anti-HLA antibodies, which can lead to higher risks of acute and chronic rejection and compromised survival in solid organ recipients. To reduce this risk, patients expected to undergo kidney, heart, or lung transplantations should receive blood that is leukocyte reduced. Leukocyte reduction can be conducted during red blood cell processing or at the bedside with a filter. Because of conflicting data in liver transplantation patients, leukocyte reduction is considered optional for this population of patients. Plasma exchange, IVIg, and rituximab have been used in patients with positive panel reactive antibodies (PRAs) or major ABO incompatibility to minimize the risk of hyperacute rejection.

The most frequent transfusion-associated infection complicating solid organ transplantation is CMV. Although this is usually due to CMV reactivation in a seropositive recipient, seronegative recipients can acquire CMV through transfusion. For this reason, seronegative recipients should receive transfusions that are documented to be CMV negative.

Transfusion-associated GVHD is a rare cause of morbidity and mortality among solid organ transplantation patients, although it is associated with a mortality that exceeds 90%. Because of the rarity of the event, irradiation of blood products is not routinely recommended for recipients of solid organ transplantations.

Posttransplantation erythrocytosis

Posttransplantation erythrocytosis occurs in 10% to 20% of patients immediately following kidney transplantation, although the incidence appears to be decreasing. Although patients with posttransplantation erythrocytosis appear to have an improved overall survival compared with patients without the disorder, graft survival is reduced in this population. The etiology of erythrocytosis after kidney transplantation is related to the renin-angiotensin system and specifically angiotensin-converting enzyme (ACE) genotype, although the precise mechanism is unknown. Patients with posttransplantation erythrocytosis respond well to either ACE inhibitors such as fosinopril or angiotensin receptor blockers (ARBs) such as losartan. The routine use of these agents in patients with a transplanted kidney is probably the reason that the incidence of posttransplantation erythrocytosis is decreasing.

Posttransplantation lymphoproliferative disorders

Posttransplantation lymphoproliferative disorders (PTLDs) constitute a group of predominantly B-cell disorders that are typically initiated by the Epstein-Barr virus (EBV) in patients who are immunosuppressed following solid organ transplantation. For the consultant, this group of disorders typically presents as unexplained cytopenias in the case of

PTLD marrow involvement or can present as lymphadenopathy similar to the presentation of other non-Hodgkin lymphomas. PTLD typically results from EBV-initiated recipient B-lymphocyte proliferation.

Risk factors for the development of PTLD include the following: (i) receipt of a solid organ from an EBV-seropositive donor by an EBV-seronegative recipient; (ii) primary activation or reactivation of EBV in the recipient; (iii) prolonged immunosuppression with antibodies to T-cell antigens or the use of calcineurin inhibitors such as cyclosporine or tacrolimus; (iv) pediatric patients; (v) hepatitis C infection; and (vi) CMV infection. PTLD is most common in heart-lung transplantation recipients followed by lung, liver, pancreas, and cadaveric kidney transplantation recipients. Prophylactic administration of acyclovir or ganciclovir in EBV-seronegative children appears to reduce the incidence of PTLD.

PTLD is classified by the World Health Organization as shown in Table 2-7. Reactive or polyclonal PTLD typically occurs within the first year of transplantation. Clonal PTLD has an incidence that increases over time. B-symptoms such as fevers, night sweats, and weight loss are common at diagnosis. Approximately half of PTLD patients have disease limited to a single extranodal site, whereas 15% have disease limited to a single nodal group. In 30% of patients, the disease is multifocal.

Treatment for PTLD involves both enhancement of the cytotoxic T-lymphocyte (CTL) response and cytotoxic therapy. CTL responses are most often enhanced by reduction of immunosuppression, which is effective in over half of PTLD patients. Alternatively, interferon alfa can be used. Cytotoxic therapy includes use of typical lymphoma regimens with rituximab and is typically reserved for patients unresponsive to a reduction in immunosuppression. Only approximately half of patients are responsive to cytotoxic therapy, and in these individuals, the 5-year survival rate is 20% to 30%.

Drug-related abnormalities

One of the most common reasons for hematologic consultation in patients after solid organ transplantation is cytopenia, which is often caused by immunosuppressant drugs. Azathioprine is particularly problematic, causing cytopenias in >10% of patients. Because azathioprine and its principal metabolite are predominantly cleared by the kidney, azathioprine-induced marrow toxicity is common following kidney transplantation rejection. Azathioprine toxicity is exacerbated by allopurinol, ACE inhibitors, and trimethoprim/sulfamethoxazole. Because these drugs are commonly prescribed, the consultant should be aware of these common drug interactions.

Thrombotic microangiopathy, which mimics TTP, is seen in occasional patients who receive a calcineurin inhibitor. Thrombotic microangiopathy can be difficult to distinguish from rejection of the transplanted kidney, and renal biopsy may be required to make the distinction. Importantly, the treatment for thrombotic microangiopathy involves withdrawal of the drug, whereas rejection may require increasing immunosuppression. Tacrolimus is often substituted for cyclosporine in patients with thrombotic microangiopathy. Systemic thrombotic microangiopathy may lead to dialysis and graft loss in a high proportion of patients, although a localized thrombotic microangiopathy diagnosed by kidney biopsy in patients with a primary manifestation of renal failure typically responds to elimination of the offending drug. Unlike in TTP, there are insufficient data documenting the utility of plasma exchange for patients with posttransplantation thrombotic microangiopathy, a situation in which the ADAMTS13 level is not low and in which an ADAMTS13 inhibitor is not detectable.

Alloimmune complications

Passenger lymphocytes in the transplanted solid organ can very rarely (<1% of transplantations) cause GVHD in patients with a single HLA class I mismatch. This is related to transmission of alloreactive T lymphocytes within the transplanted solid organ. The risk of GVHD is related to

Table 2-7 World Health Organization classification of posttransplantation lymphoproliferative disorders (PTLD).

Category	Subtype
Early lesions	Reactive plasmacytic hyperplasia
	Infectious mononucleosis–like
Polymorphic PTLD	Polyclonal
	Monoclonal
Monomorphic PTLD	B-cell lymphomas
	Diffuse large B-cell lymphoma (immunoblastic, centroblastic, anaplastic)
	Burkitt/Burkitt-like lymphoma
	Plasma cell myeloma
	T-cell lymphomas
	Peripheral T-cell lymphoma
	Other types (γ-δ, hepatosplenic, T/NK)
Other types	Hodgkin disease–like lesions
	Plasmacytoma-like lesions

Adapted from Harris NL, Jaffe ES, Diebold J, et al. The World Health Organization classification of neoplastic diseases of the haematopoietic and lymphoid tissues: report of the Clinical Advisory Committee Meeting, Airlie House, Virginia, November 1997. *Histopathology*. 2000;36:69–86.

the dose of transplanted lymphocytes. Of all the solid organ transplantations, patients receiving a small bowel transplantation receive the largest dose of passenger lymphocytes. As such, donors are typically treated with antilymphocyte antibodies or corticosteroids prior to transplantation to minimize the transplantation of donor T lymphocytes. GVHD in solid organ transplantation patients presents similarly to GVHD in bone marrow transplantation patients. Fever, rash, and diarrhea 2 to 6 weeks after transplantation are common initial complaints. Cytopenias, due to GVHD directed against host hematopoietic cells, are also common, leading to difficulty distinguishing GVHD from infection with CMV, drug reaction, or allograft rejection. Treatment of GVHD after solid organ transplantation includes supportive care, corticosteroids, and anti–T-cell antibodies.

Another alloimmune complication of solid organ transplantation that can be the cause for hematology consultation is immune hemolysis secondary to passenger lymphocytes (passenger lymphocyte syndrome). Passenger lymphocyte syndrome is also more common in transplantations containing the greatest lymphocyte numbers. The syndrome is most common in small bowel transplantations followed by heart-lung recipients and liver and kidney transplantations. Most cases are due to ABO incompatibility, but the syndrome has also been reported to occur secondary to incompatibility with Rh D, c, e, JK(a), K, and Fy(a) antigens. Hemolysis is abrupt and occurs several days after transplantation, but is generally moderate and not life threatening. Treatment involves appropriate transfusion of compatible cells and potentially the use of plasma exchange for persistent hemolysis. Fortunately, passenger lymphocyte syndrome is typically short-lived due to the short survival of donor lymphocytes in the circulation.

ITP has also been described in the posttransplantation setting and may be severe, protracted, and unresponsive to standard ITP therapies.

Key points

- PTLD most commonly occurs within the first year of a solid organ transplantation in EBV-naive patients transplanted with an organ from an EBV-infected donor.
- Cytopenias occurring after transplantation of a solid organ may be due to infection, drugs, or GVHD.
- ABO mismatch between organ donor and recipient can result in hemolysis from passenger lymphocytes in the transplanted organ.
- Post–kidney transplantation erythrocytosis responds to ACE inhibitor or ARB therapy.

Pregnancy

Clinical case

You are asked to see a 27-year-old woman who is 34 weeks pregnant. A complete blood cell count (CBC) today revealed a white blood cell (WBC) count of 6000/μL, a platelet count of 90,000/μL, and hematocrit of 38%. Her prenatal course has been relatively uncomplicated, although her platelet count began to decrease at approximately 28 weeks and has gradually declined since that time. She has had one prior pregnancy, which was uncomplicated, and does not recall being told that she was thrombocytopenic at that time. Currently, her only complaint is significant fatigue, although on occasion, she has noted a small amount of pedal edema. Physical examination reveals a gravid uterus but no hepatosplenomegaly, lymphadenopathy, or other significant physical findings. Review of the peripheral blood film reveals decreased platelets but is otherwise unremarkable, with no platelet clumping. Coagulation studies are normal. She is concerned about bleeding during delivery and the potential implications for her child. You advise her that a course of watchful waiting is most appropriate at this point and continue to monitor her platelet counts on a weekly basis.

Anemia

During normal pregnancy, the plasma volume expands by 40% to 60%, whereas the red blood cell mass expands by 20% to 50%. Thus, a physiologic anemia develops, leading to a normal hematocrit value of 30% to 32%. Hemoglobin levels <10 g/dL suggest the possibility of a pathologic process such as nutritional deficiency. Anemia is surprisingly well tolerated during pregnancy, and major fetal and maternal complications do not become frequent until the hemoglobin decreases to as low as 6 g/dL.

Iron deficiency accounts for 75% of cases of nonphysiologic anemia in pregnancy, and the incidence of iron deficiency anemia in the United States during the third trimester may exceed 50%. Current recommendations suggest that pregnant patients receive 15 to 30 mg/d of supplemental elemental iron, although studies examining the efficacy of iron supplementation during pregnancy have not shown a clear benefit to pregnancy outcomes. For patients who do not tolerate oral iron, parenteral iron may be used. Iron sucrose is categorized as pregnancy class B (presumed safe based on animal models) and is preferred over iron dextran, which is considered pregnancy class C (safety uncertain). Recent studies have demonstrated that for patients who do not respond well to parenteral iron, the addition of recombinant erythropoietin may add benefit. In a study of 40 patients with gestational iron deficiency anemia who had unsatisfactory responses to oral iron, 20 patients were randomized to receive recombinant erythropoietin (rEPO) and parenteral iron sucrose (group 1), and 20 were randomized to receive iron sucrose alone (group 2). Patients in group 1 displayed higher reticulocyte counts on day 4, greater increases in hemoglobin from day 11, and a shorter duration of therapy to reach the target hemoglobin of 11 g/dL. No abnormalities in fetal hemoglobin levels were observed, consistent with the belief that rEPO does not cross the placenta. Thus, although rEPO may function as an adjuvant to iron replacement therapy in pregnant patients with iron deficiency anemia, it should be reserved for exceptional cases, particularly given the increased risk of thrombosis during pregnancy and the fact that improved fetal outcomes have not been demonstrated. Alternative causes of anemia should also be sought in patients refractory to standard iron therapy.

The majority of macrocytic anemias during pregnancy are due to folate deficiency, whereas vitamin B_{12} deficiency is rare. Folate requirements increase from 50 μg/d in the nonpregnant female to at least 150 μg/d during pregnancy, and the Centers for Disease Control and Prevention recommend supplementation with 400 μg/d of folate to prevent neural tube defects. Folate deficiency is most precisely diagnosed by measuring plasma levels of homocysteine and methylmalonic acid.

Thrombocytopenia

Thrombocytopenia affects 10% of pregnant women and results from several disorders that may or may not be specific to pregnancy. Pregnant patients may present with isolated thrombocytopenia or develop thrombocytopenia as a component of a systemic disorder that may be unique to pregnancy. A summary of causes of pregnancy in thrombocytopenia is presented in Table 2-8.

Isolated thrombocytopenia most commonly results from "gestational" or "incidental" thrombocytopenia of pregnancy. Incidental thrombocytopenia usually develops during the second or third trimester in otherwise healthy pregnant women. The degree of thrombocytopenia is usually mild, and by definition, the platelet count does not decrease below approximately 70,000/μL. This disorder may represent an extreme example of the common 10% decrease in platelet count that occurs during normal pregnancy. Incidental thrombocytopenia does not affect pregnancy outcome, does not cause thrombocytopenia in the offspring of affected women, and requires no specific treatment. However, incidental thrombocytopenia may be impossible to distinguish from ITP or may be an early manifestation of a more serious disorder that develops later in pregnancy. Thus, patients with suspected incidental thrombocytopenia should be monitored throughout pregnancy.

ITP affects approximately 1 in 10,000 pregnancies. In contrast to gestational thrombocytopenia, ITP often becomes manifest during the first trimester. A prior history of thrombocytopenia or autoimmune disease preceding pregnancy or during previous pregnancies is useful in making a diagnosis of ITP. Patients with ITP generally present with more severe thrombocytopenia than those with incidental thrombocytopenia, but the 2 disorders may be indistinguishable when ITP is mild. Therapy of ITP in pregnant patients is similar in some respects to that in patients who are not pregnant,

Table 2-8 Differential diagnosis of thrombocytopenia in pregnancy.

	MAHA	Thrombo-cytopenia	Coagulopathy	Hypertension	Liver disease	Renal disease	CNS disease	Time of onset
ITP	–	Mild-severe	–	–	–	–	–	Anytime, common in 1st trimester
Gestational	–	Mild	–	–	–	–	–	2nd–3rd trimester
Preeclampsia	mild	Mild-moderate	Absent-mild	Moderate-severe	–	Protein	Seizures in eclampsia	Late 2nd to 3rd trimester
HELLP	Moderate-severe	Moderate-severe	May be present (mild)	Absent-severe	Moderate-severe	Absent-moderate	Absent-moderate	Late 2nd to 3rd trimester
HUS	Moderate-severe	Moderate-severe	Absent	Absent-mild	Absent	Moderate-severe	Absent-mild	Postpartum
TTP	Moderate-severe	Severe	Absent	Absent	Absent	Absent-moderate	Absent-severe	2nd to 3rd trimester
AFLP	Mild	Mild-moderate	Severe	Absent-mild	Severe	Absent-mild	Absent-mild	3rd trimester

AFLP = acute fatty liver of pregnancy; CNS = central nervous system; HELLP = hemolysis, elevated liver function tests, low platelets; HUS = hemolytic uremic syndrome; ITP = idiopathic thrombocytopenic purpura; MAHA = microangiopathic hemolytic anemia; TTP = thrombotic thrombocytopenic purpura.

although greater emphasis should be placed on avoiding corticosteroids, which may cause unique toxicities such as gestational diabetes or hypertension in pregnant individuals. Prednisone exposure in the first trimester may also be associated with an increased incidence of cleft palate. These concerns have prompted some to advocate the use of IVIg as first-line therapy in pregnant patients with ITP. Intravenous anti-D has been used successfully to treat ITP in Rh(D)-positive women, although only a few patients have been reported, and thus, the safety of this agent cannot be considered established. Similarly, there is little experience with the use of rituximab in pregnant individuals, although B-cell lymphocytopenia has been reported in the offspring of individuals treated with this agent, which is considered pregnancy class C. The thrombopoietic agents romiplostim and eltrombopag are also considered pregnancy class C, and a registry has been developed for patients taking these agents who become pregnant. The use of cytotoxic therapy is associated with teratogenicity in many cases, although azathioprine has been commonly used in pregnancy with apparent safety.

In light of these considerations, patients with severe ITP refractory to steroids and IVIg should be considered for splenectomy, which may be performed most safely in the midsecond trimester, when the risk of inducing premature labor is minimized and the gravid uterus does not yet obscure the surgical field.

Approximately 10% of the offspring of patients with ITP will also be thrombocytopenic, and 5% will have platelet counts <20,000/μL. There are no maternal laboratory studies that reliably predict whether an infant of a mother with ITP will be born thrombocytopenic; perhaps the best indicator is a prior history of thrombocytopenia at delivery in a sibling. Moreover, no maternal interventions have been convincingly shown to increase the fetal platelet count. The delivery of the offspring of mothers with ITP by cesarean section has not been shown to reduce the risk of fetal intracranial hemorrhage, a rare complication affecting <1% of these infants, at delivery; however, some continue to advocate this approach, particularly when a sibling has been previously found to be severely thrombocytopenic at delivery. These considerations and the appreciation that the risk of fetal platelet count determination by percutaneous umbilical cord blood sampling (PUBS) is likely greater than that of fetal intracranial hemorrhage during vaginal delivery explain why the utilization of PUBS has decreased significantly in recent years. All offspring of patients with ITP should be monitored closely for the development of ITP within the first 4 to 7 days after delivery, and all thrombocytopenic neonates should undergo cranial ultrasound. Severely affected offspring generally respond well to IVIg.

Thrombocytopenia may also occur in patients with preeclampsia. Preeclampsia affects 6% of all first pregnancies and usually develops in the third trimester; its diagnostic features include hypertension and proteinuria (>300 mg/24 h). Preeclampsia occurs most commonly in primagravidas who are either <20 or >30 years of age. Eclampsia, defined by the presence of grand mal seizures accompanying preeclampsia, complicates <1% of preeclamptic pregnancies. Some studies suggest that preeclampsia may be more common in patients with thrombophilia, particularly those with APLAs, although this association is not well established. Thrombocytopenia develops in up to 50% of patients with preeclampsia, with its severity generally related to that of the underlying disease. The pathogenesis of thrombocytopenia in preeclampsia is not well understood, although accelerated platelet consumption likely contributes.

The HELLP (hemolysis, elevated liver function tests, low platelets) syndrome affects 0.1% to 0.89% of all live births and is associated with a maternal mortality of 0% to 4%. HELLP and preeclampsia share many clinical features, although HELLP occurs in a slightly older population (mean age of approximately 25 years). Because approximately 10% of patients with HELLP develop hypertension and proteinuria, it is often considered a preeclampsia variant. The major diagnostic criteria for HELLP include microangiopathic hemolytic anemia, levels of serum aspartate aminotransferase exceeding 70 U/L, and thrombocytopenia, with a platelet count <100,000/μL. Microangiopathic hemolysis is accompanied by schistocytes on the peripheral blood film and an elevated lactate dehydrogenase (LDH); some experts suggest that a minimal LDH of 600 U/dL is required for diagnosis. In some cases, HELLP may be difficult to distinguish from TTP-HUS. Because many patients with HELLP may present with isolated right upper quadrant and epigastric pain in the absence of hypertension and proteinuria, patients may be misdiagnosed as having primary gastrointestinal disease and referred for surgical consideration. HELLP is associated with significant maternal and fetal morbidity and mortality, which exceeds that associated with preeclampsia; therefore, prompt diagnosis and treatment are essential. The offspring of patients with both preeclampsia and HELLP may also become thrombocytopenic, although the thrombocytopenia is usually mild.

Therapy for HELLP and preeclampsia is directed toward stabilization of the mother, followed by expeditious delivery, after which these disorders usually remit within 3 to 4 days in the majority of patients. However, HELLP, in particular, may occasionally worsen or even develop postpartum. Pre- or postnatal corticosteroids have been suggested in several small, randomized studies to hasten resolution of the biochemical abnormalities and thrombocytopenia associated with HELLP, although these studies have not been sufficiently powered to demonstrate an effect on maternal or fetal mortality. One should consider the use of such adjunctive therapies if thrombocytopenia continues to worsen or there is continuing clinical deterioration 5 to 7 days after delivery.

TTP and HUS are discussed earlier in this chapter. However, it is worth noting that the incidence of TTP is increased during pregnancy, and pregnant women comprise 10% to 20% of the patients in many large TTP series. TTP may develop in either the second or third trimesters. Whether the decreased levels of ADAMTS13 that occur in pregnancy predispose to the development of thrombotic microangiopathies is uncertain. The manifestations of TTP in pregnant and nonpregnant women are identical, and pregnant patients respond equally well to plasma exchange. A major dilemma in the management of TTP is the difficulty in its diagnosis; confusion with pregnancy-specific disorders such as HELLP may delay diagnosis and lead to increased morbidity and mortality. Although delivery of the fetus is the standard approach to management of patients with preeclampsia, this intervention does not ameliorate the course of TTP.

The incidence of HUS is also increased in association with pregnancy. Although some cases of HUS develop near term, the majority of cases develop 3 to 4 weeks postpartum, and their clinical features resemble most closely atypical HUS, with renal failure as the predominant manifestation. The prognosis of postpartum HUS is poor, with persistent renal failure in >25% of affected individuals. Although responses to plasma exchange have been reported, the overall response rate to this intervention is low; nevertheless, a trial of plasma exchange is indicated, particularly given the difficulty in distinguishing TTP and HUS and the potential role of deficiencies of complement regulatory proteins in this syndrome. There is no consensus on the risk of developing recurrent TTP or HUS in subsequent pregnancies; although the non–prospectively collected literature suggests that this risk may be relatively high (10%–20%), a recent registry report did not confirm this.

Lastly, there are several additional causes of thrombocytopenia that the hematologist must consider when evaluating pregnant patients. DIC may accompany severe preeclampsia and be initiated by processes such as retained fetal products, placental abruption, or amniotic fluid embolism. It is commonly associated with mild thrombocytopenia, and the degree of microangiopathic hemolysis is generally not as severe as that observed in preeclampsia, HELLP, or the primary thrombotic microangiopathies. Nevertheless, DIC in this setting can be severe, abrupt, and fatal if not managed appropriately. *Acute fatty liver of pregnancy* (AFLP) usually occurs in the third trimester and affects primarily primiparas and women with twin gestations. Symptoms include nausea, vomiting, right upper quadrant pain, anorexia, jaundice, and cholestatic liver dysfunction. Most patients have DIC, and diabetes insipidus and hypoglycemia are present in >50% of cases. Thrombocytopenia is usually mild, but maternal bleeding is common due to the accompanying coagulopathy resulting from diminished hepatic synthesis of coagulation proteins, as well as DIC and acquired antithrombin deficiency. Some cases of AFLP and possibly HELLP may result from fetal mitochondrial fatty acid oxidation disorders, most commonly a deficiency of long-chain 3-hydroxyacyl-coenzyme A dehydrogenase. *Drug-induced thrombocytopenia* has been discussed, and *HIV infection* may also cause an immune-mediated thrombocytopenia due to antibodies reactive with amino acids 49 to 66 of GPIIIa, which cross-react with HIV-Nef. Impaired megakaryopoiesis also occurs in HIV-infected patients due to infection of megakaryocytes by the virus, and patients with HIV are also at increased risk for the development of TTP. *Congenital thrombocytopenias,* such as the May-Hegglin anomaly or other disorders associated with mutations in the *MYH9 gene,* may occasionally escape diagnosis until adulthood. *Type 2b vWD* may induce thrombocytopenia due to platelet agglutination caused by increased levels of mutant vWF in pregnancy. The mutant vWF that is produced in patients with type 2b vWD binds its platelet receptor GPIb with increased avidity, and the resultant platelet agglutination leads to accelerated platelet clearance and thrombocytopenia.

von Willebrand disease

vWD is the most common inherited bleeding disorder and is found in approximately 1% of the general population. There are several variants. Type 1 vWD results from a partial, quantitative deficiency of vWF and accounts for 50% of all vWD cases. Type 2 vWD consists of several subtypes: type 2b, as mentioned earlier, is characterized by increased affinity of vWF binding to platelet GB1b due to a mutation in the GP1b binding region of vWF; type 2N is characterized by a loss of function mutation in the factor VIII (FVIII) binding site in vWF; type 2M is characterized by decreased affinity of vWF for its platelet receptor GPIb, and type 2a is characterized by a selective decrease in the high molecular weight multimers of vWF. Type 3 vWD is characterized by a severe deficiency in vWF resulting in a corresponding deficiency of FVIII.

Under the regulation of elevated estrogen levels that occur in pregnancy, the levels of vWF and FVIII increase, generally beginning in the early second trimester and peaking between 29 and 35 weeks. Most patients with type 1 vWD normalize their levels of vWF and FVIII during pregnancy, although those with more severe disease may not. Given the somewhat unpredictable nature of these responses, measurement of vWF levels should be performed between approximately 32 and 34 weeks; levels generally remain fairly stable through the remainder of pregnancy, and thus, levels obtained at this time allow a plan for delivery to be developed. Although levels of vWF may also increase in patients with type 2 vWD, functional levels may not be significantly enhanced due to the production of a functionally deficient protein. Levels of vWF generally do not increase during pregnancy in patients with type 3 vWD.

In most cases, the physiologic increase in vWF levels exceeds the minimum 50% recommended for the epidural anesthesia and delivery and allows these procedures to be performed without therapeutic intervention. However, the decline in vWF levels after delivery is unpredictable and subject to significant variability. Although levels may decline gradually over 1 to 2 weeks in most patients, in others, they decrease precipitously. Thus, if epidural anesthesia is used, it is generally judicious to remove the catheter as soon as possible after delivery is completed.

Although antepartum hemorrhage in patients with vWD may occasionally occur during the first trimester, before the increase in vWF levels occurs, postpartum hemorrhage may occur in up to 22% of women with vWD, most commonly those with type 2 vWD and those with vWF levels <50%. Several therapeutic options are available for therapy of postpartum hemorrhage in these patients. DDAVP is effective in raising vWF levels in patients with type 1 vWD. Although theoretical concerns about the vasoconstrictive effects of DDAVP on placental perfusion and the potential oxytocic effect of DDAVP have been raised, these have not been borne out in practice. However, because pregnant patients often receive large volumes of fluids at the time of delivery, DDAVP should be used judiciously, as significant fluid retention and hyponatremia have been reported. For patients with hemorrhage that requires replacement therapy, purified vWF-FVIII concentrates may be used. These, as well as oral contraceptives, may also be used for therapy of late postpartum hemorrhage. Some recommendations have in fact suggested the initiation of prophylactic oral contraceptives beginning immediately after delivery and continued for approximately 1 month in women with no contraindication.

Thrombophilia and thromboembolism during pregnancy

Pregnant women are at increased risk for the development of thromboembolism. The relative risk of VTE during pregnancy and the postpartum period is 4.2, with an overall incidence of 199.7/100,000 in a primarily white population. Approximately 80% of these events are deep venous thrombi (DVT), whereas 20% are pulmonary emboli. Moreover, the rate of VTE is approximately 5-fold higher in the postpartum period than during pregnancy, with one third of pregnancy-associated DVT and one half of pulmonary emboli occurring after delivery. The risk of arterial thromboembolism is also increased approximately 3- to 4-fold in pregnant women, reflecting the hypercoagulable state associated with pregnancy.

Pregnancy-associated DVT is more often proximal and massive than in the nonpregnant setting and usually occurs in the left lower extremity. In contrast, distal DVT occurs with similar frequency in the left and right lower extremities. The left-sided predominance of VTEs may reflect compression of the left iliac vein between the right iliac artery and lumbar vertebrae.

Although a number of factors, such as decreased venous capacitance and decreased venous outflow, are likely to contribute to the development of thrombosis during pregnancy, the fact that VTE is as frequent in the first trimester as during the rest of pregnancy and the increased risk of arterial thromboembolism suggest that blood hypercoagulability is the major contributor to thrombosis in pregnant women. Pregnancy is associated with increased levels of factors VII, VIII, and X; fibrinogen; and vWF, as well as increases in the levels of plasminogen activator inhibitor types 1 and 2. In parallel, a substantial decrease in the levels of free protein S occurs due to increased levels of C4b binding protein. An increase in activated protein C resistance in the absence of factor V Leiden and unexplained by the decrease in free proteins S is also observed in many pregnant patients, particularly in the third trimester.

Between 20% and 50% of all thromboembolic events that occur in pregnant women are associated with a thrombophilic disorder. A systematic review has provided estimates of the relative risks of VTE associated with various thrombophilic disorders in pregnant women. This study assigned factor V Leiden homozygosity a relative risk of 34.40, factor V Leiden heterozygosity a relative risk of 8.32, prothrombin G20210A gene mutation homozygosity a relative risk of 26.36, and prothrombin G20210A heterozygosity a relative risk of 6.8. Another study suggested a positive predictive value for pregnancy-associated thrombosis of 1:500 for factor V Leiden, 1:200 for prothrombin G20210A, and 4.6:100 for double heterozygotes of these mutations, assuming an overall thrombosis rate of 0.66/1000 pregnancies. The positive predictive value was 1:113 for protein C deficiency and 1:2.8 for type I antithrombin deficiency. These estimates of absolute risk in pregnant patients with thrombophilia are useful in developing treatment approaches and suggest the need for individualized treatment plans based on the type of thrombophilia as well as the presence of homozygous versus heterozygous mutations. APLAs, in addition to their association with poor pregnancy outcomes, are associated with an increased risk of thrombosis in pregnancy, although the exact magnitude of the risk is uncertain.

In addition to the risk of thromboembolism in a pregnant patient, several toxicities of anticoagulant therapy unique to pregnancy must also be considered when developing treatment approaches. First, the oral vitamin K antagonist (VKA) warfarin is teratogenic, causing an embryopathy consisting of nasal hypoplasia and/or stippled epiphyses. Limb hypoplasia may also be observed. Estimates of the frequency of these abnormalities in exposed infants vary widely, although an incidence of between approximately 0.6% and 6% seems most likely. The teratogenic effects occur primarily following exposure to warfarin during weeks 6 to 12 of pregnancy, whereas warfarin is probably safe during the first 6 weeks of gestation. VKAs used at any time during pregnancy have also been associated with rare CNS developmental abnormalities such as dorsal midline dysplasia and ventral midline dysplasia leading to optic atrophy. Finally, an increased risk of minor neurodevelopmental abnormalities has been suggested in the offspring of women exposed to warfarin during the second and third trimesters, although the significance of these problems is uncertain. Warfarin may also cause an anticoagulant effect in the fetus, which may lead to bleeding at delivery. Second, prophylactic UFH is associated with a substantial risk of osteoporosis and a 2% to 3% incidence of vertebral fractures when administered throughout pregnancy. Several reports suggest substantially less osteoporosis when patients receive LMWH, which also displays a better pharmacokinetic profile, and a 5- to 10-fold reduction in the incidence of HIT. Thus, LMWH is now the preferred agent for the prevention and treatment of VTE in pregnant patients. However, as pregnancy progresses and the volume of distribution increases for LMWH, dose adjustments may be required. Some recommend that LMWH be changed to UFH at the 36th week of gestation, due to the shorter half-life of the former in the setting of incipient parturition and the potential use of epidural anesthesia.

The diagnosis of VTE is difficult in the pregnant population, due to a lack of validation of standard diagnostic studies. A recent systematic review concluded, however, that an abnormal compression ultrasound (CUS) is sufficient for a diagnosis of DVT during pregnancy. By comparison, a normal CUS does not reliably exclude DVT because of the low sensitivity for isolated iliac DVT; thus, patients with a normal CUS should undergo repeat testing 6 to 8 days later, or earlier if indicated by symptoms. Negative serial CUS studies reliably exclude DVT. If doubt about the diagnosis persists, limited venography with abdominal shielding may be performed. This exposes the fetus to <0.05 mSv (1 mSv = 0.1 rad) of radiation. In patients with suspected pulmonary embolism, a negative ventilation/perfusion (V/Q) scan excludes pulmonary embolism, whereas a positive scan confirms the diagnosis. All other abnormal V/Q scans should be considered nondiagnostic, and helical computed tomography (CT) scanning, or alternatively, shielded pulmonary angiography should be pursued. There is insufficient information at this time to define accurately the utility of D-dimer testing in diagnosing DVT during pregnancy.

A number of scenarios exist concerning the prevention and treatment of primary and recurrent thrombosis in pregnant individuals. In general, several approaches to such situations are considered acceptable due to the paucity of prospective trials comparing, for example, close clinical surveillance versus anticoagulation with UFH or LMWH. Although thrombophilia is a major risk factor for thrombosis during pregnancy, the relatively low absolute risk for thrombosis in individuals with a single genetic thrombophilic trait justifies an approach of close clinical surveillance in many situations. Although addressing each of these potential scenarios in depth is beyond the scope of this chapter, evidence-based guidelines have recently been updated by the ACCP. These guidelines are summarized in Table 2-9. Despite the different approaches considered acceptable in the antenatal setting, the increased risk of thrombosis in the postnatal setting suggests that anticoagulation be considered in essentially all women with a known thrombophilic predisposition, although guidelines do not advocate routine screening of patients for such abnormalities.

Table 2-9 American College of Chest Physicians guidelines for anticoagulant treatment of VTE/thrombophilia in pregnancy.

Scenario	Recommended treatment	Comments
Acute VTE		
Acute VTE	Initial therapy with either adjusted-dose subcutaneous LMWH or adjusted-dose UFH (IV bolus, followed by continuous infusion to maintain PTT within the therapeutic range, or subcutaneous therapy adjusted to maintain the PTT 6 hours after injection in the therapeutic range) for at least 5 days Continue subcutaneous LMWH or UFH throughout pregnancy Continue anticoagulants at least 6 weeks postpartum (minimum total duration of 6 months)	For pregnant patients receiving LMWH or UFH, discontinue the heparin at least 24 hours prior to elective induction of labor

(Continued)

Table 2-9 American College of Chest Physicians guidelines for anticoagulant treatment of VTE/thrombophilia in pregnancy (*continued*)

Scenario	Recommended treatment	Comments
Prior episode of VTE		
Prior VTE associated with transient risk factor	Antepartum: close clinical surveillance	If prior event was estrogen or pregnancy related, suggest close clinical surveillance or prophylaxis antepartum
	Postpartum prophylaxis	
Single idiopathic VTE, but no thrombophilia, not receiving long-term anticoagulants	Antepartum: prophylactic LMWH/UFH, or intermediate-dose LMWH/UFH, or close clinical surveillance	
	Postpartum prophylaxis	
Single episode of VTE and thrombophilia (laboratory confirmed), not receiving long-term anticoagulants	Antepartum: prophylactic or intermediate-dose LMWH or UFH, or close clinical surveillance	
	Postpartum prophylaxis	
Higher risk thrombophilia (antithrombin deficiency, compound heterozygous prothrombin G20210A and factor V Leiden, or homozygotes for these conditions, persistent positivity for APLA), with a single prior VTE, not receiving long-term anticoagulants	Antepartum: prophylactic or intermediate-dose LMWH of UFH	
	Postpartum prophylaxis	
Multiple episodes (≥2), not receiving long-term anticoagulants	Antepartum: prophylactic, intermediate-dose, or adjusted-dose LMWH or UFH	
	Postpartum prophylaxis	
Currently on long-term anticoagulation	LMWH or UFH throughout pregnancy (adjusted-dose LMWH or UFH, 75% of adjusted-dose LMWH, or intermediate-dose LMWH)	
	Resumption of long-term anticoagulation postpartum	
All women with prior DVT	Antenatal and postpartum compression stockings	
No prior VTE		
Antithrombin deficiency	Antepartum prophylaxis	
	Postpartum prophylaxis	
Any other thrombophilia	Antepartum: close clinical surveillance, or prophylactic LMWH or UFH	
	Postpartum prophylaxis	

Definitions of anticoagulant regimens:
- Prophylactic UFH: UFH 5000 U subcutaneously every 12 hours
- Intermediate-dose UFH: UFH subcutaneously every 12 hours in doses adjusted to target an anti-Xa level of 0.1 to 0.3 U/mL
- Adjusted-dose UFH: UFH subcutaneously every 12 hours in doses adjusted to target a mid-interval activated PTT into the therapeutic range
- Prophylactic LMWH: for example, dalteparin 5000 U subcutaneously every 24 hours, tinzaparin 4500 U subcutaneously every 24 hours, or enoxaparin 40 mg subcutaneously every 24 hours (extremes of body weight may require dose modification)
- Intermediate-dose LMWH: for example, dalteparin 5000 U subcutaneously every 12 hours or enoxaparin 40 mg subcutaneously every 12 hours
- Adjusted-dose LMWH: weight-adjusted full-treatment doses of LMWH, given once or twice daily (eg, dalteparin 200 U/kg or tinzaparin 175 U/kg every day, dalteparin 100 U/kg every 12 hours, or enoxaparin 1 mg/kg every 12 hours)
- Postpartum anticoagulants: vitamin K antagonists for 4 to 6 weeks with a target INR of 2.0 to 3.0, with initial UFH or LMWH overlap until the INR is >2.0, or prophylactic LMWH for 4 to 6 weeks
- Surveillance: clinical vigilance and appropriate objective investigation of women with symptoms suspicious of deep vein thrombosis or pulmonary embolism

Adapted from Bates SM, Greer IA, Pabinger I, et al. Venous thromboembolism, thrombophilia, antithrombotic therapy, and pregnancy. American College of Chest Physicians Evidence-Based Clinical Practice Guidelines (8th Edition). *Chest*. 2008;133(Suppl 6):844S–886S.
APLA = antiphospholipid antibodies; INR = international normalized ratio; IV = intravenous; LMWH = low molecular weight heparin; PTT = partial thromboplastin time; SC = subcutaneous; UFH = unfractionated heparin; VTE = venous thromboembolism.

Thrombophilia, fetal loss, and poor pregnancy outcomes

Most studies addressing the relationship between thrombophilia and fetal loss have been small, retrospective, and uncontrolled case-control or cohort studies, and thus their findings must be interpreted cautiously. The majority of these studies have shown an association between thrombophilia, either acquired or inherited, and both recurrent fetal loss and pregnancy complications (eg, preeclampsia, intrauterine growth restriction [IUGR]). However, due to the weak design and small size of most of these studies, these associations remain hotly debated. Moreover, even if an association between thrombophilia, fetal loss, and pregnancy complications exists, causality has not been demonstrated.

The strongest evidence of an association between thrombophilia and fetal loss comes from studies in patients with APLAs. APLAs are found in approximately 15% of women with recurrent fetal loss (≥3), and these women have been reported in some studies to experience fetal loss at a rate approaching 90% in subsequent pregnancies; however, other older studies have demonstrated that normal outcomes may occur in many patients even without therapy. Although the majority of normal individuals and patients with APLA experience early fetal loss, an increased proportion of APLA-positive patients experience late fetal loss (after the 10th week of gestation). Several randomized studies, none of which were placebo controlled, have examined the effect of treatment of women with APLAs with aspirin, heparin, or both. These studies have generally demonstrated an advantage of aspirin and heparin over either aspirin or heparin alone, although a recent, randomized trial was stopped early when it became evident that LMWH and aspirin offered no advantage over aspirin alone, with almost 80% of women in both arms having successful pregnancies. Current ACCP guidelines suggest that a patient with APLAs and recurrent pregnancy loss or late pregnancy loss but no history of thrombosis should be treated with antepartum prophylactic or intermediate-dose UFH or prophylactic LMWH combined with acetylsalicylic acid.

Inherited thrombophilia is less strongly associated with pregnancy loss than APLA. Large case-control studies have come to differing conclusions as to whether such an association exists. However, several meta-analyses and a large systematic review have concluded that both hetero- and homozygous factor V Leiden and prothrombin G2021A mutations, acquired activated protein C resistance and hyperhomocysteinemia are associated with early pregnancy loss (defined as first or second trimester). For first trimester pregnancy loss alone, significant associations were seen for factor V Leiden (homo- and heterozygous grouped together), heterozygous prothrombin G20210A, anticardiolipin antibodies, acquired activated protein C resistance, and homocysteinemia, but not homozygous MTHFR mutations. For third trimester fetal loss, protein S deficiency was most strongly associated, but significant associations were also observed for factor V Leiden, heterozygous prothrombin G20210A, and APLAs. In interpreting this data, however, the limitations of meta-analyses must be considered, particularly given the poor quality of the primary data. Moreover, in most cases, the odds ratios are very low, and the confidence intervals are wide and often approaching unity, thus raising concern about the clinical relevance of the findings.

Associations of thrombophilias with pregnancy complications, in particular preeclampsia, and IUGR have also been demonstrated, although these associations are likely less strong and thus even more controversial.

These associations have led to widespread screening of patients with poor pregnancy outcomes for congenital and acquired thrombophilias and increased use of anticoagulant therapy in attempts to optimize pregnancy outcomes. However, these studies have not yielded consistent data, likely due to differences in study populations and design, as well as differences among the specific agents studied and their dosing. Most studies have not been randomized or placebo controlled, and outcomes are often compared with historical controls. Moreover, the use of historical controls has not allowed consideration of "regression toward the mean." Indeed, one study demonstrated live birth rates in the range of 90% in patients with ≥3 first trimester or ≥2 second trimester losses without anticoagulant or aspirin treatment.

Current ACCP guidelines suggest that women with recurrent early pregnancy loss (≥3 miscarriages) and women with prior severe or recurrent preeclampsia or IUGR should be screened for APLAs. Notably, screening for inherited thrombophilic traits is not recommended. For women with APLAs and recurrent (≥3) pregnancy losses and no history of venous or arterial thrombosis, antepartum administration of prophylactic or intermediate-dose UFH or prophylactic LMWH combined with aspirin is recommended. For women at high risk of preeclampsia, low-dose aspirin throughout pregnancy may decrease the development of preeclampsia by approximately 50% and is recommended. However, UFH and LMWH are not recommended for prophylaxis in patients with a previous history of preeclampsia. These recommendations are summarized in Table 2-10.

Artificial heart valves

Without anticoagulant therapy, patients with mechanical heart valves have a high risk of arterial thromboembolism. Warfarin appears to be more effective than heparin at preventing valvular thrombosis in these patients. However, debate continues as to whether the benefit to the mother in prevention of valvular thrombosis offsets the risk of

Table 2-10 American College of Chest Physicians guidelines for anticoagulant therapy of thrombophilia-related fetal loss.

Scenario	Recommended diagnostic or therapeutic intervention	Comments
Recurrent early pregnancy loss (3 or more miscarriages), or unexplained late pregnancy loss	Screen for APLA	"Early" is defined differently in various reports, but is generally considered to be first or second trimester with most losses in first
Severe or recurrent preeclampsia or IUGR	Screen for APLA	
APLA positive, recurrent (≥3) pregnancy loss or late pregnancy loss, and no history of venous or arterial thrombosis	Antepartum administration of prophylactic or intermediate-dose UFH or prophylactic LMWH combined with aspirin	
High risk for preeclampsia	Low-dose aspirin throughout pregnancy	
	For women with history of preeclampsia, UFH and LMWH are not recommended as prophylaxis in subsequent pregnancies	

Anticoagulant regimens are defined in the footnote to Table 2-8. Risk factors for preeclampsia are essential hypertension, diabetes, underlying renal disease, high body mass index (≥35 kg/m2), increased age (≥35 years), and prior preeclampsia.
Adapted from Bates SM, Greer IA, Pabinger I, et al. Venous thromboembolism, thrombophilia, antithrombotic therapy, and pregnancy. American College of Chest Physicians Evidence-Based Clinical Practice Guidelines (8th Edition). *Chest*. 2008;133(Suppl 6):844S–886S.
APLA = antiphospholipid antibodies; IUGR = intrauterine growth restriction; LMWH = low molecular weight heparin; UFH = unfractionated heparin.

warfarin-induced embryopathy and neurodevelopmental abnormalities. A systematic review assessed the merits of 3 approaches: (i) the continued use of VKAs throughout pregnancy; (ii) replacement of VKAs with heparin from 6 to 12 weeks; or (iii) use of UFH throughout pregnancy. This analysis concluded that the use of VKAs throughout pregnancy was associated with a 6.4% incidence of warfarin embryopathy; this was eliminated when heparin was substituted at or before 6 weeks. The incidence of fetal wastage and bleeding was similar in all groups. The use of VKAs throughout pregnancy led to the lowest incidence of valve thrombosis and systemic embolism (3.9%); substitution of heparin from weeks 6 to 12 increased this risk to 9.2%. The use of UFH alone throughout pregnancy was associated with a 33.3% risk of thromboembolic complications. This analysis is consistent with other retrospective studies in that VKAs were associated with a lower risk of valve thrombosis and systemic emboli; however, in many such studies, the adequacy of UFH dosing is uncertain. LMWH has also been used in pregnant patients with mechanical heart valves, although valvular thrombosis on this regimen has occurred with concerning frequency. A literature review of pregnant patients treated with LMWH found an incidence of valve thrombosis of 8.64% and an overall thromboembolic rate of 12.35%; however, further analysis of these data suggested that many patients may have received an insufficient dose of LMWH, and in those individuals in whom anti–factor Xa levels were measured, outcomes appeared to be improved. Hence, at present, there are insufficient data to make definitive recommendations concerning the use of VKAs versus heparin in pregnant patients with mechanical heart valves, and additional study is needed. Current guidelines developed by the AACP are presented in Table 2-11 and recommend stringent monitoring of both of these agents, as well as the addition of aspirin in those at highest risk for thromboembolism.

Hematologic malignancies

Malignancies are not commonly diagnosed during pregnancy. However, among the cancers diagnosed during pregnancy, hematologic malignancies are the most common. Because of the typical age of presentation of Hodgkin lymphoma and pregnancy, Hodgkin lymphoma is the most common cancer diagnosed during pregnancy. Among the hematologic malignancies, non-Hodgkin lymphoma and both acute and chronic leukemia are the other hematologic malignancies most commonly diagnosed during pregnancy. Because hematologic malignancies are rare complications of pregnancy, much of the literature on their treatment in pregnancy is anecdotal and not based on carefully constructed studies. Patient outcomes for hematologic malignancies do not appear to be different in pregnant patients, as compared with nongravid patients of the same age and health status. There are, however, some special considerations during delivery for patients with hematologic malignancies. Because there have been reports of Hodgkin lymphoma metastasizing to the placenta, it is advisable to carefully examine the placenta for malignancy after delivery. Similarly, leukemic infiltrates can be found on the maternal side of the placenta, but maternal to fetal transmission of leukemia is extremely rare.

Table 2-11 American College of Chest Physicians guidelines for anticoagulant treatment of pregnant patients with artificial heart valves.

Scenario	Recommended treatment	Comments
Pregnant women with prosthetic heart valves	Adjusted-dose, twice-daily LMWH throughout pregnancy, in doses adjusted to achieve the manufacturer's peak anti-Xa LMWH (preferable) 4 hours after injection	All patients should be assessed for additional risk factors for thromboembolism including valve type, position, and history of thromboembolism, and decision should also be influenced by the patient's preference
	Adjusted-dose UFH throughout pregnancy administered SC every 12 hours in doses adjusted to keep the mid-interval aPTT at least twice control or to attain an anti-Xa heparin level of 0.35–0.70 U/mL, or	
	UFH or LMWH (as above) until the 13th week, with warfarin substitution until close to delivery when UFH or LMWH is resumed	
Pregnant women with prosthetic heart valves at very high risk of thromboembolism in whom concerns exist about the efficacy and safety of UFH or LMWH (eg, older generation prosthesis in the mitral position or history of thromboembolism)	Vitamin K antagonists throughout pregnancy with replacement by UFH or LMWH close to delivery, after thorough discussion of the potential risks and benefits of the approach	This recommendation puts equal weight toward avoiding maternal and fetal complications
Pregnant women with prosthetic valves at high risk of thromboembolism	Addition of low-dose aspirin (75–100 mg/d) to one of the regimens above	

Adapted from Bates SM, Greer IA, Pabinger I, et al. Venous thromboembolism, thrombophilia, antithrombotic therapy, and pregnancy. American College of Chest Physicians Evidence-Based Clinical Practice Guidelines (8th Edition). *Chest.* 2008;133(Suppl 6):844S–886S.
aPTT = activate partial thromboplastin time; LMWH = low molecular weight heparin; SC = subcutaneous; UFH = unfractionated heparin.

The diagnosis and evaluation of a hematologic malignancy in pregnancy has several important considerations. Radiography for diagnosis should be used sparingly in pregnant patients, and whenever possible, abdominal shielding should be used. Because of placental uptake of 18-fluorodeoxyglucose, positron emission tomography scanning is to be avoided in pregnant patients. Magnetic resonance imaging of the chest, abdomen, or pelvis is preferable to CT scanning in pregnant patients, and ultrasonography is also safe. Bone marrow aspiration and biopsy from the posterior iliac crest are also safe in pregnancy.

In deciding treatment options for malignancy in patients during the first trimester of pregnancy, the aggressiveness of the disease, wishes of the patient and family, and potential deleterious effects of therapy on the mother and fetus must all be carefully taken into account. Because some chemotherapeutic agents and radiation have known risks of fetal teratogenicity and miscarriage, therapeutic abortion is often considered in the first trimester for patients with aggressive cancers, especially acute leukemia. Consultation with the hospital ethics committee may be helpful in making the difficult decision of pregnancy termination.

Folate inhibitors such as methotrexate, thalidomide and its derivatives, retinoic acid derivatives, and purine or pyrimidine analogs should not be used during the first trimester of pregnancy due to the increased risk for fetal malformation and death. Cytarabine, typically used to treat acute myeloid leukemia, appears to be particularly teratogenic in the first trimester. Such is also the case for alkylating agents. In pregnant patients with acute lymphoblastic leukemia, L-asparaginase has been found to be particularly prothrombotic and is best avoided. The use of all-*trans* retinoic acid to treat acute promyelocytic leukemia in pregnant patients is controversial. Although there are published case reports documenting all-*trans* retinoic acid efficacy and safety in small numbers of pregnant patients, the data are insufficient in drawing general conclusions about drug safety, especially in the first trimester. Other chemotherapy agents, including interferon alfa, doxorubicin, bleomycin, vinblastine, and dacarbazine, do not appear to be teratogenic in the first trimester. In the second or third trimester, most chemotherapeutic agents can be used to treat aggressive malignancies. When chemotherapy is used to treat malignancy during the second or third trimester, fetal development does not appear to be affected, but fetal and neonatal mortality is increased, as is the incidence of IUGR and low birth weights. Neutropenia can be seen in newborns whose mothers have been exposed to cytotoxic chemotherapy immediately before delivery.

There have been reports of successful pregnancies occurring in patients with chronic myeloid leukemia treated with newer small-molecule inhibitors such as imatinib; however, imatinib is teratogenic in animals and therefore is best avoided as initial treatment of chronic myeloid leukemia in pregnancy. Management of patients who become pregnant while on imatinib is controversial. The risk of fetal malformation must be carefully weighed against the risk of imatinib cessation. Newer tyrosine kinase inhibitors such as dasatinib have not been evaluated in pregnant patients.

When treating lymphoma, radiation therapy is contraindicated in the first trimester of pregnancy, and proper shielding of the developing fetus must be performed whenever possible in the latter 2 trimesters.

Long-term follow-up studies suggest that children born of mothers with a previous hematologic malignancy during pregnancy do not appear to be at increased risk for fetal malformations or for the development of cancers later in life.

Key points

- Iron deficiency is the most common cause of anemia during pregnancy, and routine iron supplementation should be offered. In pregnant patients with iron deficiency who do not tolerate oral iron, iron sucrose is the preferred parenteral agent.
- Thrombocytopenia in pregnant patients may result from a number of different etiologies. The most common cause is incidental thrombocytopenia of pregnancy, in which the platelet count usually does not decrease to <70,000/ L. This disorder is not associated with increased maternal or fetal morbidity.
- ITP is the most common cause of isolated thrombocytopenia during pregnancy.
- TTP-HUS, preeclampsia, and HELLP may be difficult to distinguish from one another in some patients. If TTP-HUS is suspected, a trial of plasma exchange should be initiated.
- Levels of vWF and FVIII generally increase during normal pregnancy in patients with type 1 vWD, the most common subtype. Levels should be monitored throughout pregnancy and, in particular, between weeks 32 and 34 to confirm the expected increase. However, levels of vWF may decrease precipitously after delivery in some patients, and supplementation with vWF/FVIII-containing products may be required.
- Thrombophilia is associated with an increased risk of thrombosis during pregnancy and particularly in the puerperium. The relative risks for heterozygous thrombophilic conditions are relatively small, but those for homozygous or doubly heterozygous conditions are substantial. Guidelines are available (Table 2-9) for management of pregnant individuals with thrombophilia.

Key points (continued)

- Thrombophilia is probably associated with a small but significant increased incidence of fetal loss, as well as with pregnancy complications. This association is strongest with APLAs and less so with inherited thrombophilias. Current guidelines recommend screening appropriate patients for APLAs, but not for inherited thrombophilias. Likewise, treatment of patients with APLAs and an appropriate clinical history is recommended.
- VKAs are associated with embryopathy when administered between weeks 6 and 12 of pregnancy. Use of these agents during the second and third trimester may also be associated with neurodevelopmental abnormalities. Warfarin is not present in high concentrations in breast milk, and mothers on warfarin may breast feed safely.
- The optimal anticoagulation regimen for pregnant patients with artificial heart valves is uncertain, but guidelines favor the use of adjusted-dose LMWH, with close monitoring.
- Although malignancies are uncommonly diagnosed during pregnancy, Hodgkin lymphoma is the most common.
- Most chemotherapeutic agents can be used safely in the latter 2 trimesters of pregnancy. Folate antagonists, purine and pyrimidine analogs, L-asparaginase, and alkylating agents are to be avoided during the first trimester of pregnancy.

Selected outpatient hematology topics

Mild thrombocytopenia

Although the definition of "mild" is arbitrary, patients with platelet counts in the range of 80,000/μL to 120,000/μL are commonly referred for consultation. Mild thrombocytopenia may result from less severe presentations of many of the same disorders that cause more pronounced thrombocytopenia, as well as several additional disorders.

The differential diagnosis of mild thrombocytopenia may be narrowed by determining whether it is new in onset or chronic; thus, the results of prior blood counts from as far in the past as possible should be vigorously sought. New-onset thrombocytopenia generally results from development of a new disease process or the institution of a new drug, with thrombocytopenia as either a primary (eg, ITP) or secondary (eg, HIV or other infectious process, bone marrow infiltration, myelodysplasia) manifestation. Chronic thrombocytopenia may also suggest the possibility of an inherited process (eg, variant of an *MYH9*-related disorder). Cyclic thrombocytopenia must also be considered in a patient in whom the platelet count varies over time, and splenomegaly should be assessed with close physical examination and/or ultrasound.

Mild thrombocytopenia that is not clinically important in terms of increasing bleeding risk may yet be significant as a marker of an underlying disorder. Thus, the patient should be questioned carefully for signs or symptoms of infection, autoimmune disease, or malignancy, and the physical examination should focus on the assessment of lymphadenopathy, hepatosplenomegaly, skin rashes, and musculoskeletal abnormalities.

Drug-induced thrombocytopenia has been discussed earlier in reference to acutely ill patients but should be considered in patients with mild thrombocytopenia as well. Although drugs such as sulfa-containing antibiotics often cause severe thrombocytopenia, others (for example, psychotropic agents) may cause a number of blood dyscrasias, including mild thrombocytopenia. A listing of drugs associated with thrombocytopenia and the strength of the apparent association may be found at Platelets on the Web (http://www.ouhsc.edu/platelets/index.html). However, when assessing a patient, it is often reasonable to assume that most drugs may cause thrombocytopenia; even those such as H2 blockers, which do so only rarely, are so commonly used that their overall contribution to cases of isolated thrombocytopenia may be substantial. Over-the-counter medications, in particular herbal supplements, should also be considered.

As with any hematologic disorder, examination of the peripheral blood film is an essential part of the evaluation. Clumped platelets may suggest pseudothrombocytopenia; if this is observed, the platelet count should be repeated in a citrated tube. Large platelets may be consistent with an MYH9-related disorder, such as the May-Hegglin anomaly; neutrophil inclusions would support this diagnosis. Likewise, small platelets may suggest an inherited disorder such as the Wiskott-Aldrich syndrome. Hypersegmented neutrophils and macrocytosis may suggest vitamin B_{12} deficiency. Lymphocytosis may suggest underlying chronic lymphocytic leukemia, and circulating plasma cells may be consistent with myeloma. Dysmorphic red blood cells, hypogranulated neutrophils, or Pelger-Huët cells may suggest underlying myelodysplasia, which may occasionally present with isolated thrombocytopenia.

There are no guidelines as to when, or whether, the bone marrow should be examined. Although the incidence of primary marrow disorders such as myelodysplastic syndromes increases with age, recent epidemiologic studies demonstrate that ITP is also common in elderly patients. If thrombocytopenia is isolated and there are no other abnormalities on the peripheral blood film or detected on the physical examination, bone marrow examination is not immediately necessary, and the patient may be followed with serial platelet counts. Should unexplained symptoms arise, other hematologic abnormalities appear, or the thrombocytopenia worsen, further evaluation should be considered.

In a recent study, the outcomes of 191 otherwise healthy individuals with incidentally discovered borderline thrombocytopenia (platelet count of 100,000-150,000/μL) that had been stable for 6 months were determined. With a median observation time of 64 months, 64% of the cases of thrombocytopenia either resolved spontaneously or persisted with no other disorders becoming apparent. The most common pathologic event developing during follow-up was autoimmune disease. The 10-year probability of developing ITP was 6.9%, and the 10-year probability of developing autoimmune diseases other than ITP was 12.0%.

Leukocytosis

Patients with unexplained leukocytosis are frequently referred to hematologists due to concern about a potential underlying hematologic malignancy. As with any other CBC abnormality, a careful review of the peripheral blood smear is essential in establishing the final diagnosis. Although most patients with leukocytosis are referred because of concern for leukemia, most patients with unexplained leukocytosis do not have a hematologic malignancy. Some causes of unexplained leukocytosis may be quite pedestrian such as benign neutrophilia observed in cigarette smokers.

In addition to examining the peripheral smear, a careful history and physical examination are also important. For example, a history of unexplained fever or chills with a new heart murmur may suggest an underlying infection such as bacterial endocarditis. A history of diarrhea may suggest occult infection with *Clostridium difficile*. A history of lithium use may indicate a drug-induced leukocytosis. As with a careful history, examination of the skin, lymph nodes, liver, and spleen size is also important in evaluating patients with leukocytosis. For example, patients with exudative pharyngitis, splenomegaly, and lymphocytosis may have infectious mononucleosis.

In addition to examining the peripheral smear, flow cytometry and cytogenetics may be helpful in detecting an abnormal leukocyte clone. A bone marrow aspiration and biopsy can be useful in evaluating leukocyte precursors if analysis of a specific molecular marker is necessary. Such might be the case when assaying for the PDGFR-α/FIP1-L1 transcript in a patient with unexplained eosinophilia.

Table 2-12 lists specific etiologic considerations in patients with leukocytosis.

Leukopenia

Leukopenia is defined in patients having a WBC count <2 standard deviations below the mean. In evaluating a patient with leukopenia, it is important to check previous CBCs to establish changes in the WBC count over time. Importantly, some racial groups such as Africans, African Americans, and Yemenite Jews have lower leukocyte counts than those typically reported as "normal" by most laboratories. Patients

Table 2-12 Hematology consultation for leukocytosis: etiologic considerations.

Neutrophilia	Monocytosis	Eosinophilia	Lymphocytosis
Eclampsia	Pregnancy	Allergic rhinitis	Mononucleosis syndrome
Thyrotoxicosis	Tuberculosis	Asthma	Epstein-Barr virus
Hypercortisolism	Syphilis	Tissue-invasive parasite	Cytomegalovirus
Crohn disease	Endocarditis	Bronchopulmonary aspergillosis	Primary HIV
Ulcerative colitis	Sarcoidosis	Coccidioidal infection	Viral illness
Inflammatory/rheumatologic disease	Systemic lupus erythematosus	HIV	Pertussis
Sweet's syndrome	Asplenia	Immunodeficiency	*Bartonella henselae* (cat scratch disease)
Granulomatous infections	Corticosteroids	Vasculitides	Toxoplasmosis
Bronchiectasis		Drug reaction	Babesiosis
Occult malignancy		Adrenal insufficiency	Drug reaction
Trauma/burn		Occult malignancy	Reactive large granular lymphocytosis
Severe stress		Pulmonary syndromes	
Panic		Gastrointestinal syndromes	
Asplenia		Hypereosinophilic syndrome	
Cigarette smoking			
Tuberculosis			
Chronic hepatitis			
Hereditary neutrophilia			
Corticosteroids			
β-agonists			
Lithium			

HIV = human immunodeficiency virus.

with cyclic neutropenia, due to disorders with neutrophil elastase, typically have a 21-day periodicity associated with their neutropenia. Leukopenia can be further defined by the WBC population or populations specifically affected. Leukopenia results from either decreased marrow production of leukocytes or from decreased circulation times of leukocytes due to destruction, margination, or sequestration. A list of causes of acquired leukopenias that affect neutrophils, lymphocytes, or both is included in Table 2-13.

In evaluating patients with unexplained leukopenia, it is important to take a careful medication history because many drugs, including antibiotics, anti-inflammatory drugs, and anticonvulsants, can cause leukopenia. Drug-induced leukopenia can be dose related, as is the case with phenothiazines, or can be immunologic. A wide variety of infectious disorders can also cause leukopenia, including hepatitis, mononucleosis, HIV, typhoid, and malaria.

Patients with leukopenia may be asymptomatic and may not require treatment. Patients who are profoundly leukopenic may complain of fever, mouth sores, or myalgias. Evaluation of patients with leukopenia includes a careful physical examination including examination of the mucous membranes and skin. The peripheral smear should be evaluated for the presence of blasts (acute leukemia) or Pelger-Huët cells

Table 2-13 Causes of acquired leukopenia.

Autoimmune
Marrow aplasia
Thymoma
Idiopathic
Hematologic malignancy
Infections
Sepsis
Viral (HIV, CMV, EBV, hepatitis A, B, C, influenza, parvovirus, others)
Bacterial (tuberculosis, tularemia, *Brucella*, typhoid)
Rickettsial (Rocky Mountain spotted fever, ehrlichiosis)
Fungal (histoplasmosis)
Parasitic (malaria, leishmaniasis)
Drug and chemical induced (corticosteroids, antilymphocyte globulin, carbamazepine, sulfonylureas, others)
Immunodeficiency
Nutritional
Iatrogenic
Autoimmune conditions (systemic lupus erythematosus, rheumatoid arthritis)
Acute respiratory distress syndrome
Increased neutrophil margination (hemodialysis)

CMV = cytomegalovirus; EBV = Ebstein-Barr virus; HIV = human immunodeficiency virus.

(myelodysplasia). Evaluation of the bone marrow with flow cytometry may also be helpful to look for clonal disorders. A rheumatologic evaluation including antinuclear antibody (ANA) and rheumatoid factor may help to diagnose a previously undetected collagen vascular disorder. Splenomegaly in this setting might suggest Felty syndrome, although idiopathic causes of splenomegaly may also lead to leukopenia.

Treatment of leukopenia depends on the specific etiology. Importantly, treatment with colony-stimulating factors should not be used without a definitive diagnosis requiring such intervention.

Atypical lymphoproliferative processes
Lymphadenopathy

The peak mass of lymphoid tissue occurs in adolescence. In adults, lymph nodes are normally not palpable except for the inguinal region where small nodes up to 1.5 cm are not uncommon. Although superficial enlarged nodes can be palpated, deeper nodes require imaging with CT, positron emission tomography, or magnetic resonance imaging for detection. Lymph node enlargement can be seen with a variety of disorders including infections, malignancy, and collagen vascular disorders (Table 2-14). In the primary care setting, >98% of enlarged lymph nodes are nonmalignant in etiology, whereas 50% of patients referred to a specialist for lymphadenopathy are found to have malignant disease. On physical examination, the size, location, consistency, and presence of pain in nodes is helpful in establishing a differential diagnosis. Additional laboratory testing including ANA, monospot, HIV testing, and a CBC may be helpful in evaluating patients with enlarged nodes. Of course, biopsy is typically required to determine the precise etiology of lymphadenopathy. If a hematologic malignancy is suspected, every attempt should be made to perform an excisional biopsy because fine-needle biopsy is typically inaccurate in diagnosing lymphoma. Lymph node biopsy specimens are typically sent for flow cytometry, cytogenetics, and immunohistochemistry.

Persistent polyclonal lymphocytosis

Persistent polyclonal lymphocytosis is an unusual disorder of unclear etiology characterized by stable polyclonal expansion of lymphocytes, elevated polyclonal immunoglobulin (Ig) M, predilection for woman, and the presence of binucleated lymphocytes on the peripheral smear. Although associated with cigarette smoking, lymphocytosis persists despite smoking cessation. The disorder has been associated with the +i(3q) chromosomal abnormality and with somatic mutations in the *IgV* gene. The disorder follows a benign course, with progression to malignancy being extremely rare.

Table 2-14 Causes of persistent unexplained lymphadenopathy.

Localized	Generalized
Bacterial infection	Mononucleosis syndrome
Fungal infection	Epstein-Barr virus
Tuberculosis	Cytomegalovirus
Other mycobacterial infections	Primary HIV
Bartonella henselae (cat scratch disease)	Chronic HIV
	Other viral infections
Sarcoidosis	Leptospirosis
Langerhans cell histiocytosis	Tularemia
Inflammatory pseudotumor	Miliary tuberculosis
Progressive transformation of germinal centers	Brucellosis
	Lyme disease
Malignancy (eg, NHL, HD, CLL, metastatic carcinoma)	Secondary syphilis
	Toxoplasmosis
	Histoplasmosis
	Systemic lupus erythematosus
	Rheumatoid arthritis
	Still disease
	Rosai-Dorfman disease
	Sarcoidosis
	Langerhans cell histiocytosis
	Phenytoin
	Drug-induced serum sickness
	Castleman disease
	Kikuchi disease
	Kawasaki disease
	Angioimmunoblastic lymphadenopathy
	Atypical lymphoproliferative process
	Hemophagocytic lymphohistiocytosis
	Malignancy (eg, indolent NHL, CLL)

CLL = chronic lymphocytic leukemia; HD = Hodgkin disease; HIV = human immunodeficiency virus; NHL = non-Hodgkin lymphoma.

Castleman disease

Castleman disease is a rare disorder characterized by adenopathy that is typically unicentric, although 10% of patients can have multicentric disease. Unicentric Castleman disease can be of either the hyaline vascular variant, characterized by shrunken germinal centers, increased vascularity, and expansion of the mantle zone with an "onion skin" pattern, or a plasmacytoid variant, which is more typically found in multicentric disease. The plasmablastic variant has also been described in aggressive multifocal disease. Castleman disease is a polyclonal expansion of plasma cells and B and T lymphocytes, perhaps due to elevation in interleukin 6 (IL-6) levels. Human herpes virus 8 (HHV8), which encodes a viral IL-6 protein, has been implicated in multicentric disease, especially in patients with the HIV virus, in whom it is almost always found. Unicentric disease of the hyaline vascular variant is typically treated with radiation therapy or local resection, with recurrence being uncommon. Mixed histology localized disease, plasmacytoid variants, and multicentric disease can present with B-symptoms, organomegaly, and cytopenias, as with lymphoma. These subtypes may also progress to lymphoma. Treatment for aggressive Castleman disease is similar to treatment for lymphoma. Anti–IL-6 therapy is currently under investigation. Antivirals such as ganciclovir have been investigated in HIV-positive patients with HHV8-positive disease.

Splenomegaly

The typical spleen weighs approximately 150 g and is not palpable on physical examination. Splenic enlargement is frequently not appreciated on physical examination unless the spleen size is increased by 40%. Spleen size is typically quantified by measuring the number of centimeters an enlarged spleen is identified below the costal margin. Splenic enlargement is best appreciated on physical examination when there is percussive dullness in Traube's semilunar triangle bordered by the left sternal border, the costal margin, and lower border of the 9th rib. Ultrasonography can accurately determine the precise size of an enlarged spleen. Other imaging modalities such as CT or magnetic resonance imaging can be useful in assessing architectural changes in the spleen due to infarction, infection, infiltration, or tumor. An enlarged spleen can weigh as much as several kilograms. Splenomegaly most typically is seen in patients with cirrhosis when increased portal pressure causes venous engorgement and disrupts the normal splenic architecture. Such is also the case with splenic vein thrombosis. Splenomegaly can also occur when the spleen is involved by a neoplastic process such as lymphoma. Infiltrative disorders such as Gaucher disease can also lead to splenomegaly. Table 2-15 lists the differential diagnosis of splenomegaly.

In evaluating patients with splenomegaly, it is important to review the CBC because splenomegaly can frequently lead to cytopenias from splenic sequestration. Additionally, a peripheral smear should be reviewed to check for the presence of spherocytes and to review the WBC morphology.

Massive splenomegaly may require splenectomy due to frequent pain from infarction or due to recalcitrant cytopenias. Splenectomy may also be indicated for patients with hereditary spherocytosis, ITP, or warm antibody–mediated hemolytic anemia. Because of the risk of infection with encapsulated organisms, patients undergoing splenectomy should be vaccinated for *Pneumococcus*, *Haemophilus*, and *Neisseria meningitides*, and patients who have undergone

Table 2-15 Causes of splenomegaly.

Congestive diseases
Liver disease
   Cirrhosis*
   Veno-occlusive disease
   Congenital hepatic fibrosis
Portal vein obstruction
Splenic vein obstruction*
Hepatic vein occlusion (Budd-Chiari syndrome)
Congestive heart failure*
Malignancy
Leukemia/lymphoma*
Chronic idiopathic myelofibrosis
Polycythemia vera
Essential thrombocythemia
Myeloid metaplasia
Other hematologic disease
Hemolytic anemia
Infection
Infectious mononucleosis*
Human immunodeficiency virus infection*
Cytomegalovirus*
Toxoplasmosis
Viral hepatitis
Salmonellosis
Relapsing fever
Tularemia
Syphilis
Malaria
Endocarditis*
Tuberculosis
Schistosomiasis
Storage diseases
Gaucher disease
Niemann-Pick disease
Inflammatory diseases
Felty syndrome (rheumatoid arthritis)
Systemic lupus erythematosus
Rheumatic fever
Serum sickness
Sarcoidosis
Miscellaneous
Tropical splenomegaly
Primary splenic hyperplasia
Metastatic cancer

* Diagnoses marked with an asterisk are the most common causes of splenomegaly.

splenectomy should carry an antibiotic prescription with them afterward with instructions to initiate treatment if they become febrile and cannot seek medical attention promptly. Splenectomy may be associated with a long-term increased risk of vascular complications and pulmonary hypertension, particularly when performed for treatment of disease with increased red blood cell turnover. Splenic radiation, although popular in the past, appears to have limited utility in reducing the effects of hypersplenism.

> **Key points**
> - Persistent polyclonal lymphocytosis is an unusual disorder that follows a benign course.
> - Castleman disease is associated with elevated levels of IL-6.

Consultation in pediatric patients

Many of the consultative hematology issues discussed earlier also apply to pediatric patients, particularly with respect to perioperative and intensive care questions. However, there are certain situations in which pediatric patients differ greatly from adults. Most important, and most likely to come to the attention of adult hematologists outside of a pediatric hospital setting, are the special hematologic considerations of the newborn. Developmental issues include the transition of fetal to adult red blood cell production, with associated differences in "normal" values for red blood cells. Additionally, acute maturation is required of the liver synthetic function, and normal values for coagulation parameters change rapidly during this period. Finally, alloimmune problems may result from antigenic differences between mother and infant. Later in childhood, anemia is a common problem with specific age-related considerations, and neutropenia is more common and often transient in children compared with adults. Fortunately for children, most cases of ITP in childhood resolve within 6 months and often do not require treatment. These key issues are discussed in this section, and additional annotated references are provided in the bibliography at the end of the chapter.

Anemia in the newborn

Figure 2-1 illustrates the diagnostic approach to anemia in the newborn. Newborns are relatively polycythemic and macrocytic at birth (Table 2-16), reflecting the hypoxic intrauterine environment and the characteristics of fetal red blood cell production. Mean hemoglobin and hematocrit on day 1 of life for a term newborn are 19.0 ± 2.2 g/dL and $61\% \pm 7.4\%$, respectively, with a mean reticulocyte count of $3.2\% \pm$

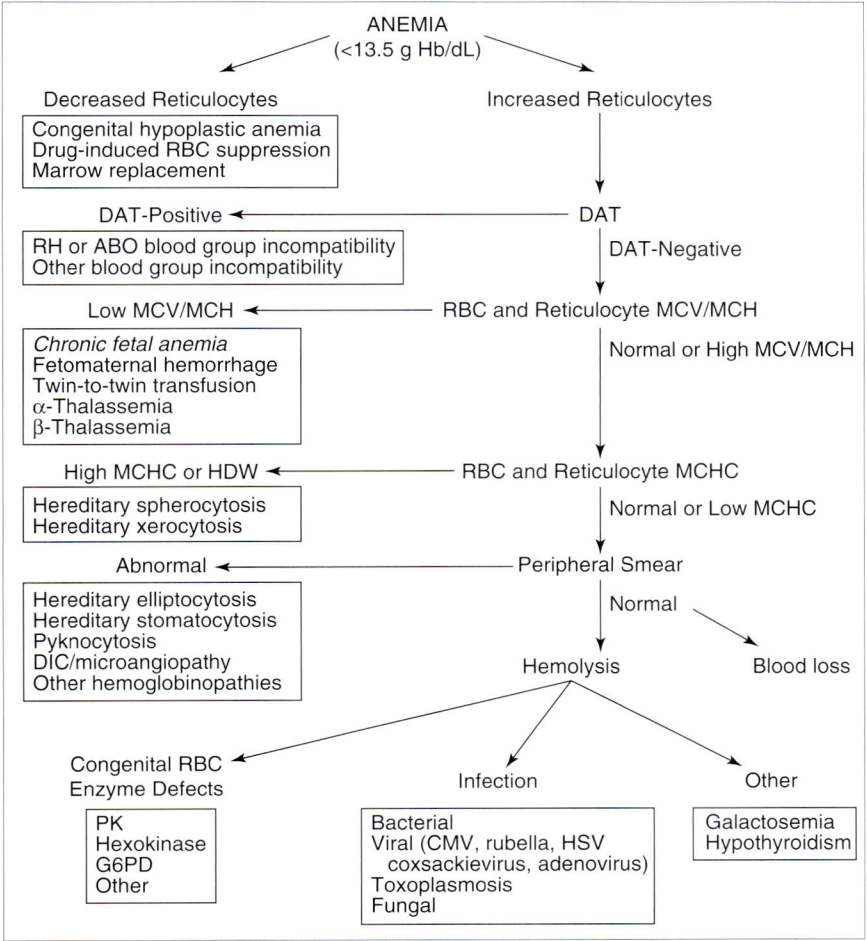

Figure 2-1 Diagnostic approach to anemia in the newborn. CMV = cytomegalovirus; DAT = direct antiglobulin test; DIC = disseminated intravascular coagulation; G6PD = glucose-6-phosphate dehydrogenase; HDW = hemoglobin distribution width; HSV = herpes simplex virus; MCHC = mean corpuscular hemoglobin concentration; MCV/MCH = mean corpuscular volume/mean corpuscular hemoglobin; PK = pyruvate kinase. From Brugnara C, Platt OS. The neonatal erythrocyte and its disorders. In: Nathan DG, Orkin SH, Ginsburg D, Look AT, eds. *Nathan and Oski's Hematology of Infancy and Childhood*. 6th ed. Philadelphia, PA: WB Saunders; 2003:19–55.

Table 2-16 Normal hematologic values for newborns.

Red blood cell parameter	Term newborn day 1 ± SD*	
Hb (g/dL)	19.0 ± 2.2	
Hct (%)	61 ± 7.4	
MCV (fL)	119 ± 9.4	
Reticulocytes (%)	3.2 ± 1.4	
Coagulation/inhibitor parameter	**Healthy term newborn cord blood**[†]	**Healthy preterm (30–38 weeks) cord blood**[†]
PT (seconds)	16.7 (12–23.5)	22.6 (16–30)
INR	1.7 (0.9–2.7)	3.0 (1.5–5.0)
aPTT (seconds)	44.3 (35–52)	104.8 (76–128)
Fibrinogen (von Clauss; g/L)	1.68 (0.95–2.45)	1.35 (1.25–1.65)
Factor II activity (%)	43.5 (27–64)	27.9 (15–50)
Factor V activity (%)	89.9 (50–140)	48.9 (23–70)
Factor VII activity (%)	52.5 (28–78)	45.9 (31–62)
Factor VIII activity (%)	94.3 (38–150)	50 (27–78)
Factor IX activity (%)	31.8 (15–50)	12.3 (5–24)
Factor X activity (%)	39.6 (21–65)	28 (16–36)
Factor XI activity (%)	37.2 (13–62)	14.8 (6–26)
Factor XII activity (%)	69.8 (25–105)	25.8 (11–50)
Antithrombin III activity (%)	59.4 (42–80)	37.1 (24–55)
Protein C activity (%)	28.2 (14–42)	14.1 (8–18)
Protein C antigen (%)	32.5 (21–47)	15.9 (8–30)
Total protein S (%)	38.5 (22–55)	21.0 (15–30)
Free protein S (%)	49.3 (33–67)	27.1 (18–40)

* From Matoth Y, Zaizov R, Varsano I. Postnatal changes in some red cell parameters. *Acta Paediatr Scand*. 1971;60:317–323.
[†] Values are means, followed by lower and upper boundaries including 95% of population. From Reverdiau-Moalic P, Delahousse B, Body G, et al. Evaluation of blood coagulation activators and inhibitors in the healthy human fetus. *Blood*. 1996;88;900–906.
aPTT = activated partial thromboplastin time; Hb = hemoglobin; Hct = hematocrit; INR = international normalized ratio; MCV = mean corpuscular volume; PT = prothrombin time.

1.4%. Thus, what is a normal hematocrit during much of childhood represents anemia in the newborn. Red blood cell production decreases shortly after birth with the abrupt decrease in erythropoietin level, such that the reticulocyte count reaches 0.5% by day 7, leading to a physiologic nadir of hemoglobin (10.7 ± 0.9 g/dL) at approximately 7 to 9 weeks of age.

The primary causes of anemia in the newborn fall into the same broad categories as in adults: blood loss, increased destruction, or decreased production. However, the common etiologies differ. Blood loss in the newborn can be the result of an obstetrical accident such as placenta previa or abruption, rupture of an abnormal umbilical cord or anomalous placental vessels, an acute or chronic fetal–maternal hemorrhage, or internal hemorrhage. In all cases but chronic fetal–maternal hemorrhage, depending on the extent of blood loss, the infant may have signs and symptoms of circulatory shock. These include pallor, tachycardia and tachypnea, hypotension, weak or absent pulses, and acidosis. Acutely, the hemoglobin may be normal or near normal, and the red blood cells will demonstrate normal newborn macrocytosis. These infants require emergency resuscitation with fluids and usually packed red blood cells. In the setting of chronic blood loss, the infant may be well compensated but pale. Congestive heart failure and hepatomegaly may be present in severe cases. The hemoglobin concentration will be low, and red blood cells will be relatively microcytic (compared with normal newborn macrocytes) due to iron deficiency. If marginally compensated, these infants may require transfusion with packed red blood cells. Fetal–maternal hemorrhage can be confirmed, and the quantity of blood loss estimated, by the Kleihauer-Betke technique on maternal blood, in which fetal cells are resistant to elution of hemoglobin in an acid medium.

An uncommon, and usually obvious, source of blood loss is the twin–twin transfusion syndrome. Estimates of frequency of this syndrome, defined as a ±5 g/dL difference in hemoglobin between twins, have ranged from 6% to 33% of pregnancies with a monochorial placenta (which represent ~70% of monozygotic twin pregnancies). Hemorrhage can be acute or chronic, with presentations varying as described previously; the potential for polycythemia with its complications must be remembered for the reciprocal twin. Although iron deficiency is extremely uncommon in the newborn, who acts as an effective and selfish "parasite" of the mother's iron supply, it is important to recognize that the majority of the newborn's total body iron at birth resides in circulating red blood cells. Thus, although an infant may be well compensated with a hematocrit in the 30% to 40% range, his or her total-body iron stores are much lower than normal. Such an infant will be at high risk of developing iron deficiency over the first several months of growth unless supplemental iron is provided.

In all cases of significant anemia from blood loss, such as those described previously, supplemental oral iron should be provided for the first several months of life. Additionally, infants born prematurely will have lower total-body iron stores than normal and should be supplemented with oral iron.

Hemolytic anemia in the newborn may be the result of inherited abnormalities of red blood cell structure or function, immune-mediated destruction by passively transferred maternal IgG, or processes external to the red blood cells, such as infection, DIC, or severe acidosis. For infants with shortened red blood cell life span but without severe anemia, the only clinical finding may be exaggerated neonatal jaundice. Although the differential diagnosis is long, it may be shortened by a careful family history (focusing in particular on other family members with neonatal jaundice, anemia, need for transfusion, splenectomy, and early gallstone formation), examination of the infant for signs of contributing illnesses, and careful review of the peripheral smear and reticulocyte count. Maternal and infant blood type and Rh should be performed along with a direct antiglobulin test (DAT) in the infant. Rh disease is now rare in developed countries, given the widespread use of prenatal screening and Rh-immune globulin administration to Rh-negative women. ABO incompatibility is most common in the setting of an A infant and O mother, given that maternal isohemagglutinin titers are usually higher for A than for B and that the density of A antigen expression on neonatal red blood cells is usually higher than that of B antigen. Because A antigen density may be low enough that the "cross-linking" required for a positive DAT may not occur, ABO incompatibility should still be suspected despite a negative DAT if mother is O and infant is A, a hemolytic anemia is present, and peripheral smear is either normal or positive for a few spherocytes. Importantly, hereditary spherocytosis may present in the neonatal period with similar clinical and laboratory features; therefore, follow-up hemoglobin, reticulocyte counts, and additional studies may be required to differentiate between these 2 processes. Maternal antibodies to red blood cell antigens other than A and B are uncommon but may cause severe disease. In particular, anti-Kell antibodies may produce severe disease in up to 40% to 50% of affected fetuses.

Red blood cell enzyme deficiencies may also cause hemolysis and jaundice in the newborn. Glucose-6-phosphate dehydrogenase (G6PD) deficiency is a relatively common cause of neonatal jaundice. Although not all infants with G6PD deficiency develop jaundice, those who do often have more jaundice than anemia. Isolated anemia with an inappropriately low reticulocyte count is suggestive of impaired red blood cell production and should raise the possibility of Diamond-Blackfan anemia (DBA). Up to a quarter of patients with DBA are anemic at birth, including hemoglobin values <10 g/dL; 5% to 10% of such infants are small for gestational age, and 25% have at least one congenital anomaly. The most common anomalies are abnormalities of the head, face, or palate, and some infants have limb anomalies including triphalangeal or other thumb defects, radial anomalies, and kidney abnormalities. The bone marrow in affected infants is normocellular with a striking paucity of erythroid precursors. Approximately 25% of DBA patients have heterozygous mutations in the ribosomal protein S19 (*RPS19*) gene, and mutations in at least 5 other ribosomal protein genes have now been identified, including *RPS17*, *RPS24*, *RPL5*, *RPL11*, and *RPL35A*. DBA can be differentiated from Fanconi anemia by the fact that only children with Fanconi anemia will have abnormal chromosomal breakage following culture of their lymphocytes with diepoxybutane or mitomycin C. Previous treatment approaches, centered on the use of prednisone shortly after diagnosis, have recently given way to support with transfusion for the first year of life to minimize the adverse effects of prednisone on growth and potential suppression of the infant's response to immunizations. A trial of prednisone can be administered near the patient's first birthday.

Neutropenia in the newborn

Neutropenia is discussed in more detail in Chapter 13. However, the pediatric hematology consultant must consider several additional factors in evaluating infants with neutropenia. The first is that the neonatal marrow capacity is limited, and transient neutropenia is relatively common in sick neonates, in whom neutrophil consumption in response to sepsis, respiratory distress, or other acute processes may exceed production capacity. In addition, transient and usually benign neutropenia is often seen in infants of mothers whose pregnancies are complicated by pregnancy-induced hypertension (PIH) and usually resolves spontaneously in 3 to 5 days.

Less commonly, neonatal alloimmune neutropenia (NAIN) results from the transplacental passage of maternal antibodies reactive with paternal antigens on the infant's neutrophils and is therefore the neutrophil equivalent of Rh disease. The resulting neutropenia can be profound, with the potential for sepsis, omphalitis, cellulitis, and other serious infections. Antibiotics are indicated in cases of severe neutropenia, and granulocyte colony-stimulating factor (5 μg/kg/dose) has resulted in rapid improvement in neutrophil counts in affected infants. The diagnosis of NAIN can generally be made by confirming antigenic differences between maternal and paternal neutrophils, most commonly the NA1 and NA2 alleles of the Fcγ receptor IIIb, and by demonstrating maternal antibodies that bind to paternal neutrophils. NAIN typically resolves in weeks to months. In contrast, autoimmune neutropenia, in which the child develops autoantibodies against neutrophil antigens, is usually diagnosed between 3 and 30 months of age and typically runs a benign course. Treatment is not usually indicated for neutropenia alone, but granulocyte colony-stimulating factor can be given if the child develops severe or recurrent infections. Often, dosing 2 to 3 days a week is adequate to prevent infection. The above situations must be differentiated from the relatively rare inherited causes of neutropenia, including severe congenital neutropenia or Kostmann disease, Shwachman-Diamond syndrome, cyclic neutropenia, glycogen storage disease Ib, Barth syndrome, and neutropenia associated with immunodeficiency syndromes.

Thrombocytopenia in the newborn

Thrombocytopenia is a fairly common problem in the newborn and presents important diagnostic and therapeutic challenges. As in the case of transient neutropenia, limited capacity of the neonatal marrow to increase platelet production in the face of rapid consumption can result in thrombocytopenia in the sick newborn, and therefore, a critical first question is whether the child is "well" or "ill." For example, infants who have suffered perinatal asphyxia, respiratory distress, sepsis, polycythemia, necrotizing enterocolitis, other acute processes, or intrauterine viral infections may have thrombocytopenia on a secondary basis. The timing of thrombocytopenia onset may also be helpful in discriminating between its potential causes, with onset in the fetal/newborn period characteristic of congenital disease, aneuploidy, congenital infections, and alloimmune and autoimmune thrombocytopenias, whereas later onset is typical for acquired disorders such as sepsis, thrombosis, DIC, growing hemangiomas, or necrotizing enterocolitis. It should be noted that, although rare, HIT has been diagnosed in the neonate.

Thrombocytopenia is seen in up to half of newborns admitted to a neonatal ICU, and up to a fifth of such infants may develop severe thrombocytopenia. Such infants can be supported with platelet transfusion as clinically indicated. In the newborn, platelet transfusion is usually recommended for platelet counts $<30 \times 10^9/L$ and for counts between 30 and $49 \times 10^9/L$ for infants <1 week of age with a birth weight of <1000 g or who are clinically unstable and have had previous major bleeding or a coexistent coagulopathy.

Maternal autoimmune disorders, including systemic lupus erythematosus and ITP, can impact the infant's platelet count by transplacental transmission of IgG reactive with common antigens on the infant's platelets. In addition, PIH can be associated with transient thrombocytopenia in the newborn. If the mother is well and has a normal platelet count, neonatal alloimmune thrombocytopenia (NAIT) should be suspected. This process results from the transplacental passage of maternal antibody reactive with paternal-derived antigens expressed by infant platelets, analogous to Rh disease. However, unlike Rh disease, where it is uncommon for first pregnancies to be affected, the smaller size of the platelet increases the frequency of entry into maternal circulation; thus, first pregnancies can result in medically significant maternal antibody production. The majority of clinical cases result from maternal antibody against human platelet antigen (HPA)-1a (~80%) and HPA-5b (10% to 15%). There is a potential for NAIT if platelet antigen typing reveals antigens that are present in the father and absent in the mother. Diagnosis is confirmed if antibodies against paternal platelets are identified in the mother, although severe thrombocytopenia in a healthy neonate born to a healthy mother should be presumed to be due to NAIT. It is important to confirm the diagnosis of NAIT for several reasons. First, optimal treatment of the infant with NAIT and severe thrombocytopenia includes transfusion of HPA-compatible platelets, if available. If the mother's clinical condition allows, maternal platelets can be collected, washed (to avoid any additional passive transmission of antibody), and used as an HPA-compatible transfusion product. Many blood banks have a cohort of HPA-1a–negative platelet donors who can be called in as needed. In a child with severe thrombocytopenia or bleeding symptoms, however, treatment should not be delayed while awaiting confirmation of the diagnosis or procurement of an HPA-compatible product, and random donor platelets should be given in the interim. Studies have demonstrated at least transient increments in the infant's platelet counts following transfusion of HPA-incompatible products. IVIg (0.5 g/kg/d for 2 days) and methylprednisone may also decrease the rate of platelet destruction and can be used as adjunctive therapy. An additional reason to confirm the diagnosis of NAIT is because of the significant implications for subsequent pregnancies. The risk of severe thrombocytopenia is higher with subsequent pregnancies and can occur as early as the second trimester. Risk stratification takes into account a history of intracranial hemorrhage occurring before or after birth and a fetal platelet count (if obtained) <20,000/μL in a prior pregnancy. Prenatal management of such pregnancies is beyond the scope of this chapter, but may include administration of steroids and IVIg to the mother and intrauterine transfusion of antigen-negative platelets to the fetus. Any mother at risk should be counseled and managed in a high-risk obstetric setting. Women who have a sister who had a child with NAIT should be offered platelet antigen typing because they may also be at risk of having an affected child.

More rarely, thrombocytopenia in newborns can be due to inherited or congenital disease. In this setting, platelet size, inheritance pattern, and associated features, if any, can be helpful in making the diagnosis. Thrombocytopenia in boys with small platelets and T-cell deficiency should raise the possibility of Wiskott-Aldrich syndrome or its variants. Macrothrombocytopenia is characteristic of *MYH9*-related disease (autosomal dominant), Bernard-Soulier syndrome (autosomal recessive), *GATA1* mutations (X-linked recessive), and gray platelet syndrome (variable inheritance). Type 2B vWD and congenital TTP are additional rare causes of familial thrombocytopenia that can present with large platelets due to increased platelet destruction. Normocytic thrombocytopenia is seen in congenital amegakaryocytic thrombocytopenia (autosomal recessive), thrombocytopenia with absent radii (variable inheritance), and thrombocytopenia with radioulnar synostosis (autosomal dominant). Although uncommon, accurate diagnosis is important to direct management and provide appropriate counseling for these families.

Coagulopathy in the newborn

An accurate assessment of hemostasis in the newborn requires knowledge of the normal range for coagulation screening tests and for specific clotting factor levels (Table 2-16). The vitamin K–dependent factors II, VII, IX, and X are physiologically low in neonates, despite the routine administration of vitamin K. Notably, the normal newborn range for factor IX activity, 15% to 50%, has occasionally led to the misdiagnosis of mild hemophilia B or incorrect identification of a female infant as being a carrier based on a low activity. The contact factors (XI, XII, prekallikrein, and high molecular weight kininogen) are also lower than normal adult levels. By contrast, several factors are at adult levels at birth, including factors VIII, V, and XIII; fibrinogen; and vWF. Because of these physiologic differences, both the median and upper limit of the PT (median, 16.7 seconds; upper limit, 23.5 seconds) and aPTT (median, 44.3 seconds; upper limit, 52 seconds) are higher than ranges established for adult patients. Coagulation factor production gradually increases over the first few months of life, reaching adult levels by approximately 6 months of age. As with other hematologic problems in sick neonates, coagulation abnormalities can result from sepsis, asphyxia, or other triggers of DIC. Unexpected bleeding in an otherwise well newborn, such as bleeding at circumcision, prolonged oozing from heelstick blood draws, or more bleeding/bruising than expected for the difficulty of delivery, should raise the possibility of a genetic coagulopathy. Almost a third of infants with severe hemophilia A represent new mutations. Thus, these patients will not have an informative family history. Additionally, many families are uncertain or unaware of a family history, particularly for mild or moderate hemophilia. Factor XIII deficiency is an autosomal recessive disorder and should be considered especially in the case of umbilical cord bleeding or unexplained intracranial hemorrhage.

In contrast to infants with moderate to severe hemophilia A or B, vWD rarely results in bleeding in the newborn unless it is severe (type 3). The hematology consultant should be aware of vitamin K deficiency, which is increasing in frequency given the move toward home deliveries and away from medical interventions in families where parents desire a "natural" birth. Bleeding from vitamin K deficiency can occur early (days 2-7 of life) and at a rate of approximately 1.5% in otherwise healthy, breast-fed infants who did not receive supplemental vitamin K. Bleeding can be intracranial, gastrointestinal, umbilical, head/neck, at injection sites, or from circumcision. Formula-fed infants are not at risk. If an infant is suspected to have vitamin K deficiency, vitamin K should be administered while confirmatory laboratory tests are pending. Because of the risk of hematoma formation with intramuscular injection in these patients, subcutaneous administration is recommended (usual dose, 1 mg). Although the onset of effect is slightly delayed as compared with intravenous administration, the risk of anaphylactoid reaction with intravenous vitamin K can be avoided.

Thrombosis in the newborn

Similar to pregnancy, the balance between hemostasis and fibrinolysis is shifted toward thrombosis in the newborn. Although antithrombin levels in neonates are mildly lower than in adults (42% to 80%), the vitamin K–dependent anticoagulants, proteins C and S, are strikingly lower; mean protein C activity is 28% (range, 14%–42%), and mean protein S activity is 38.5% (range, 22%–55%). Although evidence suggests that the fibrinolytic system is activated at birth, plasminogen levels are relatively low, so plasmin generation is somewhat decreased in response to thrombolytic agents. When added to the physiologic stresses of labor and delivery, the newborn period thus represents the greatest risk of thrombosis that a child with an underlying thrombophilic condition will face until adulthood. This is particularly true in the sick neonate.

Neonatal thrombotic complications include those associated with umbilical venous or arterial catheters, renal vein thrombosis, arterial and venous stroke, and cerebral venous sinus thrombosis. Clinically, it may be difficult to determine whether the thrombotic event occurred pre- or postnatally. Screening for inherited thrombophilia in a child with a first thrombotic event is controversial; although some recommend screening all such children, others conclude that unless it will alter acute management, such screening is not cost effective. In neonates, age-related variation in normal factor levels may complicate interpretation of results; however, the factor V Leiden and prothrombin G20210A mutations can be reliably ascertained, and severe deficiencies of ATIII, protein S, and protein C can be detected. In addition, in some cases the mother may be screened for antiphospholipid antibodies, which can cross the placenta. Special mention should be made of the rare but potentially devastating homozygous deficiencies of protein C and protein S. Infants classically present with purpura fulminans lesions at birth without an obvious other cause for DIC. Other presentations can include intrauterine ophthalmic or cerebral thrombosis. The level of protein C or S in such patients is usually undetectable. Emergency treatment should include 10 to 20 mL/kg of fresh frozen plasma every 6 to 12 hours, generally administered for 6 to 8 weeks, until all lesions have healed and until a therapeutic INR has been achieved with oral anticoagulation therapy. A protein C concentrate is now approved for use in patients who have confirmed severe protein C deficiency. Recommended dosing is 100 to 120 IU/kg every 6 to 12 hours to maintain trough protein C activity levels above 25%, but dosing varies according to concurrent clinical conditions.

Anticoagulation therapy in infants with acute thrombosis can include conventional UFH, LMWH, and warfarin. Warfarin dosing in infants can be complicated, however, by several factors, including changing levels of coagulation proteins in the first months of life, disparate levels of vitamin K in breast milk and fortified formulas, and lack of a liquid warfarin preparation. Therefore, LMWH is increasingly preferred. Newborns have rapid metabolism of LMWH; thus, the recommended dosing for enoxaparin in term newborns is 1.7 mg/kg/dose every 12 hours, and in infants <2 months, it is 1.5 mg/kg/dose; beyond 2 months of age, dosing is 1 mg/kg/dose every 12 hours as in older children. Dose adjustments should be made as needed to maintain anti-Xa activity levels of 0.5 to 1 U/mL as in adults. Anti-Xa activity testing should be performed 4 hours after administration of enoxaparin and obtained by venipuncture or through a saline-locked peripheral IV because contamination of the sample with heparin will confound results. Experience with newer anticoagulants such as the direct thrombin inhibitors in neonates and infants is limited. Thrombolytic therapy can be considered in the newborn when thrombosis poses risk to life, limb, or organ. Effective tPA dosing may be somewhat higher in newborns compared with older patients, and supplemental plasminogen (as provided by fresh frozen plasma) may be necessary to achieve optimum clot lysis.

Anemia in children

There are several important considerations in evaluating children with anemia that may be different than adults. Asymptomatic anemia is often discovered at approximately 1 year of life when many children may get hemoglobin checked as a screen for iron deficiency or lead exposure. Microcytic anemia is usually either due to iron deficiency or thalassemia. Whereas lead poisoning is an uncommon cause of anemia unless severe, iron deficiency can increase a child's risk for toxicity from lead due to pica and ingestion of contaminated dirt and increased absorption of lead in the gut. Iron deficiency is common around the ages of 1 to 2 years old. Maternal iron stores are usually exhausted after about 6 months, and thereafter, the child must take in enough dietary iron to maintain hematopoiesis. Premature infants are at increased risk because the bulk of maternal iron is transferred to the infant during the third trimester. Although the iron in breast milk is typically more bioavailable than that of cow milk, it is generally inadequate as a sole source of iron beyond 4 to 6 months of life. At 1 year of life, children typically switch from iron-fortified formulas to iron-poor cow milk, and toddlers who are fussy eaters may drink milk to the exclusion of adequate intake of solid iron-containing foods. Intolerance of cow milk proteins may exacerbate the problem through gastrointestinal irritation with consequent poor absorption and occult blood loss. Children may be remarkably asymptomatic despite significant anemia, and often it is a visiting relative who first notes that the child is pale. In addition to microcytosis, typical erythrocyte morphologic findings in iron deficiency include hypochromia, anisocytosis, and reticulocytopenia. A low ferritin indicates depletion of iron stores; however, a normal ferritin does not exclude the diagnosis of iron deficiency because ferritin, as an acute-phase reactant, can be elevated in the presence of inflammation of any cause. Occult blood in the stool, low serum albumin, or eosinophilia might raise concerns for intolerance of cow milk protein. The best confirmatory test for iron deficiency is response to a therapeutic trial of iron. Within 2 weeks of appropriate iron replacement (3-6 mg/kg/d of elemental iron), reticulocytosis and improvement of hemoglobin should be observed. The most common reasons children fail a trial of iron therapy are noncompliance and a diagnosis other than iron deficiency. Less commonly, rapid blood loss or malabsorption can negate the benefits of oral iron replacement. If there is no response to an adequate trial of iron, it should be stopped and alternative causes should be sought.

Thalassemia is most common in children of African American, Mediterranean, or Asian backgrounds. In some states, hemoglobin electrophoresis is performed as part of the newborn screen, and an abnormal hemoglobin (eg, Bart, Constant Spring, hemoglobin E, S, or C) may be identified at birth. Hemoglobin composition changes in the first 6 months of life with the diminution of hemoglobin F, and repeat electrophoresis at 6 to 12 months of life may reveal increased hemoglobin A_2 or persistence of fetal hemoglobin that is helpful in making a diagnosis of thalassemia. However, α thalassemia silent carrier or trait will not be evident on hemoglobin electrophoresis and α-globin gene sequence analysis is necessary to confirm this diagnosis. Although in many cases anemia may be mild, it is important to make the correct diagnosis so that children with thalassemia are not inappropriately treated with iron and so that they and their parents can receive genetic counseling.

Older children who develop iron deficiency anemia without an obvious dietary explanation should be evaluated for abnormal blood loss. Common sites are gastrointestinal, such as in inflammatory bowel disease or celiac disease, or menstrual in girls with undiagnosed vWD. Less common but important to exclude are anatomic abnormalities such as a Meckel diverticulum or double uterus, pulmonary hemosiderosis, or Wegener granulomatosis. Older children and teens may be inaccurate historians when it comes to describing abnormal stools or menstrual bleeding patterns, either due to embarrassment, fear, or lack of an adequate frame of reference, and therefore, direct and repetitive questioning may be required to elicit symptoms.

ITP in children

Although ITP is covered in detail in Chapter 8, certain aspects of ITP in children are worth mentioning here. In contrast to adult ITP, the majority of pediatric patients will have acute rather than chronic ITP, with 75% of patients having complete resolution of their disease by 6 months from presentation. Of patients who have thrombocytopenia beyond 6 months, a significant proportion will resolve by 1 year. In children with chronic ITP who have not responded to therapy, it is important to consider the possibility of an inherited thrombocytopenia. Most pediatric patients with acute ITP present in the toddler to young child age group, with quite sudden onset of bruising, petechiae, or bleeding. A history of a preceding viral illness and occasionally live vaccination is frequently elicited. ITP remains a clinical diagnosis, consisting of isolated thrombocytopenia in an otherwise well child without obvious secondary cause for the thrombocytopenia. Potential other causes of thrombocytopenia include nonimmune destruction (eg, hypersplenism, TTP, hemophagocytosis) or hypoproduction (eg, marrow failure syndromes or leukemia). Although a bone marrow examination is not required, it should be obtained if there are features, such as additional cytopenias, persistent fevers, or hepatosplenomegaly, that call the diagnosis of ITP into question, and many pediatric hematologists consider a marrow examination to be critical prior to initiating corticosteroids, if that is the first therapy administered for ITP.

Significant controversy exists regarding the need to treat pediatric patients with ITP without bleeding. Although recommendations for treatment continue to be based primarily on symptoms rather than platelet numbers, clinical judgment is necessary to assess bleeding risk. The most recent American Society of Hematology (ASH) international consensus report on the investigation and management of ITP (Provan et al, 2010) incorporates multiple factors in the assessment of risk for severe bleeding, including platelets $<10,000/\mu L$, bleeding symptoms if any, head injury, concomitant coagulopathy or vasculitis, ability to control activity in young children, and lifestyle and psychosocial factors. Quality of life is also increasingly being recognized as a factor affecting the management of individual patients. In part, the controversy over management of ITP in children reflects the extremely low incidence of severe or life-threatening bleeding in this population, as well as the evidence that treatment does not alter the underlying course of the disease. This is topic of ongoing study. When treatment is indicated, prospective randomized studies have demonstrated that IVIg and intravenous Rho(D) immune globulin (anti-D) lead to the most rapid increase in platelet count to $>20,000/\mu L$. Anti-D has been used with increasing frequency in Rh-positive patients because of the ease of administration. Corticosteroids may also be effective and are much less costly. Their adverse effects make them unpopular, however, with patients and families. Splenectomy is usually avoided in children, especially those who are <5 years old or have had ITP for <1 year, due to the potential for spontaneous remission and lifelong risk of sepsis in splenectomized patients. Rituximab has been used in children with chronic ITP as a means to avoid or delay splenectomy, although the long-term consequences of this treatment in children are not known. New thrombopoietin receptor agonists are approved for use in chronic ITP, but their role in pediatrics is not yet established. Adjunctive therapies such as antifibrinolytic agents and oral contraceptives may be useful for management of specific bleeding symptoms.

Lupus anticoagulants in children

Lupus anticoagulants are identified in 3 different settings in children. In the first, children who have suffered a thrombotic event or who are being evaluated for rheumatic illness are found to be positive for a lupus anticoagulant or other APLAs. In this setting, the underlying prothrombotic pathophysiology is believed to be similar to that of adults, and the clinical meaning of the anticoagulant, in terms of treatment and prognosis for the thrombosis, is similar as well. In the second setting, children with unexpected bleeding are found to have a prolonged aPTT with or without a prolonged PT, neither of which fully corrects with a 1:1 mix with normal control plasma. Further laboratory testing reveals a lupus anticoagulant and a low factor II activity. In this case, the associated bleeding is likely due to enhanced clearance of factor II by the APLAs. Thrombocytopenia can also be associated with APLAs in patients with bleeding symptoms. Immunosuppressive therapy should be considered for these bleeding children to suppress the autoantibody production and prothrombin consumption. The third and most common scenario in which a lupus anticoagulant is identified is during screening prior to a planned invasive procedure. This usually occurs in a child without any significant bleeding or clotting history who is unexpectedly found to have a prolonged aPTT. Such prolonged aPTTs are also unlikely to correct completely to the normal range with a 1:1 mix, although incubation of the mix for 1 to 2 hours may be required to demonstrate the prolongation. Specific testing should also be performed in this setting to confirm the lupus anticoagulant. Importantly, such lupus anticoagulants in asymptomatic children are not associated with an increased risk of bleeding or thrombosis, and the child can generally proceed safely to surgery without any specific intervention. Such abnormalities are frequently associated with a preceding viral infection and are almost always transient, although the aPTT may not return to normal for many months.

Bibliography
Hematology consultation

Goldman L, Lee T, Rudd P. Ten commandments for effective consultations. *Arch Intern Med*. 1983;143:1753–1755. *A summary of fundamental and time-tested practices for medical and subspecialty consultations.*

Kitchens CS, Alving BM, Kessler CM, eds. *Consultative Thrombosis and Hemostasis*. 2nd ed. New York, NY: Elsevier Science; 2007. *A textbook on coagulation disorders with a good discussion of consultations.*

Sears CL, Charlson ME. The effectiveness of a consultation. Compliance with initial recommendations. *Am J Med*. 1983;74:870–876. *This multivariate analysis of 202 general medical consultations revealed that compliance was greatest when the total number of recommendations was limited to 5 or fewer and they focused on issues central to current patient care.*

Rosenblum D. Hematology consultation. In: Handin RL, Stossel TP, Lux SE, eds. *Blood. Principles and Practice of Hematology*. 2nd ed. Philadelphia, PA: JP Lippincott Co; 2002. *A review of hematology consultation, including the role of the consultant in a multidisciplinary team.*

Surgery and invasive procedures
Preprocedure assessment for bleeding risk

Alving BM, Spivak JL, DeLoughery TG. Consultative hematology: hemostasis and transfusion issues. *Hematology*. 1998;320–341. *This review provides a concise description of presurgical planning for anticipated transfusions, thrombocytopenia in an ICU setting, and the use of newer anticoagulants.*

American College of Chest Physicians. The Eighth ACCP Conference on Antithrombotic and Thrombolytic Therapy. *Chest*. 2008:133(Suppl 6). *The most up to date and detailed evidence-based guidelines for managing antithrombotic and thrombolytic therapy. This publication is a must-read for hematology consultants.*

Dagi TF. The management of postoperative bleeding. *Surg Clin North Am*. 2005;85:1191–1213. *An authoritative overview of preoperative assessment and management of bleeding.*

Lind SE, Marks PW, Ewenstein BM. The hemostatic system. In: Handin RL, Stossel TP, Lux SE, eds. *Blood: Principles and Practice of Hematology*. Philadelphia, PA: JP Lippincott Co; 2002:959. *A condensed summary of the screening of subjects for bleeding disorders and the evaluation of abnormal coagulation tests.*

Reding MT, Key NS. Hematologic problems in the surgical patient: bleeding and thrombosis. In: Hoffman R, Benz EJ, Shattil SJ, et al, eds. *Hematology: Basic Principles and Practice*. 4th ed. Philadelphia, PA: Elsevier Inc; 2005.

Segal JB, Dzik WH. Paucity of studies to support that abnormal coagulation test results predict bleeding in the setting of invasive procedures: an evidence-based review. *Transfusion*. 2005;45:1413–1425. *Review of evidence addressing the lack of predictive value for screening test results with common outpatient invasive procedures.*

Smetana GW, Macpherson DS. The case against routine preoperative laboratory testing. *Med Clin North Am*. 2003;87: 7-40. *Addresses coagulation, hematologic, blood, and urine biochemical tests and electrocardiograms.*

Intraoperative hemorrhage, hemostatic agents, and transfusion therapy

Alten JA, Benner K, Green K, et al. Pediatric off-label use of recombinant factor VIIa. *Pediatrics*. 2009;123:1066–1072. *Study of factor VIIa in pediatric patients suggesting increased thromboembolism risk.*

Casati V, Guzzon D, Oppizzi M, et al. Tranexamic acid compared with high-dose aprotinin in primary elective heart operations: effects on perioperative bleeding and allogeneic transfusions. *J Thorac Cardiovasc Surg*. 2000;120:520–527. *A randomized, prospective, unblinded, single-institution trial (N = 1040) revealed no difference in bleeding, transfusion, hematologic values, thrombotic complications, intubation times, ICU stays, or hospital stays between tranexamic acid and aprotinin prophylaxis for elective coronary artery bypass grafting.*

Casbard AC, Williamson LM, Murphy MF, Rege K, Johnson T. The role of prophylactic fresh frozen plasma in decreasing blood loss and correcting coagulopathy in cardiac surgery. A systemic review. *Anesthesia.* 2004;59:550–558. *Systemic review detailing use of fresh frozen plasma in preoperative setting.*

Dzik WH, Corwin H, Goodnough LT, et al. Patient safety and blood transfusion: new solutions. *Transfus Med Rev.* 2003;17:169–180. *Authoritative review.*

Enomoto TM, Thorborg P. Emerging off-label uses for recombinant activated factor VII: grading the evidence. *Crit Care Clin.* 2005;21:611–632. *Concise overview of clinical reports and evidence-based guidelines for specific off-label indications of activated factor VIIa.*

Forgie MA, Wells PS, Laupacis A, Fergusson D. Preoperative autologous donation decreases allogeneic transfusion but increases exposure to all red blood cell transfusion. *Arch Intern Med.* 2000;158:610–616. *Meta-analysis including 6 randomized and 9 cohort studies. In the randomized studies (N = 933), the odds ratio of allogeneic transfusion was 0.17 and the odds ratio of transfusion (allogeneic + autologous) was 3.03.*

Goodnough LT. Autologous blood donation. *Anesthesiol Clin North Am.* 2005;23:263–270. *Review of rationale and PABD, acute normovolemic hemodilution, and intraoperative and postoperative blood salvage.*

Henry D, Carless P, Ferguson D, Laupacis A. The safety of aprotinin and lysine-derived antifibrinolytic drugs in cardiac surgery: a meta-analysis. *CMAJ.* 2009;180:183–193. *Meta-analysis purporting the benefits of aminocaproic acid over aprotinin.*

Karkouti K, Beattie WS, Dattilo KM, et al. A propensity score case-control comparison of aprotinin and tranexamic acid in high-transfusion-risk cardiac surgery. *Transfusion.* 2006;46:327–338. *Among 898 propensity score–matched patients, both agents showed similar hemostatic effectiveness, but aprotinin appeared to be associated with worsening renal function among patients with preexisting renal dysfunction.*

Levi M, Cromheecke ME, de Jonge E, et al. Pharmacologic strategies to decrease excessive blood less in cardiac surgery: a meta-analysis of clinically relevant endpoints. *Lancet.* 1999;354:1940. *A meta-analysis of 72 randomized controlled trials showed that the odds ratio of mortality was 0.55 with aprotinin compared with placebo. Both aprotinin and lysine analogs, but not desmopressin, significantly decreased perioperative blood loss and the need for transfusion without increasing MI.*

Levy JH. Hemostatic agents. *Transfusion.* 2004;44(Suppl 12):58S–62S. *Concise review of experience with DDAVP, lysine analogs, and aprotinin through 2004.*

Lodge JP, Jonas S, Jones RM, et al. Efficacy and safety of repeated perioperative doses of recombinant factor VIIa in liver transplantation. *Liver Transpl.* 2005;11:973–979. *This randomized, double-blind, placebo-controlled trial, and a similarly designed study by Planinsic et al, observed no benefit in regards to the number of perioperative red blood cell units transfused to patients with end-stage liver disease undergoing orthotopic liver transplantation after a single preoperative dose or multiple perioperative doses of rFVIIa.*

MacLaren R, Weber LA, Brake H, et al. A multicenter assessment of recombinant factor VIIa off-label usage: clinical experiences and associated outcomes. *Transfusion.* 2005;45:1434–1442. *Summary of recent data from 21 US academic medical centers on use, benefit, and potential events.*

Mangano DT, Tudor IC, Dietzel C, for the Multicenter Study of Perioperative Ischemia Research Group and the Ischemia Research and Education Foundation. The risk associated with aprotinin in cardiac surgery. *N Engl J Med.* 2006;354:353–365. *A major observational study of 4374 patients undergoing coronary revascularization with cardiopulmonary bypass and prophylaxis with tranexamic acid, aminocaproic acid, aprotinin, or no agent. Prophylaxis with any of the 3 agents resulted in significantly less perioperative blood loss. However, those who received aprotinin suffered a 1.5- to 2.5-fold increased risk of renal, cardiac, or cerebral adverse events, likely reflecting the multiple prothrombotic mechanisms of aprotinin and greater end-organ microvascular ischemic potential, especially in the kidneys.*

Mankad PS, Codispoti M. The role of fibrin sealants in hemostasis. *Am J Surg.* 2001;182(Suppl 2):21S–28S. *Review of the need for and appropriate use of fibrin sealants during surgery.*

Mayer SA, Brun NC, Begtrup K, et al. Recombinant activated factor VII for acute intracerebral hemorrhage. *N Engl J Med.* 2005;352:777–785. *Early administration of rFVIIa improved neurologic end points and mortality compared with placebo in this study; however, 7% of treated patients suffered serious thromboembolic adverse events, mainly myocardial or cerebral infarction, as compared with 2% of those given placebo. These data prompted an FDA warning about the off-label use of rFVIIa and thrombotic risk.*

O'Connell KA, Wood JJ, Wise RP, et al. Thromboembolic adverse events after use of recombinant human coagulation factor VIIa. *JAMA.* 2006;295:293–298. *The majority of thromboembolic events with rFVIIa since 1999 have occurred in patients receiving the drug for off-label indications, most commonly for surgical bleeding or prophylaxis. Arterial and venous events, which were equally prevalent, resulted in significant morbidity. These complications were the probable cause of death in roughly three fourths of the case fatalities.*

Planinsic RM, van der Meer J, Testa G, et al. Safety and efficacy of a single bolus administration of recombinant factor VIIa in liver transplantation due to chronic liver disease. *Liver Transpl.* 2005;11:973–979.

Shander A, Rijhwani TS. Acute normovolemic hemodilution. *Transfusion.* 2004;44(Suppl):26S–34S.

Spiess BD. Risks of transfusion: outcome focus. *Transfusion.* 2004;44(Suppl):4S–14S. *A review of the adverse events associated with inappropriate transfusions in perioperative and critical care patients.*

Postoperative bleeding

Aledort LM, Green D, Teitel JM. Unexpected bleeding disorders. In: Schechter GP, Broudy VC, Williams ME, eds. *Hematology.* Washington, DC: American Society of Hematology; 2001:306–321. *Case studies illustrating the diagnostic evaluation of patients* with unexpected bleeding problems following surgery including laboratory evaluation and interventions.

Dagi TF. The management of postoperative bleeding. *Surg Clin North Am.* 2005;85:1191–1213. *An overview of assessment and management of postoperative bleeding due to technical or hemostatic issues.*

Karkouti K, Beattie WS, Datillo KM, et al. A propensity score case-control comparison of aprotinin and tranexemic acid in high-transfusion-risk cardiac surgery. *Transfusion.* 2006;46:327–338. *Study showing increased renal dysfunction in cardiac surgery patients who receive aprotinin.*

McKenna R. Abnormal coagulation in the postoperative period contributing to excessive bleeding. *Med Clin North Am.* 2001;85:1277–1310. *A thorough review with 30 references.*

Postoperative thrombosis

Agnelli G, Bergqvist D, Cohen AT, Gallus AS, Gent M; PEGASUS Investigators. Randomized clinical trial of postoperative fondaparinux versus perioperative dalteparin for prevention of venous thromboembolism in high-risk abdominal surgery. *Br J Surg.* 2005;92:1212–1220. *This study showed that prophylactic fondaparinux was more effective than dalteparin in preventing perioperative VTE in cancer patients undergoing high-risk abdominal surgery.*

Anaya DA, Nathens AB. Thrombosis and coagulation: deep vein thrombosis and pulmonary embolism prophylaxis. *Surg Clin North Am.* 2005;85:1163–1177. *Concise review of VTE risk factors and prophylactic strategies for general and high-risk procedures.*

Buller HR, Agnelli G, Hull RD, et al. Antithrombotic therapy for venous thromboembolic disease: the Seventh ACCP Conference on Antithrombotic and Thrombolytic Therapy. *Chest.* 2004;126(Suppl 3):401S–428S. *Evidence-based recommendations for risk assessment, prophylaxis strategies, and special considerations.*

Douketis JD, Eikelboom JW, Quinlan DJ, et al. Short-duration prophylaxis against venous thromboembolism after total hip or knee replacement: a meta-analysis of prospective studies investigating symptomatic outcomes. *Arch Intern Med.* 2002;162:1465–1471. *This meta-analysis revealed the surprising finding that hip surgery was more often associated with symptomatic VTE (2.5% vs 1.4% P = .02) even though symptomatic venographic evidence of thromboembolic disease in 7080 patients showed that more than twice as many knee patients had thrombosis (post knee replacement 38.8%, post knee replacement 16.4%, P ≤ .001).*

Ericksson BI, Lassen MR; Pentasaccharide in Hip-Fracture Surgery Plus Investigators. Duration of prophylaxis against venous thromboembolism with fondaparinux after hip fracture surgery: a multicenter, randomized, placebo-controlled, double-blind study. *Arch Intern Med.* 2003;163:1337–1342. *This study showed that extended duration of fondaparinux, for 19 to 23 days reduced the risk of VTE by 96%, compared with therapy for only 6 to 8 days, with a nonsignificant trend toward increased bleeding.*

Geerts WH, Pineo GF, Heit JA, et al. Prevention of venous thromboembolism: the Seventh ACCP Conference on Antithrombotic and Thrombolytic Therapy. *Chest.* 2004;126(Suppl 3):338S–400S. *Evidence-based recommendations for risk assessment, prophylaxis strategies, and special considerations.*

Hirsh J, Raschke R. Heparin and low-molecular-weight heparin. *Chest.* 2004;126(Suppl 3):188S–203S. *An authoritative review of the use of UFH and LMWH.*

Horlocker TT, Wedel DJ, Benzon H, et al. Regional anesthesia in the anticoagulated patient: defining the risks (the second ASRA Consensus Conference on Neuraxial Anesthesia and Anticoagulation). *Reg Anesth Pain Med.* 2003;28:172–197. *Recommendations to minimize the risk of perispinal hematoma in the perioperative patient undergoing neuraxial anesthesia/analgesia.*

Kearon C. Duration of venous thromboembolism prophylaxis after surgery. *Chest.* 2003;124(Suppl):386S–3892S.

Mangano DT, Tudor IC, Dietzel C, for the Multicenter Study of Perioperative Ischemia Research Group and the Ischemia Research and Education Foundation. The risk associated with aprotinin in cardiac surgery. *N Engl J Med.* 2006;354:353–365. *Major observational study showing increased risk of renal, cardiac, and CNS events in patients receiving aprotinin.*

Intensive care unit
Anemia

Corwin HL, Gettinger A, Fabian TC, et al, for the EPO Critical Care Trials Group. Efficacy and safety of epoetin alfa in critically ill patients. *N Engl J Med.* 2007;357:965–976. *This is a randomized, placebo-controlled trial of recombinant erythropoietin in medical, surgical, or trauma patients admitted to the ICU. The incidence of red cell transfusion was not reduced, although a suggestion of reduced mortality in trauma patients was observed.*

Corwin HL, Gettinger A, Pearl RG, et al. Efficacy of recombinant human erythropoietin in critically ill patients. *JAMA.* 2002;288:2827–2835. *A randomized controlled trial of recombinant erythropoietin in ICU patients, demonstrating a decrease in transfusion requirement in patients randomized to receive erythropoietin.*

Gerber DR. Transfusion of packed red blood cells in patients with ischemic heart disease. *Crit Care Med.* 2008;36:1068–1074. *A comprehensive review of current literature concerning the utility of and complications associated with transfusion of packed red blood cells in medical and surgical patients with ischemic heart disease.*

Hebert PC, Wells G, Blajchman MA, et al. A multicenter, randomized, controlled clinical trial of transfusion requirements in critical care. *N Engl J Med.* 1999;340:409–417. *This is a landmark, randomized, prospective study demonstrating that a less aggressive transfusion strategy was associated with lower in-hospital mortality and similar 30-day mortality as a more aggressive strategy.*

Rawn J. The silent risks of blood transfusion. *Curr Opin Anaesthesiol.* 2008;21:664–668. *This article is a comprehensive review of the less commonly appreciated adverse effects of blood transfusion in a number of diverse clinical settings.*

Vincent JL, Baron J-F, Reinhart K, et al, for the ABC Investigators. Anemia and blood transfusion in critically ill patients. *JAMA.* 2002;288:1499–1507. *This is a careful study designed to define the incidence of anemia and utilization of blood transfusion in an ICU. The investigators found that the average total blood volume drawn daily from a patient was 41.1 mL and the average volume of blood draw was 10.3 mL.*

Zarychanski R, Turgeon AF, McIntyre L, Fergusson DA. Erythropoietin-receptor agonists in critically ill patients: a meta-analysis of randomized clinical trials. *CMAJ.* 2007;177:725–734. *A meta-analysis of 9 studies of recombinant erythropoietin in critically ill patients. The conclusion of these authors was that the reduction in red blood cell transfusions in patients receiving erythropoietin was very small and that routine therapy with erythropoietin is not supported by evidence at the present time.*

Thrombocytopenia

Aster RH. Immune thrombocytopenias caused by glycoprotein IIb/IIIa inhibitors. *Chest.* 2005;127:53S–59S. *Review of drug-induced thrombocytopenia caused by GPIIb/IIIa inhibitors.*

Aster RH, Bougie DW. Drug-induced immune thrombocytopenia. *N Engl J Med.* 2007;357:580–587. *A review of the incidence and mechanisms of drug-induced thrombocytopenia, the drugs most commonly implicated, and the management.*

Levi M, Löwenberg EC. Thrombocytopenia in critically ill patients. *Semin Thromb Haemost.* 2008;34:417–424. *An extremely useful and focused review of the mechanisms responsible for thrombocytopenia and the differential diagnosis of thrombocytopenia in critically ill patients.*

Provan D, Stasi R, Newland AC, et al. International consensus report on the investigation and management of primary immune thrombocytopenia. *Blood.* 2010;115:168–186. *The most current guidelines concerning the diagnosis and management of ITP.*

Selleng K, Selleng S, Greinacher A. Heparin-induced thrombocytopenia in intensive care patients. *Semin Thromb Haemost.* 2008;34:425–438. *A review of HIT, with special emphasis on diagnosis and management in the intensive care setting.*

Selleng S, Selleng K, Wollert HG, et al. Heparin-induced thrombocytopenia in patients requiring prolonged intensive care unit treatment after cardiopulmonary bypass. *J Thromb Hemost.* 2008;6:428–435. *A close examination of the patterns of platelet count recovery and fall after bypass surgery, and their implications for the diagnosis of HIT and management of the patient.*

Warkentin TE. An overview of heparin-induced thrombocytopenia syndrome. *Semin Thromb Haemost.* 2004;30:273–283. *A comprehensive review of the pathophysiology and clinical manifestations of HIT.*

Warkentin TE, Kelton JG. A 14-year study of heparin-induced thrombocytopenia. *Am J Med.* 1996;101:502–507. *A retrospective study examining the incidence of arterial and venous thrombosis in HIT and reporting that patients with HIT but not thrombosis may proceed to develop thrombosis even after discontinuation of heparin. This is the basis for the recommendation to use alternative anticoagulants in these patients.*

Warkentin TE, Kelton JG. Temporal aspects of heparin-induced thrombocytopenia. *N Engl J Med.* 2001;344:1286–1292. *A study of the time to development of HIT in patients preexposed to heparin at various times prior to heparin reexposure, demonstrating that patients recently exposed to heparin may develop HIT very rapidly upon reexposure.*

Infection and DIC

Levi M, Toh C, Thachill J, Watson HG. Guidelines for the diagnosis and management of disseminated intravascular coagulation. *Br J Haematol.* 2009;145:24–33. *British Committee for Standards in Haematology guidelines for diagnosing and managing DIC.*

Marks PW. Coagulation disorders in the ICU. *Clin Chest Med.* 2009;30:123–129. *A broad review of coagulation problems and their management in acutely ill patients in the intensive care setting.*

Russell JA. Management of sepsis. *N Engl J Med.* 2006;355:1699–1713. *A comprehensive review on the management of sepsis, including the use of activated protein C.*

Sharma B, Sharma M, Majumder M, Steier W, Sangal A, Kalawar M. Thrombocytopenia in septic shock patients—a prospective observations study of incidence, risk factors and correlation with clinical outcome. *Anaesth Intensive Care.* 2007;35:874–880. *An observational study assessing the incidence of thrombocytopenia in septic shock patients, as well as factors that correlate with the development of thrombocytopenia and its prognostic value.*

Taylor FB, Toh CH, Hoots WK, Wada H, Levi M. Towards definition, clinical and laboratory criteria and a scoring system for disseminated intravascular coagulation. *Thromb Haemost.* 2001;86:1327–1330. *Proposed guidelines for common criteria for the diagnosis of DIC from the International Society on Thrombosis and Haemostasis Scientific Subcommittee on DIC.*

Massive transfusion-induced thrombocytopenia

Levy JH. Massive transfusion coagulopathy. *Semin Hematol.* 2006;43:S59-S63. *Review of the coagulopathy induced by massive transfusion in refractory hemorrhage and trauma.*

Thrombotic thrombocytopenic purpura and the hemolytic uremic syndrome

Delvaeye M, Noris M, De Vriese A, et al. Thrombomodulin mutations in atypical hemolytic uremic syndrome. *N Engl J Med.* 2009;361:345–357. *An original report identifying mutations in thrombomodulin as contributors to the development of atypical*

HUS through dysregulation of the complement system. Includes a discussion of other complement regulatory proteins implicated in the development of HUS.

George JN. How I treat patients with thrombotic thrombocytopenic purpura-hemolytic uremic syndrome. *Blood.* 2000;96:1223–1229. *Practical recommendations on the approach to and management of TTP.*

McCrae KR, Sadler JE, Cines DB. Thrombotic thrombocytopenic purpura and the hemolytic uremic syndrome. In: Hoffman R, Benz EJ Jr, Shattil SJ, et al, eds. *Hematology: Basic Principles and Practice.* 5th ed. Philadelphia, PA: Elsevier, Churchill, Livingstone; 2009:2099–2112. *Comprehensive and up to date review of the pathogenesis, diagnosis, and management of the thrombotic microangiopathies in children and adults.*

Noris M, Remuzzi G. Atypical hemolytic uremic syndrome. *N Engl J Med.* 2009;361:1676–1687. *An up to date review categorizing the complement mutations that may lead to atypical hemolytic uremic syndrome and describing the mechanisms by which they do so.*

Sadler JE. Von Willebrand factor, ADAMTS13 and thrombotic thrombocytopenic purpura. *Blood.* 2008;112:11–18. *A thorough review of the pathogenesis of TTP, with emphasis on the roles of vWF and ADAMTS13.*

Zheng XL, Sadler JE. Pathogenesis of thrombotic microangiopathies. *Annu Rev Pathol.* 2008;3:249–277. *A detailed review of the pathogenesis of the thrombotic microangiopathies and implications for diagnosis and treatment.*

Catastrophic antiphospholipid syndrome

Asherson RA, Cervera R, Piette J-C, et al. Catastrophic antiphospholipid syndrome: clinical and laboratory features of 50 patients. *Medicine.* 1998;77:195–207. *Review of the clinical manifestations of the catastrophic antiphospholipid syndrome.*

Bucciarelli S, Erkan D, Espinosa G, Cervera R. Catastrophic antiphospholipid syndrome: treatment, prognosis and the risk of relapse *A review of recent data concerning the diagnosis, prognosis, and therapy of the catastrophic antiphospholipid syndrome.*

Erkan D, Lockshin M. New approaches for managing antiphospholipid syndrome. *Nat Clin Practice Rheum.* 2009;5:160–170. *Review of new approaches to management of the antiphospholipid syndrome with a section on the catastrophic antiphospholipid syndrome.*

Consultation for hematologic complications of solid-organ transplantation

Ainsworth CD, Crowther MA, Treleaven D, et al. Severe hemolytic anemia post-renal transplantation produced by donor anti-D passenger lymphocytes: case report and literature review. *Transfus Med Rev.* 2009;23:155–159. *Comprehensive review of passenger lymphocyte-induced hemolytic anemia.*

Blaes AH, Peterson BA, Bartlett N, et al. Rituximab therapy is effective for posttransplant lymphoproliferative disorders after solid organ transplantation: results of a phase II trial. *Cancer.* 2005;104:1661–1667. *Single-agent rituximab induced responses in 7 of 11 patients with PTLD, with a median time to treatment failure of 10 months.*

Buell JF, Gross TG, Hanaway MJ, et al. Chemotherapy for posttransplant lymphoproliferative disorder: the Israel Penn International Transplant Tumor Registry experience. *Transplant Proc.* 2005;37:956–957.

Capello D, Cerri M, Muti G, et al. Molecular histogenesis of posttransplantation lymphoproliferative disorders. *Blood.* 2003;102:3775–3785. *An analysis of molecular histogenesis of 52 B-cell monoclonal PTLDs showed multiple mutations that distributed unevenly among the various lymphomas but supported the premise that the proliferating cells derive from germinal center cells.*

Choquet S, Leblond V, Herbrecht R et. al. Efficacy and safety of rituximab in B-cell post-transplant lymphoproliferative disorder: results of a prospective multicenter phase 2 study. *Blood.* 2006;107:3053–3057. *In this large multicenter trial that included 43 evaluable patients, 4 weekly doses of rituximab induced responses in 44% of patients, and the 1-year overall survival rate was 67%.*

Djokic M, LeBeau MM, Swinnen LJ, et al. Post-transplant lymphoproliferative disorder subtypes correlate with different recurring chromosomal abnormalities. *Genes Chromosomes Cancer.* 2006;45:313–318.

Harris NL, Jaffe ES, Diebold J, et al. The World Health Organization classification of neoplastic diseases of the hematopoietic and lymphoid tissues: report of the clinical advisory committee meeting, Airlie House, Virginia, November 1997. *Histopathology.* 2000;36:69–86. *Contains classification schema for lymphomas, including categories for PTLD.*

Jain AB, Marcos A, Pokharna R, et al. Rituximab (chimeric anti-CD20 antibody) for posttransplant lymphoproliferative disorder after solid organ transplantation in adults: long-term experience from a single center. *Transplantation.* 2005;80:1692–1698. *Among 14 patients who received rituximab for primary or salvage therapy, 50% responded, and overall survival at 5 years was 35%.*

Kedzierska K, Kabat-Koperska J, Safranow K, et al. Influence of angiotensin 1-converting enzyme polymorphism on development of post-transplant erythrocytosis in renal graft recipients. *Clin Transplant.* 2008;22:156–161. *Study of risk factors for posttransplantation erythrocytosis and identification of the D allele as a risk factor.*

Knight JS, Tsodikov A, Cibrik DM, et al. Lymphoma after solid organ transplantation: risk, response to therapy and survival at a transplantation center. *J Clin Oncol.* 2009;10:3354–3362. *Data from the University of Michigan suggesting that the highest risk of PTLD occurs in EBV-naive recipients who receive an organ from an EBV-infected donor.*

McLeod BC. Thrombotic microangiopathies in bone marrow and organ transplant patients. *J Clin Apheresis.* 2002;17:118–123. *Cogent discussion of the pathophysiologic mechanisms of posttransplantation thrombotic microangiopathies and the reasons why plasma exchange does not appear beneficial for this disorder.*

Petz LD. Immune hemolysis associated with transplantation. *Semin Hematol.* 2005;42:145–155. *Concise review of pathophysiology, incidence, clinical manifestations, and management of donor-mediated hemolysis (passenger lymphocyte syndrome) following hematopoietic stem cell or solid organ transplantation.*

Schwimmer J, Nadasdy TA, Spitalnik PF, et al. De novo thrombotic microangiopathy in renal transplant recipients: a comparison of hemolytic uremic syndrome with localized renal thrombotic microangiopathy. *Am J Kidney Dis.* 2003;41:471–479. *Patients with thrombotic microangiopathy localized to the renal allograft did not require dialysis and did not lose the graft compared with rates of 54% and 38% for these outcomes, respectively, among patients with systemic thrombotic microangiopathy.*

Smith DM, Agura E, Netto G, et al. Liver transplant-associated graft-versus-host disease. *Transplantation.* 2003;75:118–126. *Comprehensive retrospective review of 12 cases in a single-institution experience.*

Taylor AL, Marcus R, Bradley JA. Post-transplant lymphoproliferative disorders (PTLD) after solid organ transplantation. *Crit Rev Oncol Hematol.* 2005;56:155–167. *Recent overview of pathology, incidence, clinical presentations, treatment, and potential prophylactic approaches to PTLD.*

Triulzi DJ. Specialized transfusion support for solid organ transplantation. *Curr Opin Hematol.* 2002;9:527–532. *Brief, comprehensive overview of salient issues and considerations for transfusion in organ transplantation recipients.*

Pregnancy
Anemia

Breymann C, Visca E, Huch R, Huch A. Efficacy and safety of intravenously administered iron sucrose with and without adjuvant recombinant human erythropoietin for the treatment of resistant iron-deficiency anemia during pregnancy. *Am J Obstet Gynecol.* 2001;184:662–667. *A randomized study of iron sucrose versus iron sucrose and erythropoietin in pregnant women with a suboptimal response to oral iron. Both regimens were effective, although more rapid responses were observed in patients treated with erythropoietin.*

Thrombocytopenia in pregnancy

Crary SE, Buchanan GR. Vascular complications after splenectomy for hematologic disorders. *Blood.* 2009;114(14):2861–2868. *A comprehensive review of the vascular complications of splenectomy for a number of indications.*

D'Angelo A, Fattorini A, Crippa L. Thrombotic microangiopathy in pregnancy. *Thromb Res.* 2009;123(Suppl 2):S56-S62. *A thorough review of pregnancy-associated thrombotic microangiopathies, with emphasis on pathology and differential diagnosis.*

Kelton JG. Idiopathic thrombocytopenic purpura complicating pregnancy. *Blood Rev.* 2002;16:43–46. *A classic review on the significance and management of ITP in pregnancy.*

Martin JN, Bailey AP, Rehberg JF, Owens MT, Keiser SD, May WL. Thrombotic thrombocytopenic purpura in 166 pregnancies: 1955–2006. *Am J Obstet Gynecol.* 2008;199:98–104. *A comprehensive literature review of TTP in pregnancy, with discussion of differential diagnosis and the need for rapid recognition and therapy.*

McCrae KR. Thrombocytopenia in pregnancy: differential diagnosis, pathogenesis and management. *Blood Rev.* 2003;17:7-14. *A comprehensive review of the causes and management of thrombocytopenia during pregnancy.*

Provan D, Stasi R, Newland AC, et al. International consensus report on the investigation and management of primary immune thrombocytopenia. *Blood.* 2010;115:168–186. *International consensus guidelines for the diagnosis and management of ITP.*

Rodeghiero F, Stasi R, Gernsheimer T, et al. Standardization of terminology, definitions and outcome criteria in immune thrombocytopenic purpura of adults and children: report from an international working group. *Blood.* 2009;113:2386–2393. *International consensus guidelines for the terminology and outcome criteria for ITP.*

Stavrou E, McCrae KR. Immune thrombocytopenia in pregnancy. *Hematol Oncol Clin North Am.* 2009;23:1299–1316. *A contemporary review on the differential diagnosis and management of ITP in pregnancy.*

Win N, Rowley M, Pollard C, Beard H, Hambley H, Booker M. Severe gestational (incidental) thrombocytopenia: to treat or not to treat. *Hematology.* 2005;10:69–72. *A description of 6 women with probable severe cases of gestational thrombocytopenia and their management. This article reviews gestational thrombocytopenia and the distinction from ITP in more pronounced cases.*

vWD in pregnancy

Demers C, Derzko C, David M, Douglas J. Gynaecological and obstetric management of women with inherited bleeding disorders. *Int J Gynecol Obstet.* 2006;95:75–87. *Guidelines established by the Society of Obstetricians and Gynaecologists of Canada for obstetrical management of women with bleeding disorders.*

James AH. Guidelines for bleeding disorders in women. *Thromb Res.* 2009;123(Suppl 2):S124-S128. *A summary of existing guidelines from various groups for the management of bleeding disorders in women.*

James AH. More than menorrhagia: a review of the obstetric and gynaecological manifestations of von Willebrand disease. *Thromb Res.* 2007;120:S17-S20. *Review of several gynecologic disorders that are influenced by vWD, with an emphasis on pregnancy manifestations.*

Kujovich JL. von Willebrand disease and pregnancy. *J Thromb Haemost.* 2004;3:246–253. *Detailed review of vWD and its management during pregnancy.*

Rodeghiero F, Castaman G, Tosetto A. How I treat von Willebrand disease. *Blood.* 2009;114:1158–1165. *A general, case-based discussion of vWD treatment, with discussion of a pregnant patient.*

Thrombophilia and thromboembolic disease in pregnancy

Bates SM, Greer IA, Pabinger I, Sofaer S, Hirsh J. Venous thromboembolism, thrombophilia, antithrombotic therapy, and pregnancy. *Chest* 2008;133:844S–886S. *The most recent evidence-based guidelines from the ACCP concerning thrombosis and thrombophilia in pregnancy and the indications for and proper use of anticoagulants in this setting.*

Brenner B, Hoffman R, Card H, Dulitsky M, Younis J, for the LIVE-ENOX Investigators. Efficacy and safety of two doses of enoxaparin in women with thrombophilia and recurrent pregnancy loss: the LIVE-ENOX study. *J Thromb Haemost* 2005;3:227–229. *A multicenter, randomized, prospective trial of patients with APLAs and 3 or more fetal losses in the first trimester treated with enoxaparin at doses of either 40 or 80 mg/d. There was no difference in outcomes between the two groups (successful birth rates of 84.3% and 78.3%, respectively).*

Brill-Edwards P, Ginsberg JS, Gent M, et al. Safety of withholding heparin in pregnant women with a history of venous thromboembolism. Recurrence of Clot in This Pregnancy Study Group. *N Engl J Med.* 2000;343:1439–1444. *A prospective study demonstrating that in patients with a prior venous thrombosis in pregnancy who did not have thrombophilia, heparin may be safely withheld during subsequent pregnancies.*

Heit JA, Kobbervig CE, James AH, Petterson TM, Bailey KR, Melton LJ. Trends in the incidence of venous thromboembolism during pregnancy or postpartum: a 30-year population-based study. *Ann Intern Med.* 2005;143:697–706. *A review of the epidemiology and incidence of thrombosis in pregnant patients from the Mayo Clinic.*

James AH, Abel DE, Brancazio LR. Anticoagulants in pregnancy. *Obstet Gynecol Surv.* 2005;61:59–69. *A review of the appropriate use of anticoagulants in pregnant patients, including indications.*

Laskin CA, Spitzer KA, Clark CA, et al. Low molecular weight heparin and aspirin for recurrent pregnancy loss: results from the randomized, controlled HepASA trial. *J Rheumatol.* 2009;36:279–287. *A randomized controlled trial in women with recurrent pregnancy loss and either autoantibodies or a coagulation abnormality treated with LMWH plus aspirin or aspirin alone. The trial was stopped after 4 years when no differences in the groups was observed and the live birth rate in the aspirin alone arm was higher than expected (79.1%). Bone mineral density in the femoral neck or lumbar spine did not differ between groups. This study suggests that the addition of heparin to aspirin may not improve outcomes in these patients.*

Lim W, Crowther MA, Eikelboom JW. Management of antiphospholipid antibody syndrome. *JAMA.* 2006;295:1050–1057. *A comprehensive review of the management of the antiphospholipid syndrome, with a section on management of pregnant patients.*

Lindqvist PG, Merlo J. The natural course of women with recurrent fetal loss. *J Thromb Haemost.* 2005;3:227–229. *A manuscript that should be read by anyone interested in this area, discussing the importance of regression toward the mean in clinical trials and its implications for interpreting studies of anticoagulants in patients with recurrent fetal loss that depend on historical controls.*

Nijkeuter M, Ginsberg JS, Huisman MV. Diagnosis of deep vein thrombosis and pulmonary embolism in pregnancy: a systematic review. *J Thromb Haemost.* 2006;4:496–500. *A contemporary review of the preferred methods for diagnosis of DVT and pulmonary embolism in pregnant patients.*

Noble LS, Kutteh WH, Lashey N, Franklin RD, Herrada J. Antiphospholipid antibodies associated with recurrent pregnancy loss: prospective, multicenter, controlled pilot study comparing treatment with low-molecular weight heparin versus unfractionated heparin. *Fertil Steril.* 2005;83:684–690. *A prospective, controlled (not randomized) study that demonstrated equivalent outcomes in patients with 3 or more consecutive pregnancy losses before 20 weeks treated with low-dose aspirin and either LMWH (enoxaparin 40 mg/d) or UFH (5000 U twice a day).*

Robertson L, Wu O, Langhorne P, et al, for the Thrombosis: Risk and Economic Assessment of Thrombophilia Screening (TREATS) Study. Thrombophilia in pregnancy: a systematic review. *Br J Haematol.* 2005;132:171–196. *A systematic review of the association of thrombophilia with thrombosis and adverse pregnancy outcomes. The study confirms an increased relative risk for these complications, although the absolute risk of VTE and adverse outcomes is low.*

Hematologic malignancies

Ault P, Kantarjian H, O'Brien S, et al. Pregnancy among patients with chronic myeloid leukemia treated with imatinib. *J Clin Oncol.* 2006;24:1204–1208. *This retrospective review of 19 pregnancies occurring among 18 women in hematologic remission showed that brief drug exposure during conception and pregnancy did not adversely affect the fetus but discontinuing imatinib resulted in loss of chronic myeloid leukemia response.*

Aviles A, Diaz-Maqueo JC, Talavera A, Guzman R, Garcia EL. Growth and development of children of mothers treated with chemotherapy during pregnancy: current status of 43 children. *Am J Hematol.* 1991;36:243–248. *In this moderately sized study, none of the 43 children followed for several years showed any abnormalities of growth or development, and none had any birth defects or malignancies.*

Aviles A, Neri N. Hematological malignancies and pregnancy: a final report of 84 children who received chemotherapy in utero. *Clin Lymphoma.* 2001;2:173–177. *With a median follow-up of 18.7 years, no cancer or acute leukemia was observed.*

Aviles A, Neri N, Nambo MJ. Long-term evaluation of cardiac function in children who received anthracyclines during pregnancy. *Ann Oncol.* 2006;17:286–288. *No clinical or echocardiographic cardiac toxicity was detected among 81 children with a mean follow-up of 17 years.*

Cardonick E, Iacobucci A. Use of chemotherapy during human pregnancy. *Lancet Oncol.* 2004;5:283–291. *Review of risks associated with individual drugs during various stages of fetal development, treatment regimens for specific malignancies, including leukemias and lymphomas, and considerations for delivery and breastfeeding.*

Carradice D, Austin N, Bayston K, Ganly PS. Successful treatment of acute promyelocytic leukemia during pregnancy. *Clin Lab Haematol.* 2002;24:307–311.

Chelghoum Y, Vey N, Raffoux E, et al. Acute leukemia during pregnancy: a report on 37 patients and a review of the literature. *Cancer.* 2005;104:110–127. *Among 31 patients with acute myeloid leukemia and 6 patients with acute lymphoblastic leukemia, pregnancy did not appear to affect the treatment response and course of the leukemia. Elective terminations were carried out for most first trimester cases. Aggressive chemotherapy during second and third trimesters was well tolerated, and healthy premature or term births resulted without fetal malformations.*

Chen J, Lee RJ, Tsodikov A, et al. Does radiotherapy around the time of pregnancy for Hodgkin's disease modify the risk of breast cancer? *Int J Radiat Oncol Biol Phys.* 2004;58:1474–1479.

Hurley TJ, McKinnell JV, Irani MS. Hematologic malignancies in pregnancy. *Obstet Gynecol Clin North Am.* 2005;32:595–614. *Overview of fetal and maternal risks and management of Hodgkin disease, non-Hodgkin lymphoma, and leukemias.*

Selected outpatient hematology topics

Balduini CL, Iolascon A, Savoia A. Inherited thrombocytopenias: from genes to therapy. *Haematologica.* 2002;87:860–880. *This article reviews the inherited platelet disorders.*

Brown KA. Nonmalignant disorders of lymphocytes. *Clin Lab Sci.* 1997;10:329–335. *This is a review of the causes of benign lymphocytopenia and lymphocytosis.*

Casper C. The aetiology and management of Castleman disease at 50 years: translating pathophysiology to patient care. *Br J Haematol.* 2005129:3-17. *Authoritative overview of pathobiology, histologic classification, diagnosis, and treatment of unicentric and multicentric Castleman disease.*

Casper C, Nichols WG, Huang ML, et al. Remission of HHV-8 and HIV-associated multicentric Castleman disease with ganciclovir treatment. *Blood.* 2004;103:1632–1634. *Interesting case reports of 3 subjects treated with ganciclovir who achieved clear symptomatic relief.*

Collins LS, Fowler A, Tong CYW, de Ruiter A. Multicentric Castleman's disease in HIV infection. *Int J STD AIDS.* 2006;17:19–25. *Review with an emphasis on antiviral approaches for HHV-8 in HIV-positive patients.*

Del Giudice I, Peleri SA, Rossi M, et al. Histopathological and molecular features of persistent polyclonal lymphocytosis (PPBL) with progressive splenomegaly. *Br J Haematol.* 2009;144:726–731. *Concise clinical description of this disorder.*

Dispenzieri A. Castleman disease. *Cancer Treat Res.* 2008;142:293–330. *Up to date review of the syndrome.*

Haddy TB, Rana SR, Castro O. Benign ethnic neutropenia: what is a normal absolute neutrophil count? *J Lab Clin Med.* 1999;133:15–22. *This review article stresses the frequency of "neutropenia" among people of African and Middle Eastern descent (as high as 50% in some groups), including a lack of scientific evidence that a particular neutrophil count is minimal for all ethnic groups.*

Laurence J. T-cell subsets in health, infectious disease, and idiopathic CD4$^+$ T lymphocytopenia. *Ann Intern Med.* 1993;119:55–62.

Rao VK, Straus SE. Causes and consequences of the autoimmune lymphoproliferative syndrome. *Hematology.* 2006;11:15–23.

Stasi R, Amadori S, Osborn J, Newland AC, Provan D. Long-term outcome of otherwise healthy individuals with incidentally discovered borderline thrombocytopenia. *PLoS Med.* 2006;3:e24. *A prospective study examining the long-term outcome of patients with mild thrombocytopenia, demonstrating that such individuals have a 10-year probability of 12% of developing autoimmune disease.*

Tefferi A, Hanson CA, Inwards DJ. How to interpret and pursue an abnormal complete blood cell count in adults. *Mayo Clin Proc.* 2005;80:923–936. *Concise summaries of differential diagnoses and diagnostic algorithms for anemia, thrombocytopenia, thrombocytosis, leukopenia, and leukocytosis.*

Consultation in pediatric patients

Anemia in the newborn

Bizzarro MJ, Colson E, Ehrenkranz RA. Differential diagnosis and management of anemia in the newborn. *Pediatr Clin North Am.* 2004;4:1087–1107. *An extensive review of the topic, including pathophysiology, norms, approach to diagnosis, and guidelines for transfusions, with 81 references.*

Lipton JM, Ellis SR. Diamond Blackfan anemia; diagnosis, treatment and molecular pathogenesis. *Hematol Oncol Clin Norht Am.* 2009;23:261–282. *An extensive review (97 references) of the disease incorporating data from the Diamond-Blackfan anemia registry.*

Neutropenia in the newborn

Christensen RD. Congenital neutropenia. *Clin Perinatol.* 2004;31:29–38. *This review (42 references) focuses on the more severe forms of congenital neutropenia, particularly Kostmann neutropenia, but also touches on immune-mediated neutropenia.*

Thrombocytopenia in the newborn

Berkowitz RL, Busell JB, McFarland JG. Alloimmune thrombocytopenia: state of the art 2006. *Am J Obstet Gynecol.* 2006;195:907–913. *This review summarizes current data and controversies in the antenatal management of NAIT.*

Birchall JE, Murphy MF, Kaplan C, et al. European collaborative study of the antenatal management of feto-maternal alloimmune thrombocytopenia. *Br J Hematol.* 2003;122:275–288. *This study by the European Fetomaternal Alloimmune Thrombocytopenia Study Group found that history of a previous sibling with a prenatal intracranial hemorrhage or a platelet count <20,000/μL attributable to HPA-1a alloimmunization was associated with lower platelet counts in fetuses in subsequent pregnancies. Antenatal maternal therapy improved* platelet counts to >50,000/μL in the majority of cases. These data suggest that treatment can be stratified based on the sibling history of NAIT and support the use of maternal therapy as first-line treatment.

Bussel JB, Sola-Visner M. Current approaches to the evaluation of the fetus and neonate with immune thrombocytopenia. *Semin Perinatol.* 2009;33:35–42. *This review (39 references) focuses on the diagnosis and management of the newborn with NAIT.*

Manno CS. Management of bleeding disorders in children. *Hematology Am Soc Hematol Educ Program.* 2005:416–422. *This review provides more details about NAIT (43 references).*

Roberts I, Murray NA. Neonatal thrombocytopenia: causes and management. *Arch Dis Child Fetal Neonatal Ed.* 2003;88:F359-F364. *This thorough and pragmatic review (79 references) covers causes, mechanisms, presentation, differential diagnosis, and treatment options for thrombocytopenia in the newborn.*

Roberts I, Stanworth S, Murray NA. Thrombocytopenia in the neonate. *Blood Rev.* 2008;22:173–186. *This thorough and pragmatic review (122 references) covers causes, mechanisms, presentation, differential diagnosis, and treatment options for thrombocytopenia in the newborn.*

Coagulopathy in the newborn

Chalmers EA. Neonatal coagulation problems. *Arch Dis Child Fetal Neonatal Ed.* 2004;89:F475-F478. *A review (28 references) of neonatal hemostasis and its alterations and recommended laboratory investigations.*

Thrombosis in the newborn

Kearon C, Kahn SR, Agnelli G, et al Antithrombotic therapy for venous thromboembolic disease. *Chest.* 2008;133:454S–545S. *An exhaustive review of the literature, clinical trials, and treatment recommendations, including neonate-specific guidelines, resulting from the 8th ACCP Conference on Antithrombotic and Thrombolytic Therapy (393 references).*

Manco-Johnson MJ. How I treat venous thrombosis in children. *Blood.* 2006;107:21–29. *A very thorough review (73 references) of diagnostic and therapeutic issues in childhood thrombosis, including recommendations for neonates and infants.*

Tcheng WY, Dovat S, Gurel Z, et al. Severe congenital protein C deficiency; description of a new mutation and prophylactic protein C therapy and in vivo pharmacokinetics. *J Pediatr Hematol Oncol.* 2008;30:166–171. *A case description and review (36 references) of management in purpura fulminans due to deficiency of protein C.*

Thornburg C, Pipe S. Neonatal thromboembolic emergencies. *Semin Fetal Neonatal Med.* 2006;11:198–206. *Summary of evaluation and treatment of thrombosis in the neonate (51 references).*

Anemia in childhood

Ferrara M, Coppola M, Coppola A, et al. Iron deficiency in childhood and adolescence: a retrospective review. *Hematology.* 2006;11:183–186. *This review summarizes the reasons for iron deficiency identified in 238 children from 7.5 months to 16 years of age. In addition to correction of anemia, it is important consider underlying disorders that may present with iron deficiency (4 references).*

Orkin, S. Fisher D, Lux S, et al. *Nathan and Oski's Hematology of Infancy and Childhood.* 7th ed. Philadelphia, PA: Saunders Elsevier; 2009. *This textbook serves as a basic reference for the pathophysiology of common and rare disorders of red blood cells in childhood.*

Richardson M. Microcytic anemia. *Pediatr Rev.* 2007;28:5-14. *This review provides a summary of diagnostic considerations for the child who presents with microcytic anemia (9 references).*

ITP in children

Beck CE, Nathan PC, Parkin PC, Blanchette VS, Macarthur C. Corticosteroids versus intravenous immune globulin for the treatment of acute immune thrombocytopenic purpura in children: a systematic review and meta-analysis of randomized controlled trials. *J Pediatr.* 2005;4:521–527. *Exhaustive meta-analysis concluding that corticosteroid-treated children with acute ITP are 26% less like to achieve >20 × 10^9/L platelet count by 48 hours after treatment, as compared with IVIg (31 references).*

Crary SE, Buchanan GR. Vascular complications after splenectomy for hematologic disorders. *Blood.* 2009;114:2861–2868.

Provan D, Stasi R, Newland AC, et al. International consensus report on the investigation and management of primary immune thrombocytopenia. *Blood.* 2010;115:168–186. *Recommendations for diagnosis and treatment of both adult and pediatric ITP (207 references).*

Rodeghiero F, Stasi R, Gernsheimer T, et al. Standardization of terminology, definitions and outcome criteria in immune thrombocytopenic purpura of adults and children: report from an international working group. *Blood.* 2009;113:2386–2393. *Consensus statement for development of standard terminology and definitions for primary ITP and criteria for grading severity and clinically meaningful response to therapy, with the goal to facilitate improved randomized studies (75 references).*

Segel GB, Feig SA. Controversies in the diagnosis and management of childhood acute immune thrombocytopenic purpura. *Pediatr Blood Cancer.* 2009;53:318–324. *Discussion of practice consensus and supporting data (74 references).*

Tarantino MD. The pros and cons of drug therapy for immune thrombocytopenic purpura in children. *Hematol Oncol Clin North Am.* 2004;18:1301–1314. *Up-to-date discussion that reviews recent trials and rationale for using, or withholding, available treatments for ITP (99 references).*

Lupus anticoagulant in children

Briones M, Abshire T. Lupus anticoagulants in children. *Curr Opin Hematol.* 2003;10:375–379. *A summary of literature regarding symptomatic and asymptomatic lupus anticoagulants in children.*

Thrombocythemia in children

Provan D, Newland A, Norfolk D, et al. Guidelines for the investigation and management of idiopathic thrombocytopenic purpura in adults, children and in pregnancy. *Br J Haematol.* 2003;120:574–596. *British guidelines for the management of ITP, with a discussion of what constitutes a "safe" platelet count in a variety of situations.*

Randi ML, Putti MC, Scapin M, et al. Pediatric patients with essential thrombocythemia are mostly polyclonal and V617FJAK2 negative. *Blood.* 2006;108:3600–3602. *A comparison of JAK2V671F mutation frequency and clonality in pediatric and adult essential thrombocythemia (24 references).*

Strauss RG. Pretransfusion trigger platelet counts and dose for prophylactic platelet transfusions. *Curr Opin Hematol.* 2005;12:499–502. *A discussion of the requirement for platelet transfusions in patients with thrombocytopenia, and the minimal platelet count that should trigger transfusion.*

Teofili L, Giona F, Martini M, et al. Markers of myeloproliferative diseases in childhood polycythemia vera and essential thrombocythemia. *J Clin Onol.* 2007;25:1048–1053. *A comparison of markers used in the diagnosis of myeloproliferative diseases between children and adults (34 references).*

CHAPTER 03

Hematopoietic growth factors

David C. Dale and Gary H. Lyman

Myeloid growth factors, 75
Erythroid growth factors, 81
Platelet growth factors, 86
Other HGFs, 88
Bibliography, 88

The hematopoietic growth factors (HGFs) and their receptors play essential roles in regulating hematopoiesis (see Chapter 2). For each hematopoietic lineage, specific factors are critical for producing and maintaining circulating levels of the cells. For example, granulocyte colony-stimulating factor regulates neutrophil production; granulocyte-macrophage colony-stimulating factor enhances production of neutrophils, monocytes, and eosinophils; erythropoietin regulates red blood cell production; and thrombopoietin regulates platelet production. This chapter focuses on results of clinical trials and approved uses for these HGFs and provides an overview of other factors at early stages in development.

Myeloid growth factors

Granulocyte colony-stimulating factor (filgrastim, lenograstim)

Granulocyte colony-stimulating factor (G-CSF) is a myeloid growth factor produced by monocytes, macrophages, fibroblasts, endothelial cells, and many other types of cells. Normally, circulating levels of G-CSF are very low or undetectable.

Conflict-of-interest disclosure: *Dr. Dale:* consultancy: Amgen, Biota, Regeneron, Schering-Plough, Tarix, Telik; research funding: Amgen, Genzyme, Merck, Schering-Plough, Telik, Barth Foundation, National Institutes of Health, University of Washington; honoraria: Amgen, Biota, Caremark, Cellerant, Regeneron, Schering-Plough, Tarix, Telik, BCDecker, Wolters Kluwer Health (Lippincott Williams & Wilkins), American College of Physicians, US Department of Health and Human Services; patents and royalties: book chapters and editing for Wolters Kluwer Health (Lippincott Williams & Wilkins); speakers' bureau: Amgen; membership on board of directors or advisory committee: Cellerant (Scientific Advisory Board), Schering Plough (Data Safety Monitoring Board). *Dr. Lyman:* research funding: Amgen; speakers' bureau: Amgen.

Table 3-1 FDA-approved indications for filgrastim.

Accelerate neutrophil recovery after acute myelogenous leukemia induction or consolidation chemotherapy
Mobilize peripheral blood stem cells
Accelerate neutrophil recovery in patients receiving myelosuppressive chemotherapy
Severe chronic neutropenia (idiopathic, cyclic, congenital)

Infections, endotoxin administration, and inflammatory mediators such as interleukin-1 (IL-1) or tumor necrosis factor (TNF) dramatically increase the circulating levels of G-CSF.

G-CSF plays the central role in regulating neutrophil formation and deployment. Its biologic effects are mediated through the G-CSF receptor, which is expressed both on mature neutrophils and their progenitors. Mice with a targeted disruption of the G-CSF receptor (G-CSF "knockouts") have severe neutropenia but normal hematocrit levels and platelet counts. Acquired mutations in the G-CSF receptor (most are truncations of the cytoplasmic tail of the receptor) are found in children with severe congenital neutropenia in transition to myelodysplasia or acute myelogenous leukemia (see Chapter 7), but not in neutropenia associated with other conditions.

Filgrastim is a recombinant form of G-CSF produced in *Escherichia coli* by introduction of the human G-CSF gene. It is identical to native human G-CSF except for the addition of an amino-terminal methionine. Filgrastim is licensed for use in the United States and in many other countries (Table 3-1). Lenograstim is G-CSF produced in a mammalian cell line and is in clinical use outside the United States.

Pegylated methionyl G-CSF (pegfilgrastim)

Pegfilgrastim is methionyl G-CSF (filgrastim) with polyethylene glycol covalently bound to the amino-terminal methionine residue. Pegylation reduces the renal clearance of G-CSF and prolongs the duration of its effects. Trials comparing pegylated G-CSF and G-CSF show similar biologic activities and clinical benefits to reduce the occurrence of chemotherapy-induced febrile neutropenia. There have been no observed differences in pegfilgrastim pharmacokinetics that relate to sex or older age. The pharmacokinetic profile of pegfilgrastim is not expected to be affected by hepatic insufficiency but has not been sufficiently assessed in this setting. Likewise, the pharmacokinetics, safety, and efficacy of pegfilgrastim have not been fully established in pediatric patients. The approved indications for pegfilgrastim are shown in Table 3-2.

Granulocyte-macrophage colony-stimulating factor (sargramostim, molgramostim)

Granulocyte-macrophage colony-stimulating factor (GM-CSF) is a glycoprotein constitutively produced by monocytes, macrophages, endothelial cells, and fibroblasts. Inflammatory cytokines such as IL-1 or TNF increase GM-CSF production. GM-CSF promotes the growth of myeloid colony-forming cells (CFU-GM), increases the number of circulating neutrophils and monocytes, and enhances the phagocytic function and microbicidal capacity of mature myeloid cells. GM-CSF stimulates dendritic cell maturation, proliferation, and function and increases antigen presentation by macrophages and dendritic cells. Knockout of GM-CSF in mice results in a normal complete blood count and a normal number of progenitor cells in the marrow, indicating that GM-CSF is not essential for hematopoiesis. However, mice that lack GM-CSF have lung pathology consistent with pulmonary alveolar proteinosis. Some cases of human pulmonary alveolar proteinosis are due to a defect in the common β chain of the receptor for GM-CSF, interleukin-3 (IL-3), and interleukin-5 (IL-5). These infants have decreased alveolar macrophage function and accumulate surfactant in the alveoli. Thus, GM-CSF does play a key role in the function of pulmonary macrophages.

Two recombinant forms of GM-CSF are currently in clinical use: sargramostim (yeast-expressed GM-CSF) and molgramostim (E coli–expressed GM-CSF). Only sargramostim

Table 3-2 FDA-approved indications for pegfilgrastim.

Reduce the risk of febrile neutropenia after myelosuppressive chemotherapy
Decrease the incidence of infection as manifested by febrile neutropenia in patients with nonmyeloid malignancies receiving myelosuppressive anticancer drugs associated with a clinically significant incidence of febrile neutropenia

Table 3-3 FDA-approved indications for GM-CSF/sargramostim.

Reduce the risk of death due to infection in patients ≥55 years old undergoing induction chemotherapy for AML
Mobilize autologous peripheral blood stem cells and enhance neutrophil recovery after transplantation
Promote neutrophil recovery after autologous or allogeneic bone marrow transplantation
Improve neutrophil production in patients with delayed engraftment or graft failure after autologous or allogeneic bone marrow transplantation

is approved for clinical use by the US Food and Drug Administration (FDA) (Table 3-3). The sequence of sargramostim differs from that of native GM-CSF by a single amino acid substitution at position 23.

Clinical use of G-CSF and GM-CSF
Prevention of chemotherapy-induced febrile neutropenia

Febrile neutropenia represents the major dose-limiting toxicity of cancer chemotherapy and is associated with considerable morbidity, mortality, and costs. The main uses of G-CSF and GM-CSF are for the prevention of febrile neutropenia in patients receiving cancer chemotherapy. G-CSF is used predominantly, based on results of randomized controlled trials, clinical guidelines, and FDA-approved indications. The original FDA approval of G-CSF for prevention of febrile neutropenia was based on 2 randomized controlled trials in patients with small-cell lung cancer. The patients in these trials received combination chemotherapy causing severe neutropenia that lasted for an average of 6 days. Treatment with G-CSF reduced the duration of severe neutropenia to approximately 3 days and reduced the occurrence of febrile neutropenia (temperature >38.3°C with neutrophils <0.5 × 10^9/L) and infections by approximately 50%. Other controlled trials have demonstrated a similar effect with G-CSF started in the first chemotherapy cycle within the first 3 days after chemotherapy and continued for up to 10 days (primary prophylaxis). If G-CSF treatment is further delayed, for example, until patients develop neutropenia (secondary prophylaxis), it is ineffective or far less effective. Although all individual studies are too small to demonstrate an effect of G-CSF on survival, a meta-analysis combining the results of randomized trials has demonstrated a reduction in infection-related and all-cause mortality. It has also been demonstrated that G-CSF will allow a greater percentage of patients to receive full courses of standard-dose chemotherapy on schedule through avoidance of neutropenia and febrile neutropenia and preemptive dose reductions to avoid these complications. Some data now suggest a benefit of G-CSF to improve long-term outcomes through maintenance of chemotherapy doses and schedules. However, additional studies of long-term outcomes are needed to determine the consistency and magnitude of this effect.

Pegfilgrastim for prevention of febrile neutropenia

A phase III, double-blind, placebo-controlled clinical trial of primary prophylaxis with pegfilgrastim was conducted in patients with breast cancer receiving docetaxel 100 mg/m^2 every 3 weeks to determine the efficacy of pegfilgrastim when given with less myelosuppressive regimens. Patients were randomly assigned to pegfilgrastim 6 mg or placebo on the day following chemotherapy. Patients in the pegfilgrastim arm experienced significantly lower incidence of febrile neutropenia (1% vs 17%), hospitalizations (1% vs 14%), and anti-infective use (2% vs 10%; all $P < .001$).

Pegfilgrastim is FDA approved to reduce the risk of febrile neutropenia in patients undergoing chemotherapy (Table 3-2). Based on the prolonged half-life of pegfilgrastim, it has been recommended that chemotherapy not be given sooner than 14 days after a dose of pegfilgrastim. The safety profile of pegfilgrastim is otherwise similar to that of other forms of G-CSF.

GM-CSF for prevention of febrile neutropenia

The use of GM-CSF to prevent chemotherapy-induced febrile neutropenia is now relatively uncommon. GM-CSF is not FDA approved for this indication except to reduce the risk of death from infections in patient >55 years old undergoing induction therapy for acute myeloid leukemia (Table 3-3).

Clinical guidelines for the use of the myeloid growth factors

The American Society of Clinical Oncology (ASCO), the National Comprehensive Cancer Network (NCCN), and other organizations have developed guidelines for the use of use of myeloid growth factors to prevent febrile neutropenia.

In brief, current ASCO guidelines (Table 3-4) include the following:

1. Primary prophylaxis is recommended for patients at high risk (>20%) of febrile neutropenia due to age, medical history, disease characteristics, or the myelotoxicity of the chemotherapy regimen.

Table 3-4 ASCO guidelines.

Setting/indication	Recommended	Not recommended
General circumstance	Febrile neutropenia risk in the range of 20% or higher	
Special circumstances	Clinical factors dictate use	
Secondary prophylaxis	Based on chemotherapy reaction among other factors	
Therapy of afebrile neutropenia		Not to be used routinely
Therapy of febrile neutropenia	If high risk for complications or poor clinical outcomes	Not to be used routinely as adjunctive treatment with antibiotic therapy
Acute myeloid leukemia	After induction therapy, patients >55 years old most likely to benefit	Not to be used for priming effects
	After the completion of consolidation chemotherapy	
Myelodysplastic syndrome		Intermittent administration for a subset of patients with severe neutropenia and recurrent infection
Acute lymphocytic leukemia	After the completion of initial chemotherapy of first postremission course	
Radiotherapy	Consider if receiving radiation therapy alone and prolonged delays are expected	Avoid in patients receiving concomitant chemotherapy and radiation therapy
Older patients	If >65 years old with diffuse aggressive lymphoma and treated with curative chemotherapy	
Pediatric populations	For the primary prophylaxis of pediatric patients with a likelihood of febrile neutropenia and the secondary prophylaxis or therapy for high-risk patients	G-CSF use in children with ALL should be considered carefully

2. Primary prophylaxis should be given with "dose-dense" chemotherapy regimens.
3. Secondary prophylaxis after a neutropenia-related event has occurred is generally recommended if reduced dosing or dose-intensity will compromise disease-free or overall survival or expected treatment outcome.

The NCCN guidelines recommend the following:

1. Primary prophylaxis is recommended for patients in whom the expected risk of febrile neutropenia is >20% when treatment is given with a curative intent, to prolong survival, to maintain quality of life, or to avoid symptoms and complications associated with febrile neutropenia.
2. Myeloid growth factor support is not recommended for patients for whom the risk of febrile neutropenia is <10%. Use for the 10% to 20% risk group is to be considered based on patient-specific factors, disease-related factors, and the specifics of the chemotherapy regimen.

Specific factors predisposing to febrile neutropenia and serving as current indications for considering use of myeloid growth factors are listed in Table 3-5.

Febrile neutropenia

All patients with febrile neutropenia should be treated empirically with antibiotics, after a thorough physical examination directed at identifying a site of infection and after appropriate cultures are obtained. A number of studies have addressed whether patients with febrile neutropenia benefit from initiation of a myeloid growth factor in addition to broad-spectrum antibiotics. A meta-analysis of 13 randomized clinical trials compared the use of G-CSF or GM-CSF plus antibiotics to the use of antibiotics alone in patients with chemotherapy-induced febrile neutropenia. The meta-analysis showed that the use of a myeloid growth factor accelerated the time to neutrophil recovery and shortened hospital stay but did not affect overall survival. ASCO guidelines recommend that the myeloid growth factors should not be routinely used as adjuncts to antibiotics for patients with febrile neutropenia. These guidelines recommend that the myeloid growth factors should be considered for patients expected to have prolonged (>10 days) and profound neutropenia (<0.1×10^9/L); use should also be considered for those over age 65 with pneumonia, hypotension, invasive fungal infections, or sepsis.

Acute myelogenous leukemia

Neutropenia, anemia, and thrombocytopenia are common presenting features of acute myelogenous leukemia (AML) and also important complications in its treatment. There are many studies of the use of myeloid growth factors to sensitize leukemic cells to increase the effectiveness of chemotherapy and to prevent infectious complications. Although G-CSF and GM-CSF may shorten the duration of neutropenia during the induction phase of chemotherapy, neither consistently reduces the occurrence of febrile neutropenia or infections or the duration of hospitalization. Results for sensitization of the leukemic cells to chemotherapy are also inconsistent, and use of the myeloid growth factors in this way is not recommended except for research studies.

During the consolidation phase of treatment, the marrow is more responsive, and 2 large randomized trials have demonstrated significant decreases in the duration of severe neutropenia with an associated decrease in infections requiring antibiotics with G-CSF therapy. No consistent favorable impact of G-CSF or GM-CSF on treatment response and survival has been observed.

Acute lymphoblastic leukemia

Neutropenia is a common consequence of treatment in patients with acute lymphoblastic leukemia (ALL). Eight randomized control trials including more than 700 adults and children demonstrated that neutrophil recovery is accelerated with myeloid growth factor therapy mostly using G-CSF. No consistent therapeutic benefits in reducing infections, shortening hospitalizations, or improving the overall treatment outcomes were observed.

Mobilization of autologous peripheral blood stem cells and enhancement of neutrophil recovery after transplantation

Autologous peripheral blood stem cells are now routinely collected from cancer patients by leukapheresis after cytoreductive chemotherapy or after cytoreductive chemotherapy followed by G-CSF or GM-CSF. Mobilization with G-CSF has been demonstrated to involve several steps. First, G-CSF markedly enhances neutrophil production. G-CSF administration also releases neutrophil elastase and

Table 3-5 Risk factors for febrile neutropenia.

Age >65 years
Previous chemotherapy or radiation therapy
Bone marrow involvement of tumor
Preexisting neutropenia, infections, open wounds, or recent surgery
Poor performance status
Decreased renal function
Decreased liver function, particularly increased bilirubin level

Adapted from NCCN Clinical Practice Guidelines (see Crawford J, Armitage J, Balducci L, et al. Myeloid growth factors. *J Natl Compr Canc Netw.* 2009;7:64–83).

cathepsin G from the granules of the developing marrow neutrophils. When released, these proteases cleave adhesion molecules expressed on the surfaces of the marrow stromal cells. Cleavage of the bond of chemokine receptor-4 (CXCR4), expressed on hematopoietic progenitor cells, and its ligand chemokine ligand 12 (CXCL12; also known as stromal-derived factor 1 [SDF1]), expressed on marrow stromal cells, is thought to be the principal the principal mechanism for progenitor cell release into the circulation.

As discussed in Chapter 12, transplantation of autologous peripheral blood stem cells results in marrow engraftment after myeloablative therapy. Clinical trials of autologous peripheral blood stem cell transplantation have shown that the use of a myeloid cytokine after stem cell infusion accelerates neutrophil recovery by 2 to 4 days. However, neutrophil recovery to $>0.5 \times 10^9$/L is so rapid (median, 11–14 days) without a myeloid growth factor that it has been difficult to demonstrate a meaningful clinical benefit of G-CSF or GM-CSF, including reduced risk of sepsis or death due to infection in patients receiving a peripheral blood stem cell product. Recent studies have shown that a CXCR4 antagonist called AMD3100 (also called plerixafor) acts synergistically with G-CSF to yield greater numbers of CD34$^+$ stem cells. AMD3100 is now FDA approved as an adjunct to G-CSF for stem cell mobilization in certain conditions, particularly in patients who are expected to mobilize poorly with G-CSF alone.

Mobilization of peripheral blood stem cells from normal donors for allogeneic transplantation

G-CSF treatment of normal donors effectively mobilizes stem cells for use in subsequent allogeneic transplantation and has an excellent safety profile.

Acceleration of neutrophil recovery after bone marrow transplantation

Currently, most transplantation programs use peripheral blood stem cells in preference to bone marrow because of the ease of collection of peripheral blood stem cells and their more rapid neutrophil and platelet engraftment. When bone marrow transplantation is performed, a myeloid growth factor after bone marrow stem cell infusion significantly accelerates neutrophil recovery. In a pivotal study, patients undergoing autologous bone marrow transplantation for lymphoid malignancy were randomized to GM-CSF versus placebo after marrow infusion. Neutrophils recovered to 0.5×10^9/L faster with GM-CSF. G-CSF had a similar effect. A meta-analysis of 18 clinical trials totaling 1198 patients showed no change in the risk of acute or chronic graft-versus-host disease after allogeneic stem cell transplantation with either GM-CSF or G-CSF, compared with patients who did not receive a myeloid growth factor.

Improvement of neutrophil production in patients with delayed engraftment or graft failure after bone marrow transplantation

Patients who do not achieve a neutrophil count of 0.1×10^9/L by day 21 after transplantation or whose neutrophil counts drop below 0.5×10^9/L after engraftment often respond to a myeloid growth factor with improvement in neutrophil production.

Severe chronic neutropenia (idiopathic, cyclic, congenital)

Severe chronic neutropenia is a heterogeneous group of inherited and acquired disorders characterized by a persistent neutrophil count of $<0.5 \times 10^9$/L and recurrent bacterial infections. Recently, the genetic and molecular causes for the inherited forms of severe chronic neutropenia have been discovered. Kostmann syndrome, autosomal recessive severe congenital neutropenia, is due to mutations in the *HAX1* gene, which encodes the HCLS1-associated protein X-1. It is usually diagnosed in an infant from a consanguineous marriage. The child will have a neutrophil count of $<0.2 \times 10^9$/L, an arrest in myeloid maturation at the promyelocyte–myelocyte stage in the marrow, and recurrent infections. Sporadic and autosomal dominant severe congenital neutropenia is a similar and more common condition and usually attributable to mutations in the gene for neutrophil elastase, the *ELA2* or *ELANE* gene. Mutations in *G6PC3*, the gene encoding glucose-6-phosphatase, catalytic subunit 3; *WAS*, the gene for the Wiscott-Aldrich protein; and, rarely, the gene for the G-CSF receptor (*G-CSFR* or CD114) may have a similar clinical phenotype. Cyclic neutropenia is another form of congenital neutropenia. These patients have neutrophil counts that oscillate on a 21-day cycle and have recurrent tissue infections during the periods of neutropenia. Cyclic neutropenia is also due to mutations in the narrow portion of the *ELA2* gene. Laboratory and clinical studies suggested that the neutropenia in all of these conditions is attributable to accelerated apoptosis of neutrophil precursors in the marrow.

Most patients with congenital and cyclic neutropenia respond well to treatment with G-CSF. Treatment significantly improves neutrophil counts, dramatically decreases the incidence and severity of bacterial infections, and appears to improve survival. Responses can be maintained over many years with daily or alternate-day G-CSF. Patients with cyclic neutropenia maintained on G-CSF continue to have regular fluctuations in the neutrophil count, but the depth of the nadir is less and lasts for fewer days. Patients with severe congenital neutropenia attributable to mutations in *ELANE*, *HAX1*, or *WAS* or to as yet unknown mutations are at risk of developing AML. The lifetime risk is estimated to be as high as 30%. In contrast, there is no apparent risk of AML in patients with cyclic neutropenia.

The Severe Chronic Neutropenia International Registry is a useful source for additional information about the diagnosis and treatment of severe chronic neutropenia (http://depts.washington.edu/registry/).

Myelodysplasia

Myelodysplasia is an acquired neoplastic hematopoietic stem cell disorder. Ineffective hematopoiesis results in decreased production of mature neutrophils, red blood cells, and platelets; the neutrophils and platelets often have functional defects that further impair their ability to ward off bacterial infection or staunch bleeding. A number of clinical trials have investigated treatment of myelodysplasia with the HGFs. Treatment with G-CSF or GM-CSF can normalize the neutrophil count in most patients with myelodysplasia, but whether this translates into reduced mortality from bacterial or fungal infection is less clear. G-CSF or GM-CSF appears to enhance the effects of erythropoietin in the treatment of anemia and myelodysplastic patients. There is no convincing evidence at present that growth factor therapy accelerates progression from myelodysplasia to AML.

Other potential clinical uses of G-CSF
Human immunodeficiency virus

Neutropenia is common in advanced human immunodeficiency virus (HIV) infection. This complication was far more common before the availability of the highly effective antiviral drugs for this disease. Treatment with G-CSF promptly increases the neutrophil count to the normal range in most patients. A large, randomized, multicenter trial in HIV-positive patients with a low CD4 count (0.2×10^9/L) and ANC (0.75–1.0×10^9/L) showed that G-CSF–treated patients (dose adjusted to increase the ANC to 2.0-10.0×10^9/L) had fewer bacterial infections, less antibiotic use, and fewer hospital days, but no change in viral load, compared with the control group.

Leukapheresis

Large numbers of neutrophils can be collected by leukapheresis from normal donors pretreated with G-CSF plus dexamethasone, and these neutrophils exhibit normal function in vitro. Transfusion of G-CSF–stimulated neutrophil leukapheresis products into severely neutropenic stem cell transplantation recipients can transiently increase the peripheral neutrophil count to the normal range ($<2.0 \times 10^9$/L). Whether neutrophil transfusions will increase survival in patients with profound sustained neutropenia who have an active bacterial or fungal infection is under investigation.

Diabetes

A recent meta-analysis summarized the potential benefits of G-CSF as an adjunctive therapy for the treatment of diabetic foot infections. Based on an analysis of 5 trials with a total of 167 patients, this review showed that G-CSF did not significantly affect the likelihood of resolution of the infection or wound healing but its use was associated with significantly reduced likelihood of lower extremity surgical interventions including amputation. G-CSF treatment appears to reduce the duration of hospital stay but not the duration of systemic antibiotic treatment. The evidence suggests benefit, but it is unclear exactly which patients will be helped by adjunctive G-CSF.

Pneumonia

A number of clinical trials have explored the use of G-CSF in nonneutropenic adults with community-acquired pneumonia or hospital-acquired pneumonia. In an evidence-based review, 6 studies with a total of 1984 people were identified. G-CSF use appeared to be safe, with no increase in the incidence of serious adverse events. However, the use of G-CSF was not associated with improvement in mortality at 28 days.

Myocardial infarction

Studies have suggested that G-CSF–mobilized stem cells may improve cardiac function after myocardial infarction, presumably by stimulating angiogenesis. In one small prospective clinical study, G-CSF therapy with intracoronary infusion of peripheral blood stem cells showed improved cardiac function and promoted angiogenesis in patients with myocardial infarction. However, aggravation of in-stent restenosis led to early termination of the study. Although studies such as these are intriguing for utilization of G-CSF–mobilized stem cells for a variety of new applications, no conclusive evidence exists at present supporting these applications.

Adverse effects of G-CSF

The major adverse effect of G-CSF is bone pain in the hips, which usually coincides with marrow recovery and may be due to expansion of hematopoiesis within the marrow cavity. Medullary bone pain occurs in approximately 30% of patients treated with G-CSF, and osteoporosis has been observed in some patients administered G-CSF. Other adverse effects of G-CSF include headache and fatigue. G-CSF should not be used in patients with sickle cell disease; case reports document precipitation of sickling and severe pain crisis in these individuals. Other rare adverse effects include splenic rupture and adult respiratory distress syndrome.

Adverse effects of GM-CSF

The major adverse effect of GM-CSF is a flu-like illness characterized by fever (22% of patients) and myalgias and arthralgias (15%). A fraction of patients treated with GM-CSF experience fluid retention (8%) or dyspnea (13%). GM-CSF should not be used concurrently with chemoradiotherapy. A case report details abrupt onset of sickle cell pain crisis in a patient who received GM-CSF injections around a chronic leg ulcer.

Risk of leukemia with G-CSF and GM-CSF

Because G-CSF and GM-CSF can stimulate proliferation of leukemic blasts, there have been concerns that these agents might cause leukemia. At present, there is no convincing evidence that treatment outcomes for AML are worsened by myeloid growth factor treatments used in conjunction with appropriate chemotherapy. In patients receiving myelotoxic chemotherapy agents for other types of cancer, there is a significant risk of secondary leukemias. This risk probably is directly related to specific leukemogenic chemotherapy agents and regimens. Recent analysis of data from randomized trials suggests that the risk of AML may be increased in those receiving chemotherapy supported by the myeloid growth factors, but the interpretation of the results is made difficult by the observation that patients treated with myeloid growth factor usually receive larger doses and longer courses of chemotherapy.

New versions of G-CSF and GM-CSF

Because of the potency and effectiveness of G-CSF and GM-CSF, there have been many efforts to identify additional myeloid growth factors and to make new derivatives from the parent molecules. Several new products with a prolonged duration of their stimulatory effects, similar to pegylated G-CSF, are in development. A key issue is whether or not the new molecules are immunogenic. The development of antibodies to a growth factor can be hazardous because they can block the activity of the administered drug and also neutralize the effects of the naturally produced, endogenous growth factors, thus worsening neutropenia.

The number of laboratories and biopharmaceutical companies producing myeloid growth factors is also increasing rapidly. Their products are molecularly similar to the approved products and are called "biosimilars." Testing and introduction of biosimilars is proceeding rapidly.

Erythroid growth factors

Erythropoietin (epoetin alfa)

Erythropoietin is a glycoprotein that stimulates red blood cell production. Mice engineered to lack the erythropoietin gene die in utero with severe anemia. Early and late erythroid colony-forming cells (burst-forming unit–erythroid [BFU-E] and colony-forming unit–erythroid [CFU-E]) are present in these mice, indicating that commitment to the erythroid lineage does not require erythropoietin, but CFU-E proliferation and terminal maturation into red blood cells are dependent on erythropoietin. Mutations in the genes encoding for the erythropoietin receptor or for molecules involved in the regulation of erythropoietin production have been identified in some cases of familial polycythemia.

During adult life, erythropoietin is made predominantly in the kidney with a smaller component produced in the liver. Production of erythropoietin is increased by hypoxia and diminished by polycythemia. Erythropoietin circulates in the blood at levels measurable by a clinically available enzyme-linked immunosorbent assay (ELISA). Erythropoietin acts by binding to high-affinity receptors expressed on erythroid progenitor cells. Activation of signaling cascades downstream of the receptor stimulates survival, proliferation, and differentiation of erythroid precursors. Erythropoietin also binds to neural cells, including astrocytes, and to endothelial cells.

Epoetin alfa is a recombinant form of erythropoietin (rhEPO) that is produced by a mammalian cell line into which the human erythropoietin gene has been introduced. It contains the identical amino acid sequence of the native compound and is FDA approved for use in the United States for a number of indications (Table 3-6).

Chronic renal failure

The anemia of chronic renal failure is a normocytic, normochromic anemia with underproduction of red blood cells primarily due to inadequate erythropoietin production by the diseased kidneys. Erythropoietin deficiency can be seen with creatinine values of ≥ 2 mg/dL, and as renal function declines, the likelihood of anemia increases. Erythropoietin treatment causes a marked improvement in hemoglobin and hematocrit levels, a reduction in transfusion requirement, improved quality of life, and increased exercise capacity. Epoetin alfa doses of approximately 100 to 150 U/kg body weight 3 times per week are usually required.

Table 3-6 FDA-approved indications for epoetin alfa.

Anemia of chronic renal failure, both predialysis and dialysis patients
Anemia associated with zidovudine treatment in HIV-positive patients
Chemotherapy-induced anemia
To reduce the need for allogeneic transfusion in patients undergoing elective noncardiac nonvascular surgery

ASCO/American Society of Hematology guideline recommendations for erythropoietin

For patients with chemotherapy-associated anemia, the Committee continues to recommend initiating an erythropoiesis-stimulating agent (ESA) as hemoglobin (Hb) approaches or falls below 10 g/dL, to increase Hb and decrease transfusions. ESA treatment continues to be recommended for patients with low-risk myelodysplasia for similar reasons. There is no evidence showing increased survival as a result of ESA treatment. Conclusive evidence is lacking that, absent clinical circumstances necessitating earlier treatment, initiating ESAs at Hb levels greater than 10 g/dL either spares more patients from transfusion or substantially improves their quality of life. Starting doses and dose modifications based on response or lack thereof should follow the package insert. Continuing ESAs beyond 6 to 8 weeks in the absence of response, assuming appropriate dose increase has been attempted in non-responders as per US Food and Drug Administration guidelines, does not seem to be beneficial, and ESA therapy should be discontinued. The Committee recommends monitoring iron stores and supplementing iron intake for ESA-treated patients. ESAs should be used cautiously with chemotherapy, or in clinical states, associated with elevated risk for thromboembolic complications. The Committee also cautions against ESA use for patients with cancer who are not receiving chemotherapy, since recent trials report increased thromboembolic risks and decreased survival under these circumstances.

Other uses of epoetin alfa

Two strategies use epoetin alfa to reduce the need for allogeneic red blood cell transfusion in elective orthopedic surgery: preoperative use of epoetin alfa to increase the hematocrit and preoperative use of epoetin alfa to facilitate autologous blood donation. In one study, patients were randomized to 15 days of treatment with epoetin alfa or placebo, starting 10 days before elective hip or knee surgery. The use of epoetin alfa reduced the proportion of patients receiving allogeneic red blood cell transfusions and the number of units transfused. The greatest benefit was in the patients who had anemia (hemoglobin, 10-13 g/dL) at the first preoperative visit. These mildly anemic patients had a 13% chance of allogeneic transfusion if treated with epoetin alfa and a 45% chance of allogeneic transfusion if treated with placebo. For patients who had an initial hemoglobin of >13 g/dL, the risk of allogeneic transfusion was low and not statistically different in the epoetin alfa and the placebo groups. Weekly epoetin alfa (600 U/kg) is as effective as a lower dose of daily epoetin alfa. Orthopedic surgery patients are at risk for deep venous thrombosis, and epoetin alfa therapy, particularly in patients with an initial hemoglobin >13 g/dL, may increase the risk of thrombosis compared with placebo-treated patients.

An alternative approach is to use epoetin alfa to facilitate autologous blood donation. Most patients who have a normal hematocrit can donate enough units of red blood cells to avoid allogeneic transfusion. However, having a low hematocrit at the first preoperative visit or a small body size are risk factors for requiring allogeneic transfusion. One study randomized patients with mild anemia (hematocrit <39%) to treatment with epoetin alfa versus placebo. The epoetin alfa–treated patients donated an average of 4.5 units of red blood cells, and the placebo-treated patients donated 3 units of red blood cells. Thus, epoetin alfa increased the number of units donated and diminished the usual decrease in hematocrit from autologous donation. However, a national survey of orthopedic surgeons in the United States revealed that approximately 45% of autologous units donated before elective surgery were not used. This substantially increases the cost per autologous unit transfused. Additionally, a very low risk of bacterial contamination or clerical error attends the use of autologous blood, just as with allogeneic blood. Whether a patient is treated with epoetin alfa alone or epoetin alfa to facilitate autologous donation, it is essential to provide iron supplementation to keep the ferritin ≥100 ng/dL and the transferrin saturation ≥20% to optimize the erythropoietic response.

Epoetin alfa treatment should be considered preoperatively in Jehovah's Witnesses or other individuals who will not accept transfusion. Critically ill patients in the intensive care unit have serum erythropoietin levels that are inappropriately low for their degree of anemia. Randomized clinical trials showed that epoetin alfa treatment increased the reticulocyte count and decreased the number of red blood cell transfusions compared with placebo-treated patients with a similar Acute Physiologic and Chronic Health Evaluation II (APACHE II) score. However, there was no difference in mortality in the 2 groups, and epoetin alfa is more expensive than transfusions in this setting.

Sustained anemia of any etiology can cause congestive heart failure. An intriguing small study randomized patients with severe congestive heart failure and anemia to treatment with epoetin alfa (to increase the hemoglobin to 12.5 g/dL) or placebo. Epoetin alfa treatment resulted in a marked improvement in New York Heart Association functional class and a modest improvement in left ventricular ejection fraction. These findings need to be tested in a larger double-blind randomized clinical trial. Epoetin alfa has also been used to enhance athletic performance in endurance sports, such as bicycling; this use of epoetin alfa is dangerous, unethical, and banned by the International Olympic Committee. Preclinical studies suggest that epoetin alfa may cross the blood–brain barrier and be neuroprotective after a stroke; this is an area of active research.

Adverse effects associated with the use of erythropoietin

The main adverse effect of rhEPO is its potential to exacerbate hypertension in patients with chronic renal failure. The cause of rhEPO–related hypertension is not well understood. Hypertension is not seen in patients with normal renal function receiving rhEPO for other indications. Pure red cell aplasia (PRCA) due to the development of antierythropoietin antibodies has been described predominantly in patients with chronic renal failure but is extremely rare.

An increased risk of venous thromboembolic complications has been observed in cancer patients receiving erythropoiesis-stimulating agents (ESAs), along with recent evidence from some clinical trials of an increased risk of early mortality. As noted earlier, concerns regarding tumor progression with the use of epoetin alfa arose when the results of 2 randomized clinical trials, one involving patients with head and neck cancer undergoing radiotherapy and the other in women with metastatic breast cancer receiving first-line chemotherapy, were reported. In the head and neck trial, an increased rate of locoregional progression was noted in the epoetin alfa–treated arm. In the metastatic breast cancer trial, use of epoetin alfa to maintain a high hemoglobin target in patients, most of whom did not have anemia at the start of treatment, was associated with decreased survival.

Darbepoetin alfa

Darbepoetin alfa is an erythropoiesis-stimulating protein, structurally related to erythropoietin (Figure 3-1), also produced by recombinant DNA technology. However, it has 5 N-linked oligosaccharide chains, whereas erythropoietin has 3 chains attached to the molecule peptide backbone, and as a result, darbepoetin alfa has a higher molecular weight than erythropoietin and a 3-fold longer half-life in vivo. It binds to the same receptor as erythropoietin, so its biologic activities are similar.

The advantage of darbepoetin alfa is that it can be administered less frequently than erythropoietin to achieve the same increment in hematocrit. Darbepoetin alfa is FDA approved for use in patients with anemia of chronic renal failure and for treatment of chemotherapy-induced anemia in patients with nonmyeloid malignancies.

Darbepoetin alfa for chronic renal failure

In dialysis patients, darbepoetin alfa effectively maintains the hemoglobin in the target range established by the National Kidney Foundation guidelines. The recommended starting dose of darbepoetin alfa is 0.45 µg/kg administered as a single subcutaneous or intravenous injection once weekly; doses

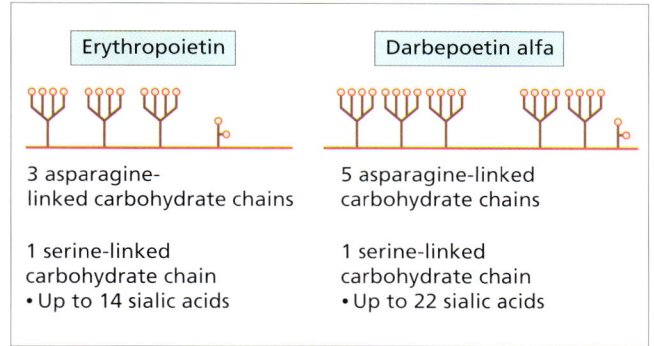

Figure 3-1 Like erythropoietin, darbepoetin alfa is a 165–amino acid polypeptide. However, 5 amino acids have been altered to permit the attachment of 2 additional carbohydrate side chains. This modification prolongs the half-life in vivo.

should be titrated not to exceed a target hemoglobin concentration of 12 g/dL.

In predialysis patients with anemia due to chronic renal insufficiency, darbepoetin alfa administered as infrequently as once every 2 to 4 weeks maintains the hemoglobin in the target range. Recently, PRCA associated with neutralizing antibodies to erythropoietin has been reported in patients treated with darbepoetin alfa.

The same safety concerns mentioned earlier for epoetin alpha apply to darbepoetin alpha.

Darbepoetin alfa for anemia associated with chemotherapy

Phase III clinical trials in patients receiving chemotherapy for lung cancer show that darbepoetin alfa given once per week maintains the hemoglobin, reduces the need for red blood cell transfusion, and improves quality of life (assessed by the Functional Assessment of Cancer Therapy–Fatigue scale), compared with placebo-treated patients. Darbepoetin alfa is effective when given once per week, once every 2 weeks, once every 3 weeks, or once every 4 weeks. Thus, darbepoetin alfa can be administered once per chemotherapy cycle. The recommended starting dose is 2.25 µg/kg weekly or 500 µg every 3 weeks, given as a subcutaneous injection.

Other uses of darbepoetin alfa

A clinical trial in congestive heart failure patients is examining whether long-term treatment with darbepoetin alfa to increase the hemoglobin will result in better exercise tolerance. Other studies focus on the use of darbepoetin alfa in HIV-positive patients with anemia. Darbepoetin is being evaluated in patients with myelodysplasia at different dose levels, with responses that are comparable to those achieved by epoetin alfa.

Adverse effects associated with the use of darbepoetin alfa

Darbepoetin alfa has essentially the same safety profile as epoetin alfa with the same concerns expressed regarding an increased mortality seen in some of the randomized controlled trials (see earlier section on adverse effects of epoetin alfa). An individual patient data meta-analysis of 6 randomized controlled trials of darbepoetin alfa versus placebo in patients with chemotherapy-induced anemia found an increased risk of thromboembolic complications but no increased risk of death (hazard ratio [HR] = 0.97; 95% confidence interval [CI], 0.85–1.10) or disease progression (HR = 0.93; 95% CI, 0.84–1.04).

Platelet growth factors

Thrombopoietin

Thrombopoietin (TPO) is the primary regulator of platelet production. Mice engineered to lack either TPO or its receptor Mpl have platelet counts that are approximately 10% to 15% of normal values and have a normal hematocrit and white blood cells (WBCs). The numbers of hematopoietic progenitor cells and stem cells are reduced by 50% to 90% in these mice, indicating that TPO also acts directly and/or indirectly at the progenitor cell and stem cell level. TPO enhances stem cell survival, colony-forming unit–megakaryocyte (CFU-Meg) proliferation, and megakaryocyte nuclear endo-reduplication and maturation and modestly potentiates platelet activation in the presence of other platelet activators. Mutations in Mpl cause a rare pediatric disorder, congenital amegakaryocytic thrombocytopenia. These children present with severe thrombocytopenia and virtually absent megakaryocytes and progress to pancytopenia. Conversely, specific mutations in the 5′ region of the TPO gene result in overproduction of TPO and are a cause of familial thrombocythemia.

The liver is the primary site of TPO production in vivo, although TPO is also made by bone marrow microenvironmental cells. TPO is constitutively produced and circulates in the blood at measurable levels. Platelets and megakaryocytes bind, internalize, and degrade TPO, and thus regulate the quantity of TPO in the circulation. When platelet counts are high, TPO levels are usually low. Conversely, in diseases in which there is reduced platelet production such as aplastic anemia, TPO levels are high. Immune thrombocytopenic purpura (ITP) is characterized by increased platelet turnover. In ITP, TPO levels are not markedly elevated, likely because of binding and degradation of TPO by the expanded number of megakaryocytes in the marrow or by immune destruction of platelet precursors.

The effect of TPO is mediated through the TPO receptor on megakaryocytes and platelets, with TPO levels regulated mostly by the quantity of receptors available for binding. After the unfortunate experience with a previous recombinant TPO with the development of cross-reacting antibodies resulting in severe thrombocytopenia, TPO agonists have been developed with no sequence homology with endogenous TPO. The new products include TPO peptide mimetics, nonpeptide mimetics, and agonist antibodies. Romiplostim is a peptide mimetic representing a recombinant fusion protein with 2 identical subunits, each with 2 TPO binding domains and covalently bound to the Fc domain of a human immunoglobulin G molecule.

Romiplostim was the first TPO receptor agonist to receive approval by the US FDA based on thrombocytopenia in patients with ITP with poor response to corticosteroids, immunoglobulins, or splenectomy. Approval was based on durable platelet response in 2 phase III double-blind, randomized, placebo-controlled trials in patients receiving at least one prior treatment for ITP. There was no significant increase in serious adverse events reported in the romiplostim arm, and most adverse events were mild to moderate. Data from these trials have also shown that romiplostim is associated with significant improvements in patient-reported quality of life. Although no neutralizing antibodies to TPO were found, FDA approval was accompanied by considerable pharmacovigilance, including a Risk Evaluation and Mitigation Strategy (REMS). Reticulin formation was found in 10 patients but with no progression to marrow fibrosis in the 2 phase III studies. Severe thrombocytopenia was reported in 4 patients after discontinuation of romiplostim, which resolved in 2 weeks.

Eltrombopag is an orally administered, small-molecule agonist of the TPO receptor. It selectively binds the transmembrane domain of the receptor on platelets, megakaryocytes, and their precursors. It acts via the Janus kinase/signal transducers and activators of transcription (JAK/STAT) pathway to stimulate megakaryocyte proliferation and differentiation. It was approved by the FDA based on randomized, double-blind, placebo-controlled, multicenter phase II and III trials. After 6 weeks, eltrombopag at 50 mg/d significantly improved platelet counts in the majority of patients, and the proportion achieving a platelet count >200,000/μL was approximately 8-fold higher than with the placebo. Eltrombopag was well tolerated, and the adverse events were not significantly different for the drug and placebo in the pivotal trial.

Eltrombopag is FDA approved for the treatment of thrombocytopenia in patients with chronic immune (idiopathic) thrombocytopenic purpura who have had an insufficient response to corticosteroids, immunoglobulins, or splenectomy. It should be used only in patients whose degree of thrombocytopenia and clinical condition increase the risk for bleeding. It should not be used in an attempt to normalize platelet counts.

Currently the best strategy for treatment of ITP and other causes of chronic thrombocytopenia are under review, and a number of clinical trials of these new agents and others are currently ongoing.

Chemotherapy-induced thrombocytopenia

Initial clinical trials of a TPO (recombinant TPO or pegylated megakaryocyte growth and development factor [Peg-MGDF]) focused on amelioration of chemotherapy-induced thrombocytopenia. Treatment with a TPO in patients undergoing outpatient chemotherapy for lung cancer, gynecologic malignancy, sarcoma, or other tumors increased the platelet count nadir and shortened the duration of thrombocytopenia. There was no evidence of platelet activation or excess thrombosis in the patients treated with a TPO. When used after myelosuppressive chemotherapy, such as induction chemotherapy for AML, treatment with a TPO did not shorten the duration of thrombocytopenia or diminish the number of platelet transfusions compared with placebo. Early trials of a TPO given after high-dose chemotherapy and stem cell transplantation have not shown clinically meaningful benefit. There are no data yet available on the potential role of eltrombopag and romiplostim for this indication, although clinical trials are under way.

Interleukin-11 (oprelvekin)

Interleukin-11 (IL-11) is a 178–amino acid nonglycosylated growth factor produced by marrow stromal cells. IL-11 is a member of the family of cytokines that use gp130 as the signaling component of the receptor. IL-11 promotes CFU-Meg growth and increases the size and ploidy of megakaryocytes, particularly in conjunction with other cytokines, and modestly increases the platelet count in vivo. It is unlikely that IL-11 plays a significant role in normal hematopoiesis because targeted disruption of the IL-11 receptor α-subunit in mice does not alter the WBC, hematocrit, platelet count, or ability of the mice to recover from myelosuppressive chemotherapy. Oprelvekin is a recombinant form of IL-11 expressed in *E coli* that differs from the native protein by deletion of one amino acid from the amino terminus.

Primary prevention of chemotherapy-induced thrombocytopenia

A randomized clinical trial examined oprelvekin use for primary prevention of chemotherapy-induced thrombocytopenia. In this trial, women with breast cancer treated with dose-intensive outpatient doxorubicin and cyclophosphamide chemotherapy with filgrastim support were randomized to receive oprelvekin 50 μg/kg/d subcutaneously for 10 to 17 days or placebo after each of the first 2 chemotherapy cycles. The oprelvekin-treated patients had a 68% chance of avoiding platelet transfusion, whereas the placebo-treated patients had a 41% chance of avoiding platelet transfusion. Oprelvekin treatment accelerated platelet recovery in subsequent cycles of chemotherapy, compared with placebo-treated patients. There was no difference in the duration of neutropenia in the oprelvekin and placebo groups. This trial demonstrated that oprelvekin is effective for primary prevention of chemotherapy-induced thrombocytopenia in patients receiving moderately dose-intensive chemotherapy (Table 3-7). Oprelvekin does not significantly enhance platelet recovery or decrease the need for platelet transfusions after autologous stem cell transplantation.

Secondary prevention of chemotherapy-induced thrombocytopenia

A multicenter randomized placebo-controlled clinical trial evaluated oprelvekin treatment in patients who had required a platelet transfusion during the prior cycle of chemotherapy. The majority of the patients had breast cancer or non-Hodgkin lymphoma, and all were receiving outpatient chemotherapy. The patients were randomized to receive oprelvekin or placebo daily for 14 to 21 days after chemotherapy. The oprelvekin-treated patients had a 30% chance of avoiding a platelet transfusion after the subsequent cycle of chemotherapy, whereas the placebo-treated patients had a 4% chance of avoiding a platelet transfusion. There was no difference in the duration of neutropenia or the number of red blood cell transfusions. The conclusion from this clinical trial was that oprelvekin treatment is effective for secondary prevention of platelet transfusion in patients who required a platelet transfusion after a prior cycle of chemotherapy.

Adverse effects of oprelvekin

In a phase I dose-escalation trial of oprelvekin, 16 women with breast cancer received oprelvekin for 14 days during the month prior to chemotherapy. Oprelvekin treatment in the absence of chemotherapy resulted in an approximate doubling of the platelet count. The hematocrit decreased by 20% within 2 to 3 days of starting oprelvekin. The anemia resolved 1 to 2 weeks after stopping the drug. Oprelvekin increases renal sodium reabsorption, resulting in a 20% increase in the plasma volume. Common symptoms include peripheral edema, shortness of breath, and occasionally exacerbation of preexisting pleural effusion. In one clinical trial, 10% of the oprelvekin-treated patients had transient atrial tachyarrhythmias, usually atrial

Table 3-7 FDA-approved indications for oprelvekin.

To prevent severe thrombocytopenia and reduce the need for platelet transfusion after myelosuppressive chemotherapy fibrillation or atrial flutter. Acute-phase proteins, including C-reactive protein and fibrinogen, increase during oprelvekin treatment. At higher dose levels, patients experience myalgias and arthralgias. Fever is not an adverse effect of oprelvekin.

Other HGFs

Stem cell factor (ancestim)

Stem cell factor is an HGF constitutively produced by endothelial cells and fibroblasts and in the testes and ovaries. Stem cell factor is normally present in both a transmembrane and a soluble form and is critical for normal hematopoiesis, mast cell production and function, melanocyte production, germ cell function, and gut motility. Absence of stem cell factor in mice (the *Sl* mutation) or lack of cell surface expression of its receptor Kit (the *W* mutation) results in intrauterine death due to severe anemia, demonstrating that stem cell factor plays a critical nonredundant role in hematopoiesis. Activating mutations in the cytoplasmic domain of Kit play a role in the biogenesis of systemic mastocytosis and gastrointestinal stromal tumors. There are no FDA-approved indications for this factor, but its effects have been studied extensively.

Mobilization of peripheral blood stem cells

Ancestim is a recombinant full-length soluble form of stem cell factor expressed in *E coli*. Ancestim is not FDA approved in the United States but is approved in Canada and Australia for use with G-CSF to enhance peripheral blood stem cell mobilization. Ancestim use in Australia is targeted for patients at risk for inadequate stem cell collection. In one study, patients with NHL or Hodgkin disease who had been extensively pretreated were randomized to receive G-CSF or G-CSF plus ancestim and then underwent leukapheresis. By day 5 of leukapheresis, 17% of the patients mobilized with G-CSF alone and 47% of the patients mobilized with G-CSF plus ancestim had achieved the $CD34^+$ cell collection target. Similarly, ancestim increased the yield of $CD34^+$ cells and decreased the number of leukaphereses when used together with G-CSF and mobilization chemotherapy.

Adverse effects of ancestim

Adverse effects after ancestim administration have included both local cutaneous reactions at the injection site and, rarely, systemic allergic (anaphylaxis-like) reactions. Melanocyte hyperplasia can occur at injection sites, resulting in pigmentation. Mast cell infiltration of the injection site may cause transient local edema with a ring of erythema. Ancestim promotes both mast cell production and activation, which is the likely cause of the occasional systemic allergic reaction (urticaria, pruritus, dyspnea, cough, hoarseness, and throat tightness). Premedications including inhaled albuterol, ranitidine, and either diphenhydramine or cetirizine are used with ancestim to decrease the risk of a systemic allergic reaction. Any patient with a systemic allergic reaction should not receive ancestim again.

Bibliography

Guidelines for the uses of the myeloid growth factors

Crawford J, Armitage J, Balducci L, et al. Myeloid growth factors. *J Natl Compr Canc Netw*. 2009;7:64–83.

Smith TJ, Khatcheressian J, Lyman GH, et al. 2006 update of recommendations for the use of white blood cell growth factors: an evidence-based clinical practice guideline. *J Clin Oncol*. 2006;24:187–205.

Prevention of chemotherapy-induced febrile neutropenia with G-CSF or GM-CSF

Crawford J, Ozer H, Stoller R, et al. Reduction by granulocyte colony-stimulating factor of fever and neutropenia induced by chemotherapy in patients with small-cell lung cancer. *N Engl J Med*. 1991;325:164–170.

Kuderer NM, Dale DC, Crawford J, Cosler LE, Lyman GH. Mortality, morbidity, and cost associated with febrile neutropenia in adult cancer patients. *Cancer*. 2006;106:2258–2266.

Kuderer NM, Dale DC, Crawford J, Lyman GH. Impact of primary prophylaxis with granulocyte colony-stimulating factor on febrile neutropenia and mortality in adult cancer patients receiving chemotherapy: a systematic review. *J Clin Oncol*. 2007;25:3158–3167.

Lyman GH. Impact of chemotherapy dose intensity on cancer patient outcomes. *J Natl Compr Canc Netw*. 2009;7:99–108.

Sung L, Nathan PC, Alibhai SM, Tomlinson GA, Beyene J. Meta-analysis: effect of prophylactic hematopoietic colony-stimulating factors on mortality and outcomes of infection. *Ann Intern Med*. 2007;147:400–411.

Sung L, Nathan PC, Lange B, Beyene J, Buchanan GR. Prophylactic granulocyte colony-stimulating factor and granulocyte-macrophage colony-stimulating factor decrease febrile neutropenia after chemotherapy in children with cancer: a meta-analysis of randomized controlled trials. *J Clin Oncol*. 2004;22:3350–3356.

Trillet-Lenoir V, Green J, Manegold C, et al. Recombinant granulocyte colony stimulating factor reduces the infectious complications of cytotoxic chemotherapy. *Eur J Cancer*. 1993;29A:319–324.

Wittman B, Horan J, Lyman GH. Prophylactic colony-stimulating factors in children receiving myelosuppressive chemotherapy: a meta-analysis of randomized controlled trials. *Cancer Treat Rev*. 2006;32:289–303.

Pegfilgrastim for prevention of febrile neutropenia

Green MD, Koelbl H, Baselga J, et al. A randomized double-blind multicenter phase III study of fixed-dose single-administration pegfilgrastim versus daily filgrastim in patients receiving myelosuppressive chemotherapy. *Ann Oncol*. 2003;14:29–35.

Holmes FA, O'Shaughnessy JA, Vukelja S, et al. Blinded, randomized, multicenter study to evaluate single administration pegfilgrastim once per cycle versus daily filgrastim as an adjunct to chemotherapy in patients with high-risk stage II or stage III/IV breast cancer. *J Clin Oncol*. 2002;20:727–731.

Skarlos DV, Timotheadou E, Galani E, et al. Pegfilgrastim administered on the same day with dose-dense adjuvant chemotherapy for breast cancer is associated with a higher incidence of febrile neutropenia as compared to conventional growth factor support: matched case-control study of the Hellenic Cooperative Oncology Group. *Oncology*. 2009;77: 107–112.

Vogel C, Wojtukiewicz M, Carroll R, et al. First and subsequent cycle use of pegfilgrastim prevents febrile neutropenia in patients with breast cancer: a multicenter, double-blind, placebo-controlled phase III study. *J Clin Oncol*. 2005;23: 1178–1184.

Vose JM, Crump M, Lazarus H, et al. Randomized, multicenter, open-label study of pegfilgrastim compared with daily filgrastim after chemotherapy for lymphoma. *J Clin Oncol*. 2003;21:514–519.

Whitworth JM, Matthews KS, Shipman KA, et al. The safety and efficacy of day 1 versus day 2 administration of pegfilgrastim in patients receiving myelosuppressive chemotherapy for gynecologic malignancies. *Gynecol Oncol*. 2009;112:601–604.

Treatment of chemotherapy-induced febrile neutropenia with G-CSF or GM-CSF

Clark OA, Lyman GH, Castro AA, Clark LG, Djulbegovic B. Colony-stimulating factors for chemotherapy-induced febrile neutropenia: a meta-analysis of randomized controlled trials. *J Clin Oncol*. 2005;23:4198–4214.

Acute myelogenous leukemia

Heil G, Hoelzer D, Sanz MA, et al. A randomized, double-blind, placebo-controlled, phase III study of filgrastim in remission induction and consolidation therapy for adults with de novo acute myeloid leukemia. The International Acute Myeloid Leukemia Study Group. *Blood*. 1997;90:4710–4718.

Löwenberg B, van Putten W, Theobald M, et al. Effect of priming with granulocyte colony-stimulating factor on the outcome of chemotherapy for acute myeloid leukemia. *N Engl J Med*. 2003;349:743–752.

Rowe JM, Andersen JW, Mazza JJ, et al. A randomized placebo-controlled phase III study of granulocyte-macrophage colony-stimulating factor in adult patients (>55–70 years of age) with acute myelogenous leukemia: a study of the Eastern Cooperative Oncology Group (E1490). *Blood*. 1995;86:457–462.

Stem cell mobilization

Anderlini P, Przepiorka D, Körbling M, Champlin R. Blood stem cell procurement: donor safety issues. *Bone Marrow Transplant*. 1998;21(suppl 3):S35–S39.

Anderlini P, Rizzo JD, Nugent ML, et al. Peripheral blood stem cell donation: an analysis from the International Bone Marrow Transplant Registry (IBMTR) and European Group for Blood and Marrow Transplant (EBMT) databases. *Bone Marrow Transplant*. 2001;27:689–692.

Bonig H, Chudziak D, Priestley G, Papayannopoulou T. Insights into the biology of mobilized hematopoietic stem/progenitor cells through innovative treatment schedules of the CXCR4 antagonist AMD3100. *Exp Hematol*. 2009;37:402–415.

DiPersio JF, Stadtmauer EA, Nademanee A, et al. Plerixafor and G-CSF versus placebo and G-CSF to mobilize hematopoietic stem cells for autologous stem cell transplantation in patients with multiple myeloma. *Blood*. 2009;113:5720–5726.

Kobbe G, Bruns I, Fenk R, Czibere A, Haas R. Pegfilgrastim for PBSC mobilization and autologous haematopoietic SCT. *Bone Marrow Transplant*. 2009;43:669–677.

Schmitz N, Linch DC, Dreger P, et al. Randomised trial of filgrastim-mobilized peripheral blood progenitor cell transplantation versus autologous bone-marrow transplantation in lymphoma patients. *Lancet*. 1996;347:353–357.

Vose JM, Ho AD, Coiffier B, et al. Advances in mobilization for the optimization of autologous stem cell transplantation. *Leuk Lymphoma*. 2009;50:1412–1421.

Willis F, Woll P, Theti D, et al. Pegfilgrastim for peripheral CD34+ mobilization in patients with solid tumours. *Bone Marrow Transplant*. 2009;43:927–934.

Accelerate neutrophil recovery after bone marrow transplantation

Bensinger WI, Martin PJ, Storer B, et al. Transplantation of bone marrow as compared with peripheral-blood cells from HLA-identical relatives in patients with hematologic cancers. *N Engl J Med*. 2001;344:175-181.

Ho VT, Mirza NQ, Junco Dd D, Okamura T, Przepiorka D. The effect of hematopoietic growth factors on the risk of graft-vs-host disease after allogeneic hematopoietic stem cell transplantation. *Bone Marrow Transplant*. 2003;32:771–775.

Nemunaitis J, Rabinowe SN, Singer JW, et al. Recombinant granulocyte-macrophage colony-stimulating factor after autologous bone marrow transplantation for lymphoid cancer. *N Engl J Med*. 1991;324:1773-1778.

Severe chronic neutropenia (idiopathic, cyclic, congenital)

Dale DC, Bolyard AA, Schwinzer BG, et al. The Severe Chronic Neutropenia International Registry: 10-year follow-up report. *Support Cancer Ther*. 2006;3:220–231.

Dale DC, Link DC. The many causes of severe congenital neutropenia. *N Engl J Med*. 2009;360:3–5.

Rosenberg PS, Alter BP, Link DC, et al. Neutrophil elastase mutations and risk of leukaemia in severe congenital neutropenia. *Br J Haematol.* 2008;140:210–213.

Welte K, Zeidler C, Dale DC. Severe congenital neutropenia. *Semin Hematol.* 2006;43:189–195.

Other potential clinical uses of G-CSF and GM-CSF

Cruciani M, Lipsky BA, Mengoli C, de Lalla F. Granulocyte-colony stimulating factors as adjunctive therapy for diabetic foot infections. *Cochrane Database Syst Rev.* 2009;3:CD006810.

Dale DC, Price TH. Granulocyte transfusion therapy: a new era? *Curr Opin Hematol.* 2009;16:1–2.

Gotlib J, Lavori P, Quesada S, Stein RS, Shahnia S, Greenberg PL. A phase II intra-patient dose-escalation trial of weight-based darbepoetin alfa with or without granulocyte-colony stimulating factor in myelodysplastic syndromes. *Am J Hematol.* 2009;84:15–20.

Greenberg PL, Sun Z, Miller KB, et al. Treatment of myelodysplastic syndromes patients with erythropoietin with or without granulocyte colony-stimulating factor: results of a prospective randomized phase 3 trial by the Eastern Cooperative Oncology Group (E1996). *Blood.* 2009;114:2393–2400.

Joseph J, Rimawi A, Mehta P, et al. Safety and effectiveness of granulocyte colony stimulating factor in mobilizing stem cells and improving cytokine profile in advanced chronic heart failure. *Am J Cardiol.* 2006;97:681–684.

Kang HJ, Kim HS, Zhang SY, et al. Effects of intracoronary infusion of peripheral blood stem-cells mobilised with granulocyte-colony stimulating factor on left ventricular systolic function and restenosis after coronary stenting in myocardial infarction: the MAGIC cell randomised clinical trial. *Lancet.* 2004;363:1735–1736.

Kuritzkes DR. Neutropenia, neutrophil dysfunction, and bacterial infection in patients with human immunodeficiency virus disease: the role of granulocyte colony-stimulating factor. *Clin Infect Dis.* 2000;30:256–260.

Kuritzkes DR, Parenti D, Ward DJ, et al. Filgrastim prevents severe neutropenia and reduces infective morbidity in patients with advanced HIV infection: results of a randomized, multicenter, controlled trial. G-CSF 930101 Study Group. *AIDS.* 1998;12:65–74.

Orlic D, Kajstura J, Chimenti S, et al. Mobilized bone marrow cells repair the infarcted heart, improving function and survival. *Proc Natl Acad Sci USA.* 2001;98:10344–10349.

Park S, Grabar S, Kelaidi C, et al. Predictive factors of response and survival in myelodysplastic syndrome treated with erythropoietin and G-CSF: the GFM experience. *Blood.* 2008;111:574–582.

Price TH, Bowden RA, Boeckh M, et al. Phase I/II trial of neutrophil transfusions from donors stimulated with G-CSF and dexamethasone for treatment of patients with infections in hematopoietic stem cell transplantation. *Blood.* 2000;95:3302–3309.

Biosimilars and new myeloid growth factors

Dale DC. Neutrophil biology and the next generation of myeloid growth factors. *J Natl Compr Canc Netw.* 2009;7:92–98.

Huston A, Lyman GH. Agents under investigation for the treatment and prevention of neutropenia. *Expert Opin Investig Drugs.* 2007;16:1831–1840.

Erythropoietin (epoetin alfa)

Guidelines

Rizzo JD, Somerfield MR, Hagerty KL, et al. Use of epoetin and darbepoetin in patients with cancer: 2007 American Society of Clinical Oncology/American Society of Hematology clinical practice guideline update. *J Clin Oncol.* 2008;26:132–149.

Chronic renal failure

Casadevall N, Nataf J, Viron B, et al. Pure red-cell aplasia and anti-erythropoietin antibodies in patients treated with recombinant erythropoietin. *N Engl J Med.* 2002;346:469–475.

Cody J, Daly C, Campbell M, et al. Recombinant human erythropoietin for chronic renal failure anaemia in pre-dialysis patients. *The Cochrane Collaboration.* New York, NY: Wiley; 2006.

Verhelst D, Rossert J, Casadevall N, et al. Treatment of erythropoietin induced pure red cell aplasia: a retrospective study. *Lancet.* 2004;363:1768–1771.

Anemia in preterm infants

Bishara N, Ohls RK. Current controversies in the management of the anemia of prematurity. *Semin Perinatol.* 2009;33:29–34.

Ohls RK. The use of erythropoietin in neonates. *Clin Perinatol.* 2000;27:681–696.

Shannon KM, Keith JF III, Mentzer WC, et al. Recombinant human erythropoietin stimulates erythropoiesis and reduces erythrocyte transfusions in very low birth weight preterm infants. *Pediatrics.* 1995;95:1–8.

Anemia associated with HIV infection

Abrams DI, Steinhart C, Frascino R. Epoetin alfa therapy for anaemia in HIV-infected patients: impact on quality of life. *Int J STD AIDS.* 2000;11:659–665.

Henry DH, Beall GN, Benson CA, et al. Recombinant human erythropoietin in the treatment of anemia associated with immunodeficiency virus (HIV) infection and zidovudine therapy: overview of four clinical trials. *Ann Intern Med.* 1992;117:739–748.

Saag MS, Bowers P, Leitz GJ, Levine AM; Community HIV Anemia Management Protocol Sites (CHAMPS) Study Group. Once-weekly epoetin alfa improves quality of life and increases hemoglobin in anemic HIV+ patients. *AIDS Res Hum Retroviruses.* 2004;20:1037–1045.

Volberding PA, Levine AM, Dieterich D, et al. Anemia in HIV infection: clinical impact and evidence-based management strategies. Anemia in HIV Working Group. *Clin Infect Dis.* 2004;38:1454–1463.

Anemia in patients with cancer receiving chemotherapy or radiation therapy

Bohlius J, Schmidlin K, Brillant C, et al. Recombinant human erythropoiesis-stimulating agents and mortality in patients with cancer: a meta-analysis of randomised trials. *Lancet.* 2009;373:1532–1542.

Gabrilove JL, Cleeland CS, Livingston RB, et al. Clinical evaluation of once-weekly dosing of epoetin alfa in chemotherapy patients: improvements in hemoglobin and quality of life are similar to three-times-weekly dosing. *J Clin Oncol.* 2001;19:2875–2882.

Glaspy J, Bukowski R, Steinberg D, et al. Impact of therapy with epoetin alfa on clinical outcomes in patients with nonmyeloid malignancies during cancer chemotherapy in community oncology practice. Procrit Study Group. *J Clin Oncol.* 1997;15:1218–1234.

Henke M, Laszi R, Rube C, et al. Erythropoietin to treat head and neck cancer patients with anemia undergoing radiotherapy: randomized, double-blind, placebo-controlled trial. *Lancet.* 2003;362:1255–1260.

Leyland-Jones B, Semiglazov V, Pawlicki M, et al. Maintaining normal hemoglobin levels with epoetin alfa in mainly nonanemic patients with metastatic breast cancer receiving first-line chemotherapy: a survival study. *J Clin Oncol.* 2005;23:5865–5868.

Ludwig H, Crawford J, Osterborg A, et al. Pooled analysis of individual patient-level data from all randomized, double-blind, placebo-controlled trials of darbepoetin alfa in the treatment of patients with chemotherapy-induced anemia. *J Clin Oncol.* 2009;27:2838–2847.

Wun T, Law L, Harvery D, et al. Increased incidence of symptomatic venous thrombosis in patients with cervical carcinoma treated with concurrent chemotherapy, radiation, and erythropoietin. *Cancer.* 2003;98:1514–1520.

Reduction in allogeneic transfusion in surgery patients

de Andrade JR, Jove M, Landon G, Frei D, Guilfoyle M, Young DC. Baseline hemoglobin as a predictor of risk of transfusion and response to epoetin alfa in orthopedic surgery patients. *Am J Orthop.* 1996;25:533–542.

Price TH, Goodnough LT, Vogler WR, et al. The effect of recombinant human erythropoietin on the efficacy of autologous blood donation in patients with low hematocrits: a multicenter, randomized, double-blind, controlled trial. *Transfusion.* 1996;36:29–36.

Darbepoetin alfa

Bohlius J, Schmidlin K, Brillant C, et al. Erythropoietin or darbepoetin for patients with cancer: meta-analysis based on individual patient data. *Cochrane Database Syst Rev.* 2009;3:CD007303.

Egrie JC, Browne JK. Development and characterization of novel erythropoiesis stimulating protein (NESP). *Br J Cancer.* 2001;84(suppl 1):3–10.

Smith RE Jr, Tchekmedyian NS, Chan D, et al. A dose- and schedule-finding study of darbepoetin alpha for the treatment of chronic anaemia of cancer. *Br J Cancer.* 2003;88:1851–1858.

Steurer M, Sudmeier I, Stauder R, et al. Thromboembolic events in patients with myelodysplastic syndrome receiving thalidomide in combination with darbepoetin-alpha. *Br J Haematol.* 2003;121:101–103.

Suranyi M, Lindberg JS, Navarro J, et al. Treatment of anemia with darbepoetin alfa administered de novo once every other week in chronic kidney disease. *Am J Nephrol.* 2003;23:106–111.

Vansteenkiste J, Pirker R, Massuti B, et al. Double-blind placebo-controlled, randomized phase III trial of darbepoetin alfa in lung cancer patients receiving chemotherapy. *J Natl Cancer Inst.* 2002;94:1211–1220.

Thrombopoietin

Bussel JB, Kuter DJ, George JN, et al. AMG 531, a thrombopoiesis-stimulating protein, for chronic ITP. *N Engl J Med.* 2006;355:1672–1681.

George JN, Mathias SD, Go RS, et al. Improved quality of life for romiplostim-treated patients with chronic immune thrombocytopenic purpura: results from two randomized, placebo-controlled trials. *Br J Haematol.* 2009;144:409–415.

Kaushansky K. The molecular mechanisms that control thrombopoiesis. *J Clin Invest.* 2005;15:3339–3347.

Kuter DJ, Bussel JB, Lyons RM, et al. Efficacy of romiplostim in patients with chronic immune thrombocytopenic purpura: a double-blind randomised controlled trial. *Lancet.* 2008;371:395–403.

Nurden AT, Viallard JF, Nurden P. New-generation drugs that stimulate platelet production in chronic immune thrombocytopenic purpura. *Lancet.* 2009;373:1562–1569.

Wang B, Nichol JL, Sullivan JT. Pharmacodynamics and pharmacokinetics of AMG 531, a novel thrombopoietin receptor ligand. *Clin Pharmacol Ther.* 2004;76:628–638.

Interleukin-11 (oprelvekin)

Ellis M, Zwaan F, Hedström U, et al. Recombinant human interleukin 11 and bacterial infection in patients with haematological malignant disease undergoing chemotherapy: a double-blind placebo-controlled randomised trial. *Lancet.* 2003;361:275–280.

Ghalib R, Levine C, Hassan M, et al. Recombinant human interleukin-11 improves thrombocytopenia in patients with cirrhosis. *Hepatology.* 2003;37:1165–1171.

Gordon MS, McCaskill-Stevens WJ, Battiato LA, et al. A phase I trial of recombinant human interleukin-11 (neumega rhIL-11 growth factor) in women with breast cancer receiving chemotherapy. *Blood.* 1996;87:3615–3624.

Isaacs C, Robert NJ, Bailey FA, et al. Randomized placebo-controlled study of recombinant human interleukin-11 to prevent chemotherapy-induced thrombocytopenia in patients with breast cancer receiving dose-intensive cyclophosphamide and doxorubicin. *J Clin Oncol.* 1997;15:3368–3377.

Stem cell factor (ancestim)

Broudy VC. Stem cell factor and hematopoiesis. *Blood.* 1997;90:1345–1364.

Facon T, Harousseau JL, Maloisel F, et al. Stem cell factor in combination with filgrastim after chemotherapy improves peripheral blood progenitor cell yield and reduces apheresis requirements in multiple myeloma patients: a randomized, controlled trial. *Blood.* 1999;94:1218–1225.

Stiff P, Gingrich R, Luger S, et al. A randomized phase 2 study of PBPC mobilization by stem cell factor and filgrastim in heavily pretreated patients with Hodgkin's disease or non Hodgkin's lymphoma. *Bone Marrow Transplant.* 2000;26:471–481.

# Chapter 04

Iron metabolism, iron overload, and the porphyrias

Alice D. Ma and Victor R. Gordeuk

Regulation of iron homeostasis, 93
Hereditary hemochromatosis and other iron overload syndromes, 96
The porphyrias, 101
Bibliography, 107

Iron is a mineral required by every living cell for DNA synthesis, oxygen transport, and respiration. Iron's ability to accept and donate electrons allows it to shuttle between ferrous (Fe^{2+}) and ferric (Fe^{3+}) oxidation states and is essential for its participation in a number of enzymatic reactions.

Despite the importance of iron to living cells, it can also be toxic. Iron catalyzes the formation of free radical ions, and therefore under physiologic states does not exist unbound to proteins or heme. Causes of iron overload include the repeated blood transfusions that are required to manage certain chronic anemias, the ineffective erythropoiesis that characterizes certain chronic anemias, and mutations in a number of genes that lead to decreased production of hepcidin or resistance to hepcidin and consequently increased iron absorption. This chapter will focus on iron metabolism in the normal host and in iron overload states including hemochromatosis. Iron deficiency anemia will be discussed with the underproduction anemias in Chapter 5. This chapter will also discuss the porphyrias as a model of disorders of synthesis of the iron-containing heme molecule.

Regulation of iron homeostasis

The average content of iron in men is 35 to 45 mg/kg; menstruating women have lesser amounts. Most of the iron in the body is present in the hemoglobin molecule of the red blood cells, each milliliter of which contains about 1 mg of iron (Figure 4-1). Men and women have approximately 2 g and 1.5 g of erythrocyte iron, respectively. Iron is stored as ferritin or hemosiderin, predominantly in the macrophages of the spleen, bone marrow, and liver. At steady state, the serum ferritin level is a good reflection of total body iron stores. Total iron storage is approximately 1 g in men and 600 mg in women. Substantial amounts of iron are found as myoglobin in muscle, and much smaller amounts are found as cytochromes and other enzymes in all cells of the body. The smallest amount of iron is in the plasma bound to transferrin. Each molecule of transferrin can bind 2 molecules of iron. Transferrin-bound iron is constantly turning over as iron is used by body tissues, especially developing red blood cells in the bone marrow. Dietary iron usually amounts to 15 to 25 mg daily, of which 5% to 10% is absorbed. This proportion can be increased up to 5-fold in states of iron deficiency. At steady-state conditions, the body requires 1 mg of iron daily to compensate for normal obligatory losses through desquamation of cells and trace amounts in urine and bile.

Iron metabolism is carefully regulated such that the amount of iron absorbed equals the amount of iron lost. There is no physiologic pathway for iron excretion. During the past 15 years, much has been learned concerning the molecular mechanisms underlying the absorption, transport, utilization, and storage of iron. Regulation of iron balance relies on the function of a number of key proteins (listed in Table 4-1). The major processes discussed in this section are shown schematically in Figure 4-1.

In food, iron is found as inorganic iron (both Fe^{2+} and Fe^{3+}) and as heme (iron complexed to protoporphyrin IX).

Conflict-of-interest disclosure: *Dr. Ma* declares no competing financial interest. *Dr. Gordeuk:* consultancy: Merck, Amgen, Ikaria; research funding: Merck, TRF Pharma, Biomarin; speakers' bureau: Novartis.

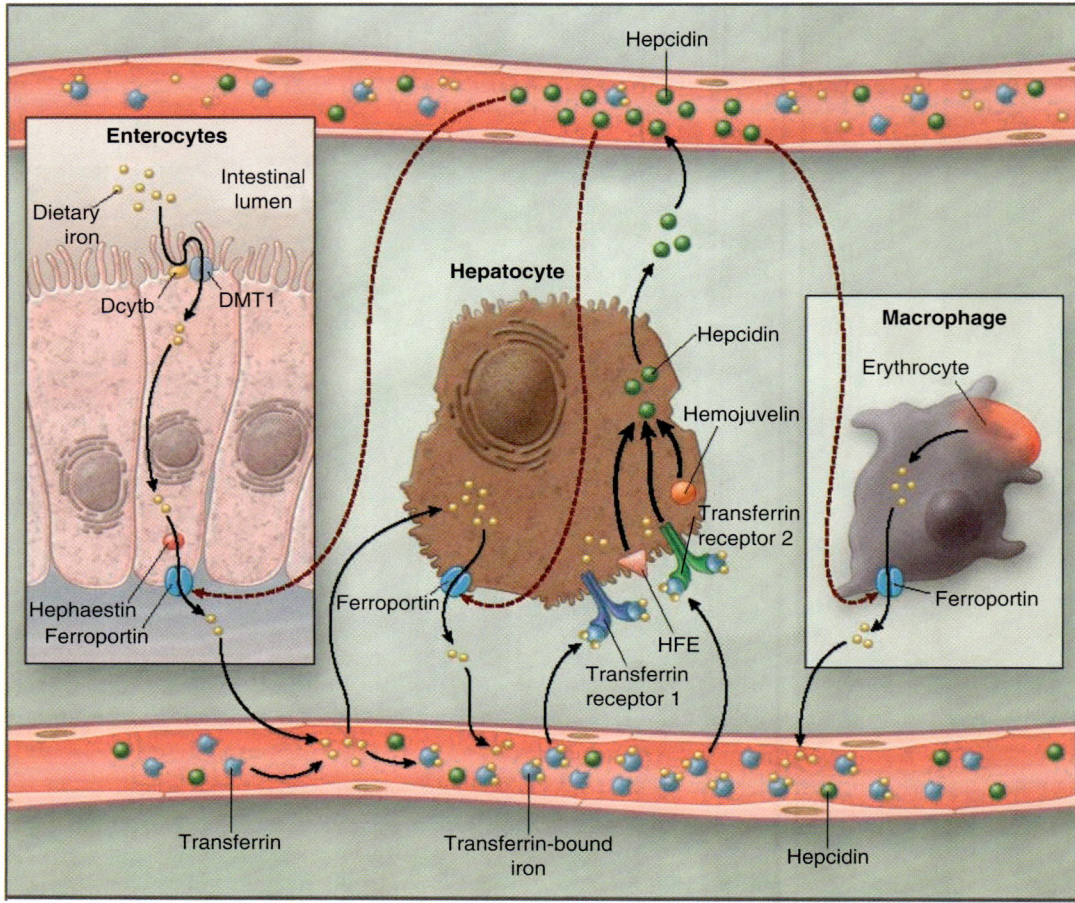

Figure 4-1 Regulators of iron balance. Dietary iron enters the enterocyte after being reduced to the ferrous state by duodenal cytochrome b (Dcytb) and being transported by divalent metal transporter 1 (DMT1). Hephaestin facilitates iron export by ferroportin. Hepatocytes take up either free or transferrin-bound iron and release it back into the circulation via the action of ferroportin. Ferroportin also releases iron from macrophages. Ferroportin-mediated release of iron is inhibited by hepcidin. From Fleming RE, Bacon BR. Orchestration of iron homeostasis. *N Engl J Med*. 2005;352:1742, with permission.

The typical diet consists of 90% inorganic iron and 10% heme iron, although diets in the developed world can comprise >50% heme iron, mainly in the form of meat. Heme iron is the most bioavailable iron, and its absorption tends to remain constant, regardless of diet composition. In contrast, inorganic iron absorption depends on other items in the diet, being enhanced by ascorbic acid and inhibited by compounds such as phytates and polyphenols in cereals and plants.

The rate of iron absorption is influenced by a number of factors, including the body's iron stores, the degree of erythropoietic activity, the concentration of hemoglobin in the blood, the blood oxygen content, and inflammatory cytokines. When iron stores are low or when there is increased erythropoietic activity, anemia, or hypoxemia, iron absorption increases.

Iron is mainly absorbed in the duodenum through 2 distinct pathways. One pathway exists for the absorption of iron in the form of the Fe^{2+} ferrous ion, and a second pathway is for iron bound to heme. Nonheme iron must be maintained in its ferrous Fe^{2+} state by duodenal ferric reductase (Dcytb) to be absorbed. It is transported into the enterocyte through the apical membrane by the divalent metal transporter 1 (DMT1). The pathway for the absorption of heme iron is not known.

Iron may be stored within the enterocyte, which is sloughed in the feces, or it may be transported into the portal plasma by ferroportin at the basolateral membrane. Ferroportin is the sole iron exporter in mammalian tissues. The transport activity of enterocyte ferroportin is enhanced by the ferroxidase activity of hephaestin. Iron released into the circulation is bound by transferrin and transported to sites of iron use, predominantly erythroid precursors in the bone marrow.

The hereditary hemochromatosis (HFE) protein is mutated in the majority of cases of hereditary hemochromatosis in

Table 4-1 Major proteins involved in iron homeostasis.

Regulation of iron balance relies on the function of a number of key proteins. Among these are:

Ferritin, the major cellular iron storage protein

Transferrin (Tf), the major transport protein for iron in the circulation

Transferrin receptor 1 (TfR1), which is responsible for delivering iron from the plasma into erythroid precursors in the bone marrow and other cells of the body

Transferrin receptor 2 (TfR2), which is expressed on hepatocytes and helps to regulate the expression of hepcidin

Iron responsive protein (IRP) 1 and 2, which regulate synthesis of a number of proteins including apoferritin and TfR1

Duodenal ferric reductase (Dcytb), which reduces intestinal luminal ferric iron to the ferrous form that can be transported by DMT1

Divalent metal transporter 1 (DMT1), which transports ferrous iron from the gut lumen into the enterocyte

Ferroportin, the protein responsible for iron export out of enterocytes and macrophages to Tf in the plasma; ferroportin bound to hepcidin is rapidly internalized and degraded

Hephaestin, a ceruloplasmin analog whose ferroxidase activity enhances the export activity of enterocyte ferroportin

Ceruloplasmin, a plasma and macrophage protein whose ferroxidase activity enhances the export activity of macrophage ferroportin

Hepcidin, a 25–amino acid peptide that regulates iron absorption and release of iron from macrophages

HFE, a protein mutated in the majority of cases of hemochromatosis that is expressed on hepatocytes and helps to regulate hepcidin production

Hemojuvelin, a protein that regulates hepcidin production in concert with TfR2 and HFE

Caucasians. Normally, the HFE protein is expressed on the hepatocyte and cooperates with transferrin receptor 2 (TfR2) and hemojuvelin (HJV) in regulating the production of hepcidin. Mutated HFE has a disruption in a disulfide bond, leading to a conformational change in its structure and a decrease in its ability to bind β_2-microglobulin. Mutated HFE leads to a deficiency in the production of hepcidin, and iron overload occurs because of increased iron transport by enterocyte ferroportin to plasma transferrin.

Transferrin-bound iron is transported to erythroblasts, where holotransferrin binds to the transferrin receptor (TfR) and enters the cells by endocytosis. Within the developing erythron, the regulation of the synthesis of TfR and apoferritin is controlled at the level of translation (Figure 4-2). Messenger RNA (mRNA) for these proteins contains iron response elements (IREs) that have a conserved nucleotide sequence and a stem loop structure. mRNA for apoferritin has a single IRE in the 5′ untranslated region. mRNA for TfR has multiple IREs in the 3′ untranslated region. Iron response protein-1 (IRP-1) is formed when aconitase, an important enzyme in the Krebs cycle, undergoes a conformational change. In the presence of iron, this enzyme functions as a Krebs cycle enzyme. In low iron states, the conformational change causes the enzyme to function as IRP-1. As such, IRP-1 can bind to IREs and modulate iron absorption. When IRP-1 binds to apoferritin mRNA IRE, it inhibits translation of apoferritin. When IRP-1 binds to the TfR mRNA IREs, it stabilizes the mRNA and increases translation of this receptor. Thus, when cytosolic iron is low, there is decreased synthesis of apoferritin and increased synthesis of TfRs, which in turn localize on the developing red blood cell membrane. Similarly, when iron is readily available, IRP-1 undergoes a conformational change and will no longer bind to IREs. As a result, the number of TfRs on the red blood cell membrane is decreased, and translation of apoferritin is increased.

Most of the iron in the erythron couples with protoporphyrin to form the heme molecule. Heme forms a complex with the globin proteins, thus forming hemoglobin. Erythrocytes survive in the circulation for approximately 120 days, at which point the aging red blood cell is phagocytized by macrophages in the reticuloendothelial system. Within these macrophages, hemoglobin is catabolized, and iron is released to plasma transferrin by the action of ferroportin, which is the same as the iron export protein found within the gut enterocyte. When iron is once again released to plasma transferrin, the cycle repeats itself. Any iron not released to

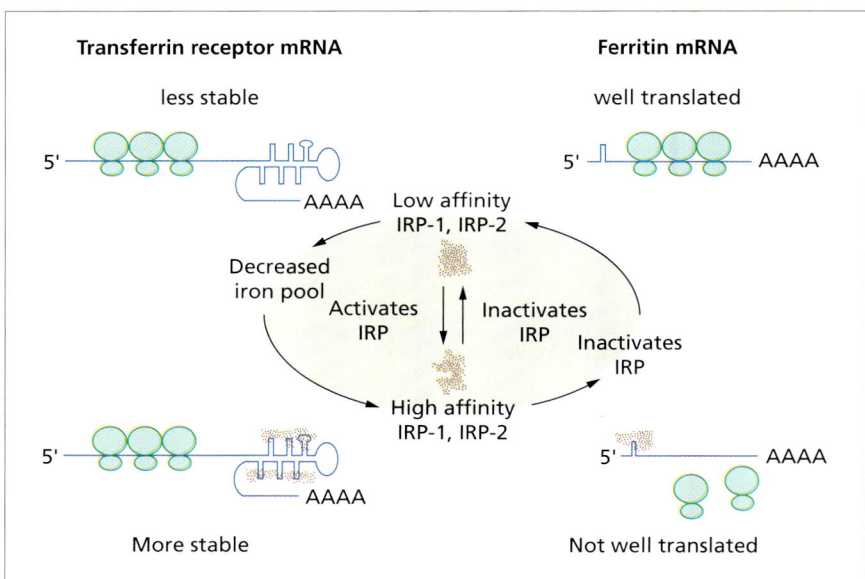

Figure 4-2 Coordinate regulation of transferrin receptor and ferritin synthesis by the iron regulatory proteins iron response protein (IRP)-1 and IRP2. Because both IRPs seem to respond to changes in cellular iron similarly and seem to bind to iron response elements (IREs) indistinguishably, only a single IRP is shown in the figure. Transferrin receptor synthesis is controlled by adjusting the amounts of cytoplasmic transferrin receptor messenger RNA (mRNA). The 3′ untranslated region (3′ UTR) of transferrin receptor mRNA contains 5 IREs. Binding of IRPs to the IREs in the 3′ UTR retards cytoplasmic degradation, increasing the concentration of cytoplasmic transferrin receptor mRNA and the rate of transferrin receptor synthesis. With an increased number of cellular transferrin receptors, iron uptake is enhanced. By contrast, ferritin synthesis is controlled without changes in the amount of ferritin mRNA present by repressing translation of ferritin mRNA. The 5′ untranslated regions (5′ UTR) of ferritin mRNA contain a single IRE. Binding of an IRP to the IRE in the 5′ UTR arrests translation of ferritin mRNA, so less ferritin is produced and iron sequestration is diminished. Redrawn from Brittenham GM. Disorders of iron metabolism: deficiency and overload. In: Hoffman R, Benz EJ, Shattil SJ, Furie B, Cohen HJ, Silberstein LE, eds. *Hematology: Basic Principles and Practice*. New York, NY: Churchill Livingstone; 1994:492–523, with permission.

plasma transferrin may be stored within macrophages as ferritin or hemosiderin.

Hepcidin, a 25–amino acid peptide with bactericidal properties, is the major regulator of iron absorption and storage. Hepcidin regulates ferroportin activity by binding to ferroportin and leading to its internalization and degradation. Thus, elevated levels of hepcidin lead to decreased iron absorption from the gut and increased storage of iron within the hepatocyte and macrophage. Hepcidin production is increased 100-fold in inflammatory anemias, being induced by interleukin (IL)-6 and IL-1. Thus, hepcidin is an acute-phase reactant and is responsible for the anemia of inflammation. Hepcidin levels are downregulated by anemia and iron deficiency. Additionally, interactions between HJV and the bone morphogenetic protein (BMP)/Smad signaling pathway, in concert with TfR2 and HFE, regulate hepcidin levels. The full mechanisms of the regulation of hepcidin levels are still being investigated. Mutations of *HFE* are responsible for the majority of hereditary hemochromatosis cases, and mutations of *TFR2*, *HJV*, and *HAMP* (the gene for hepcidin) also lead to hemochromatosis.

Hereditary hemochromatosis and other iron overload syndromes

Clinical case

A 48-year-old male is sent for evaluation of abnormal iron studies. For the past 3 years, he has complained of chronic fatigue and progressive arthralgias of the second and third metacarpophalangeal joints. He has recently been diagnosed with glucose intolerance. He is otherwise healthy and takes no medications. He drinks a moderate amount of alcohol. His father died of cryptogenic cirrhosis at age 63. On examination, his skin is bronze colored, and his liver is palpated 3 cm below the costal margin. His complete blood count is normal. Fasting blood glucose is 184 mg/dL. Iron saturation is 73% with a ferritin value of 1997 ng/mL. The patient has a healthy teenage son who has not seen a physician for many years.

The term iron overload (hemosiderosis) is nonspecific and refers to a state of iron deposition in various body tissues or organs. Hemochromatosis refers to the clinical expression of iron-induced injury in affected body tissues. Hereditary hemochromatosis is a relatively common congenital cause of iron overload secondary to increased gastrointestinal absorption of iron at the level of the enterocyte. Other etiologies of hemochromatosis also exist and are discussed in the following sections (Table 4-2).

HFE hemochromatosis
Epidemiology and pathophysiology

HFE hemochromatosis results from a genetic defect that leads to increased absorption of dietary iron (as described earlier). Inheritance is autosomal recessive. The C282Y mutation (discussed later) accounts for the majority of the genotypic and phenotypic expression of hereditary hemochromatosis in Caucasians. In contrast to the prevalence in the Caucasian population, the C282Y mutation is not common in African Americans or Asians with iron overload. Tremendous variation exists between the genotypic and phenotypic expression of hereditary hemochromatosis. The true penetrance varies depending on whether biochemical, tissue biopsy, or clinical parameters are used to define the syndrome.

A G to A mutation at nucleotide 845 of *HFE* leads to a cysteine to tyrosine substitution at amino acid position 282 (C282Y). Approximately 15% of Caucasians of European descent are heterozygotes and 5 in 1000 are homozygotes for this mutation. Homozygotes for the C282Y mutation (C282Y/C282Y) account for 60% to 90% of clinical cases of hereditary hemochromatosis. Although biochemical abnormalities such as an elevated transferrin saturation or ferritin may rarely be present in heterozygotes (C282Y/WT), very few will develop clinical features of iron overload in the absence of other risk factors, such as alcohol, hepatitis, chronic hemolysis, transfusion, or exogenous iron administration.

A second mutation involves a G to C substitution at nucleotide 187 of *HFE*, leading to a histidine to aspartic acid substitution at amino acid position 63 (H63D). Up to 30% of the Caucasian population are heterozygotes for this more common mutation. The H63D defect is less penetrant, and only a small minority of homozygotes (H63D/H63D) will develop clinical features of iron overload. Heterozygotes for the H63D mutation (H63D/WT) rarely develop biochemical or clinical evidence of iron overload.

Compound heterozygotes for the 2 mutations (C282Y/H63D) may occasionally develop mild subclinical iron overload and should be evaluated for coexisting risk factors if hemochromatosis is expressed clinically. In the United States, 15% to 30% of patients with clinical hemochromatosis have no identifiable *HFE* mutation. The prevalence of different genotypic combinations among clinically affected individuals is listed in Table 4-3.

Although homozygosity for the C282Y mutation accounts for up to 90% of clinical hereditary hemochromatosis, there remains much debate concerning the true phenotypic penetrance. In a population screening study by Olynyk et al (1999), approximately 50% of all homozygotes for the C282Y mutation developed phenotypic expression consistent with the disease, typically by the age of 60. In a pedigree study by Bulaj et al (2000), which investigated homozygous family members of known hemochromatosis probands, 85% of

Table 4-2 Causes of hemochromatosis and iron overload.

1. *Hereditary conditions affecting the hepcidin/ferroportin axis*
   HFE hemochromatosis in Caucasians
   TFR2 hemochromatosis
   Hemojuvelin hemochromatosis
   Hepcidin hemochromatosis
   Ferroportin disease
2. *Conditions of ineffective erythropoiesis*
   β thalassemia major and intermedia
   Hemoglobin E/β thalassemia
   Hemoglobin H disease
   Congenital dyserythropoietic anemias
   Hereditary and acquired sideroblastic anemias
3. *Multiple blood transfusions*
   Aplastic anemia
   Diamond-Blackfan anemia
   Thalassemia major
   Sickle cell anemia
   Myelodysplasia
4. *Other hereditary conditions*
   African iron overload
   Melanesian iron overload
   Aceruloplasminemia
   Atransferrinemia

Table 4-3 Prevalence *HFE* genotypes among patients with hereditary hemochromatosis.

Genotype	Prevalence among patients with hereditary hemochromatosis
C282Y/C282Y	60%–90%
C282Y/H63D	0%–10%
C282Y/WT	Rare
H63D/H63D	0%–4%
H63D/WT	Rare
WT/WT	15%–30%

C282Y refers to a cysteine to tyrosine substitution at amino acid position 282. H63D refers to a histidine to aspartic acid substitution at amino acid position 63.
Adapted from Cogswell ME, Burke W, McDonnell SM, Franks AL. Screening for hemochromatosis. A public health perspective. *Am J Prev Med*. 1999;2:134–140.
WT = wild type.

males and 65% of females had biochemical evidence of iron overload. Despite these findings, only 38% of males and 10% of females had disease-related symptoms, and only 15% had fibrosis or cirrhosis on liver biopsy. With increasing age, disease-related morbidity increased, especially in homozygous men older than 40 years of age. A controlled study by Beutler et al (2002) suggested that the clinical penetrance of homozygous hereditary hemochromatosis is much lower than previously predicted. In this study, the most common symptoms of hereditary hemochromatosis were no more prevalent in homozygotes (C282Y/C282Y) than in an unaffected control population. The penetrance of individuals homozygous for the C282Y mutation was estimated to be <1%. Other subsequent studies also suggested a low clinical penetrance of homozygous hemochromatosis. The true clinical penetrance of homozygous hemochromatosis is uncertain but probably lies somewhere between 1% and 25%. Much of the variability in these estimates involves the different populations studied (blood donors vs preventive care clinics vs general population vs family members of affected probands) and how clinical penetrance was defined (iron studies vs liver function tests vs clinical symptoms vs liver biopsy specimens).

Diagnosis

The transferrin saturation in patients with homozygous hemochromatosis is higher than in normal individuals but shows considerable variability. A transferrin saturation >50% in males or >45% in females should be repeated and also prompt a serum ferritin measurement. Ferritin values, although imperfect, are a surrogate marker for total body iron stores. Ferritin values can be elevated in several conditions other than iron overload, including the metabolic syndrome, inflammatory conditions, acute or chronic hepatitis, alcoholic liver disease, and the hyperferritinemia-cataract syndrome. In a population-based screening program performed through the Centers for Disease Control and Prevention, only 11% to 22% of individuals with an elevated serum transferrin had a concurrent elevation in serum ferritin (Figure 4-3).

Molecular genotyping of the *HFE* locus, now a readily available test, should be considered if the diagnosis remains in question after secondary causes of iron overload have been ruled out or if at-risk family members exist. Before genotyping is performed, a detailed discussion with the patient concerning the possible clinical, emotional, and financial implications of making such a diagnosis should be undertaken.

A liver biopsy is the gold standard in making the diagnosis of iron overload. Liver biopsy provides information on iron content, iron distribution, and whether fibrosis or cirrhosis has developed. Liver biopsy has been recommended *HFE*^{C282Y} homozygotes with abnormal liver function tests or ferritin >1000 mg/L to evaluate for cirrhosis. Liver biopsy also has

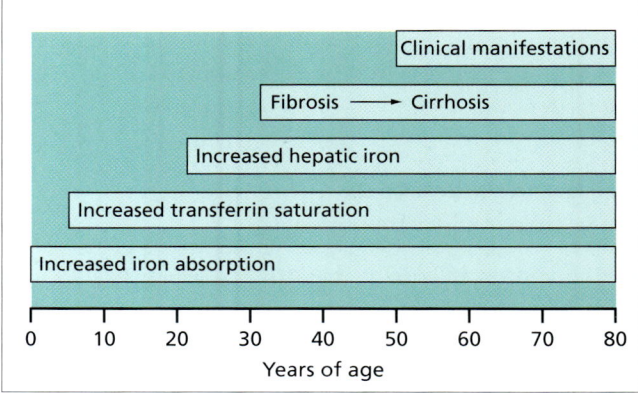

Figure 4-3 The natural history of hemochromatosis. An increase in the percent saturation of transferrin can be detected in children homozygous for hemochromatosis. Increased liver iron stores can generally be detected in homozygous men by the end of the second decade. The serum ferritin concentration increases as hepatic iron stores increase. Hepatic fibrosis can be detected early in the fourth decade. Clinical manifestations generally occur in the fifth decade or later.

been considered if a strong suspicion of pronounced iron overload exists despite a negative evaluation for *HFE* mutations or other primary or secondary causes. Cirrhosis is rare on liver biopsy if serum ferritin is <1000 μg/L regardless of age or serum liver enzyme levels. In hereditary hemochromatosis, if liver biopsy is performed, the distribution of iron is primarily parenchymal, whereas Kupffer cell iron loading is prominent in transfusional iron overload. A Perls stain of grade 3 or 4, a hepatic iron concentration of >80 mmol/g (4.5 mg/g) dry weight, or a hepatic iron index score ≥1.9 all confirm the presence of increased body iron stores. An additional method of estimating total body storage iron is by phlebotomy. If >4 g of iron (16 U) can be mobilized by phlebotomy without the patient becoming iron deficient, body iron stores are at least 4 times greater than normal. Liver biopsy is being performed less frequently in the evaluation of hereditary hemochromatosis now that confirmatory genotyping has become readily available. Techniques including hepatic magnetic resonance imaging (MRI) or superconducting quantum interference device (SQUID) susceptometry are other noninvasive methods currently being investigated. MRI for quantifying the amount of iron deposition in liver and heart is becoming available in increasing numbers of centers. SQUID is available in only a few centers.

Clinical presentation

The classic finding of a male with skin bronzing, hepatomegaly, and diabetes is an advanced and now rare presentation of the disease. Patients often present to hematologists for evaluation of abnormal iron studies initially identified during health physicals, as part of screening when affected relatives are identified, or when iron panels are drawn for a variety of other indications. Early diagnosis is essential to alter the disease course and avoid end-organ complications. The clinical presentation is varied and often consists of nonspecific findings such as chronic fatigue, weakness, nonspecific abdominal pain, arthralgias, and mild elevation of liver enzymes, all of which may be noted years before the correct diagnosis is made. Patients may be mistakenly diagnosed with seronegative arthritis or pseudogout. Endocrine organs are commonly affected. Diabetes, hypothyroidism, and gonadal failure may occur. Both the mechanical and conduction systems of the heart can be affected, and patients may present with heart failure or arrhythmias. An increased frequency of depression has been noted. Iron-induced liver damage remains the most recognized and feared complication of untreated disease. As the disease advances and iron deposition goes untreated, hepatic fibrosis and cirrhosis may develop. Once cirrhosis develops, a >200-fold increased risk of hepatocellular carcinoma has been documented.

Treatment

Prompt and aggressive treatment before end-organ complications occur is the key to management. Life expectancy of patients can be normal if this goal is met. Phlebotomy is the key therapeutic modality. Removal of 1 unit of blood (200–250 mg iron) should be initiated at weekly intervals until ferritin levels decrease to 20 to 50 ng/mL, provided the hematocrit is maintained above 33% to 35%. Normal adults would become iron deficient after 4 to 6 phlebotomies on such a program because the typical 1.0 g of iron stores would be depleted. Patients with 4 g of storage iron will not become iron deficient until 16 to 20 phlebotomies have been performed. In more advanced cases, total body iron burden can be >20 g, requiring weekly phlebotomy for >1 year. After the ferritin value has decreased to 20 to 50 ng/mL, lifelong maintenance phlebotomy may be required. Typically, phlebotomy is required every 2 to 4 months to maintain the ferritin level at the aforementioned target.

Therapeutic phlebotomy is often effective at improving a patient's overall sense of well-being, including resolving fatigue and malaise, normalizing skin pigmentation, and reducing elevated liver enzymes. The effect of phlebotomy on improving arthralgias, diabetes, and hypogonadism is less successful. Phlebotomy may not reverse cirrhosis or its attendant risk for hepatocellular carcinoma.

Phlebotomy is usually not indicated and only infrequently performed during adolescence. If an isolated increase in transferrin saturation is identified during screening, ferritin values should be monitored at 3- to 6-month intervals. Phlebotomy should be initiated only when ferritin values reach >300 ng/mL in males or >200 ng/mL in nonpregnant females of reproductive age. Avoidance of alcohol and exogenous medicinal iron or iron-containing vitamins should be stressed. Dietary change aimed at avoiding iron-containing foods is often impractical and not necessary as long as patients are compliant with phlebotomy. Patients should be warned about the risks of eating raw seafood because the incidence of *Vibrio vulnificus* and *Yersinia enterocolitica* infections is increased. Patients with iron overload are also at risk for mucormycosis, especially as they begin chelation therapy. Treatment of cardiac, hepatic, and other complications of iron overload is essential. Liver transplantation has been performed in the setting of end-stage liver disease. Iron chelation should be considered if phlebotomy is contraindicated.

Historically, patients with hemochromatosis have been excluded from donating blood. As the nation's blood supply has diminished, this exclusionary criterion has been reconsidered. It is estimated that in this country, 635,000 individuals between the ages of 20 and 74 years have hemochromatosis and could serve as potential blood donors. The US Food and Drug Administration (FDA) has recently announced a guideline that allows patients with hemochromatosis, in the absence of other exclusionary criteria, to serve as blood donors. The blood, however, must be identified as coming from a patient with hemochromatosis and, despite its increased iron content, is often never transfused to a recipient. On a case-by-case basis, the FDA will exempt donor centers from labeling hemochromatosis blood units, but only if the center provides therapeutic phlebotomy free of charge, even if the patient is excluded from donation for other reasons. The American Association of Blood Banks has reported that hemochromatosis blood donors could boost the US blood supply by anywhere from 200,000 to 3 million units annually.

Screening

Controversy exists concerning the role of population screening for hereditary hemochromatosis. Currently, population-based screening is not recommended. Early screening of at-risk individuals or families should be stressed. Measurement of transferrin saturation and serum ferritin concentration and genotyping of the *HFE* locus are appropriate screening methods in high-risk individuals. Issues of genetic discrimination need to be considered; some authorities recommend against genetic screening during childhood or adolescence. First-degree relatives of affected individuals should be screened for iron overload, but whether genotyping should be performed in these at-risk first-degree relatives to definitively rule in or rule out homozygous C282Y hemochromatosis is controversial. Both the pros and cons of genotypic screening should be discussed, and further evaluation should proceed based on the desires of each individual family member.

Other forms of hemochromatosis

A juvenile form of hereditary hemochromatosis exists in which iron overload develops at a young age, and the genes encoding hemojuvelin and or hepcidin are mutated in the majority of these cases. Patients with this disease may die by the age of 30 years, after the development of endocrine complications and heart failure. Hemochromatosis resulting from mutations of TfR2 are quite rare and indistinguishable clinically from *HFE* hemochromatosis. Like *HFE* hemochromatosis, these conditions are inherited in an autosomal recessive fashion and are associated with low levels of hepcidin, suggesting a common mechanism for disease. Neonatal hemochromatosis with perinatal liver failure has been described. The pathophysiology and possible genetic defect underlying this disorder have not been well worked out.

Ferroportin disease

Iron overload resulting from mutations of *FPN1* is known as ferroportin disease. Ferroportin disease is inherited as autosomal dominant and, compared with classical hemochromatosis, may be characterized by early increase in ferritin in the presence of a low-normal transferrin saturation and early decrease in serum iron concentration and hemoglobin levels during phlebotomy. The disease is typically less severe than classical hemochromatosis, although all clinical features including organ dysfunction may appear.

Other causes of iron overload

Many chronic anemias are associated with clinically significant iron overload. Thalassemia is the most recognized cause worldwide (Table 4-2). There are likely 2 causes of iron overload in these syndromes. First, ineffective erythropoiesis, the intramedullary death of developing red blood cells, leads to inappropriately increased iron absorption related to secretion of growth differentiation factor-15 by erythroblasts and related suppression of hepcidin production by hepatocytes. Second, blood transfusions administered for causes other than blood loss leads to the inexorable accumulation of the iron in the transfused red blood cells. Ineffective erythropoiesis may be a prominent cause of increased iron stores in thalassemia major, congenital dyserythropoietic anemias, and sideroblastic anemias, but blood transfusions also usually contribute. Blood transfusions are the predominant cause of iron overload in patients with aplastic anemia, pure red cell aplasia, myelodysplasia, and sickle cell anemia. Because each unit of red blood cells contains 200 to 250 mg of iron, lifetime blood transfusion of 50 to 100 U (a common occurrence in sickle cell anemia) would result in storage of 10 to 20 g of iron, similar to patients with advanced hemochromatosis.

An endemic form of nutritional iron overload has been noted in rural Africans who consume a traditional fermented beverage prepared at home in steel containers. However, not all individuals with high dietary iron develop iron overload, and heterozygosity for an unidentified iron-regulating gene may contribute. Nutritional iron overload is otherwise rare.

Less severe forms of iron overload have been described in association with alcoholic cirrhosis, hepatitis C, nonalcoholic steatohepatitis (NASH), porphyria cutanea tarda, and chronic medicinal iron intake. It has been noted that in some of these disorders, the frequency of *HFE* mutations is higher than would be predicted and likely contributes to the risk of iron overload. Hereditary atransferremia is characterized by the development of iron deposition secondary to inefficient utilization of iron by erythroid cells. Hereditary aceruloplasminemia may mimic hemochromatosis but is characterized by normal transferrin saturation and the presence of neurologic deficits. Ceruloplasmin has ferroxidase activity that is important for release of iron from macrophages; therefore, patients with a mutated gene may accumulate excess iron.

Iron chelation therapy

The management of secondary causes of hemochromatosis is difficult. Anemia often exists, and red blood cell transfusion may be required, making phlebotomy impractical. Rarely, erythropoietin can be used to increase hematocrit values to a range safe for phlebotomy. Splenectomy may decrease transfusion requirements in thalassemic patients as well as in other selected cases of chronic hemolytic anemias. Therapy aimed at treating the underlying condition, as in aplastic anemia for example, should be strongly considered. Avoiding unnecessary transfusions in patients with sickle cell disease and thalassemic syndromes is essential.

Deferoxamine is an effective iron-chelating agent used extensively in these conditions. When initiated early in the disease course, negative iron balance can be achieved and organ damage prevented. Deferoxamine is administered by nightly continuous subcutaneous infusion (up to 40 mg/kg) over an 8- to 12-hour period. Ascorbic acid 100 mg/d increases urinary iron excretion in deferoxamine-treated thalassemic patients but should be used with caution in heavily iron-loaded patients because of the possibility of increasing cardiac toxicity of iron overload. Local skin complications of deferoxamine are frequent and include pain, swelling, and pruritus at the injection site. These complications can be minimized by rotation of injection sites, addition of hydrocortisone to the solution containing deferoxamine, antihistamines, or local measures. Potential ocular and auditory complications secondary to deferoxamine mandate annual audiologic and ophthalmologic evaluation. Chronic deferoxamine therapy is arduous and expensive, and poor compliance often diminishes potential therapeutic benefits. Most experience with deferoxamine has been in patients with thalassemia major or sickle cell anemia who require chronic transfusion and thus have transfusional iron overload.

Deferasirox is the first oral iron chelator to receive FDA approval for treatment of transfusion-related iron overload in adults and children older than 2 years of age. A phase III trial showed that 20 to 30 mg/kg of deferasirox daily was sufficient to reduce liver iron concentrations and serum ferritin levels. Potential adverse effects included nausea, vomiting, diarrhea, abdominal pain, skin rash, agranulocytosis, and increases in serum creatinine or liver function tests. It is recommended that serum creatinine, liver function tests, and complete blood count be assessed before initiating therapy and monitored monthly thereafter to determine whether dose modification or discontinuation is necessary. Approximately one third of deferasirox-treated patients experienced dose-dependent increases in serum creatinine, although most of the creatinine concentrations remained within normal range. Liver function should be monitored monthly, and if there is an unexplained, persistent, or progressive increase in serum transaminase levels, deferasirox should be interrupted or discontinued. The complete blood count should be monitored as well, and deferasirox therapy should be interrupted if there is a decrease in the granulocyte count below the normal range. As with deferoxamine, cases of ocular and auditory disturbances have been reported.

Clinical case (continued)

The patient presented in this section has laboratory evidence suggesting iron overload. He has clinical manifestations consistent with hemochromatosis including diabetes, skin bronzing, hepatomegaly, and arthritis. Given the markedly elevated serum ferritin, a liver biopsy should be considered to evaluate for cirrhosis and to confirm the diagnosis. Secondary causes of iron overload should be ruled out. *HFE* genotyping could be considered. The patient should be counseled on alcohol cessation. Upon documentation of iron overload, an aggressive phlebotomy program should be initiated. Annual screening for hepatocellular carcinoma by liver ultrasound and measurement of α-fetoprotein should be performed if there is evidence of cirrhosis on liver biopsy. The patient's son should undergo initial screening with measurement of transferrin saturation and serum ferritin concentration and should then be monitored on a yearly basis for the development of iron overload. If his father has genotypic evidence of hereditary hemochromatosis, the son can also undergo genotyping to better predict his future risk. If elevated serum ferritin concentration develops in the son, a regular phlebotomy program should be recommended to minimize the risk for future complications of iron overload.

Key points

- The absorption of iron is highly regulated at the level of the enterocyte by hepcidin and ferroportin.
- Iron overload may be due to hereditary or acquired causes or blood transfusions.
- The $HFE^{C282Y/C282Y}$ genotype is the most common and most penetrant mutation leading to clinical iron overload in hereditary hemochromatosis.
- The true clinical penetrance of the $HFE^{C282Y/C282Y}$ genotype is debated but is likely <30%.
- Clinical manifestations of iron overload are similar regardless of etiology.
- Phlebotomy to remove excess iron is the primary treatment for homozygous hemochromatosis.
- Iron chelation therapy with deferoxamine or deferasirox is an option when phlebotomy is not possible. Annual audiologic and ophthalmologic examinations are required.
- Some clinical manifestations of hemochromatosis are reversible, but liver cirrhosis and the risk for hepatocellular carcinoma are not.
- Population screening is controversial, but high-risk individuals should be screened.

The porphyrias

Clinical case

A 52-year-old woman is referred for evaluation of lifelong cutaneous photosensitivity that has prompted the patient to exercise routine measures to protect herself from sunlight. The patient is G0P0 and postmenopausal. Past history reveals a splenectomy at age 29 for unknown cause. There is no exposure to alcohol or medicinal drugs. Physical examination shows no chronic skin changes, hepatomegaly, or stigmata of portal hypertension. The hemoglobin level is 12.0 g/dL (normal, 12.0–16.0 g/dL), and the mean corpuscular volume is 89 fL (normal, 80–100 fL). Liver function tests show a total bilirubin level of 0.6 mg/dL (normal, 0.1–1.2 mg/dL), an aspartate aminotransferase level of 96 U/L (normal, <41 U/L), and an alkaline phosphatase level of 115 U/L (normal, 33–115 U/L). Urine concentrations of δ-aminolevulinic acid, porphobilinogen (PBG), and uroporphyrin are normal. Erythrocyte protoporphyrin concentration is 18,900 μg/dL (normal, <90 μg/dL), and stool protoporphyrin level is 5100 μg/24 h (normal <1800 μg/24 h).

The porphyrias are a group of metabolic disorders characterized by inherited defects in the heme biosynthetic pathway (Figure 4-4). Eight enzymes are involved in the biosynthesis of heme. A defect in the first step, δ-aminolevulinic acid (ALA) synthetase, is associated with X-linked sideroblastic anemia. Defects in the 7 subsequent steps in heme synthesis result in distinct clinical porphyric syndromes due to the buildup of porphyrin precursors proximal to the enzymatic

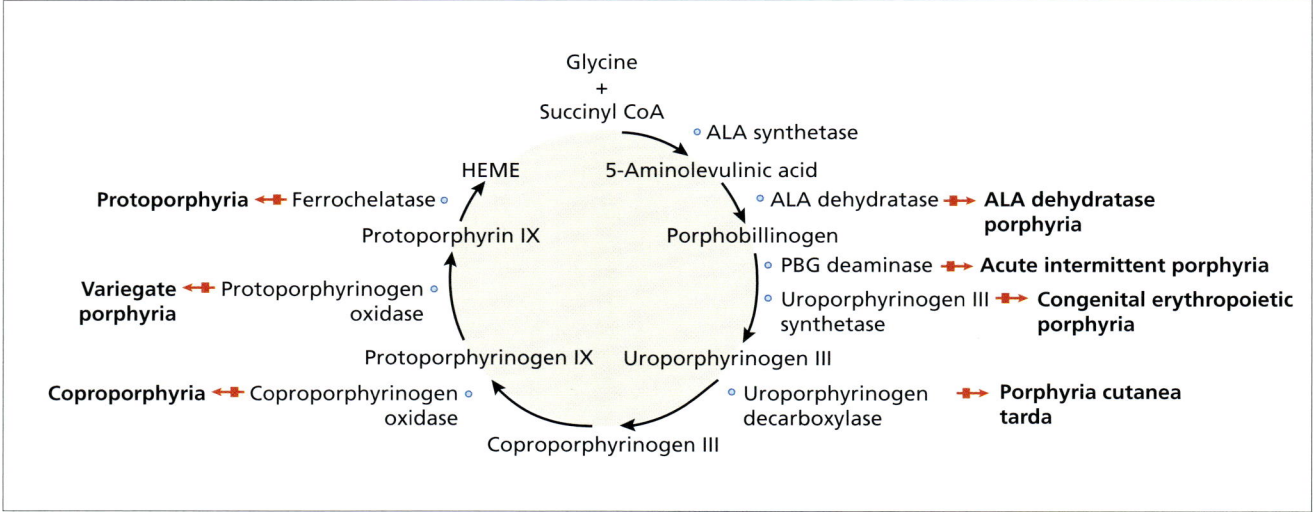

Figure 4-4 Heme biosynthetic pathway and associated porphyric syndromes. Porphyric syndromes are in boldface. Arrows point to the affected enzyme associated with each disorder.

defect. ALA may mediate neurologic toxicity via interaction with γ-aminobutyric acid (GABA) receptors. Porphyrin intermediates after PBG are photoreactive and potential oxidants. The clinical findings of each porphyria are dependent on the specific enzymatic defect as well as the characteristics of the accumulated intermediates of heme metabolism.

The porphyrias can be described as acute or chronic depending on the pattern of manifestation. Porphyrias may also be grouped according to whether the clinical presentation consists of neurovisceral changes, photosensitivity, or both (Table 4-4).

The phenotypic expression of each distinct porphyria is affected by many factors. Multiple molecular mutations have been identified for most of the enzyme defects. Environmental and metabolic factors are also important contributors to clinical expression. The clinical penetrance of the most common types of porphyria, porphyria cutanea tarda (PCT) and acute intermittent porphyria (AIP), is low in the absence of environmental or metabolic exposures.

Porphyrins or their precursors accumulate above normal trace amounts and are excreted into the urine or feces, depending on water solubility. The excretion profiles of the porphyrins and their precursors reflect the enzymatic defect in the heme synthetic pathway and are diagnostic for each specific disorder (Table 4-4). Abnormalities can thus be detected through measurement of the accumulated porphyrin or its precursors in the appropriate body fluid. Measurement can be difficult. Proper timing of collection and meticulous handling of the specimen including appropriate measures to minimize light exposure are required to obtain valid laboratory data. Specimens are best collected during an acute exacerbation. Mild elevations in precursor porphyrins are common and nonspecific. Levels approximating >5 to 10 times the normal values in the appropriate body fluid are

Table 4-4 Genetic, clinical, and biochemical features of the porphyrias.

	Inheritance	Clinical manifestations	Major excretory routes and intermediates of heme metabolism
Acute porphyrias			
Acute intermittent porphyria	AD	Neurovisceral	Urine ALA + PBG
Hereditary coproporphyria	AD	Neurovisceral; cutaneous	Urine ALA + PBG; fecal coproporphyrins
Variegate porphyria	AD	Neurovisceral; cutaneous	Urine ALA + PBG; fecal protoporphyrins
ALA dehydratase deficiency	AR	Neurovisceral	Urine ALA
Nonacute or cutaneous porphyrias			
Porphyria cutanea tarda	AD	Blistering cutaneous lesions	Urine uroporphyrins
Erythropoietic protoporphyria	AD	Painful cutaneous lesions; hepatic	Fecal protoporphyrin; red blood cell protoporphyrin
Congenital erythropoietic porphyria	AR	Disfiguring cutaneous lesions, skeletal changes, anemia	Urine uroporphyrin I

AD = autosomal dominant; ALA = δ-aminolevulinic acid; AR = autosomal recessive; PBG = porphobilinogen.

necessary to be considered diagnostic. These levels may not be evident between episodes of the acute porphyrias. Enzymatic measurements or DNA studies may be necessary to identify disease in asymptomatic individuals.

Acute porphyrias
Metabolic defects

Defects in each of 4 different enzymes account for the characteristics of the acute porphyrias. Penetrance is incomplete, and only a minority of individuals with each genetic defect may have phenotypic expression of the disease. The clinical sequelae of the acute porphyrias are often unmasked only in the presence of endogenous or exogenous factors that promote heme biosynthesis and lead to further accumulation of porphyrins and their precursors.

Acute intermittent porphyria

AIP is the most common of the acute porphyrias and is due to a deficiency in PBG-deaminase activity. Inheritance is autosomal dominant. The genetic defect affects approximately 1 in 10,000 persons in the United States and Europe. Clinical expression of the disease occurs in <10% of carriers. PBG-deaminase activity approximating 50% of normal is seen in red blood cells of patients with AIP. Extensive molecular heterogeneity exists, and >100 mutations have been noted in the *PBG-deaminase* gene in patients with AIP. During a severe attack, the urine may appear a "port wine" color due to markedly elevated levels of ALA and PBG. Urinary ALA and PBG levels are variable between attacks and at times may be normal. Red blood cell PBG-deaminase levels remain low at all times (~50%) confirming an individual carries the mutation and may be at risk for clinical sequelae. PBG-deaminase has 2 isoforms (erythroid and nonerythroid) resulting from alternative splicing of mRNA. Approximately 10% of AIP patients have a normal red blood cell PBG-deaminase level but have diminished PGB-deaminase activity in the liver due to a mutation in the nonerythroid isoform.

Hereditary coproporphyria

Hereditary coproporphyria is much less common and is due to a deficiency of coproporphyrinogen oxidase activity (~50%). Inheritance is autosomal dominant. Homozygotes with <5% activity have also been described. Excessive amounts of coproporphyrins accumulate in the stool, along with ALA and PBG in the urine, during acute attacks.

Variegate porphyria

Variegate porphyria is due to a deficiency of protoporphyrinogen oxidase. Inheritance is autosomal dominant. Although variegate porphyria appears worldwide, it is most prevalent in South Africans of Dutch ancestry, where it is theorized to have arisen as a founder gene mutation from a Dutch settler. Rare homozygous cases have been described. Protoporphyrins and coproporphyrins in the stool, as well as ALA and PBG in the urine, are the major intermediates excreted.

ALA dehydratase deficiency

ALA dehydratase deficiency is the least common porphyria, with only 4 cases described in the literature. It is unique among the acute porphyrias in its autosomal recessive mode of inheritance. A defect in ALA dehydratase leads to accumulation of large amounts of ALA in the urine without much PBG. ALA dehydratase is also inhibited in tyrosinemia and plumbism (lead toxicity). In addition to ALA dehydratase, lead inhibits coproporphyrinogen oxidase and ferrochelatase. Lead poisoning causes abdominal pain, constipation, nausea, and neuropathy and thus can be confused with acute porphyria. Urine excretion of ALA exceeds that of PBG in plumbism, but measurements of lead levels and the finding of a microcytic anemia with basophilic stippling of red blood cell will help to differentiate it from porphyria. Lead inhibition of ALA dehydratase can be reversed by addition of zinc and dithiothreitol.

Clinical features

The 4 types of acute porphyria present with similar acute neurovisceral presentations and may be indistinguishable during an acute attack. Acute abdominal pain, nausea, vomiting, and constipation are the most common symptoms, likely secondary to autonomic dysfunction. The presentation can resemble an acute surgical abdomen, and unnecessary exploratory laparotomy has been performed. Peripheral motor neuropathy may occur, leading to wide variations in presentation. Respiratory paralysis can ensue, requiring prolonged mechanical ventilation due to cranial nerve involvement or bulbar paralysis. Sensory nerve involvement is less frequent. Hyponatremia secondary to inappropriate secretion of antidiuretic hormone can be profound. Varying degrees of neuropsychiatric abnormalities have been described ranging from anxiety and depression to agitation, delirium, and seizures. Concomitant psychiatric illness may lead to a delay in diagnosis. The length and severity of individual attacks are extremely variable and poorly predicted. Symptoms may also vary substantially within a given patient during separate attacks.

Metabolic and environmental factors are important contributors to the clinical expression of each porphyria. The acute porphyrias rarely present prior to puberty, and gonadal hormones are thus thought to play a contributing role. Certain medications are believed to be common precipitating factors through induction of ALA synthetase or cytochrome P450 activity. The barbiturates, other anticonvulsants, sulfonamides, oral contraceptives, and alcohol are best described. Several Web sites are available that define which individual drugs are safe, unsafe, or unproven in patients with porphyria (www.porphyria-europe.com and www.porphyriafoundation.com). Decreased carbohydrate intake, stress, and dehydration are also thought to be precipitating factors.

Cutaneous photosensitivity leading to blistering skin lesions occurs in 20% to 30% of cases of hereditary coproporphyria and 40% to 70% of cases of variegate porphyria due to accumulation of photosensitive porphyrin substrates. Skin damage is not seen in AIP or ALA dehydratase deficiency because the porphyrin precursors are not activated by ultraviolet sunlight.

Diagnostic algorithm

A diagnostic algorithm for the evaluation of patients with a suspected acute porphyric syndrome is illustrated in Figure 4-5. Initial rapid testing for urine PBG should be considered for patients presenting with symptoms of acute porphyria using the Trace PBG Kit (Thermo Trace/DMA, Arlington, TX) or other qualitative test such as Watson-Schwarz or Hoersch test. Samples for quantitative measurement of porphyrins should be collected during an acute attack and not exposed to sunlight during collection, shipping, or evaluation. Enzymatic activity measurement and DNA testing are recommended to confirm the type of acute porphyria and to enable identification of asymptomatic relatives who may be at risk. Erythrocyte PBG-deaminase determinations are readily available, although 10% of AIP patients will have a normal level because their defect is in the non-erythroid form of this enzyme. PBG-deaminase deficiency

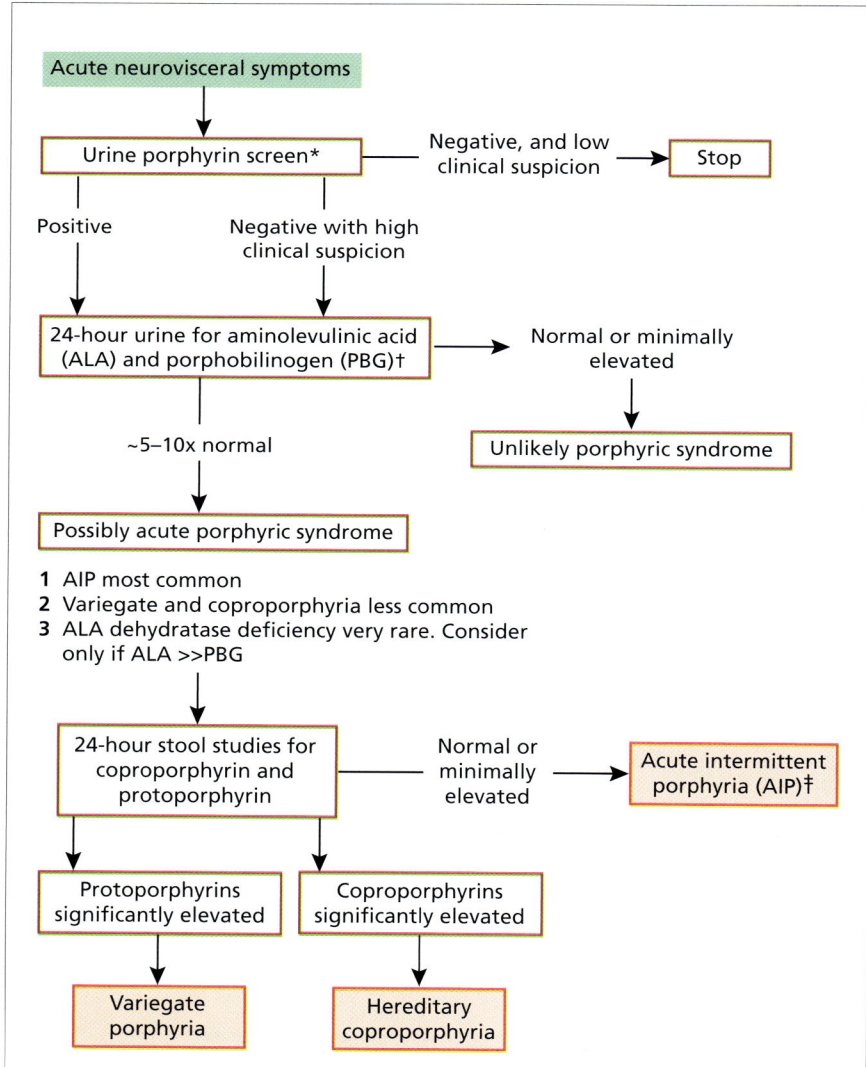

Figure 4-5 Diagnostic algorithm for patients with suspected acute porphyric syndrome. *Qualitative tests such as Watson-Schwarz test, Hoersch test, or Trace PBG Kit can be considered. †Collected without exposure to sunlight and during acute crisis. ‡Consider checking red blood cell porphobilinogen deaminase for confirmation.

may also escape detection because of the overlap between high carrier and low normal values, greater activity in young red blood cells when reticulocytosis is present, or improper processing of the blood sample. Mutation analysis is available at the Mount Sinai School of Medicine, Department of Human Genetics and in several European laboratories.

Treatment

The treatment of choice for all but mild attacks of acute porphyria is intravenous hemin therapy. Hemin, formed when heme is dissociated from its apoprotein and the Fe^{2+} iron is oxidized to Fe^{3+} iron, can inhibit ALA synthetase, the rate-limiting step of heme biosynthesis. Hemin is available as hematin (Panhematin; Ovation Pharmaceuticals, Deerfield, IL) in the United States and as heme arginate (Normosang; Orphan Europe, Paris, France) in Europe. Both agents are given intravenously 3 to 4 mg/kg once daily for 4 days. Potential adverse effects include disseminated intravascular coagulation, phlebitis at the infusion site, and renal failure. These complications may be minimized by reconstituting hemin with albumin. Biochemical precursors should be followed and clinical examinations should be performed to gauge the effectiveness of therapy. Glucose is known to suppress the induction of ALA synthetase, the initial step in heme synthesis. Carbohydrate loading consisting of 500 g of dextrose daily can be used for mild attacks (absence of weakness and hyponatremia) and while waiting for hemin to be available for a more severe attack. During acute attacks, correction of dehydration and hyponatremia is essential, as is monitoring the expiratory flow rate. Intravenous narcotics may be necessary to control acute pain.

Supportive care is also integral to the management of acute porphyrias. Prevention of precipitating factors or avoidance of offending drugs is of paramount importance. Avoidance of smoking, caffeine, alcohol, and stress is thought to be helpful in minimizing acute attacks. Women with frequent premenstrual attacks may benefit from treatment with gonadotropin-releasing hormone analogs. Long-term consequences of acute porphyria include hypertension and end-stage renal failure. A 60- to 70-fold increase in the incidence of mortality due to hepatoma has been observed in acute porphyria patients, indicating the need for periodic determination of α-fetoprotein levels and hepatic imaging studies. In rare individuals with severe, unremitting disease, liver transplantation has been performed with success.

Nonacute or cutaneous porphyrias

PCT, erythropoietic protoporphyria, and congenital erythropoietic porphyria are considered among the chronic porphyrias. These disorders are similar in that they do not present with acute neurovisceral attacks. The clinical presentation of these disorders is chronic in nature, even though the severity may wax and wane over time.

Porphyria cutanea tarda
Metabolic defect

PCT is due to a partial deficiency in the enzyme uroporphyrinogen decarboxylase (UROD). PCT is the most common porphyria, and both sporadic (type I) and familial (type II) forms exist. In heterozygous individuals, half-normal enzyme activity is noted. A rare homozygous form termed hepatoerythropoietic porphyria also exists. The diagnosis of PCT is confirmed by the presence of excessive amounts of urine uroporphyrins in the presence of typical blistering skin lesions. Increased iron stores are common and may be related to downregulation of hepcidin.

Clinical features

Clinical manifestations of PCT are limited to the skin; neurovisceral symptoms never occur. Patients typically present in the spring and summer months with painless blistering erosions or scarring in sun-exposed areas such as the hands, chest, and feet (Figure 4-6). Uroporphyrins are phototoxic when exposed to sunlight and disrupt the dermal–epidermal junction in the face of even minor trauma, causing the typical blistering skin lesions. Typically heterozygotes are clinically asymptomatic. However, the phenotypic expression of PCT is often triggered by conditions leading to excess iron and environmental exposures such as alcohol or estrogen. Increased iron is thought to impair residual UROD function

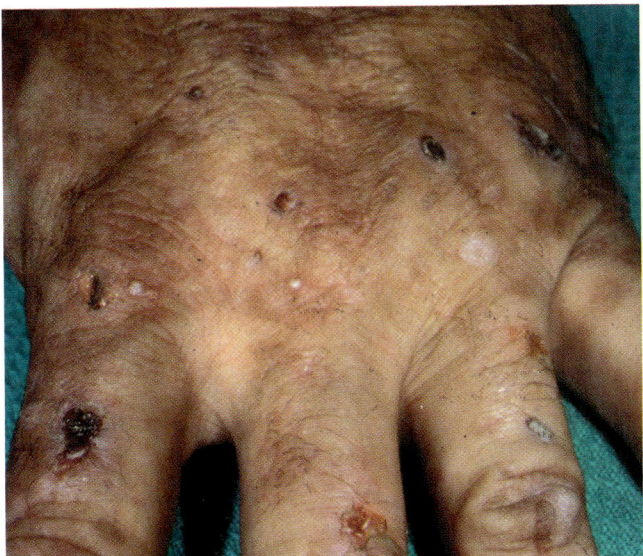

Figure 4-6 Typical scarring and blistering skin lesions on sun-exposed areas in a patient with porphyria cutanea tarda (PCT).

in hepatocytes, leading to further uroporphyrin accumulation. The genetic mutations leading to hereditary hemochromatosis are seen with greater than expected frequencies in patients with symptoms, because excess iron likely plays a role in the phenotypic expression of PCT. In fact, increased iron is found in up to 80% of liver biopsy specimens in patients with PCT. PCT may be associated with liver damage ranging from mild elevations of hepatic transaminases to cirrhosis and subsequent risk for hepatoma. PCT may also be associated with polymorphisms in cytochromes (CYP1A2) and the TfR1 gene (*TFRC*). Susceptible dialysis patients may also develop clinical manifestations due to transfusional iron overload. The mechanism whereby exogenous estrogen precipitates PCT is not entirely clear. Hepatitis C, human immunodeficiency virus (HIV), and certain environmental toxic compounds are also associated with PCT.

Treatment

Removal of iron through phlebotomy therapy is the mainstay of treatment and is highly effective in inducing remission. Often a limited number of procedures removing 400 to 500 mL of blood with each phlebotomy can lead to clinical remission within a few months. Phlebotomy should be continued until ferritin values decrease to <50 μg/L. Remissions may be permanent if known precipitating factors are avoided and iron does not reaccumulate. However, if the precipitating factor cannot be removed or modified, then maintenance phlebotomy may be required to ameliorate skin damage and symptoms. Iron chelation therapy can be considered if the patient cannot tolerate phlebotomy.

The identification, modification, and avoidance of precipitating factors are also important. If an underlying disease, such as hepatitis C, is identified, an attempt at treatment should be made. The patient should avoid excessive sunlight and cover sun-exposed areas of the skin. Sunscreen containing zinc oxide, which forms an opaque film, is the preferred sun-blocking agent. Typical sunscreens are not effective because light absorption by porphyrins is maximal around 400 nm and extends into the visible range. Chloroquine given at low doses may be a useful second-line agent when phlebotomy is contraindicated. Patients with cirrhosis should be monitored for the potential development of hepatocellular carcinoma.

Erythropoietic protoporphyria
Metabolic defect

Erythropoietic protoporphyria is characterized by the autosomal dominant inheritance of a defect in ferrochelatase, the terminal enzyme of the heme biosynthetic pathway. Levels of ferrochelatase are approximately 30% of normal in patients with the disease, suggesting that the disease is expressed when the patient has a mutant allele in combination with a low-expression wild-type allele. Molecular analysis has identified a variety of mutations that lead to a decrease in ferrochelatase production. Massive accumulation of protoporphyrin is seen in erythrocytes and in the plasma and feces.

Clinical features

Large amounts of protoporphyrins can accumulate in early life and lead to marked photosensitivity in sun-exposed areas of skin. Even with limited exposure to sun or fluorescent light, painful burning of the skin is followed by erythema and edema. These findings are in contrast to the small painless blistering skin lesions that occur with sun exposure in patients with PCT. Photoexcitation of protoporphyrin can also generate oxygen free radicals, which damage cell membranes and lead to excess fibroblast activity. Chronic skin changes and progressive liver failure secondary to fibrosis have been noted. A mild microcytic hypochromic anemia may also be present.

Therapy

Avoidance of sunlight and use of opaque topical sunscreens, as in PCT, are indicated. β-Carotene has been used to increase tolerance to the sun. Liver transplantation has been performed in a few patients who had significant hepatic involvement and hepatic failure. Bone marrow transplantation is potentially curative.

Congenital erythropoietic porphyria (Gunther disease)
Metabolic defect

Congenital erythropoietic porphyria is an extremely rare autosomal recessive deficiency of the enzyme uroporphyrin III synthetase. Multiple mutations leading to this defect have been identified. Homozygous individuals have massive accumulation and excretion of uroporphyrin I.

Clinical features

Patients with severe disease develop mutilating photodermatitis early in life, although milder forms do exist. Increased skin fragility ultimately leads to ulceration and necrosis of the hands and feet. Alopecia is common. Historically, it is thought that references to werewolves may have actually described patients with chronic erythropoietic porphyria. Anemia secondary to a combination of hemolysis, hypersplenism, and ineffective erythropoiesis has been noted. Skeletal changes including vertebral collapse, short stature, and pathologic fractures are common and thought to be secondary to compensatory bone marrow expansion. Teeth may appear pink or brown due to high porphyrin content.

Treatment

The only curative treatment described to date is bone marrow transplantation. Sunscreen and β-carotene are typically poorly tolerated and ineffective. Prompt treatment of bacterial skin infections is of paramount importance. Hypertransfusion of red blood cells is effective in reducing endogenous porphyrin biosynthesis, but subsequent iron overload is a concern. Other therapies have been investigated but have not proved successful.

> **Clinical case (continued)**
>
> The patient presented in this section has a history of lifelong dermal photosensitivity without blistering and without a history of neurovisceral complications. This history is suggestive of erythropoietic protoporphyria. The markedly elevated protoporphyrin levels in red blood cells and stool and the normal urinary uroporphyrin concentration confirm the diagnosis of erythropoietic protoporphyria. Rarely erythropoietic protoporphyria is complicated by hemolysis and splenomegaly, but we do not know whether these findings are what led to splenectomy in this patient. The patient continued to protect herself from sun exposure and was treated with β-carotene, but progressive hepatic dysfunction was observed, with the alkaline phosphatase increasing to 239 U/L. A liver biopsy demonstrated cirrhosis and hepatocellular accumulation of crystalline pigment.

> **Key points**
>
> - The porphyrias are a heterogeneous group of disorders characterized by defects in enzymes of the heme biosynthetic pathway.
> - Patients with exacerbations of acute porphyria have 5- to 10-fold increases in metabolic precursors such as ALA and PBG. Minor elevations of these precursors are nonspecific and not diagnostic of disease.
> - Clinical manifestations including neurovisceral symptoms, photosensitivity, or the combination are due to the specific nature of each porphyrin or precursor that accumulates.
> - The clinical presentation of each type of porphyria is due to the combination of an underlying genetic defect modified by various metabolic, environmental, and epigenetic factors.
> - Clinical features of AIP include neurovisceral symptoms, but skin damage is not seen. PBG-deaminase is decreased in red blood cells in most, but not all, patients. Treatment of acute attacks may require infusion of hemin. Long-term follow-up includes screening for hepatocellular carcinoma.
> - In PCT, patients present with skin damage, but without neurovisceral symptoms. Patients should be evaluated for iron overload, hepatitis C, HIV, and other risk factors. Phlebotomy to reduce iron burden is a key element of treatment.
> - Treatment is unique to each porphyria but generally involves minimizing exposure to inciting agents such as sun exposure in PCT or causative drugs or dehydration in AIP. Phlebotomy is indicated in PCT, whereas caloric loading is indicated in AIP.

Bibliography

Regulation of iron homeostasis

Bleackley MR, Wong AY, Hudson DM, Wu CH, Macgillivray RT. Blood iron homeostasis: newly discovered proteins and iron imbalance. *Transfus Med Rev.* 2009;23:103–123. *A review of iron metabolism and associated disorders.*

Casey JL, Hentze MW, Koeller DM, et al. Iron-responsive elements: regulatory RNA sequences that control mRNA levels and translation. *Science.* 1988;240:924–928. *The classic paper showing the relationship between mRNA sequences and iron regulation.*

Fleming MD. The regulation of hepcidin and its effects on systemic and cellular iron metabolism. *Hematology Am Soc Hematol Educ Program.* 2008:151–158. *A review discussing the mechanisms underlying the regulation of hepcidin levels, including a discussion of HJV and the BMP/Smad pathways.*

Fleming RE, Bacon BR. Orchestration of iron homeostasis. *N Engl J Med.* 2005;352:1741–1744. *A pithy review of iron balance.*

Kuhn LC, Hentze MW. Coordination of cellular iron metabolism by post-transcriptional gene regulation. *J Inorg Biochem.* 1992;47:183–195. *Excellent discussion of the role of IRPs in iron metabolism.*

Pietrangelol A. The ferroportin disease. *Blood Cells Mol Dis.* 2004;32:131–138. *A review of ferroportin disease.*

Roy CN, Enns CA. Iron homeostasis: new tales from the crypt. *Blood.* 2000;96:4020–4027. *An updated proposed model of iron absorption.*

Weiss G, Goodnough LT. Anemia of chronic disease. *N Engl J Med.* 2005;352:1011–1023. *Recent review of this topic, including the role of hepcidin on iron balance.*

Hereditary hemochromatosis and other iron overload syndromes

Ajioka RS, Kushner JP. Clinical consequences of iron overload in hemochromatosis homozygotes. *Blood.* 2003;101:3351–3353. *Expert opinion arguing that the true penetrance of hereditary hemochromatosis is likely higher than recently suggested by some experts. Part of back-to-back articles with differing opinions on this subject.*

Beutler E. Hemochromatosis: genetics and pathophysiology. *Annu Rev Med.* 2006;57:331–347. *A concise review and update on hereditary hemochromatosis.*

Beutler E. The HFE Cys282Tyr mutation as a necessary but not sufficient cause of clinical hereditary hemochromatosis. *Blood.* 2003;101:3347–3350. *Expert opinion arguing that the true penetrance of hereditary hemochromatosis is likely much lower than recently stated. Part of back-to-back articles with differing opinions on this subject.*

Beutler E, Felitti VJ, Koziol JA, Ho NJ, Gelbart T. Penetrance of 845G→A (C282Y) HFE hereditary haemochromatosis mutation in the USA. *Lancet.* 2002;359:211–218. *A population screening study that compares symptoms of individuals with hereditary hemochromatosis to a control population. The penetrance of homozygous hereditary hemochromatosis is predicted to be much less than previously considered.*

Brittenham GM, Badman DG; National Institute of Diabetes and Digestive and Kidney Diseases (NIDDK) Workshop. Noninvasive measurement of iron: report of an NIDDK workshop. *Blood.* 2003;101:15–19. *Review of noninvasive measurement of iron including MRI and SQUID.*

Bulaj ZJ, Ajioka RS, Phillips JD, et al. Disease-related conditions in relatives of patients with hemochromatosis. *N Engl J Med.* 2000;343:1529–1535. *Genotypic and phenotypic frequencies of hemochromatosis in family members of probands with clinical disease.*

Cogswell ME, Burke W, McDonnell SM, Franks AL. Screening for hemochromatosis. A public health perspective. *Am J Prev Med.* 1999;16:134–140. *Summary of screening recommendations for hereditary hemochromatosis.*

Deugnier YM, Loreal O, Turlin B, et al. Liver pathology in genetic hemochromatosis: a review of 135 homozygous cases and their bioclinical correlations. *Gastroenterology.* 1992;102:2050–2059. *A description of the evaluation of iron content in liver biopsy specimens.*

Feder JN, Gnirke A, Thomas W, et al. A novel MHC class I-like gene is mutated in patients with hereditary haemochromatosis. *Nat Genet.* 1996;13:399–408. *A description of the identification of the HFE gene and associated mutations.*

Ganz T. Hepcidin, a key regulator of iron metabolism and mediator of anemia of inflammation. *Blood.* 2003;102:783–788. *Review of hepcidin biochemistry.*

Lee PL, Beutler E, Rao SV, Barton JC. Genetic abnormalities and juvenile hemochromatosis: mutations of the HJV gene encoding hemojuvelin. *Blood.* 2004;103:4669–4671. *A description of 2 kindreds of patients with juvenile hemochromatosis with mutations in the HJV gene.*

McDonnell SM, Phatak PD, Felitti V, Hover A, McLaren GD. Screening for hemochromatosis in primary care settings. *Ann Intern Med.* 1998;129:962–970. *Population-based screening study of hemochromatosis.*

Morrison ED, Brandhagen DJ, Phatak PD, et al. Serum ferritin level predicts advanced hepatic fibrosis among U.S. patients with phenotypic hemochromatosis. *Ann Intern Med.* 2003;138:627–633. Erratum in: *Ann Intern Med.* 2003;139:235. *Cross-sectional study investigating serum ferritin levels, liver enzymes, and age as predictors of cirrhosis and the need for liver biopsy in patients with hereditary hemochromatosis.*

Olynyk JK, Cullen DJ, Aquilia S, Rossi E, Summerville L, Powell LW. A population-based study of the clinical expression of the hemochromatosis gene. *N Engl J Med.* 1999;341:718–724. *Population-based screening study of hemochromatosis.*

The porphyrias

Ajioka RS, Phillips JD, Weiss RB, et al. Down-regulation of hepcidin in porphyria cutanea tarda. *Blood.* 2008;112:4723–4728. *A clinical study suggesting that downregulation of hepcidin may underlie hepatic iron loading in PCT.*

Anderson KE, Bloomer JR, Bonkovsky HL, et al. Recommendations for the diagnosis and treatment of the acute porphyrias. *Ann Intern Med.* 2005;142:439–450. *Guidelines for diagnosis and management of the acute porphyrias developed by an expert panel.*

Anderson KE, Sassa S, Bishop DF, Desnick RJ. Disorders of heme biosynthesis: X-linked sideroblastic anemia and the porphyrias. In: Scriver CR, Beaudet A, Sly WS, Valle D, eds. *The Metabolic and Molecular Bases of Inherited Disease.* 8th ed. New York, NY: McGraw-Hill; 2001:2991–3062. *A comprehensive treatise on heme metabolism and its related disorders; an online version is available through many libraries.*

Bonkovsky HL. Neurovisceral porphyrias: what a hematologist needs to know. *Hematology Am Soc Hematol Educ Program.* 2005:24–30. *A good review of the acute porphyrias with useful tables and diagrams.*

Daniell WE, Stockbridge HL, Labbe RF, et al. Environmental chemical exposures and disturbances of heme synthesis. *Environ Health Perspect.* 1997;105(Suppl 1):37–53. *Role of drugs and chemicals in induction of the acute porphyrias.*

Dhar GJ, Bossenmaier I, Petryka ZJ, Cardinal R, Watson CJ. Effects of hematin in hepatic porphyria. Further studies. *Ann Intern Med.* 1975;83:20–30. *Description of the role of hematin in treatment of severe attacks of acute porphyria.*

Egger NG, Goeger DE, Payne DA, Miskovsky EP, Weinman SA, Anderson KE. Porphyria cutanea tarda: multiplicity of risk factors including HFE mutations, hepatitis C, and inherited uroporphyrinogen decarboxylase deficiency. *Dig Dis Sci.* 2002;47:419–426. *The many factors associated with PCT.*

Grandchamp B, Picat C, Mignotte V, et al. Tissue-specific splicing mutation in acute intermittent porphyria. *Proc Natl Acad Sci USA.* 1989;86:661–664. *Description of alternative isoforms of PBG deaminase.*

Kauppinen R. Porphyrias. *Lancet.* 2005;365:241–252. *Excellent brief review of the porphyric syndromes.*

Linet MS, Gridley G, Nyren O, et al. Primary liver cancer, other malignancies, and mortality risks following porphyria: a cohort study in Denmark and Sweden. *Am J Epidemiol.* 1999;149:1010–1015. *Description of the increased risk for liver cancer in AIP and PCT in a Scandinavian population.*

Najahi-Missaoui W, Dailey HA. Production and characterization of erythropoietic protoporphyric heterodimeric ferrochelatases. *Blood.* 2005;106:1098–1104. *A consideration of the factors that lead to clinical expression of erythropoietic protoporphyria in patients heterozygous for a ferrochelatase mutation.*

Sarkany RPE. The management of porphyria cutanea tarda. *Clin Exp Dermatol.* 2001;26:225–232. *Review of the diagnosis and clinical management of PCT.*

CHAPTER 05

Acquired underproduction anemias

Michal G. Rose and Cindy A. Leissinger

Underproduction anemias resulting from nutritional deficiencies, 110
Megaloblastic anemias, 115
Underproduction anemias resulting from organ dysfunction, 121
Marrow failure states leading to underproduction anemias, 125
Anemia secondary to marrow infiltration or abnormalities in the marrow microenvironment, 127
Complex/multifactorial anemias, 128
Bibliography, 130

Erythrocyte production requires the presence of bone marrow stem cells, erythropoietin (EPO), elemental iron, vitamins, cytokines, and a suitable marrow microenvironment. Deficiency or unavailability of any of these key components may lead to the underproduction of erythrocytes and result in anemia. Normal erythropoiesis follows an ordered progression from the pluripotent colony-forming unit–granulocyte erythroid-monocyte macrophage (CFU-GEMM), to the burst-forming units–erythroid (BFU-E), to colony-forming units–erythroid (CFU-E), to proerythroblasts, to erythroblasts, and finally to mature erythrocytes (see Figure 12-1). Red blood cell (RBC) maturation is dependent on the presence of EPO, a 165–amino acid glycoprotein produced by the kidney. EPO acts via cross-linkage of its receptor. The resulting receptor dimers initiate a sequence of signaling reactions that both prevent apoptosis and stimulate proliferation and maturation of erythroid cells. EPO production is increased by hypoxia and is regulated at the level of transcription. A complete discussion of iron metabolism is presented in Chapter 4 and will be only briefly reviewed in this chapter. Iron utilization is critical in the formation of erythrocytes because iron is a necessary component of heme, and the majority of total body iron is found in the RBC mass. Although ingested iron is absorbed throughout the gastrointestinal (GI) mucosa, it is most efficiently absorbed in the distal duodenum and proximal jejunum.

Absorbed iron is complexed with transferrin and ultimately either incorporated into the erythroblast or stored as ferritin. Iron utilization is regulated at the messenger RNA (mRNA) level such that when cytoplasmic iron is low, there is increased translation of the transferrin receptor and decreased translation of apoferritin (ferritin devoid of iron). Conversely, when cytoplasmic iron is high, translation of apoferritin is increased and translation of the transferrin receptor is decreased. Other key nutrients such as folic acid and cobalamin are also critical to the developing RBC. The marrow microenvironment is similarly important to erythropoiesis as a source of cytokines, vascular supply, and adhesion molecules.

The production and maintenance of a suitable RBC mass are necessary to ensure survival. The average man has an RBC mass of 26 to 32 mL/kg, whereas the average female has an RBC mass of 23 to 29 mL/kg. Values are slightly lower in children. The average erythrocyte has a life span of 120 days. Senescent erythrocyte clearance occurs via macrophages in the marrow, liver, and spleen. The precise signaling mechanisms responsible for this clearance are not known.

The etiologies of anemia are diverse and range from external blood loss, to underproduction of RBCs, to the accelerated destruction of developing or mature RBCs. In addition, anemia may be either inherited or acquired. This chapter will focus on anemia due to the acquired underproduction of RBCs. Although diverse in etiology, the underproduction anemias are characterized by a hypoproliferation of RBCs and by a low or inappropriately "normal" reticulocyte count. This chapter divides the underproduction anemias into those that are secondary to vitamin or nutrient deficiencies, organ

---

Conflict-of-interest disclosure: *Dr. Rose* declares no competing financial interest. *Dr. Leissinger* declares no competing financial interest.

dysfunction, bone marrow failure states, and abnormalities in the bone marrow microenvironment. Many anemias are multifactorial and complex in etiology, yet some of these are so commonly seen in clinical practice that they deserve separate consideration. Thus, anemia associated with pregnancy, aging, cancer, and human immunodeficiency virus (HIV) infection will be covered as separate topics in this chapter. An outline of the acquired underproduction anemias covered in this chapter is depicted in Table 5-1.

Underproduction anemias resulting from nutritional deficiencies

Iron
Iron deficiency anemia

> **Clinical case**
>
> A 52-year-old woman presents 4 years after gastric bypass with fatigue and dyspnea on exertion. Her only medication is intramuscular 1000 μg vitamin B$_{12}$ each month. She denies GI bleeding and is postmenopausal. Her physical examination is significant for skin pallor and pale conjunctivae. Stool is guaiac negative. Laboratory evaluation reveals a hypoproliferative microcytic anemia with hemoglobin of 7.4 g/dL, mean cell volume (MCV) of 74 fL, and reticulocyte count of 1%. White blood cell count is normal, and the platelet count is slightly elevated at 502,000/μL. Iron studies reveal a low serum iron, elevated total iron-binding capacity (TIBC), and a markedly reduced ferritin of 9 ng/mL (normal range, 15–400 ng/mL). Serum cobalamin, folic acid, homocysteine (HCY), and methylmalonic acid (MMA) levels are normal. A colonoscopy and esophagogastroduodenoscopy fail to reveal any source of bleeding. Oral iron replacement does not correct her anemia, although she rapidly responds to the administration of intravenous iron gluconate.

Iron deficiency remains the most common cause of anemia worldwide. Using anemia as an indirect indicator for iron deficiency, it is estimated that close to 50% of preschool children and pregnant women in nonindustrialized countries and 30% to 40% in industrialized countries are iron deficient. However, iron deficiency anemia is less common in the United States, with approximately 5%, 1%, and 7% of toddlers, preschool children, and females aged 12 to 49 years, respectively, affected. Chapter 4 describes iron metabolism in detail. Table 5-2 lists common causes of iron deficiency. In developing countries, hookworm infection leading to chronic intestinal blood loss is the most common cause of iron deficiency. In the developed world, nonparasitic GI blood loss is the most common cause of iron deficiency in adult males, whereas menstrual blood

Table 5-1 Selected acquired causes of underproduction anemias.

Vitamin/nutrients
  Iron
    Deficiency
    Dysregulation (anemia of chronic inflammation/disease)
  Megaloblastic anemias
    Cobalamin deficiency
    Folate deficiency
    Other deficiencies
  Trace elements
  Sideroblastic anemias (nonmyelodysplastic)
  Starvation

Organ dysfunction
  Renal disease
  Endocrine deficiency (pituitary, thyroid, adrenal, testis, other)
  Gastrointestinal disorders
  Liver disease

Marrow failure states
  Pure red cell aplasia
    Immune
    Infection
    Drug
    Other

Abnormalities in the marrow microenvironment
  Infiltrative processes
    Malignant
    Storage diseases (ie, Gaucher disease)
    Hemophagocytic syndrome

Complex/multifactorial etiologies
  Anemia associated with pregnancy
  Anemia of aging
  Anemia of cancer
  Anemia associated with HIV infection

HIV = human immunodeficiency virus.

loss is the most common cause in premenopausal females. Iron deficiency should not be considered a diagnosis but a secondary outcome due to an underlying medical condition. During infancy, iron deficiency usually results from excessive intake of whole cows' milk or prolonged breast-feeding without iron supplementation. In premenopausal women in the United States, excessive menstrual bleeding (typically >80 mL/month) is the most common etiology of iron deficiency. Iron deficiency may be a physiologic response to rapid growth in body size during infancy and adolescence, but it still requires treatment. In any case, once the diagnosis of iron deficiency anemia is made, a search for the precise cause is necessary. In fact, iron deficiency may be the first clue to a myriad of diverse diseases such as celiac disease, paroxysmal nocturnal hemoglobinuria, and GI malignancies.

Iron deficiency is usually a late result of an extended period of negative iron balance. Iron deficiency follows a typical

Table 5-2 Causes of iron deficiency anemia.

Increased iron requirements
  Blood loss
    Hookworm infestation
    Gastrointestinal disorders (esophageal varices, hemorrhoids, peptic ulcer disease, malignancies)
    Extensive and prolonged menstruation
    Pulmonary (hemoptysis, pulmonary hemosiderosis), urologic, or nasal disorders
    Chronic blood donations
    Dialysis
    Factitious removal
  Intravascular hemolysis with hemoglobinuria
    Paroxysmal nocturnal hemoglobinuria
    Cardiac valve prostheses
  Rapid growth in body size between 2 and 36 months of age
  Pregnancy and lactation
Inadequate iron supply
  Poor nutritional intake in children (not a common independent mechanism in adults but may be a contributing factor)
  Malabsorption
    Gastric bypass surgery
    Diseases affecting the stomach or duodenum (eg, Crohn disease)
    Achlorhydria, *Helicobacter pylori* infection
    Celiac sprue
  Abnormal transferrin function
    Congenital atransferrinemia
    Autoantibodies to transferrin receptors

progression of events. Initially, iron stores in the bone marrow, liver, and spleen are depleted as reflected by a decreased serum ferritin. As iron stores become exhausted, the TIBC begins to rise and serum iron saturation begins to fall. Anemia and microcytosis are present only in the later stages in the development of iron deficiency anemia.

Iron deficiency in adult men and postmenopausal women in the United States is often a consequence of GI bleeding, which can arise from either upper or lower GI tract sources. Common causes include peptic ulcer disease, esophageal varices, gastritis, and angiodysplasia. GI malignancy, especially colon cancer, should be considered in all adults with unexplained iron deficiency. Less common causes in the United States include hookworms, amebiasis, and Meckel diverticulum. Uncommonly, anemia may occur due to bleeding from the respiratory tract. In 2 rare conditions, idiopathic pulmonary hemosiderosis and Goodpasture syndrome, iron may accumulate in the pulmonary macrophages, making it unavailable for use in hematopoiesis, even without overt hemoptysis. Iron can also be lost from the genitourinary tract as menstrual loss or urinary loss. During the average menstrual cycle, women lose between 10 and 15 mg of iron. It takes approximately 10 mg of dietary iron to absorb 1 mg of elemental iron; consequently, it is difficult to replace menstrual iron loss with dietary iron alone, making menstruation the most common cause of iron deficiency in premenopausal women. Iron deficiency can also develop after chronic blood donation or can be iatrogenic secondary to other reasons (eg, hospitalized patients undergoing frequent blood draws or self-phlebotomy in patients with underlying psychiatric disorders).

Pregnancy and lactation increase the demand for iron by 3-fold. During pregnancy, iron is diverted to the developing fetus, which accumulates about 250 mg of iron from maternal sources. Moreover, the typical expansion of blood volume and growth of other maternal tissues further increase maternal demands for iron. Blood loss during delivery also compromises iron stores and contributes to iron deficiency. It is estimated that approximately 1200 mg of iron must be acquired from the body's iron stores or from the diet by the end of a term pregnancy. Additionally, iron is secreted in breast milk for use by the developing infant. In fact, nearly all lactating women will become iron deficient if not treated with supplemental iron.

Iron deficiency from poor dietary intake is most notable in infants and children. It is rare for an adult to become iron deficient solely due to insufficient oral intake. Iron endowment at birth is a major determinant of iron deficiency in early infancy. Total body iron at birth is dependent on 2 factors: birth weight and hemoglobin concentration. Accordingly, preterm infants and babies who experience perinatal blood loss are predisposed to develop early iron deficiency anemia. The daily iron requirement in normal term infants is 1 mg/kg, whereas it is 2 mg/kg in premature infants. Infants who drink cows' milk as a sole source of nutrition are particularly susceptible to iron deficiency because cows' milk has little iron (0.5 mg/L) and its bioavailability (absorption) is poor. In addition, consumption of cows' milk has been associated with GI bleeding in some infants due to the toxic effects on the intestinal mucosa of a heat-labile protein present in cows' milk, but not in cows' milk–based formulas. It is estimated that 20% to 40% of infants who are fed primarily cows' milk or nonfortified formula develop iron deficiency.

Most adults consume about 5 mg of iron per 1000 calories. Dietary iron exists in 2 forms: inorganic iron and heme iron. Although most iron in the diet is inorganic, heme iron is best absorbed. Meats and liver are particularly rich sources of heme iron. Spinach, once thought to be high in iron, contains unabsorbable iron chelates. Legumes have moderate amounts of iron, whereas most other vegetables are low in iron. Iron fortification of grains, a common practice, has limited value as a means of increasing dietary iron because most grains contain phytates that chelate iron. In addition, ferrous salts cause an unpleasant flavor in baked goods. Ascorbic acid helps facilitate the absorption of nonheme iron.

Iron deficiency due to malabsorption can occur in patients with celiac disease, Crohn disease, chronic giardiasis, or any infiltrative processes affecting the proximal small bowel. Patients, as presented in the clinical case provided earlier, may develop iron deficiency after gastric or small bowel resection. Celiac disease, which may affect up to 1% of the population, accounts for up to 20% of refractory iron deficiency anemia. The classic presentation of abdominal pain, diarrhea, and malabsorption is seen only in the minority of cases. Noninvasive testing using serologic assays for endomysial antibodies and tissue transglutaminase antibodies have sensitivities and specificities >95%. Diagnosis should be confirmed with a duodenal biopsy. Although adherence is difficult, patients with celiac disease often respond to a gluten-free diet.

Gastric acid is necessary for the maintenance of inorganic iron in the ferric form. Therefore, achlorhydria, which is seen in up to 30% of the elderly, is a common cause of iron deficiency, and the association of iron deficiency and pernicious anemia is well documented. *Helicobacter pylori* infection is known to reduce both iron and ferritin levels in adults and children. Iron deficiency may occur as a result of occult GI bleeding, competition for dietary iron by the bacteria, and the increase in intragastric pH, resulting in decreased iron absorption. Treating *H pylori* in infected individuals with refractory iron deficiency has been shown to result in an appropriate response to oral iron therapy and normalization of hemoglobin levels. Patients with refractory iron deficiency should be tested for celiac disease, autoimmune atrophic gastritis, and *H pylori* infection.

Iron-deficient individuals may have no symptoms. Excessive fatigue and other nonspecific signs of anemia become more pronounced as iron deficiency and anemia become worse. Ice eating (pagophagia) and other forms of pica are seen in only a minority of patients. Findings on physical examination become more pronounced as the iron deficiency worsens and include pallor, stomatitis, glossitis, koilonychia of the nails, and other symptoms due to the effects of iron on rapidly dividing cells. Esophageal webs as seen in the Plummer-Vinson syndrome are present only in a minority of cases and may respond to oral iron replacement. Infants with iron deficiency are often irritable and inattentive. A number of studies have shown that iron-deficient infants exhibit myriad behavioral and neurodevelopmental abnormalities. This is not surprising because iron is part of a number of important oxidative enzymes in the brain and other tissues. Severe iron deficiency has also been associated with increased risk of premature birth, increased maternal and infant mortality, and impaired work capacity.

Figure 5-1 shows a typical peripheral smear from a patient with severe iron deficiency. The erythrocytes in iron deficiency anemia are microcytic and hypochromic, although

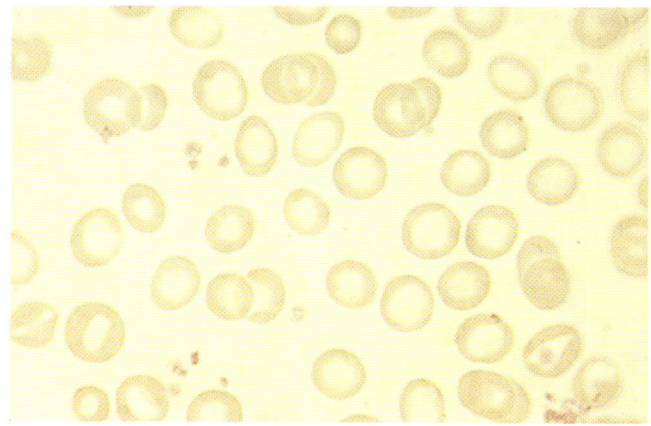

Figure 5-1 Peripheral smear in a patient with iron deficiency anemia. From ASH Image Bank (2002); doi:10.1182/ashimagebank-2002-100325.

they may be normocytic early in the course prior to the development of anemia. Frequently, the RBC distribution width (RDW) is increased, and in advanced states, the peripheral blood smear shows anisopoikilocytosis and bizarrely shaped erythrocytes, including characteristic cigar-shaped or pencil-shaped cells. Target cells may be seen but are infrequent and are more likely indicative of a thalassemia syndrome (which may also present with microcytic anemia). Thrombocytopenia is rarely seen, whereas thrombocytosis is more common, especially in patients with active blood loss.

The diagnosis of iron deficiency anemia is not always straightforward. The serum iron level, a poor reflection of iron stores, is low to normal in iron deficiency but is subject to diurnal variation, being highest later in the day, and fluctuates with dietary iron intake. The TIBC is usually increased or in the high normal range in iron deficiency. The iron saturation (the ratio of serum iron to TIBC) is usually low (<10%). Very low serum ferritin values of <15 μg/L are diagnostic of iron deficiency. Because ferritin is an acute-phase reactant, ferritin levels increase with inflammatory diseases. Therefore, ferritin levels may be normal in patients with iron deficiency and acute or chronic infection, active inflammatory diseases, or cancer. However, a serum ferritin of >100 μg/L is unusual in iron-deficient patients. A summary of selected standard results and investigational laboratory results seen in iron deficiency, as compared with the anemia of chronic inflammation/disease (to be discussed later), is presented in Table 5-3. Iron stores are usually normal or elevated in thalassemia, which also causes microcytic anemia. As opposed to the RDW in iron deficiency, the RDW is usually normal in thalassemia, and target RBCs are often seen on review of the peripheral blood smear. Erythrocyte zinc protoporphyrin (ZPP) levels are increased in iron deficiency when, in the absence of iron, zinc is inserted into the protoporphyrin ring in the last stage of hemoglobin synthesis. This well-established assay is conducted on a drop of

Table 5-3 Laboratory parameters in iron deficiency anemia as compared with AOCD.

	Fe deficiency	AOCD
Standard		
Serum Fe	↓ to Nl	↓ to Nl
TIBC	High Nl to ↑	↓ to low Nl
% iron saturation	↓↓	↓
Serum ferritin	↓↓*	Nl to ↑↑
MCV	↓ to ↓↓	↓ to Nl
RDW	↑	Nl to ↑†
Investigational		
sTfR	↑	Nl
Hepcidin	↓	↑

*In the absence of concomitant inflammation, infection, or malignancy.
†Dependent on the underlying disease process.
AOCD = anemia of chronic inflammation disease; Fe = iron; TIBC = total iron-binding capacity; MCV = mean corpuscular volume; Nl = normal; RDW = red blood cell distribution width; sTfR = soluble serum transferrin receptor.

blood using a dedicated portable instrument and is suited for population studies and in pediatric and obstetric clinics. However, ZPP levels also increase in lead poisoning. Measurement of the soluble serum transferrin receptor (sTfR) can also help diagnose iron deficiency. In iron-deficient states, levels of this receptor are increased, but they remain normal in anemia of chronic inflammation/disease. Measurement of the ratio of sTfR to serum ferritin (R/F ratio) has been reported to increase the utility of this assay. However, sTfR levels correlate with the total mass of erythroid precursors and thus also increase in patients with hemolysis, myelodysplasia, and thalassemia and with the use of erythropoietic stimulating agents. The test, although commercially available, lacks standardization, and values vary between laboratories and assays. The percentage of circulating hypochromic erythrocytes and the reticulocyte hemoglobin concentration (CHr) are newer measures of early iron-deficient erythropoiesis that require specific automated analyzers not available in most laboratories. Serum hepcidin, the primary regulator of iron homeostasis in the body, decreases in iron deficiency. A serum hepcidin assay is not yet commercially available but may prove a useful aid to the diagnosis of iron disorders in the future. Evaluation of the bone marrow for stainable iron had been considered the gold standard for the diagnosis of iron deficiency. Unfortunately, it is relatively expensive and invasive, has questionable sensitivity, and is suboptimal in children due to the pain associated with the procedure. Patient samples should be compared with adequate positive controls before the diagnosis of iron deficiency is made based on a tissue specimen. An improvement in hemoglobin in response to iron supplementation is often the simplest way to diagnose iron deficiency.

The treatment of uncomplicated iron deficiency is best accomplished with oral iron salts. There is little difference in effectiveness among various oral iron preparations, but the ferrous iron salts are preferred due to increased solubility at the pH of the duodenum and jejunum. Ferrous sulfate is the cheapest iron replacement salt, costing less than US $1.00 per gram of iron. Typical replacement doses of oral iron are approximately 200 mg of elemental iron daily in adults and 3 to 6 mg/kg/d in infants and children (split into divided doses). Because ferrous sulfate contains 66 mg of elemental iron per 325-mg tablet, one tablet 3 times daily is an appropriate replacement dose, although many patients only tolerate 1 or 2 tablets daily. Oral iron salts are best absorbed on an empty stomach but best tolerated with foods. If a patient has excessive epigastric pain, heartburn, nausea, or other GI symptoms when taking iron on an empty stomach, a trial of iron taken with meals should be recommended. Patients should be alerted that iron may turn their stools a darker color. Liquid iron preparations are available for infants and young children (25 mg/mL of iron as drops and 44 mg/5 mL as elixir). These preparations may stain the teeth and should therefore be taken through a straw if possible. Children younger than 5 years of age typically are treated with Feosol (GlaxoSmithKline, London, United Kingdom; 44 mg of elemental iron) in daily divided doses, whereas children aged 5 to 12 years can be treated with one tablet of ferrous sulfate daily. Adolescents are treated with 1 to 2 tablets of iron salts each day. Sustained-release iron formulations and polysaccharide–iron complexes are reported to have fewer GI adverse effects than iron salts, although some contain less iron, and absorption may be compromised. Ascorbic acid can facilitate iron absorption, but its addition to the replacement regimen is not clearly cost effective and may increase the adverse effects of iron replacement therapy. It is simpler to instruct patients to take oral iron supplements with orange juice. Antacids, the tannins found in tea, calcium supplementation, bran, and whole grains, if taken concurrently with oral iron, can all decrease iron absorption. True malabsorption of ferrous sulfate is rare but can be diagnosed by administering an oral dose of liquid ferrous sulfate in a fasting state while obtaining serum iron levels before and 1 and 2 hours after administration. If the serum iron does not increase by at least 100 mg/100 mL, malabsorption is likely.

Oral iron supplementation is the preferred replacement route in most uncomplicated cases of iron deficiency. Indications for parenteral iron supplementation include iron malabsorption due to resection or disease of the stomach or bowel (as presented in the previous clinical case), conditions with high iron requirements such as chronic GI blood loss, and failure of oral iron therapy due to poor tolerance or adherence. Parenteral iron is best given intravenously because intramuscular iron is painful and has been associated with development of soft tissue sarcomas. For years, high molecular weight iron dextran was the only form of parenteral iron available in the United States. Its use is complicated by a low but significant risk of anaphylaxis (11.3/million), and a 25-mg test dose should be given to all patients prior to infusion. Four other parenteral iron preparations are now available: low molecular weight iron dextran, which is considerably safer than its high molecular weight counterpart; iron sucrose; ferumoxytol; and iron gluconate. The advantages of iron dextran include its low cost and the ability to give total iron replacement of 2 g or more with a single infusion, although it is often given in 2-mL (100-mg) aliquots. Iron sucrose and iron gluconate have a very low incidence of anaphylaxis, no fatal cases have been reported, and their administration does not require a test dose. They cause arthralgias and myalgias, which are usually mild. Disadvantages of these newer formulations include greater cost and the inability to give total replacement doses in a single infusion because they cause GI and vasoactive reactions at doses above 200 to 400 mg. Newer iron preparations have been developed to enable more rapid high-dose bolus injections. Ferumoxytol enables a bolus injection of 510 mg to be administered in 17 seconds and was recently approved by the US Food and Drug Administration. Ferric carboxymaltose was recently licensed in Europe, and it enables 1000 mg of iron to be given as an intravenous infusion over 15 minutes.

Patients should respond to iron replacement with a reticulocytosis occurring between 4 and 7 days following iron therapy. A hemoglobin response may be seen as early as 1 to 2 weeks following parenteral iron replacement; however, it may take several weeks for the full effects to be realized. An increase in hemoglobin is usually apparent within 1 to 2 weeks of initiation of oral iron, and the anemia usually resolves within 4 to 6 weeks. Iron therapy should be continued for several months following correction of anemia to replete iron stores. Serum ferritin can be used as an estimate of storage iron and to help gauge the length of iron replacement therapy. Failure of response to oral iron should lead to speculation about ongoing bleeding, poor patient compliance, poor iron absorption, or appropriateness of the diagnosis.

Iron deficiency during infancy and early childhood is preventable. The introduction of iron-fortified formula and resurgence of interest in breast-feeding has reduced iron deficiency in some patient populations. However, the introduction of whole cows' milk into the diet before 12 months of age, excessive cows' milk intake during the second year of life irrespective of earlier feeding practices, and failure to provide an extra source of iron to infants exclusively breast-fed beyond 6 months of age all contribute to iron deficiency remaining an important public health problem. Pregnant women should be encouraged to take prenatal vitamins containing iron. There is some evidence that the motor and intelligence quotient (IQ) deficits that may occur in iron-deficient infants are not fully reversible even following iron replacement.

> **Key points**
>
> - Iron deficiency is the most common cause of anemia worldwide, and when present, the underlying cause must be investigated.
> - A hypoproliferative hypochromic microcytic anemia, often with an elevated RDW, is typical of iron deficiency anemia.
> - Newer assays for the diagnosis of iron deficiency have been developed, but they are not in routine clinical use.
> - Serum iron, percent iron saturation, and ferritin are typically low, whereas TIBC is typically elevated in classic iron deficiency.
> - Iron replacement should begin with oral ferrous salts unless the patient cannot absorb or tolerate oral iron formulations.
> - Iron sucrose and iron gluconate are safer than iron dextran for parenteral replacement but are more costly and cannot be given as a total-dose iron infusion.
> - Iron deficiency during infancy and childhood should be diagnosed and treated to prevent developmental delays.

Anemia of chronic disease/inflammation (dysregulation of iron)

> **Clinical case**
>
> A 44-year-old woman is referred for evaluation of a hypoproliferative normocytic anemia with a hemoglobin of 8 g/dL. Her past medical history is significant for a mitral valve replacement 1 year earlier. Recently, she has developed low-grade fevers, malaise, and generalized fatigue. Her examination is unremarkable except for a temperature of 38.5°C and a 2/6 systolic ejection murmur over the mitral valve. Laboratory evaluation reveals a decreased serum iron, low TIBC, and low percent iron saturation. Serum ferritin is 55 ng/mL, and the Westergren sedimentation rate (WESR) is elevated at 92 mm/hr. Blood cultures subsequently return positive for methicillin-resistant *Staphylococcus aureus*. Transesophageal echocardiogram confirms subacute bacterial endocarditis of the prosthetic mitral valve. The patient is placed on vancomycin and ferrous sulfate 365 mg 3 times per day. Four weeks later, the hemoglobin increases to 11 g/dL.

Anemia is common in patients with chronic inflammatory conditions such as malignancy, autoimmune diseases, and chronic infections. The resulting anemia is termed anemia of chronic disease or anemia of inflammation. In this chapter, the terms anemia of chronic disease/inflammation are represented by the often-used abbreviation AOCD. In hospitalized medical patients, AOCD is thought to be the most common cause of anemia, surpassing iron deficiency anemia in frequency. It is now recognized that patients with illnesses not traditionally thought to be inflammatory in origin, such as trauma, postsurgery, and prolonged critical illness, may also develop AOCD. AOCD is generally a sign of underlying disease activity, rather than a disease in and of itself (as in the clinical case provided at the beginning of this section). Thus, an aggressive search for an underlying disorder should be performed when diagnosing AOCD as the cause of anemia.

Patients with AOCD typically have hemoglobin levels in the range of 7 to 11 g/dL. The anemia in AOCD is hypoproliferative, normochromic, and normocytic. However, over time, the anemia may become more severe with microcytic, hypochromic indices. The reticulocyte count is reduced. Although laboratory values overlap and may not be discriminating, iron studies are often used to differentiate AOCD from iron deficiency anemia. Typically, iron levels are low to normal, iron-binding capacity is low to low normal, and ferritin is normal or elevated in AOCD (Table 5-3). In many but not all conditions, an elevated WESR or C-reactive protein (CRP) may be a clue to the diagnosis of AOCD.

Multiple processes are involved in the pathogenesis of AOCD, and cytokines, such as tumor necrosis factor α (TNFα), interleukin 1 (IL-1), interleukin 6 (IL-6), and interferons, play a central role in the abnormalities observed in these patients. These cytokines cause a reduction in the proliferation of erythroid precursors in response to EPO, a decrease in the production of EPO relative to the degree of anemia, and a moderate decrease in RBC survival. However, the hallmark of AOCD is alterations in iron metabolism. Inflammatory cytokines, especially IL-6, cause an increase in the hepatic synthesis of hepcidin, the key regulator of iron transmembrane transport. Hepcidin blocks iron absorption in the intestine and blocks iron release from enterocytes and macrophages. This in turn results in low plasma iron levels and iron-deficient erythropoiesis.

In infants and children, inflammatory anemia does not require the presence of an underlying chronic inflammatory disorder. Even minor bacterial or viral infections, when recurrent, can cause a mild normocytic anemia with blunted reticulocyte response within a few weeks. These anemias exhibit a pathophysiology similar to AOCD. This "anemia of inflammation" is self-limited and resolves when the infant is free of infection.

In most patients with AOCD, the anemia is mild and improves with the treatment of the underlying disorder. Patients may have concomitant iron deficiency, as suggested in the presented case by a low normal ferritin level in the presence of a chronic infection, and should be repleted. If treatment becomes necessary, EPO at doses ranging from 10,000 units 3 times weekly to 40,000 to 60,000 units weekly or darbepoetin at doses ranging from 100 IU weekly or 200 IU biweekly have been shown to be beneficial in some patients. Patients with EPO levels >500 IU/mL (or >100 IU/mL in some studies) are unlikely to respond to supplemental EPO replacement. Usually, if supplemental EPO is effective, an increase in hemoglobin is seen within several weeks. Better responses are seen in patients with lower endogenous EPO levels. Iron stores should be monitored in patients treated with EPO because iron deficiency may develop as erythropoiesis is increased. Typically, iron saturation should be maintained at >20% and ferritin values maintained >100 ng/mL during therapy with EPO.

> **Key points**
>
> • AOCD is the most common cause of anemia in patients with underlying inflammatory diseases.
> • AOCD is characterized by a hypoproliferative normocytic or microcytic anemia with decreased serum iron, TIBC, and percent saturation of iron and increased serum ferritin.
> • The pathophysiology of AOCD is multifactorial, but the sequestration of iron secondary to elevated hepcidin levels plays a central role.
> • Treatment should be directed at the underlying medical condition.
> • If anemia is severe and the patient is symptomatic, EPO can be considered. Iron stores should be monitored during EPO supplementation.

Megaloblastic anemias

The hallmark of megaloblastic anemia is the identification of abnormalities in the peripheral smear and bone marrow reflecting the nuclear/cytoplasmic dyssynchrony caused by impaired DNA synthesis. Megaloblastic anemia may be the result of multiple etiologies, including cobalamin or folate deficiency or drugs that impair DNA synthesis. Although RBCs and RBC precursors are most often the first cell line affected, eventual abnormalities affect leukocytes and platelets as well, often resulting in pancytopenia as the megaloblastic process progresses. RBC morphology is characterized by large, often oval cells (macro-ovalocytes) that may contain remnants of the mitotic spindle apparatus (Cabot rings) (Figure 5-2) or nuclear remnants (Howell-Jolly bodies). In very severe cases, RBCs with megaloblastic nuclei, including promegaloblasts, may be seen in the peripheral blood. Slight macrocytosis may be the earliest sign of megaloblastic anemia. Neutrophils are hypersegmented (Figure 5-3), with at least 5% of the neutrophils having 5 lobes and some with 6 lobes or more. Although the majority of patients with megaloblastic anemia will have a markedly increased MCV, the MCV may be within normal limits or even decreased in patients with concurrent iron deficiency or thalassemia. Basophilic stippling may also be present. The bone marrow shows megaloblastic changes in all cell lines, with the most striking changes seen in the erythrocyte lineage. The myeloid

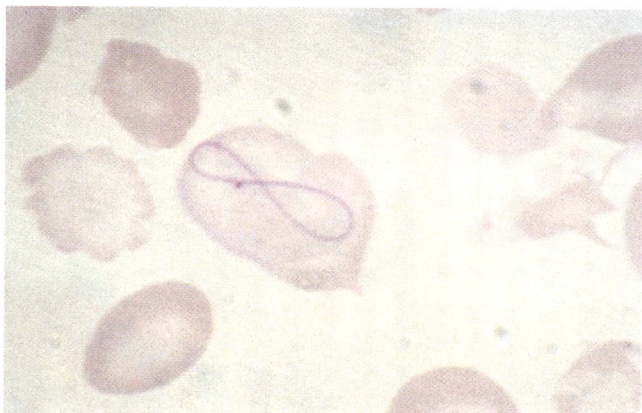

Figure 5-2 Cabot rings. From ASH slide bank #993.

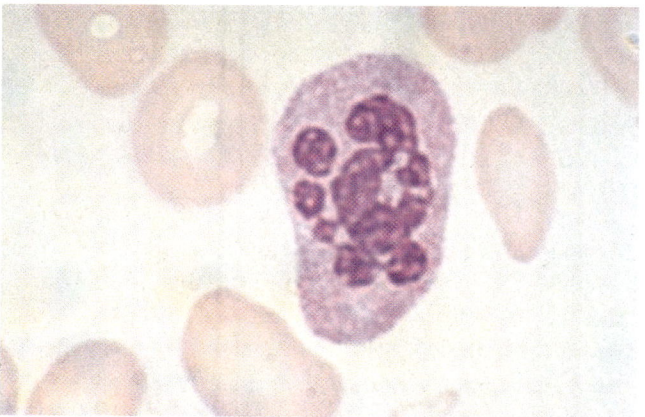

Figure 5-3 Peripheral smear from a patient with cobalamin deficiency. From ASH slide bank #987.

to erythroid (M:E) ratio may be decreased, and there may be increased ringed sideroblasts. Because there is ineffective hematopoiesis with intramedullary cell destruction, lactate dehydrogenase (LDH) is typically elevated. Unconjugated bilirubin and urate may also be elevated.

Cobalamin (vitamin B$_{12}$) deficiency

> **Clinical case**
>
> A previously healthy 45-year-old woman presents for evaluation of weakness, fatigue, and easy bruising that has progressively increased over the past year. She is on no medications. Her history is significant for gastric bypass surgery 15 years earlier due to morbid obesity. Her physical examination is significant for tachycardia, pallor, multiple bruises of the extremities, and trace pedal edema bilaterally. On neurologic examination, she is noted to have somewhat slowed mentation, although she is fully alert and oriented; she has minimal loss of position and vibratory sense in the feet bilaterally. Laboratory evaluation reveals a hemoglobin of 5.1 g/dL, MCV of 115 fL, neutrophil count of 960/μL, and platelet count of 35,000/μL. A serum cobalamin level is <100 pg/mL, serum folate is normal, and RBC folate is mildly depressed. She is begun on daily parenteral cobalamin replacement, with symptomatic improvement and brisk reticulocytosis noted within 1 week.

Although some microorganisms synthesize cobalamin (vitamin B$_{12}$), humans, like most animals, must eat cobalamin-containing foods to survive. Cobalamin has 2 parts: a porphyrin-like cobalt-containing molecule and a nucleotide. Cobalamin is a coenzyme for 2 enzymes, methylmalonyl coenzyme A (CoA) mutase and methyltetrahydrofolate-homocysteine methyltransferase. The first enzyme is important in disposing of propionate formed when valine and isoleucine are metabolized. In this reaction, methylmalonyl CoA is formed and is converted to succinyl CoA, which becomes part of the Krebs cycle (Carmel et al, 2003, Figure 3). The second enzyme is important in both the formation of methionine and the conversion of methyltetrahydrofolate to tetrahydrofolate, which in turn must be conjugated with glutamate to remain intracellular and allow folate to enter the cell.

Dietary, or food-bound, cobalamin, such as that found in meat products, is released from foods by gastric proteases. In the stomach, cobalamin is bound to R-binders (found in gastric secretions and saliva), which stabilize cobalamin in the acidic environment. Upon entering the alkaline environment of the small intestine, cobalamin is released from R-binders and in turn binds to intrinsic factor (synthesized in gastric parietal cells), which is necessary for cobalamin absorption. Intrinsic factor–bound cobalamin moves through the small intestine to the terminal ileum where the complex is bound to its receptor, cubulin, and undergoes endocytosis. Cobalamin is bound to transcobalamin II and transported in the blood for uptake at the tissue level. Although transcobalamin II–bound cobalamin is responsible for cobalamin utilization, transcobalamin I is the principal cobalamin-binding protein in the blood. Transcobalamin I is likely important for cobalamin excretion and may also play a role as a storage protein. Transcobalamin III has also been identified and likely represents a group of transcobalamins with different abilities to bind cobalamin. There is a pronounced enterohepatic circulation of cobalamin, which is responsible for the fact that it takes years to become cobalamin deficient from decreased dietary intake alone. In addition to the highly regulated processing of ingested cobalamin, it appears that very small amounts (ie, 1%–5%) of free cobalamin may be absorbed from the intestine by passive diffusion, which may account for the benefit of oral cobalamin even in patients who have a failure in one or more of the steps of regulated absorption.

Pernicious anemia (PA), the most common cause of cobalamin deficiency, is an autoimmune disorder characterized by the destruction of gastric parietal cells, which synthesize intrinsic factor. PA typically begins after the age of 40 years. It is more common in individuals with histocompatibility (human leukocyte antigen [HLA]) types A2, A3, B7, and B12, and with blood type A. It is more prevalent in Northern Europeans, especially Scandinavians, and in African Americans. In PA, there is atrophy of the gastric parietal cells that secrete intrinsic factor, acid, and pepsin. Antiparietal cell antibodies, directed against the H^+/K^+ adenosine triphosphatase (ATPase), occur in 90% of persons with PA compared with 5% of the general population. However, it is believed that they are not responsible for the gastric atrophy seen in PA because the luminal location of the H^+/K^+-ATPase makes it inaccessible to the antibodies. Rather, there is evidence from mouse models that the parietal cells are destroyed by autoimmune $CD4^+$ T cells that recognize the H^+/K^+-ATPase. In addition, antibodies to intrinsic factor or to the intrinsic factor–cobalamin complex that are found in 70% of patients with PA may contribute to the disease. PA is associated with other autoimmune disorders including autoimmune thyroid disease and diabetes mellitus. In addition, patients with PA are at increased risk of gastric carcinoma and carcinoid tumors. Cobalamin deficiency may also occur after total gastrectomy or in the presence of atrophic gastritis, due to lack of functioning parietal cells. Less commonly, other disorders such as Crohn disease, small bowel resection, or bacterial overgrowth can interfere with the ileal absorption of intrinsic factor–cobalamin complexes. Rarely, cobalamin deficiency can occur in patients with hypersecretion of gastric acid such as in the Zollinger-Ellison syndrome. In this situation, there is insufficient alkalinization in the duodenum to neutralize excess acid, so pancreatic proteases are not inactivated and cobalamin cannot be transferred from R-binders to intrinsic factor for absorption. Causes of cobalamin deficiency are listed in Table 5-4.

The prevalence of cobalamin deficiency increases with advancing age, most likely due to a decreased ability to separate cobalamin from food protein due to decreased gastric acidity. Cobalamin deficiency can result from intestinal disorders that lead to faulty cobalamin absorption, such as in regional enteritis or lymphoma, or following ileal resection. Patients who have had surgery to create blind intestinal loops can develop bacterial overgrowth that leads to cobalamin deficiency through preferential uptake of cobalamin by enteric bacteria. The fish tapeworm, *Diphyllobothrium latum*, found in Canada, Alaska, and the Baltic Sea, competes with the host for cobalamin, which can lead to cobalamin deficiency.

Because alkalinization is important for the transfer of cobalamin from R-binders to intrinsic factor, patients with pancreatic deficiency may not absorb cobalamin. However, frank deficiency of cobalamin in pancreatic deficiency is rare.

Table 5-4 Selected causes of cobalamin deficiency.

Reduced dietary intake
  Vegetarians who avoid dairy products and eggs (strict vegans)

Impaired absorption
  Hypochlorhydria (inability to separate cobalamin from food)
    Age
    Atrophic gastritis
    Medications (proton-pump inhibitors, H_2 antagonists)
  Inadequate pancreatic protease (inability to transfer cobalamin from R-binders to IF)
    Severe pancreatic insufficiency
    Zollinger-Ellison syndrome
  Competition for luminal cobalamin (inadequate binding of cobalamin to IF)
    Bacterial overgrowth due to blind-loop syndromes
    Fish tapeworm
  Deficiency of IF
    Pernicious anemia
    Gastric resection
  Decreased ileal absorption of cobalamin–IF
    Ileal resection or bypass
    Ileal dysfunction caused by sprue, Crohn disease, or infiltration of bowel wall
    Medications (cholestyramine, metformin, colchicine)

Rare congenital disorders
  Congenital IF deficiency
  Defective IF–cobalamin receptors
    Imerslund-Grasbeck syndrome
  Abnormal plasma cobalamin transport
    Deficiency of transcobalamin II
    Defective transcobalamin II
  Inborn errors of intracellular cobalamin metabolism (cobalamin mutant syndromes)
    Defects lead to methylmalonic aciduria and/or homocystinuria

IF = intrinsic factor.

Acute megaloblastic anemia is a rare occurrence following nitrous oxide anesthesia, which disrupts intracellular cobalamin metabolism and can lead to megaloblastosis and pancytopenia in as little as 12 to 24 hours. Although the effects disappear spontaneously, fatalities have been reported in instances where nitrous oxide was chronically administered to tetanus patients. Recreational users of nitrous oxide have developed neuropsychiatric problems thought to be related to combined system degeneration.

Patients with cobalamin deficiency can have severe neuropsychiatric complications. These are presumed secondary to abnormal methyl group metabolism and are prevented by methionine, a precursor of S-adenosylmethionine, a potent methylator. These neurologic defects may not reverse with therapy and may occur without evidence of anemia. The neurologic syndrome begins with loss of vibratory sensation in the toes and fingers and can progress to spastic ataxia caused by demyelinization of the dorsal and lateral columns of the spinal cord. In addition, psychiatric changes including psychosis and dementia can develop. Importantly, replacement of folate alone may improve the anemia in patients with cobalamin deficiency, thereby masking underlying cobalamin deficiency and allowing progression of neurologic deficits. Therefore, cobalamin levels should always be measured prior to initiation of folate in patients at risk for concomitant vitamin B_{12} deficiency.

Low serum cobalamin levels are diagnostic of deficiency in most patients with megaloblastic anemia and/or classic neurologic symptoms due to cobalamin deficiency. Over 95% of patients with clinically evident cobalamin deficiency will have cobalamin levels <200 ng/L. In early cobalamin deficiency, serum levels of both MMA and HCY become elevated before cobalamin levels decrease beneath the lower limits of the normal range (200–250 ng/L). This has allowed the detection of a "subclinical" cobalamin deficiency state in which cobalamin levels are in the low normal range of 250 to 350 ng/L but MMA and HCY levels are elevated (Table 5-5). There is some debate about the clinical importance of identifying such asymptomatic patients because the majority do not progress to symptomatic cobalamin deficiency. The incidence of subclinical cobalamin deficiency may be as high as 15% in some groups (such as the elderly). At present, routine screening of asymptomatic individuals is not recommended. If an individual is identified as having subclinical cobalamin deficiency based on metabolic testing, careful follow-up with or without cobalamin replacement is warranted.

Low cobalamin levels alone are not diagnostic of clinical cobalamin deficiency in the absence of overt megaloblastic anemia or typical neurologic changes and can be seen in association with a variety of other clinical conditions including folate deficiency and use of certain drugs such as anticonvulsants. True cobalamin deficiency in these situations can be confirmed by elevations in MMA and HCY levels, although it is important to be aware that other pathophysiologic states can occasionally lead to false-positive metabolite elevations (Carmel et al, 2003, Table 2). Elevated HCY levels associated with cobalamin deficiency may increase a patient's risk of vascular thrombosis, but this topic is controversial. Currently, an evaluation for cobalamin deficiency should include a serum cobalamin level and at least one of the other metabolic tests, unless other clinical signs and symptoms support the diagnosis of cobalamin deficiency. In the introductory case, the diagnosis of cobalamin deficiency was made from the cobalamin level and the associated clinical findings. Of note is that some patients with megaloblastic anemia will progress to pancytopenia, as in the case provided. The RBC folate level is low in >50% of patients with cobalamin deficiency and megaloblastic anemia, as in the previous clinical scenario, so it cannot be used to distinguish between these 2 deficiencies.

Ascertaining the etiology of cobalamin deficiency is becoming more difficult as the classic Schilling test is no longer available in many centers. The presence of either anti-intrinsic factor antibodies or antiparietal cell antibodies supports the diagnosis of PA. However, confirmation of ileal malabsorption syndromes as the cause of cobalamin deficiency can only be confirmed by a Schilling test.

Parenteral cobalamin is used for replacement in deficient patients and is recommended for patients with significant symptomatology. It is necessary to saturate tissue stores as well as compensate for daily losses. Typical treatment is 1000 μg intramuscularly daily for 2 weeks, then 1000 μg weekly until the anemia resolves, followed by 1000 μg monthly thereafter. Excess cobalamin is excreted in the urine, so toxicity due to excessive vitamin replacement does not occur. Recent studies suggest that oral cobalamin may be a safe and effective treatment in some patients, even when intrinsic factor is present at low levels. The initial oral replacement dose begins at 1000 to 2000 μg daily. Patients treated with oral cobalamin should be observed carefully to ensure that laboratory parameters are correcting and cobalamin levels are replete. For those who respond to oral therapy, lifelong replacement can be accomplished with 1000 μg daily. In nonresponders, parenteral cobalamin should replace oral supplementation.

Following replacement, the marrow shows resolution of megaloblastic changes within hours and reticulocytes appear in the peripheral blood, usually peaking approximately 1 week after starting replacement therapy. Hypersegmentation of neutrophils may persist for up to 2 weeks. Blood counts and MCV return to normal in 2 to 3 months. Failure to respond to cobalamin replacement may indicate concomitant iron

Table 5-5 Laboratory findings in cobalamin and folate deficiency.

	Clinical cobalamin deficiency	Subclinical cobalamin deficiency	Folate deficiency
Cobalamin level (serum)	<200 ng/L	200–350 ng/L	>300 ng/L*
Folate level (serum)	>4 ng/ml	>4 ng/ml	<2 ng/ml
Homocysteine (serum)	↑↑	↑	↑
Methylmalonic acid (serum)	↑↑	↑	Normal

*Although most patients with folate deficiency will have normal levels of cobalamin, approximately one third will have falsely low serum cobalamin levels (ie, <200 ng/L).

deficiency or thyroid insufficiency. Neurologic abnormalities usually resolve within 3 months, although in some patients, this may take as long as 6 to 12 months. In rare patients, neurologic abnormalities may be irreversible. Lifelong cobalamin treatment is usually necessary.

Cobalamin deficiency in infants and children is uncommon. Congenital PA, which does not present until 18 to 36 months of age (due to vitamin B_{12} stores accumulated in the liver during fetal life), results from inability of parietal cells to secrete intrinsic factor. In older children, PA, similar to the disease seen in adults, may present in isolation or be associated with other immunologic disorders. The Imerslund-Gräsbeck syndrome results from impaired absorption of the vitamin B_{12}–intrinsic factor complex by the terminal ileum. This autosomal recessively inherited receptor defect also causes proteinuria. Transcobalamin II deficiency is also inherited as an autosomal recessive trait that presents in early infancy with severe megaloblastic anemia despite normal intrinsic factor secretion, cobalamin absorption, and cobalamin levels.

> **Key points**
> - Although diverse in its etiology, impaired absorption is the most common cause of cobalamin deficiency.
> - Cobalamin deficiency may lead to neuropsychiatric and hematologic manifestations.
> - Subclinical cobalamin deficiency can be diagnosed by elevated MMA and HCY levels.
> - Debate exists concerning the clinical importance of asymptomatic cobalamin deficiency.
> - Oral cobalamin may be a safe and effective route of replacement, but careful follow-up is required to determine efficacy.
> - Treatment is usually effective but often must be continued lifelong.

Folic acid deficiency

Folate exists in nature as a conjugate with glutamic acid residues. Folate is important biologically as a transporter of single carbon fragments, but to do so it must be reduced to tetrahydrofolate. It is used in the synthesis of both purines and pyrimidines and participates in the conversion of uracil to thymidine. Folates are maintained intracellularly by conjugation with glutamic acid residues. Folate must be deconjugated to contain only one glutamic acid residue to be absorbed from the duodenum and proximal jejunum. Once it is in its monoglutamate form, cells can take up folate.

Folate deficiency may result from decreased intake, impaired absorption, increased utilization, and various drug interactions. Unlike cobalamin deficiency, the major cause of folate deficiency is decreased dietary intake. Folate is found in green vegetables such as asparagus, broccoli, lima beans, spinach, and lettuce and in fruits such as lemons, bananas, and melons. Recently, the US Department of Agriculture increased the supplementation of folate in all grain products. The recommended amount of dietary folate is 400 μg daily. Persons who consume inadequate amounts of folate will become anemic in several months. Dietary folate deficiency is most common in alcoholics, persons on parenteral nutrition who are not adequately replaced, and elderly patients with nutritionally poor diets ("tea and toast" diets). In addition, excessive cooking of vegetables can destroy the folate, leading to deficiency. Because folate is absorbed in the duodenum and jejunum, abnormalities of the small bowel as with celiac disease, regional enteritis, extranodal lymphoma, or amyloidosis can lead to malabsorption of folate. Because the growing fetus has a high avidity for folate, pregnancy greatly increases folate requirements. Folate supplementation should be part of routine prenatal care to reduce the risks of neural tube defects. Hemolytic anemia can also lead to folate deficiency because of excessive RBC turnover and increased folate utilization and demand. Folate supplementation should be considered in patients with chronic hemolytic states such as sickle cell anemia, especially those with severe anemia. Other conditions of rapid cell turnover such as exfoliative dermatitis can also produce folate deficiency. Dialysis patients can become folate deficient due to loss through the dialysis membrane.

Folate deficiency is often asymptomatic aside from the symptoms due to the resultant anemia. Although neuropsychiatric symptoms have been seen in persons with folate deficiency, they are not nearly as severe or common as those seen in persons with cobalamin deficiency. Folate deficiency has been associated with neural tube defects in the fetus. Folate deficiency is also associated with high levels of HCY (but not MMA), which may lead to increased risk of vascular disease and thrombosis (Table 5-5). A recent population-based study suggested that oral mucosal changes may be the earliest sign of folate deficiency. As with cobalamin deficiency, the prevalence of folate deficiency increases with age.

Folate-deficient persons may develop a megaloblastic anemia. The peripheral smear of folic acid deficiency is similar to that found in cobalamin deficiency and cannot be used to differentiate these 2 conditions.

The RBC folate level is a better measurement of tissue folate stores than the serum folate level, which reflects recent folate intake. Comparatively, the RBC folate level is proportional to an individual's folate stores over the previous 120 days or the life span of the erythrocytes. Care must be taken with interpretation of this laboratory measurement, however, because RBC folate levels may also be low in persons with cobalamin deficiency.

Folate-deficient persons are treated with high doses (1-5 mg daily) of oral folate. Concomitant cobalamin deficiency should be ruled out prior to beginning treatment with folate because anemia may improve but the neurologic symptoms due to cobalamin deficiency will progress and the diagnosis may be missed. Folate replacement is inexpensive and effective even in persons with malabsorption.

> **Key points**
>
> - As opposed to cobalamin deficiency, the most common cause of folate deficiency is decreased dietary intake.
> - Folate replacement should be part of routine prenatal care. Patients with chronic hemolytic anemia should also receive daily folate supplementation.
> - Elevated HCY, but not MMA, is associated with folate deficiency.
> - RBC folate is a better indicator of tissue folate stores, but levels may be depressed with cobalamin deficiency.
> - Cobalamin deficiency should be ruled out prior to treatment with folate.

Other causes of megaloblastic anemia

In addition to folate and cobalamin deficiency, there are other causes of megaloblastic anemia that look identical on the peripheral smear to these vitamin-deficient states. These include the use of drugs such as the pyrimidine analog 5-fluorouracil, which also inhibits DNA synthesis; drugs such as azathioprine that act as purine analogs and also inhibit DNA synthesis; agents such as methotrexate that act as antifolates; drugs such as hydroxyurea that act as RNA-reductase inhibitors; anticonvulsant drugs; H^+/K^+-ATPase inhibitors; and others. Nitrous oxide is associated with an acute megaloblastic anemia secondary to destruction of methylcobalamin, and abuse of this compound has been associated with psychosis and other neurologic defects. Zidovudine therapy for HIV characteristically produces a megaloblastic anemia.

Finally, myelodysplastic conditions, erythroleukemia, and rare recessively inherited disorders (ie, orotic aciduria) are often associated with morphologic changes that resemble (but are not identical to) megaloblastosis.

Nonmyelodysplastic sideroblastic anemias

The presence of ringed sideroblasts in the marrow is the hallmark of sideroblastic anemia (Figure 5-4). Sideroblasts are erythroid precursors with excess mitochondrial iron that surrounds or "rings" the nucleus. This iron is in the form of mitochondrial ferritin, which may be a specific marker for sideroblastic anemias. Sideroblastic anemia may be secondary to myelodysplasia (Chapter 15), inherited conditions,

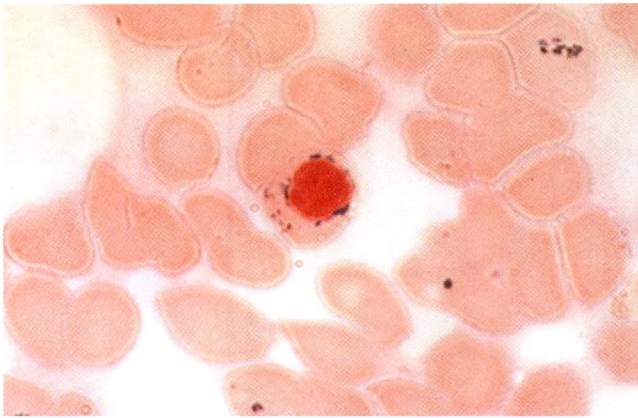

Figure 5-4 Marrow from a patient with sideroblastic anemia. From ASH slide bank #1531.

drugs, or toxins or due to mutations in the δ-aminolevulinic acid (ALA) synthase gene (*ALAS*). Excessive intake of alcohol or treatment with isoniazid (INH), chloramphenicol, or cycloserine has led to cases of acquired sideroblastic anemia. Copper deficiency, as seen with chronic zinc ingestion or chronic total parenteral nutrition without copper supplementation, can also lead to sideroblastic anemia. The mechanism of anemia in patients with sideroblastic conditions is ineffective erythropoiesis.

Hereditary sideroblastic anemia is less common than acquired causes. The disorder is usually X-linked and, although heterogeneous, may be related to mutations in either *ALAS* or in the promoter region for ALA synthase, the first enzyme in porphyrin synthesis. In addition, defects in a mitochondrial adenosine triphosphate–binding gene, *ABC7*, have been connected to X-linked sideroblastic anemias. Using pyridoxine as a cofactor, ALA synthase allows for the formation of ALA from glycine and succinyl CoA. Because the enzyme is dependent on pyridoxine, it should not be surprising that some patients with hereditary sideroblastic anemia respond to 50 to 200 mg of pyridoxine daily. A trial of pyridoxine is reasonable in all patients with nonmyelodysplastic sideroblastic anemia, although only a proportion of patients will respond.

Pearson syndrome is a rare hereditary disorder characterized by refractory sideroblastic anemia with vacuolization of marrow precursors and dysfunction of the exocrine pancreas. It is caused by mitochondrial DNA deletions and duplications. It usually presents in infancy with pancytopenia and progresses to multiorgan failure.

Anemia from malnutrition and trace element deficiencies

Data from survivors of World War II concentration camps have provided evidence that prolonged starvation can lead

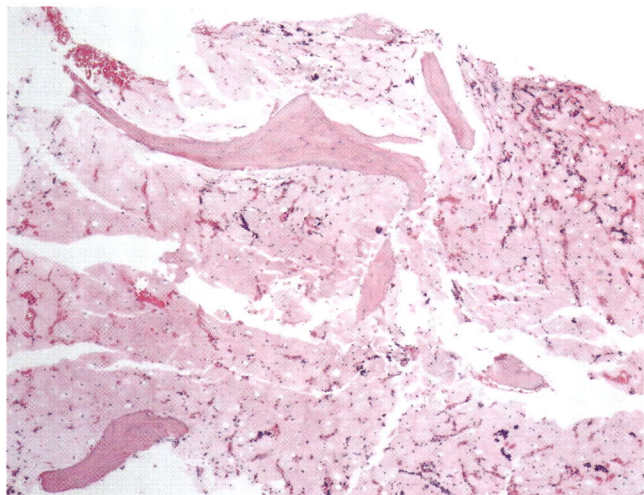

Figure 5-5 Bone marrow biopsy specimen from a patient with anorexia nervosa. Note the almost complete replacement of the marrow by the hyaluronic acid extracellular matrix material. Hematopoietic elements and fat cells are markedly decreased. From ASH image bank #100972, case 4.

to a normochromic normocytic anemia. The bone marrows of such patients are often hypocellular. Rarely, patients with severe starvation or anorexia nervosa can have gelatinous transformation of the marrow due to severe marrow necrosis (Figure 5-5). The bone marrow in these patients may reveal a proteinaceous matrix that does not resemble a normal marrow specimen. Histologically, very few marrow-derived cells are seen.

Deficiency of trace elements is also associated with anemia. For example, copper deficiency may be associated with a sideroblastic microcytic anemia that is not responsive to iron supplementation and should be differentiated from myelodysplasia. Copper is part of the molecule hephaestin, which converts iron to its ferric (Fe^{3+}) state, a step necessary for transport by transferrin. Copper deficiency most frequently occurs in malnourished infants or persons on total parenteral nutrition but has also been reported following gastric resection. Excess dietary zinc can impair copper absorption and can lead to a similar physiologic state. Zinc is found in some over-the-counter cold remedies, and case reports of copper deficiency have been described in individuals who chronically abuse these cold formulations.

Deficiencies of vitamins A, B_6, and E have been associated with anemia. Replacement of these vitamins leads to rapid correction of the anemia. Anemia due to various vitamin deficiencies remains a significant problem in the non-Western world, and routine supplementation for at-risk young children should be implemented whenever possible.

Underproduction anemias resulting from organ dysfunction

Kidney disease

> **Clinical case**
>
> A 72-year-old man presents to his primary care provider complaining of increasing dyspnea, exertional angina, and fatigue. He can no longer play golf, which he has enjoyed for several years. He is found to have a hypoproliferative normocytic anemia with a hemoglobin of 8.4 g/dL. White blood cell count with differential and platelet count are normal. He is referred for further evaluation. As part of the evaluation, a serum creatinine returns at 2.2 mg/dL. The glomerular filtration rate is subsequently measured at 23 mL/min/1.73 m², indicating stage IV renal disease. Iron studies are normal, and serum ferritin is 223 ng/mL. EPO is begun at 50 U/kg weekly along with oral iron replacement. Within 4 weeks, the patient experiences a good clinical and laboratory response. Two months later, the patient returns with fatigue and exertional dyspnea. Initial laboratory studies reveal a hemoglobin of 9.3 g/dL with an MCV of 77 fL. Iron studies are performed and return consistent with iron deficiency. A workup for GI bleeding including upper and lower endoscopy reveals only angiodysplastic lesions of the large bowel. Intravenous iron gluconate is administered with good clinical response.

The anemia of kidney disease is the most common and best understood of the underproduction anemias resulting from organ dysfunction. The most important cause of anemia in these patients is the underproduction of EPO secondary to a decrease in the number of renal cortical cells available to produce the hormone. The accumulation of uremic toxins may also cause reduced synthesis of EPO. The ability of the kidney to secrete EPO deteriorates as renal function worsens; however, a direct correlation to the degree of renal dysfunction varies greatly between patients. For example, patients with diabetes often have anemia out of proportion to the apparent reduction in renal function. Approximately 25% of dialysis patients have a relative resistance to EPO therapy, which is usually associated with the presence of inflammation. Multiple markers of inflammation, including IL-6, CRP, TNFα, fibrinogen, and ferritin, are found in patients with end-stage renal disease and EPO resistance, with IL-6 levels demonstrating the strongest correlation with the required EPO dose. Some causes of inflammation in patients with end-stage renal disease include uremia, release of cytokines by exposure to dialysis membranes, impaired renal clearance of cytokines, recurrent infections, and reduced antioxidant capacity of plasma and RBCs.

Other causes of anemia in patients with renal failure include concomitant blood loss secondary to uremic platelet dysfunction and, in patients undergoing dialysis, blood loss in the dialysis circuit and from the frequent phlebotomies needed to monitor electrolytes and blood levels. These losses may amount to up to a 2-g loss of iron annually. Blood loss from angiodysplasia of the GI tract is also more common in uremic patients. Folic acid may also be removed with dialysis and should be supplemented in all patients undergoing renal replacement therapy. Secondary hyperparathyroidism may also contribute to the anemia of renal failure through suppression of the bone marrow.

Erythrocyte survival may also be mildly to moderately decreased in a subset of patients with renal insufficiency. In the setting of uremia, RBCs become less deformable and are more susceptible to mechanical destruction and clearance by macrophages. Metabolically, uremia causes the erythrocyte to have decreased activity of enzymes involved in the hexose-monophosphate shunt and decreased ATPase activity. This leads to increased susceptibility to oxidative stress and abnormal membrane permeability, which can in turn lead to decreased erythrocyte life span. Hemodialysis may introduce RBC toxins such as copper, formaldehyde, chlorine, nitrates, and chloramines, which can damage RBCs and decrease survival. The mechanical process of dialysis can lead to RBC fragmentation.

The anemia of chronic kidney failure is usually normochromic and normocytic unless complicated by iron deficiency or vitamin deficiencies. The reticulocyte count is low. The peripheral smear is often normal, but in patients with severe kidney failure, it may show erythrocytes with short cytoplasmic extensions termed *burr cells* or *echinocytes* (Figure 5-6). The bone marrow usually is normocellular in renal failure, but hypoplasia with relative erythroid hypoproduction and marrow fibrosis (osteitis fibrosa) related to secondary hyperparathyroidism have been described. Iron studies are usually normal but may show low serum iron levels in the case of blood loss or may be accompanied by low serum transferrin levels and high ferritin as seen in AOCD. Because of the multifactorial nature of the anemia in renal disease, there is a wide range of possible hemoglobin concentrations for any given degree of renal dysfunction (Figure 5-7). Studies have demonstrated that the prevalence of anemia is greater in persons with creatinine clearances <60 mL/min/1.73 m^2; however, this population-based trend cannot be applied to individual patients. Anemia may also be present at higher levels of creatinine clearance, underscoring the importance of measuring hemoglobin in persons with renal disease and the need for individualized assessment of anemia.

The treatment of anemia in patients with chronic kidney disease has been transformed by the development and use of recombinant human EPO and other erythroid-stimulating agents (ESAs) (see Chapter 3). However, the target hemoglobin/hematocrit for patients with chronic kidney disease and dialysis patients treated with erythropoietic agents has been a topic of much debate over the past few years. Recent studies have shown that targeting normal or near-normal hemoglobin values is associated with increased risk of adverse cardiovascular events and mortality compared with lower target hemoglobin levels. Potential explanations for the increased risk of cardiovascular events include increases in blood viscosity, a procoagulant effect of the higher hemoglobin, higher blood

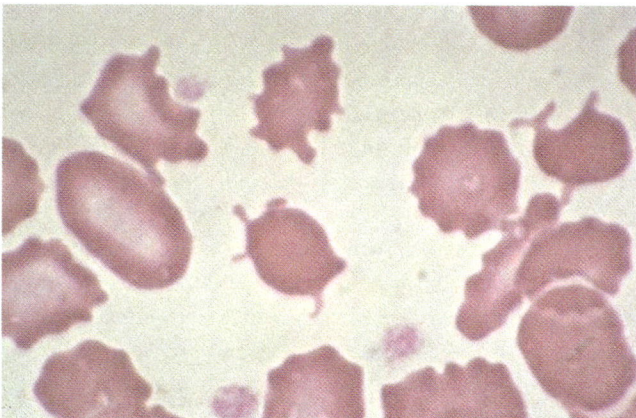

Figure 5-6 Peripheral blood smear of a patient with uremia. Note the erythrocytes with short cytoplasmic extensions (echinocytes). ASH Image Bank (2008); doi:10.1182/ashimagebank-2008-8-00154.

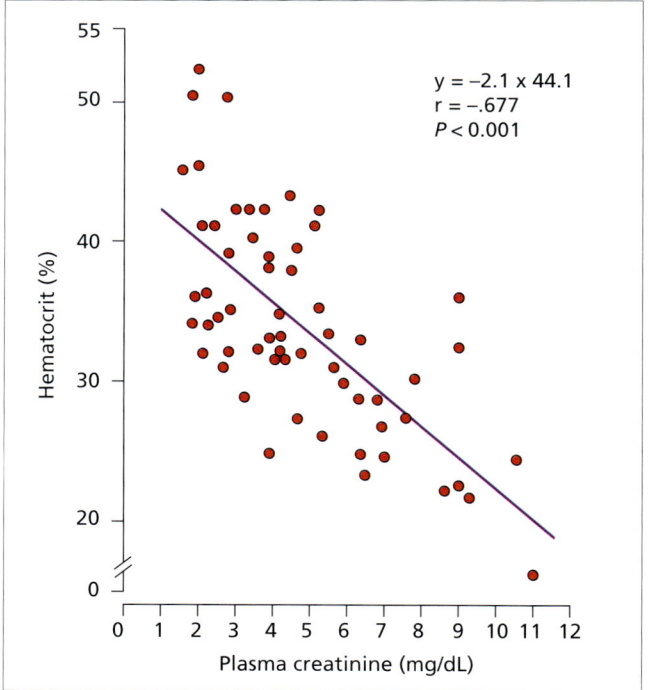

Figure 5-7 Relationship between hematocrit and plasma creatinine concentration in 60 patients with varying degrees of renal insufficiency. The severity of anemia is directly related to the level of reduced renal function. Reprinted with permission from McGonigle RJS, Wallin JD, Shadduck RK, et al. Erythropoietin deficiency and inhibition of erythropoiesis in renal insufficiency. *Kidney Int*. 1984;25:437–444.

pressure, and direct toxicities of high, nonphysiologic doses of ESA. Current guidelines adopted by American and many other professional groups recommend target hemoglobin levels in the range of 11 to 12 g/dL and not to exceed 13 g/dL. EPO dose should not exceed 20,000 units per week, and workup for other causes of anemia and EPO resistance should be initiated in patients who do not achieve target hemoglobin with this dose of EPO.

In patients with chronic kidney disease who are not on dialysis and in patients receiving peritoneal dialysis, EPO should be given at a subcutaneous dose of 50 to 100 U/kg once a week with monitoring of the hemoglobin and blood pressure every 2 to 4 weeks. Darbepoetin alfa, an EPO moiety with increased sialic acid groups resulting in a longer half-life and greater affinity for the EPO receptor, can be dosed less frequently. Recommended starting doses of darbepoetin in nondialysis patients are 0.45 μg/kg/wk administered subcutaneously or 60 μg subcutaneously every 2 weeks. Hemodialysis patients are usually treated intravenously for ease of administration, despite the fact that intravenous therapy requires on average approximately 30% more ESA than with the subcutaneous route. The usual starting dose of EPO is 50 to 100 U/kg intravenously 3 times a week after dialysis.

ESA therapy is generally well tolerated. The main adverse effects include hypertension and an increase in the incidence of seizures and thrombosis if the hemoglobin is raised too high. As discussed in a later section in this chapter ("Marrow failure states leading to underproduction anemias"), antibodies directed against the naturally occurring hormone EPO have been described after exogenous supplementation.

Iron stores must be evaluated in all chronic kidney failure and dialysis patients. Nephrologists routinely supplement patients with iron to maintain serum transferrin saturation >20% and serum ferritin >100 ng/dL. Many dialysis centers have standing protocols for monitoring and replacing iron. Intravenous iron replacement can improve hemoglobin response in some chronic kidney patients. Iron can be replaced parenterally as iron dextran, iron gluconate, or iron sucrose, the latter 2 being less prone to anaphylaxis and being used most frequently in many dialysis centers. Common causes of EPO failure in persons with renal disease include iron or folate deficiency, ongoing blood loss, hyperparathyroidism, or aluminum toxicity. The patient in the clinical case presented in this section developed iron deficiency while on ESA supplementation and oral iron therapy. Intravenous iron gluconate was effective in replenishing iron stores and improving his anemia.

Anemia from endocrine abnormalities

In general, the anemia accompanying most endocrine disorders is typically mild, often asymptomatic, and likely overshadowed by the clinical effects of the specific hormone deficiency. In fact, in some cases, the anemia may actually be considered physiologic due to the decreased oxygen requirements accompanying some of these hormone deficiencies.

Pituitary deficiency may be associated with a mild normochromic normocytic anemia. The bone marrow of such patients is usually hypoplastic and resembles that seen in other marrow failure states. Anemia is most likely due to secondary deficiency of hormones produced by endocrine organs that are normally stimulated by the anterior lobe of the pituitary (thyroid hormone, androgens, or cortisol) and modulate EPO production. The anemia responds to appropriate hormone replacement.

Patients with primary hypothyroidism may be anemic. The anemia is felt to be secondary to an absence of EPO-stimulated erythroid colony formation from lack of triiodothyronine (T_3), thyroxine (T_4), and reverse triiodothyronine (rT_3). The anemia is usually normochromic and normocytic, and hemoglobin values are usually not less than 8 g/dL. Macrocytosis may occur in patients with autoimmune hypothyroidism, particularly if there is coexistent B_{12} deficiency, folate deficiency, or hemolysis. Conversely, microcytosis can occur in women with concomitant iron deficiency from menorrhagia, which may be seen in myxedema. There is a well-recognized association between hypothyroidism and PA, so patients with either disorder should be screened for the other. The response to thyroid replacement is typically sluggish, and it may take months before the anemia resolves. Unlike patients with hypothyroidism, patients with hyperthyroidism are only rarely anemic, and anemia in this condition is typically microcytic and poorly understood.

Patients with Addison disease may have a normochromic normocytic anemia that is responsive to EPO or glucocorticoids. However, the mild decrease in RBC mass may be masked by a concomitant decrease in plasma volume, leading to a normal hemoglobin concentration. When replacement with glucocorticoid therapy is initially begun, the anemia may become apparent as the plasma volume is restored.

Hypogonadism usually results in a 1- to 2-g/dL decrease in hemoglobin concentration. Androgens stimulate increased EPO production and can increase the effects of EPO on the developing erythron. Thus, men typically have higher hemoglobin concentrations than age-matched women. The hemoglobin values of castrate men typically fall to within the normal range for age-matched women. Androgens are sometimes used to correct anemias due to marrow hypoproduction in conditions such as myelodysplasia and myelofibrosis.

Anemia is a rare complication of early primary hyperparathyroidism. In more severe forms, excess parathyroid hormone may be toxic to the marrow and can lead to myelosclerosis. Anemia is more commonly seen in secondary hyperparathyroidism, contributing to the anemia seen in patients with renal disease. However, it is difficult to determine the relative importance of parathyroid excess, as compared with EPO deficiency. Blood abnormalities in the setting of hypoparathyroidism are likely due to accompanying PA or part of a type 1 endocrinopathy syndrome.

Although insulin likely does not affect EPO, anemia is more severe and occurs at an earlier stage in patients with diabetic nephropathy compared with patients with renal failure from other causes. The exact mechanism for this finding remains uncertain. Small studies have suggested that recombinant human EPO treatment may be effective in these patients even if the renal insufficiency is only mild.

Anemia associated with GI abnormalities

The gut is the main entry point for nutrients essential for hematopoiesis, as well as toxins that may suppress it. Compromise of intestinal integrity by way of surgery, medical illness, or drugs can result in the malabsorption of essential vitamins and minerals such as iron, B_{12}, and folate, as discussed earlier. Patients who have had compromise to the segments of alimentary tract (ie, Crohn disease affecting the terminal ileum) necessary for absorbing and processing specific vitamins should be screened for deficiency, and empiric replacement should be considered before deficiency occurs. Occult GI blood loss is a common cause of iron deficiency anemia and may be the first sign of severe underlying diseases. Protein deprivation, whether voluntary or due to malabsorption, can lead to decreased EPO production.

Anemia associated with liver disease

Anemia, as well as other hematopoietic abnormalities, is frequently seen in patients with liver disease. The true incidence of anemia is dependent on the cause of liver disease but has been reported in up to 75% of patients with chronic liver disease. The etiology of anemia is multifactorial and likely reflects underproduction, blood loss, and increased destruction of RBCs. In alcoholic liver disease, concomitant folic acid deficiency may be seen and should be evaluated. Alcohol-induced pancreatitis may lead to decreased B_{12} absorption. Ethanol and its metabolites have been shown to inhibit erythroid production directly and may lead to acute or chronic anemia even in the absence of severe liver disease. In addition, EPO production and erythropoiesis are suppressed by alcohol. Viral hepatitis may be associated with pure red cell aplasia. GI blood loss is common in liver disease, especially in patients with esophageal varices. Shortened RBC survival is also noted in chronic liver disease. The decreased life span of RBCs in liver disease is at least partially explained by congestive splenomegaly, abnormal erythrocyte metabolism, and alterations in RBC membrane lipids. Changes in cholesterol composition lead to alterations in RBC surface area characterized by the target cells typically seen on review of the peripheral blood smear. Marked hemolytic anemia may develop in alcoholics with relatively mild liver disease. This condition, when accompanied by jaundice and hyperlipidemia, is termed *Zieve syndrome*. This syndrome may be self-limiting if the patient abstains from alcohol. Marked spur cells are noted on the blood smear in this condition, which has also been termed *spur cell anemia* (Figure 5-8). In the presence of underlying cirrhosis, spur cell anemia is likely irreversible without liver transplantation.

The typical anemia of liver disease is usually mild to moderate but may become more severe as cirrhosis, splenomegaly, and portal hypertension develop. The anemia is usually normocytic or macrocytic, but the MCV rarely exceeds 115 fL in the absence of megaloblastic changes in the bone marrow. The reticulocyte count is often minimally to moderately increased in liver disease but may be suppressed by alcohol or concomitant iron deficiency. More marked reticulocytosis may be seen with hemorrhage or in spur cell anemia. Bone marrow cellularity is often increased, and erythroid hyperplasia is observed. The peripheral blood smear will often show acanthocytes and target cells as the disease severity increases. Megaloblastosis may be seen in up to 20% of subjects.

The treatment of anemia in liver disease is primarily supportive. If present, iron, B_{12}, and folate deficiencies should be corrected. If ongoing hemolysis is noted, folate should be supplemented. Alcohol and other toxins should be avoided. Supplementation with exogenous EPO can be considered if the anemia is severe and the patient symptomatic. Splenectomy should not be routinely performed but can be considered only if the anemia is severe, the patient is symptomatic, the spleen is markedly enlarged, and bone marrow production is adequate.

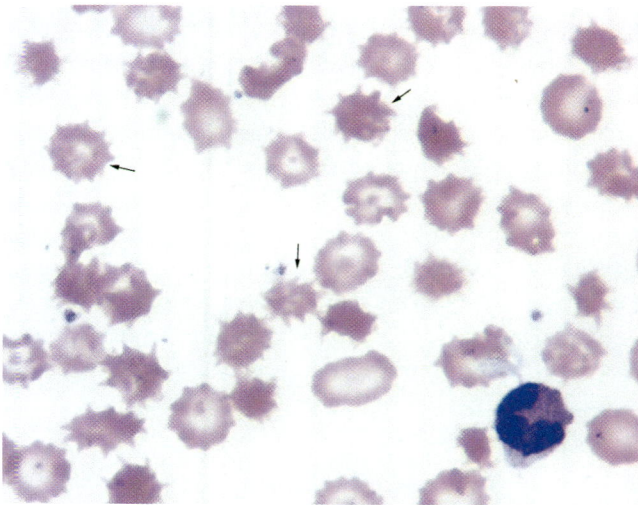

Figure 5-8 Spur cell anemia in a patient with severe liver disease and hemolytic anemia. Arrows point to spur cells. Target cells are also seen. From ASH slide bank case #100507.

> **Key points**
>
> - Renal disease is the prototypical disorder of EPO deficiency. Supplemental replacement of EPO is effective treatment of anemia in patients with kidney disease.
> - Patients with kidney disease who fail to respond to EPO may have either true or functional iron deficiency, folic acid deficiency, aluminum toxicity, or ongoing bleeding.
> - Anemia associated with other endocrinopathies is often mild to moderate as compared with the symptoms from the endocrine deficiency itself. Appropriate hormone replacement usually leads to resolution of anemia.
> - Anemia associated with GI diseases and liver disease is often multifactorial with elements of bone marrow underproduction, blood loss, and shortened RBC survival. Treatment is usually supportive and aimed at the underlying disease process.

Marrow failure states leading to underproduction anemias

A variety of different hematopoietic disorders can affect the bone marrow and lead to the underproduction of RBCs and resultant anemia. Much of the time, the anemia is only part of a more global disorder affecting the bone marrow. Many of these disorders such as aplastic anemia (Chapter 15), acute leukemia (Chapters 16 and 17), myelodysplastic syndrome, and dyserythropoietic anemias (Chapter 15) are discussed elsewhere. In this section, we will focus on pure red cell aplasia as a bone marrow disorder leading exclusively to anemia.

Pure red cell aplasia

> **Clinical case**
>
> A 64-year-old female presents with fatigue and dyspnea on exertion, which has been progressive over the last 2 months. She is on no medications and has no significant past medical history. Previous blood counts reportedly have been normal. Physical examination is significant for skin pallor and pale conjunctivae. Stool is guaiac negative. Laboratory evaluation reveals hemoglobin of 6.4 g/dL, MCV of 99 fL, and corrected reticulocyte count of 0.3%. White blood cell and platelet counts are normal. Bone marrow examination reveals a lack of erythroid precursors and lack of erythroid maturation, but otherwise is unremarkable. Flow cytometry does not reveal a lymphoproliferative disorder, and cytogenetic evaluation results are normal. Computed tomography (CT) scan of the chest fails to identify a thymoma. Prednisone 1 mg/kg daily is prescribed, and within 2 weeks, a partial response is seen. After 6 weeks, a complete response is seen, and a slow taper of prednisone is begun. The patient relapses after prednisone withdrawal. She is begun on cyclosporin A at 4 mg/kg daily with a gradual, but complete, response in her blood counts.

Pure red cell aplasia (PRCA) refers to a diverse group of disorders characterized by severe progressive anemia, reticulocytopenia, and either a lack of RBC precursors or arrest in the differentiation of RBC progenitors, typically at the proerythroblast stage. A representative bone marrow from a patient with PRCA, showing a marked decrease in RBC progenitors, is shown in Figure 5-9. PRCA can be congenital or acquired and may be the result of abnormal stem cells or autoimmune, viral, or chemical inhibition of erythroblastosis (Table 5-6). This chapter will cover acquired causes of PRCA. Diamond-Blackfan anemia, the prototypical congenital cause of PRCA, is covered in Chapter 15.

Acquired causes of PRCA can be divided into those that are acute and those that are chronic. Acute RBC aplasia may occur in the setting of a chronic hemolytic anemia and is

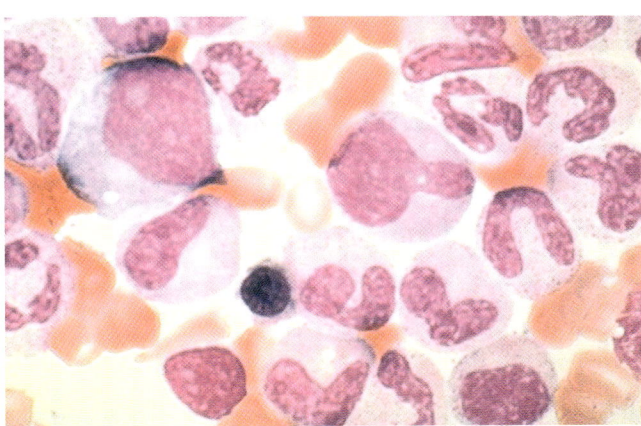

Figure 5-9 Bone marrow biopsy showing marked erythroid hypoplasia in a patient with acquired pure red cell aplasia. From ASH slide bank #1528.

Table 5-6 Classification of pure red cell aplasia.

Congenital (discussed in Chapter 15)
   Diamond-Blackfan anemia

Acquired
   Acute
      Human parvovirus and other viral infections
      Drugs
         Erythropoietin
         Other (ie, phenytoin, chloramphenicol, gold salts, isoniazid)
      Transient erythroblastemia of childhood (TEC)
   Chronic
      Idiopathic
      Thymoma
      Lymphoproliferative diseases
      Collagen vascular and other autoimmune diseases
      Solid tumors
      ABO-mismatched bone marrow transplantation
      Associated with other primary bone marrow disorders

most commonly caused by acute infection with human parvovirus, the agent responsible for erythema infectiosum or fifth disease in children. Human parvovirus is a common infection, with 50% of children having detectable immunoglobulin G (IgG) to human parvovirus and 90% of the elderly having evidence of previous infection. The virus binds to the P antigen on the surface of RBC progenitors and destroys proliferating erythroid progenitor cells. In patients with an underlying hemolytic process requiring greater than normal production of erythrocytes to maintain an adequate circulating RBC mass, severe anemia can quickly result in the presence of human parvovirus infection. The majority of infected patients who have a normal RBC life span remain asymptomatic, despite the transient decrease in erythropoiesis. Human parvovirus infection may result in the appearance of giant pronormoblasts in the marrow, as shown in Figure 5-10. Treatment of human parvovirus-induced RBC aplasia is usually supportive (ie, packed RBC transfusion for symptomatic anemia) because the virus is rapidly cleared by the immune system. However, human parvovirus may be particularly problematic in HIV or other immunosuppressed individuals, such as those after organ transplantation, because the virus may not be effectively cleared by the host immune system, leading to chronic infection. Immunocompromised patients may therefore not be able to mount an effective immune response, and standard IgG and immunoglobulin M (IgM) titers against human parvovirus may remain negative even in the face of active infection. Polymerase chain reaction (PCR) studies for human parvovirus DNA are thus recommended in this patient population. Patients with HIV, as well as other immunosuppressed patients, typically respond to intravenous immunoglobulin (IVIg), which contains high titers of antibodies to human parvovirus. Reticulocytosis is often seen 3 to 5 days after infusion, with resolution of anemia occurring later. Relapses may occur and should be investigated if anemia recurs. Hepatitis and mononucleosis have also rarely been associated with RBC aplasia.

Many different drugs have been reported to cause PRCA, although it remains unknown why only a minority of patients administered these drugs become affected. Drugs such as diphenylhydantoin and other antiseizure medications, chloramphenicol, gold salts, lindane, dapsone, INH, rifampin, and sulfasalazine have been associated with PRCA. The anemia typically resolves upon discontinuing the offending drug. PRCA has been described due to the development of antierythropoietin antibodies during treatment with recombinant human EPO. Although rare, this syndrome has occurred primarily after administration of Eprex (Janssen-Ortho, Toronto, Ontario, Canada), an EPO alfa product marketed outside of the United States. The number of cases of EPO-associated PRCA peaked in 2001 and has since declined due to changes in the manufacturing, distribution, storage, and administration of Eprex. In addition to the discontinuation of Eprex, many affected patients were also prescribed immunosuppression with variable results. A more detailed discussion of anti-EPO antibodies can be found in Chapter 3.

A unique form of transient PRCA observed in infants and young children is transient erythroblastopenia of childhood. Affected patients are between 6 and 36 months of age and present only with the insidious onset of pallor. The degree of anemia is variable but may be quite severe and necessitate RBC transfusion. The differential diagnosis includes Diamond-Blackfan anemia and parvovirus infection. Although the pathophysiology is not well characterized, most cases appear to be due to an IgG antibody directed against erythroblasts. The condition resolves spontaneously within several months with no sequelae.

Chronic acquired PRCA is more common than acute causes and is usually immunologic in origin, as in the clinical case provided. Chronic PRCA may be idiopathic in origin or secondary to other underlying diseases such as thymoma, lymphoproliferative disorders, solid tumors, and collagen vascular disorders. Immunologic mechanisms implicated in the suppression of erythroid precursors in these varied disorders include autoantibodies, natural killer cell–mediated toxicity, and T-lymphocyte–mediated toxicity. The connection between thymoma and PRCA has long been known but is less common than previously thought. Recent studies have shown that only 10% to 15% of patients with PRCA have a detectable thymoma. The pathophysiology is presumed to be T-cell–mediated erythroid colony destruction. The response to thymectomy in these cases is variable; a minority of patients achieves a complete remission after thymoma resection. PRCA may also be found in patients with lymphoproliferative disorders such as large granular lymphocytic (LGL)

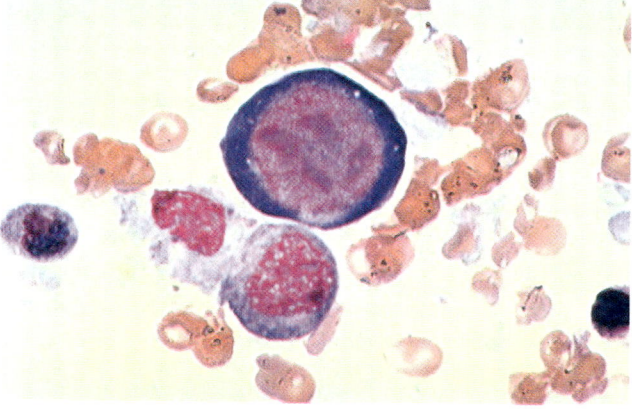

Figure 5-10 Giant pronormoblast in a patient with human parvovirus infection. From ASH slide bank #4608.

leukemia, chronic lymphocytic leukemia (CLL), and lymphoma. It was recently recognized that LGL leukemia may be the most common underlying cause of secondary PRCA. Because LGL leukemia may be present even in the absence of significant lymphocytosis, it is recommended that patients with idiopathic PRCA undergo lymphocyte immunophenotyping and T-cell receptor gene rearrangement analysis to look for LGL leukemia. Treatment aimed at the underlying disorder may prove effective in treating PRCA. Approximately 20% of patients receiving ABO-mismatched bone marrow transplantation develop a prolonged RBC aplasia due to recipient isohemagglutinins, especially anti-A, against the donor RBCs; generally, the condition improves over time or with the development of graft-versus-host disease. When the anemia is severe or life threatening, treatment with plasma exchange using donor-type plasma and high doses of EPO has been effective in some patients.

Many treatment modalities have been instituted for patients with chronic acquired PRCA, but therapy should initially be directed against an underlying disorder such as human parvovirus or lymphoproliferative disorders if identified. Transfusion therapy remains important in patients with severe symptomatic anemia. Iron overload and alloantibody formation limit this therapy as a long-term approach. Supplemental EPO therapy is seldom effective but has been used in certain instances such as after ABO-incompatible bone marrow transplantation. In the presence of a thymoma, thymectomy has been helpful, but response is not uniform and may require additional immunosuppressive therapy. There does not appear to be any benefit to the removal of a normal thymus gland in patients with PRCA who do not have a thymoma or thymic hyperplasia identified. Glucocorticoids and other immunosuppressive agents such as antithymocyte globulin and/or cyclosporine may be effective to treat PRCA, especially in idiopathic cases. As in the case presented, prednisone is often the initial treatment of choice with second-line immunosuppression reserved for refractory or relapsing cases. Cytotoxic therapy such as oral cyclophosphamide has also been used with some success, especially in cases associated with lymphoproliferative disorders. Responding patients are generally treated for 3 to 6 months before immunosuppression is slowly withdrawn. The majority of patients will respond to one or more of the treatment modalities, which are generally used sequentially until a response is achieved; however, many patients will relapse after withdrawal of therapy and will require a long-term approach to immunosuppression, particularly if an underlying disorder (lymphoproliferative disorder or collagen vascular disease) persists. Both anti-CD20 monoclonal antibody (rituximab) and anti-CD52 antibody (alemtuzumab) have been reported to induce remissions in some patients with treatment resistant PRCA; anti-CD20, in particular, has effectiveness that may be limited to patients with underlying B-cell lymphoproliferative disorders or other autoantibody-mediated disorders. Causes of death in nonresponding patients include infection, iron overload, or cardiovascular events. The median survival time for patients with chronic acquired PRCA is >10 years.

Key points

- PRCA may be an acute, chronic, or congenital disorder.
- Human parvovirus is a frequent cause of acquired acute PRCA in patients with shortened RBC life span. The suppression of erythropoiesis remains clinically silent in most patients with normal RBC survival.
- Parvovirus infection may become chronic in immunosuppressed individuals. IVIg may be effective therapy.
- Acquired causes of PRCA may be idiopathic or secondary to underlying disorders such as lymphoproliferative or collagen vascular diseases.
- Patients should be evaluated for thymoma, although it is found in only a small minority of cases. If discovered, thymectomy should be considered.
- Idiopathic acquired PRCA in adults is often responsive to immunosuppressive therapy, such as prednisone. In children, the condition is generally transient and self-limited, often requiring no specific therapy.

Anemia secondary to marrow infiltration or abnormalities in the marrow microenvironment

Myelophthisic anemia is characterized by teardrop-shaped erythrocytes, immature leukocytes, nucleated erythrocytes, and large megakaryocyte fragments on the peripheral smear (Figure 5-11), often referred to as a *leukoerythroblastic* peripheral smear. Secondary myelophthisis occurs in response to infiltration of the marrow by tumor, macrophages in lipid storage disease (ie, Gaucher disease), fibrosis, or granulomas. These conditions may be accompanied by extramedullary hematopoiesis leading to organomegaly and the presence of marrow elements in the spleen, liver, or other affected tissues. Rarely, carcinocythemia (cancer cells in the circulating blood) can be demonstrated.

Myelophthisis is believed to occur as a result of the release of cytokines, which stimulate fibroblastic proliferation and fibrosis in the marrow. Myelophthisis does not usually occur in leukemias, with the exception of acute megakaryoblastic leukemia, but is common in myelofibrosis (see Chapter 14) or when small-cell lung cancer, breast cancer, or prostate cancer spread to the bone marrow.

Bone marrow biopsy showing frank tumor cells, Gaucher disease, or other infiltrating disorders in the presence of

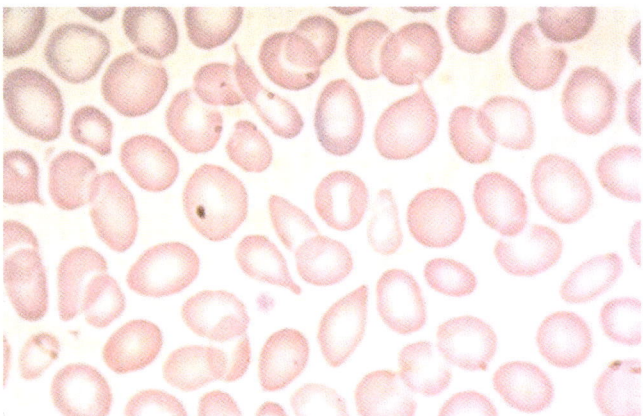

Figure 5-11 Teardrop cells on the peripheral smear. From ASH slide bank #1462.

marked marrow fibrosis is diagnostic of these secondary causes of myelophthisis. T1-weighted magnetic resonance imaging (MRI) may demonstrate areas of abnormal signal consistent with marrow infiltration.

Treatment of this disorder involves treatment of the underlying disease processes. Supplemental EPO is effective for some patients. Unfortunately, life expectancy in most patients with marrow invasive tumors is limited. Lifelong treatment with imiglucerase is effective in the treatment of Gaucher disease.

During infancy, myelophthisic anemia can be seen in the setting of osteopetrosis or marble bone disease. These conditions vary in their severity, but infants affected with the autosomal recessive form present within the first few months of life with pancytopenia, hepatosplenomegaly, and cranial nerve palsies. Osteopetrosis is caused by failure of osteoclast development or function, and mutations in at least 10 genes have been identified, accounting for 70% of cases. Severe cases are treated by bone marrow transplantation.

Complex/multifactorial anemias

Anemia associated with pregnancy

Beginning during the first trimester of pregnancy, the plasma volume increases out of proportion to the RBC mass. Throughout pregnancy, the plasma volume may increase 40%, whereas the RBC mass usually increases only approximately 20%. The result of this imbalance is the so-called dilutional anemia of pregnancy. Typically, the reduction in the hematocrit plateaus between the 16th and 22nd week of pregnancy. The average hemoglobin and hematocrit values during pregnancy are 11 g/dL and 33%, respectively. In the puerperium, the blood volume quickly returns to a new baseline, initially reflecting blood loss at delivery and iron utilization during the pregnancy.

As discussed in the subsection on iron deficiency anemia, iron requirements increase during pregnancy, and iron deficiency is common, especially in the non-Western world. Oral iron supplementation is initially preferred for replacement, but intravenous iron has been given safely in those who are intolerant to or do not respond to oral iron. Folate requirements also increase during pregnancy, and megaloblastic anemia has been reported, especially during the third trimester. Prenatal vitamins containing both iron and folate can help reduce, but not eliminate, these risks. Vitamin B_{12} deficiency due to a lack of intrinsic factor has been reported in pregnancy and should be considered in the differential diagnosis of a macrocytic anemia. Serum B_{12} levels may be less reliable during pregnancy, and HCY and MMA levels should be checked to confirm true deficiency. Aplastic anemia and hemolytic anemia may be seen more commonly during pregnancy.

Pregnant patients are also susceptible to the same diseases that afflict nonpregnant women. Although iron deficiency and folate deficiency have been stressed, the clinician should keep an open mind while evaluating anemia in pregnant women. The evaluation and workup of pregnant patients with anemia should therefore mirror that of nonpregnant women, although the differences in normal hemoglobin values between pregnant and nonpregnant women need to be kept in mind. Treatment will depend on the etiology of anemia and is often similar to that of nonpregnant individuals. Special scenarios do exist, such as the use of chemotherapeutic agents for primary bone marrow disorders. Because any treatment has effects on both the mother and developing fetus, care should be closely coordinated between the hematologist, obstetrician, and neonatologist.

> **Key points**
> - Anemia in pregnancy is due in part to an imbalance between the expansion of the plasma volume and the RBC mass.
> - Iron deficiency and folate deficiency are important causes of anemia in pregnancy.
> - The evaluation of anemia in pregnancy should be similar to that in nonpregnant individuals.

Anemia of the elderly

Recently, findings from the National Health and Nutrition Examination Study (NHANES III) indicated that 11.0% of men and 10.2% of women over the age of 65 were anemic (based on the definition of anemia as hemoglobin <13 g/dL for men and <12/dL for women). Other studies have supported this finding, as well as the higher prevalence rates of anemia in elderly African Americans. Anemia is an independent risk factor for cognitive decline and is associated with decreased bone density, decreased muscle strength, and decreased physical performance in elderly patients. The presence of anemia, either with or without other chronic illnesses, is associated with increased hospitalization, morbidity, and mortality.

Analysis of data from NHANES III showed that approximately two thirds of the cases of anemia were attributable to iron deficiency, other nutritional deficiencies, chronic inflammatory illnesses, and renal insufficiency. However, 34% of cases were unexplained based on the information available in the database. Several studies have attempted to elucidate the mechanisms for this group of unexplained anemias. Investigators have suggested that a variety of age-related physiologic changes may contribute to this process including blunting of the hypoxia-driven EPO response, decrease in sex steroids, and alterations in bone marrow stem cells and cellularity. Because it is likely that anemia is multifactorial in a given individual, a thorough clinical and laboratory evaluation is justified to identify those causes of anemia that are amenable to therapy. A reasonable approach to evaluation is given in Table 5-7.

Key points

- The NHANES III study demonstrated that anemia is prevalent in the elderly with incidences that increase with age.
- Approximately one third of the cases of anemia in the elderly remain unexplained after laboratory investigation.
- Functional impairment and increased morbidity and mortality have been demonstrated in elderly anemic patients.

Anemia of cancer

Anemia is among the most common hematologic manifestations of cancer. The incidence of anemia in cancer patients is highly dependent on many variables, including cancer type, stage, and both present and past anticancer therapy, but may exceed 90% in patients with advanced disease receiving chemotherapy. The mechanisms underlying anemia of malignancy are complex, and numerous factors contribute to its development. Cytokine-mediated changes cause a relative decrease in EPO production and a decrease in the response of erythroid precursors to EPO. As in AOCD, cytokines cause elevated hepcidin levels and a functional iron deficiency (see earlier section on AOCD). Other causes of anemia in patients with cancer include effects of chemotherapy and radiotherapy, bone marrow infiltration, blood loss, autoimmune and microangiopathic hemolysis, and nutritional deficiencies.

A major change in the supportive care of cancer patients occurred with the availability of recombinant EPO. Numerous studies have demonstrated a decrease in transfusion requirements among cancer patients receiving ESA, with some studies also showing improvement in quality of life in treated patients. However, cumulative data suggest that ESAs cause tumor growth and shortened survival in patients with advanced breast, head and neck, lymphoid, and non–small-cell cancer, especially when dosed to a hemoglobin >12 g/dL. The presence of EPO receptors has been suggested in a number of human cancers, and studies have suggested that exogenous ESA may stimulate proliferation of tumor cells or may promote tumor growth through effects on the tumor microenvironment and angiogenesis. Further doubt

Table 5-7 Evaluation of anemia in the elderly for the clinical hematologist: a practical approach.

Always useful
1. Anemia-oriented history and physical examination, with particular emphasis on comorbid conditions associate with anemia and drug history
2. CBC/differential/platelet, absolute reticulocyte count, smear review
3. Tests of iron stores (Fe, TIBC, ferritin)
4. Serum cobalamin and folate levels
5. Chemistry panel (including calculated creatinine clearance)
6. TSH

Sometimes useful
1. Serum testosterone
2. Serum erythropoietin (with caveat for what represents a "normal" erythropoietin in an elderly person)
3. Tests of inflammation (ESR, C-reactive protein)
4. Methylmalonic acid, serum homocysteine
5. RBC folate level
6. Bone marrow aspiration and biopsy, cytogenetics

Modified from Guralnik JM, Ershler WB, Schrier SL, et al. Anemia in the elderly: a public health crisis in hematology. *Hematology Am Soc Hematol Educ Program.* 2005:531.

CBC = complete blood count; ESR = erythrocyte sedimentation rate; Fe = iron; RBC = red blood cell; TIBC = total iron-binding capacity; TSH = thyroid-stimulating hormone.

regarding the safety of ESA for the treatment of the anemia of cancer was raised in a recent large meta-analysis. In this study, individual patient data were analyzed from 13,933 patients with cancer treated on 53 randomized controlled trials using ESA versus standard of care. The analysis demonstrated a 17% increase in mortality in ESA-treated patients during the active study period. There was a 10% increase in mortality when the analysis was restricted to the studies that included patients treated with chemotherapy. Other studies have suggested that ESA treatment increases the risk of venous thromboembolism in patients with cancer. The current Food and Drug Administration guidelines state that ESAs should not be used in cancer patients who are not receiving chemotherapy and are not indicated for patients receiving myelosuppressive therapy when the anticipated outcome is cure.

> **Key points**
>
> - Anemia is frequent in cancer patients and leads to a decreased quality of life.
> - The mechanisms leading to the anemia of cancer are complex and likely multifactorial, including the effects of tumor-driven cytokine production, anticancer therapy, bone marrow infiltration, bleeding, EPO deficiency, and hemolysis.
> - Erythropoietic agents increase mortality and venous thromboembolism in patients with cancer and should be avoided.

Anemia associated with HIV

Anemia is the most prevalent hematologic abnormality associated with HIV infection. Not surprisingly, anemia prevalence increases with HIV disease progression. Several studies have shown that anemia is independently associated with decreased survival and decreased quality of life in HIV-infected patients. Anemia in HIV-infected patients is usually multifactorial, and the most likely etiologies depend on the stage of the HIV infection and the medications the patient is receiving. Zidovudine and trimethoprim-sulfamethoxazole are commonly associated with bone marrow suppression and macrocytosis. Infections associated with anemia include Mycobacterium avium complex, tuberculosis, histoplasmosis, cytomegalovirus, Epstein-Barr virus, and human parvovirus (see the earlier section "Pure red cell aplasia"). Malignant disorders, mainly non-Hodgkin lymphoma, can infiltrate the bone marrow and cause anemia. Nutritional deficiencies, including vitamin B_{12}, folate, and iron, are common in HIV patients and are related to blood loss, malabsorption, and poor nutrition. Patients with HIV are at risk for hemolysis due to a variety of mechanisms, including microangiopathic hemolysis, antibody-mediated mechanisms, and drug-induced mechanisms, especially in patients with glucose-6-phosphate dehydrogenase deficiency.

Hypogonadism is a frequent finding in patients with advanced HIV and is associated with a mild anemia. The HIV virus itself infects bone marrow cells and may interfere with hematopoiesis.

The use of highly active antiretroviral therapy (HAART) has been shown to reduce the prevalence of anemia in several population studies. Even the inclusion of zidovudine in the regimen does not appear to diminish the beneficial effect of HAART on anemia. In addition to HAART, the management of anemia in HIV patients should include correction of nutritional deficiencies and treatment of infections. ESAs have been shown to reduce transfusion requirements in HIV patients with baseline EPO levels of <500 mU/mL, in whom nutritional deficiencies and other causes have been corrected.

> **Key points**
>
> - Anemia is common in patients with HIV and correlates with disease severity.
> - Anemia in patients with HIV is often multifactorial. Causes include drugs, infections (including the HIV virus), lymphoma, and nutritional deficiencies.
> - HAART therapy improves anemia through reduction of the HIV viral load.
> - EPO therapy has proven effective in a subset of patients with HIV.

Bibliography

Iron deficiency anemia

Alleyne M, Horne MK, Miller JL. Individualized treatment for iron-deficiency anemia in adults. *Am J Med.* 2008;121:943–948. *Practical approach to diagnosis and treatment of iron deficiency in adults.*

Auerbach M, Ballard H, Glaspy J. Clinical update: intravenous iron for anaemia. *Lancet.* 2007;369:1502–1504. *A review of parenteral iron formulations available with their adverse effects and recommended doses and modes of administration.*

Clark SF. Iron deficiency anemia. *Nutr Clin Pract.* 2008;23: 128–141. *A comprehensive review of the etiology, diagnosis, and treatment of iron deficiency anemia.*

Cook JD. Diagnosis and management of iron-deficiency anemia. *Best Pract Res Clin Haematol.* 2005;18:319–332. *Overview of diagnosis, treatment, and classification of isolated iron deficiency in the presence of other diseases.*

Halfdanarson TR, Litzow MR, Murray JA. Hematologic manifestations of celiac disease. *Blood.* 2007;109:412–421. *A review of the causes of anemia and other hematologic abnormalities in patients with celiac disease.*

Richardson M. Microcytic anemia. *Pediatr Rev.* 2007;28:5–14. *A review of causes of microcytic anemia in childhood including iron deficiency, thalassemia, and lead toxicity.*

Umbriet J. Iron deficiency: a concise review. *Am J Hematol.* 2005;78:225–231. *Detailed up-to-date review of iron deficiency.*

Anemia of chronic disease

Andrews NC. Forging a field: the golden age of iron biology. *Blood.* 2008;112:219–230. *A concise review of the new findings in iron metabolism and their clinical applications.*

Raj DSC. Role of interleukin-6 in the anemia of chronic disease. *Semin Arthritis Rheum.* 2009;38:382–388. *Review of the pathogenesis of AOCD with emphasis on end-stage renal failure and rheumatoid arthritis.*

Weiss G, Goodnough LT. Anemia of chronic disease. *New Engl J Med.* 2005;352:1011–1023. *Review of the etiology, pathogenesis, and treatment of AOCD.*

Cobalamin deficiency

Birn H, Verroust PJ, Nexo E, et al. Characterization of an epithelial approximately 460-kDa protein that facilitates endocytosis of intrinsic factor-vitamin B12 and binds receptor-associated protein. *J Biol Chem.* 1997;272:26497–26504. *Report identifying the intrinsic factor–cobalamin receptor.*

Carmel R. How I treat cobalamin (vitamin B12) deficiency. *Blood.* 2008;112:2214–2221. *Update on the significance of metabolic testing in cobalamin deficiency states and on the ability to discriminate true deficiency states from clinically irrelevant biochemical abnormalities.*

Carmel R, Green R, Rosenblatt DS, et al. Update on cobalamin, folate, and homocysteine. *Hematology Am Soc Hematol Educ Program.* 2003:62–81.

Oh R, Brown DL. Vitamin B12 deficiency. *Am Fam Physician.* 2003;67:979–986. *Update on testing and therapy for cobalamin deficiency.*

Wolters M, Strohle A, Hahn A. Cobalamin: a critical vitamin in the elderly. *Prev Med.* 2004;39:1256–1266. *Review of causes and diagnostic challenges associated with cobalamin deficiency in the elderly.*

Folic acid deficiency

Krishnaswamy K, Madhavan Nair K. Importance of folate in human nutrition. *Br J Nutr.* 2001;85(Suppl 2):S115–S124. *Concise review of the importance of folic acid in human nutrition.*

Snow C. Laboratory diagnosis of vitamin B12 and folate deficiency: a guide for the primary physician. *Arch Intern Med.* 1999;159:1289–1298. *Comprehensive, well-organized review of laboratory tests and diagnostic algorithms.*

Anemia secondary to malnutrition and starvation

Smith RR, Spivak JL. Marrow cell necrosis in anorexia nervosa and involuntary starvation. *Br J Hematol.* 1985;60:525–530. *Report of marrow necrosis in a patient with a severe eating disorder.*

Nonmyelodysplastic sideroblastic anemia

Cotter PD, Rucknagel DL, Bishop DF. X-linked sideroblastic anemia: identification of the mutation in the erythroid-specific δ-aminolevulinate synthase gene (*ALAS2*) in the original family described by Cooley. *Blood.* 1994;84:3915–3924. *Report of molecular defect in a family with X-linked sideroblastic anemia.*

Muraki K, Sakura N, Ueda H, et al. Clinical implications of duplicated mtDNA in Pearson syndrome. *Am J Med Genet.* 2001;22:205–209. *Description of genetic defect in Pearson syndrome.*

Anemia of renal disease

Eschbach JW, Egrie JC, Downing MR, et al. Correction of the anemia of end-stage renal disease with recombinant human erythropoietin. Results of a combined phase I and II clinical trial. *N Engl J Med.* 1987;316:73–78. *First paper documenting efficacy of recombinant erythropoietin to treat anemia in patients with renal failure.*

KDOQI Work Group. KDOQI Clinical Practice Guidelines and Clinical Practice recommendations for anemia in chronic kidney disease: 2007 update of hemoglobin target. *Am J Kidney Dis.* 2007;50:471–530.

Liangos O, Pereira BJ, Jaber JL. Anemia in acute renal failure: role for erythropoiesis-stimulating proteins? *Artif Organs.* 2003;27:786–791.

Rosner MH, Bolton WK. The mortality risk associated with higher hemoglobin: is the therapy to blame? *Kidney Int.* 2008;74:695–697.

Tarumoto T, Imagawa S, Ohmine K, et al. N^G-monomethyl-L-arginine inhibits erythropoietin gene expression by stimulating GATA-2. *Blood.* 2000;96:1716–1722. *Paper showing molecular basis for erythropoietin suppression in patients with end-stage kidney disease.*

Anemia of endocrine, gastrointestinal, and liver disorders

Golde DW, Bersch N, Chopra IJ, et al. Thyroid hormones stimulate erythropoiesis in vitro. *Br J Hematol.* 1977;37:173–177. *Paper describing the role of thyroid hormone function on erythropoiesis.*

Peschle C, Rappaport IA, Magli MC, et al. Role of hypophysis in erythropoietin production during hypoxia. *Blood.* 1978;5:1117–1124. *Paper describing the effects of pituitary function on erythropoiesis.*

Spivak JL. The blood in systemic disorders. *Lancet.* 2000;355:1707–1712. *Overview of hematologic abnormalities in various systemic conditions.*

Zingraff J, Drueke T, Marie P, et al. Anemia and secondary hyperparathyroidism. *Arch Intern Med.* 1978;138:1650–1652. *Paper describing the role of parathyroid hormone as an inhibitor of erythropoiesis.*

Pure red cell aplasia

Bennett CL, Cournoyer D, Carson K, et al. Long-term outcome of individuals with pure red cell aplasia and antierythropoietin antibodies in patients treated with recombinant epoetin: a follow-up report from the Research on Adverse Drug Events and Reports (RADAR) Project. *Blood.* 2005;106:3343–3347. *Long-term follow up of patients developing antierythropoietin antibodies.*

Bennett CL, Luminari S, Nissenson AR, et al. Pure red-cell aplasia and epoetin therapy. *N Engl J Med.* 2004;351:1403–1408. *Review of epoetin-induced PRCA, including review of cases presented to the Food and Drug Administration.*

Djaldetti M, Blay A, Bergman M, et al. Pure red cell aplasia—a rare disease with multiple causes. *Biomed Pharmacother.* 2003;57:326–332. *Review of the etiologies, laboratory and clinical findings, and treatment of PRCA.*

Sawada K, Fujishima N, Hirokawa M. Acquired pure red cell aplasia: updated review of treatment. *Br J Hematol.* 2008;142:505–514. *Recent review of immunosuppressive therapy in the treatment of PRCA.*

Young NS, Abkowtiz JL, Luzzatto L. New insights into the pathophysiology of acquired cytopenias. *Hematology Am Soc Hematol Educ Program.* 2000:18–38. *Overview of acquired cytopenias, including PRCA, from the 2000 American Society of Hematology meeting.*

Myelophthisic anemia

Oster W, Herrmann F, Gamm H, et al. Erythropoietin for the treatment of anemia of malignancy associated with neoplastic bone marrow infiltration. *J Clin Oncol.* 1990;8:956–962. *Description of use of erythropoietin to treat anemia of bone marrow infiltration.*

Anemia of pregnancy

Whittaker PG, Macphail S, Lind T. Serial hematologic changes and pregnancy outcome. *Obstet Gynecol.* 1996;88:33–39. *Overview of the changes in plasma volume and RBC mass during pregnancy.*

Williams MD, Wheb MS. Anemia in pregnancy. *Med Clin North Am.* 1992;76:631–647. *Review of the causes and evaluation of anemia in pregnancy.*

Anemia of the elderly

Culleton BF, Manns BJ, Zhang J, et al. Impact of anemia on hospitalization and mortality in older adults. *Blood.* 2006;107:3841–3846. *Longitudinal study showing higher mortality as well as both cardiovascular and noncardiovascular hospital admissions associated with anemia.*

Denny SD, Kuchibhatla MN, Cohen HJ. Impact of anemia on mortality, cognition, and function in community-dwelling elderly. *Am J Med.* 2006;119:327–334. *In a community-based study, elderly African Americans were 3 times more likely to be anemic than whites; for all races and genders, anemia was associated with declining cognitive functioning and increased mortality.*

Guralnik J, Eisenstaedt R, Ferruci L, et al. Prevalence of anemia in persons 65 years and older in the United States: evidence for a high rate of unexplained anemia. *Blood.* 2004;104:2263–2268. *Analysis of NHANES III data demonstrating a high prevalence of unexplained anemias in the elderly.*

Penninx B, Pahor M, Cesari M, et al. Anemia is associated with disability and decreased physical performance and muscle strength in the elderly. *J Am Ger Soc.* 2004;52:719–724. *Studies demonstrating the impact of anemia on physical functioning measures equivalent to activities of daily living.*

Price E. Aging and erythropoiesis: current state of knowledge. *Blood Cells Mol Dis.* 2008;41:158–165. *Review of known pathophysiology involved in the anemia of ageing.*

Anemia of cancer

Bennett CL, Silver SM, Djulbegovic B, et al. Venous thromboembolism and mortality associated with recombinant erythropoietin and darbepoetin administration for the treatment of cancer-associated anemia. *JAMA.* 2008;299:914–924. *A meta-analysis demonstrating increased risk of venous thromboembolism in patients with cancer who are treated with ESA.*

Bohlius J, Schmidlin K, Brillant C, et al. Recombinant human erythropoiesis-stimulating agents and mortality in patients with cancer: a meta-analysis of randomised trials. *Lancet.* 2009;373:1532–1542. *A meta-analysis of data from 13,933 patients with cancer in 53 trials demonstrating that ESA increased mortality.*

Hardee ME, Arcasoy MO, Blackwell KL, Kirpatrick JP, Dewhirst MW. Erythropoietin biology in cancer. *Clin Cancer Res.* 2006;12:332–339. *A review of EPO and EPO-receptor biology in regard to their effects on tumor cells and other nonhematopoietic tissues.*

Anemia of HIV

Berhane K, Karim R, Cohen MH, et al. Impact of highly active antiretroviral therapy on anemia and relationship between anemia and survival in a large cohort of HIV-infected women. *J Acquir Immune Defic Syndr.* 2004;37:1245–1252. *Prospective longitudinal epidemiologic study showing that HAART use for 12 months was protective against development of anemia in women; also demonstrated that anemia was independently associated with decreased survival.*

Calis JCJ, van Hensbroek MB, de Haan RJ, et al. HIV-associated anemia in children: a systematic review from a global perspective. *AIDS.* 2008;22:1099–1112. *A review of 36 studies of anemia in HIV-infected children.*

Fangman JJ, Scadden DT. Anemia in HIV-infected adults: epidemiology, pathogenesis, and clinical management. *Curr Hematol Rep.* 2005;4:95–102. *Review of issues surrounding the etiology and treatment of anemia in HIV.*

Sloand E. Hematologic complications of HIV infection. *AIDS Rev.* 2005;7:187–196. *Overview of cytopenias in HIV-affected individuals, including the role of HAART therapy.*

CHAPTER 06

Hemolytic anemias

Charles T. Quinn and Charles H. Packman

Overview, 133
Hemolysis due to intrinsic abnormalities of the RBC, 134
Hemolysis due to extrinsic abnormalities of the RBC, 160
Bibliography, 175

Overview

Hemolysis is the accelerated destruction, and hence decreased life span, of red blood cells (RBCs). The bone marrow's response to hemolysis is increased erythropoiesis, evidenced by reticulocytosis. If the rate of hemolysis is modest and the marrow is able to completely compensate for the decreased RBC life span, then hemoglobin concentration may be normal; this is called compensated hemolysis. If the bone marrow is unable to completely compensate for hemolysis, then anemia occurs. This is called incompletely compensated hemolysis.

Clinically, hemolytic anemia produces variable degrees of fatigue, pallor, and jaundice. Splenomegaly occurs in some conditions. The complete blood count shows anemia and reticulocytosis that depend on the severity of hemolysis and the degree of bone marrow compensation. Secondary chemical changes include indirect hyperbilirubinemia, increased urobilinogen excretion, and elevated lactate dehydrogenase (LDH). Decreased serum haptoglobin levels and increased plasma free hemoglobin may also be detected. Because free hemoglobin scavenges nitric oxide, esophageal spasm or vascular sequelae such as nonhealing skin ulcers can occur. Chronic intravascular hemolysis produces hemosiderinuria, and chronic extravascular hemolysis increases the risk of pigmented (bilirubinate) gallstones.

The hemolytic anemias can be classified in different, complementary ways (Table 6-1). They can be inherited (eg, sickle cell disease or hereditary spherocytosis) or acquired (eg, autoimmune or microangiopathic). Alternatively, they

Table 6-1 Methods of classification of hemolytic anemias.

Classification	Example
Inheritance	
Inherited	Sickle cell anemia
Acquired	Autoimmune hemolytic anemia
Site of RBC destruction	
Intravascular	Paroxysmal nocturnal hemoglobinuria
Extravascular	Hereditary spherocytosis
Origin of RBC damage	
Intrinsic	Pyruvate kinase deficiency
Extrinsic	Thrombotic thrombocytopenic purpura

RBC = red blood cell.

can be characterized by the anatomic site of RBC destruction: extravascular or intravascular. Extravascular hemolysis, erythrocyte destruction by macrophages in the liver and spleen, is more common. Intravascular hemolysis refers to RBC destruction occurring primarily within blood vessels. The distinction between intravascular and extravascular hemolysis is not absolute because both occur simultaneously, at least to some degree, in the same patient, and the manifestations of both overlap. The site of RBC destruction in different conditions can be conceptualized to occur in a spectrum between pure intravascular and pure extravascular hemolysis. Some hemolytic anemias are predominantly intravascular (eg, paroxysmal nocturnal hemoglobinuria), and some are predominantly extravascular (eg, hereditary spherocytosis). Others have substantial components of both, such as sickle cell anemia in a young child with an intact spleen.

The hemolytic anemias can also be classified according to whether the cause of hemolysis is intrinsic or extrinsic to the RBC—whether the damage occurs from within or without.

Conflict-of-interest disclosure: *Dr. Quinn* declares no competing financial interest. *Dr. Packman* declares no competing financial interest.

Intrinsic causes of hemolysis include abnormalities in hemoglobin structure or function, the RBC membrane, or RBC metabolism (enzymes). Extrinsic causes may be due to an RBC-directed antibody, a disordered vasculature, or the presence of infecting organisms or toxins. In general, intrinsic causes of hemolysis are inherited and extrinsic causes are acquired, but there are notable exceptions. Paroxysmal nocturnal hemoglobinuria (PNH) is an acquired intrinsic RBC disorder, and congenital thrombotic thrombocytopenia purpura (TTP) is an inherited cause of extrinsic hemolysis. In this chapter, hemolytic anemias will be divided into intrinsic and extrinsic forms.

Hemolysis due to intrinsic abnormalities of the RBC

Intrinsic causes of hemolysis include abnormalities of hemoglobin structure or function, the RBC membrane, or RBC metabolism (enzymes). Most intrinsic forms of hemolysis are inherited conditions.

Abnormalities of hemoglobin

Hemoglobin (Hb) is the oxygen-carrying protein within RBCs. It is composed of 4 globular protein subunits, called globins, and 4 oxygen-binding heme groups, which are attached to each globin. The 2 main types of globins are the α globins and the β globins, which are made in essentially equivalent amount in precursors of RBCs. Normal adult Hb (Hb A) has 2 α globins and 2 β globins ($\alpha_2\beta_2$). Genes on chromosomes 16 and 11 encode the α globins and β globins, respectively. There are also distinct embryonic, fetal, and minor adult analogs of the α globins and β globins, all of which are encoded by separate genes.

Hb production

The gene cluster for the non-α (β-like) globins is on chromosome 11 and includes an embryonic ε-globin gene, the 2 fetal globin genes γ ($^A\gamma$ and $^G\gamma$), and the 2 adult δ and β globin genes. The cluster of α-like globin genes is on chromosome 16 and includes the embryonic ζ globin gene and the duplicated α globin genes (α_2 and α_1), which are expressed in both fetal and adult life. Both clusters also contain nonfunctional genes (pseudogenes) designated by the prefix ψ. The θ globin gene downstream of α_1 has unknown functional significance.

The expression of each globin gene cluster is under the regulatory influence of a distant upstream locus control region (LCR). The LCR for the β cluster resides several kilobases upstream. A similar regulatory region, called HS-40, exists upstream of the α cluster. The LCRs contain DNA sequence elements that bind erythroid-specific and nonspecific DNA binding proteins and serve as a "master switch" inducing expression within the downstream gene cluster. In addition to binding specific transcriptional regulatory proteins, the LCRs also facilitate the binding and interaction of transcriptional regulatory proteins in proximity to the specific genes within the downstream cluster. These regulatory proteins influence the promoter function of the α globin and β globin genes to achieve a high level of erythroid- and development-specific gene expression.

Figure 6-1 details the organization of the α and β clusters with the associated upstream regulatory elements and the normal Hb species produced during the developmental stages from intrauterine to adult life. Note that the genes are expressed developmentally in the same sequence in which they are organized physically in these clusters (left to right; 5′ to 3′). The process of developmental changes in the type and site of globin gene expression is known as Hb switching. Switching within the cluster is influenced by differential

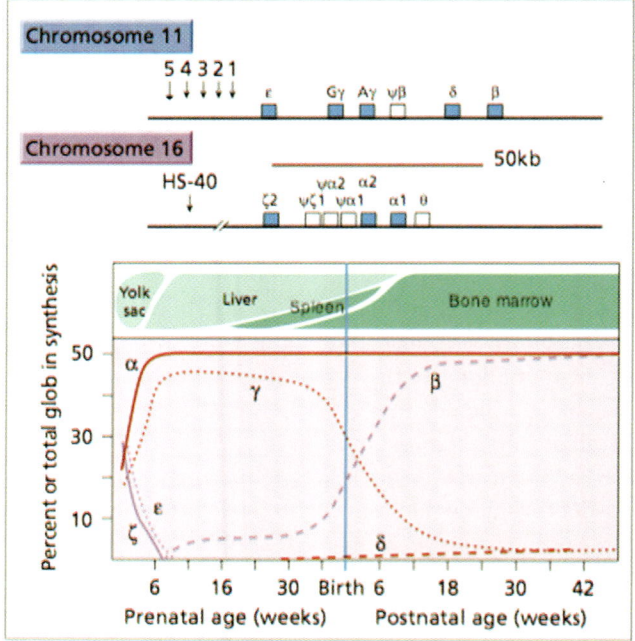

Figure 6-1 Hemoglobin (Hb) gene clusters and developmental hematopoiesis. The organization of the α- and β-globin gene clusters are shown at the top of the figure. The bottom portion of the figure illustrates the developmental changes in Hb production, both by the site of production of blood and changes in the proportions of the different globins. Modified with permission from Stamatoyannopoulos G, Majerus PW, Perlmutter RM, et al, eds. *The Molecular Basis of Blood Diseases*. 3rd ed. Philadelphia, PA: WB Saunders; 2001.

enhancing and gene-silencing effects imparted by the combination of the LCR and local regulatory proteins, but the entire process of regulatory determination remains incompletely defined. The ability to modulate the switch from the synthesis of γ to β globin chains has long been of interest because "reversing the switch" to enhance expression of fetal Hb at the expense of adult Hb might provide a means of therapeutic intervention for sickle cell disease and thalassemia.

Hb structure

Hb is a tetramer consisting of 2 pairs of globin chains. Heme, a complex of ferrous iron and protoporphyrin, is covalently linked to each globin monomer and can reversibly bind 1 oxygen molecule. The molecular weight of Hb is approximately 64 kd. The α chains contain 141 amino acids, and the β chains contain 146 amino acids, as do the β-like globins, δ and γ, which differ from β by 10 and 39 amino acids, respectively. The compositions of normal Hb species throughout development are depicted in Figure 6-1. The postembryonic Hbs are Hb A ($\alpha_2\beta_2$), Hb A_2 ($\alpha_2\delta_2$), and Hb F ($\alpha_2\gamma_2$).

When Hb is deoxygenated, there are substantial changes in the structures of the individual globins and the Hb tetramer; the iron molecule rises from the plane of its heme ring, and there is a significant rotation of each globin chain relative to the others. In the deoxy conformation, the distance between the heme moieties of the β chains increases by 0.7 nm. This conformation is stabilized in a taut (T) conformation by salt bonds within and between globin chains and by the binding of allosteric modifiers such as 2,3-bisphosphoglycerate (2,3-BPG) and of protons. The binding of oxygen to Hb leads to disruption of the salt bonds and transition to a relaxed (R) conformation.

Hb function

Hb enables RBCs to deliver oxygen to tissues by its reversible oxygen binding. With the sequential binding of 1 oxygen molecule to each of the 4 heme groups, the salt bonds are progressively broken, which increases the oxygen affinity of the remaining heme moieties. Cooperativity between the heme rings results in the characteristic sigmoid-shaped oxygen affinity curve. This phenomenon accounts for the release of relatively large amounts of oxygen with small decreases in oxygen tension.

Deoxygenation of Hb is modulated by certain biochemical influences. For example, deoxyhemoglobin binds protons with greater avidity than oxyhemoglobin, which results in a direct dependence of oxygen affinity on pH over the physiologic pH range. This Bohr effect has 2 major physiologic benefits: (i) the lower pH of metabolically active tissue decreases oxygen affinity, which accommodates oxygen delivery; and (ii) the higher pH level resulting from carbon dioxide elimination in the lungs increases oxygen affinity and oxygen loading of RBCs. An additional important influence on oxyhemoglobin dissociation is temperature. Hyperthermia decreases affinity, providing the opportunity to deliver more oxygen at the tissue level. 2,3-BPG, a metabolic intermediate of anaerobic glycolysis, is another physiologically important modulator of oxygen affinity. When 2,3-BPG binds in the pocket formed by the amino termini of the β chains, it stabilizes the deoxy conformation of Hb, thereby reducing its oxygen affinity. The intraerythrocytic molar concentrations of 2,3-BPG and Hb are normally about equal (5 mM). When 2,3-BPG levels increase during periods of hypoxia, anemia, or tissue hypoperfusion, oxygen unloading to tissues is enhanced.

Carbon dioxide reacts with certain amino acid residues in the β chain of Hb; however, this does not play a significant role in carbon dioxide transport. It has recently been reported that Hb binds nitric oxide in a reversible manner. The participation of Hb in modifying regional vascular resistance through this mechanism has been proposed.

Disorders of Hb

Disorders of Hb can be classified as qualitative or quantitative disorders. Qualitative abnormalities of Hb arise from mutations that change the amino acid sequence of the globin, thereby producing structural and functional changes in the Hb. There are 4 ways in which Hb can be qualitatively abnormal: (i) decreased solubility, (ii) instability, (iii) altered oxygen affinity, and (iv) altered oxidation state of the heme-coordinated iron. Qualitative Hb disorders are often referred to as hemoglobinopathies, even though the term can technically apply to both qualitative and quantitative disorders. Quantitative Hb disorders result from the decreased and imbalanced production of generally structurally normal globins. For example, if β-globin production is diminished by a mutation, there will be a relative excess of α globins. Such imbalanced production of α and β globins damages RBCs and their precursors in the bone marrow. These quantitative Hb disorders are called thalassemias. Both qualitative and quantitative disorders of Hb can be subdivided by the particular globin that is affected; for example, there can be α thalassemias and β hemoglobinopathies. We will begin this chapter with a review of the thalassemias and end with a discussion of several of the common qualitative Hb disorders.

Thalassemia

> **Clinical case**
>
> PC is a healthy 48-year-old female of African descent who is referred to you for evaluation of refractory microcytic anemia. She has been treated with oral iron formulations many times throughout her life. Hemoglobin values have always ranged from 10 to 11 g/dL with a mean corpuscular volume (MCV) ranging from 69 to 74 fL. She has no other prior medical history. Her examination is entirely unremarkable. Peripheral blood smear is significant for microcytosis, mild anisopoikilocytosis, and a small number of target cells. The Hb concentration is 10 g/dL with an MCV of 71 fL and mean corpuscular Hb (MCH) of 23 pg. Additional laboratory studies include a transferrin saturation of 32% and ferritin of 490 ng/mL. Hemoglobin electrophoresis reveals Hb A 98% and Hb A_2 1.8%.

Thalassemia occurs when there is quantitatively decreased synthesis of generally structurally normal globin proteins. Mutations that decrease the synthesis of α globins cause α thalassemia; mutations that decrease the synthesis of β globins cause β thalassemia.

Heterozygous thalassemia (thalassemia trait) appears to confer protection from *Plasmodium falciparum* malarial infection. As a result of this selective advantage, a wide variety of independent mutations leading to thalassemia have arisen over time and have been selected for in populations residing in areas where malaria is endemic. In general, α thalassemias are caused by deletions of DNA, whereas β thalassemias are caused by point mutations. If a mutation decreases the synthesis of one globin, α or β, it produces a relative excess of the other and an imbalance between the 2. For example, if β globin synthesis is diminished by a mutation, there will be a relative excess of α globins. Such imbalanced production of α and β globins results in damage to precursors of RBCs in the bone marrow. This damage occurs largely because the excess unpaired globin is unstable, and it precipitates within early RBC precursors in the bone marrow and oxidatively damages the cellular membrane. If the α/β globin imbalance is severe, most of the RBC precursors in the bone marrow are destroyed before they can be released into the circulation. A severe microcytic anemia is the result. The body attempts to compensate for the anemia by increasing erythropoietic activity throughout the marrow and sometimes in extramedullary spaces, although this effort is inadequate and compensation is incomplete. This pathophysiologic process is called ineffective erythropoiesis.

The thalassemias can be described simply by 2 independent nomenclatures: genetic and clinical. The genetic nomenclature denotes the type of causative mutation, such as α thalassemia or β thalassemia. The clinical nomenclature divides the thalassemias into the asymptomatic, carrier or trait state (thalassemia minor), severe transfusion-dependent anemia (thalassemia major), and everything in between (thalassemia intermedia). The 2 systems can be used together, giving α thalassemia major or β thalassemia intermedia, for example.

β Thalassemias

β Thalassemia is prevalent in the populations of the Mediterranean region, the Middle East, India, Pakistan, and Southeast Asia. It is somewhat less common in Africa. It is rarely encountered in Northern European Caucasians.

Molecular basis

β Thalassemia results from >150 different mutations of the β globin gene complex (Figure 6-2). Abnormalities have been identified in the promoter region, messenger RNA (mRNA) cap site, 5′ untranslated region, splice sites, exons, introns, and polyadenylation signal region of the β gene. Gene deletions are infrequent except in δβ and ελδβ thalassemias. A variety of single–base pair mutations or insertions/deletions of nucleotides represent the majority of described mutations. Thus, defects in transcription, RNA processing, and translation or stability of the β-globin gene product have been observed. Mutations within the coding region of the globin gene allele may result in nonsense or truncation mutations of the corresponding globin chain, leading to complete loss of globin synthesis from that allele ($β^0$ thalassemia). Alternatively, abnormalities of transcriptional regulation or mutations that alter splicing may cause markedly decreased, but not absent, globin gene synthesis ($β^+$ thalassemia). The clinical phenotype of patients with β thalassemia

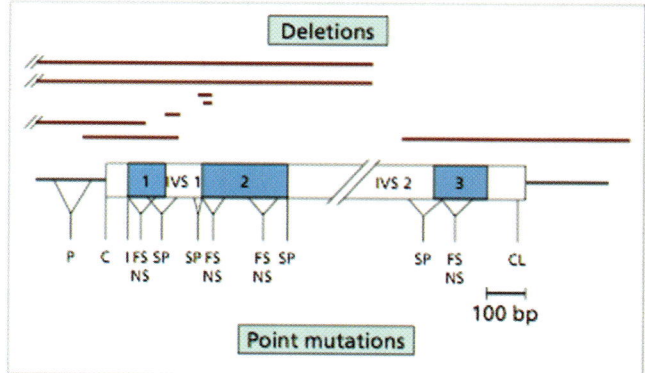

Figure 6-2 Common β thalassemia mutations. The major classes and locations of mutations that cause β thalassemia are shown. C = CAP site; CL = RNA cleavage [poly(A)] site; FS = frameshift; I = initiation codon; NS = nonsense; P = promoter boxes; SP = splice junction, consensus sequence, or cryptic splice site. From Stamatoyannopoulos G, Majerus PW, Perlmutter RM, et al, eds. *The Molecular Basis of Blood Diseases*. 3rd ed. Philadelphia, PA: WB Saunders; 2001.

is therefore determined by the number and severity of the abnormal alleles they inherit. β Thalassemia major (Cooley anemia) is almost always caused by homozygous $β^0$ thalassemia. Patients who are compound heterozygotes for thalassemic alleles, at least one of which is $β^+$, will usually have thalassemia intermedia. Patients with thalassemia minor usually are heterozygous, carrying a single β thalassemia allele (thalassemia trait), but some patients who are compound heterozygotes for very mild $β^+$ alleles may also have a thalassemia minor phenotype.

Pathophysiology

In β thalassemia, decreased β chain synthesis leads to impaired production of the $α_2β_2$ tetramer of Hb A. The reduction in Hb A in each of the circulating RBCs results in hypochromic, microcytic RBCs with target cells, a characteristic finding in all forms of β thalassemia. In addition, aggregates of excess α chains precipitate and form inclusion bodies, leading to premature destruction of erythroid precursors in the bone marrow (ineffective erythropoiesis). In more severe forms, circulating RBCs may also contain inclusions, leading to early clearance by the spleen. Splenomegaly, due to extramedullary hematopoiesis, may further contribute to the shortened RBC survival. The precipitated α-globin chains and products of degradation may also induce changes in RBC metabolism and membrane structure, leading to shortened RBC survival. In severe β thalassemia, an increased level of Hb F is distributed to varying degrees within the erythrocytes, yielding a heterogeneous pattern that persists past early infancy. It has been suggested that these cells have less α chain precipitation due to formation of $α_2γ_2$ tetramers (Hb F). Therefore, this cell population survives longer in the bone marrow and circulation. RBC membrane damage with increased surface expression of anionic phospholipids, platelet activation, and changes in hemostatic regulatory proteins contribute to a hypercoagulable state in thalassemia.

Clinical features

The clinical manifestations of β thalassemia are quite heterogeneous and depend on the extent of β-globin chain production as well as the coinheritance of any other abnormalities affecting α- or γ-globin synthesis and/or structural abnormalities of Hb (eg, Hb S). Thalassemia major, the clinical syndrome denoted *Cooley anemia*, results from homozygous or compound heterozygote genotypes that lead to absent or severe deficiency in β chain synthesis. Symptoms are usually evident within the first 6 months of life as the Hb F level begins to decline. In the absence of adequate RBC transfusions, the infant will experience failure to thrive and a variety of clinical findings. Erythroid expansion leads to widening of the bone marrow space, thinning of the cortex, and osteopenia, predisposing to fractures. Growth retardation, progressive hepatosplenomegaly, gallstone formation, and cardiac disease are common. Most homozygotes do not survive without transfusions beyond the age of 5 years. RBC transfusions may ameliorate severe anemia and suppress ineffective erythropoiesis. Chronic transfusion can reduce growth retardation and skeletal abnormalities, but with less intensive regimens, splenomegaly is still observed. Iron overload may occur secondary to increased intestinal absorption as well as RBC transfusions. Iron chelation therapy has improved patient outcome by avoiding or delaying the substantial morbidity and mortality of iron overload. Ineffective chelation will result in iron overload and consequent heart, liver, and endocrine organ failure. An increased occurrence of *Yersinia enterocolitica* bacteremia is associated with iron overload and chelation therapy.

Patients with β thalassemia intermedia are moderately anemic but usually do not require transfusion. Their disease usually results from the inheritance of 2 thalassemic genes, at least one of which is a $β^+$ allele. These patients exhibit a spectrum of clinical findings. Many have splenomegaly and prominent bony expansion. Some patients require intermittent transfusion support, whereas others are asymptomatic despite significant anemia. The patients experience significant ineffective erythropoiesis and, as a result, may have increased intestinal absorption of iron. Consequently, even in the absence of transfusion, these patients may have iron overload. An increased incidence of cerebral thrombosis and venous thromboembolism has been reported in β thalassemia major and β thalassemia intermedia following splenectomy.

Thalassemia minor is usually asymptomatic and is characterized by mild microcytic anemia. Most commonly, it arises from heterozygous β thalassemia (β thalassemia trait). Neonates with β thalassemia trait have no anemia or microcytosis; these develop with increasing age as the transition from fetal to adult Hb production progresses.

Heterozygotes with the rare εγδβ deletion present with moderately severe microcytic anemia in the neonatal period that improves during the first several months of life. In the adult, the hematologic findings are those of β thalassemia trait, with the Hb electrophoresis revealing normal Hb A_2 levels (see Laboratory findings).

Laboratory findings

A child with β thalassemia major who is not receiving transfusions will have severe anemia. Peripheral blood smear findings include anisopoikilocytosis, target cells, severe hypochromia, and basophilic stippling. The reticulocyte count is slightly increased, and nucleated RBCs are abundant. These findings are exaggerated after splenectomy. Hemoglobin electrophoresis reveals persistent elevation of Hb F ($α_2γ_2$) and variable levels of Hb A_2 ($α_2δ_2$).

Hb A will be absent in homozygous β^0 thalassemia. A variable degree of anemia with hypochromic, microcytic cells and targets is observed in β thalassemia intermedia. Patients with β thalassemia trait usually have Hb values between 9 and 11 g/dL, and microcytic, hypochromic RBCs and target cells are usually seen. Basophilic stippling is variable. The MCV is usually below 70 fL, the MCH is reduced, and the reticulocyte count can be mildly elevated. Hb A_2 levels are elevated above 3.5% (usually 4%-7%), and Hb F levels may be mildly increased. In $\delta\beta$ thalassemia trait, the Hb A_2 level is normal, but the Hb F level is elevated (typically 5%-10%).

Management of the β thalassemias

RBC transfusion has been the mainstay in the management of β thalassemia major. With initiation of a chronic transfusion regimen early in childhood, devastating clinical manifestations can be avoided. A program maintaining pretransfusion Hb levels at 9.5 g/dL can be as effective as more aggressive regimens (ie, those maintaining Hb levels >11 g/dL). Iron chelation therapy with deferoxamine is usually initiated when serum ferritin levels reach approximately 1000 μg/dL following 12 to 18 months of regular transfusions. Vitamin C supplementation can enhance iron excretion. Splenectomy is performed to alleviate abdominal symptoms or increased transfusion requirements but is usually delayed until after the age of 5 years due to the risk of sepsis secondary to encapsulated organisms. Allogeneic bone marrow transplantation from a histocompatibility (human leukocyte antigen [HLA])-compatible sibling has been performed in >1000 patients and is now curative in most. The outcome has been influenced by the age of the patient, the presence of liver disease, and the extent of iron overload. Graft-versus-host disease represents the most common long-term complication. Recent studies exploring nonmyeloablative or unrelated donor transplantation are encouraging, even in patients with prior iron loading (for whom chelation therapy prior to transplantation is advised) or concomitant hepatitis C virus (HCV) infection. Many adults with thalassemia major have chronic HCV infection resulting from contaminated RBC products that they received prior to the early 1990s. Treatment with γ-interferon and ribavirin may be complicated by hemolysis resulting from ribavirin. Investigational approaches include using erythropoietin, hydroxyurea, decitabine, and butyrate compounds to increase Hb F levels. Children with β thalassemia intermedia suffering adverse consequences of significant anemia and bony expansion may also benefit from RBC transfusions. Individuals with β thalassemia trait do not require therapy but should be identified to reduce the risk of inappropriate iron supplementation.

α Thalassemias

There is a high prevalence of α thalassemia in Africa, the Mediterranean region, Southeast Asia, and, to a lesser extent, the Middle East.

Molecular basis

Duplicated copies of the α genes are normally present on each chromosome 16, making the defects in α thalassemia more heterogeneous than in β thalassemia. The α^0 thalassemias result from loss of linked α genes on the same chromosome, denoted as $--/\alpha\alpha$. Deletions of the α genes or a deletion in HS-40, the upstream regulatory region, account for most of the α^0 thalassemia mutations. The α^+ thalassemias result from deletion of one of the linked genes, $-\alpha/\alpha\alpha$, or impairment due to a point mutation, designated $\alpha^T\alpha/\alpha\alpha$. The deletion type of α^+ thalassemia is due to unequal crossover of the linked genes, whereas the nondeletion type includes mutations resulting in abnormal transcription or translation or the production of unstable α globin. The $-\alpha/\alpha\alpha$ genotype (the silent carrier state) occurs in approximately 1 in 3 African Americans. The $--/\alpha\alpha$ genotype of α thalassemia trait (deletions in the *cis* configuration) is more common in individuals of Asian descent, whereas the $-\alpha/-\alpha$ genotype (deletions in the *trans* position) is more common in individuals of African or Mediterranean descent. Hb Constant Spring is a common nondeletion α^+ thalassemia, common in Southeast Asia, resulting from a mutation that affects termination of translation and results in abnormally elongated α chains.

Pathophysiology

As in the β thalassemias, the imbalance of globin chain synthesis results in decreased Hb synthesis and microcytic anemia. Excess γ and β chains form tetramers termed Hb Bart and Hb H, respectively. These tetramers are more soluble than unpaired α globins and form RBC inclusions only slowly. Consequently, although α thalassemia is associated with a hemolytic anemia, it does not lead to significant ineffective erythropoiesis. The homozygous inheritance of α^0 thalassemia ($--/--$) results in the total absence of α chains, death in utero, or hydrops fetalis. Unpaired γ chains form Hb Bart (γ_4), and there may be persistence of embryonic Hb. Hb Bart is soluble and does not precipitate; however, it has a very high oxygen affinity and is unable to deliver oxygen to the tissues. This leads to severe tissue hypoxia, resulting in edema, congestive heart failure, and death. Hb H disease results from the coinheritance of α^0 thalassemia and α^+ thalassemia or α^0 thalassemia and a nondeletional form of α thalassemia, such as Hb Constant Spring ($--/-\alpha$, $--/\alpha^T\alpha$, or $--/\alpha^{CS}\alpha$). The excess β chains form Hb H (β_4) that is unstable, causing precipitation within circulating cells and hemolysis. Patients have moderately severe hemolytic anemia.

Clinical features

In contrast to β thalassemias, α thalassemias can manifest in both fetal and postnatal life. The clinical manifestations of α thalassemia are related to the number of functional α globin genes (Figure 6-3). Homozygous α^0 thalassemia (– –/– –) results in the Hb Bart hydrops fetalis syndrome. The lack of Hb F due to the absence of α chains produces intrauterine hypoxia, resulting in marked expansion of bone marrow and hepatosplenomegaly in the fetus and enlargement of the placenta. There is usually in utero death between 30 and 40 weeks or soon after birth. Moreover, the mother often experiences morbidity from polyhydramnios. The clinical manifestations are variable in Hb H disease (– –/–α), with severe forms demonstrating transfusion dependence and other individuals having a milder course. As in β thalassemia, splenomegaly occurs commonly in the anemic patient. The homozygous state for Hb Constant Spring results in moderate anemia with splenomegaly. Hb H–Constant Spring (– –$\alpha^{CS}\alpha$) is typically more severe than classical Hb H disease (– –/–α). Thalassemia trait (2-gene deletion α thalassemia) occurs in 2 forms: α^0 thalassemia trait (– –/αα) or homozygosity for α^+ thalassemia (–α/–α). Individuals with thalassemia trait have a lifelong mild microcytic anemia. Heterozygotes for α^+ thalassemia (–α/αα), so-called silent carriers, are clinically normal.

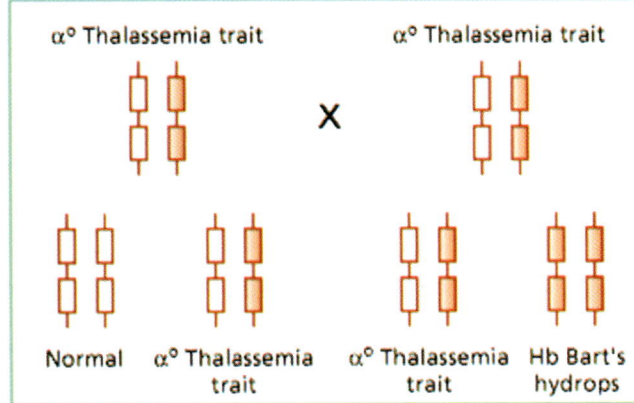

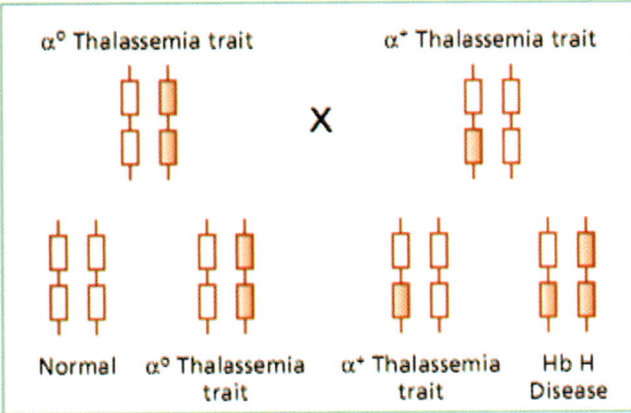

Figure 6-3 Genetics of α thalassemia. The α-globin genes are represented as boxes. The red α-globin genes represent deletions or otherwise inactivated α genes. The open boxes represent normal α genes. The terms α^0 and α^+ thalassemia are defined in the text. The potential offspring of 2 parents with α^0 thalassemia trait is shown in the upper panel. The potential offspring of one parent with α^0 thalassemia trait and the other with α^+ thalassemia trait is shown in the lower panel (note the lack of hemoglobin [Hb] Bart hydrops fetalis in these offspring). From Stamatoyannopoulos G, Majerus PW, Perlmutter RM, et al, eds. *The Molecular Basis of Blood Diseases*. 3rd ed. Philadelphia, PA: WB Saunders; 2001.

Laboratory features

The blood smear in Hb Bart hydrops fetalis syndrome reveals markedly abnormal RBC morphology with anisopoikilocytosis, hypochromia, targets, basophilic stippling, and nucleated RBCs. The Hb electrophoresis reveals approximately 80% Hb Bart and the remainder Hb Portland ($\zeta_2\gamma_2$). Hb H disease is characterized by anisopoikilocytosis and hypochromia with elevated reticulocyte counts. Hb electrophoresis reveals 5% to 40% of the rapidly migrating Hb H. Supravital staining with brilliant cresyl blue will reveal inclusions representing in vitro precipitation of Hb H. In newborns with α^0 thalassemia trait, the Hb electrophoresis reveals 2% to 5% Hb Bart and microcytosis (<95 fL). Children and adults heterozygous for α^0 thalassemia (– –/αα) or homozygotes for deletion forms of α^+ thalassemia (–α/–α) have mild anemia with hypochromic, microcytic RBCs and target cells. The RBC indices are similar to those of β thalassemia trait, but the Hb electrophoresis is normal (or shows a reduction in Hb A_2). The high prevalence of the –α/–α genotype in African Americans is noteworthy. About 2% to 3% of all black persons in the United States have asymptomatic microcytosis and borderline anemia (often mistaken for iron deficiency) due to this condition. Minimal or no anemia or morphologic abnormalities of RBCs are observed with heterozygous α^+ thalassemia (–α/αα), and the Hb electrophoresis is normal.

Management of the α thalassemias

A fetus with homozygous α^0 thalassemia can be rescued with intrauterine transfusion, followed by postnatal chronic transfusions or stem cell transplantation. Patients with Hb H disease usually require no specific interventions. For those patients with splenomegaly and significant anemia, splenectomy may prove useful. Some patients, especially those with Hb H–Constant Spring, require intermittent or chronic RBC transfusions. Due to the high prevalence of the α^0 genotype in Southeast Asian and certain Mediterranean populations, screening programs and genetic counseling can serve to reduce the occurrence of births resulting in Hb Bart hydrops fetalis and Hb H disease.

Clinical case (continued)

The patient (PC) presented in this case likely has the homozygous state for α^+ thalassemia ($-\alpha/-\alpha$). Patients with this condition usually have mild microcytic, hypochromic anemia. Targeted RBC forms suggest the presence of thalassemia in an otherwise healthy person. With single or double α gene deletions, the Hb electrophoresis is typically normal, unlike in β thalassemia. α Thalassemia is often a diagnosis of exclusion, and identification of similar findings in family members supports the diagnosis. Iron deficiency should be ruled out. Exogenous iron should not be prescribed because it is unnecessary and potentially harmful. Patients are generally asymptomatic, require no treatment, and have a normal life expectancy.

Key points

- The thalassemias are characterized by a reduced rate of synthesis of one of the globin subunits of the Hb molecule.
- The intracellular precipitation of the excess, unpaired globin chains in thalassemia damages RBC precursors and circulating RBCs, resulting in ineffective erythropoiesis and hemolysis.
- The β thalassemias are caused by >150 different mutations, usually point mutations, with a wide variety of genetic abnormalities documented.
- Patients with thalassemia major require transfusion support, experience iron overload, and may benefit from splenectomy. A spectrum of clinical manifestations is observed in thalassemia intermedia, whereas the carrier state has no associated symptoms.
- The Hb electrophoresis in β thalassemia reveals increased levels of Hb A_2 and variably increased Hb F.
- The α thalassemias are primarily due to DNA deletions. Four α genes are normally present, so multiple phenotypes are possible when gene deletions occur.
- Homozygous α^0 thalassemia manifests in fetal life with the formation of Hb Bart (γ_4) and hydrops fetalis.
- The clinical manifestations in Hb H disease are variable, with some affected individuals requiring transfusions and others being less symptomatic.
- α Thalassemia trait is characterized by mild anemia with microcytic indices and a normal Hb electrophoresis.

Sickle cell disease

Clinical case

A 17-year-old African American male with homozygous SS sickle cell disease is admitted to the hospital with a 4-day history of a typical painful episode involving his arms and legs. There is no recent febrile illness. Past medical history is remarkable for few hospital admissions for pain crises and RBC transfusion once as a young child. He is in severe pain and ill appearing, and vital signs are remarkable for a pulse of 129 and temperature of 38.5°C. Scleral icterus and moderate jaundice are noted. Laboratory data include Hb of 7.2 g/dL (baseline 9.1 g/dL), corrected reticulocyte count of 2%, and platelet count of 72,000/μL. Liver function tests are elevated above baseline and include a direct bilirubin of 4.8 mg/dL, aspartate aminotransferase (AST) of 1200 U/L, and alanine aminotransferase (ALT) of 1550 U/L. His creatinine is elevated at 4.3 mg/dL. Abdominal ultrasound is nondiagnostic. He is immediately started on intravenous fluids and opioid analgesics. Broad-spectrum antibiotics are empirically administered. Over the next 24 hours, he becomes tachypneic and slightly confused. Hypoxemia develops despite oxygen supplementation, and anuria ensues. Serum creatinine has increased to 6.4 mg/dL, direct bilirubin to 7.8 mg/dL, AST to 2725 U/L, and creatine phosphokinase (CPK) to 2200 IU/L, and Hb has decreased to 5.8 g/dL. The patient undergoes simple transfusion and subsequently RBC exchange. Acute dialysis is required. He slowly improves during a prolonged 3-week hospitalization. No infectious etiology was identified.

Sickle Hb (Hb S) was the first Hb variant discovered. It has been well characterized on a biochemical and molecular level. Heterozygosity for the sickle cell gene (β^S), called sickle cell trait, occurs in >20% of individuals in equatorial Africa, up to 20% of individuals in the eastern provinces of Saudi Arabia and central India, and approximately 5% of individuals in parts of the Mediterranean region, the Middle East, and North Africa. In Hb S, a hydrophobic valine is substituted for the normal, more hydrophilic glutamic acid at the 6th residue of the β-globin chain (Figure 6-4). This substitution is due to a single nucleotide mutation (GAG/GTG) in the sixth codon of the β-globin gene. Heterozygous inheritance of Hb S offers a degree of protection from severe malaria infection. This has been offered as an explanation for the evolutionary selection of the Hb S gene despite the devastating effect of homozygous inheritance of Hb S. The β^S gene is inherited in an autosomal codominant fashion. That is, heterozygous inheritance does not cause disease but is detectable (sickle cell trait); homozygous inheritance or compound heterozygous inheritance with another mutant β-globin gene results in disease. The *sickle cell syndromes* include all conditions in which β^S is inherited (including sickle cell trait). In contrast, the term *sickle cell disease*

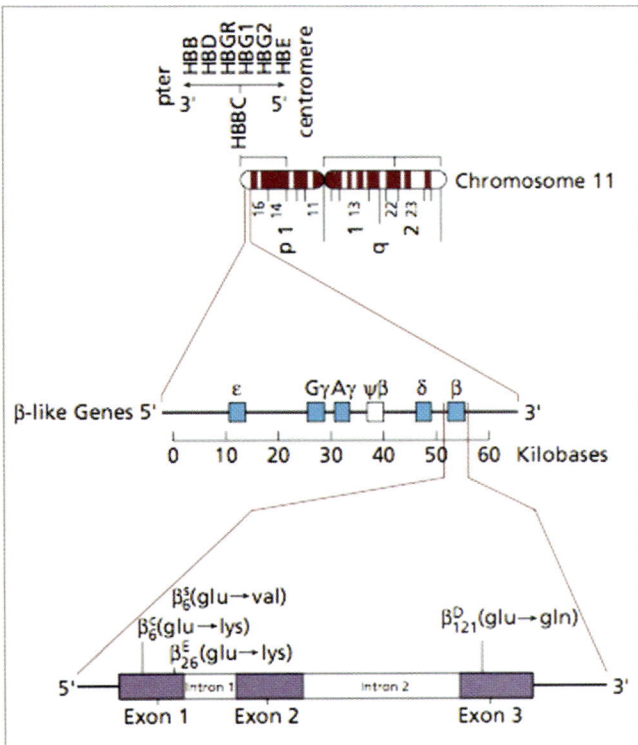

Figure 6-4 Common β-globin variants. The locations of the mutations within the chromosome (top), the β-globin cluster (middle), and the β-globin gene itself (bottom) are shown for 4 common β-globin variants.

includes only those genotypes associated with chronic hemolytic anemia and vaso-occlusive pain (not sickle trait): homozygous sickle cell anemia (Hb SS), sickle-Hb C disease (Hb SC), sickle-β^0 thalassemia (Hb Sβ^0), and sickle-β^+ thalassemia (Hb Sβ^+). Less common Hb mutants such as O^{Arab}, D$^{Los Angeles}$, or E may be inherited in compound heterozygosity with β^S to result in sickle cell disease.

Sickle cell trait (Hb AS) occurs in 8% to 9% of the African American population and is best regarded as a benign condition, despite rare complications of hematuria, renal papillary necrosis, pyelonephritis during pregnancy, and risk of splenic infarction at high altitude. Sickle trait is also associated with the extremely rare medullary carcinoma of the kidney and an increased risk of sudden death during extreme conditions of dehydration and hyperthermia. This simple heterozygous state generally has an Hb A:S ratio of approximately 60:40, due to the greater electrostatic attraction of α chains to β^A rather than β^S chains. When the availability of α chains is limited by coinherited α thalassemia, the A:S ratio is further increased.

Pathophysiology

The sine qua non of sickle cell pathophysiology is the intra-erythrocytic polymerization of deoxyhemoglobin S. When deoxygenation of Hb S occurs, the normal conformational change of the tetramer exposes on its external surface a hydrophobic β_6 valine (instead of the hydrophilic glutamate of Hb A), resulting in decreased solubility and a tendency of deoxyhemoglobin S tetramers to aggregate or polymerize. The rate and degree of this polymerization determines the rheologic impairment of sickle erythrocytes and the change in morphology for which the condition was named. Polymerization rate and extent are related to the intracellular concentration of Hb S, the type and fractional content of other Hbs present (particularly Hb F), and percent oxygen saturation. These variables correlate with the rate of hemolysis in sickle cell syndromes.

Multiple factors determine the clinical manifestations of sickle cell disease. In addition to physiologic changes such as tissue oxygenation and pH, multiple genetic polymorphisms and mutations may modify the presentation of the disease. This is best appreciated by examining the influence of the coinheritance of other Hb abnormalities on the effects of Hb S. For example, the coexistence of α thalassemia reduces the hemolytic severity as well as the risk of cerebrovascular accidents. High levels of fetal Hb (Hb F) may substantially reduce symptoms and clinical consequences. Compound heterozygosity for a second abnormal Hb (eg, Hb C, D, or E) or β thalassemia also modifies some of the manifestations of disease (discussed later in this section) (Table 6-2).

Table 6-2 Typical clinical and laboratory findings of the common forms of sickle cell disease after 5 years of age.

Disease	Clinical severity	S (%)	F (%)	A$_2$ (%)*	A (%)	Hemoglobin (g/dL)	MCV (fL)
SS	Usually marked	[mt]90	[lt]10	[lt]3.5	0	6–9	[mt]80
Sβ^0	Marked to moderate	[mt]80	[lt]20	[mt]3.5	0	6–9	[lt]70
Sβ^+	Mild to moderate	[mt]60	[lt]20	[mt]3.5	10–30	9–12	[lt]75
SC	Mild to moderate	50	[lt]5	0†	0	10–15	75–85
S–HPFH‡	Asymptomatic	[lt]70	[mt]30	[lt]2.5	0	12–14	[lt]80

*Hemoglobin A$_2$ can be increased in the presence of hemoglobin S, even in the absence of β thalassemia. The classical findings are shown here.
†There will be 50% hemoglobin C that migrates near hemoglobin A$_2$ on alkaline gel electrophoresis or isoelectric focusing.
HPFH = hereditary persistence of fetal hemoglobin; MCV = mean corpuscular volume.

Several restriction fragment length polymorphisms (RFLP) may be identified in the vicinity of a known gene and define the genetic background upon which a disease-causing mutation has arisen. For example, the coinheritance of a defined set of RFLPs around the β-globin gene can define a disease-associated "haplotype" that marks the sickle mutation within a specific population. These β-globin haplotypes have also been associated with variations in disease severity. This association is probably not related to the RFLPs themselves but mediated through linked differences in γ chain (Hb F) production. The $β^S$ gene has been found to be associated with 5 distinct haplotypes, referred to as the Benin (Ben), Senegal (Sen), Central African Republic (CAR or Bantu), Cameroon (Cam), and Arab-Indian (Asian) haplotypes. This is evidence that the $β^S$ gene arose by 5 separate mutational events. In general, the Asian and Sen haplotypes are associated with a milder clinical course, and CAR is associated with a worse course.

Although the deoxygenation/polymerization/sickling axiom provides a basic understanding of sickle cell disease, there is an increasing appreciation that interactions of sickle cells with other cells and proteins contribute to the hemolytic and vaso-occlusive processes. There are in vitro data showing that sickle erythrocytes exhibit abnormally increased adherence to vascular endothelial cells as well as to subendothelial extracellular matrix proteins. There is apparent endothelial damage, as demonstrated by the increased number of circulating endothelial cells in sickle cell disease patients and the increase in such cells during vaso-occlusive crises. The disruption of normal endothelium results in the exposure of extracellular matrix components including thrombospondin, laminin, and fibronectin. Endothelial cell receptors include the vitronectin receptor $α_vβ_3$ integrin and the cytokine-induced vascular cell adherence molecule-1 (VCAM-1). RBC receptors include CD36 (glycoprotein IV), the $α_4β_1$ integrin, the Lutheran blood group glycoproteins, and sulfatides. Vaso-occlusion may thus be initiated by adherence of sickle erythrocytes to endothelial cells and extracellular matrix molecules exposed during the process of endothelial damage and completed by trapping of sickled, nondeformable cells behind this nidus of occlusion. Activation of blood coagulation resulting in enhanced thrombin generation and evidence for platelet hyperreactivity have been demonstrated in patients with sickle cell disease during steady-state and vaso-occlusive episodes. It has been suggested that the exposure of RBC membrane phosphatidylserine and circulating activated endothelial cells in sickle cell disease patients contributes to the hypercoagulability by providing procoagulant surfaces. The correlation of elevated white blood cell counts to increased mortality and adverse outcomes identified by epidemiologic studies of sickle cell disease patients suggests that neutrophils also participate in vaso-occlusion. This concept has been further supported by the precipitation of vaso-occlusive episodes with markedly increased neutrophil counts associated with the administration of granulocyte colony-stimulating factor (G-CSF). These findings together support the concept that the products of multiple genes as well as inflammatory cytokines contribute to the pathology of sickle cell disease.

Laboratory features

The diagnosis of the sickle cell syndromes is made by the identification of Hb S in erythrocyte hemolysates. Historically, cellulose acetate electrophoresis at alkaline pH was used to separate Hb A, Hb A_2, and Hb S, and citrate agar electrophoresis at acidic pH was used to separate comigrating Hb D and Hb C from Hb S and Hb A_2, respectively. Currently, high-performance liquid chromatography (HPLC) and isoelectric focusing are used in most diagnostic laboratories to separate Hbs. In both Hb SS and $Sβ^0$ thalassemia disease, no Hb A is present. However, in Hb SS, the MCV is normal, whereas in Hb $Sβ^0$ thalassemia, the MCV is reduced. Hb A_2 is elevated in $Sβ^0$ thalassemia, but it can also be nonspecifically elevated in the presence of Hb S, so an elevation of A_2 cannot reliably distinguish Hb SS from $Sβ^0$ thalassemia alone. In sickle cell trait and $Sβ^+$ thalassemia, both Hb S and Hb A are identified. The A:S ratio is 60:40 in sickle trait (more A than S) and approximately 15:85 in $Sβ^+$ thalassemia (more S than A). Microcytosis, target cells, anemia, and clinical symptoms occur only in $Sβ^+$ thalassemia, not sickle trait (Table 6-2). Review of the peripheral smear will reveal the presence of irreversibly sickled cells in Hb SS and Hb $Sβ^0$ thalassemia, but rarely in $Sβ^+$ thalassemia (Figure 6-5) and Hb SC. Turbidity tests (for Hb S) are positive in all sickle cell syndromes, including Hb AS. The classic sickle cell slide test or "sickle cell prep" (using sodium metabisulfite or dithionite) and turbidity tests only detect the presence of Hb S, so they do not differentiate sickle cell disease from sickle cell trait. Therefore, they have limited utility. Sickle cell disease can be diagnosed by DNA testing of the preimplanted zygote in the first trimester of pregnancy using chorionic villus sampling, in the second trimester using amniocentesis, or after birth using peripheral blood.

Clinical manifestations

Two major physiologic processes, shortened RBC survival (hemolysis) and vaso-occlusion, account for most of the clinical manifestations of sickle cell disease. The erythrocyte life span is shortened from the normal 120 days to approximately 10 to 25 days, resulting in moderate to severe hemolytic anemia, with a steady-state mean Hb concentration of

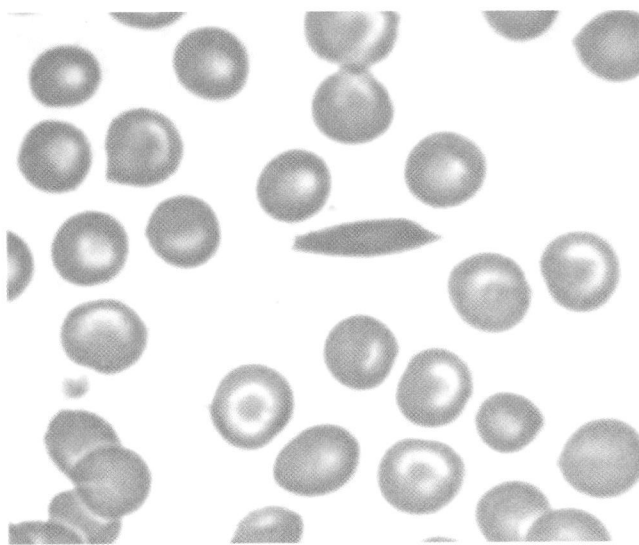

Figure 6-5 Irreversibly sickled cell. This peripheral blood film shows an irreversibly sickled cell (ISC) that occurs in sickle cell anemia (SS), Sβ^0 thalassemia. ISCs are rare in hemoglobin SC and Sβ^+ thalassemia. Also note the target cells in this view.

8 g/dL (range from 6% to 9%) in Hb SS disease. The anemia is generally well tolerated because of compensatory cardiovascular changes and increased levels of 2,3-BPG. However, several conditions are associated with acute or chronic declines in the Hb concentration, which may lead to symptomatic anemia (Table 6-3). Sudden "aplastic crises" due to erythroid aplasia resulting from parvovirus B19 infection and lesser degrees of bone marrow suppression may be associated with other infections or marrow infarction. Sudden anemia unrelated to marrow suppression may be due to splenic sequestration (including adults with Hb SC or Sβ^+ thalassemia) or, less frequently, hepatic sequestration or superimposed autoimmune hemolysis or glucose-6-phosphate dehydrogenase (G6PD) deficiency. Chronic exacerbations of anemia may be the result of folate or iron deficiency or of reduced erythropoietin levels related to concurrent renal insufficiency. Because of the chronic erythrocyte destruction, patients with sickle cell disease have a high incidence of pigmented gallstones, which are often asymptomatic.

Acute painful "vaso-occlusive" crises are the most common complications. These often unpredictable episodes are thought to be caused by obstruction of the microcirculation by erythrocytes and other blood cells, leading to painful tissue hypoxia and microinfarction. They most commonly affect the long bones, back, chest, and abdomen. Acute pain crises may be precipitated by dehydration, cold temperatures, exercise (in particular swimming), pregnancy, infection, or stress. Often no precipitating factor can be identified. Painful episodes may or may not be accompanied by low-grade fever.

One of the first manifestations of sickle cell disease, acute dactylitis (hand–foot syndrome), results from bone marrow necrosis of the hands and feet. The first attack generally occurs between 6 and 18 months of life, when the Hb F level declines; attacks become uncommon after age 6 years when the site of hematopoiesis shifts from the peripheral to the axial skeleton. Long-bone infarcts with pain and swelling may mimic osteomyelitis. Other skeletal complications of sickle cell disease include osteomyelitis, particularly due to salmonella and staphylococci, and avascular necrosis, especially of the femoral and humeral heads.

Sickle cell disease is a multisystem disorder. Organ systems subject to recurrent ischemia, infarction, and chronic dysfunction include the lungs (acute chest syndrome, pulmonary fibrosis, pulmonary hypertension, hypoxemia), central nervous system (cerebral infarction, subarachnoid and intracerebral hemorrhage, seizure disorders, cognitive impairment), cardiovascular system (cardiomegaly, congestive heart failure), genitourinary system (isosthenuria, hematuria, papillary necrosis, glomerulonephritis, priapism), spleen (splenomegaly, splenic sequestration, splenic infarction and involution, hyposplenism), eyes (retinal artery occlusion, proliferative sickle retinopathy, vitreous hemorrhage, retinal detachment), and skin (leg ulcerations). The risk of life-threatening septicemia and meningitis due to encapsulated organisms, such as *Streptococcus pneumoniae*, is markedly increased in children with sickle cell disease. This susceptibility is related to functional and anatomic asplenia and decreased opsonization due to deficient production of natural antibodies. The risk for such infections persists into adulthood.

Table 6-3 Causes of acute exacerbations of anemia in sickle cell disease.

Cause	Comment
Aplastic crisis	Caused by human parvovirus; does not recur
Acute splenic sequestration crisis	Often recurrent in childhood before splenic involution
Acute chest syndrome	Anemia may precede the onset of respiratory signs and symptoms
Vaso-occlusive crisis	Minimal decline only
Hypoplastic crisis	Mild decline; accompanies many infections
Accelerated hemolysis	Infrequent; accompanies infection of concomitant G6PD deficiency
Hepatic sequestration	Rare
Folate deficiency (megaloblastic crisis)	Rare, even in the absence of folate supplementation

G6PD = glucose-6-phosphate dehydrogenase.

There are many important clinical differences among the genotypes that cause sickle cell disease (Table 6-2). Hemoglobin SS is associated with the most severe anemia, most frequent pain, and shortest life expectancy (median age, 42 years for men and 48 years for women in one large, old study), although there is tremendous heterogeneity in these variables even within this group. Hemoglobin Sβ^0 thalassemia can closely mimic Hb SS, despite the smaller sickle cells, lower MCH concentrations, and higher levels of Hb F and Hb A_2 associated with this genotype. Patients with Hb SC generally live longer lives (median age, 60 years for men and 68 years for women) and have less severe anemia (~20% are not anemic at all), higher MCH concentrations, and less frequent pain, but more frequent ocular and bone complications. Although Hb C does not enter into the deoxyhemoglobin S polymer, patients with Hb SC have symptoms, whereas those with sickle cell trait do not. This is thought to be caused by 2 important consequences of the presence of Hb C: the Hb S content in Hb SC is 10% to 15% higher than that seen in sickle trait (Hb S of approximately 50% vs 40%), and the absolute intraerythrocytic concentration of total Hb is increased. The latter phenomenon results from persistent loss of cellular K^+ and water from these cells induced by the toxic effect of Hb C on cell membranes. Another effect of this dramatic cellular dehydration is the generation of target cells, which are far more prevalent on the peripheral smear than sickled forms (Figure 6-6). Finally, in Hb SC disease, the increased hematocrit combined with the higher MCH concentration (MCHC) and cellular dehydration results in higher whole blood viscosity, which may increase the likelihood of vaso-occlusion. Patients with Hb Sβ^+ thalassemia have less severe anemia and pain than patients with Hb Sβ^0 thalassemia. This is the result of smaller cells, lower MCHC, increased content of Hb F and Hb A_2, and, most important, the presence of significant amounts (10%-30%) of Hb A that interferes with polymerization.

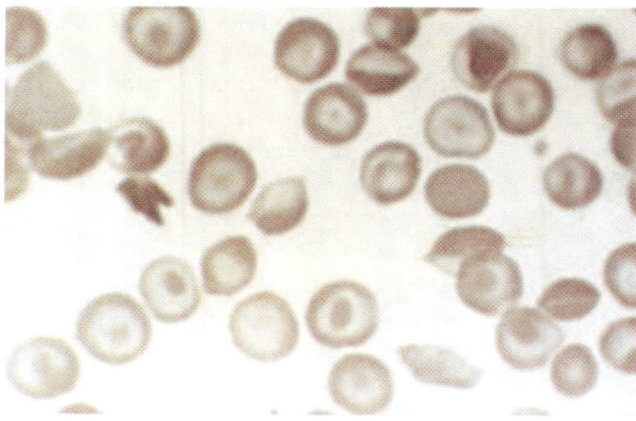

Figure 6-6 Sickle-hemoglobin C disease. This peripheral blood film shows no irreversibly sickled cells, as expected for hemoglobin SC, but shows instead a large number of target cells and several dense, contracted, and folded cells containing aggregated and polymerized hemoglobin.

Treatment

Treatment of sickle cell disease includes general preventive and supportive measures, as well as treatment of specific complications. The updated National Institutes of Health monograph entitled *The Management of Sickle Cell Disease* (Publication No. 02-2117) is an excellent resource for addressing the spectrum of treatment issues. Table 6-4 summarizes the results of major clinical trials influencing current clinical practice.

Preventive interventions

Children should receive the heptavalent pneumococcal conjugate vaccine as well as the 23-valent pneumococcal polysaccharide, *Haemophilus influenzae*, and hepatitis B vaccines, in addition to twice-daily penicillin prophylaxis at least until

Table 6-4 Randomized clinical trials in sickle cell disease.

Clinical trial	Outcome
Penicillin Prophylaxis in Sickle Cell Disease (PROPS)	Oral penicillin greatly reduces the incidence of invasive pneumococcal infections in children
Penicillin Prophylaxis in Sickle Cell Disease II (PROPS II)	Penicillin prophylaxis can be discontinued at 5 years of age
Multicenter Study of Hydroxyurea in Patients with Sickle Cell Anemia (MSH)	Hydroxyurea reduces the frequency of painful episodes and appears to reduce the frequency of acute chest syndrome, transfusions, and hospitalizations
National Preoperative Transfusion Study	Simple transfusion to increase the Hb concentration to 10 g/dL is as effective as exchange transfusion to reduce Hb S to [lt]30%
Stroke Prevention Trial in Sickle Cell Anemia (STOP)	First overt stroke can be prevented with red blood cell transfusions in high-risk children identified by transcranial Doppler (TCD) ultrasonography
Optimizing Primary Stroke Prevention in Sickle Cell Anemia (STOP 2)	Discontinuation of prophylactic red blood cell transfusions after 30 months results in a high rate of reversion to abnormal TCD velocities and stroke

Hb = hemoglobin.

the age of 5 years. Vaccinations against influenza on an annual basis and pneumococcus at 3- to 5-year intervals should be administered to all patients. Folic acid supplements are used by some to prevent depletion of folate stores and megaloblastic anemia related to chronic hemolysis, but this is probably unnecessary in developed countries, where diets are better and flour is fortified with folate. Ophthalmologic examinations should be performed periodically after age 10 years. Genetic counseling services by trained individuals should be available for families with members having sickle cell syndromes.

Painful episodes

Acute pain unresponsive to rest, hydration, and oral analgesics at home requires prompt attention and represents the leading cause for hospital admission. Painful episodes can be associated with serious complications, and a high frequency of pain is a poor prognostic factor for survival. It is essential to exclude infectious and other etiologies of pain in the febrile patient. A complete blood count should be obtained. Because some degree of negative fluid balance is often present, oral or intravenous hydration is an important therapeutic modality. Caution must be used with intravenous hydration of adults having decreased cardiac reserve. A monograph produced by the American Pain Society providing comprehensive guidelines for management of sickle cell pain including graded evidence for specific interventions is a valuable reference source (*Guideline for the Management of Acute and Chronic Pain in Sickle Cell Disease*, 1999). Prompt administration of analgesics is a priority, and the selection of agents should be individualized based on previous experience. Parenteral opioids, preferably morphine or hydromorphone, are often necessary for both children and adults. The addition of nonsteroidal anti-inflammatory drugs (NSAIDs) such as ibuprofen or ketorolac may decrease the requirement for opioid analgesics but should be used with caution in sickle cell disease due to nephrotoxic effects. Maintenance analgesia can be achieved with patient-controlled analgesia (PCA) pumps or with administration at fixed intervals. Constant infusion of opioids requires close monitoring because the hypoxia or acidosis resulting from respiratory suppression is particularly dangerous. Meperidine is discouraged because of its short half-life and the accumulation of the toxic metabolite normeperidine, which lowers the seizure threshold. Use of pain assessment instruments and attention to the level of sedation at regular intervals are necessary. Oxygen supplementation is not required unless hypoxemia is present. The use of incentive spirometry has been shown to reduce pulmonary complications in patients presenting with chest or back pain. It has been demonstrated that the number of hospitalizations for painful events can be reduced by prompt intervention in an outpatient setting dedicated to sickle cell disease management. Nonpharmacologic management techniques should be considered as well as evaluation for depression for the patient with frequent episodes or chronic pain. Blood transfusion is not indicated in the treatment of routine painful episodes.

RBC transfusion

Patients with sickle cell disease often receive transfusions unnecessarily. However, RBC transfusions may be effective for certain complications of the disease. Transfusion is indicated as treatment of specific acute events, including splenic sequestration, symptomatic aplastic crisis, cerebrovascular accident (occlusive or hemorrhagic), acute ocular vaso-occlusive events, and acute chest syndrome with hypoxemia. Although the first 2 events only require correction of anemia and thus are treated with simple transfusion, stroke, ocular events, and severe acute chest syndrome are best treated with exchange transfusion aimed at decreasing the percentage of Hb S to <30% and increasing the Hb level to 9 to 10 g/dL. In addition, transfusions are indicated for the prevention of recurrent strokes as well as for the treatment of high-output cardiac failure and, on occasion, as part of therapy for osteomyelitis. A randomized controlled trial of prophylactic transfusion for children with abnormal transcranial Doppler (TCD) results showed a reduced risk of the first stroke in patients receiving transfusions. Transfusion has also been advocated for patients with severe pulmonary hypertension and chronic nonhealing leg ulcers and to prevent recurrences of priapism. When chronic transfusion is indicated, RBCs may be administered as a partial exchange transfusion, which may offer a long-term advantage of retarding iron accumulation. The goal of chronic transfusion is usually to achieve a nadir total Hb level of 9 to 10 g/dL with the Hb S under 30% to 50%. It is important to avoid the hyperviscosity associated with Hb levels above 11 to 12 g/dL in the presence of 30% or more Hb S. Patients with Hb SC requiring transfusion pose special challenges, with the need to avoid hyperviscosity usually necessitating exchange transfusion to ensure the Hb concentration does not exceed 11 to 12 g/dL.

Preoperative transfusion in preparation for surgery under general anesthesia may afford protection against perioperative complications and death but is probably not indicated in all cases, particularly minor procedures. In a recent study, simple transfusion to a total Hb level of 10 g/dL afforded protection equal to partial exchange and was associated with fewer complications. However, patients undergoing prolonged surgery, regional compromise of blood supply (eg, during orthopedic surgery), or hypothermia or patients with a history of pulmonary or cardiac disease may do better with preoperative exchange transfusion. Transfusions also may be useful in preparation for intravenous ionic contrast studies, chronic intractable pain, and complicated pregnancy. Transfusions are not indicated for the treatment of steady-state anemia, routine pain crises, uncomplicated pregnancy, most leg ulcers, or minor surgery not requiring general anesthesia.

Up to 30% of patients with sickle cell disease who repeatedly undergo transfusion will become alloimmunized to RBC antigens (especially E, C, and Kell), and this risk increases with increasing exposure. Alloimmunization predisposes patients to delayed transfusion reactions. Severe painful crises with a decrease in the Hb level within days to weeks of a transfusion should alert the clinician to consider this diagnosis. Identification of a new alloantibody may not be made acutely, and reticulocytopenia can be an associated finding. In this situation, additional transfusions are hazardous and should be avoided if at all possible. Universal RBC phenotyping and matching for the antigens of greatest concern (eg, C, D, E, and Kell) can minimize alloimmunization.

Acute chest syndrome
The diagnosis of acute chest syndrome is based on finding a new radiographic pulmonary infiltrate associated with symptoms such as fever, cough, and chest pain. Typically there are abnormalities on the chest examination. As the term implies, various causes can contribute to the findings. Young age, low Hb F, high steady-state Hb, and elevated white blood cell count in steady state have been identified as risk factors. In a recent multicenter prospective study, bacterial or viral infections accounted for approximately 30% of episodes, whereas fat emboli from the bone marrow were responsible for approximately 10% of events, with pulmonary infarction as another common cause. In children, fever is a common presenting symptom, whereas chest pain is more common in adults. Acute chest syndrome often develops in patients initially presenting with a vaso-occlusive episode or other clinical problems. Early recognition of the condition is of utmost importance because acute chest syndrome has been recognized as the leading cause of mortality for both adults and children with sickle cell disease. Management includes maintaining adequate oxygenation and administration of antibiotics to address the major pulmonary pathogens and community-acquired atypical organisms. Fluid management needs particular attention to limit oral and intravenous administration to 1.0 to 1.5 times maintenance. Pain control to avoid excessive chest splinting and the use of incentive spirometry are key adjunctive measures. Bronchodilator therapy is effective if there is associated reactive airway disease, which is particularly common in children. Transfusion of RBCs should be considered if there is hypoxemia despite adequate oxygen supplementation.

Exchange techniques are often necessary to reduce the proportion of Hb S rapidly and should be used before respiratory failure. Patients with acute chest syndrome are at risk for recurrences as well as subsequent chronic lung disease. Preventive measures include hydroxyurea therapy and chronic RBC transfusions.

Central nervous system disease
Overt symptomatic stroke may occur in 11% of young sickle cell anemia patients (but is rare in SC disease and Sβ^+ thalassemia), accounting for significant morbidity and mortality. The more frequent use of neuroimaging has identified a substantial incidence of subclinical cerebrovascular disease, with at least 25% of children having covert or "silent" strokes. The majority of overt strokes result from ischemic events involving large arteries with associated vascular endothelial damage, including intimal and medial proliferation. Hemorrhagic events are more common in adults and may result from rupture of collateral vessels (moyamoya) near the site of previous infarction. Suspicion of a neurologic event requires emergent imaging with computed tomography (CT) followed by magnetic resonance imaging (MRI). The acute management of overt stroke includes transfusion, usually by an exchange technique, to reduce the Hb S percentage to <20% to 30%. Chronic transfusion therapy to maintain the Hb S <30% decreases the chance of recurrent overt stroke but does not eliminate it. After 3 to 5 years of such transfusions and no recurrent neurologic events, some physicians "liberalize" the transfusion regimen to maintain the Hb S <50%. The optimal duration of transfusions is not known, and they are often continued indefinitely, but at least one report suggests the possibility of using hydroxyurea for long-term secondary stroke prevention. A randomized controlled trial (SWiTCH) to study this strategy has completed enrollment, and results are expected in late 2011. The use of hydroxyurea is also currently being explored as means of primary stroke prevention in a phase III multicenter randomized controlled trial for children with abnormal TCD velocities (TWiTCH). As mentioned earlier, an abnormal TCD velocity can identify children with Hb SS at high risk of primary overt stroke.

Pregnancy
Pregnancy poses some risk to the mother as well as to the fetus. Spontaneous abortions occur in approximately 5% of pregnancies in sickle cell anemia, and preeclampsia occurs at an increased frequency in sickle cell disease. Preterm labor and premature delivery are common. All patients should be followed in a high-risk prenatal clinic, ideally at 2-week intervals with close consultation with a hematologist. Patients should receive folic acid 1 mg/d, in addition to the usual

prenatal vitamins, and should be counseled regarding the additional risks imposed by poor diet, smoking, alcohol, and substance abuse. Data do not support the routine use of prophylactic transfusions. However, simple or exchange transfusions should be instituted for the indications outlined previously, as well as for pregnancy-related complications (eg, acute toxemia). Close follow-up is also indicated postpartum when the patient is still at high risk for complications. Contraception with an intrauterine device, subcutaneous implant, oral low-dose estrogen pills, or condoms should be discussed with all women of childbearing age.

Modifying the disease course

In addition to chronic transfusions, 2 other disease-modifying treatments are currently available: hydroxyurea is ameliorative, and hematopoietic stem cell transplantation is curative. Based on the knowledge that patients with high Hb F levels have less severe disease, many investigators tested a variety of experimental strategies for pharmacologic induction of Hb F production and identified hydroxyurea as efficacious and practical. A multicenter, randomized, placebo-controlled trial then found that daily oral administration of hydroxyurea significantly reduced the frequency of pain episodes, acute chest syndrome, and transfusions in adult Hb SS patients. No serious short-term adverse effects were observed, although monitoring of blood counts was required to avoid potentially significant cytopenias. Interestingly, the therapeutic response to hydroxyurea sometimes occurs in the absence of a change in Hb F levels, suggesting that a reduction in white blood cell count and other mechanisms may be beneficial. Laboratory studies revealed that hydroxyurea reduced adherence of RBCs to vascular endothelium, improved RBC hydration, and increased the time to polymerization. Follow-up at 9 years indicates that patients taking hydroxyurea seem to have reduced mortality without evidence for an increased incidence of malignancy. Indications for hydroxyurea are frequent painful episodes, recurrent acute chest syndrome, severe symptomatic anemia, and other severe vaso-occlusive events. Pregnancy should be avoided while taking this agent. Ongoing trials of hydroxyurea in children are yielding encouraging results. Hematopoietic stem cell transplantation has been primarily used for children with stroke or other severe disease manifestations, with an event-free survival rate of >80%. In most centers, few patients meet the criteria, which include identification of an HLA-matched sibling donor. Alternative donor sources such as umbilical cord blood are now being used. As novel approaches, such as nonmyeloablative conditioning regimens, undergo further development, stem cell transplantation for patients with sickle cell disease may be expanded.

Clinical case (continued)

The case in this section describes a patient with sickle cell anemia who has experienced pain episodes but not other major complications related to his disease. He is admitted for a pain crisis, and multiorgan failure ensues. Acute multiorgan failure is a well-described complication of sickle cell disease. High baseline Hb levels may represent a key risk factor. It often is precipitated by a severe acute pain crisis and is thought to be secondary to widespread intravascular sickling and subsequent ischemia within affected organs. Aggressive transfusion therapy can be lifesaving and result in complete recovery.

Key points

- The clinical manifestations of sickle cell disease are primarily due to hemolysis and vaso-occlusion.
- Multiple cellular and genetic factors contribute to the phenotypic heterogeneity of sickle cell disease.
- The Hb F level is a major determinant of clinical manifestations and outcomes.
- Pneumococcal sepsis is now uncommon, but it remains a potential cause of death in infants and young children, so universal newborn screening, compliance with penicillin prophylaxis, and vaccination remain a priority.
- Human parvovirus infection is the cause of aplastic crisis.
- Splenic sequestration is a consideration in the differential diagnosis of a sudden marked decrease in the Hb concentration.
- There are differences in frequency of clinical events and survival among the various genotypes of sickle cell disease.
- Sickle cell disease is a leading cause of stroke in young individuals, and a substantial incidence of covert or "silent" infarctions has recently been appreciated.
- A randomized clinical trial has demonstrated efficacy of RBC transfusion in preventing first stroke in children with abnormal TCD velocity.
- A randomized clinical trial demonstrated that preoperative simple transfusion was as effective as exchange transfusion. The preoperative management of the older patient, particularly with cardiac or pulmonary dysfunction, has not been defined.
- A randomized placebo-controlled clinical trial has established the efficacy of hydroxyurea in reducing the frequency of painful episodes and acute chest syndrome. A follow-up study suggests a reduction in mortality for patients taking hydroxyurea.
- The causes of acute chest syndrome include infection, fat embolism, and pulmonary infarction.

Hemoglobin E

Hb E is one of the 2 most prevalent Hb mutants. It has become more common in the United States during the past 20 to 30 years as a result of immigration. Hb E is found with highest frequency in Southeast Asians and has its highest prevalence in Burma and Thailand, where the gene frequency may approach 30%. The gene frequency is also high in Laos, Cambodia, and Vietnam. The structural change is a substitution of glutamic acid by lysine at the 26th position of the β-globin chain (Figure 6-4). A thalassemia-like defect is related to the single base GAG/AAG substitution creating a new potential splicing site, which results in abnormal mRNA processing and reduction of mRNA that can direct translation. Hb E is also slightly unstable in the face of oxidant stress.

Patients heterozygous for Hb E (Hb E trait) have no anemia, mild microcytosis (MCV approximately 71-75 fL in adults and as low as 65 fL in children), target cells, and 30% to 35% Hb E. The Hb E concentration will be lower with the coinheritance of α thalassemia. Homozygotes (Hb E disease) may have mild anemia, microcytosis (MCV approximately 65-69 fL in adults and 55-65 fL in children), and substantial numbers of target cells. The compound heterozygous state, Hb E-β thalassemia, is now one of the more common forms of thalassemia intermedia and thalassemia major in the United States. Hb E-$β^0$ thalassemia is associated with mostly Hb E, with increased amounts of Hb F and Hb A_2; the electrophoretic pattern in Hb E-$β^+$ thalassemia is similar except for the presence of approximately 15% Hb A. Hb E comigrates with Hb C and Hb A_2 on cellulose acetate.

Patients with Hb E disease are usually asymptomatic and do not require specific therapy. However, patients who coinherit Hb E and β thalassemia, especially those with Hb E-$β^0$, may have significant anemia. Some need intermittent or chronic RBC transfusions, and some may benefit from splenectomy.

Hemoglobin C

Hb C is the third most common mutant Hb after Hb S and Hb E. The Hb C mutation arose in West Africa. The prevalence in African Americans is 2% to 3%. The Hb mutant results from the substitution of lysine for glutamic acid as the 6th amino acid of β globin, the consequence of a single nucleotide substitution (GAG/AAG) in the 6th codon (Figure 6-4). The resultant positive-to-negative charge difference on the surface of the Hb C tetramer results in a molecule with decreased solubility of both the oxy and deoxy forms that may undergo intraerythrocytic aggregation and crystal formation. Hb C stimulates the K:Cl cotransport system, promoting water loss and resulting in dehydration and poorly deformable RBCs that have a predilection for entrapment within the spleen. Consequently, patients with Hb CC and patients with Cβ thalassemia have mild chronic hemolytic anemia and splenomegaly. Patients may develop cholelithiasis, and the anemia may be more exaggerated in association with infections. Heterozygous individuals (Hb C trait) are clinically normal. The coinheritance of Hb S and Hb C results in significant pathologic consequences (see Sickle cell disease).

Hb CC results in mild hemolytic anemia and slightly elevated reticulocyte counts. The MCHC is elevated because of the previously mentioned effect of Hb C on cellular hydration. The MCV is generally reduced. The blood smear shows prominent target cells. RBCs containing Hb crystals may also be seen on the blood smear, particularly in patients who have had splenectomy. Individuals with Hb C trait have normal Hb levels but may have target cells on the peripheral smear. Confirmation of the diagnosis requires identification of Hb C, which comigrates with Hb A_2, Hb E, and Hb O_{Arab} on cellulose acetate. Thus, Hb C must be distinguished by acid agar gel electrophoresis, isoelectric focusing gel electrophoresis, or HPLC.

Specific treatment of patients with Hb CC is neither available nor required.

Hemoglobin D

Hb D is usually diagnosed incidentally. Hb D^{Punjab} (also called Hb $D^{Los\ Angeles}$) results from the substitution of glutamine for glutamic acid at the 121st position of the β chain (Figure 6-4). This mutant has a prevalence of approximately 3% in the Northwest Punjab region of India but is also encountered in other parts of the world. Patients with homozygous (Hb DD) or heterozygous (Hb AD) do not have hemolysis. The major clinical relevance of Hb D is that its compound heterozygous inheritance with Hb S results in sickle cell disease, perhaps as a result of the low-affinity Hb D promoting Hb deoxygenation. The diagnosis of Hb AD (D trait) or DD is made by Hb electrophoresis. Hb S and Hb D have similar electrophoretic mobilities on alkaline cellulose acetate electrophoresis. They can be differentiated by acid citrate agar electrophoresis, isoelectric focusing, HPLC, or solubility studies; this distinction is important for genetic and prognostic counseling.

> **Key points**
>
> - Hb C, Hb D, and Hb E are common mutant Hbs that can have significant consequences when coinherited with Hb S.
> - Homozygosity for Hb E (EE) is a mild condition, but compound heterozygosity for Hb E and β thalassemia can be a clinically significant thalassemia syndrome.

Unstable Hb

Unstable Hb mutants are inherited in an autosomal dominant pattern, and affected individuals are usually heterozygotes. Unstable Hbs constitute one of the largest groups of

Hb variants, although individually, each is rare. In Hb Köln, the most prevalent unstable Hb, the β_{98} Val/Met substitution destabilizes the heme pocket. In Hb Zurich, the β_{63} His/Arg also disrupts the heme pocket. Other mechanisms that destabilize Hb include (i) alteration of the $\alpha_1\beta_1$ interface region (eg, Hb Tacoma, β_{30} Arg/Ser); (ii) distortion of the helical configuration of structurally important regions (eg, Hb Bibba, α_{136} Leu/Pro); and (iii) introduction of the interior polar amino acid (eg, Hb Bristol, β_{67} Val/Asp). Unstable γ chain variants (eg, Hb Poole, γ_{130} Trp/Gly) can cause transient hemolytic anemia in the neonate that will spontaneously resolve.

These abnormal Hbs precipitate spontaneously or with oxidative stress. Precipitated Hb inclusions (Heinz bodies) impair erythrocyte deformability, resulting in premature erythrocyte destruction by macrophages of the liver and spleen. The severity of the hemolysis varies with the nature of the mutation but may be accelerated by fever or ingestion of oxidant drugs.

An unstable hemoglobinopathy should be suspected in a patient with hereditary nonspherocytic hemolytic anemia. The Hb level may be normal or decreased. Hypochromia of the RBCs (resulting from loss of Hb due to denaturation and subsequent pitting), "bite cells," and basophilic stippling may occur. The evaluation includes Hb electrophoresis (which is often normal), crystal violet Heinz body staining, and the isopropanol stability test. The isopropanol test may be falsely positive in the neonate due to high fetal Hb levels, so the heat stability test should be used during the first months of life. Management includes avoidance of oxidant agents, and many recommend supplementation with folic acid. Splenectomy may be useful for patients with severe hemolysis and splenomegaly.

Oxygen affinity mutants

The Hb variants with altered ligand (oxygen) affinity can be classified into 3 categories: (i) those with increased oxygen affinity, (ii) those with decreased oxygen affinity, and (iii) M Hbs. These conditions have an autosomal dominant inheritance pattern.

Increased oxygen affinity variants should be considered in patients with familial erythrocytosis. The mutations usually result from amino acid substitutions at the critical $\alpha_1\beta_2$ contact region (eg, Hb Chesapeake, α_{92} Arg/Leu) or at the carboxyl terminus of the β chain (eg, Hb Bethesda, β_{145} Tyr/His). There may also be amino acid substitutions at the 2,3-BPG binding site. There usually are no changes in RBC morphology or hemolysis. Measurement of oxygen dissociation will reveal increased oxygen affinity. Mutants with decreased oxygen affinity should be considered in patients with familial asymptomatic anemia. These variants also tend to result from amino acid substitutions in the $\alpha_1\beta_2$ contact region (eg, Hb Kansas). In contrast to the high-affinity variants, these mutants result in decreased oxygen affinity and dissociation of the Hb tetramer into 2 symmetric dimers. The net effect in some of these variants is that tissue oxygen delivery is facilitated. This results in decreased erythropoietin production and "physiologic" anemia.

The diagnosis of M hemoglobinopathies should be considered in patients with asymptomatic cyanosis and no desaturation of their Hb. In these disorders, the ferrous iron (Fe^{2+}) of heme is vulnerable to oxidation to the ferric state (Fe^{3+}). This methemoglobin (M Hb) is incapable of binding oxygen, which leads to cyanosis. Certain M Hb mutations also render the molecule unstable, accounting for a clinical picture of both cyanosis and hemolysis.

The diagnosis of oxygen affinity mutants is established by determination of the P_{50} of the Hb, which is the partial pressure of oxygen at which the Hb is 50% saturated, along with Hb electrophoresis, which often is normal. Diagnosis should be established to avoid further inappropriate, often invasive diagnostic workup. Treatment is neither available nor warranted.

Acquired hemoglobinopathies

Many substances when ingested or inhaled may undergo chemical reactions with Hb, leading to the formation of abnormal Hb adducts. These toxic modifications of Hb can impair its primary function in tissue respiration. Clinical manifestations become evident when compensatory mechanisms are no longer able to overcome the rate or extent of the noxious damage. Abnormal glycation of Hb (Hb A_{1C}) in diabetes has no functional detriment.

Carboxyhemoglobinemia

The most common acquired abnormality is carboxyhemoglobinemia. Carbon monoxide is a tasteless, odorless, nonirritating gas produced by incomplete combustion of organic materials, particularly petroleum, tobacco tar, wood, and cotton. Its toxic effects in humans result from its binding to Hb at the same site as oxygen, but with an affinity approximately 200 times greater. Compared with oxyhemoglobin, carboxyhemoglobin less readily dissociates, which results in functional hypoxemia and tissue hypoxia predominantly of the organs most sensitive to oxygen deprivation, the central nervous and cardiovascular systems.

Clinical manifestations roughly correlate with carboxyhemoglobin levels but also depend on the duration and intensity of exposure. Chronic occupational exposure or heavy cigarette smoking may produce substantial carboxyhemoglobin levels that can lead to erythrocytosis. Sudden elevation of carboxyhemoglobin results in rapid progression from loss of consciousness to coma, seizures, and death. Prompt removal from the offending site is the first goal of therapy, and inhalation of 100% oxygen is used to improve the partial pressure of oxygen in the blood and reduce the half-life of clearance of carboxyhemoglobin. When there are severe cardiopulmonary or central nervous system symptoms, hyperbaric oxygen may be required to reduce levels of carboxyhemoglobin rapidly.

Methemoglobinemia

When the iron in Hb is oxidized from the ferrous (Fe^{2+}) to the ferric state (Fe^{3+}), Hb is converted to methemoglobin, which is unable to bind and transport oxygen. Normally, methemoglobin produced in the RBC is maintained at a level of <1% by 2 enzyme-dependent processes. Reduced nicotinamide adenine dinucleotide (NADH) diaphorase (cytochrome b5 reductase), when coupled with oxidation of NADH to nicotinamide adenine dinucleotide (NAD), reduces methemoglobinemia and susceptibility to oxidative stress. The nicotinamide adenine dinucleotide phosphate (NADPH)–dependent methemoglobin reductase system requires an exogenous electron carrier (such as methylene blue) and thus is normally quiescent. Exposure to a number of drugs or toxic substances that oxidize the heme iron directly or indirectly can overwhelm the NADH diaphorase system and generate methemoglobin (Table 6-5). Methemoglobinemia levels of 10% to 20% result in visible cyanosis; levels >30% result in headache, dizziness, dyspnea, tachypnea, or tachycardia; levels >50% lead to progressive stupor and obtundation; and levels >70% are lethal. Methemoglobinemia should be considered in a patient presenting with asymptomatic cyanosis or cyanosis refractory to oxygen inhalation. When the patient's blood appears brown and does not turn red when exposed to oxygen, methemoglobinemia is likely. A normal oxygen tension (PaO_2) with a decreased oxygen saturation measured by pulse oximetry or co-oximetry indicates the presence of methemoglobin.

In pediatric patients, acquired methemoglobinemia is seen most often in babies between 1 and 4 months of age with diarrhea and metabolic acidosis. The presumed mechanism is abnormal absorption from the inflamed bowel of nitrites and other potent oxidants. A contributing cause is low erythrocyte NADH-diaphorase activity during the neonatal period. Methylene blue, administered intravenously, 1 mg/kg over 5 minutes, is the treatment of choice for the toxic type of methemoglobinemia, especially for levels >40% or in the presence of central nervous system symptoms. This dose may be repeated in 1 hour, and then every 4 to 6 hours, not to exceed a total dose of 7 mg/kg. Methylene blue therapy should be avoided in the presence of G6PD deficiency because it is ineffective and may precipitate hemolysis. Additional measures include the use of high-flow oxygen therapy and even hyperbaric oxygen treatment in severe cases, especially those involving nitrite exposure.

Congenital methemoglobinemia due to homozygous deficiency of NADH-diaphorase activity will cause generally asymptomatic cyanosis that can be successfully treated with oral ascorbic acid (300-600 mg daily in 3-4 divided doses) or more effectively treated with oral methylene blue, 60 mg 3 to 4 times daily. These drugs activate the latent NADPH-dependent methemoglobin reductase system.

Sulfhemoglobinemia

Sulfhemoglobinemia results from irreversible oxidation of Hb by certain chemicals and drugs, notably sulfonamides, acetanilide, and phenacetin. It is produced chemically by the addition of hydrogen sulfide to Hb and can be distinguished from methemoglobin by its spectral characteristics in the presence of cyanide. In contrast to methemoglobin, sulfhemoglobin production is not reversible; it remains in the RBCs until they are destroyed. Fortunately, sulfhemoglobinemia is rarely symptomatic, even with levels exceeding 30% to 40%. Thus, treatment consists of withdrawal of the offending agent.

Hemoglobin H

Hb H disease is a common, inherited form of α thalassemia, classically caused by the constitutional deletion of 3 of the 4 α-globin genes. Hb H can also be produced as an acquired phenomenon in the setting of myelodysplastic syndromes and some myeloid leukemias, in which somatic mutations of the *ATRX* gene down-regulate α-globin production and cause globin chain imbalance. This condition is called the α thalassemia–myelodysplastic syndrome

Table 6-5 Agents that induce methemoglobinemia.

Acetanilide
Acetaminophen
Aniline dye derivatives
Dapsone
Phenacetin
Primaquine
Naphthalene
Nitrates, nitrites
Nitroprusside
Local anesthetics (eg, benzocaine, lidocaine)
Sulfonamides

(ATMDS). The X-linked *ATRX* gene encodes a chromatin remodeling factor (X-linked helicase 2) that regulates α-globin production. Constitutional deletions of this gene produce the α thalassemia–mental retardation syndrome.

Abnormalities of the RBC membrane

> **Clinical case**
>
> A 36-year-old woman is referred for evaluation of moderate anemia. She has been told she is anemic for as long as she can remember, and she has intermittently been prescribed iron. She occasionally has mild fatigue but is otherwise asymptomatic. Her past history is significant only for intermittent jaundice and a cholecystectomy for gallstones at age 22 years. She takes no medications. A cousin and an aunt have also had anemia and jaundice. Her examination is significant for mild splenomegaly. Prior laboratory data reveal hematocrit values between 29% and 33%. Today's hematocrit is 27%, MCV is 98 fL, and MCHC is 38 g/dL. Corrected reticulocyte count is 7%. Review of the peripheral blood smear reveals numerous spherocytes.

Hereditary spherocytosis (HS), hereditary elliptocytosis (HE), and hereditary pyropoikilocytosis (HPP) are a heterogeneous group of disorders with a wide spectrum of clinical manifestations. This group of disorders is characterized by abnormal shape and flexibility of RBCs due to a deficiency or dysfunction of one or more of the membrane proteins, which leads to shortened RBC survival (hemolysis). Multiple genetic abnormalities, including deletions, point mutations, and defective mRNA processing, have been identified as underlying causes. The HS syndromes are generally due to private mutations unique to each kindred. In contrast, some HE syndromes are due to specific mutations in individuals from similar locales (eg, Melanesian elliptocytosis), suggesting a founder effect.

RBC membrane protein composition and assembly

The RBC membrane consists of a phospholipid/cholesterol lipid bilayer intercalated by integral membrane proteins such as band 3 (the anion transport channel) and the glycophorins (Figure 6-7). This relatively fluid layer is stabilized by attachment to a membrane skeleton. Spectrin is the major protein of the skeleton, comprising approximately 75% of its mass. The skeleton is organized into a hexagonal lattice. The hexagon arms are formed by fiber-like spectrin tetramers, whereas the hexagon corners are composed of small oligomers of actin that, with the aid of other proteins (4.1 and adducin), connect the spectrin tetramers into a 2-dimensional lattice. The membrane cytoskeleton and its fixation to the lipid/protein bilayer are the major determinants of the shape, strength, flexibility, and survival of RBCs. When any of these constituents are altered, RBC survival may be shortened.

A useful model to understand the basis for RBC membrane disorders divides membrane protein–protein and protein–lipid associations into 2 categories. Vertical interactions are perpendicular to the plane of the membrane and involve a spectrin–ankyrin–band 3 association facilitated by protein 4.2 and attachment of spectrin–actin–protein 4.1 junctional complexes to glycophorin C. Horizontal interactions, which are parallel to and underlying the plane of the membrane, involve the assembly of α and β spectrin chains into heterodimers, which self-associate to form tetramers. Because the distal ends of spectrin bind to actin, with the aid of protein 4.1 and other minor proteins (Figure 6-7), a contractile function of the cytoskeleton may

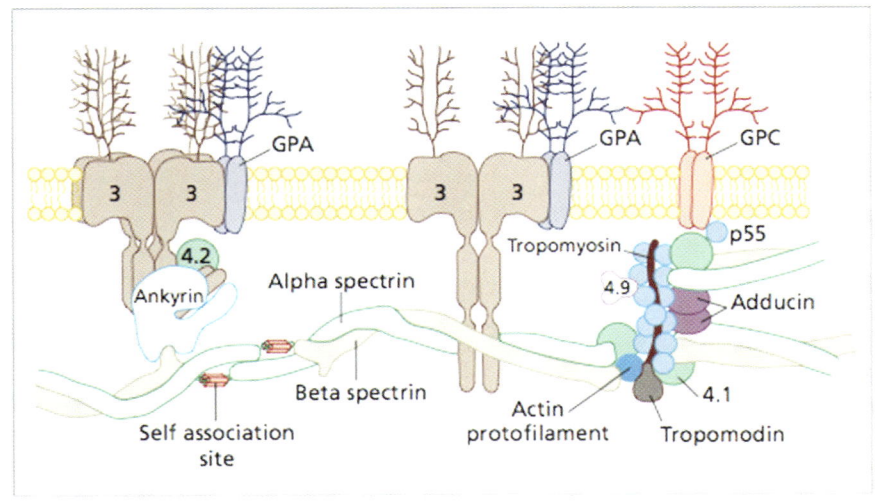

Figure 6-7 The red blood cell membrane. A model of the red blood cell membrane is shown in which the relative positions of the various proteins are correct, but the proteins and lipids are not drawn to scale. From Handin RI, Lux RJH, Stossel T. *Blood: Principles and Practice of Hematology*. Philadelphia, PA: Lippincott-Raven; 1995.

be important for normal RBC survival. Generally, HS is caused by defects in vertical interactions, whereas HE is caused by defects in the horizontal interactions.

Hereditary spherocytosis

HS is common in individuals of Northern European descent with an occurrence of approximately 1 in 2000. Penetrance is variable, and the prevalence of a clinically recognized disorder is much lower. In 75% of cases, the inheritance pattern is autosomal dominant with sporadic cases representing the remaining 25%, half of which represent an autosomal recessive inheritance pattern and the other half de novo mutations. HS is characterized by spherocytic, osmotically fragile RBCs and is both clinically and genetically heterogeneous.

Pathophysiology

The pathophysiology of HS generally involves aberrant interactions between the skeleton and the overlying lipid bilayer ("vertical interactions"). A common epiphenomenon in HS RBCs is a varying degree of spectrin loss, which is usually due to a defect in one of the membrane proteins involved in the attachment of spectrin to the membrane rather than a primary defect in the spectrin molecule itself. Spectrin as the major protein of the skeleton forms a nearly monomolecular submembrane layer that covers most of the inner membrane surface; therefore, the density of this skeletal layer in HS erythrocytes is reduced. Consequently, the lipid bilayer is destabilized, leading to loss of membrane lipid and thus surface area through microvesiculation. The result of these changes is a spheroidal-shaped RBC. The inherent reduced deformability of spherocytes leads to their inability to traverse the unique constraining apertures that characterize splenic vascular walls. The spleen "conditions" RBCs, enhancing membrane loss. Retained and further damaged by the hypoxic and acidic environment in the spleen, they are ultimately prematurely destroyed.

The molecular basis of HS is heterogeneous (Table 6-6). A deficiency or defect of the ankyrin molecule represents the most common cause of dominant HS. In 30% to 45% of cases, the defect comprises both ankyrin and spectrin deficiency, in 30% spectrin only, and in 20% band 3 mutations. Various mutations of the ankyrin gene have been identified. Multiple band 3 mutations have also been described. Although less frequent, mutations of the β spectrin gene have been found in autosomal dominant HS, whereas α spectrin gene abnormalities have been identified only in recessively inherited HS. Mutations in the protein 4.2 gene have been found primarily in Japanese patients with autosomal recessive HS.

Clinical manifestations

The clinical expression ranges from an asymptomatic and often undiagnosed condition with nearly normal Hb levels (*compensated hemolysis*) to severe hemolysis and anemia. Patients with mild HS have a relatively uneventful course, although some may develop pigmented gallstones in adolescence and early adult life. Mildly anemic patients may be diagnosed later in adult life during evaluation for unrelated conditions. Patients with moderately severe disease may present with several additional complications. Aplastic crisis, which may be the presentation for some patients, requires emergent attention. The cause of aplastic crisis is human parvovirus infection that produces selective suppression of erythropoiesis, resulting in reticulocytopenia and inability to compensate for ongoing RBC destruction. The "hyperhemolytic crisis" characterized by accelerated hemolysis leading to increased jaundice and splenic enlargement is a common problem in affected children. Other complications include the rare megaloblastic crisis

Table 6-6 Defects of red blood cell membrane proteins in hereditary spherocytosis, elliptocytosis, and pyropoikilocytosis.

Class of defect	Hereditary spherocytosis	Hereditary elliptocytosis and pyropoikilocytosis
Protein deficiency	Spectrin	Spectrin*
	Ankyrin†	Protein 4.1
	Band 3	Glycophorin C
	Protein 4.2	
Protein dysfunction	β spectrin abnormality affects β spectrin–protein 4.1 interaction†	Defective spectrin dimer self-association due to spectrin mutations
		Protein 4.1 abnormality affects β spectrin–protein 4.1 interaction

*Seen in patients with hereditary pyropoikilocytosis, where it coexists with a spectrin mutation that affects spectrin self-association.
†Red blood cells of the patients are also partially deficient in spectrin.

secondary to acquired folic acid deficiency usually associated with high-demand situations such as pregnancy. Leg ulcerations have been rarely reported. Patients with severe hemolysis and resulting expansion of the erythroid compartment in the bone marrow can develop maxillary hyperplasia interfering with dentition or extramedullary hematopoietic masses that may mimic malignancy. Patients may manifest a variety of symptoms attributable to splenomegaly, including early satiety, left upper quadrant fullness, and hypersplenism. HS may be diagnosed in the neonatal period based on a positive family history or marked jaundice. The diagnosis should also be considered in patients of all ages with intermittent jaundice, mild refractory anemia, and/or splenomegaly. Rare associated syndromes suggest that mutant RBC membrane proteins may also reside in other tissues. Thus, distal renal tubular acidosis may occur in HS patients harboring mutant band 3 (the anion channel protein).

Laboratory evaluation

In addition to the usual laboratory abnormalities indicating hemolysis, the principal diagnostic feature is the identification of spherocytes on the peripheral blood smear (Figure 6-8A). HS should be considered in the differential diagnosis of direct antiglobulin test (DAT)-negative hemolytic anemia. The extent of spherocytosis is variable and, in mild cases, may be missed even by the experienced clinician. Additional morphologic abnormalities, including spiculated cells and elliptocytes, may be observed. The RBC indices may provide a clue, with an increase in the MCHC (due to cellular dehydration) even in the context of minimal anemia. The osmotic fragility test using increasingly hypotonic saline solutions will support the diagnosis with the finding of increased RBC lysis compared with normal RBCs. Sensitivity of the test is enhanced by 24-hour incubation at 37°C, but mild cases can still be missed by the test. A newer and increasingly used test for HS and related cytoskeleton-associated hemolytic anemias is the eosin-5-maleimide (EMA) binding test. EMA binds to band 3 on RBCs, and a reduction in binding, measured by fluorescence intensity, corresponds to a quantitative reduction in erythrocyte band 3, consistent with HS. The EMA binding test has a higher predictive value for HS than osmotic fragility. Review of the complete blood count, reticulocyte count, and peripheral smear from family members may prove helpful. The differential diagnosis for spherocytes and increased osmotic fragility includes autoimmune hemolytic anemia, so a DAT should be performed as part of the evaluation when the family history is negative.

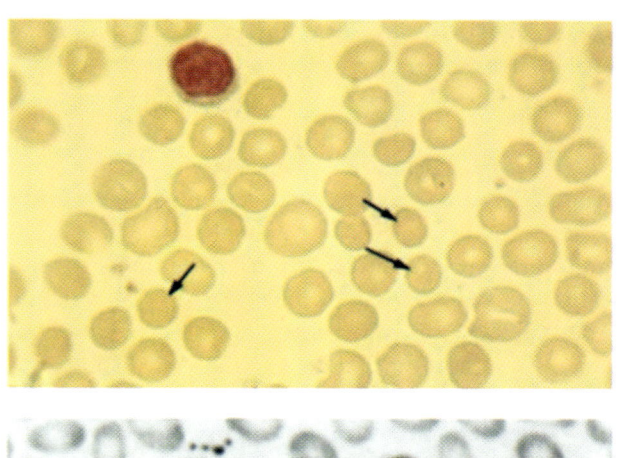
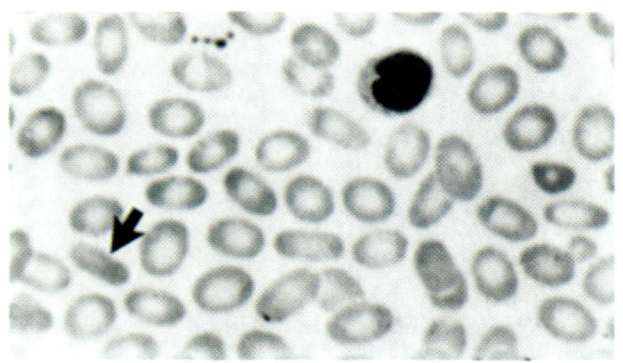
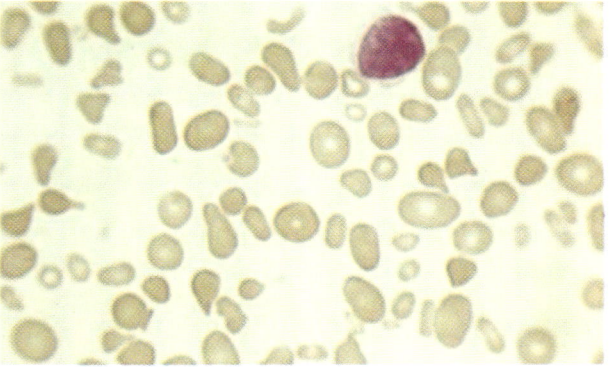

Figure 6-8 Peripheral blood findings in inherited disorders of the red blood cell membrane. A, Numerous spherocytes (*arrows*). B, Numerous elliptocytes and a rod-shaped cell (*arrow*). C, Marked poikilocytosis.

Treatment

As with other hemolytic anemias, folic acid supplementation should be considered for patients with severe anemia even though overt folic acid deficiency is rarely encountered. Patients need to be aware of the signs and symptoms of aplastic and hyperhemolytic crises to seek prompt medical attention. The definitive treatment of HS is splenectomy, which ameliorates the hemolytic anemia in almost all patients, although the underlying intrinsic defect of the circulating RBCs is not altered. In rare patients with HS and severe hemolysis, the procedure markedly diminishes the hemolytic rate but may not fully correct the anemia. Controlled clinical trial data are not available to provide guidelines in making the decision to recommend splenectomy. Thus, the indications for splenectomy are somewhat controversial, but the prevailing view advocates surgery for patients with symptomatic hemolytic anemia or its complications, particularly gallstones. Additional considerations for splenectomy in the pediatric population include failure to thrive, recurrent hyperhemolytic episodes, or symptoms from chronic anemia including a hypermetabolic state. The laparoscopic technique is often preferred to open splenectomy. Accessory spleens are common, so a thorough search should be performed at the time of splenectomy. The patient should receive pneumococcal, *H influenzae* type b, and meningococcal vaccines before the procedure, and pediatric patients usually receive prophylactic penicillin for at least several years thereafter to reduce the risk of bacterial sepsis. Thromboembolic events may also exist following splenectomy, although data are limited. Because of the increased frequency of post-splenectomy infections in young children, splenectomy should not be performed before the age of 5 years except in patients with severe disease manifested by the need for periodic or regular transfusions.

The patient presented in this section should be suspected of having HS. It is not uncommon for the diagnosis to be made in adulthood, as patients with mild or moderate disease are often well compensated. An elevated reticulocyte count, elevated MCHC, intermittent jaundice, history of gallstones, and spherocytes on peripheral smear all support the diagnosis. The diagnosis should be confirmed by demonstrating increased osmotic fragility of RBCs and a negative DAT. Family members should be evaluated for anemia.

Key points

- HS is the most common inherited hemolytic anemia of individuals from Northern Europe.
- Abnormalities in ankyrin, spectrin, band 3, and protein 4.2 that result in a reduction in the quantity of spectrin account for the RBC membrane loss characteristic of HS.
- HS should be suspected in cases of DAT-negative hemolytic anemia when spherocytes are identified on the peripheral blood smear. The diagnosis can be supported with the osmotic fragility test, the sensitivity of which is increased with incubation at 37°C. A positive family history is also supportive of the diagnosis.
- Clinical manifestations of HS vary from a lack of symptoms to severe hemolysis.
- Splenectomy decreases hemolysis and reduces gallstone formation for most affected patients.

Hereditary elliptocytosis and hereditary pyropoikilocytosis

The clinical presentation, inheritance, alteration in RBC shape and physical properties, and underlying molecular defects are considerably more heterogeneous in HE than in HS. Three distinct subtypes are distinguished: (i) common HE, characterized by biconcave elliptocytes and, in more severe forms, rod-shaped cells, poikilocytes, and fragments (Figure 6-8B); (ii) spherocytic HE, a phenotypic hybrid between HE and HS; and (iii) Southeast Asian ovalocytosis with unique spoon-shaped erythrocyte morphology. In most cases, the inheritance of HE is autosomal dominant. The exception is HPP, a rare and severe variant of common HE that is recessively inherited (Figure 6-8C). The clinical expression of common HE, the most prevalent form of elliptocytosis, is highly variable, ranging from an asymptomatic carrier state to a severe hemolytic disease with poikilocytosis and erythrocyte fragmentation.

Pathophysiology

The underlying defects involve horizontal interactions between proteins of the membrane skeleton, especially spectrin–spectrin and spectrin–protein 4.1 interactions. These defects weaken the skeleton; under the influence of shear stress in the microcirculation, the cells progressively lose the ability to regain the normal disc shape and are stabilized in the elliptocytic or poikilocytic shape. In severely affected patients, the weakening of the skeleton grossly diminishes membrane stability, leading to RBC fragmentation.

Different underlying molecular defects have been identified in common HE, consistent with the heterogeneous nature of the disorder (Table 6-6). In the majority of cases, patients have mutant α or β spectrin, resulting in defective self-association and an increased percentage of spectrin heterodimer in the membrane. A partial or complete absence or dysfunction of protein 4.1 occurs in some patients with missense and deletion mutations. Patients with HPP appear to be compound heterozygotes. Coinheritance of a mutation leading to spectrin deficiency and a mutation of spectrin resulting in a qualitatively defective molecule has been identified in some patients with the condition. Southeast Asian ovalocytosis is prevalent among certain ethnic groups in Malaysia, the Philippines, Papua New Guinea, and probably other Pacific countries as well. It is an asymptomatic condition characterized by rigid RBCs of a unique spoon-shaped morphology. Affected individuals are heterozygous for a mutation of band 3.

Clinical manifestations, laboratory evaluation, and treatment

HE must be differentiated from a variety of other conditions in which elliptocytes and poikilocytes are commonly found on the peripheral blood smear, including iron deficiency, thalassemia, megaloblastic anemia, myelofibrosis, and myelodysplasia. However, as opposed to HE, the percentage of elliptocytes in these other conditions usually does not exceed 60%. The presence of elliptocytes and evidence of dominant inheritance of elliptocytosis in other family members differentiate HE from the previous conditions. Whereas most patients with common HE are asymptomatic, occasional patients who are homozygotes or compound heterozygotes for 1 or 2 molecular defects have more severe hemolytic disease. African American neonates with common HE may have severe hemolysis, with striking RBC abnormalities, which abate during the initial months of life. The most severe form of elliptocytosis, HPP, is typically recessively inherited and is characterized by a striking micropoikilospherocytosis and fragmentation with some elliptocytes. A markedly low MCV, typically in the range of 50 to 60 fL, may be observed. In HPP, RBCs are thermally unstable and fragment at temperatures of 46°C to 48°C, reflecting the presence of mutant spectrin in the cells. Additional specialized laboratory investigation includes separation of solubilized membrane proteins by polyacrylamide gel electrophoresis, which may reveal either an abnormally migrating spectrin or a deficiency or abnormal migration of protein 4.1. An increased fraction of unassembled dimeric spectrin in the extract can be detected by electrophoresis of extracts under nondenaturing conditions.

Treatment is not necessary for most individuals with common HE. Splenectomy may be of benefit for patients with symptomatic hemolytic anemia or its complications (see Hereditary spherocytosis).

tions that vary in width, length, and surface distribution. Several conditions are associated with this morphology. In severe liver disease, acanthocyte formation is a 2-step process involving the transfer of free nonesterified cholesterol from abnormal plasma lipoproteins into the erythrocyte membrane and then the subsequent remodeling of abnormally shaped erythrocytes by the spleen. Rapidly progressive hemolytic anemia is seen in association with advanced and often end-stage alcoholic cirrhosis, sometimes referred to as Zieve syndrome, or other conditions such as metastatic liver disease, cardiac cirrhosis, Wilson disease, and fulminant hepatitis.

In abetalipoproteinemia, the primary molecular defect involves a congenital absence of apolipoprotein B in plasma. Consequently, all plasma lipoproteins containing this apoprotein as well as plasma triglycerides are nearly absent. Plasma cholesterol and phospholipid levels are also markedly reduced. The role of these lipid abnormalities in producing acanthocytes is not well understood. The most striking abnormality of the acanthocyte membrane in abetalipoproteinemia is an increase in membrane sphingomyelin. Abetalipoproteinemia is an autosomal recessive disorder that manifests in the first month of life with steatorrhea. Retinitis pigmentosa and progressive neurologic abnormalities, such as ataxia and intention tremors, develop between 5 and 10 years of age and progress to death by the second or third decade of life.

Acanthocytes have also been described in patients with the McLeod phenotype, a condition in which the erythrocytes have reduced surface Kell antigen because the Kx protein needed for its expression is absent. The Kx antigenic protein is encoded by the X chromosome, so males are affected with mild compensated hemolysis, whereas asymptomatic carrier females may be identified by flow cytometric analysis of Kell blood group antigen expression.

> **Key points**
>
> - HE is due to defects in the interactions of RBC cytoskeleton proteins ("vertical interactions"), with spectrin abnormalities accounting for most of the cases.
> - The majority of patients with HE are not symptomatic and require no therapy.
> - HPP is a rare condition with apparent coinheritance of spectrin defects leading to markedly abnormal RBCs characterized by increased thermal instability.

Other RBC membrane disorders
Acanthocytosis

Spur cells, or acanthocytes (from the Greek *acantha*, or thorn; Figure 6-9), are erythrocytes with multiple irregular projec-

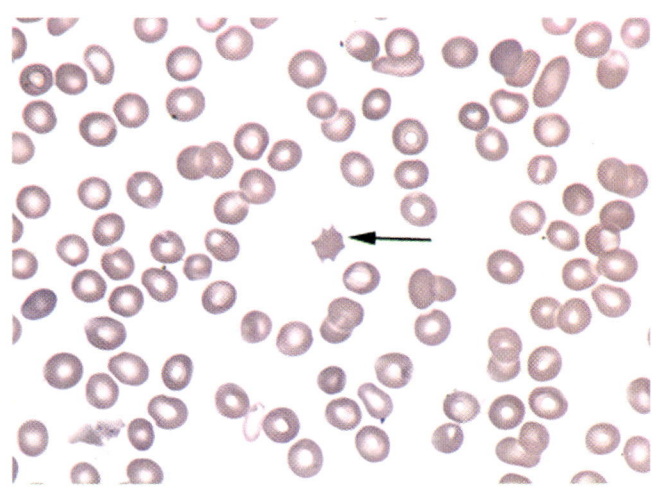

Figure 6-9 Acanthocyte (*arrow*).

Stomatocytosis

Stomatocytes have a wide transverse slit or stoma toward the center of the RBC (Figure 6-10). A few stomatocytes (between 3% and 5%) are found on blood smears of healthy individuals. Several inherited and acquired disorders are associated with stomatocytosis. The inherited forms are associated with abnormalities in erythrocyte cation permeability and volume, which is either increased (hence, the designation hydrocytosis), decreased (xerocytosis), or near normal. The specific molecular defects are unknown. Of significant clinical importance is the recognition that patients with hereditary stomatocytosis have an increased risk of developing thrombotic events after splenectomy. Acquired stomatocytosis can be seen in acute alcoholism and hepatobiliary disease (although target cells are more common) and occasionally in malignant neoplasms and cardiovascular disorders. Stomatocytes may also occur as an artifact.

Rh deficiency (null) syndrome

This term is used to designate rare cases of either absent (Rh_{null}) or markedly reduced (Rh_{mod}) expression of the Rh antigen in association with mild to moderate hemolytic anemia. Three proteins (RhCE, RhD, and Rh50) comprise the Rh protein family. This disorder arises through autosomal recessive inheritance of either a suppressor gene unrelated to the Rh locus or a silent allele at the locus itself. The normal complexed structure forms an integral membrane protein; its loss disrupts membrane architecture. Rh_{null} cells have increased rates of cation transport and sodium–potassium membrane ATPase activity that results in dehydrated RBCs. Stomatocytes and occasional spherocytes are the result of this dehydration and can be identified on the peripheral blood smear. Laboratory evaluation shows increased RBC osmotic fragility, reflecting a marked reduction of the membrane surface area. The relationship between the absence of the Rh antigen proteins and RBC alterations leading to hemolysis presumably involves membrane microvesiculation, leading to diminished erythrocyte flexibility. Splenectomy results in improvement of the hemolytic anemia.

Abnormalities of RBC enzymes

> **Clinical case**
>
> A 23-year-old African American male who recently underwent cadaveric renal transplantation for end-stage renal disease is referred for evaluation of anemia. His past history is significant for an episode of hemolytic-uremic syndrome (HUS) that led to renal failure 2 years prior to referral. He had no further relapses of HUS or TTP. His posttransplantation course has been unremarkable with good graft function and no rejection. When he left the hospital, his hematocrit was 31%. His discharge medications included prednisone, cyclosporine, trimethoprim/sulfamethoxazole, and acyclovir. He complains of increasing fatigue and dyspnea over the 10 days since discharge. Friends have noted yellowing of his eyes. He denies any fever or infectious symptoms. On physical examination, he has a heart rate of 112, blood pressure of 89/45, and scleral icterus. Otherwise, the examination is unremarkable. Current hematocrit is 20%, corrected reticulocyte count is 10%, and LDH is 1543 U/L. Serum creatinine is 1.8 mg/dL, and the platelet count is 302,000/μL, similar to hospital discharge. On review of the peripheral blood smear, polychromatophilia is noted. A moderate number of bite and blister cells are identified.

Normal metabolism of the mature RBC involves 2 principal pathways of glucose catabolism: the glycolytic pathway and the hexose-monophosphate shunt. The 3 major functions of the products of glucose catabolism in the erythrocyte are (i) maintenance of protein integrity, cellular deformability, and RBC shape; (ii) preservation of Hb iron in the ferrous form; and (iii) modulation of the oxygen affinity of Hb. These functions are served by the regulation of appropriate production of 5 specific molecules: adenosine triphosphate (ATP), reduced glutathione, reduced NADH, reduced NADPH, and 2,3-BPG. Maintenance of the biochemical and structural integrity of the RBC depends on the normal function of >20 enzymes involved in these pathways as well as the availability of 5 essential RBC substrates: glucose, glutathione, NAD, NAD phosphate (NADP), and adenosine diphosphate (ADP).

The primary function of the glycolytic pathway is the generation of ATP, which is necessary for the ATPase-linked

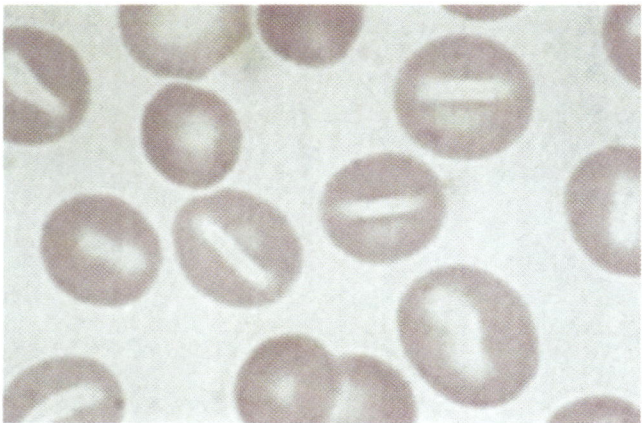

Figure 6-10 Stomatocytes.

sodium–potassium and calcium membrane pumps essential for cation homeostasis and the maintenance of erythrocyte deformability. The production of 2,3-BPG is regulated by the Rapoport–Luebering shunt, which is controlled by bisphosphoglyceromutase, the enzyme that converts 1,3-BPG to 2,3-BPG. Concentration of 2,3-BPG in the RBC in turn regulates Hb oxygen affinity, thus facilitating the transfer of oxygen from Hb to tissue-binding sites. The major function of the hexose-monophosphate shunt pathway is preservation and regeneration of reduced glutathione, which protects Hb and other intracellular and membrane proteins from oxidant injury.

Abnormalities of the glycolytic pathway

Defects in the glycolytic pathway lead to a decrease in the production of ATP or a change in the concentration of 2,3-BPG. Deficiencies of erythrocyte hexokinase, glucose phosphate isomerase, phosphofructokinase, and pyruvate kinase (PK) all lead to a decrease in ATP concentration. Although genetic disorders involving nearly all of the enzymes of the glycolytic pathway have been described, PK accounts for >80% of the clinically significant hemolytic anemias. With the exception of phosphoglycerate kinase deficiency, which is X-linked, all other glycolytic enzyme defects exhibit autosomal recessive inheritance patterns.

PK deficiency is the most common congenital nonspherocytic hemolytic anemia caused by a defect in glycolytic RBC metabolism. The syndrome is both genetically and clinically heterogeneous. PK deficiency has a worldwide distribution but is more common among those of northern and eastern European heritage. Severe cases can present either with neonatal jaundice or in early childhood with jaundice, splenomegaly, and failure to thrive. Alternatively, a mild presentation with fully compensated hemolytic anemia has been described. Osmotic fragility of the patient's RBCs is typically normal and may be helpful in differentiating this condition from HS. Several screening tests have been developed to diagnose PK deficiency, but often they lack sensitivity to diagnose specific PK variants. Reference laboratories can perform quantitative measurement of the erythrocyte enzyme level necessary to diagnose this condition accurately.

Both glucose phosphate isomerase and hexokinase deficiencies produce nonspherocytic hemolytic anemia associated with decreased erythrocyte ATP and 2,3-BPG content. These disorders are rare; patients often present in childhood with mild to moderate anemia and reduced exercise tolerance. A form of acquired hexokinase deficiency occurs in Wilson disease, in which elevated copper levels in the blood inhibit hexokinase in a fluctuating fashion that may lead to intermittent brisk intravascular hemolysis. Phosphofructokinase deficiency was first described as a muscle glycogen storage disease; some patients with this deficiency have a chronic hemolytic anemia. In phosphofructokinase deficiency, low levels of erythrocyte ATP lead to low-grade hemolysis, but the limiting symptoms are usually weakness and muscle pain on exertion. Children with phosphoglycerate kinase have associated neuromuscular manifestations including seizures, spasticity, and mental retardation.

These enzymopathies are associated with anemia of variable severity. Peripheral blood smears from patients with PK deficiency show small dense crenated cells (echinocytes) (Figure 6-11). In the more severe cases, marked reticulocytosis, nucleated RBCs, and substantial anisopoikilocytosis can be seen. The MCV is usually normal or increased, reflecting the contribution of reticulocytes. An increase in the reticulocyte count (up to 70%) is observed after splenectomy.

Patients with severe hemolysis should receive folate supplementation. Splenectomy is generally reserved for patients with poor quality of life, chronic transfusion requirements, need for cholecystectomy, and persistent severe anemia. The response is variable, but most patients with PK deficiency benefit with an increase in the Hb level. Splenectomy may be complicated by postoperative thromboembolic phenomena.

Abnormalities of the hexose-monophosphate shunt

G6PD deficiency is the most frequently encountered abnormality of RBC metabolism, affecting >200 million people worldwide. A survival advantage has been noted in G6PD-deficient patients infected with *P falciparum* malaria, possibly accounting for its high gene frequency,

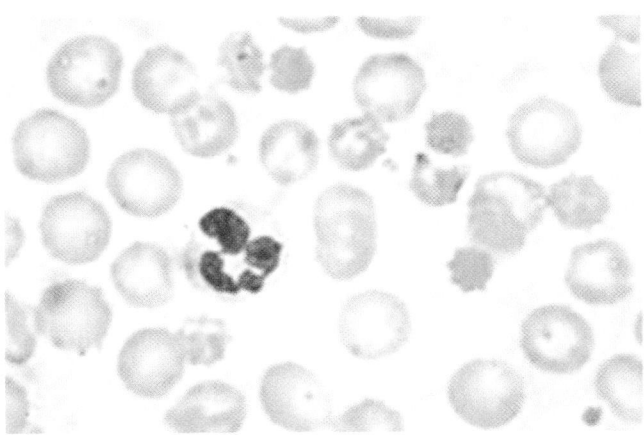

Figure 6-11 Pyruvate kinase deficiency. The peripheral blood film shows many small dense crenated cells (echinocytes).

especially in endemic regions. The gene for G6PD is carried on the X chromosome and exhibits extensive polymorphism. Enzyme deficiency is observed in males carrying a variant gene. Females with a variant gene have 2 clonal RBC populations, 1 normal and 1 deficient; the clinical presentation depends on the extent of inactivation ("lyonization") of the affected X chromosome bearing the abnormal gene. Worldwide, >300 genetic variants of G6PD have been described and are categorized according to whether the defect leads to normal activity, moderately deficient activity, or severely deficient activity, and whether it is associated with hemolytic anemia. G6PD enzyme variants are distinguished based on electrophoretic mobility. G6PD B, the wild-type enzyme, and G6PD A$^+$, a common variant in the African American population, demonstrate normal enzyme activity and are not associated with hemolysis. G6PD A$^-$ is present in approximately 10% to 15% of African American males. This variant is an unstable enzyme, which results in a decrease in enzyme activity in aged RBCs. In contrast, other G6PD variants have reduced catalytic activity and marked instability or are produced at a decreased rate, rendering both reticulocytes and older cells susceptible to hemolysis. Enzymatic deficiency of this type is seen in up to 5% of persons of Mediterranean or Asian ancestry, as well as Ashkenazi Jews. The common example of this deficiency is the G6PD B variant, G6PD Mediterranean.

Hemolysis in G6PD-deficient RBCs is due to a failure to generate adequate NADPH, leading to insufficient levels of reduced glutathione. This renders erythrocytes susceptible to oxidation of Hb by oxidant radicals such as hydrogen peroxide. The resulting denatured Hb aggregates and forms intraerythrocytic Heinz bodies, which bind to membrane cytoskeletal proteins. Membrane proteins are also subject to oxidation, leading to decreased cellular deformability. Cells containing Heinz bodies are entrapped or partially destroyed in the spleen, resulting in loss of cell membranes through pitting of Heinz bodies and leading to hemolysis.

The severity of hemolytic anemia in patients with G6PD deficiency depends on the type of defect, the level of enzyme activity in the erythrocytes, and the severity of the oxidant challenge. Ingestion of an oxidant drug is sometimes the precipitating cause (Table 6-7). Hemolytic anemia in patients with G6PD deficiency may first be recognized during an acute clinical event that induces oxidant stress, such as infection, diabetic ketoacidosis, or severe liver injury. In children, either infection or exposure to naphthalene (moth balls) is a common precipitating event. Individuals with G6PD A$^-$ do not manifest anemia until they are exposed to an oxidant drug or other oxidant challenge. Such an exposure may provoke an acute hemolytic episode with intravascular hemolysis. In the G6PD A$^-$ variant, an adequate reticulocyte response can result in restoration of the hematocrit even if the offending drug is continued because the newly formed reticulocytes are relatively resistant to oxidant stress given their higher G6PD levels. Women heterozygous for G6PD A$^-$ usually experience only mild anemia because a population of G6PD normal cells coexists. Men and heterozygous women with the G6PD Mediterranean variant can experience severe hemolysis in face of oxidant stress, and the offending agent must be removed because the reticulocytes have low enzyme levels and are prone to hemolysis.

Table 6-7 Agents that cause clinically significant hemolysis in patients with G6PD deficiency.

Acetanilide	Pentaquine
Dapsone	Phenylhydrazine
Dimercaptosuccinic acid	Phenazopyridine
Furazolidone	Primaquine
Glibenclamide	Sulfacetamide
Isobutyl nitrite	Sulfamethoxazole
Methylene blue	Sulfanilamide
Nalidixic acid	Sulfapyridine
Naphthalene	Thiazolesulfone
Niridazole	Toluidine blue
Nitrofurantoin	Trinitrotoluene (TNT)
Pamaquine	Urate oxidase

Data from Beutler E. Glucose-6-phosphate dehydrogenase deficiency. In: Starbury JB, Wyngaarden JB, Frederickson DS, et al, eds. *The Metabolic Basis of Inherited Disease*. 5th ed. New York, NY: McGraw-Hill; 1983. Updated from Beutler E. Glucose-6-phosphate dehydrogenase deficiency and other red cell enzyme abnormalities. In: Beutler E, Lichtman MA, Coller BS, et al, eds. *Williams Hematology*. 6th ed. New York, NY: McGraw-Hill; 2001.
G6PD = glucose-6-phosphate dehydrogenase.

Certain G6PD variants may result in a congenital nonspherocytic hemolytic anemia with persistent splenomegaly. Affected individuals are extremely susceptible to the oxidant stress associated with the drugs and disorders mentioned previously and may also exhibit severe hemolysis ("favism") after ingestion of fava beans. Hemolytic anemia due to favism may be severe or even fatal, particularly in children. Newborns with G6PD Mediterranean or other variants can exhibit jaundice. The G6PD A$^-$ variant is not usually associated with an increased risk of pathologic jaundice in term infants, but in premature infants, significant jaundice can occur.

When hemolytic anemia occurs after the ingestion of an oxidant drug or in association with the clinical states leading to oxidant stress, the patient should be evaluated for G6PD

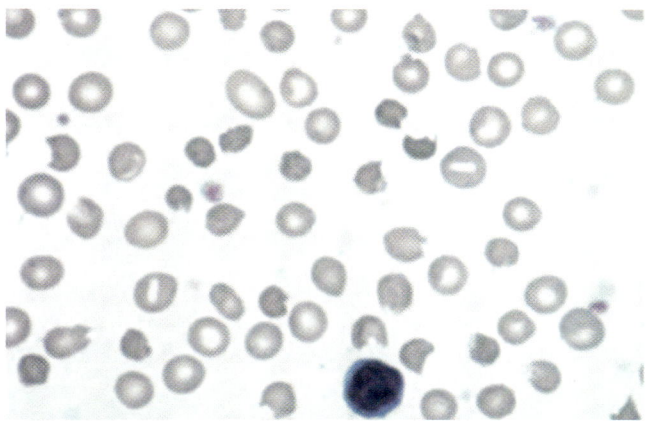

Figure 6-12 Glucose-6-phosphate dehydrogenase deficiency. The peripheral blood smear shows several red blood cells with the hemoglobin confined to one side of the cells with the remainder appearing as a hemoglobin-free ghost (eccentrocytes).

deficiency. There may be significant anemia, hyperbilirubinemia, elevated plasma Hb, and hemoglobinuria due to brisk intravascular hemolysis. G6PD deficiency should also be considered in an individual with evidence of chronic DAT-negative hemolysis. The peripheral blood smear reveals RBCs with the Hb confined to one side of the cells, with the remainder appearing as an Hb-free ghost (eccentrocytes) (Figure 6-12). The morphology has previously been described as bite or blister cells, interpreted as the result of removal of denatured Hb by the spleen; however, it appears that the accumulated oxidized Hb actually remains and is adherent to the RBC membrane. Brilliant cresyl blue staining may reveal Heinz bodies. Screening or quantitative biochemical assays can be used to make the diagnosis. In the G6PD A⁻ variant, during an acute hemolytic episode, an elevated reticulocyte count will raise the mean level of erythrocyte G6PD and render a false-negative result. G6PD levels should therefore be checked several months after the acute event when there will be RBCs of varying ages. Although defects of other hexose-monophosphate shunt enzymes (eg, phosphogluconate dehydrogenase, glutathione reductase) are rare, they should be considered in cases of oxidant-induced hemolysis in which G6PD levels are normal.

Abnormalities of nucleotide metabolism

Pyrimidine-5'-nucleotidase deficiency is an enzymatic abnormality of pyrimidine metabolism associated with hemolytic anemia. The peripheral blood smear in patients with this defect often shows RBCs containing coarse basophilic stippling. Lead intoxication also inactivates the enzyme, leading to an acquired variant of pyrimidine-5'-nucleotidase deficiency.

Adenosine deaminase (ADA) excess is an unusual abnormality. It is caused by a genetically determined increase in the activity of a normal erythrocyte enzyme. The excessive deaminase activity prevents normal salvage of adenosine and causes subsequent depletion of ATP and hemolysis.

> **Clinical case (continued)**
>
> The patient presented in this section should be suspected of having G6PD deficiency. Patients with the African American variant (G6PD A⁻) are often asymptomatic until they ingest medication or experience an infection, which leads to oxidant stress of the RBCs. Trimethoprim/sulfamethoxazole may be an offending agent. During the early phases of hemolysis, bite cells can be seen on review of the peripheral blood smear. A Heinz body preparation will show the typical inclusions, which consist of denatured Hb. G6PD levels should not be measured in the acute setting, because values may be normal, given the reticulocytosis. Treatment is primarily supportive. Offending drugs should be discontinued, and alternative agents should be chosen. However, if the prescribed agent is necessary and cannot be substituted, a trial of continuation is reasonable because hemolysis is often compensated in the G6PD A⁻ variant even if drug administration is continued.

> **Key points**
>
> - The glycolytic pathway provides the erythrocyte with the ATP necessary for maintenance of membrane integrity, preservation of ferrous Hb, and oxygen affinity. Additional products of the pathway are NADH for methemoglobin reduction and 2,3-BPG for regulating the oxygen affinity of Hb.
> - Glucose metabolism through the hexose-monophosphate shunt produces NADPH to maintain the antioxidative activity of the RBC.
> - Enzymopathies represent a major consideration in the differential diagnosis of inherited DAT-negative nonspherocytic hemolytic anemias.
> - PK deficiency is the most common defect of the glycolytic pathway. The echinocyte is the characteristic abnormality observed on the peripheral blood smear.
> - The most common enzyme deficiency is G6PD, with >300 genetic variants. Oxidant stress in the presence of deficient G6PD activity results in hemolysis with the generation of bite cells (eccentrocytes).
> - In the G6PD A⁻ deficiency, a quantitative measurement of the enzyme levels should be delayed until after the acute hemolytic episode. In the G6PD B variant, levels are low in RBCs of all ages.
> - Defects of purine and pyrimidine metabolism are infrequent. The peripheral blood smear in pyrimidine-5'-nucleotidase deficiency shows RBCs with coarse basophilic stippling.

Hemolysis due to extrinsic abnormalities of the RBC

> **Clinical case**
>
> A 68-year-old male is admitted to the hospital with complaints of weakness, shortness of breath, and chest pain. Over the prior year, he experienced weight loss and intermittent night sweats and generally felt poorly. His prior history is significant for diet-controlled diabetes and elevated cholesterol. He is taking no medications. On examination, he appears chronically ill and pale. Scleral icterus is noted. Axillary adenopathy and splenomegaly are appreciated. His fingertips are mildly cyanotic appearing. Laboratory data are significant for a spun hematocrit of 24% and an MCV of 143 fL. LDH is elevated at 2321 U/L, indirect bilirubin at 2.1 mg/dL, and reticulocyte count at 13%. The peripheral blood smear shows agglutinated RBCs. The blood bank reports a direct Coombs test positive for complement (3+) but negative for immunoglobulin (Ig) G. Serum protein electrophoresis reveals a monoclonal IgM. Abdominal CT scan reveals splenomegaly and diffuse adenopathy.

Hemolytic anemia due to immune injury to RBCs

In autoimmune hemolytic anemia (AHA), shortened RBC survival is mediated by autoantibodies. AHA is classified by the temperature at which autoantibodies bind optimally to the patient RBCs. In adults, the majority of cases (80%-90%) are mediated by antibodies that bind to RBCs at 37°C (warm autoantibodies). In the cryopathic hemolytic anemias, the autoantibodies bind most avidly to RBCs at temperatures <37°C (cold autoantibodies). Some patients exhibit both warm and cold reactive autoantibodies. These cases are classified as mixed AHA.

The warm- and cold-antibody classifications are further divided by the presence or absence of an underlying related disease. When no underlying disease is recognized, the AHA is termed *primary* or *idiopathic*. *Secondary* cases are those in which the AHA is a manifestation or complication of an underlying disorder. In general, the secondary classification should be used in preference to idiopathic only when the AHA and the underlying disease occur together more often than random and when the AHA resolves with successful treatment of the underlying disease. The connection is strengthened when the underlying disease has a component of immunologic aberration. Using these criteria, primary (idiopathic) AHA and secondary AHA occur with approximately equal frequency.

Certain drugs may also cause immune destruction of RBCs by 3 different mechanisms. Some drugs induce formation of true autoantibodies directed against RBC antigens. The hapten-drug adsorption mechanism is characterized by the presence of antidrug antibodies in the blood. These antibodies bind only to RBC membranes that are coated with tightly bound drug. In a third type of drug-immune hemolytic anemia, antibodies recognize a neoantigen formed by a drug or its metabolite and an epitope of a specific membrane antigen. This is termed *ternary* or *immune complex mechanism*. In some, if not all, cases mediated by the ternary (immune) complex mechanism, antibodies may recognize both a drug or its metabolite and an epitope of a specific RBC antigen. The classification of the immune hemolytic anemias is shown in Table 6-8.

Pathophysiology
Warm AHA

The most common type of AHA is mediated by warm-reactive autoantibodies of the IgG isotype. Warm-reacting IgG antibodies bind optimally to antigens on RBCs at 37°C and may or may not fix complement, but they typically do not cause direct agglutination of RBCs due to their small size. Enhanced destruction of antibody-coated RBCs is mediated by Fc receptor–expressing macrophages, primarily located in the spleen. Partial phagocytosis results in the formation of spherocytes that may circulate for a time but eventually become entrapped in the spleen, resulting in enhanced RBC destruction.

Cold AHA

In contrast to warm-reactive autoantibodies, cold-reactive autoantibodies bind optimally to RBCs at temperatures <37°C. Cold autoantibodies are typically of the IgM isotype, and because of their large, pentameric conformation, they are able to span the distance between several RBCs to cause direct agglutination. Their ability to injure RBCs is dependent on their ability to fix complement. The consequence of complement fixation is clearance of C3b-coated cells by attachment to complement receptors on macrophages, primarily in the spleen, and Kupffer cells in the liver. Direct lysis by completion of the terminal complement sequence may also occur. Cold autoantibodies are characteristic of AHA associated with *Mycoplasma* infection, as well as with Epstein-Barr virus–related disease. In addition, cold agglutinin disease is typically seen in the elderly, almost always associated with B-cell lymphoproliferative disorders; it is caused by a monoclonal IgM antibody that binds to carbohydrate I antigens or i antigens at temperatures below body temperature. Cold-reacting IgG (Donath-Landsteiner) autoantibodies, seen in paroxysmal cold hemoglobinuria, may cause significant intravascular lysis of RBCs as a result of their ability to fix complement. Donath-Landsteiner hemolytic anemia

Table 6-8 Classification of immune injury to red blood cells.

  I. Warm-autoantibody type: autoantibody maximally active at 37°C
   A. Primary or idiopathic warm AHA
   B. Secondary warm AHA
   1. Associated with lymphoproliferative disorders (eg, Hodgkin disease, lymphoma)
   2. Associated with the rheumatic disorders (eg, SLE)
   3. Associated with certain nonlymphoid neoplasms (eg, ovarian tumors)
   4. Associated with certain chronic inflammatory diseases (eg, ulcerative colitis)
   5. Associated with ingestion of certain drugs (eg, α-methyldopa)
 II. Cold-autoantibody type: autoantibody optimally active at temperatures [lt]37°C
   A. Mediated by cold agglutinins
   1. Idiopathic (primary) chronic cold agglutinin disease (usually associated with clonal B-lymphocyte proliferation)
   2. Secondary cold agglutinin hemolytic anemia
   a. Postinfectious (eg, *Mycoplasma pneumoniae* or infectious mononucleosis)
   b. Associated with malignant B-cell lymphoproliferative disorder
   B. Mediated by cold hemolysins
   1. Idiopathic (primary) paroxysmal cold hemoglobinuria
   2. Secondary
   a. Donath-Landsteiner hemolytic anemia, usually associated with an acute viral syndrome in children (relatively common)
   b. Associated with congenital or tertiary syphilis in adults
III. Mixed cold and warm autoantibodies
   A. Primary or idiopathic mixed AHA
   B. Secondary mixed AHA
   1. Associated with the rheumatic disorders, particularly SLE
 IV. Drug-immune hemolytic anemia
   A. Hapten or drug adsorption mechanism
   B. Ternary (immune) complex mechanism
   C. True autoantibody mechanism
   D. Nonimmunologic protein adsorption (probably does not cause hemolysis)

Adapted from Packman CH. Hemolytic anemia resulting from immune injury. In: *Williams Hematology*. 7th ed. New York, NY: McGraw-Hill; 2006. AHA = autoimmune hemolytic anemia; SLE = systemic lupus erythematosus.

accounts for almost one third of AHA cases in children. Donath-Landsteiner autoantibodies bind to antigens in the P system.

Mixed AHA

Some cases of AHA are associated with the presence of both IgM and IgG autoantibodies. Hemolysis is generally more severe in these cases. AHA due to IgA antibodies is rare. IgA autoantibodies are usually accompanied by IgG autoantibodies. The mechanisms for RBC destruction appear to be similar to those for IgG.

Drug-induced immune hemolytic anemia

The clinical and laboratory features of drug-induced and idiopathic hemolytic anemia are similar, so a careful history of drug exposure should be obtained in the initial evaluation. The number of drugs that can cause immune hemolytic anemia is large and encompasses a broad spectrum of chemical classes (Table 6-9). Three basic mechanisms of drug-induced immune RBC injury are recognized. A fourth mechanism may lead to nonimmunologic deposition of multiple serum proteins, including immunoglobulins, albumin, fibrinogen, and others, on RBCs, but RBC injury does not occur. The mechanisms of drug-induced immune hemolytic anemia and positive DATs are summarized in Table 6-10.

Hapten or drug adsorption mechanism

This mechanism applies to drugs that bind firmly to proteins on the RBC membrane. The classic setting is very high-dose penicillin therapy, but other drugs such as cephalosporins and semisynthetic penicillins are also implicated. The antibody responsible for hemolytic anemia by this mechanism is of the IgG class and directed against epitopes of the drug itself. Other manifestations of drug sensitivity, such as hives or anaphylaxis, are not usually present. The antibody binds to drug molecules attached to the RBC membrane.

Table 6-9 Drugs associated with immune injury to red blood cells or a positive direct antiglobulin test.

Hapten or Drug Adsorption Mechanism
- Carbromal
- Cephalosporins
- Cianidanol
- Hydrocortisone
- 6-Mercaptopurine
- Oxaliplatin
- Penicillins
- Tetracycline
- Tolbutamide

Ternary-Immune Complex Mechanism
- Amphotericin B
- Antazoline
- Cephalosporins
- Chlorpropamide
- Diclofenac
- Diethylstilbestrol
- Doxepin
- Etodolac
- Hydrocortisone
- Metformin
- Nomifensine
- Oxaliplatin
- Pemetrexed
- Probenecid
- Quinine
- Quinidine
- Rifampicin
- Stibophen
- Thiopental
- Tolmetin

Autoantibody Mechanism
- Cephalosporins
- Cianidanol
- Cladribine
- Diclofenac
- l-Dopa
- Efalizumab
- Fludarabine
- Glafenine
- Latamoxef
- Lenalidomide
- Mefenamic acid
- α-Methyldopa
- Nomifensine
- Oxaliplatin
- Pentostatin
- Procainamide
- Teniposide
- Tolmetin

Nonimmunologic Protein Adsorption
- Carboplatin
- Cephalosporins
- Cisplatin
- Oxaliplatin

Uncertain Mechanism of Immune Injury
- Acetaminophen
- p-Aminosalicylic acid
- Carboplatin
- Chlorpromazine
- Efavirenz
- Erythromycin
- Fluorouracil
- Ibuprofen
- Insecticides
- Isoniazid
- Melphalan
- Mephenytoin
- Nalidixic acid
- Omeprazole
- Phenacetin
- Streptomycin
- Sulindac
- Temafloxacin
- Thiazides
- Triamterene

Antibodies eluted from patients' RBCs or present in their sera react in the indirect antiglobulin test (IAT) only against drug-coated RBCs, which distinguishes these drug-dependent antibodies from true autoantibodies. Destruction of RBCs coated with drug and IgG antidrug antibody occurs mainly through sequestration by splenic macrophages. Hemolytic anemia typically occurs 7 to 10 days after the drug is started and ceases a few days to 2 weeks after the patient discontinues taking the drug.

Ternary or immune complex mechanism: drug–antibody–target cell interaction

Drugs in this group exhibit only weak direct binding to blood cell membranes. A relatively small dose of drug is capable of triggering destruction of blood cells. Blood cell injury is mediated by a cooperative interaction among 3 reactants to generate a ternary complex consisting of the drug or a drug metabolite, a drug-binding membrane site (an antigen) on the target cell, and a drug-dependent antibody. The drug-dependent antibody is thought to bind, through its Fab domain, to a compound neoantigen consisting of loosely bound drug and a blood group antigen intrinsic to the RBC membrane. The pathogenic antibody recognizes the drug only in combination with a particular membrane structure of the RBC (eg, a known alloantigen). Binding of the drug itself to the target cell membrane is weak until the attachment of the antibody to *both* drug and cell membrane is stabilized. Yet the binding of the antibody is drug dependent. RBC destruction occurs intravascularly after completion of the whole complement sequence, often resulting in hemoglobinemia and hemoglobinuria. The DAT is positive usually only for complement.

Autoantibody mechanism

Several drugs, by unknown mechanisms, induce the formation of autoantibodies reactive with RBCs in the absence of the instigating drug. The most studied drug in this category has been α-methyldopa, but levodopa and other drugs also have been implicated. Patients with chronic lymphocytic leukemia treated with pentostatin, fludarabine, or cladribine may have severe and sometimes fatal autoimmune hemolysis, although the mechanisms of autoantibody induction are likely different, most likely involving dysregulation of T lymphocytes.

Nonimmunologic protein adsorption

A small proportion (~5%) of patients receiving cephalosporin antibiotics, cisplatin and carboplatin, develop positive antiglobulin reactions due to nonspecific adsorption of plasma proteins to their RBC membranes. This process may occur within 1 to 2 days after the drug is instituted. Multiple plasma proteins, including immunoglobulins, complement, albumin, fibrinogen, and others, may be detected on RBC membranes in such cases. Hemolytic anemia resulting from this mechanism does not occur. However, this phenomenon may complicate crossmatch procedures unless the drug history is considered.

Table 6-10 Immune hemolytic anemia and positive direct antiglobulin reactions caused by drugs.

	Hapten or drug adsorption	Ternary immune complex formation	Autoantibody formation	Nonimmunologic protein adsorption
Prototype drug	Penicillin	Third-generation cephalosporins	α-Methyldopa	Cephalothin
Role of drug	Binds to red blood cell membrane	Forms 3-way complex with antibody and red blood cell membrane component	Induces antibody to native red blood cell antigen	Possibly alters red blood cell membrane
Drug affinity to cell	Strong	Weak	None demonstrated	Strong
Antibody to drug	Present	Present	Absent	Absent
Antibody class predominating	IgG	IgM or IgG	IgG	None
Proteins detected by direct antiglobulin test	IgG, rarely complement	Complement	IgG, rarely complement	Multiple plasma proteins
Dose of drug associated with positive antiglobulin test	High	Low	High	High
Mechanism of red blood cell destruction	Splenic sequestration	Direct lysis by complement plus splenic sequestration	Splenic sequestration	None

Modified from Packman CH. Hemolytic anemia resulting from immune injury. In: *Williams Hematology*. 7th ed. New York, NY: McGraw-Hill; 2006. Ig = immunoglobulin.

Clinical manifestations and laboratory findings

Several clinical features of AHA are common to both warm- and cold-antibody types. Patients may present with signs and symptoms of anemia (eg, weakness, dizziness), jaundice, abdominal pain, and fever. Mild splenomegaly is common. Hepatomegaly and lymphadenopathy may be evident at presentation depending on the etiology. Anemia may vary from mild to severe, usually with either normocytic or macrocytic cells. Patients most frequently present with reticulocytosis. However, reticulocytopenia may initially be present up to one third of the time as a result of intercurrent folate deficiency, infection, involvement of the marrow by a neoplastic process, or nonidentifiable causes. Indirect bilirubin and LDH are elevated to varying degrees, and the haptoglobin is depressed. The blood smear often demonstrates spherocytes (Figure 6-13). Nucleated RBCs may also be present.

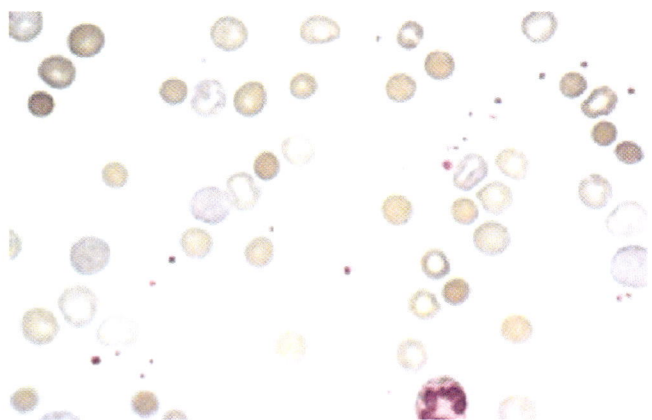

Figure 6-13 Warm-antibody autoimmune hemolytic anemia. Note the small round spherocytes and the large, gray polychromatophilic erythrocytes.

The onset of warm-antibody AHA may be rapid or insidious, but rarely is it so severe as to cause hemoglobinuria. Presenting symptoms are usually related to anemia or jaundice. In secondary cases, the presenting complaint is usually related to the underlying disease.

Patients with idiopathic or primary cold agglutinin disease usually have mild to moderate chronic hemolysis. Acute exacerbations can be associated with cold exposure. Spontaneous autoagglutination of RBCs at room temperature may be seen as clumps of cells on the blood smear (Figure 6-14). Occasionally spurious marked elevations in the MCV and MCHC measurements and decrease in the RBC count are observed due to simultaneous passage of 2 or 3 agglutinated RBCs through the aperture of the automated cell counter.

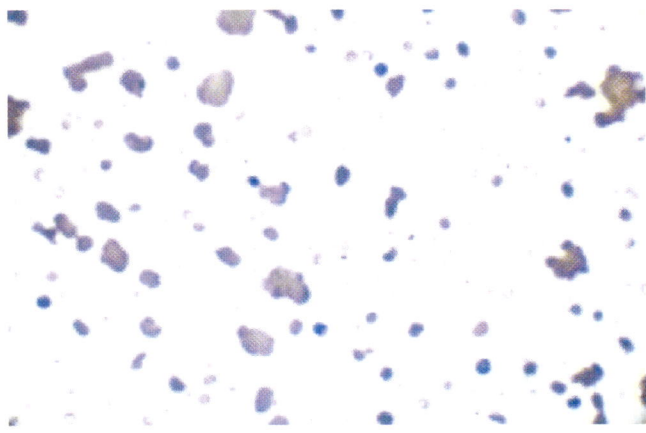

Figure 6-14 Cold agglutinin disease.

Drug-immune hemolytic anemia due to the hapten or true autoantibody mechanism is usually mild. In contrast, hemolysis due to the ternary or immune complex mechanism can be acute in onset, severe, and sometimes fatal.

The DAT (Coombs test) is usually positive in AHA but may be negative in some patients. The threshold of detection of commercial antiglobulin reagents, which detect mainly IgG and fragments of C3, is approximately 200 to 500 antibody molecules per cell. However, <100 molecules of IgG per cell may significantly shorten RBC survival in vivo. IgM cold agglutinins are usually removed from RBCs during washing and are not usually detected. IgA is usually not detected by most commercial reagents. When monospecific anti-IgG and anti-C3 reagents are used, 30% to 40% of patients with AHA will have only IgG on their RBCs; a slightly larger number will have both IgG and C3; and only approximately 10% will have C3 alone. The major reaction patterns of the DAT and their differential diagnosis are summarized in Table 6-11.

The strength of the direct Coombs test has poor clinical correlation with severity of hemolysis among patients, but in a given patient over time, the degree of hemolysis correlates fairly well with the current strength of the antiglobulin reaction. In the rare case of direct Coombs test–negative hemolytic anemia suspected of having an immune etiology, the diagnosis can sometimes be confirmed by using more sensitive assays for RBC-bound immunoglobulin, such as an enzyme-linked immunoadsorbent assay (ELISA) or radiolabeled anti-immunoglobulin. Specific assays for cell-bound IgA may also be worthwhile. In cold agglutinin disease, the DAT is positive with anti-C3 only.

Table 6-11 Differential diagnosis of reaction patterns of the direct antiglobulin test.

Reaction pattern	Differential diagnosis
IgG alone	Warm-antibody autoimmune hemolytic anemia
	Drug-immune hemolytic anemia: hapten/drug adsorption type or autoantibody type
Complement alone	Warm-antibody autoimmune hemolytic anemia with subthreshold IgG deposition
	Cold agglutinin disease
	Paroxysmal cold hemoglobinuria
	Drug-immune hemolytic anemia: ternary immune complex type
IgG plus complement	Warm-antibody autoimmune hemolytic anemia
	Drug-immune hemolytic anemia: autoantibody type (rare)

IgG = immunoglobulin G.

Approximately 1 in 10,000 healthy blood donors have a positive DAT. The positive DAT in these individuals is usually due to warm-reacting IgG autoantibodies, indistinguishable from those occurring in AHA. Many of these individuals never develop AHA, but some do. It is not known how many of these normal individuals with a positive DAT may eventually develop AHA.

Treatment

Asymptomatic patients develop anemia over a period sufficient to allow for cardiovascular compensation and do not require RBC transfusions. However, for patients with symptomatic coronary artery disease or patients who rapidly develop severe anemia with circulatory failure, as in paroxysmal cold hemoglobinuria or ternary (immune) complex drug-immune hemolysis, transfusions can be lifesaving.

Transfusion of RBCs in immune hemolytic anemia is often problematic. Finding a serocompatible donor blood is rarely possible. It is most important to identify the patient's ABO type to find either ABO-identical or ABO-compatible blood for transfusion to avoid a hemolytic transfusion reaction. The difficult technical issue relates to detection of RBC alloantibodies masked by the presence of the autoantibody.

Clinicians and blood bank physicians no longer speak of "least incompatible" blood for transfusion because all units will be serologically incompatible. However, units incompatible due to autoantibody are less dangerous to transfuse than units incompatible due to alloantibody. Patients with a history of pregnancy, abortion, or prior transfusion are at risk of harboring an alloantibody. Patients who have never been pregnant or transfused with blood products are unlikely to harbor an alloantibody. Consultation between the clinician and the blood bank physician should occur early to allow for informed discussion and confident transfusion of mismatched blood if the situation demands.

The selected RBCs should be transfused slowly while the patient is monitored carefully for signs of a hemolytic transfusion reaction. Even if transfused cells are rapidly destroyed, the increased oxygen-carrying capacity provided by the transfused cells may maintain the patient during the time required for other modes of therapy to become effective.

In AHA, therapy is aimed at decreasing the production of autoantibody and at decreasing clearance of RBCs from the circulation. For warm-antibody IgG-mediated hemolysis, glucocorticoids such as prednisone are usually the first-line treatment in all but drug-induced syndromes (for which removal of the offending agent is the principal treatment). Glucocorticoids decrease the ability of macrophages to clear IgG- or complement-coated erythrocytes and reduce autoantibody production. After remission is achieved with prednisone at approximately 60 to 100 mg/d (or 1 mg/kg/d), the dose should be decreased by 10 mg/d each week until a dose of 30 mg/d is reached. Subsequent dose reduction should then proceed more slowly (at 5 mg/d per week), with the goal of either maintaining remission with prednisone at 20 to 40 mg every other day or complete weaning of prednisone if the DAT becomes negative; this goal is not always achievable. Approximately two thirds of adult patients respond to prednisone, with approximately 20% achieving complete remission. Pulses of high-dose glucocorticoids (eg, 1 g methylprednisolone intravenously) are effective in some patients in whom standard therapy has failed.

Splenectomy is often considered if hemolysis remains severe for 2 to 3 weeks at prednisone doses of 1 mg/kg, if remission cannot be maintained on low doses of prednisone, or if the patient has intolerable adverse effects or contraindications to glucocorticoids. Removing the spleen results in a reduced rate of clearance of IgG-coated cells. Although not usually recommended in children, splenectomy in patients past adolescence appears relatively safe. Patients should receive pneumococcal, *H influenzae*, and meningococcal vaccines before splenectomy. Approximately two thirds of patients will have complete or partial remission with splenectomy, but relapses are common.

Other therapies may be effective for patients with refractory hemolysis or for those who relapse after glucocorticoids or splenectomy. Monoclonal anti-CD20 (rituximab) has been useful in refractory cases, including adults and children, with response rates ranging from 40% to 100%. Immunosuppressive drugs such as cyclophosphamide, azathioprine, mycophenolate mofetil, and cyclosporine, as well as the nonvirilizing androgen, danazol, have been used with varying degrees of success. Intravenous Ig has been less successful in treatment of AHA than in immune thrombocytopenic purpura.

For patients with idiopathic cold agglutinin disease, maintaining a warm environment may be all that is needed to avoid symptomatic anemia. Cold agglutinin disease usually does not respond to glucocorticoids. Recently, rituximab has demonstrated efficacy in treating cold agglutinin disease, with response rates approaching 50%. Chlorambucil and cyclophosphamide have been beneficial in selected cases. Chemotherapy is indicated if the disorder is associated with a lymphoproliferative disorder. Splenectomy is usually not indicated because cells are usually cleared by intravascular hemolysis or hepatic Kupffer cells. Intravenous Ig does not have a role in management. Plasmapheresis may be temporarily effective in acute situations by removing IgM cold agglutinin from the circulation.

AHA during childhood tends to occur suddenly, during or after an acute infection. As many as one third of cases are associated with intravascular hemolysis due to a Donath-Landsteiner antibody directed against the erythrocyte P antigen. Usually these patients exhibit only a single paroxysm of hemolysis. In warm-antibody hemolytic anemia, acute management is similar to that for adults. Approximately two thirds of children recover completely within a matter of weeks. Only a small percentage of children (but a larger proportion of adolescents) exhibit more chronic refractory disease that warrants consideration of other pharmacologic agents or splenectomy.

Clinical case (continued)

The patient presented in this section has cold agglutinin disease, likely secondary to underlying lymphoma. Automated techniques reveal that the RBC count is artifactually low and the MCV and MCHC are falsely elevated secondary to RBC agglutination. Warming of the blood tube with immediate measurement and slide preparation will minimize agglutination. The DAT is positive only for complement. Lymphoproliferative disorders are well-identified underlying etiologies. The patient should be maintained in a warm environment. Amelioration of the anemia can be anticipated with cytotoxic therapy for the lymphoma.

Key points

- Warm antibody–induced immune hemolytic anemia is typically IgG mediated and results in spherocytic RBCs.
- Cold agglutinin disease is IgM mediated with associated complement activation. The peripheral blood smear reveals RBC agglutination and spherocytes.
- A variety of drugs cause immune hemolytic anemia. Clinical laboratory support of the diagnosis may not be available. Discontinuation of the suspected offending drug is indicated.
- Symptoms due to AHA are typically indistinguishable from other causes of hemolysis.
- The DAT is the primary tool for diagnosing AHA. It is rarely positive in healthy individuals and may be negative in AHA.
- Warm antibody–mediated AHA is treated with glucocorticoids, other immunosuppressive agents such as rituximab, and splenectomy.
- Avoidance of cold environments may be sufficient to avoid complications of cold agglutinin disease. Chemotherapy and rituximab have a role, and plasmapheresis can occasionally be helpful in the acute and temporary management of symptomatic cases by physically removing the antibody.
- Immune-mediated hemolytic anemia is uncommon in children. Most cases are acute and transient, following viral infection.
- Transfusion therapy can be difficult in patients with AHA. Consultation with the blood bank is important. A history of prior pregnancy, abortion, or transfusion of blood products should be obtained because these patients are at risk of harboring dangerous alloantibodies. No patient with AHA should be allowed to die because serologically "compatible" RBCs are not available.

Paroxysmal nocturnal hemoglobinuria

> **Clinical case**
>
> A previously healthy 37-year-old female is admitted to the hospital for evaluation of severe abdominal pain. Workup reveals mesenteric vein thrombosis. The patient is treated with thrombolytic therapy and anticoagulated with heparin, leading to clinical improvement. She has no prior or family history of thrombosis. She is currently taking an oral contraceptive. Her examination is significant for mild scleral icterus and jaundice. There is no abdominal tenderness. Mild splenomegaly is noted. Laboratory studies are significant for a hematocrit of 32% with a corrected reticulocyte count of 8%. White blood cell count and platelet count are slightly depressed. Indirect bilirubin is elevated at 4 mg/dL, but AST, ALT, and alkaline phosphatase are normal. LDH is also increased at 1024 U/L. Blood bank evaluation confirms a Coombs-negative hemolytic anemia. A bone marrow aspirate and biopsy are hypocellular and reveal findings concerning for early myelodysplasia.

PNH should be considered in the patient with unexplained hemolysis, pancytopenia, or unprovoked thrombosis. PNH is an acquired clonal disorder of hematopoietic stem cells occurring in both children and adults with no apparent familial predisposition.

Pathophysiology

Hemolysis in PNH is due to the action of complement on abnormal RBCs. Compared with normal RBCs, PNH RBCs lyse more readily in the presence of activated complement. Earlier tests to diagnose PNH (eg, Ham test or acid hemolysis test; sucrose hemolysis test) were based on this property of PNH RBCs. It is now known that PNH granulocytes and platelets are sensitive to complement as well.

The biochemical basis of complement sensitivity was initially elusive. Early on, PNH blood cells were found to be deficient in leukocyte alkaline phosphatase and erythrocyte acetylcholinesterase. However, neither of these deficiencies explained the complement sensitivity or the clinical manifestations in PNH. Subsequently, 2 complement regulatory proteins, CD55 (decay accelerating factor [DAF]) and CD59 (homologous restriction factor or membrane inhibitor of reactive lysis [MIRL]), were also found to be missing from PNH blood cells, helping to explain the unusual sensitivity of RBCs to the hemolytic action of complement. Of these, CD59, whose action is to inhibit the terminal complement sequence leading to hemolysis, seems to be the most important.

The approximately 20 proteins missing from the hematopoietic cells in PNH are all attached to the membrane by a glycosylphosphatidylinositol (GPI) anchor. Defective synthesis of the GPI anchor is due to somatic mutations in the *pig-A* gene in hematopoietic stem cells. Whereas a *pig-A* gene mutation appears to be necessary for the development of PNH and its clinical manifestations, it is not sufficient because *pig-A* mutations can be found in small numbers of hematopoietic stem cells in normal individuals. Patients with aplastic anemia exhibit a larger proportion of stem cells with *pig-A* mutations.

A multistep process seems necessary for PNH to develop. It is thought that in aplastic anemia and likely in PNH that immunologic processes suppress proliferation of normal hematopoietic precursors more efficiently than proliferation of precursors lacking GPI-anchored proteins. Resistance to apoptotic death may partly explain the "survival advantage" of these GPI-negative cells. The abnormal clones are thus able to expand until the numbers of abnormal progeny are sufficient to cause the clinical manifestations of PNH.

Two missing GPI-linked proteins may contribute to the increased incidence of thrombosis in PNH—urokinase plasminogen activator receptor, the lack of which may decrease local fibrinolysis, and tissue factor pathway inhibitor, the lack of which may increase the procoagulant activity of tissue factor. PNH platelets, which are sensitive to the lytic activity of complement, are hyperactive. RBC phospholipids released during intravascular hemolysis may also serve to initiate clotting.

Most of the clinical manifestations of the disease are due to the lack of the complement-regulating protein CD59. The monoclonal antibody eculizumab, which binds the complement component C5, thereby inhibiting terminal complement activation, decreases hemolysis of RBCs and the tendency to thrombosis as well. The drug does not seem to alter the defect in hematopoiesis. Thus, although deficient hematopoiesis is probably related to deficiency of GPI-anchored proteins, it is not related to complement sensitivity.

Laboratory findings

There are no specific morphologic abnormalities of the RBCs in PNH. RBCs may be macrocytic, normocytic, or microcytic, being the latter when iron deficiency develops because of chronic urinary iron loss from intravascular hemolysis. With or without iron deficiency, the reticulocyte count may not be as elevated as expected for the degree of anemia. This is due to underlying bone marrow dysfunction that often accompanies the PNH. Leukopenia and thrombocytopenia are often present. Serum LDH is usually elevated and may suggest the diagnosis in the patient with minimal anemia. Iron loss may amount to 20 mg/d, and urine hemosiderin is often identified. Bone marrow examination reveals erythroid hyperplasia unless there are associated bone marrow disorders.

Laboratory diagnosis

The laboratory diagnosis of PNH formerly relied on the demonstration of abnormally complement-sensitive erythrocyte populations. Ham first described the acidified serum lysis test in 1938. In that test, acidification of the serum activates the alternative pathway of complement, and increased amounts of C3 are fixed to RBCs lacking complement regulatory proteins. Complement sensitivity of PNH RBCs can also be demonstrated in high-concentration sucrose solutions, the basis for the "sugar water" or sucrose hemolysis test. These tests are primarily of historical interest and are not used routinely in the clinical laboratory because flow cytometry techniques aimed specifically at demonstrating the deficiency in expression of GPI-anchored proteins in PNH are readily available. Using commercially available monoclonal antibodies, blood cells can be analyzed for expression of the GPI-anchored proteins CD55 (DAF) and CD59 (MIRL). These methods have the sensitivity to detect small abnormal populations; because monocytes and granulocytes have short half-lives and their numbers are not affected by transfusion, analysis of GPI-anchored proteins on neutrophils or monocytes rather than RBCs is preferred.

A new assay is being used increasingly to detect GPI-deficient blood cells. The fluorescein-labeled aerolysin (FLAER) assay exploits a property of aerolysin, the principle virulence factor of the bacterium *Aeromonas hydrophila*, which binds selectively with high affinity to the GPI anchor of most cell lineages. FLAER is most useful to assay the GPI anchor on granulocytes because aerolysin binds weakly to glycophorin on RBCs.

Clinical manifestations

Although chronic hemolytic anemia is a common manifestation, only a minority of patients report nocturnal hemoglobinuria. The degree of anemia seen in PNH varies in affected individuals from minimal to quite severe. Symptoms related to episodes of hemolysis include back and abdominal pain, headache, and fever. Exacerbations of hemolysis can occur with infections, surgery, or transfusions. Several symptoms in PNH may be related to the ability of free plasma Hb to scavenge nitric oxide. These include esophageal spasm, male erectile dysfunction, renal insufficiency, and thrombosis.

Aplastic anemia has been diagnosed both before and after the identification of PNH. PNH clones are present in approximately 20% of patients with severe aplastic anemia. Approximately 20% of patients with myelodysplastic syndromes have PNH clones. Hemolysis in the setting of bone marrow hypoplasia or myelodysplastic and/or myeloproliferative disorders should suggest the diagnosis of PNH. Infections associated with leukopenia and bleeding due to thrombocytopenia contribute to increased mortality. An increased incidence of acute leukemia has also been reported.

Patients frequently have thrombotic complications that can be life threatening and may represent the initial manifestation of PNH. In addition to venous thrombosis involving an extremity, there is a propensity for thrombosis of unusual sites such as hepatic veins (Budd-Chiari syndrome), other intra-abdominal veins, cerebral veins, and venous sinuses. Thus, complaints of abdominal pain or severe headache should alert the clinician to the consideration of thrombosis in the patient with PNH. The thrombotic tendency is particularly enhanced during pregnancy.

Treatment

The clinical manifestations of PNH are highly variable among patients. For patients with PNH clones numbering <10%, no clinical intervention is needed. However, because expansion of the clone may occur, the size of the clone should be monitored every 6 to 12 months. Anemia is often the dominant issue in PNH. Glucocorticoids can reduce complement activation and decrease the hemolysis; however, high doses are frequently necessary, and every-other-day administration has been recommended to reduce the adverse effects. Iron may be required to replace the large urinary losses seen in PNH. Folate supplementation is also usually recommended. Erythropoietin (10,000-20,000 U 3 times weekly) may be helpful for patients with inadequate reticulocyte responses. Transfusion may be necessary when these measures fail to maintain adequate Hb levels.

Eculizumab is a humanized monoclonal antibody that was engineered to reduce its immunogenicity; importantly, it is unable to bind Fc receptors on cells or to activate complement. It binds to C5 and blocks the terminal complement sequence. Its use in PNH to treat hemolysis was approved by the US Food and Drug Administration based on its efficacy in 2 phase III clinical trials. Eculizumab reduces intravascular but not extravascular hemolysis, eliminates or reduces transfusion requirement in almost all patients, improves quality of life, and decreases the risk of thrombosis. It does not treat the marrow failure. It must be used indefinitely because it does not treat the underlying cause of PNH.

Although eculizumab is generally well tolerated, its most serious complication is sepsis due to *Neisseria* organisms.

Patients congenitally lacking one of the terminal complement components, C5 to C9, are known to be at risk for *Neisseria* infection. Patients receiving eculizumab are at risk because of its inhibition of the terminal complement sequence. Vaccination against *Neisseria meningitidis* is recommended 2 weeks before starting therapy. Revaccination every 3 to 5 years may be important because eculizumab is given for an indefinite period. Because vaccination does not eliminate the risk completely, patients should be told to seek medical attention for any symptoms consistent with *Neisseria* infection.

Allogeneic hematopoietic stem cell transplantation is the only known cure for PNH. However, because of the high risk for serious complications including death, such treatment should be reserved for patients with severe pancytopenias or the rare individuals whose hemolysis or thrombosis is not controlled by eculizumab. For patients with PNH and marrow failure who lack an HLA-matched sibling donor, immunosuppressive therapy may be attempted.

Thrombosis is the leading cause of death in PNH patients. Thrombosis should be treated promptly with anticoagulation. Thrombolytic therapy may be considered as well, depending on the extent and location of the clot. In contrast to anticoagulation as treatment, prophylactic anticoagulation is controversial. In one large, nonrandomized trial, primary prophylaxis with warfarin decreased the risk of thrombosis in patients with large PNH clones (>50% PNH granulocytes). However, because eculizumab also decreases the risk of thrombosis, prophylactic anticoagulation is not indicated in these patients based on the current state of knowledge. The bigger question concerns prophylaxis in patients who do not require eculizumab; in general, lacking a randomized trial, it is probably not indicated until further studies are available. The exception may be pregnant women who are at particularly increased risk for thrombosis; low molecular weight heparin may be useful in these patients during pregnancy and the puerperal period. Eculizumab is a pregnancy category C pharmaceutical and its use in pregnancy is not established. Also, patients with PNH undergoing surgery should receive prophylactic anticoagulation in the perioperative period. The recommended duration of either prophylactic or therapeutic anticoagulation has not been established.

Prognosis

The median survival for PNH is 10 to 15 years. Thrombotic events, progression to pancytopenia, and age >55 years at diagnosis are poor prognostic factors. The development of a myelodysplastic syndrome or acute leukemia markedly shortens survival. Patients without leukopenia, thrombocytopenia, or other complications can anticipate long-term survival.

Clinical case (continued)

The patient presented in this section likely has PNH. She has evidence of hemolysis and marrow failure. The diagnosis can be confirmed by flow analysis for CD55 and CD59 on granulocytes, revealing a population of cells with absence of GPI-linked proteins. Treatment is aimed at the major clinical presentation. Eculizumab is effective in decreasing hemolysis and thrombosis but not marrow failure. Thrombosis is treated with anticoagulation; thrombolytic therapy may be used if the thrombosis is acute. There are no randomized studies to support anticoagulation for prophylaxis of thrombosis, but it is prudent to use prophylaxis in high-risk situations for thrombosis such as pregnancy or surgery. If pancytopenia is marked, immunosuppressive therapy such as antithymocyte globulin and cyclosporine have been used. Allogeneic marrow transplantation has been performed in selected cases, primarily those with severe marrow failure and an HLA-matched sibling donor. Marrow transplantation is the only potentially curative therapy of PNH.

Key points

- PNH is an acquired clonal hematopoietic stem cell disorder caused by a somatic mutation of the *PIG-A* gene that results in hematopoietic cells lacking GPI-linked proteins.
- Patients may experience chronic hemolytic anemia, cytopenias, and/or a thrombotic tendency.
- Flow cytometric techniques to identify cell populations lacking GPI-linked proteins (CD55 and CD59) have replaced the sucrose hemolysis and Ham tests.
- PNH clones have been identified in individuals without hematologic abnormalities.
- Bone marrow failure often precedes or follows clinical PNH.
- Steroid therapy along with supportive measures can ameliorate the hemolytic anemia.
- Eculizumab, a monoclonal antibody directed against C5, eliminates or reduces hemolysis, improves quality of life, and decreases the risk of thrombosis.
- *Neisseria* sepsis is a potentially fatal complication of eculizumab therapy. Vaccination against *Neisseria* should be given 2 weeks prior to initiation of eculizumab.
- Prompt evaluation is indicated for symptoms of thrombosis, particularly at unusual sites. Anticoagulation is indicated for documented thrombosis, and thrombolytic therapy may be useful, depending on the location and size of the clot.
- Prophylactic warfarin seems to prevent thrombosis in patients with large PNH clones, but its use for this purpose is controversial, at least in patients who respond to eculizumab.
- Allogeneic hematopoietic cell transplantation has curative potential. Because of the risk of serious or fatal complications, its use should be reserved for those patients with severe cytopenias or patients with severe hemolysis or thrombosis refractory to eculizumab.

Fragmentation hemolysis

> **Clinical case**
>
> A 63-year-old male is referred for evaluation of anemia. His past history is significant for oxygen-dependant chronic obstructive pulmonary disease, coronary artery disease, a mechanical aortic valve placed in 1986, and mild heart failure. On examination, he has distant breath sounds and a grade 3/6 systolic ejection murmur heard at the left upper sternal border. Mild scleral icterus is noted. Laboratory data are significant for a hematocrit of 21% (normal 2 years prior). Corrected reticulocyte count is elevated at 3%, LDH is 1686 IU/dL, and indirect bilirubin is 3.4 mg/dL. Examination of the blood smear reveals schistocytes, hypochromic RBCs, and a few cigar-shaped RBCs.

Fragmentation hemolysis takes place within the vasculature. Laboratory features common to both intra- and extravascular hemolysis include increased concentrations of plasma bilirubin and LDH and decreased concentration of plasma haptoglobin. Additional features characteristic of extravascular as opposed to intravascular hemolysis include the presence of free Hb in the plasma and urine, resulting in red urine and pink plasma. If the hemolysis is chronic, urine hemosiderin may be present. In fragmentation hemolysis, schistocytes are a prominent feature of the blood smear (Figure 6-15).

Pathophysiology

Among the several causes of fragmentation hemolysis, the common thread is mechanical damage to RBCs, resulting in the presence of fragmented RBCs or schistocytes on the blood smear. When microvascular or endothelial injury is present, the process is termed microangiopathic hemolytic anemia. When thrombosis is part of the picture, the term thrombotic microangiopathy is used. In disseminated intravascular coagulation (DIC), the microangiopathic hemolytic anemia is accompanied by activation and consumption of soluble clotting factors, resulting in prolongation of the prothrombin time and activated partial thromboplastin time, whereas TTP-HUS is associated with activation of platelets, but not soluble clotting factors. In both processes, thrombocytopenia accompanies the hemolytic anemia, and both thrombosis and bleeding may occur.

Injury to blood vessel endothelium, intravascular clotting, and primary platelet activation all result in formation of fibrin strands in the circulation. The shearing force generated as the RBCs pass through the fibrin strands causes the RBCs to be cut into small irregular pieces. RBCs may also be broken into pieces by direct mechanical trauma as may occur in march hemoglobinuria or with a dysfunctional mechanical heart valve in which high-velocity jets of blood strike an unendothelialized surface. The resulting small RBC fragments are self-sealing and continue to circulate, albeit with shortened survival. This is due in part to their decreased deformability that results in accelerated removal by the spleen.

Etiology
Cardiac valve hemolysis

Hemolysis may occur with calcific or stenotic native heart valves, although it is usually very mild and well compensated in the absence of severe valvular disease. Mechanical heart valves have a smaller diameter than the native heart valve. Normally, the hemodynamic consequences are minimal. However, prosthetic valve dysfunction or perivalvular regurgitation may result in intravascular hemolysis. An aged or damaged valve surface may become irregular, leading to thrombus formation. In a high-flow state such as exists across the aortic valve or across a regurgitant mitral valve, the formation of jets and turbulent flow results in high shear stress that may exceed the stress resistance of the normal RBC. Hemolysis may be made worse with concomitant cardiac failure or high-output states. Recently designed bioprosthetic heart valves have a significantly decreased risk of thrombus formation and a lower rate of traumatic hemolysis. A recent prospective study reported a 25% rate of mild subclinical hemolysis with a mechanical prosthesis and a 5% rate with a bioprosthesis.

Ruptured chordae tendinae, aortic aneurysm, and patch repair of cardiac defects, as well as intraventricular assist devices and aortic balloon pumps used in the management of severe heart failure, have been associated with traumatic hemolysis. Intravascular hemolysis has also been described

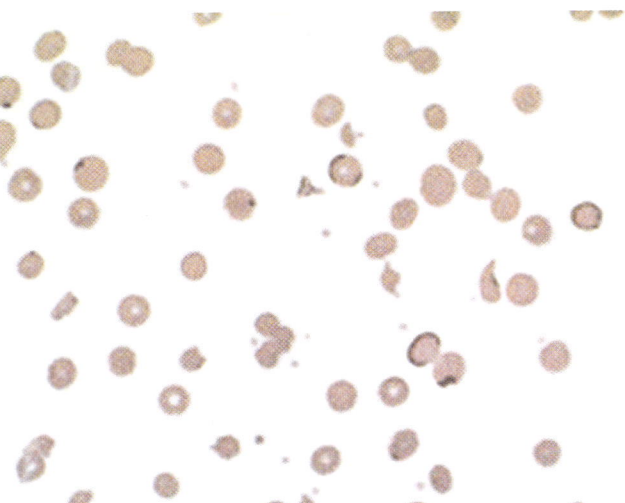

Figure 6-15 Schistocytes.

after cardiopulmonary bypass and is thought to be secondary to both physical damage and complement activation.

Anemia is variable in patients with prosthetic valve hemolysis. The blood smear may include abnormal erythrocytes with schistocytes and cells with abnormal membrane projections.

With chronic hemolysis, Hb is lost in the urine, leading to iron deficiency. Iron-deficient RBCs are mechanically fragile, which can worsen hemolysis, exacerbate anemia, and lead to further hemodynamic compromise that itself may increase the rate of hemolysis. At times, this cycle may be abated by correction of iron deficiency or by RBC transfusion. The addition of erythropoietin to increase RBC production may also help to compensate for ongoing hemolysis. If anemia is severe or fails to respond to the conservative measures, valve replacement may become necessary.

Hemolytic-uremic syndrome–thrombotic thrombocytopenia purpura

TTP and HUS are due to deposition of platelet microthrombi along the endothelium of small vessels of multiple organs. The classic clinical presentation consists of microangiopathic hemolytic anemia and thrombocytopenia. In advanced stages, fever, renal failure, and waxing mental status changes are seen. TTP may be confused with eclampsia, the HELLP syndrome (*h*emolysis, *e*levated *l*iver enzymes, *l*ow *p*latelets), and acute fatty liver of pregnancy, all of which can present with microangiopathic anemia. A critical distinguishing feature between TTP-HUS and DIC is the presence of consumptive coagulopathy in the latter. Malignant hypertension and sclerodermal renal crisis may resemble TTP-HUS, presenting with microangiopathic hemolysis, thrombocytopenia, and renal insufficiency. Rapid control of the hypertension is important in these patients. (TTP and the HUS are covered in detail in Chapter 19.)

> ### Clinical case (continued)
>
> The patient presented in this section has evidence of a moderate hemolytic anemia. The blood smear is consistent with both traumatic hemolysis and iron deficiency because schistocytes and hypochromic and cigar-shaped cells were noted on review of the peripheral blood smear. Valve structure and function should be investigated with an echocardiogram or other imaging studies. Other causes for hemolysis should be ruled out. The patient should be evaluated for iron deficiency. If further evaluation confirms iron deficiency, the patient should receive oral iron. Erythropoietin administration should also be considered. He appears to be a poor surgical candidate, but valve replacement may become necessary if conservative treatment fails.

Certain drugs, especially antineoplastic agents, can cause microangiopathic hemolysis that resembles TTP and HUS. Mitomycin, a chemotherapeutic agent used in the treatment of gastrointestinal malignancies, has been best described. Gemcitabine, another chemotherapeutic agent, has also been implicated. The mechanism has been proposed to be direct endothelial injury. Both tacrolimus and cyclosporine used to prevent and treat graft-versus-host disease can cause a similar syndrome. Ticlopidine and clopidogrel, antiplatelet agents, have both been associated paradoxically with TTP- or HUS-like syndromes.

Disseminated intravascular coagulation

DIC is associated with many disorders including sepsis, obstetrical catastrophes, and malignancy. The disorder is characterized by activation of coagulation and generation of excess thrombin leading to deposition of fibrin strands in arterioles, venules, and capillaries. Microangiopathic hemolytic anemia may be present but is often not severe enough to cause morbidity. Disseminated malignancy presents with microangiopathic anemia and DIC in approximately 5% of cases. Fibrin deposition and vascular disruption by the malignancy itself have both been noted. Mucin-producing adenocarcinomas are frequent offenders. Promyelocytic leukemia characteristically presents with DIC due, at least in part, to the release of tissue factor from promyelocytic granules. If treatment is effective at reversing the underlying condition causing DIC, hemolysis and the coagulopathy often resolve.

HELLP syndrome

The HELLP syndrome (microangiopathic *h*emolysis, *e*levated *l*iver enzymes, and a *l*ow *p*latelet count) is a serious complication of late pregnancy that is part of a spectrum with preeclampsia. Thrombocytopenia and microangiopathic hemolytic anemia with or without renal failure may also occur in pregnancy due to TTP-HUS and acute fatty liver of pregnancy (AFLP). It is important to distinguish TTP-HUS and AFLP from HELLP and preeclampsia for therapeutic reasons. However, the clinical features are quite similar, and the correct diagnosis is often elusive.

Although not absolute, the timing of onset during the pregnancy may be helpful. In general, TTP-HUS occurs earlier in gestation than AFLP, preeclampsia, or HELLP; approximately two thirds of TTP cases in pregnancy occur in the first or second trimester. Most cases of AFLP, preeclampsia, and HELLP occur after 20 weeks of gestation, the great majority in the third trimester. A history of proteinuria and hypertension prior to onset of hemolysis, liver abnormalities, and thrombocytopenia favors the diagnosis of preeclampsia or HELLP, whereas a high LDH level with only modest elevation of AST favors TTP-HUS. Severe liver dysfunction or liver failure favor AFLP.

The characteristics of the coagulopathy are different as well. Whereas both TTP-HUS and HELLP are characterized by thrombocytopenia, in HELLP and more so in AFLP, there may also be DIC with evidence of consumptive coagulopathy. In TTP-HUS, only thrombocytopenia is seen without evidence of consumption of soluble clotting factors. Treatment of HELLP and AFLP consists of prompt delivery of the fetus. The use of dexamethasone in HELLP, previously supported by small studies, has not proved helpful in subsequent randomized trials.

Kasabach-Merritt syndrome

Kasabach-Merritt syndrome occurs in young children. It is characterized by consumptive coagulopathy occurring in the capillaries of a large kaposiform hemangioendothelioma. Microangiopathic hemolytic anemia accompanies evidence of DIC. A number of treatments including glucocorticoids, chemotherapy, interferon alfa, embolization, and surgical removal have been tried with some success.

Foot strike hemolysis

Foot strike hemolysis, also known as *march hemoglobinuria*, has been described in soldiers subjected to long foot-stomping marches in rigid-soled boots, long-distance runners, conga drummers, pneumatic hammer operators, and karate enthusiasts. Hemoglobinuria occurs shortly after the episode of exercise. The hemolysis is caused by direct trauma to RBCs in the blood vessels of the extremities. This condition has become much less common as shoe technology has improved. Cessation of the activity always leads to resolution of the hemolysis.

Hemolytic anemia due to chemical or physical agents

> ### Clinical case
>
> A 23-year-old female is referred for evaluation of mild anemia noted during a workup of liver function test abnormalities. Her recent history has been significant for bizarre schizophrenic-like behavior and arthritis. She has not had a menstrual period in several months. Recent slit lamp examination by an ophthalmologist revealed golden brown pigmentation of the cornea. Physical examination is otherwise unremarkable. Laboratory data suggest a Coombs-negative hemolytic anemia. Liver enzymes are moderately elevated. A ceruloplasmin level returns low at 11 mg/dL.

The use of primaquine and dapsone to prevent or treat *Pneumocystis jiroveci* in acquired immunodeficiency syndrome (AIDS) patients has become fairly common. Both drugs may cause methemoglobinemia in high doses in normal patients and may precipitate hemolysis in patients with G6PD deficiency. Most AIDS clinics screen their patients for G6PD deficiency before starting either of these drugs. Methemoglobinemia and G6PD deficiency are covered in detail earlier in this chapter.

Ribavirin, used to treat HCV infection, is a frequent cause of hemolysis by an unknown mechanism. The hemolysis is dose dependent and decreases or resolves with decreased ribavirin dose or discontinuation of the drug. However, the rate of sustained HCV response also decreases with dose reduction. Erythropoietin has been used as an adjunct to maintain ribavirin therapy at full dose.

Phenazopyridine is a bladder analgesic that is used to treat the symptoms of cystitis. In high doses, it has been associated with oxidative hemolysis. It is recommended that patients be treated for no more than 2 days. Overdoses, prolonged administration, and renal insufficiency have led to methemoglobinemia and severe hemolysis, occasionally severe enough to induce acute renal failure.

Lead intoxication can lead to a modest shortening of RBC life span, although the anemia is more often due to an abnormal heme synthesis and decreased production of erythrocytes. On the blood smear, RBCs are normocytic, hypochromic, with prominent basophilic stippling in young polychromatophilic cells.

Copper causes hemolysis through direct toxic effects on RBCs and has been observed in association with hemodialysis. Copper accumulates in RBCs and disrupts normal metabolic function through a variety of mechanisms including oxidation of intracellular reduced glutathione, Hb, and NADPH and inhibition of multiple cytoplasmic enzymes. Wilson disease, due to a mutation of the *ATP7B* gene, leads to absence or dysfunction of a copper-transporting ATPase encoded on chromosome 13. This subsequently results in lifelong copper accumulation. Hemolytic anemia may be an early manifestation. The hemolytic process in Wilson disease varies in severity and duration. Kayser-Fleischer rings due to the deposition of copper around the periphery of the cornea are a key diagnostic finding. Diagnosis can be made by quantitative ceruloplasmin measurements or by liver biopsy with assessment of the copper concentration. Treatment consists of penicillamine, which mobilizes copper stores. Acute hemolysis in Wilson disease has been treated successfully with plasmapheresis.

Certain spider bites may be associated with traumatic RBC fragmentation. In the southern United States, the brown recluse spider (*Loxosceles reclusa*) is the most common species causing hemolysis. The toxin proteolyzes the RBC membrane through damage to protein band 3 and other integral proteins. In the northwestern United States, hemolysis has been noted after hobo spider (*Tegenaria agrestis*) bites. Microangiopathic hemolysis may occur after the bite of pit vipers (eg, rattlesnakes, cottonmouth moccasins, copperheads) associated with DIC induced by the venom. Cobra venom contains phospholipases that may cause hemolysis. Massive bee and wasp stings have rarely been associated with intravascular hemolysis.

Fragmentation hemolysis has been described after injury from a variety of physical agents. Thermal injury can lead to severe intravascular hemolysis. This is best described in patients suffering from extensive third-degree burns. At temperatures above 47°C, irreversible injury occurs to the RBC membrane. Shortened RBC survival has been noted after ionizing radiation exposure.

> **Clinical case (continued)**
>
> The patient presented in this section displays the classic historical and physical findings of Wilson disease. The low ceruloplasmin level is diagnostic. Hemolytic anemia has been well described in this disease. Once the severity of her liver disease is further evaluated, treatment with penicillamine should be considered. The hemolytic anemia is likely to resolve as excess copper is removed.

Hemolytic anemia due to infection

> **Clinical case**
>
> A 21-year-old man went to the emergency department of his local hospital complaining of fever and shaking chills. He had just returned from a 6-month deployment in eastern Afghanistan with the US Army. He has been home for 2 weeks on leave prior to reporting for his next duty assignment in the United States. He states that he faithfully took his malaria prophylaxis consisting of mefloquine 250 mg weekly while in Afghanistan; he was instructed to continue the weekly mefloquine for 4 more doses after deployment, plus primaquine 15 mg daily for the first 2 weeks. On examination, he appeared acutely ill. Vital signs were as follows: blood pressure 126/66, pulse 110, respirations 20, and temperature 39°C. The remainder of the examination was unremarkable. There was no splenomegaly. A Wright-Giemsa–stained thick blood smear confirmed the diagnosis of *Plasmodium vivax* malaria.

Infection may lead to hemolysis through a variety of mechanisms. Parasites may directly invade RBCs, leading to premature removal by macrophages of the liver and spleen. Alternatively, hemolytic toxins may be produced by the organism and lead to damage of the RBC membrane. Development of antibodies to RBC surface antigens has been well described with certain viral and bacterial illness, especially infectious mononucleosis and *Mycoplasma pneumoniae* infections. Hypersplenism may ensue, which can further decrease RBC life expectancy. In addition, the antibiotic drugs used to treat a variety of these infections may lead to further hemolysis in G6PD-deficient individuals. Anemia that occurs with concomitant acute or chronic infection is likely to be multifactorial, with the anemia of chronic inflammation often coexisting and predominating.

RBC membrane injury caused by bacteria
Clostridial sepsis

Clostridial sepsis is seen in patients with anaerobic subcutaneous infections, in body areas of impaired circulation, after trauma, after septic abortion or postpartum sepsis, and in patients with acute cholecystitis with gangrene of the gallbladder or bowel necrosis. Severe neutropenia of any cause may also be a significant risk factor. The α toxin of *Clostridium* is a lecithinase (phospholipase C) that disrupts the lipid bilayer structure of the RBC membrane, leading to membrane loss and hemolysis. Brisk intravascular hemolysis with spherocytosis seen on the peripheral blood smear is accompanied by hemoglobinemia, hemoglobinuria, and severe anemia. The plasma may be a brilliant red color, and there may be dissociation between the Hb and hematocrit values due to plasma Hb levels reaching several grams per deciliter. Acute renal failure may ensue secondary to excessive hemoglobinuria, but the exact mechanism remains disputed. Renal failure and hepatic failure contribute to the high mortality in clostridial sepsis.

Hemolytic anemias with gram-positive and gram-negative organisms

Septicemia and endocarditis caused by gram-positive bacteria such as streptococci, staphylococci, *S pneumoniae*, and *Enterococcus faecalis* are often associated with hemolytic anemia. The anemia in patients with infections due to gram-positive cocci appears to result from the direct toxic effect of a bacterial product on erythrocytes. *Salmonella typhi* infection may be accompanied by severe hemolytic anemia with hemoglobinemia. In typhoid fever, the onset of hemolysis may occur during the first 3 weeks of illness, with anemia lasting from several days to >1 week. *Salmonella* and other microorganisms can cause direct agglutination of RBCs in vitro, but it is not known whether this phenomenon contributes to in vivo hemolysis. In approximately one third of patients with typhoid fever, a positive DAT develops, but hemolytic anemia is not manifest in all cases.

Immune hemolysis associated with infections

Pneumonia caused by *M pneumoniae* can be associated with production of cold agglutinins, IgM antibodies directed against the RBC I antigen. Hemolytic anemia associated with *M pneumoniae* may occur during the second or third week of the illness. The onset of the hemolysis may be rapid, usually occurring after recovery from respiratory symptoms. The clinical presentation often includes dyspnea or fatigue and the presence of pallor and jaundice. The blood smear shows RBC agglutination with or without spherocytosis and with polychromatophilia (Figure 6-14). When ethylenediaminetetraacetic acid (EDTA)-anticoagulated blood is cooled in a test tube, RBC agglutination can be seen; disagglutination occurs when the blood is warmed. Cold agglutination titers at the onset of hemolysis usually exceed 1:256 and may reach higher levels, although they are typically lower than in monoclonal cold agglutinin disease. The DAT is positive for complement deposition on RBCs. The hemolytic anemia associated with *Mycoplasma* pneumonia is self-limited, transient, and usually mild, although severe cases requiring corticosteroid therapy or plasmapheresis have been reported.

Infectious mononucleosis caused by Epstein-Barr virus infection may also be associated with hemolytic anemia due to cold agglutination. The cold agglutinin in this case is an IgM antibody directed against the i antigen. Severe hemolytic anemia associated with infectious mononucleosis is unusual, although anti-i antibodies are frequently present. When hemolytic anemia occurs, the mechanism involves fixation of complement on the RBC membrane by IgM antibody. Hemolysis proceeds either by completion of the complement cascade through C9 or by opsonization of RBCs with fragments of C3 leading to phagocytosis of RBCs by macrophages in the liver or spleen.

Several other viral infections have been associated with AHA. These include cytomegalovirus, herpes simplex, rubeola, varicella, influenza A, and human immunodeficiency virus. Postviral acute hemolytic anemia in children may be due to the formation of a cold-reactive hemolytic IgG antibody of the Donath-Landsteiner type, which induces complement lysis of RBCs.

Microangiopathic hemolytic anemias associated with infection include bacteremia with gram-negative organisms, staphylococci, meningococci, and pneumococci, all of which can lead to DIC with endothelial damage and fibrin thrombi within the microcirculation. RBC injury results from mechanical fragmentation by fibrin strands in the vasculature. Microvascular damage induced by meningococcal and rickettsial infections (eg, Rocky Mountain spotted fever) may be associated with DIC, thrombocytopenia, microvascular thrombi, and fragmentation hemolytic anemia. Patients with either congenital or tertiary syphilis may develop paroxysmal cold hemoglobinuria. Whereas paroxysmal cold hemoglobinuria used to be fairly common in the late 19th and earlier 20th centuries, it is rare today due to the disappearance of congenital and tertiary syphilis.

Hemolytic anemia associated with parasitic infestation of RBCs
Malaria

Malaria is the most common cause of hemolytic anemia worldwide. Transmitted by the bite of an infected female *Anopheles* mosquito, sporozoites that are injected from the mosquito make their way to liver cells. Merozoites enter into the bloodstream 1 to 2 weeks later. Hemolysis in malaria results directly from erythrocytic infestation by *Plasmodium* organisms (Figures 6-16 and 6-17). Noninfected RBCs may also be hemolyzed by

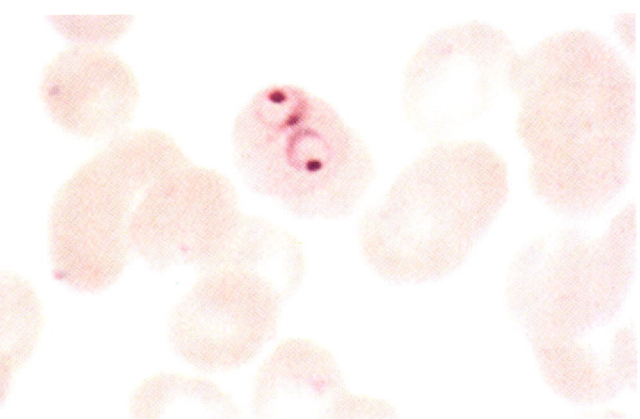

Figure 6-16 Intraerythrocyte parasite *Plasmodium falciparum*.

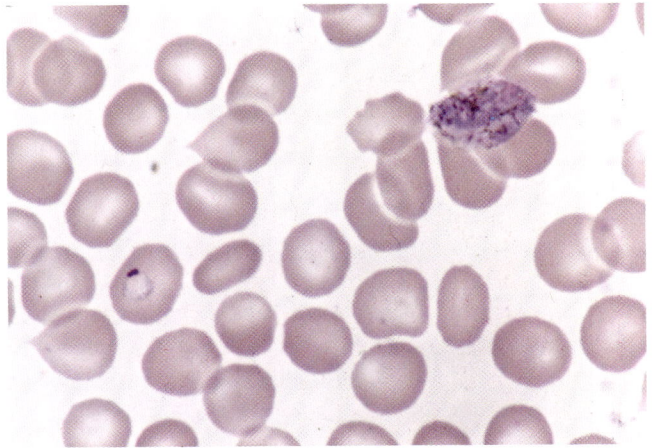

Figure 6-17 Intraerythrocyte parasite *Plasmodium vivax*. Trophozoite (ring form) and female gametocyte. Used with permission from *Lichtman's Atlas of Hematology*, http://www.accessmedicine.com.

poorly understood mechanisms. Infested erythrocytes are selectively removed from the circulation by the spleen, with some RBCs reentering circulation after splenic pitting of parasites. Previously infested erythrocytes manifest membrane and metabolic abnormalities along with decreased deformability. In addition, the *Plasmodium* species digests the host RBC Hb for its own use as a nutrient.

The severity of the hemolytic process is often out of proportion to the degree of parasitemia. *P vivax* and *Plasmodium ovale* invade only reticulocytes, whereas *Plasmodium malariae* invades only mature erythrocytes. *P falciparum* invades erythrocytes of all ages and is associated with more severe hemolysis. In areas where malaria has been a frequent cause of death for many centuries, a number of genetic polymorphisms are prevalent, including G6PD deficiencies, thalassemias, and hemoglobinopathies. These polymorphisms have in common the ability to interfere with the ability of the malaria parasites to invade RBCs.

With *P falciparum* infection, intravascular hemolysis may be severe and associated with hemoglobinuria (blackwater fever). Another potentially lethal complication of *P falciparum* infection, cerebral malaria, results from expression of *P falciparum* erythrocyte protein 1 on the membranes of infected RBCs. These RBCs adhere to receptors on vascular endothelium in various organs including the central nervous system, resulting in vaso-occlusion and neurologic manifestations.

Diagnosis of malaria is based on identification of parasite-infected RBCs on a thick Wright-stained blood smear. The distinction of *P falciparum* infection from the other species is important because its treatment may constitute a medical emergency. The findings of 2 or more parasites per RBC and infestation of >5% of RBCs are characteristic of *P falciparum* infection.

Chemoprophylaxis should be offered to all people planning travel to known endemic areas. The hemolytic anemia of malaria resolves after successful therapy with quinine, chloroquine, artemisinin, and other drugs, depending on the species of malaria. Many of these agents may be associated with drug-induced hemolysis in patients with G6PD deficiency.

Babesiosis

Babesiosis is a protozoan infection caused by *Babesia microti*. Once thought to be rare, outbreaks have been described with increasing frequency on Nantucket Island, Cape Cod, northern California, and several other North American locations. The organism is transmitted by the bite of the *Ixodides* tick, which infects many species of wild birds and domestic animals and occasionally humans. Babesiosis may rarely be transmitted by transfusion with fresh or frozen-thawed RBCs. Infection leads to a clinical syndrome of fever, lethargy, malaise, and hemoglobinuria 1 to 4 weeks after the bite. Hemolytic anemia due to intravascular hemolysis occurs, and renal and liver function tests are frequently abnormal. The disease is often asymptomatic in persons with intact spleens; patients who have undergone splenectomy are at high risk for severe symptomatic infection. Babesia infection can be diagnosed by demonstrating typical intraerythrocytic parasites on a thin blood smear (Figure 6-18). Standard treatment has consisted of clindamycin and quinine. Recent studies have suggested that atovaquone plus azithromycin is an equally efficacious regimen, yet better tolerated.

Bartonellosis

Bartonellosis, caused by *Bartonella bacilliformis*, manifests 2 clinical stages: an acute hemolytic anemia and a chronic granulomatous phase. The micro-organism enters the blood following the bite of an infected sand fly. The infective *Bartonella* agent adheres to the membrane of RBCs that are then removed by the spleen. The hemolytic anemia of bartonellosis develops rapidly and may be severe, with hemoglobinemia and hemoglobinuria. When untreated, this disorder is associated with high mortality. Survivors manifest a second stage of the disease with cutaneous granulomas. Bartonellosis is common in South America and has been reported in the Peruvian Andes and parts of Brazil, where it is also known as Oroya fever. On Giemsa-stained blood films, red-violet rods of varying length can be identified on RBCs and represent the bacteria. Effective treatment exists and consists of penicillin, streptomycin, chloramphenicol, or tetracycline.

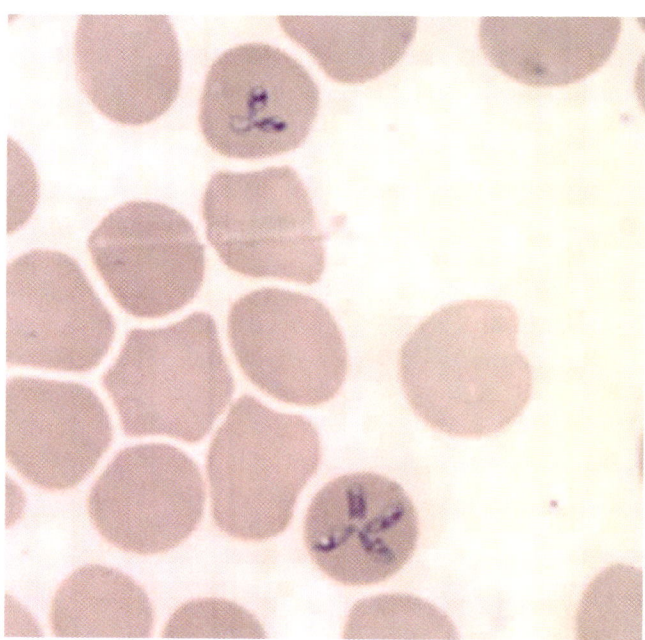

Figure 6-18 Intraerythrocyte parasite *Babesia microti*.

> **Clinical case (continued)**
>
> The patient described earlier in this section was admitted for treatment. The Centers for Disease Control and Prevention Malaria Hotline (770-488-7788) was called, and the regimen of chloroquine and primaquine was recommended for *P vivax* malaria acquired in Afghanistan. The patient made a full recovery. He ultimately admitted that he had forgotten to take his prophylactic medications after leaving Afghanistan. The most common cause of failure of malaria prophylaxis in military or civilian populations is noncompliance. Because of the importance of primaquine in terminal prophylaxis and treatment of vivax malaria, it is currently the policy of the US military to screen all personnel for G6PD deficiency.

> **Key points**
>
> - RBC fragmentation syndromes are diverse in etiology.
> - In all suspected cases of hemolytic anemia, the blood smear should be examined carefully for schistocytes. Their presence can direct differential diagnosis.
> - RBC destruction can be at the macrovascular or microvascular (microangiopathic) level of the circulatory system. Classic examples include heart valve hemolysis, DIC, and TTP.
> - Various chemical exposures or physical agents can cause fragmentation hemolysis.
> - Infection can cause accelerated RBC destruction through a variety of mechanisms including direct invasion, toxin production, and immune mechanisms.
> - Malaria, the most common infectious disease worldwide, causes hemolysis through both direct parasitic invasion of RBCs and alterations in noninfected cells. Malaria can be diagnosed by thorough review of a thick Wright-stained peripheral blood smear.

Bibliography

Thalassemia

Cunningham MJ, Macklin EA, Neufeld EJ, et al. Complications of beta thalassemia major in North America. *Blood*. 2004;194:34-39. *A well-written overview of complications affecting 342 patients with thalassemia intermedia and major followed at institutions participating in the Thalassemia Clinical Research Network.*

Neufeld EJ. Oral chelators deferasirox and deferiprone for transfusional iron overload in thalassemia major: new data, new questions. *Blood*. 2006;107:3436–3441. *This commentary very nicely summarizes the many recent developments in management of iron overload in thalassemia and other anemias where iron overload is problematic.*

Rund D, Rachmilewitz E. Beta-thalassemia. *N Engl J Med*. 2005;353:1135–1146. *A well-written overview of the pathophysiology and management of thalassemia.*

Vichinsky EP, MacKlin EA, Waye JS, et al. Changes in the epidemiology of thalassemia in North America: a new minority disease. *Pediatrics*. 2005;116:818–825. *A review from the National Institutes of Health–supported Thalassemia Clinical Research Network that highlights the fact that most young thalassemia patients are from Asia or the Middle East, not Greece or Italy, and that the clinical heterogeneity within the thalassemia population is far greater than in years past.*

Weatherall DJ. Disorders of globin synthesis: the thalassemias. In: Lichtman MA, Beutler E, Kipps TJ, et al, eds. *Williams Hematology*. 7th ed. New York, NY: McGraw-Hill; 2006:633–666. *A lucid comprehensive summary of genetics, pathophysiology, screening, and clinical aspects of the thalassemias.*

Sickle cell disease

Adams RJ, McKie VC, Hsu L, et al. Prevention of a first stroke by transfusions in children with sickle cell anemia and abnormal results on transcranial Doppler ultrasonography. *N Engl J Med*. 1998;339:5-11. *A prospective randomized clinical trial demonstrating that a chronic transfusion program can reduce the risk of stroke in children with abnormal transcranial Doppler results.*

Bakanay SM, Dainer E, Clair B, et al. Mortality in sickle cell patients on hydroxyurea therapy. *Blood*. 2005;105:545–547. *A concise review of a single institution's experience with hydroxyurea in 226 adults with sickle cell disease, indicating substantial mortality in older patients with substantial preexisting organ damage.*

Benjamin LJ, Dampier CD, Jacox AK, et al. *Guideline for the Management of Acute and Chronic Pain in Sickle-Cell Disease*. Glenview, IL: American Pain Society; 1999. APS Clinical Practice Guidelines Series, No. 1. *A comprehensive evidence-based approach to the evaluation and treatment of sickle cell pain.*

Charache S, Terrin ML, Moore RD, et al. Effect of hydroxyurea on the frequency of painful crises in sickle cell anemia. Investigators of the Multicenter Study of Hydroxyurea in Sickle Cell Anemia. *N Engl J Med*. 1995;332:1317–1322. *A multicenter phase III randomized study that established the efficacy of hydroxyurea in the treatment of adults with sickle cell disease.*

Gladwin M, Sachdev V, Jison ML, et al. Pulmonary hypertension as a risk factor for death in patients with sickle cell disease. *N Engl J Med*. 2004;350:886–895. *Pulmonary hypertension is common in sickle cell disease and predisposes to high risk of premature death.*

National Heart, Lung, and Blood Institute and Division of Blood Diseases and Resources. *The Management of Sickle Cell Disease*. 4th ed. Bethesda, MD: National Institutes of Health; revised June 2002. NIH publication 02–2117. *A useful monograph addressing diagnosis, counseling, health maintenance, and treatment of sickle cell disease.*

The Optimizing Primary Stroke Prevention in Sickle Cell Anemia (STOP 2) Trial Investigators. Discontinuing prophylactic transfusions used to prevent stroke in sickle cell disease. *N Engl J Med*. 2005;353:2769–2778. *A follow-up study to the 1998 STOP trial showing that discontinuation of transfusions for primary stroke prevention results in a high rate of abnormal transcranial Doppler abnormalities and clinical stroke.*

Platt OS, Brambilla DJ, Rosse WF, et al. Mortality in sickle cell disease. Life expectancy and risk factors for early death. *N Engl J Med*. 1994;330:1639–1644. *A landmark prospective study of >3000 patients addressing survival and risk factors for mortality in sickle cell disease.*

Quinn CT, Rogers ZR, Buchanan GR. Survival of children with sickle cell disease. *Blood*. 2004;103:4023–4027. *A review of the Dallas Newborn Cohort characterizing contemporary timing and causes of mortality of children with sickle cell disease diagnosed by newborn screening and receiving penicillin prophylaxis and care in a comprehensive sickle cell center.*

Steinberg MH, Barton F, Castro O, et al. Effect of hydroxyurea on mortality and morbidity in adult sickle cell anemia: risks and benefits up to 9 years of treatment. *JAMA*. 2003;289:1645–1651. *Follow-up of the Multicenter Study of Hydroxyurea in Sickle Cell Anemia (MSH) revealing reduced mortality for patients taking hydroxyurea.*

Vichinsky EP, Haberkern CM, Neumayr L, et al. A comparison of conservative and aggressive transfusion regimens in the perioperative management of sickle cell disease. The Preoperative Transfusion in Sickle Cell Disease Study Group. *N Engl J Med*. 1995;333:206–213. *A multicenter randomized clinical trial comparing simple transfusion (conservative arm) with a regimen to reduce Hb S below 30% (aggressive arm) in >600 surgical procedures. The number of serious clinical complications was similar to a reduction in transfusion-associated complications in the conservative arm.*

Vichinsky EP, Neumayr LD, Earles AN, et al. Causes and outcomes of the acute chest syndrome in sickle cell disease. National Acute Chest Syndrome Study Group. *N Engl J Med*. 2000;342:1855–1865. *A prospective multicenter trial analyzing 671 episodes of acute chest syndrome. Clinical presentation, causes, and outcomes are addressed.*

Wanko SO, Telen MJ. Transfusion management in sickle cell disease. *Hematol Oncol Clin North Am*. 2005;19:803–826. *An up-to-date overview of the risks and benefits of blood transfusion in persons with sickle cell disease.*

Weatherall D, Hofman K, Rodgers G, et al. A case for developing North-South partnerships for research in sickle cell disease. *Blood*. 2005;105:921–923. *This short essay makes the case for the need for close collaboration between developed and poor countries to successfully address unanswered questions regarding the pathophysiology and management of sickle cell disease.*

Weatherall MW, Higgs DR, Weiss H, et al. Phenotype/genotype relationships in sickle cell disease: a pilot twin study. *Clin Lab Haem*. 2005;27:384–390. *A fascinating study of identical twin pairs with sickle cell disease showing concordance in many hematologic and some clinical features but discordance in many disease manifestations.*

RBC membrane disorders

Bolton-Magge PH, Stevens RF, Dodd NJ, et al. Guidelines for the diagnosis and management of hereditary spherocytosis. *Br J Haematol*. 2004;126:455–474. *Well-written and practical management recommendations, based on scientific evidence when possible, from the British Society of Haematology.*

Cartron JP. Rh-deficiency syndrome. *Lancet*. 2001;358(suppl):S57. *Concise, single-page review on Rh-deficiency syndrome.*

Tse WT, Lux SE. Red blood cell membrane disorders. *Br J Hematol*. 1999;104:2-13. *An update on biochemical and genetic abnormalities accounting for HS and HE/HPP.*

Enzymopathies

Beutler E. G6PD deficiency. *Blood*. 1994;84:3613–3636. *A comprehensive review of clinical manifestations, genetics, diagnosis, and treatment of G6PD deficiency.*

Rees DC, Duley JA, Marinaki AM. Pyrimidine 5′ nucleotidase deficiency. *Br J Hematol*. 2003;120:375–383. *A recent comprehensive review of 5′ pyrimidine nucleotidase deficiency.*

Van Wijk R, van Solinge WW. The energy-less red blood cell is lost: erythrocyte enzyme abnormalities of glycolysis. *Blood*. 2005;106:4034–4042. *A comprehensive review of RBC glycolytic enzyme abnormalities.*

Zanella A, Bianchi P. Red cell pyruvate kinase deficiency: from genetics to clinical manifestations. *Best Pract Res Clin Hematol*. 2000;13:57–81. *A comprehensive review of the most common glycolytic pathway deficiency that causes hemolytic anemia.*

Immune-mediated hemolysis

Garratty G, Petz LD. Approaches to selecting blood for transfusion to patients with autoimmune hemolytic anemia. *Transfusion*. 2002;42:1390–1392. *Outlines the approach to transfusion in patients with immune hemolytic anemia, with emphasis on selection of blood units and early consultation between the clinician and the blood bank physician.*

Garratty, G. Drug-induced immune hemolytic anemia. *Hematology 2009*. Washington, DC: American Society of Hematology; 2009: 73–79.

Garvey B. Rituximab in the treatment of autoimmune haematological disorders. *Br J Haematol*. 2008;141:149–169. *Overview of the use and efficacy of rituximab in autoimmune blood diseases.*

Ness PM. How do I encourage clinicians to transfuse mismatched blood to patients with autoimmune hemolytic anemia in urgent situations? *Transfusion*. 2006;46:1859–1862. *Outlines the approach to transfusion in patients with immune hemolytic anemia, with emphasis on selection of blood units and early consultation between the clinician and the blood bank physician.*

Packman CH. Hemolytic anemia due to immune injury. In: *Williams Hematology*. 8th ed. McGraw Hill; 2010. *A concise review of the clinical presentation, laboratory evaluation, and therapeutic approaches to autoimmune hemolysis and drug-immune hemolytic anemia.*

Petz LD. "Least incompatible" units for transfusion in autoimmune hemolytic anemia: should we eliminate this meaningless term? A commentary for clinicians and transfusion medicine professionals. *Transfusion*. 2003;42:1503–1507. *Outlines the* approach to transfusion in patients with immune hemolytic anemia, with emphasis on selection of blood units and early consultation between the clinician and the blood bank physician.

Schollkopf C, Kjeldsen L, Bjerrum OW, et al. Rituximab in chronic cold agglutinin disease: a prospective study of 20 patients. *Leuk Lymphoma*. 2006;47:253–260. *Prospective study of rituximab in cold agglutinin disease.*

Paroxysmal nocturnal hemoglobinuria

Brodsky RA. How I treat paroxysmal nocturnal hemoglobinuria. *Blood*. 2009;113:6522–6527. *An excellent, well-referenced review on the management of PNH.*

Brodsky RA, Mukhina GL, Li S, et al. Improved detection and characterization of paroxysmal nocturnal hemoglobinuria using fluorescent aerolysin. *Am J Clin Pathol*. 2000;114:459–466. *Describes the use of fluorescent aerolysin to diagnose PNH.*

Brodsky RA, Young NS, Antonioli E, et al. Multicenter phase 3 study of the complement inhibitor eculizumab for the treatment of patients with paroxysmal nocturnal hemoglobinuria. *Blood*. 2008;111:1840–1847. *Eculizumab reduces intravascular hemolysis and thrombosis and improves quality of life in patients with PNH.*

Dunn DE, Tanawattanacharoen P, Boccuni P, et al. Paroxysmal nocturnal hemoglobinuria cells in patients with bone marrow failure syndromes. *Ann Intern Med*. 1999;131:401–408. *A clinical investigation revealing the occurrence of PNH identified by flow cytometry in approximately 20% of patients with aplastic anemia and myelodysplasia.*

Hall C, Richards S, Hillmen P. Primary prophylaxis with warfarin prevents thrombosis in paroxysmal nocturnal hemoglobinuria (PNH). *Blood*. 2002;102:3587–3591. *Prospective, nonrandomized trial describing the use of warfarin to prevent thrombosis in high-risk patients with PNH.*

Hillmen P, Lewis SM, Bessler M, et al. Natural history of paroxysmal nocturnal hemoglobinuria. *N Engl J Med*. 1995;333:1253–1258. *A long-term follow-up study of patients with PNH revealing a median survival after diagnosis of 10 years and evidence that spontaneous remission can occur.*

Rosse WF. Paroxysmal nocturnal hemoglobinuria as a molecular disease. *Medicine (Baltimore)*. 1997;76:63–93. *An authoritative review of the pathophysiology and clinical manifestations of PNH.*

RBC fragmentation

Antman KH, Skarin AT, Mayer RJ, et al. Microangiopathic hemolytic anemia and cancer. *Medicine (Baltimore)*. 1979;58:377–384. *An early description of microangiopathy in the cancer patient.*

Brawley RK, Donahoo JS, Gott VL. Current status of the Beall, Bjork-Shiley, Braunwald-Cutter, Lillehei-Kaster and Smeloff-Cutter cardiac valve prostheses. *Am J Cardiol*. 1975;35:855–865. *A comparison of the physiology and complications of several different types of valve prosthesis.*

Conrad ME. Pathophysiology of malaria. Hematologic observations in human and animal studies. *Ann Intern Med*. 1969;70:134–141. *A description of the pathophysiology and the hematologic changes associated with malaria.*

Goldstein DJ. Worldwide experience with the MicroMed DeBakey Ventricular Assist Device as a bridge to transplantation. *Circulation*. 2003;108(suppl 1):II272-II277. *Prospective study on the functioning of intraventricular assist devices with data on incidence of hemolysis.*

Gordon LI, Kwaan HC. Thrombotic microangiopathy manifesting as thrombotic thrombocytopenic purpura/hemolytic uremic syndrome in the cancer patient. *Semin Thromb Hemost*. 1999;25:217–221. *Review of thrombotic microangiopathies in cancer patients with special consideration of cancer type, chemotherapy, and treatment options.*

Mecozzi G, Milano AD, De Carlo M, et al. Intravascular hemolysis in patients with new-generation prosthetic heart valves: a prospective study. *J Thorac Cardiovasc Surg*. 2002;123:550–556. *Recent prospective study investigating the incidence of subclinical and clinical hemolysis with new-generation prosthetic heart valves.*

Chemical or physical agent

Deiss A, Lee GR, Cartwright GE. Hemolytic anemia in Wilson's disease. *Ann Intern Med*. 1970;73:413–418. *Review of the occurrence of hemolytic anemia in Wilson disease.*

Infection

Miller LH, Baruch DI, Marsh K, Doumbo OK. The pathogenic basis of malaria. *Nature*. 2002;415:673–679. *Good review of malaria pathogenesis.*

Spach DH, Liles WC, Campbell GL, et al. Tick-borne diseases in the United States. *N Engl J Med*. 1993;329:936–947. *A review of tick-borne diseases, including babesiosis, with emphasis on physiology, life cycle, diagnosis, and treatment.*

CHAPTER 07

Thrombosis and thrombophilia

Stephan Moll and Janna M. Journeycake

Pathophysiology of thrombosis, 179	Venous thromboembolism, 202	Acknowledgment, 212
Thrombophilias, 180	Arterial thromboembolism, 210	Bibliography, 212
Antithrombotic drugs, 195		

This chapter gives an overview of the pathophysiologic contributors to thrombosis; describes the mechanisms, epidemiology, testing issues, and clinical relevance of inherited and acquired thrombophilias; discusses the drugs used as antithrombotics; and reviews various clinical, diagnostic, and therapeutic aspects of thrombosis.

Pathophysiology of thrombosis

Thrombosis, defined as excessive clotting, has 3 main causes, referred to as Virchow's triad: reduced blood flow (stasis), blood hypercoagulability, and vascular wall abnormalities. Blood in the vasculature is kept in a fluid state by the delicate balance of multiple procoagulant and anticoagulant factors (ie, coagulation proteins [coagulation factors], platelets, leukocytes, erythrocytes, and components of the vessel wall). If blood vessel integrity is interrupted, coagulation takes place and a blood clot (ie, thrombus) forms to prevent excessive bleeding. Thrombus formation is a tightly controlled mechanism to prevent excessive and pathologic thrombus formation (ie, thrombosis). Natural anticoagulants, such as antithrombin, protein C, and protein S, serve as "police proteins," controlling and limiting thrombin formation. Once a thrombus has formed, its growth is limited by clot lysis, which eventually leads to thrombus resolution. This is part of the mechanism that leads to vascular wall healing and reestablishment of intravascular blood flow.

Thrombosis is often multifactorial, caused by both genetic and acquired risk factors. The degree of contribution to thrombosis of the 3 components of Virchow's triad varies between arterial and venous thrombosis, as well as between thrombotic events in individual patients. Stasis of blood is a well-known predisposing factor for venous thrombosis. However, the events that trigger an episode of unprovoked (formerly called *idiopathic*) venous thromboembolism (VTE) in a specific location and at a certain time are not well understood. A pathophysiologic model suggests that each individual has a baseline thrombosis risk, which increases as the person ages (Figure 7-1A). Transient risk factors, such as major surgery or estrogen therapy, temporarily increase a person's thrombosis risk, but the threshold of thrombosis formation is often not reached (Figure 7-1B). Most people, therefore, never reach the thrombosis threshold and never develop a VTE. However, the individual who has a higher baseline thrombosis risk, such as the individual with an inherited or acquired thrombophilia, may cross the thrombosis threshold while exposed to a transient risk factor and, thus, develop a VTE (Figure 7-1B).

In general, venous thrombosis is caused by disturbances in the plasma coagulation system, with platelet participation playing a minor role, whereas in arterial thrombosis, platelets play the predominant role, with some participation of the plasma coagulation system. This paradigm helps explain why coagulation protein abnormalities, such as factor V Leiden, the prothrombin 20210 mutation, and deficiencies of protein C, protein S, and antithrombin, predominantly

Conflict-of-interest disclosure: *Dr. Moll:* consultancy: Bayer, Roche Diagnostics, International Technidyne Corp., Lundbeck, GTC Biotherapeutics, Talecris, Ortho McNeil-Janssen Pharmaceuticals; research funding: International Technidyne Corp.; honoraria: Lundbeck, Talecris; grant support: CDC grant # 1U01DD000292-0. *Dr. Journeycake:* honoraria: Baxter Healthcare; membership on board of directors or advisory committee: Physicians Advisory Council of Baxter Healthcare; grant support, NIH K23 Career Development Award (K23 HL0840970).
Off-label drug use: *Dr. Moll:* new oral anticoagulants rivaroxaban, apixaban, dabigatran. *Dr. Journeycake:* anticoagulant agents in children.

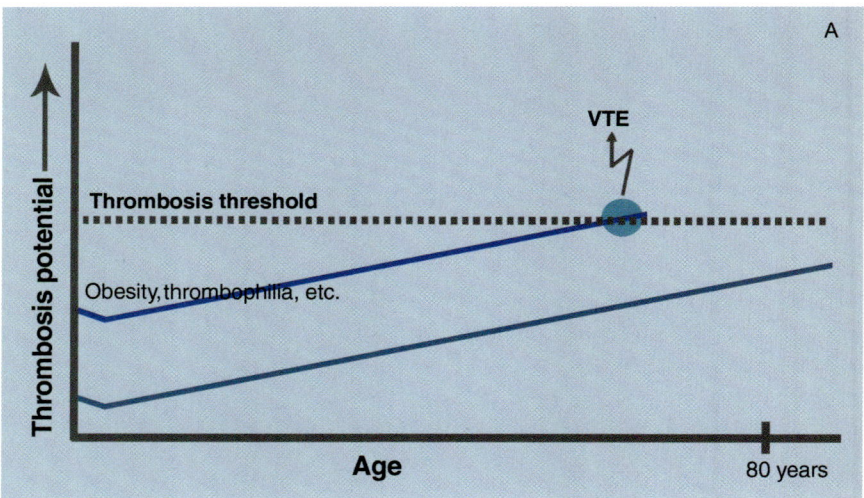
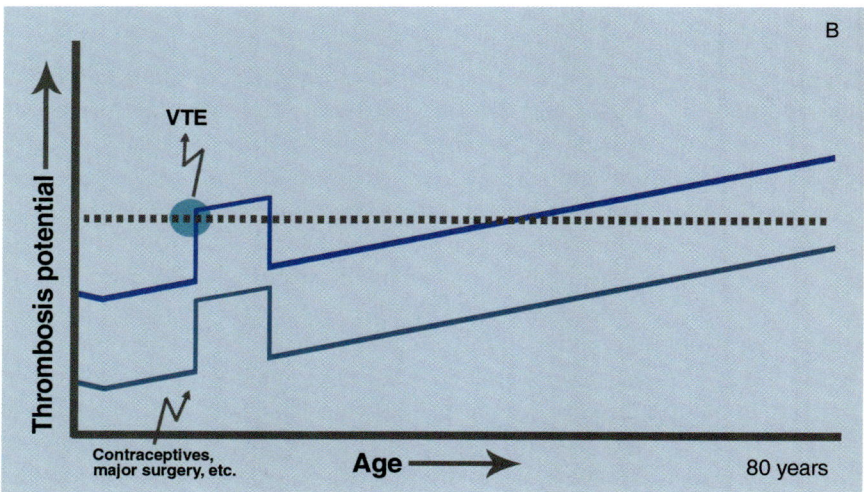

Figure 7-1 Threshold model of thrombosis risk. VTE = venous thromboembolism. This figure was created with the help of illustrator Marie Dauenheimer. Modified after Rosendaal FR. *Lancet.* 1999;353:1167–73.

lead to VTE. It also helps explain why antiplatelet drugs are effective in the prevention of arterial thrombosis but less effective, if at all, in preventing VTE. Thrombus formation in the cardiac ventricles and atria is often caused by stagnant blood flow in the kinetic, dyskinetic, or aneurysmal parts of the heart chambers or in fibrillating atria. Arising in a slow-flow environment, these thrombi are more likely caused by mechanisms similar to the ones that lead to venous thrombosis.

Arterial clots usually form in areas of atherosclerotic vascular damage. The events leading to atherosclerosis, mainly lipid disturbances, oxidative stress, and inflammation, have been relatively well studied. The composition and vulnerability of plaque, rather than its volume, and the severity of stenosis are the most important determinants for the development of arterial ischemic syndromes. Plaques have a high content of tissue factor, expressed on monocytes and macrophages. Disruption of the fibrous cap or endothelium overlying an atheromatous plaque leads to exposure of collagen and tissue factor, leading to platelet adhesion and aggregation and local thrombin formation, with subsequent thrombus formation.

Overall, there is a significantly better understanding of the pathophysiologic events that lead to arterial thrombosis than those leading to VTE. However, from a thrombophilia point of view, more is known about thrombophilias predisposing to VTE than those leading to arterial thrombosis.

Thrombophilias

Factor V Leiden
General information

Activated protein C (APC) is a potent inhibitor of the coagulation system, cleaving the activated forms of factor V (factor Va) and VIII (factor VIIIa) (Figure 7-2A and 7-2B).

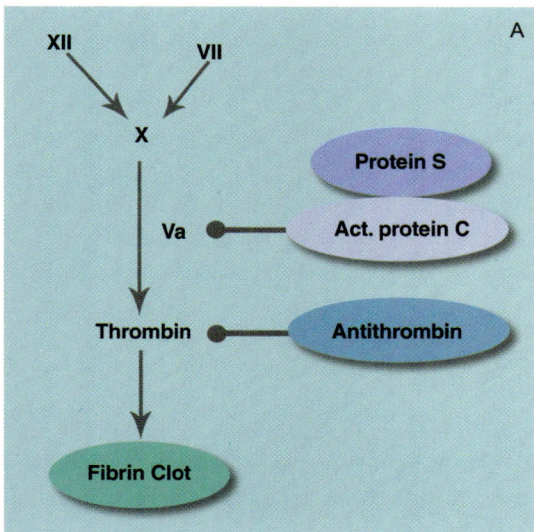

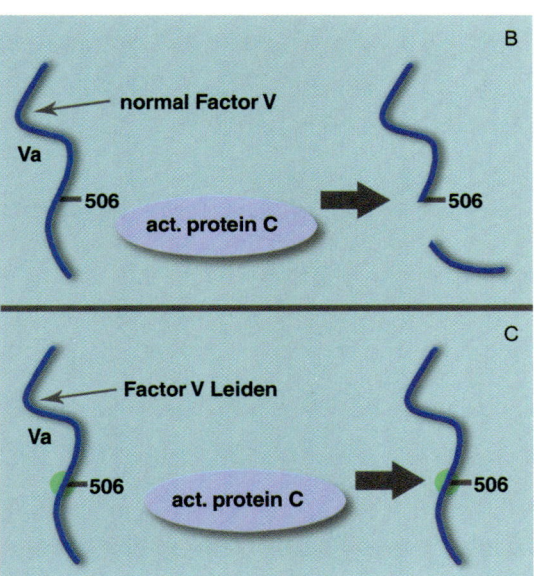

Figure 7-2 A, Sites of action of the natural anticoagulants; B, method of inactivation of factor V; and C, demonstration of the inability of activated protein C, to inactive factor Va when the factor V Leiden mutation is present. This figure was created with the help of illustrator Marie Dauenheimer.

The factor V Leiden (FVL) mutation is a point mutation (G1691A) in the factor V gene, leading to a factor V molecule with an arginine-to-glutamine substitution at position 506 (Arg506Gln, R506Q). This abolishes a cleavage site of APC and makes activated factor V less susceptible to inactivation (Figure 7-2C). Based on the initial observation that APC did not appropriately prolong the activated partial thromboplastin time (aPTT) in a dose-dependent fashion, this defect was termed *APC resistance*. FVL accounts for >90% of APC resistance. Other causes of APC resistance include less common genetic mutations of factor V (eg, factor V Cambridge, factor V Liverpool) and acquired causes of APC resistance, including antiphospholipid antibodies, pregnancy, and cancers. FVL is inherited in an autosomal dominant fashion. The high prevalence of FVL in the general population suggests that it has led to evolutionary selection advantages, including less blood loss during delivery and improved survival during sepsis.

Prevalence

FVL is the most common known inherited thrombophilia, with a prevalence of 3% to 8% in the white US population and 1.2% in African Americans. It is rarely found in native African and Asian populations. Homozygous FVL occurs in 1 in 500 to 1600 whites.

Testing

The diagnosis of FVL is made by genetic testing (ie, polymerase chain reaction testing of the *FVL* gene). However, one can also use an APC resistance assay first, which is an aPTT-based coagulation assay using factor V–deficient plasma. The currently used second-generation APC resistance assays are very sensitive and relatively specific for the detection of the FVL mutation if the right cutoff values are used. However, abnormal APC resistance test results may be due to causes other than FVL and should, therefore, be followed by the genetic FVL test. A normal APC resistance test result, however, rules out the presence of FVL and does not need to be confirmed by genetic testing. Although clinicians often consider genetic testing to be infallible, false-positive and false-negative results can occasionally occur. These may be due to sample labeling or handling errors or mistakes in reporting or interpreting the results. A patient's lack of understanding of the test performed and the result obtained or an error in recall of what the health care provider explained may also lead to misinterpretation and misunderstanding by the patient. Lastly, technical aspects of test performance and rare genetic variations (mutations close to the FVL 506 mutation) may also lead to incorrect results.

Risk for thrombosis

Heterozygosity for FVL is mildly thrombophilic, leading to a 2.7-fold increased risk of VTE. Homozygosity confers an 18-fold increased risk compared with individuals without the FVL mutation. Additional VTE risk factors, such as age, smoking, obesity, and use of estrogens, increase the risk further. In a landmark population-based study, the lowest and highest absolute 10-year risks for VTE were 1% and 10%, respectively, in heterozygotes, and 3% and 51%, respectively, for homozygotes, depending on age, smoking status, and obesity. A recent systematic review demonstrated that FVL heterozygosity is only weakly associated with an increased risk of VTE recurrence (odds ratio 1.56; 95% confidence interval 1.14–2.12) compared with individuals without FVL. The risk of recurrence in individuals with homozygous FVL compared with those without FVL is 2.65-fold (95% confidence interval 1.2–6.0) increased. There is no association between FVL and arterial thromboembolic events; a meta-analysis demosntrated the risk to be 1.21 (95% confidence interval 0.99–1.49) in FVL carriers compared with noncarriers.

Management

Because heterozygosity for FVL confers only a mildly increased risk of VTE recurrence compared with individuals without FVL, its finding alone should not alter anticoagulation treatment decisions. Because heterozygous FVL is also barely a risk factor for arterial thromboembolism, its presence should not influence management decisions. Furthermore, asymptomatic family members of persons with FVL heterozygosity do not need to be tested unless they are considering estrogen therapy or pregnancy, in which case testing could be considered. However, even in this situation, there is no strong evidence-based reason for testing, because solid management decisions can typically be made without the knowledge of the mutational status. Finding the homozygote state in a patient with an unprovoked VTE may be one of the arguments to treat with longer term anticoagulation.

Pediatric considerations

As in adults, heterozygosity is also associated with an increased risk of first VTE. However, FVL alone does not increase the risk of recurrent VTE. In the homozygous state or if combined with other thrombophilias, the risk for recurrent events is increased. Although FVL is not a clinically relevant risk factor for arterial disease in adults, several pediatric studies have demonstrated an association with stroke, particularly perinatal stroke.

Prothrombin 20210 mutation
General information

A point mutation in the factor II gene in the noncoding region in nucleotide position 20210 (G20210A) is the second most common known inherited risk factor for venous thrombosis. Individuals who are heterozygous for this polymorphism have slightly higher levels of circulating prothrombin. It is inherited in an autosomal dominant fashion.

Prevalence

The mutation is found most commonly in individuals of southern European ancestry, with a prevalence throughout Europe of 0.7% to 4%. In the United States, it occurs in 2% of the general population and in 0.5% of the African American population. The prothrombin 20210 mutation is very rare in non-Caucasian populations. Homozygosity for the prothrombin 20210 mutations occurs, by calculation, in approximately 1 in 4000 individuals of Caucasian heritage.

Testing

Testing is done using genetic testing. Although the mutation leads to higher circulating factor II levels, it is not helpful to use factor II activity or antigen levels as screening tests because there is a wide overlap of levels between people with and without the mutation. As discussed earlier for FVL, false-positive and false-negative results with polymerase chain reaction genetic testing can occur.

Risk for thrombosis

Heterozygosity for the prothrombin 20210 mutation is mildly thrombophilic, conferring a 3-fold increased risk of VTE compared with noncarrier status. A systematic review showed that heterozygosity for the prothrombin 20210 mutation, compared with the absence of the mutation, is not associated with a higher risk of recurrence. Thus, treatment decisions on length of anticoagulant therapy are typically not based on the presence or absence of the prothrombin 20210 mutation. Population-based data regarding the risk of thrombosis for homozygotes for the prothrombin gene mutation are not available. A summary of 70 cases of homozygous individuals published in the medical literature indicates a marked phenotypic heterogeneity. Data on the risk of recurrence of VTE in individuals with homozygous prothrombin 20210 mutations do not exist. Meta-analysis has not demonstrated any clinically meaningful association between the prothrombin mutation and arterial thromboembolism; the risk for an arterial event is only 1.32-fold (95% confidence interval 1.03–1.69) increased in carriers of the mutation compared with noncarriers. However, there is some suggestion of a somewhat stronger association between the prothrombin 20210 mutation and stroke and myocardial infarction in younger patients.

Management

Because heterozygosity for the prothrombin 20210 mutation confers only a mild risk of VTE recurrence, its finding alone typically does not alter anticoagulation treatment decisions.

Because the heterozygous prothrombin 20210 mutation is only a very mild risk factor for arterial thromboembolism, its presence should not influence management decisions. Furthermore, similar to the discussion earlier about FVL, family members of persons who are heterozygous need not be tested unless they are considering estrogen therapy or pregnancy, in which case testing can be considered.

Pediatric considerations

A recent meta-analysis showed that presence of the prothrombin 20210 mutation leads to an increased risk of recurrent VTE in children, with an odds ratio of 2.15 (95% confidence interval, 1.12–4.10).

Protein C deficiency
General information

Protein C is a vitamin K–dependent protein converted during the coagulation process to APC. APC acts as a natural anticoagulant. In complex with the cofactor protein S, it inactivates coagulation factors Va and VIIIa, making them unavailable as cofactors during the coagulation process (Figure 7-2A). Protein C deficiency as a cause of thromboembolism was first described in 1981. Two types of deficiency are known, but their distinction is clinically not important in regard to the thrombotic risk they confer. Type I deficiency is defined as a quantitative deficiency with low functional protein C (activity) and immunologic (antigen) level, and type II is defined as a qualitative deficiency with low activity but normal antigen level. Approximately 85% of the reported cases have type I deficiency, whereas 15% have type II deficiency. More than 160 mutations causing protein C deficiency have been described.

Prevalence

The prevalence of inherited protein C deficiency in the general population is approximately 1 in 500 to 600. By calculation, homozygous or double heterozygous protein C deficiency occurs in a fetus in approximately 1 in 1,000,000 pregnancies.

Testing

When evaluating an individual for protein C deficiency, a protein C functional (activity) test should be performed because obtaining only antigen levels will miss type II deficiencies. Outside of research studies, there is no need to obtain protein C antigen levels. Because laboratory reports may only report results as "protein C normal," leaving it unclear whether an activity or antigen test was done, a physician needs to clarify with the laboratory which test was actually done to avoid missing a type II deficiency. Falsely low protein C activity values may be seen with high levels of factor VIII and with lupus anticoagulants. The most common reason for low protein C levels is treatment with vitamin K antagonists (VKAs) (Tables 7-1 and 7-2). Some authors have advocated the use of a ratio of protein C activity or antigen and levels of other vitamin K–dependent factors to help diagnose protein C deficiencies in patients on VKAs. Although such calculations may suggest a deficiency, the poor correlation of coagulation factor levels to one another during VKA treatment makes this an error-prone approach. The authors of this chapter do not advocate the use of such ratios for clinical practice. Patients should be off VKAs for 2 to 3 weeks before testing is performed. It is not known how many patients who carry a diagnosis of protein C deficiency truly have a congenital deficiency and how many patients have an erroneous diagnosis of protein C deficiency due to testing at an inappropriate time (ie, while on VKAs). Thus, the hematologist should always question the diagnosis in a patient with an "established" diagnosis, until review of records and laboratory results has clarified that the timing of testing was correct and no confounding issues led to a transient decrease in protein C. Repeat confirmatory testing of a low protein C level at a separate time point is also recommended.

Risk for thrombosis

Protein C deficiency is considered to be one of the higher risk thrombophilias. It is a risk factor mainly for VTE. Rates of thrombosis vary widely among individuals and families

Table 7-1 Conditions associated with acquired coagulation factor deficiencies.

Factor	Conditions associated with decreased factor levels
Protein C	• Acute thrombosis
	• Warfarin therapy
	• Liver disease
	• Protein-losing enteropathy
Protein S	• Acute thrombosis
	• Warfarin therapy
	• Liver disease
	• Inflammatory states
	• Estrogens (contraceptives, pregnancy, postpartum state, hormone replacement therapy)
	• Protein-losing enteropathy
Antithrombin	• Acute thrombosis
	• Heparin therapy
	• Liver disease
	• Nephrotic syndrome
	• Protein-losing enteropathy

Table 7-2 Influence of acute thrombosis, heparin, and vitamin K antagonists on thrombophilia test results.

Test	Acute thrombosis	Unfractionated heparin	Low molecular weight heparin	Vitamin K antagonists
Factor V Leiden genetic test	Reliable	Reliable	Reliable	Reliable
APC resistance assay	Reliable*	???*	???†	Reliable*
Prothrombin 20210 genetic test	Reliable	Reliable	Reliable	Reliable
Protein C activity or antigen	???‡	Reliable	Reliable	Low
Protein S activity or antigen	May be low	Reliable	Reliable	Low
Antithrombin activity	May be low	May be low	May be low	Reliable
Lupus anticoagulant	Reliable§	???‖	???‖	May be false positive
Anticardiolipin antibodies	Reliable§	Reliable	Reliable	Reliable
Anti–β_2-glycoprotein I antibodies	Reliable§	Reliable	Reliable	Reliable
Homocysteine	Reliable	Reliable	Reliable	Reliable

*Reliable if the assay is performed with factor V–depleted plasma; thus, clinician needs to inquire how the individual laboratory performs the assay.
†Depending on the way the assay is performed, results may be unreliable; the health care provider needs to contact the laboratory and ask how the specific test performs on heparin.
‡Probably reliable, but limited data are available in literature.
§Test is often positive or elevated at time of acute thrombosis, but subsequently negative.
‖Although many test kits used for lupus anticoagulant testing contain a heparin neutralizer, making these tests reliable on unfractionated heparin (UF) and possibly low molecular weight heparin (LMWH), clinicians need to ask their laboratory how their individual test kit performs in samples with UF and LMWH.
APC = activated protein C resistance.

with protein C deficiency. A large family cohort study found that presence of protein C deficiency in asymptomatic relatives of probands with protein C deficiency and a first VTE conferred a 24-fold increased risk compared with family members without the deficiency. The annual incidence of VTE is 1.52% in protein C–deficient individuals, compared with approximately 0.1% in the general population. Protein C deficiency also confers an increased risk for recurrent VTE, which is 37% over 5 years off anticoagulation. A recent study of thrombophilic families showed that deficiency of protein C is a risk factor for arterial thromboembolism in patients <55 years old. Rates of fetal loss after 28 weeks of gestation are increased in individuals with protein C deficiency.

Management

Patients with protein C deficiency initiated on vitamin K antagonists (VKA) are at risk for warfarin-induced skin necrosis. This transient hypercoagulable state is related to abrupt decline in protein C activity after the initiation of VKA. Any patient with acute VTE who is initiated on VKA needs concurrent anticoagulation with a parenteral anticoagulant for at least 5 days and until the international normalized ratio (INR) is >2.0, but this is particularly important in the person with known protein C and S deficiency. Because of the increased association with recurrent thrombosis and protein C deficiency, consideration of long-term anticoagulation after a first unprovoked thrombotic event is appropriate in these patients. Whether the patient with protein C deficiency and a nonarteriosclerotic arterial thrombotic event would best be treated with antiplatelet or anticoagulant therapy is not known.

Pediatric considerations

Homozygous or double heterozygous protein C deficiency is associated with catastrophic thrombotic complications at birth, manifested by purpura fulminans and, frequently, death of the neonate. Treatment with protein C concentrate should be considered in these newborns. It is important to remember that the levels of natural anticoagulant proteins change with development. Protein C activity is very low when compared with adults at the time of birth. This reduction of activity can persist until adolescence. When interpreting the results of thrombophilia screening in children, it is imperative that they are compared with pediatric normative ranges and not adult ranges.

Protein S deficiency
General information

Protein S is also a vitamin K–dependent protein. Forty percent of protein S exists in a free form, and the remaining 60% exists in a complex with the transport protein called *C4b-binding protein* (C4b-BP). It is mostly free protein S that functions as a natural anticoagulant, by being a cofactor for APC for the inactivation of factors Va and VIIIa (Figure 7-2A).

Protein S deficiency was first described in 1984. More than 131 different mutations have been identified leading to protein S deficiency. Protein S deficiency is an autosomal dominant disorder. Severe protein S deficiency due to homozygous or double heterozygous mutations can lead to early onset of VTE or severe neonatal purpura fulminans and death.

Protein S deficiency is classified as type I, a quantitative deficiency in which both free and total protein S antigen levels are decreased; type II, a qualitative defect due to a dysfunctional protein in which protein S activity is low but free and total antigen levels are normal; or type III, a quantitative deficiency in which free protein S antigen level is low and the total antigen level is normal. Type III deficiency is either due to a high C4b-BP plasma concentration or an abnormal binding of protein S to this carrier protein. The majority of the known mutations (~93%) lead to quantitative deficiencies (ie, type I and III).

Prevalence

Reported prevalence in the general population varies between 1 in 800 and 1 in 3000, but due to difficulties in establishing the normal range of protein S concentrations in the general population and the difficulties in making an accurate diagnosis, the true prevalence of is not known.

Testing

A reliable test for quantitative protein S deficiency is the determination of free protein S antigen levels. However, if only antigen levels are determined, a type II protein S deficiency can be missed. If only activity is determined, some patients with quantitative and also qualitative protein S deficiency may not be discovered because some activity assays have been shown to give falsely normal results. Therefore, it is advisable to always include functional testing (protein S activity) and immunologic testing (free protein S antigen) in the laboratory evaluation of protein S deficiency. Obtaining a total protein S antigen is only helpful to determine the subtype of protein S deficiency, but for clinical purposes, such classification is not needed or helpful. High factor VIII levels, the presence of the FVL mutation, or presence of a lupus anticoagulant may give falsely low protein S activity values.

Protein S levels are low in the setting of estrogen therapy, pregnancy, liver disease, nephrotic syndrome, disseminated intravascular coagulation, and therapy with VKAs (Tables 7-1 and 7-2). Congenital protein S deficiency cannot be diagnosed in these circumstances. A patient needs to have been off VKAs for 3 weeks before protein S levels can be considered reliable. Thus, as with protein C deficiency, timing of the testing is essential to make a correct diagnosis, and repeat confirmatory testing on a new plasma sample is advisable. Critical questioning as to whether a patient said to have protein S deficiency truly has the disorder is appropriate.

Risk for thrombosis

Protein S deficiency is considered to be one of the higher-risk thrombophilias. Because of the genetic diversity of mutations associated with protein S deficiency, rates of thrombosis vary widely among individuals and families with known defects. A large family cohort study found that presence of protein S deficiency in asymptomatic relatives of probands with protein C deficiency and a first VTE conferred a 31-fold increased risk compared with family members without the deficiency. The annual incidence of VTE is 1.90% in protein S–deficient individuals, compared with approximately 0.1% in the general population. Interestingly, some authors have not found an increased risk of thrombosis in individuals with inherited protein S deficiency. Nevertheless, protein S deficiency is overall considered to be a higher risk thrombophilia because the risk of recurrent VTE off anticoagulation has been shown to be high, reaching 44% over 5 years. A large family study showed that protein S deficiency is a risk factor for arterial thromboembolism in individuals <55 years of age. Clearly, there is heterogeneity in the clinical phenotype of patients with protein S deficiency, and this needs to be taken into consideration when making decisions on anticoagulant treatment and family counseling.

Management

The implications of finding inherited protein S deficiency in an individual are similar to those discussed earlier for the person found to have protein C deficiency. Diligent overlap of parenteral anticoagulants upon initiation of VKAs for at least 5 days and until the INR is >2.0 is important to avoid warfarin-induced skin necrosis. Individuals with a first unprovoked episode of VTE are often treated long term with VKAs because of an increased risk for recurrent VTE if the patient is not on VKAs. Whether the patient with protein S deficiency and an otherwise unexplained arterial thromboembolic event would best be treated with antiplatelet or anticoagulant therapy is not known. No pharmacologic protein S concentrate exists.

Pediatric considerations

Purpura fulminans can occur in the rare newborn with severe protein S deficiency due to homozygous or double heterozygous mutations. Children are born with physiologically lower levels of total protein S than adults. However, because the amount of C4b-BP is also reduced, the free protein S level is almost the same as found in adults. Any reduction of protein S level or activity in healthy newborns should normalize by early childhood (after 6 months of age). Screening asymptomatic children for thrombophilia should be delayed until after this time so that testing does not need to be repeated.

Antithrombin deficiency
General information

Antithrombin (AT) is an enzyme that interrupts the coagulation process mostly by inhibiting thrombin (Figure 7-2A), activated factor X (factor Xa), and activated factor IX (factor IXa). It used to be referred to as antithrombin III (ATIII). AT deficiency was first described in 1965. Qualitative (type I) and quantitative (type II) defects exist. Type II deficiencies consist of defects affecting the thrombin-binding region, the heparin-binding region, and a variety of other AT molecule regions, thus termed pleiotropic defects. More than 130 different genetic mutations are known.

Prevalence

Inherited AT deficiency occurs in 1 in 500 to 5000 people. Deficiencies are typically heterozygous, because homozygous deficiencies are almost always incompatible with life. In the general population, type II deficiencies are the more prevalent subtype, accounting for 88% of all AT deficiencies. However, a majority of these type II deficiencies are heparin-binding defects, which are not very thrombogenic. Acquired low AT levels are associated with sepsis, disseminated intravascular coagulation, liver disease, nephrotic syndrome, asparaginase, chemotherapy, and acute fatty liver of pregnancy.

Testing

Testing for AT deficiency should be performed using a functional assay to detect both quantitative and qualitative defects. Heparin therapy can decrease AT levels by 30% (Tables 7-1 and 7-2). Warfarin can increase AT levels, possibly by stimulating synthesis of AT or by decreasing consumption of AT by decreasing low-grade activation of the coagulation process. Testing is best performed a few weeks after the initial thrombotic event. No one should be diagnosed as having AT deficiency based on one single abnormal test result. An abnormal result should lead to repeat testing on a new blood sample. Because type II AT deficiency due to a heparin-binding defect appears to be much less thrombogenic than type I and other type II subtypes, differentiation of the AT deficiency subtype may be important for clinical purposes. Specialized AT assays—AT activity in the absence of heparin—or gene sequencing need to be used for that purpose but are not widely available.

Risk for thrombosis

AT deficiency overall is considered to be one of the higher risk thrombophilias. Type I and II mutations affecting the thrombin-binding domain can be associated with VTE in nearly 50% of affected family members. The prevalence of VTE in individuals with a defect in the heparin-binding site is much lower; only 6% of such individuals will develop a VTE. Once anticoagulation is stopped, the risk of recurrent VTE in individuals with AT deficiency is high, between 10% and 17% per year. Although some cases of arterial thromboembolism in AT-deficient individuals have been reported, this association is much weaker than with VTE and possibly not present at all. A large family study showed no association between AT deficiency and arterial thromboembolism. The risk for fetal loss is slightly increased in women with AT deficiency.

Management

Asymptomatic individuals with AT deficiency are typically not started on long-term anticoagulation. However, they need thorough deep vein thrombosis (DVT) prophylaxis in risk situations. AT concentrate is available, either derived from the plasma of human donors or transgenically produced in goat milk. Only one guideline or consensus statement exists as to when to use AT concentrates. In view of the scarcity of solid clinical study data, this guideline consists only of level IIIC recommendations (ie, "opinions of respected authorities, based on clinical experience, descriptive studies"). The guideline provides detailed recommendations on how to dose with plasma-derived AT concentrate but lacks specifics on whom to treat and for how long. Because the risk of recurrent VTE is high, it is typically recommended that a patient with AT deficiency who has had an unprovoked VTE should be considered for long-term anticoagulation. It is not known whether the same recommendation should apply to patients with AT deficiency due to a defect in the heparin-binding site. AT deficiency occasionally confers resistance to anticoagulation with heparin. Large doses of unfractionated heparin can be required to achieve appropriate prolongation of the aPTT. In cases of severe thrombosis and inadequate anticoagulation, AT concentrate can be given.

Pediatric considerations

AT levels are reduced at birth and normalize by approximately 6 months of age. Screening of asymptomatic children should be delayed until this time to avoid needing repeat testing.

Antiphospholipid antibodies
General information

Antiphospholipid antibodies (APLAs) are acquired autoantibodies targeted against phospholipids and phospholipid-binding proteins, such as β_2-glycoprotein I and prothrombin. They are associated with arterial thromboembolism and VTE, as well as pregnancy loss. A variety of different mechanisms leading to thrombosis have been described, including effects of the antibodies on platelets, endothelial cells, monocytes, and trophoblasts and interference with complement activation, the protein C pathway, and fibrinolysis. Clinical classification of the APLA syndrome requires a history of venous or arterial thrombosis, unexplained recurrent early pregnancy loss, or one or more late pregnancy losses, together with persistent laboratory evidence of APLA at least 12 weeks apart. The criteria for definite APLA syndrome have been described as the so-called Sapporo criteria. The syndrome occurs as primary APLA syndrome not associated with any other diseases or as secondary APLA syndrome associated with autoimmune diseases, malignancy, or drugs.

Prevalence

The prevalence of APLA syndrome is poorly defined, but APLAs of some titers are found in nearly 50% of patients with systemic lupus erythematosus and 1% to 5% of the general population. Nearly 40% of patients with systemic lupus erythematosus will meet diagnostic criteria for the APLA syndrome.

Testing

The Sapporo criteria recognize the following antibodies as fulfilling criteria for APLA syndrome: (i) moderately or highly positive immunoglobulin G (IgG) and immunoglobulin M (IgM) anti–β_2-glycoprotein I antibodies; (ii) moderately or highly positive IgG and IgM anticardiolipin antibodies; and (iii) lupus anticoagulant (Figure 7-3). Lupus anticoagulants are detected by various functional coagulation assays because the APLA antibodies react with the phospholipids needed for the ex vivo coagulation process and, thus, prolong clotting times. False-positive lupus anticoagulant tests are not uncommon, occurring more

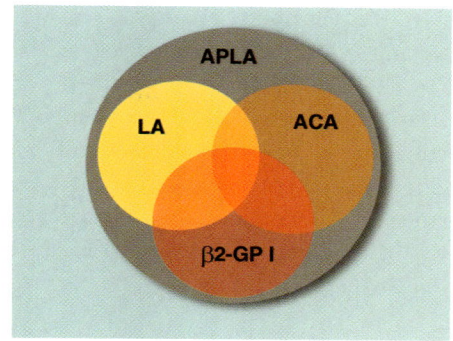

Figure 7-3 Antiphospholipid antibodies (APLAs) with their different subtypes. ACA = anticardiolipin antibody; β2-GPI = β_2-glycoprotein I; LA = lupus anticoagulant.

frequently in patients who (i) are on oral anticoagulants, (ii) are older, and (iii) have mildly positive lupus anticoagulant test results (Table 7-2). False-negative results may occur if the blood sample is suboptimally centrifuged and the prepared plasma is not platelet poor. APLA titers at the time of an acute thrombotic event may be temporarily decreased, thought to be due to consumption, but may also be transiently positive. Thus, the time of the acute thrombotic event is a suboptimal time for testing, and it may be better if testing is delayed for a few weeks. Because APLA can be transient, the Sapporo criteria require repeatedly positive tests at least 12 weeks apart to confirm a diagnosis of APLA syndrome.

A number of other APLA tests are not part of the Sapporo criteria because their association with thrombosis or pregnancy loss has not been established, including immunoglobulin A (IgA) anticardiolipin and anti–β_2-glycoprotein I antibodies, anti-phosphatidylserine antibodies, anti-phosphatidylethanolamine antibodies, and anti-phosphatidylinositol antibodies. There is presently no clear indication for testing for these additional APLA antibodies in routine clinical practice. In fact, evidence to support anticardiolipin IgG and IgM antibody elevation alone as a risk factor for thrombosis is also lacking. Nevertheless, they are part of the empirically derived Sapporo criteria. The different anticardiolipin and anti–β_2-glycoprotein I antibody test kits available for clinical practice are suboptimally standardized. Also, lupus anticoagulant reporting is not standardized, and laboratory reports can be difficult to read and interpret. Thus, critical and diligent reading of the report is advised, when interpreting a laboratory lupus anticoagulant report.

The INR determined from plasma is occasionally invalid in orally anticoagulated patients because of a lupus anticoagulant effect on the INR. Furthermore, INR determinations by point-of-care INR monitors can be inaccurate and significantly overestimate a patient's level of anticoagulation. Alternative tests, such as chromogenic factor X or clot-based factor II or X activity, to measure the oral anticoagulant effect are indicated in these patients. The target ranges for these tests depend on the reagents and instruments used for their determination, but an INR range of 2.0 to 3.0 in a non-APLA patient on warfarin corresponds to factor II activity of approximately 31% to 15% and chromogenic factor X activity of approximately 42% to 21%.

Risk for thrombosis

The APLA syndrome is highly thrombophilic and is associated with both arterial and venous thrombosis. Positivity for all 3 APLA tests (ie, lupus anticoagulant, anticardiolipin, and anti–β_2-glycoprotein I antibody tests) is associated with the highest risk for thrombosis and pregnancy loss. Review of patients with the APLA syndrome demonstrates occurrence of DVT in 32%, pulmonary embolism in 9%, stroke in 13%, transient ischemic attack in 7%, and fetal loss in 8%. APLA syndrome is also implicated in recurrent VTE once anticoagulation is discontinued. However, limited data exist on the extent of risk of recurrence. Finally, there is a 5% to 15% failure rate of warfarin therapy in preventing recurrent thrombosis.

Management

Because of the previously mentioned limitations of laboratory APLA testing and interpretation of test results, as well as the transient nature of antibodies in many patients, it is advisable to always question a diagnosis of APLA syndrome until the previous laboratory test results have been reviewed and, if necessary, repeat testing has been performed. Because of the high rate of recurrent VTE, patients with true APLA syndrome with a history of unprovoked VTE should be maintained on anticoagulation indefinitely. Randomized trials have shown that a target INR range of 2.0 to 3.0 is equally effective in preventing recurrent thrombosis as a target range of 3.0 to 4.0. This probably holds true as long as the INR is reliable and indicates a patient's true level of anticoagulation. If the aPTT is prolonged at baseline due to a lupus anticoagulant, then anti–factor Xa levels need to be used to monitor unfractionated heparin therapy. If the prothrombin time is prolonged at baseline, then the validity of the patient's INR should be checked once the patient is on warfarin, by comparing the INR to either a factor II activity or a chromogenic factor Xa assay. It can then be determined whether the INR is a reliable measure of that patient's anticoagulation and can be used for VKA monitoring. It is not known whether patients with arterial thrombosis and APLA syndrome are more effectively treated with antiplatelet or warfarin anticoagulation therapy. In the absence of prospective randomized trial data, no consensus on this topic exists. Rituximab has been shown to decrease APLA titers in some patients, but whether lowering or disappearance of APLA leads to a decreased thrombosis risk has not been studied. The management of pregnant women with APLA is discussed in Chapter 2.

Pediatric considerations

Studies of children who present for surgery, especially tonsillectomy, show a 2% prevalence of transient lupus anticoagulant with no apparent pathologic consequence due to the fact that these postinfectious APLAs more commonly bind cardiolipin in a non–β_2-glycoprotein I–dependent manner. The prognostic significance of the transient lupus anticoagulant in children who present with thrombosis in the setting of concurrent infection is probably similar to that of children who have an asymptomatic lupus anticoagulant. The only reliable indicator of significant morbidity is the diagnosis of APLA, which persists for >12 weeks in the presence of thrombosis.

Factor VIII elevation
General information

Elevated plasma levels of factor VIII are an independent and dose-dependent risk factor for VTE. Elevations in factor VIII have a familial-inherited component, but they do not follow a simple Mendelian inheritance pattern.

Prevalence

Elevated factor VIII levels have been operationally defined as values found in the top decile of a given population. Factor VIII is an acute-phase reactant, and baseline levels vary considerably. In the Leiden Thrombophilia Study, 25% of patients with a first episode of VTE had elevations in factor VIII without elevations in C-reactive protein. Elevations in factor VIII are seen commonly in patients of African ancestry with venous thrombosis.

Testing

Factor VIII clotting (functional) assays are available but have not been standardized to define the top decile of the local reference population.

Risk for thrombosis

Population-based, controlled studies have demonstrated that elevations in factor VIII >150% confer a 4.8-fold greater risk of first-episode venous thrombosis than if levels are <100%. Some studies have shown that elevated factor VIII levels are also a risk factor for recurrent VTE, but this has not been uniformly found.

Management

Because the role of elevated factor VIII levels in recurrent VTE is controversial, decisions on duration and intensity of anticoagulation should be made independent of factor VIII levels. Consequently, there is, at present, no role for routine clinical testing for factor VIII levels as part of a thrombophilia workup.

Pediatric considerations

There is suggestion that persistently elevated factor VIII activity, particularly when associated with persistently elevated D-dimer levels, has prognostic significance in children. These children have higher rates of postthrombotic syndrome and recurrent thrombotic events. It may be beneficial to treat these patients with extended anticoagulation, but this has not yet been investigated.

Homocysteine and methylenetetrahydrofolate reductase
General information

Homocystinuria is a rare autosomal recessive defect in the homocysteine pathway (Figure 7-4), most commonly in the cystathionine-β-synthase enzyme, and is associated with markedly elevated homocysteine levels (>100 μM/L). Affected individuals have a high rate of arterial and venous thrombotic events before the age of 30 years. A number of associated symptoms and signs occur, most commonly dislocation of the lens. Mild to moderately elevated homocysteine levels, on the other hand, are common and are referred to as hyperhomocysteinemia. Elevated levels may be due to deficiency of vitamin B_6, vitamin B_{12}, or folate; renal impairment; polymorphisms in the genes involved in the synthesis of the enzymes of the homocysteine metabolism; or unknown causes. In hyperhomocysteinemia, the associated signs and symptoms seen in homocystinuria do not occur.

Elevated levels of plasma homocysteine have been shown to be associated with an increased risk of venous and arterial thrombosis. From available data, it is not clear whether this association is independent of confounding effects or causal in nature. A number of prospective studies have demonstrated that lowering of homocysteine levels does not decrease the risk of primary venous and arterial thromboembolic events or of recurrent venous and arterial thrombosis. This is also true for patients with elevated homocysteine levels secondary to chronic renal disease. This implies that hyperhomocysteinemia may not be causatively contributing to the thrombotic process, but rather may act as a marker for an increased risk. The methylenetetrahydrofolate reductase (MTHFR) enzyme is a regulator of homocysteine metabolism (Figure 7-4). Polymorphisms in the *MTHFR* gene may lead to elevated plasma homocysteine levels but do not always do so.

Prevalence

A common MTHFR mutation is the C677T or "thermolabile" mutation, for which approximately 34% to 37% of US whites are heterozygous and 12% homozygous. The A1298C polymorphism occurs in most ethnic groups and is present in the heterozygous state in 9% to 20% of the population. Elevated homocysteine levels may be seen in an individual with homozygous C677T mutation or double heterozygous C677T plus A1298C mutation, but may also occur in the absence of these polymorphisms.

Testing issues

Homocysteine levels may change after food intake, but the change is typically <10% from baseline, which, for practical purposes outside of clinical studies, is not relevant.

Risk for thrombosis

Meta-analyses show that the MTHFR polymorphisms in North America, where food is supplemented with folic acid, are neither a risk factor for venous and arterial thromboembolism nor a risk factor for pregnancy complications.

Management

Because the presence of MTHFR polymorphisms is not a thrombophilic state, there is no indication to screen for these mutations. Because lowering of homocysteine levels has no demonstrated clinical benefit on thrombotic risk, there is no indication for treatment of elevated homocysteine levels with B vitamin or folic acid supplementation. Finally, because finding elevated homocysteine levels has no clinical consequences, there is no rationale to measure homocysteine levels in thrombophilia evaluations. The exception is the younger individual (<30 years old) with arterial thromboembolism or VTE, in whom there is a suspicion for homocystinuria.

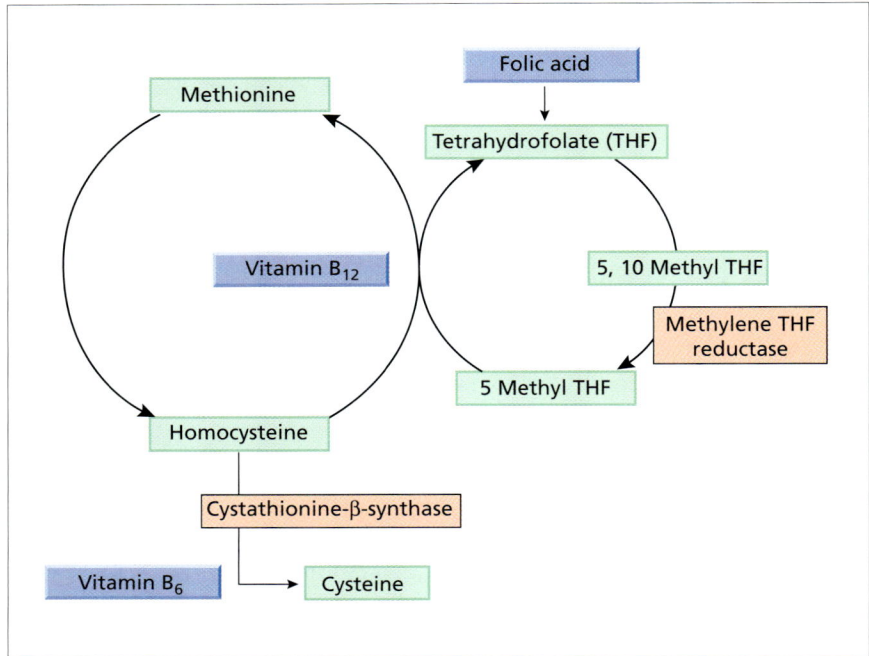

Figure 7-4 Homocysteine pathway.

Myeloproliferative disorders
General information

Essential thrombocytosis (ET) and polycythemia vera are associated with a substantial risk for thrombosis (arterial more commonly than venous). A gain-of-function mutation of the Janus kinase 2 (JAK2) enzyme, the *JAK2* V617F mutation, is found in nearly 100% of patients with polycythemia vera and in 50% of those with ET. Meta-analyses show that the presence of the *JAK2* V617F mutation is associated with an increased risk of thrombosis, either arterial or venous, in patients with ET. However, at present, there are no data to suggest that therapeutic anticoagulation decisions should be based on the presence or absence of the mutation.

Splanchnic vein thrombosis and *JAK2* V617F mutation

The *JAK2* V617F mutation is commonly found in patients with splanchnic vein thrombosis (Budd-Chiari syndrome, and portal, mesenteric, and splenic vein thrombosis), occurring in approximately a third of such patients. Only approximately half of these *JAK2* V617F mutation–positive patients have an overt myeloproliferative disorder at the time of the diagnosis of their thrombotic event. *JAK2* V617F mutation–positive patients with splanchnic vein thrombosis are more likely to develop a myeloproliferative disorder during follow-up than patients with splanchnic vein thrombosis without the mutation. Thus, patients with splanchnic vein thrombosis who are found to have the *JAK2* V617F mutation should be followed very closely to facilitate early detection of the development of clinical signs of a myeloproliferative disorder. However, one can similarly argue that *JAK2* V617F mutation–negative patients should be just as closely followed, because up to 10% of these patients will also develop a myeloproliferative disorder.

Other VTEs and *JAK2* V617F mutation

In patients with non–splanchnic vein thrombosis, the prevalence of the *JAK2* V617F mutation is <1%. Presence of the *JAK2* V617F mutation without symptoms of a myeloproliferative disorder is not associated with increased risk of recurrent venous thrombosis or progression to a myeloproliferative disorder over a 4-year follow-up period. This argues against screening patients with non–splanchnic vein thrombosis for the *JAK2* V617F mutation.

Paroxysmal nocturnal hemoglobinuria
General information

Paroxysmal nocturnal hemoglobinuria (PNH) is a clonal bone marrow disorder resulting from an acquired mutation of the phosphatidylinositol glycan class A (*PIG-A*) gene in a hematopoietic stem cell, leading to absent or decreased cell surface expression of glycoprotein (GP) I–anchored proteins on the surface of blood cells. PNH is associated with increased venous thrombosis, which most often occurs in intra-abdominal veins, particularly the hepatic veins (Budd-Chiari syndrome). Cerebral and peripheral vein thromboses also occur, but less commonly. The pathophysiology of thrombosis is not entirely understood, and no consistent abnormalities have been found. A number of etiologies have been hypothesized, including the following: (i) episodic hemolysis leading to an increase in circulating procoagulant microparticles derived from complement-injured CD55- and CD59-deficient monocytes and macrophages or from platelets and endothelial cells; (ii) complement-mediated platelet activation; and (iii) decreased fibrinolytic activity. Until recently, prevention and treatment of PNH-associated thrombosis were limited to anticoagulation. Long-term treatment with the complement inhibitor eculizumab (Soliris; Alexion Pharmaceuticals, Cheshire, CT), which was approved by the US Food and Drug Administration (FDA) in March 2007, has been demonstrated to reduce the risk of clinical thromboembolism in patients with PNH.

Management

Screening for PNH by peripheral blood flow cytometry for CD55 and CD59 is warranted in thrombophilia evaluations of patients with venous thrombosis and unexplained hemolysis or peripheral blood cytopenias. The various options in preventing and treating thrombosis in this rare disorder have recently been discussed in detail.

Abnormalities in fibrinolysis

A variety of parameters of fibrinolysis (Figure 7-5) have been investigated as potential causes of thrombophilia. Investigation of these parameters has been challenging because coagulation assays do not reliably reflect fibrinolysis of formed thrombi. Studies have often yielded conflicting or indecisive results regarding an association between antigen levels, enzyme activity, or certain polymorphisms and the risk for arterial or venous thrombosis. Given the variability of data associating impaired fibrinolysis to arterial and venous thrombosis, workup for abnormalities in the fibrinolytic pathway (ie, testing for plasminogen, tissue plasminogen activator [tPA], plasminogen activator inhibitor-1 [PAI-1], and thrombin-activatable fibrinolysis inhibitor [TAFI]) is, with the knowledge we have at present, not meaningful. Results neither explain the etiology of a thrombotic event in an individual patient nor influence decision making regarding length of anticoagulant therapy.

Plasminogen

Although plasminogen deficiency was initially believed to be a risk factor for thrombosis, more recent and cumulative data indicate that it does not lead to an increased risk for arterial or venous thrombosis. Thus, at present, plasminogen deficiency should not be considered a hypercoagulable state. Accordingly, there is no role for including plasminogen antigen or activity determination in a thrombophilia workup. Homozygous or double heterozygous defects in the plasminogen gene are associated with severe plasminogen deficiency and ligneous deposits in various tissues, such as the conjunctiva.

Tissue plasminogen activator

Increased tPA antigen levels have been found to increase the risk for arterial thrombosis in some, but not all, studies. No relationship with venous thrombosis has been detected. The observation that elevated tPA levels are associated with arterial thrombosis appears paradoxical. However, it has been speculated that this association may reflect an association of high PAI-1 levels with arterial thrombosis, which is the principal inhibitor of tPA. Surprisingly, though, the association between PAI-1 levels and arterial thrombosis has been conflicting and unconvincing. Several polymorphisms in the tPA gene have been described, but no clear association between these changes and arterial thromboembolism or VTE has been found.

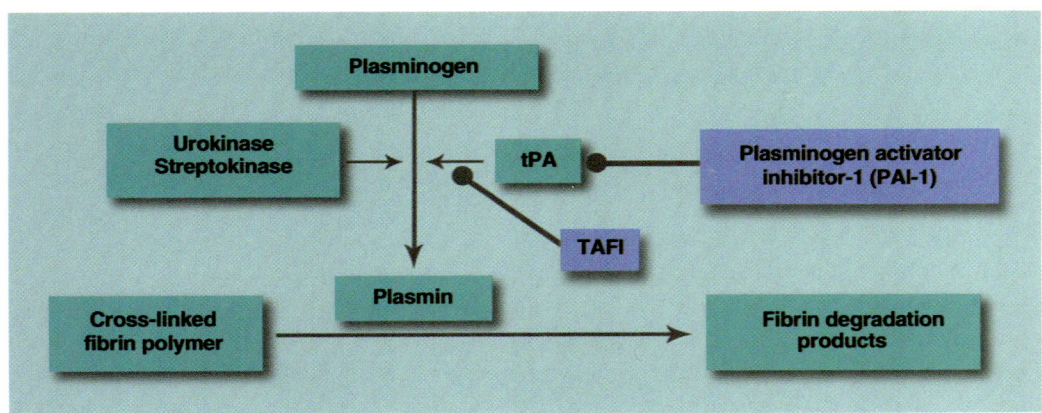

Figure 7-5 Fibrinolysis. TAFI = thrombin activatable fibrinolysis inhibitor; tPA = tissue plasminogen activator.

Plasminogen activator inhibitor-1

Although some inconsistent study findings exist regarding the association of elevated levels of PAI-1, the principal inhibitor of tPA, and the risk of VTE, overall it appears that increased levels are not a risk factor for VTE. The 4G/5G I/D polymorphism of the PAI-I gene promoter is the most frequently studied polymorphism of PAI-1 and has been shown to be associated with elevated PAI-1 antigen levels. Data on the association of the polymorphism with VTE have been inconsistent. Results of studies on the relationship between PAI-1 and arterial thrombosis are also conflicting and unconvincing. At this point, there is no clinical utility in obtaining PAI-1 activity or antigen levels or looking for PAI-1 polymorphisms when performing a thrombophilia workup in routine clinical practice.

Thrombin-activatable fibrinolysis inhibitor

TAFI suppresses fibrinolysis by cleaving residues from fibrin, thus interfering with the binding of plasmin to fibrin. Although a number of studies have shown an association between elevated TAFI levels and first or recurrent VTE and arterial thrombosis, not all studies have shown consistent results. There is no role for routine clinical testing for TAFI levels.

Other factors
Lipoprotein(a)

Lipoprotein(a) [Lp(a)], which is involved in cholesterol metabolism, competes with plasminogen for binding to fibrin due to its structural similarity with plasminogen. This impairs plasminogen activation, plasmin generation, and fibrinolysis. Lp(a) also binds to macrophages and promotes foam cell formation and the deposition of cholesterol in atherosclerotic plaques. Elevations in Lp(a) are associated with coronary heart disease and stroke in adults, as well as ischemic stroke in children. Although individual studies in adults on the association of Lp(a) and VTE have not shown consistent findings, a recent meta-analysis demonstrated that elevated levels are a mild risk factor for VTE. Similarly, studies of children show an association of elevations in Lp(a) with VTE.

Family history of VTE

Simply having a family history of VTE is a risk factor for VTE, no matter whether a thrombophilia is detectable or not. This additional risk is due to unknown or unmeasured risk factors. Having 1 first-degree relative with a history of VTE increases an individual's risk of VTE 2.2-fold; having ≥2 affected relatives increases the risk 3.9-fold. Young age of the affected relative and the number of affected relatives more strongly indicate a predisposition to develop VTE. Thus, in clinical practice, family history is an inexpensive and useful tool for risk assessment.

Others

Increased plasma coagulation factors IX and XI and fibrinogen have been shown to be risk factors for a first episode of VTE, but whether they influence the risk of recurrent VTE is not clear. Similarly, having a non-O blood group is a VTE risk factor. Dysfibrinogenemias are rare disorders, leading to either a thrombotic or a bleeding tendency. Elevated fibrinogen is a risk factor for arterial thromboembolism. Platelet glycoprotein polymorphisms have not been consistently shown to be risk factors for arterial thromboembolism.

Acquired conditions

A number of environmental and medical conditions lead to an increased risk for VTE.

Cancer

Approximately 20% of all VTEs occur in patients with cancer. The risk for VTE in cancer is determined by a number of coexisting factors that can broadly be divided into general risk factors (eg, age, obesity, past history of VTE, family history of VTE, coexisting medical conditions, inherited and acquired thrombophilias) and cancer-specific risk factors (eg, cancer type, stage, type of chemotherapy, hormonal therapy, surgery). Approximately 6% of patients with unprovoked VTE have a previously undiagnosed cancer at the time of the VTE, and approximately 10% of patients with unprovoked VTE will be diagnosed with a cancer in the year following the VTE diagnosis. It is not known whether extensive screening for cancer of the patient with unprovoked VTE is beneficial and leads to decreased cancer-associated morbidity or improved survival. Cancer should be considered in selected patients, such as the elderly and those with recent weight loss, but routine extensive screening for underlying cancer in all patients with unprovoked VTE is not recommended.

Contraceptive pills and patches

Estrogen contraceptives, no matter whether oral contraceptive pills (OCPs) or patches, increase the risk for VTE. In the overall female population, OCPs increase the risk of VTE 3- to 5-fold. However, the absolute risk is low (~1 in 3000 per year in a woman on OCPs) because VTE in the general young and healthy female population is low (~1 in 12,500 per year). Although it is mostly the estrogen component in contraceptives that determines the thrombotic risk, the type of progestin also plays a role; third-generation pills (ie, those containing the progestin desogestrel) and the estrogen/progestin contraceptive patch have twice the risk for VTE as second-generation pills. Limited data are available on the risk for VTE with progestins. It appears that they may increase the risk for VTE if given orally or as depot subcutaneous or intramuscular applications but appear to be without VTE risk if released at low doses from intrauterine devices.

The risk of VTE associated with estrogen contraceptives is further increased by a number of risk factors, such as obesity, smoking, a family history of VTE, and the presence of thrombophilias. For example, obese women who use OCPs have a 24-fold higher thrombotic risk compared with women of normal weight not taking OCPs (ie, absolute risk is 1 in 500 per year). Similarly, women who have heterozygous FVL and take OCPs have a 20- to 30-fold increased risk for VTE (ie, an absolute risk of ~1 in 500 per year). A significantly higher absolute risk is likely present in the woman on estrogen contraceptives who is obese, smokes, and has FVL. Risk factors are often not simply additive but multiplicative. For clinical practical consultative purposes, when counseling a woman with previous VTE, thrombophilia, or a family history of VTE, the woman's individual risk factors and her absolute risk for VTE need to be considered. The question is not whether estrogen-containing contraceptives are safe or contraindicated, but rather what is a patient's absolute risk and what risk is acceptable to an individual woman. General screening of all women prior to initiating contraceptives is not indicated.

Other conditions

Thrombosis may occur as a complication of systemic or local infection. Head and neck infections may trigger cerebral and sinus vein thrombosis. Liver disease will lead not only to a coagulopathy with bleeding diathesis due to decreased synthesis of procoagulant factors, but also to an increased risk for thrombosis due to decreased synthesis of anticoagulants (eg, AT, protein C and S) and fibrinolytic factors. In children, complex congenital heart disease is highly associated with both venous and arterial thrombotic events, either due to the disorders themselves or due to the need for cardiac catheterizations, hospitalization, and major surgeries.

Whom to test
Consensus guidelines

No general consensus exists as to which patients and family members should be tested for thrombophilias. At least 4 guidelines or consensus statements exist, created by the American College of Medical Geneticists, the College of American Pathologists, the British Committee for Standards in Hematology, and the European Genetics Foundation. A fifth one, by the Thrombosis Interest Group of Canada, is in development. These guidelines vary markedly in their recommendations as to who should or should not be tested, suggesting very limited testing, very widespread testing, or some intermediate level.

Reasons to test or not test

A variety of reasons for and against testing can be quoted (Table 7-3). In the United States, health insurance and employment discrimination based on a person's genetic testing results is illegal, as signed into law in May 2008 (Genetic Information Nondiscrimination Act [GINA]). However, life insurance discrimination—denial of insurance or higher premiums to be paid—based on genetic results is not included in GINA and therefore may occur. Thus, critical consideration should be given regarding which individuals should be tested for the genetic thrombophilias. The American College of Chest Physicians (ACCP) guidelines neither use the results of inherited thrombophilia screening as a factor in type, duration, or intensity of anticoagulant therapy in individuals who have had a VTE, nor for treatment decisions

Table 7-3 Reasons for performing or not performing thrombophilia testing.

Reasons for testing
Patient with thrombosis
  Influence on length of VKA therapy
  Explanation (for patient and physician) why thrombosis occurred
Asymptomatic individual (family member)
  Start VKA therapy?
  VTE prophylaxis in risk situations: higher doses, different length of therapy?
  Different choice regarding birth control or hormonal therapy?
  Different management during pregnancy?
  Lifestyle changes (weight loss, smoking cessation, increased physical activity)

Reasons for not testing
  Lack of therapeutic consequences even if test is positive/abnormal
  Suboptimal performance of tests (false-positive or false-negative results) and/or misinterpretation of tests
  Poor medical advice based on test results
  Life insurance implications
  Anxiety if test is positive
  False sense of security that thrombosis risk is low if test result is normal/negative.
  Cost of testing and consultations

INR = international normalized ratio; VKA = vitamin K antagonist; VTE = venous thromboembolism.

regarding who should receive VTE prophylaxis. It is important to realize that negative thrombophilia testing in an individual with a family history of thrombophilia does not guarantee protection from thrombotic events, because it has been shown that family history of VTE by itself is a risk factor for VTE.

Authors' approach

In view of the absence of generally accepted testing guidelines, the approach presented here is that of the authors of this chapter.

The adult hematologist's approach (S.M.)

The main reason why I test patients is to detect a higher risk thrombophilia (eg, APLA syndrome, AT deficiency, homozygous FVL, double heterozygous FVL plus prothrombin 20210 mutation, protein C deficiency, and protein S deficiency, and perhaps homozygous prothrombin 20210 mutation). Although there is no agreed-upon definition of higher risk thrombophilia, one could define it as an annual VTE incidence of >0.5% or a VTE recurrence rate, if off warfarin, of >30%. The finding of a higher risk thrombophilia has a number of consequences in my practice: (i) it decreases my threshold to recommend long-term anticoagulation in a patient who has had an episode of spontaneous VTE; (ii) it leads to discussion with the patient with an unexplained arterial, nonarteriosclerotic thromboembolic event whether anticoagulant or antiplatelet therapy might be the preferred treatment for secondary prevention; and (iii) it prompts recommendation for testing of the identified thrombophilia(s) in asymptomatic female family members (Table 7-4) and prompts advice against the use of estrogen birth control methods and for anticoagulation prophylaxis during the postpartum and, possibly, the antepartum period. I do not test for parameters of fibrinolysis or for the MTHFR polymorphisms. I limit homocysteine testing to the individual <30 years of age with thrombosis to assess for the presence of homocystinuria. Table 7-5 lists the thrombophilia tests

Table 7-5 Tests the author (SM) considers if decision on thrombophilia workup is made.

Arterial thromboembolism
- Complete blood count
- Protein C activity
- Protein S activity, free protein S antigen
- Antithrombin activity
- Anticardiolipin IgG and IgM antibodies
- Anti–β_2-glycoprotein I IgG and IgM antibodies
- Lupus anticoagulant

Venous thromboembolism
- Complete blood count
- Factor V Leiden
- Prothrombin 20210 mutation
- Protein C activity
- Protein S activity, free protein S antigen
- Antithrombin activity
- Anticardiolipin IgG and IgM antibodies
- Anti–β_2-glycoprotein I IgG and IgM antibodies
- Lupus anticoagulant
- *JAK2* V617F and PNH in splanchnic vein thrombosis
- Lipoprotein(a) (in pediatrics)

IgG = immunoglobulin G; IgM = immunoglobulin M; PNH = paroxysmal nocturnal hemoglobinuria.

that I order when evaluating a patient for thrombophilia. Table 7-6 lists the type of patients in whom I consider thrombophilia testing. However, individual decisions, often in discussion with the patient, need to be made when deciding on whom to test and how extensively to test.

The pediatric hematologist's approach (J.J.)

The incidence of thromboembolism in children who are younger than 15 years of age with confirmed thrombophilia, even with one of the stronger thrombophilias, is low. The need for thrombophilia screening in asymptomatic children is subject to debate. Finding a higher risk thrombophilia might argue for pharmacologic DVT prophylaxis in risk situations where otherwise such prophylaxis would not be

Table 7-4 Author's (SM) recommendation when to consider family testing of a patient (= proband) with thrombophilia.

	Male		Female	
Proband's thrombophilia	Proband's sons	Proband's brothers	Proband's daughters	Proband's sisters
Hetero FVL or hetero II20210	No testing	No testing	No testing	No testing
Homo FVL or homo II20210	No testing	Reasonable to test	No testing	Test
Double hetero or compound thrombophilia	Reasonable to test	Reasonable to test	Test	Test
Protein C, S, or AT deficiency	Reasonable to test	Reasonable to test	Test	Test

For a detailed discussion, see the text. "Reasonable to test": consider VTE prophylaxis with airline travel, cast, nonmajor surgery; prolonged prophylaxis after major surgeries. "Test": advise against estrogen therapy; give ante- and postpartum anticoagulation, if strong thrombophilia found.

Table 7-6 When to consider thrombophilia testing.

- VTE occurring at a younger age (ie, <50 years)
- Unprovoked VTE
- Recurrent VTE
- Thrombosis at an unusual site (splanchnic, sinus/cerebral, or renal veins)
- Unusually extensive spontaneous VTE
- Family history of VTE
- Asymptomatic individual with family history of strong thrombophilia (see Table 7-5):
  ○ Antithrombin deficiency
  ○ Protein C deficiency
  ○ Protein S deficiency
  ○ Homozygous factor V Leiden
  ○ Homozygous prothrombin mutation
  ○ Compound thrombophilias
- Recurrent VTE while adequately anticoagulated
- Unexplained arterial thromboembolism in a young person (ie, no arteriosclerosis risk factors, no cardioembolic source)
- ≥3 unexplained pregnancy losses before week 10 or ≥1 loss after week 10

VTE = venous thromboembolism.

given. Those opposing screening asymptomatic family members argue that knowing about the tendency for thrombosis has the same benefits as laboratory screening because a negative screening test in an individual with a significant family history of VTE does not guarantee protection from thrombotic events. For children with documented thromboembolic disease, there is also no consensus about when and what to screen. There is some rationale for testing children with severe or progressive thrombus in an acute setting for deficiencies of the natural anticoagulant proteins because replacement of these proteins may aid in the management of the patient. Although a recent meta-analysis in children with inherited thrombophilia demonstrated that inherited thrombophilia, with the exceptions of FVL and Lp(a) elevation, increases a child's risk for recurrent VTE, there is no evidence that screening and identifying the inherited thrombophilia, rather than practicing standard DVT prophylaxis, in any person who has had one event will reduce the rate of recurrence or postthrombotic syndrome.

Interpreting test results and educating patients

When interpreting thrombophilia laboratory test results, it is important to be aware of the circumstances that lead to abnormal test results without a true thrombophilia being present. Several results are temporarily abnormal in the patient with acute thrombosis receiving therapy with heparin and VKAs (Tables 7-1 and 7-2). When a thrombophilia is identified, educating the patient and the patient's family members is important. Online education and support resources on a variety of thrombophilias and the genetic aspects of family testing exist (www.stoptheclot.org; www.fvleiden.org; and others). Patient advocacy can be a powerful tool to promote public awareness, better health care delivery, and more research. Therefore, patients with thrombosis and thrombophilia should consider getting involved in patient advocacy, and health care providers should make their patients aware of opportunities to get involved.

Antithrombotic drugs

Venous thrombosis occurs mostly via activity of the plasma coagulation system, with only minor platelet participation. In contrast, platelets play a major role in arterial thrombus formation, with the plasma coagulation system participating some. This paradigm helps explain why drugs that block the plasmatic coagulation reaction (ie, anticoagulants) are very active in prevention of venous thrombosis and also effective in preventing arterial thrombosis, whereas antiplatelet drugs, which successfully prevent arterial thrombosis, are less or not at all effective in venous disease. As discussed in detail in Chapter 7, thrombus formation involves 3 steps: (i) platelet adhesion, (ii) platelet aggregation, and (iii) plasmatic coagulation. The natural anticoagulant system (AT, proteins C and S, and tissue factor pathway inhibitor) prevents excessive thrombus formation. The fibrinolytic system (tPA and plasminogen) degrades fibrin, prevents excessive clot formation, and facilitates clot breakdown (Figure 7-5). The group of antithrombotic drugs consists of anticoagulants, antiplatelet agents, and fibrinolytics.

Antiplatelet agents
Aspirin

Aspirin (acetylsalicylic acid) inhibits the enzyme cyclooxygenase-1 (COX-1), which is needed to form thromboxane A_2 in platelets. Thromboxane A_2 is normally released from platelet granules upon platelet adhesion and during platelet aggregation and serves as an agonist to activate and, thus, recruit other platelets to the platelet plug. Because platelets do not synthesize new cyclooxygenase and aspirin binds irreversibly to COX-1, aspirin's action lasts for the life span of a platelet (ie, 7–10 days). Complete inactivation of platelet COX-1 is typically achieved with a daily dose of aspirin of 160 mg. When used as an antithrombotic drug, aspirin is maximally effective at doses between 50 and 325 mg/d. Higher doses do not improve efficacy. However, there is considerable interindividual variability in aspirin's ability to inhibit COX-1, giving rise to biochemical and clinical aspirin resistance in a number of patients.

Phosphodiesterase inhibitors
Dipyridamole

Dipyridamole (Persantine) leads to an increase in intraplatelet cyclic adenosine monophosphate (cAMP) levels, which inhibits platelet aggregation to several agonists. However, dipyridamole by itself has little or no effect as an antithrombotic drug. Its platelet aggregation inhibitory effect is reversible. The combination of aspirin 25 mg and dipyridamole 200 mg in a sustained-release formulation is available as Aggrenox. Dipyridamole also has vasodilatory effects and should, therefore, be used with caution in patients with severe coronary artery disease, in whom episodes of angina may increase due to the steal phenomenon. Aggrenox has its major indication in secondary stroke prevention.

Cilostazol

Cilostazol (Pletal) is a selective inhibitor of the phosphodiesterase-3 isoenzyme and leads to inhibition of agonist-induced platelet aggregation, granule release, and thromboxane A_2 production. It also has vasodilatory effects and should not be used in patients with congestive heart failure. Cilostazol has its major indication in disabling claudication, particularly when revascularization cannot be performed.

Pentoxifylline

Pentoxifylline (Trental) is a phosphodiesterase inhibitor that has been shown to have some beneficial effects in ischemic disease states. Its inhibitory action on phosphodiesterase in erythrocytes leads to increased cAMP levels and improved erythrocyte flexibility, and reduction of blood viscosity may be the result of decreased plasma fibrinogen concentrations and inhibition of red blood cell and platelet aggregation. The major indication for pentoxifylline is peripheral arterial disease with claudication.

Adenosine diphosphate receptor antagonists
Clopidogrel and ticlopidine

Clopidogrel (Plavix) and ticlopidine (Ticlid) inhibit the platelet adenosine diphosphate (ADP) receptor $P2Y_{12}$ by irreversibly altering its structure. Both drugs are closely related, but clopidogrel has a more favorable adverse effect profile with less frequent thrombocytopenia and leukopenia and has, therefore, replaced ticlopidine in clinical use. Because maximal inhibition of platelet aggregation is not seen until day 8 to 11 after starting therapy, loading doses of these drugs are often given to achieve a more rapid onset of action. Inhibition of platelet aggregation persists for the life span of the platelet. In all indications, clopidogrel appears to be equally effective as aspirin, except in peripheral arterial disease, where it has been shown to be slightly more effective than aspirin for the prevention of ischemic events.

Prasugrel

A number of new ADP receptor agonists are in development. These are $P2Y_{12}$ antagonists that, compared with clopidogrel, are more rapid in onset and lead to less variable platelet response and more complete inhibition of platelet function. Prasugrel (Effient) was FDA approved in July 2009 for use in patients with unstable angina or myocardial infarction who are to be managed with percutaneous coronary intervention; it demonstrated increased efficacy compared with clopidogrel but was associated with an increased rate of major bleeding. Other agents in late stages of clinical development, but not FDA approved as of June 2010, are ticagrelor, cangrelor, and elinogrel.

GPIIb/IIIa receptor antagonists

The platelet GPIIb/IIIa receptor is the site where fibrinogen binds during platelet aggregation, resulting in cross-linking of platelets and platelet plug formation. Several inhibitors of this receptor have been developed and are in clinical use.

Abciximab

Abciximab (ReoPro) is the Fab fragment of a chimeric human–murine monoclonal antibody against the GPIIb/IIIa receptor. The drug is given as a bolus, followed by a continuous infusion for 12 hours or longer. Unbound drug is cleared from the circulation with a half-life of approximately 30 minutes. Drug bound to the GPIIb/IIIa receptor inhibits platelet aggregation for 18 to 24 hours, measured in vitro, but bound drug is demonstrable in the circulation for up to 10 days. Ex vivo platelet clumping in ethylenediaminetetraacetic acid (EDTA)-containing blood tubes can be seen in patients treated with the drug, leading to pseudothrombocytopenia when platelets are counted by an automatic blood cell counter. This phenomenon is clinically irrelevant and does not require discontinuation of the drug. However, true thrombocytopenia also occurs and, if severe enough, can require drug discontinuation.

Eptifibatide

Eptifibatide (Integrilin) is a synthetic peptide inhibitor of the so-called RGD binding site of the GPIIb/IIIa receptor. It mimics the geometric and charge characteristics of the RGD sequence of fibrinogen, thus occupying the GPIIb/IIIa receptor and preventing binding of fibrinogen and, in turn, preventing platelet aggregation. It is given as a bolus, followed by a continuous infusion for up to 3 days. The platelet aggregation inhibitory effect lasts for 6 to 12 hours after cessation of infusion.

Tirofiban

Tirofiban (Aggrastat) is a nonpeptide (peptidomimetic), small-molecule inhibitor of the GPIIb/IIIa receptor, which also binds to the RGD receptor site, similar to eptifibatide.

Oral GPIIb/IIIa antagonists

Oral GPIIb/IIIa antagonists, such as orbofiban, sibrafiban, and xemilofiban, were associated with a surprising excess in mortality. Development of these drugs was stopped. They are not clinically available.

Pediatric considerations

Aspirin dose in children is generally 1 to 5 mg/kg daily, but there is variability in the dose required to inhibit platelet aggregation. The primary adverse effect of long-term aspirin therapy is bleeding, but it is rarely seen, except in neonates who have slower clearance, patients with concurrent bleeding disorders, or children receiving anticoagulation therapy. There is also theoretical risk of developing Reye syndrome in children with intercurrent influenza or varicella infection, but this complication is not usually seen unless the dose of aspirin is >40 mg/kg, a high dose necessary for an anti-inflammatory effect. Dipyridamole in doses of 2 to 5 mg/kg is an alternative to aspirin therapy. Drugs that selectively inhibit ADP-induced platelet aggregation have not been well studied in children.

Anticoagulants
Heparins
Mechanism of action

Heparins are extracted from porcine intestine or bovine lung and consist of glycosaminoglycans of different lengths. Unfractionated heparins have a mean length of 40 monosaccharide units. Low molecular weight heparins (LMWHs) are made from unfractionated heparin through chemical and physical processes and have a mean of 15 monosaccharide units. A pentasaccharide structure within these polysaccharide molecules binds to and enhances the action of AT, which inactivates thrombin and factor Xa. Molecules of 18 monosaccharide units or more are required to bind thrombin and AT simultaneously, leading to the inactivation of thrombin.

The 5 sugars of the pentasaccharide structure, however, are sufficient to lead to a conformational change of AT that can then inactivate factor Xa. Therefore, LMWHs inactivate mostly factor Xa, whereas unfractionated heparin acts mostly against thrombin. Fondaparinux (Arixtra) is a synthetic pentasaccharide that binds to AT, leading to specific inactivation of factor Xa.

Management of bleeding

If bleeding occurs in a patient on unfractionated heparin, intravenous protamine can be given, which binds to and neutralizes heparin. Protamine can impair platelet function and interact with coagulation factors, causing an anticoagulant effect of its own. Therefore, the minimal amount of protamine to neutralize heparin should be given. LMWH is only partially reversed by protamine. However, in case of significant bleeding on LMWH, protamine should be considered, and for major bleeding, recombinant factor VIIa (NovoSeven) should be given. Protamine is likely not successful at reversing fondaparinux. Recombinant factor VIIa can be used in major bleeding associated with fondaparinux. Fresh frozen plasma (FFP) likely has little, if any, effect on bleeding associated with heparin, LMWH, and fondaparinux and is not indicated unless there is also evidence of a coagulopathy from factor depletion.

Heparin-induced thrombocytopenia

Heparin-induced thrombocytopenia (HIT) is defined as the occurrence of thrombocytopenia and a positive test for heparin-associated antibodies in a patient treated with heparin. Arterial thromboembolism and VTE can result. Strict criteria for HIT include a platelet count decrease to <100,000/μL or of >50% from baseline. However, less strict definitions for HIT are a platelet count decrease to <150,000/μL or a decrease of >30% from baseline. The clinical picture of HIT (ie, thrombosis and demonstration of heparin-associated antibodies) in patients treated with heparin can occur even with platelet counts remaining normal or, rarely, unchanged counts (termed *HIT without thrombocytopenia*). Classically, the onset of thrombocytopenia is between days 5 and 10 after the initiation of heparin therapy, but it can occur in <1 day if the patient has had heparin exposure within the preceding 100 days. The *4T score* has been evaluated as a tool to aid in the likelihood assessment that a patient has HIT. The 4 T's are as follows: (i) degree of **t**hrombocytopenia, (ii) **t**iming of thrombocytopenia, (iii) new **t**hrombosis during heparin therapy, and (iv) al**t**ernative reason is present for the thrombocytopenia. Each of these 4 components is ranked from 0 to 2 based on defined criteria, and the total score allows an assessment as HIT unlikely, moderate suspicion for HIT, or HIT likely. Confirmatory HIT antibody tests are heparin–platelet factor-4 antibody (HIT-PF4) enzyme-linked immunosorbent assay (ELISA), heparin-induced platelet aggregation study, and heparin-induced serotonin release assay. The HIT-PF4 ELISA is the most sensitive assay but the least specific. Many patients exposed to high doses of heparin, such as after cardiopulmonary bypass surgery, develop HIT-PF4 antibodies, which often do not lead to thrombocytopenia or thrombosis and appear to be clinically irrelevant. The HIT-PF4 ELISA is the test most widely used for the diagnosis of HIT. The heparin-induced platelet aggregation test and heparin-induced serotonin release assay are functional assays and are more specific for the pathogenic antibodies that actually cause the clinical picture of HIT.

HIT most commonly occurs in the patient on unfractionated heparin but can also develop on LMWH. It more commonly occurs with intravenous heparin therapy but can also be seen with subcutaneous dosing. In the patient with a moderate or high suspicion for HIT, heparin should be discontinued, and alternative anticoagulants should be started. The FDA-approved drugs for use in HIT are hirudins (lepirudin and bivalirudin) and argatroban. Desirudin is another hirudin derivative, available as a subcutaneous preparation, but it is not FDA approved for HIT. Danaparoid also has been used in HIT but was not FDA approved for that indication and is unavailable in the United States. Fondaparinux has rarely been associated with HIT and is sometimes used in HIT because HIT antibodies generally do not cross-react with the drug. A lack of systematic studies has precluded the authors of the ACCP 2008 guidelines from making recommendations about the use of fondaparinux in HIT, and it is not FDA approved for HIT.

VKAs should not be used before the platelet count has increased to 150,000/μL. The alternate anticoagulant drug (ie, a direct thrombin inhibitor or fondaparinux) should overlap with the VKA for a minimum of 5 days. Because there is cross-reactivity of the HIT-PF4 antibody between unfractionated heparin and LMWH, the latter is not a treatment alternative when HIT on unfractionated heparin has been diagnosed. Detailed recommendations for platelet count monitoring while on heparin and for the diagnosis and treatment of HIT are available in the 2008 guidelines of the ACCP.

Heparin resistance

Heparin resistance is a term used when patients require unusually high doses of unfractionated heparin to prolong the aPTT into the therapeutic range or prolong the activated clotting time above the value (typically >400 or 450 seconds) at which extracorporeal circulation on heparin is thought to be safe from an anticoagulant point of view. Causes can be AT deficiency; increased heparin clearance; significantly low baseline aPTT, such as due to elevations of factor VIII and fibrinogen; or increased nonspecific heparin-binding proteins. Occasionally, AT concentrate is considered for heparin resistance, but no detailed guidelines exist as to who should receive it, in what doses, and for how long.

Unfractionated heparin

Unfractionated heparin at therapeutic doses typically needs to be monitored with the aPTT. The therapeutic aPTT range depends on the heparin sensitivity of the aPTT reagent and the instrument used by a laboratory. A therapeutic aPTT is considered that which corresponds to a plasma anti-Xa heparin level of 0.3 to 0.7 U/mL. Optimally, a coagulation laboratory should provide clinicians with the therapeutic aPTT range for the reagent–instrument combination used in that laboratory. If a laboratory has not provided a therapeutic aPTT range for aPTT determinations, then an aPTT ratio of 2.0 to 2.5 of the mean aPTT of the normal range is often considered to be therapeutic. However, with some aPTT reagents, this range is subtherapeutic, and underdosing of a patient may occur. Heparin is mostly cleared by the reticuloendothelial system and to a smaller degree by the kidney. Patients with renal failure may require less heparin to prolong their aPTT into the therapeutic range. The half-life of heparin in plasma depends on the dose given. It is 60 minutes with a 100 U/kg bolus. A patient on continuous infusion intravenous unfractionated heparin at therapeutic doses will likely have a return to the baseline aPTT within 3 to 4 hours after discontinuation of heparin.

A nomogram needs to be used for heparin dosing. In many patients at average risk for bleeding, a loading dose of 80 U/kg heparin intravenous, followed by a continuous infusion of 18 U/kg/h is appropriate for full anticoagulation. However, this dosing may have to be modified in the patient at higher risk for bleeding. The aPTT should be determined 6 hours after initiation of heparin and after each dose change, and once every 24 hours once the aPTT is in the therapeutic range. In the occasional patient in whom the aPTT is invalid, such as a patient with a lupus anticoagulant or coagulation factor XII deficiency, anti-Xa levels need to be used for heparin monitoring. Neonates may require higher doses of heparin because the clearance is more rapid secondary to a large volume of distribution and they have lower AT levels. Long-term use of unfractionated heparin leads to an increased risk of osteoporosis. There is also a potential risk of osteoporosis with long-term LMWH use, but the risk is less than with unfractionated heparin.

Low molecular weight heparin

The various LMWH drugs differ in their composition and, thus, in their degree of antithrombin and anti-Xa activity. Therefore, dose recommendations for DVT prophylaxis and for treatment doses vary for the various LMWHs. The lack of significant binding of LMWH to plasma proteins gives them a more predictable anticoagulant effect compared with unfractionated heparin, so that fixed or weight-adjusted dosing is possible without the need for routine anticoagulant laboratory monitoring. The peak plasma effect is reached 3 to 4 hours after injection. The half-lives of the various agents differ, ranging between 3 and 7 hours. Once- or twice-daily dosing regimens are available for the different drugs. Because the LMWHs are renally cleared, dose reduction and anti-Xa monitoring is needed in patients with renal impairment. However, because the pharmacokinetic effect of impaired renal function may differ among LMWHs, there is no single creatinine clearance cutoff value below which dose reduction is clearly needed. A value of <30 mL/min is likely an appropriate cutoff threshold in most patients and with most LMWH drugs. In severe renal impairment and dialysis dependence, unfractionated heparin should be chosen over LMWH. In obese patients, an increase in prophylaxis doses is recommended for patients with morbid obesity (body mass index >40 kg/m^2). For full-dose LMWH use, dosing should be based on absolute body weight, and anti-Xa monitoring is generally not necessary for patients weighing up to 150 kg. Anti-Xa monitoring can be considered in patients with morbid obesity. Twice-daily dosing may be preferable over once-daily dosing.

A therapeutic anti-Xa level is approximately 1.0 to 2.0 U/mL for once-daily dosing and approximately 0.6 to 1.2 U/mL for twice-daily dosing, obtained 3 to 4 hours after subcutaneous injection. Anti-Xa levels should be determined if a patient on LMWH has a recurrent thrombosis or a significant bleed, to document whether the patient had sub- or supratherapeutic anti-Xa levels, which could explain the clotting or bleeding event. Many neonates (especially preterm) have minimal subcutaneous tissue, making injection impractical; thus, intravenous anticoagulation with LMWH can be considered. In children treated with therapeutic doses of LMWH, routine monitoring with anti-Xa levels is advocated, particularly because LMWH therapy is often instituted in critically or chronically ill children.

Fondaparinux

Fondaparinux (Arixtra) is a synthetic pentasaccharide, AT dependent, consisting of the key 5 monosaccharides of heparin that bind to AT and inhibit factor Xa. It is a specific anti-Xa agent without any antithrombin activity. It is given subcutaneously, reaches its peak plasma level in 2 hours, and, because of a half-life of approximately 17 hours, is dosed once daily. Because it does not bind significantly to plasma proteins, it can be given without laboratory monitoring as a fixed dose for prophylaxis of VTE or in body weight–adjusted fashion for therapy of VTE. It is cleared by the kidney and thus should not be used in patients with renal failure.

Thrombin inhibitors

Hirudins

Natural hirudin is a 65–amino acid direct thrombin inhibitor derived from the saliva of the leech *Hirudo medicinalis*. It does not require the presence of AT to exert its anticoagulant effect. Several derivatives and recombinant products have been developed. Lepirudin (Refludan) is a recombinant hirudin consisting of 65 amino acids that is administered intravenously and monitored by the aPTT. A therapeutic aPTT range is considered to be 1.5 to 2.5 times the median of the laboratory's normal aPTT range. The drug is renally cleared and has a half-life of approximately 80 minutes. It should not be used in patients with renal impairment. It is FDA approved for HIT. Desirudin (Iprivask) is also a 65–amino acid recombinant hirudin administered subcutaneously. Peak plasma levels are reached 1 to 3 hours after injection. It is primarily metabolized by the kidney, and dose reductions are needed in patients with moderate and severe renal impairment. It is FDA approved for postsurgical DVT prophylaxis. Bivalirudin (Angiomax) is a synthetic, 20–amino acid polypeptide that directly binds to and inhibits thrombin. It is given intravenously and has a half-life of 25 minutes. Dose adjustment for severe renal impairment is necessary. It is FDA approved for use during percutaneous transluminal coronary angioplasty, HIT, and DVT prophylaxis.

Argatroban

Argatroban (Novastan) is a small synthetic molecule that binds to and inhibits thrombin at its catalytic site. It is given intravenously. Because it is metabolized in the liver, dosage reductions in patients with impaired liver function are necessary. Serum tests for liver function should always be obtained prior to its use. Its half-life is 40 to 50 minutes. The drug can be started without the need for an initial bolus. The dosing is adjusted to an aPTT of 1.5 to 3 times the initial baseline value (not to exceed 100 seconds). It is FDA approved for HIT.

Vitamin K antagonists

Mechanism of action

All coagulation factors are synthesized in the liver, although von Willebrand factor and factor VIII are also produced in extrahepatic sites. Factors II, VII, IX, and X and protein C and protein S need to be carboxylated in a final synthetic reaction to become biologically active. This step requires the presence of vitamin K (Figure 7-6). The oral anticoagulants presently available in the United States for routine clinical use are VKAs. The half-lives of the vitamin K–dependent coagulation factors are 4 to 6 hours for factor VII, 24 hours for factor IX, 36 hours for factor X, 50 hours for factor II, 8 hours for protein C, and 30 hours for protein S. Because of the long half-lives of some of these factors, particularly factor II, the full antithrombotic effect of VKAs is not reached until several days after having started these drugs. Because protein C has a relatively short half life and decreases early, its lowering renders the patient hypercoagulable during the first few treatment days, before factor II, with its longer half-life, decreases and protects the patient from thrombosis. Thus, VKAs create a prothrombotic state in the first 5 days, putting the patient at risk for coumarin-induced skin necrosis and progression of thrombosis, unless a parenteral anticoagulant is given overlapping with the VKA in these first few days. The parenteral anticoagulant should be given for at least 5 days and until the INR is >2.0 on two subsequent days.

Monitoring and dose requirement

VKAs are monitored with the prothrombin time (PT). Because results of the PT depend on the sensitivity of the PT reagent used in the laboratory, PT measurements are converted to an INR by a calculation that includes a reagent's sensitivity (international sensitivity index). Coumarin VKAs are metabolized by the cytochrome P450 enzyme complex, mostly the enzymes CYP2C9 and CYP1A2 (Figure 7-6). Because of a high degree of interindividual variability in the activity of these enzymes, there is a high degree of variability in the daily drug dose that patients need to maintain their INR in the therapeutic range. Polymorphisms in the genes transcribing enzymes involved in the metabolism of VKAs, such as *CYP2C9* (cytochrome P2C9 enzyme) and *VKORC1* (vitamin K epoxide reductase complex-1), contribute to the variability in dose requirements. Finger stick whole blood INR monitors are available and yield equally reliable results as plasma-based INRs from phlebotomies. INR home monitoring by appropriately selected patients is safe and effective and a good treatment option. In some patients with fluctuating INRs, daily supplementation with vitamin K, such as 100 to 150 μg/d, has been shown to decrease INR fluctuations.

Available oral anticoagulants

Two classes of VKAs exist: coumarin derivates (warfarin, phenprocoumon, acenocoumarol, and tioclomarol), which are the most widely used VKAs; and the indandione derivatives (fluindione, anisindione, and phenindione), which are used in some countries outside the United States. The only FDA-approved VKAs are warfarin (approved in 1954) and anisindione (approved in 1957). Warfarin (Coumadin, Jantoven) has a half-life of 1 to 2.5 days, with a mean of approximately 40 hours.

The typical loading dose of warfarin in the hospitalized patient is 5 mg daily on days 1 and 2, with subsequent dosing based on the INR measurement after the first 2 doses. In children, this will equate to initial doses of 0.1 to 0.2 mg/kg. A frail or elderly patient or one who has been treated with prolonged antibiotics, has liver disease, or has undergone intestinal resection, will need a lower dose in the first few days. Some clinicians prefer using higher loading doses of 7.5 to 10 mg, particularly in a nutritionally repleted outpatient. For maintenance dosing, the highest

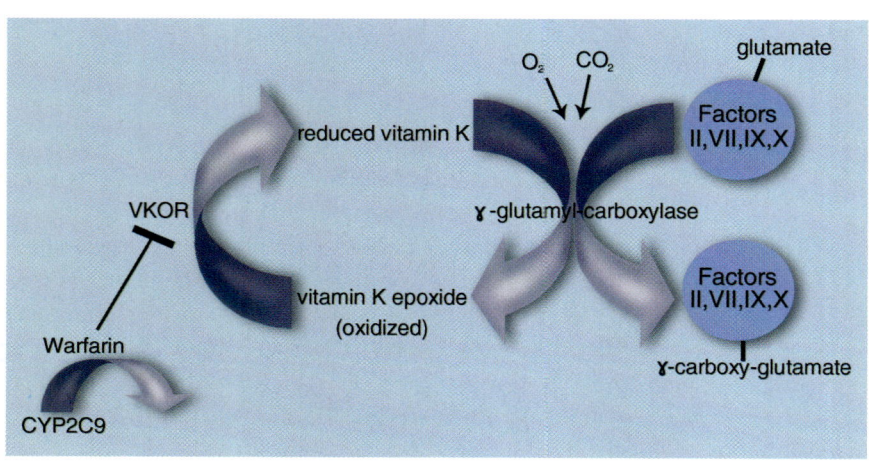

Figure 7-6 Role of vitamin K, point of activation of warfarin, and enzymes involved in vitamin K and warfarin metabolism.

dose requirements for keeping a patient in the therapeutic range are in men <50 years old (median dose, 6.4 mg/d), and the lowest requirements are in women >70 years old (median dose, 3.1 mg/d). Occasionally, patients need doses as high as 20 or 30 mg/d. Genetic testing for polymorphisms of the *CYP2C9* and *VKORC1* enzyme genes is available and helps predict, to some degree, warfarin doses needed to reach therapeutic INR ranges, but the clinical utility of these tests has not been clearly demonstrated.

Management of elevated INRs and bleeding

Several options exist to manage elevated INRs and bleeding that occur on VKAs, and the choice depends on the degree of INR elevation and the presence or absence of risk factors for bleeding and of active bleeding itself. These options have been published as recommendations from the ACCP (Table 7-7) and encompass holding the next anticoagulant dose(s) and giving vitamin K. Giving too high a dose of vitamin K should be avoided if there is no major bleeding, because it will reverse the INR completely and may make reanticoagulation of the patient more difficult. FFP can lower the INR some but not completely or markedly, because the short half-life of coagulation factor VII of 4 to 6 hours would require large and clinically impractical doses of FFP to be given for full reversal. If complete or immediate INR reversal is needed, such as when treating a major bleeding episode, a prothrombin complex concentrate (PCC) can be given. PCCs are plasma products from human donors and consist of the vitamin K–dependent factors (ie, factors II, VII, IX, and X). They exist as so-called *4-factor PCCs*, containing nearly 100% of these coagulation factors, and as *3-factor PCCs* (eg, Bebulin, Profilnine), which contain relatively low concentrations of factor VII. The 4-factor products are not FDA approved and not available in the United States. Therefore, in the United States, if a patient with VKA-associated bleeding or in whom VKA reversal is the goal is being treated with PCCs, additional FFP should also be given to increase the patient's plasma levels of factor VII.

Periprocedural interruption of oral anticoagulant therapy

Whether there is a need to stop oral anticoagulant therapy prior to a surgical or radiologic procedure depends on the bleeding risk associated with the procedure. How soon before the procedure the drug should be stopped depends on the INR. Whether bridging therapy with a subcutaneous or intravenous anticoagulant needs to be given before and after the procedure depends on the thromboembolic risk of the patient. Guidelines have been created by the ACCP to address these issues (Table 7-8).

Pediatric considerations

VKA therapy is problematic in very young children because newborns have reduced levels of the vitamin K–dependent proteins; infant formulas containing vitamin K supplements can cause resistance to VKAs, whereas breastfed infants will be very sensitive to VKAs because there is a negligible amount of vitamin K in breast milk; infants and even some older children have inadequate venous access for the frequent monitoring of INR that is required; and VKA therapy and INR values are affected by febrile illnesses, dehydration, concurrent use of antibiotics for common childhood infections, dietary changes, and weight gain. The major complication of VKA use is bleeding, occurring in 3% to 12% of patients. Reported nonhemorrhagic complications in children treated with VKA therapy for over a year include hair loss, tracheal calcification, and loss of bone density. Point-of-care whole blood monitors have made regulating VKA therapy more convenient for families because they can perform the test regularly at home via fingerstick.

Drugs in development

A large number of new anticoagulant agents are in development and being tested in clinical trials, most prominently a number of new oral agents that have a wide therapeutic window and predictable anticoagulant effect, so that in most

Table 7-7 Recommendations for management of elevated INRs and/or bleeding in patients on vitamin K antagonists (ACCP 2008 guidelines).

INR	Bleeding?	Risk factor for bleeding?	Intervention
Supratherapeutic, but < 5,0	No	No/yes	Lower or omit next VKA dose. Reduce subsequent dose
5,0 - 9,0	No	No	Omit next VKA doses. Reduce subsequent dose
5,0 - 9,0	No	Yes	Vitamin K 1–2.5 mg p.o.
> 9,0	No	No/yes	Vitamin K 2.5–5 mg p.o.
Serious bleed at any INR	Yes		Vitamin K 10 mg i.v. + FFP or PCCs or recombinant factor VIIa

*FFP = fresh frozen plasma; PCCs = prothrombin complex concentrates; VKA = vitamin K antagonist.

Table 7-8 Recommendations* when interrupting warfarin therapy for invasive procedures (ACCP 2008 guidelines).

Risk of thrombosis	Before surgery	After surgery
Low	• d/c warfarin ca. 5 d pre-op • No LMWH or low dose LMWH	• Restart warfarin 12-24 hrs after surgery • No LMWH or low dose LMWH
Intermediate	• d/c warfarin ca. 5 d pre-op • Prophylactic or full dose LMWH, or full-dose i.v. UFH	• Restart warfarin 12–24 hrs after surgery • Prophylactic or full dose LMWH, or full-dose i.v. UFH
High	• d/c warfarin ca. 5 d pre-op • Full-dose LMWH or i.v UFH	• Restart warfarin 12–24 hrs after surgery • Full-dose LMWH or i.v UFH

*These recommendations are all so-called "grade C" recommendations (ie, very weak recommendations). Other alternatives may be equally reasonable.

patients no monitoring is required. Most of these drugs are small-molecule inhibitors of coagulation factor Xa (anti-Xa drugs) and thrombin (anti-IIa drugs). These drugs do not exert their anticoagulant effect through interference with the vitamin K pathway; thus, there are no dietary restrictions for the patient regarding vitamin K intake. The thrombin inhibitor ximelagatran (Exanta) was approved in Europe for short-term use in orthopedic DVT prophylaxis, but was voluntarily withdrawn from the market in 2006; its development was stopped because of concerns about drug-induced liver toxicity. The thrombin inhibitor dabigatran and the anti-Xa agent rivaroxaban are approved for orthopedic DVT prophylaxis in a number of countries, but not in the United States. Dabigatran, rivaroxaban, and the direct anti-Xa inhibitor apixaban are presently in phase III clinical trials for a number of indications. Several other compounds are in phase I and II clinical trials.

Idraparinux is a pentasaccharide anticoagulant agent in development that has not been FDA approved as of June 2010 and is given subcutaneously. It resembles fondaparinux, but modifications of several of its side chains have led to a longer half-life, so that it is dosed once weekly. A biotinylated version of the molecule (idrabiotaparinux) has been created, the anticoagulant effect of which can be rapidly neutralized by the administration of avidin.

Thrombolytic agents

A number of different thrombolytic (fibrinolytic) drugs are in clinical use, including streptokinase, urokinase, recombinant tPA, and tPA variants. All of them activate plasminogen to plasmin, which can then exert its thrombolytic effect on fibrin (Figure 7-5). In clinical practice, they are used in various FDA-approved and non–FDA-approved indications for the management of thrombotic clinical disorders. Streptokinase is derived from culture of β-hemolytic streptococci, and urokinase is derived from tissue culture of human neonatal kidney cells. Alteplase (Cathflow, Activase) is a recombinant full-length wild-type human tPA molecule of 527 amino acids.

By deletion or substitution of functional domains and/or altering the molecules' carbohydrate composition, mutants of tPA have been produced. Reteplase (Retavase) is such a mutant recombinant tPA molecule, modified to be only 355 amino acids long, leading to a longer-half life and better penetrance into clots. Tenecteplase (TNKase) is a recombinant full-length tPA molecule with 3 modifications, leading to increased binding of the molecule to thrombus-bound plasminogen compared with native tPA, as well as greater resistance to inactivation by its endogenous inhibitor (PAI-1). In neonates and children <12 months of age, there is a need for plasminogen supplementation (using FFP) prior to administration of tPA because plasma concentrations of plasminogen in the first year of life are 50% lower than adults, making thrombolytic therapy less effective.

Venous thromboembolism

VTE encompasses superficial thrombophlebitis, DVT, and pulmonary embolism (PE). Estimates indicate that at least 350,000 and as many as 600,000 people in the United States develop DVT/PE each year and that at least 100,000 deaths each year are due to VTE. Two thirds of DVT/PE episodes are hospital associated, and one third occur in the community. VTE in children is uncommon, but hospitalization increases the risk; VTE occurs in 1 in every 200 to 300 hospitalized children. There is a bimodal peak in infants and children, with the highest rates found in neonates and adolescents.

Superficial thrombophlebitis

Superficial thrombophlebitis may occur unprovoked and unexplained (also called idiopathic) or in the setting of varicose veins, trauma, intravenous catheters or phlebotomy, underlying hypercoagulable states, and cancer, or as septic thrombophlebitis with infections. It also occurs in association with inflammatory bowel disease, thromboangiitis obliterans (Buerger disease), and Behçet disease.

Superficial thrombophlebitis typically has a benign course. LMWH and nonsteroidal anti-inflammatory drugs (NSAIDs) reduce the incidence of clot extension. Thrombophlebitis that is not very extensive requires only symptomatic therapy, consisting of analgesics, anti-inflammatory medications, and warm or cold compresses for symptom relief. Patients with extensive or recalcitrant superficial thrombophlebitis may benefit from a short course of out-of-hospital anticoagulant therapy, such as 4 weeks of subcutaneously administered unfractionated heparin, LMWH, or fondaparinux. Neither optimal dosing of these drugs (full dose, intermediate dose, or prophylactic low dose) nor duration of therapy is known, and it has not been determined whether the combination of anticoagulants with NSAIDs is more effective. Extension of superficial thrombophlebitis into the deep venous system occurs in approximately 1 in 6 patients with extensive superficial thrombophlebitis. To rule out extension, ultrasonography should be considered in all patients with extensive superficial thrombophlebitis.

The term *Trousseau syndrome* is often used for migratory thrombophlebitis in patients who subsequently are diagnosed with cancer, but the term is not well or uniformly defined. It is sometimes used for any VTE (ie, superficial thrombophlebitis, DVT, or PE) occurring in patients with known or yet unknown cancer, particularly when the VTE events are recurrent. Mondor disease is the term used for thrombophlebitis of the superficial veins of the breast and anterior chest wall, typically occurring after breast cancer surgery and mammoplasties.

Deep vein thrombosis and pulmonary embolism
Prevention

Prophylaxis against VTE should be considered in every hospitalized patient based on an individual patient's risk stratification (Table 7-9). Detailed prophylaxis guidelines for all types of patients have been published in the medical literature, most notably the ACCP 2008 guidelines. Formal DVT prophylaxis guidelines should be in use in all hospitals.

Mechanical methods of prophylaxis with graduated compression stockings or intermittent pneumatic compression devices are typically recommended for patients who are at high risk for bleeding or as an adjunct to anticoagulant-based prophylaxis. They have been studied less intensely than anticoagulant-based methods. They are generally less efficacious than the latter. Although there is some evidence that aspirin and other antiplatelet agents provide some protection against VTE in hospitalized patients at risk, they are inferior to other methods of VTE prophylaxis. Therefore, a very strong recommendation has been made in the 2008 ACCP guidelines against the use of aspirin alone as prophylaxis against VTE for any patient group.

The mainstay of VTE prophylaxis is anticoagulant drugs. Several options are available: (i) unfractionated heparin at 8- or 12-hour dosing intervals; (ii) LMWHs at once- or twice-daily intervals; (iii) fondaparinux once daily; or (iv) VKAs. Prophylaxis may only be given during the hospitalization or, if the VTE risk persists after discharge home, for an extended period of time, such as for patients after hip fracture and replacement surgery, in whom up to 5 weeks of prophylaxis are recommended.

Symptoms

DVT of the pelvic and leg veins presents with varying degrees of leg swelling, pain, warmth, and skin discoloration. Symptoms are typically diffuse. Localized symptoms are more suggestive of a superficial thrombophlebitis. A palpable subcutaneous cord-like firmness is also indicative of a superficial thrombophlebitis. The onset of symptoms of DVT can be sudden or subacute over days to weeks. DVT is not infrequently missed or misdiagnosed because the symptoms can be very nonspecific. PE presents with varying degrees of severity of shortness of breath, chest pain that is

Table 7-9 Thromboprophylaxis.

Risk level	Type of patient or procedure	DVT risk without prophylaxis	Options*
Low	Minor surgery in mobile patients; fully mobile medical patients	<10%	Ambulation
Moderate	Most general surgeries; bedridden or sick medical patients	10%–40%	LMWH, UFH bid or tid, fondaparinux
High	Hip or knee arthroplasty; major trauma, spinal cord injury	40%–80%	LMWH, fondaparinux, oral VKA (INR 2-3)

*If there is a moderate or high risk and high bleeding risk, use intermittent pneumatic compression.
bid = twice a day; DVT = deep vein thrombosis; INR = international normalized ratio; LMWH = low molecular weight heparin; tid = three times a day; UFH = unfractionated heparin; VKA = vitamin K antagonist.

classically respiratory dependent, nonproductive cough, and hemoptysis. A massive PE can lead to sudden death. Small PEs are often asymptomatic. The onset of symptoms can be sudden or subacute over several weeks, months, or years. There is no uniform definition for the severity or degree of PE. The definition can either be anatomic or physiologic. The physiologic definition is preferred for treatment decision making because it is a better predictor of mortality. Any PE that causes hemodynamic instability (hypotension) is referred to as *massive PE*. *Submassive PE* is the term for PE associated with normal arterial blood pressure but right ventricular dysfunction.

Diagnosis

Scoring systems based on a patient's VTE risk factors and clinical symptoms and findings have been established to determine how likely it is that a patient presenting with leg or lung symptoms has DVT or PE. The grouping into low and intermediate or high pretest probability helps guide which further diagnostic tests to perform. The whole blood or plasma D-dimer tests are well evaluated and useful in the diagnostic workup for DVT and PE. In outpatients with a low pretest probability for DVT or PE, a negative test with a sensitive D-dimer assay reliably rules out VTE, and no further imaging study is needed. However, outpatients with a low pretest probability for DVT or PE and a positive D-dimer test and any patients with moderate or high pretest probability for DVT or PE need to undergo imaging studies. The generalized application of D-dimer testing is, however, limited by the large number of different assays available, some highly sensitive and others less sensitive, and a lack of standardization of assays. Because clinicians are often not aware of the type of D-dimer assay used by their laboratory or the predictive value of the particular assay available to them, reliance on D-dimer results for clinical decision making for the exclusion of VTE can be unsafe, unless the test has been locally validated. In children, the D-dimer test as a diagnostic tool for VTE has not been well studied.

Venous Doppler ultrasound is the most widely used imaging study to look for DVT of the legs. Sensitivity and specificity of the test are operator dependent and an experienced ultrasound technician or physician is key in obtaining reliable results. Magnetic resonance venogram of leg or pelvic veins is a sensitive test to detect leg DVTs, but is expensive and not widely available. Imaging with magnetic resonance or computed tomography (CT) venogram may be necessary for upper extremity DVT, particularly catheter-related events, because ultrasound may miss occlusion within the superior vena cava and brachiocephalic and subclavian veins due to interference of the clavicles and ribs.

To diagnose PE, several imaging modalities exist, including ventilation/perfusion (VQ) scanning, PE-protocol chest CT angiography (also known as spiral CT or helical CT), chest magnetic resonance angiography, and conventional intravenous contrast pulmonary angiogram. The VQ scan is a well-validated imaging study. However, PE-protocol chest CTs have widely replaced VQ scans as the diagnostic method of choice because they are easier and faster to perform and have good performance characteristics. Their predictive value with a concordant clinical assessment is high, but additional testing is necessary when the clinical probability is inconsistent with the imaging results. Conventional intravenous contrast pulmonary angiography, once considered the gold standard for the diagnosis of PE, is rarely done now because the test is invasive and not widely available and has diagnostic limitations. In the patient with PE and significant clinical symptoms or extensive clot on imaging study, an echocardiogram should be performed to assess for right ventricular dysfunction. Biologic serum markers, such as cardiac troponin and brain natriuretic peptide levels, are also helpful in determining degree of right heart strain.

Acute therapy

Outpatient management of patients with DVT and PE has been shown to be safe, feasible, and cost effective and is, if possible, the preferred treatment of choice. Hospital admission is appropriate if the patient is too sick to be managed at home or if social and financial circumstances make this the safer and more feasible option.

Patients with acute VTE need to be anticoagulated to prevent extension of thrombus and decrease mortality. Intravenous unfractionated heparin and subcutaneous LMWH and fondaparinux are all effective and acceptable treatment options and need to be given for at least 5 days and until the INR is ≥2.0 for 24 hours. In young children, appropriate dosing and monitoring of fondaparinux has not been studied. In patients who are potentially unstable due to significant PE, unfractionated heparin is preferable over LMWH or fondaparinux because it has a short half-life and can easily be dose adjusted, discontinued, or reversed (with protamine) if bleeding occurs or thrombolytic therapy has to be given. In selected patients with extensive acute proximal DVT with symptom duration of <14 days and with low bleeding risk, catheter-directed thrombolysis with or without mechanical thrombus fragmentation and aspiration can be considered to reduce acute symptoms and potentially decrease the risk of developing postthrombotic syndrome. However, whether thrombolytic therapy with or without mechanical thrombectomy decreases the incidence or severity of postthrombotic syndrome has not yet been demonstrated.

May-Thurner syndrome is the term used for the chronic compression of the left common iliac vein between the overlying right common iliac artery and the fifth lumbar vertebral body posteriorly. Varying degrees of vein narrowing with this anatomic variant are common in the general population. If a May-Thurner syndrome is demonstrated on venography or magnetic resonance imaging (MRI) in the patient with left leg proximal DVT who has successfully received thrombolytic therapy, correction of the stenosis using balloon angioplasty and stenting can be considered.

Thrombolytic therapy in PE is indicated for massive life-threatening PE (ie, PE with hypotension). Selected high-risk PE patients without hypotension and at low risk for bleeding may receive thrombolytics. However, in a prospective randomized trial in patients with submassive PE, thrombolytic therapy did not decrease mortality compared with no thrombolytic therapy. It is not known whether thrombolytic therapy decreases the long-term risk of pulmonary hypertension. Although thrombolytic therapy does carry a risk of severe bleeding, in carefully selected patients, it has been shown to be relatively safe and not lead to more serious bleeding events than treatment with unfractionated heparin alone. If thrombolytic therapy is given to a patient with PE, it should be given systemically via a peripheral vein and with short infusion time, such as 2 hours. If no thrombolytics are given, oral VKAs can be started on the day of presentation. Educating the patient about VTE and VKA therapy with all its facets is important.

Duration of anticoagulant therapy

The risk of recurrent VTE in patients with a VTE secondary to a transient (reversible) risk factor is low. Therefore, time-limited anticoagulation for 3 months with a VKA is recommended. For patients with unprovoked proximal DVT as their first VTE and in whom risk factors for bleeding are absent and for whom good anticoagulation control is achievable, long-term VKA therapy is recommended by the 2008 ACCP guidelines. However, in clinical practice, this is a complex issue. Several parameters can be used in the discussion with the patient about the individual risk of recurrence (Table 7-10; Figure 7-7), and a decision about continuation or discontinuation can be made based on patient-individual risk factors for recurrence and bleeding, as well as patient preference. For patients whose first episode of unprovoked DVT is in a distal vein, 3 months of VKA therapy is sufficient, rather than indefinite therapy. In patients who are unexpectedly found to have asymptomatic DVT, the same initial and long-term anticoagulation is recommended as for comparable patients with symptomatic DVT.

In most patients, a target INR of 2.0 to 3.0 is appropriate and protects to a large degree from recurrent VTE. In patients

Table 7-10 Considerations when discussing time-limited versus long-term anticoagulation therapy in patients with unprovoked VTE.

Reasons contributing to a decision for long-term VKA therapy
- Recurrent VTE
- Strong thrombophilia present (ie, APLA syndrome, antithrombin deficiency, protein C or S deficiency, homozygous factor V Leiden, double heterozygous state for factor V Leiden and prothrombin 20210 mutation)
- Male gender
- Patient had a PE ± DVT, not just a DVT
- D-dimer result on VKA therapy positive at 3 or 6 months
- D-dimer positive after having been off VKA for 4 weeks
- VKA well tolerated with good control of INR and no bleeding complications
- Little or no impact of anticoagulant therapy on patient's lifestyle (profession, hobbies)
- Patient's preference is to stay on VKA

Reasons contributing to a decision against long-term VKA therapy
- VTE was associated with estrogen excess (estrogen contraceptives, hormone replacement therapy, pregnancy)
- Female gender
- Distal DVT only
- D-dimer result on VKA therapy negative at 3 or 6 months
- D-dimer negative after having been off VKA for 4 weeks
- VKA poorly tolerated with widely fluctuating INRs
- Occurrence of bleeding complications or significant risk for bleeding
- Significant impact of anticoagulant therapy on patient's lifestyle
- Patient's preference is to come off VKA

APLA = antiphospholipid antibody; DVT = deep vein thrombosis; INR = international normalized ratio; PE = pulmonary embolism; VKA = vitamin K antagonist; VTE = venous thromboembolism.

with cancer, the risk of recurrent VTE on VKA is high, even if the INR is in the 2.0 to 3.0 range. LMWH has been shown to be more effective than VKA in preventing recurrences in these patients and is the preferred treatment, if feasible from a financial and insurance point of view. The anticoagulant treatment options, if recurrent VTE occurs despite documented therapeutic INRs, are to either to continue VKA but increase the target INR or to switch to long-term LMWH or fondaparinux.

Postthrombotic syndrome

Postthrombotic syndrome is caused by an interplay between incompetent venous valves damaged by the thrombus or associated inflammatory mediators and impairment of venous return due to residual venous obstruction from incompletely cleared thrombus. Approximately a third to half of DVT patients will develop postthrombotic syndrome (sometimes also referred to as postphlebitic syndrome), in most cases within 1 to 2 years of the acute DVT. Symptoms

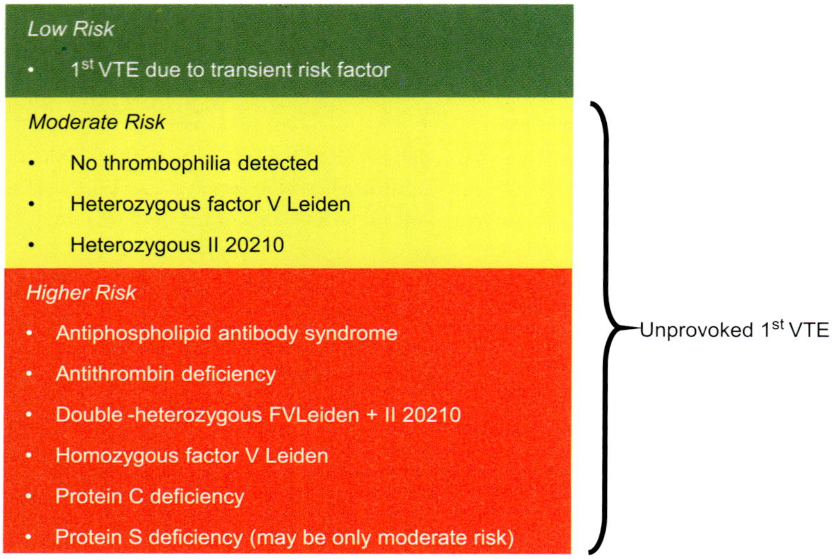

Low Risk
- 1st VTE due to transient risk factor

Moderate Risk
- No thrombophilia detected
- Heterozygous factor V Leiden
- Heterozygous II 20210

Higher Risk
- Antiphospholipid antibody syndrome
- Antithrombin deficiency
- Double-heterozygous FVLeiden + II 20210
- Homozygous factor V Leiden
- Protein C deficiency
- Protein S deficiency (may be only moderate risk)

(Moderate Risk and Higher Risk categories apply to) Unprovoked 1st VTE

Figure 7-7 Risk of recurrence of venous thromboembolism (VTE) (proximal deep vein thrombosis and/or pulmonary embolism).

and signs are chronic extremity swelling, pain, heaviness, fatigue, paresthesias, skin induration, dryness, pruritus, erythema, chronic dark pigmentation, and, in more severe cases, skin ulcers. The risk for developing postthrombotic syndrome is probably decreased if graduated compression stockings (40 mm at ankle, 30 mm at mid calf) are worn for 2 year after the acute DVT. Treatment options for patients with postthrombotic syndrome are limited. Compression stockings should be worn. In patients with significant leg swelling, imaging of leg veins with Doppler ultrasound and of the pelvic veins with CT venography or magnetic resonance venography can be considered to evaluate for focal pelvic vein obstruction or narrowing due to May-Thurner syndrome or postthrombotic scarring that might be amenable to pelvic vein angioplasty and stenting. Also, a home compression pump with compression sleeve for the affected leg should be considered for patients with significant symptoms.

Pulmonary hypertension

Pulmonary hypertension due to VTE, termed *chronic thromboembolic pulmonary hypertension*, is defined as an elevated mean pulmonary artery pressure at rest of >25 mm Hg and occurs in 1% of patients with acute PE after 6 months, 3.1% after 1 year, and 3.8% after 2 years. The patient who experiences chronic shortness of breath or significant generalized malaise after a large PE should be evaluated for pulmonary hypertension. A formal walk test with pre- and postexercise pulse oximetry measurements is appropriate. It is important to realize that chest CT angiogram findings may be minimal with chronic distal PE. A VQ scan is the screening test of choice and is indicated. Right heart catheterization with pulmonary artery pressure measurements then defines the degree of hypertension, and pulmonary arteriography helps define the etiology and allows assessment of whether potentially curative pulmonary endarterectomy is indicated. Long-term VKA therapy is indicated. Pharmacologic therapy specific for pulmonary hypertension, such as bosentan, an endothelin receptor antagonist, can be considered in the inoperable patient or the patient in whom surgery did not result in improvement.

Inferior vena cava filters

The 2008 ACCP guidelines recommend against the use of inferior vena cava (IVC) filters in trauma and spinal injury patients. Clear indications for an IVC filter are (i) acute pelvic or proximal leg DVT but inability to anticoagulate because of active bleeding or very high bleeding risk, and (ii) recurrent pelvic or proximal leg DVT despite therapeutic anticoagulation. When IVC filters are placed, retrievable filters should be considered, unless the intention at the time of placement is that they stay in permanently. Retrievable filters can be left in place for weeks to months or can remain permanently, if necessary. For patients with acute VTE who have an IVC filter inserted because of a contraindication to anticoagulation, it is recommended that they should subsequently receive a conventional course of anticoagulant therapy if their risk of bleeding resolves. Presence of a permanent IVC filter increases a patient's risk for recurrent DVT. When making a decision on length of anticoagulant therapy in a patient with a permanent IVC filter, the presence of the IVC filter should be viewed as one of the risk factors for recurrent VTE. A decision on whether to continue anticoagulants should be based on the sum of all prothrombotic risk factors, balanced against the risk factors for bleeding, as well as the implications that long-term anticoagulation may have on a patient's quality of life. With the knowledge presently available from limited clinical studies, having a permanent IVC filter should not be viewed as the sole reason for keeping a patient on long-term anticoagulant therapy.

Venous stents

Venous stents may be placed in various locations of the venous system, most commonly into the left common iliac vein due to May-Thurner syndrome, the right and left pelvic veins due to postthrombotic vessel narrowing and scarring, and the superior vena cava and central upper chest veins in central venous catheter–associated venous strictures. The best long-term management of patients who have venous stents is not known because of a lack of good-quality prospective studies examining their long-term patency with and without antiplatelet drugs or anticoagulants. Because stents are foreign bodies in the venous system and may lead to flow disturbances, it is possible that they have some prothrombotic risk. In view of the limited data available, it may be best to view the presence of a venous stent as a potential risk factor for recurrent VTE. After venous stent placement, it may be reasonable to keep a patient on anticoagulants for 3 months and then make an assessment on need for long-term anticoagulation versus no further anticoagulation based on a comprehensive assessment of the patient's risk factors for recurrent VTE and bleeding. Whether a patient who has a venous stent but is not on long-term anticoagulants may benefit from long-term antiplatelet therapy is not known.

Unusual venous thromboses
Upper extremity DVT

The superficial veins of the arm include the antecubital, cephalic, and basilic veins. The deep venous system includes the brachial vein, which becomes the axillary vein, followed by the subclavian and brachiocephalic veins, and finally the superior vena cava. Upper extremity DVTs make up 1% to 4% of all DVTs. Approximately 80% are secondary to central venous catheters and cancer, and 20% are primary events; however, these data depend largely on what patient population is studied. Doppler ultrasound (sensitivity of 78%–100% and specificity of 82%–100%), contrast venography (gold standard), and magnetic resonance venography are the diagnostic tools used to diagnose upper extremity thrombosis. PE occurs in 2% to 35% of patients. Postthrombotic syndrome is frequent, occurring in 7% to 46% of patients, and residual thrombosis and axillo-subclavian vein thrombosis appear to be associated with a higher risk, whereas catheter-associated DVT may be associated with a lower risk. The 2008 ACCP guidelines state that anticoagulation management for DVT of the upper extremity should be similar to that for DVT of the leg: (i) LMWH, unfractionated heparin, or fondaparinux in the acute setting; (ii) no thrombolytic therapy for most patients; (iii) VKA for at least 3 months and decision on duration of VKA therapy similar to that in lower extremity DVT; and (iv) no catheter removal in DVT associated with a central venous catheter if the catheter is functional and still needed. It is noteworthy to know, though, that there are no randomized studies on the duration of anticoagulant therapy for the prevention of recurrent VTE in patients with upper extremity DVT, and that there is little evidence to support indefinite anticoagulant therapy for a first unprovoked upper extremity DVT.

Upper extremity DVTs may be due to thoracic outlet syndrome, also referred to as effort thrombosis, thoracic outlet syndrome, or Paget-Schroetter syndrome. This is due to compression of the axillary vein by pressure from the clavicle, an extra rib, or enlarged or aberrantly inserted muscles, often provoked or potentiated by abduction of the arm and repetitive arm movements. There is no uniform approach to treatment of these patients. Management options include anticoagulation, thrombolytic therapy, angioplasty, thoracic outlet surgery with rib or soft tissue resection, and surgical resection of the focally narrowed vein with vein reconstruction. Individual treatment decisions need to be made, and a team approach that includes vascular surgery and vascular interventional radiology may be appropriate.

Catheter-related thrombosis

Catheter-related thrombosis can occur in several forms: (i) fibrin sleeves, (ii) catheter tip thrombosis, and (iii) catheter-related DVT. The first 2 types may lead to catheter malfunction with inability to infuse or withdraw blood and fluids. tPA is FDA approved for this indication, and an instillation of 2 mg into the catheter leads to catheter clearance in 75% of cases. The cumulative patency rate after 2 doses is 85%. In children and neonates, as many as 60% and 90% of thrombotic events, respectively, are catheter associated. Thromboprophylaxis is not routinely recommended in patients with central venous catheters because recent large and well-designed studies have not demonstrated efficacy of low-dose warfarin or aspirin in preventing catheter-associated DVT.

Hepatic vein thrombosis

Hepatic vein thrombosis, also referred to as Budd-Chiari syndrome, has varied clinical presentations, ranging from asymptomatic to fulminant liver failure. A cause can be identified in approximately 84% of patients. Similar to other venous thromboembolic disorders, Budd-Chiari syndrome also often has a multifactorial etiology. Most patients (84%) have at least 1 thrombotic risk factor, and many (46%) have >1 risk factor; the most common are myeloproliferative disorders (49% of patients). Polycythemia vera accounts for 27% of cases; ET and myelofibrosis are less prevalent causes. The *JAK2* mutation is frequently present in patients with the syndrome (29% of cases), even if no hematologic abnormalities suggestive of a myeloproliferative disorder are present. This is discussed in detail earlier in the section of this chapter on "thrombophilias." Any of the inherited and acquired thrombophilias can contribute to the development of Budd-Chiari syndrome, as can estrogens and pregnancy. PNH, although an uncommon disorder, can be detected in almost one-fifth of patients with Budd-Chiari syndrome.

The diagnosis is made by Doppler ultrasonography, contrast-enhanced CT scanning, or MRI. In the acute setting of fulminant thrombosis, thrombolytic therapy can be considered. Angioplasty of narrowed or occluded hepatic veins can be performed, shunt procedures may be required, and liver transplantation may be necessary. Anticoagulation is usually appropriate and is often given long term, typically with VKAs. However, INR monitoring may be problematic because liver synthetic dysfunction may lead to a baseline elevation of INR even before VKA therapy. Alternative monitoring tests for VKAs, such as factor II or X activity, may have to be used. Also, treatment with LMWH or fondaparinux instead of VKAs can be considered.

Portal vein thrombosis

Portal vein thrombosis is often silent and may only be discovered upon evaluation of a variceal gastrointestinal bleed. It is associated with the inherited and acquired thrombophilias, myeloproliferative disorders, *JAK2*-positive status without overt myeloproliferative disorders, PNH, intra-abdominal neoplasia, infection, trauma, surgery, and neonatal umbilical vein catheterization. It occurs in 0.6% to 26% of patients with cirrhosis of the liver. As with other venous thromboembolic disorders, often multiple contributors are identified. In a number of cases, no predisposing factor is found. Diagnosis is typically made by Doppler ultrasonography. Cavernous transformation of the portal vein reflects old portal vein thrombosis. In the patient with acute portal vein thrombosis, extension of thrombus into the mesenteric veins may occur and lead to intestinal infarction and need for surgical bowel resection. The patient with acute portal vein thrombosis is typically anticoagulated for at least 3 to 6 months to prevent progression of thrombosis. As for long-term VKA therapy in these patients, as well as in patients with incidentally discovered portal vein thrombosis, the risk of bleeding has to be individually balanced against the risk of rethrombosis. The factors to be considered before long-term anticoagulation is prescribed include identification of the triggering factor for the thrombotic event, the extent of thrombosis, the presence of persistent prothrombotic factors, the extent of esophageal and gastric varices, the presence and degree of thrombocytopenia due to hypersplenism, and history of bleeding.

Mesenteric vein thrombosis

Venous drainage of the intestine is via the superior mesenteric vein (SMV) and inferior mesenteric vein (IMV) into the portal vein. The SMV drains the small intestine and ascending colon, whereas the IMV drains mostly the sigmoid colon. The transverse and descending colon can drain through the middle and left colic veins either into the SMV or IMV. SMV thrombosis, if diagnosed late, leads mostly to small bowel ischemic changes. The very rare IMV thrombosis may lead to ischemia in the sigmoid colon. Mesenteric vein thrombosis may be caused by trauma, surgery, intra-abdominal infections, inflammatory bowel disease, pancreatic disease, and progression of portal vein thrombosis, but may also occur spontaneously, particularly in patients with inherited or acquired thrombophilias, myeloproliferative disorders, presence of the *JAK2* V617F mutation, and PNH. Symptoms are vague, often leading to a delay in diagnosis. Nonspecific abdominal pain is common, and nausea may be present. Gastrointestinal bleeding and peritonitis are seen when transmural ischemia has occurred. Symptoms may be present for days to weeks before a diagnosis is made, which often may occur only when the patient presents as a surgical emergency with ischemic bowel. The principal cause of a high mortality rate in mesenteric vein thrombosis is a delay in diagnosis. The surgical findings are typically those of a dusky but not frankly gangrenous intestine, unless full bowel wall infarction has already occurred. Areas of viability of intestine are not as sharply demarcated as they are in arterial mesenteric ischemic disease. A mesenteric artery pulse is typically felt. Preoperative diagnosis is made by CT angiography. Doppler ultrasound may also be diagnostic but is operator dependent and may have limited sensitivity in the obese patient. Once diagnosed, patients are managed with anticoagulation alone or in combination with surgical intervention. Most patients improve. Decisions on length of VKA therapy depend, as with most of the other VTE disorders, on the triggers for the thrombotic episode and the presence of thrombophilias or other permanent risk factors. Length of treatment is at least 3 months but may have to be long term. No data exist on the risk of recurrent mesenteric vein thrombosis.

Splenic vein thrombosis

Due to the intimate anatomic contact of the splenic vein with the pancreas, the main causes of splenic vein thrombosis are pancreatitis and pancreatic malignancies. Similar to mesenteric vein thrombosis, intra-abdominal problems (infection, surgery, and trauma) and thrombophilias also play a role in the etiology. Symptoms are often subtle, and the diagnosis is not infrequently a coincidental discovery on abdominal imaging studies done for other reasons. Length of anticoagulant treatment depends on the triggering factors and the persistent thrombophilic risk factors.

Cerebral and sinus vein thrombosis

Blood from the brain drains via cerebral and cortical veins into the dural sinuses, which then drain into the internal jugular veins. Thrombosis of the cerebral, cortical, and sinus veins is often referred to as *cerebral and sinus vein thrombosis* or *cerebral sinovenous thrombosis*. It is seen much more commonly in the neonatal period than in any other age group and occurs in 3 to 4 cases per 1 million in the general population, in up to 7 cases per 1 million in children, and in approximately 120 cases in the peri- and postpartum period per 1 million deliveries. Although the outcome is relatively good in adults, half of neonates die. As with other VTE events, cerebral and sinus vein thrombosis is often multifactorial, and the inherited and acquired thrombophilias play a role in its etiology, as do estrogen therapy and pregnancy. Infections such as mastoiditis, otitis, sinusitis, and meningitis are risk factors, and in neonates dehydration and perinatal complications are contributors. A cause for cerebral and sinus vein thrombosis is identified in 85% of patients. In adults, the most frequent but least specific symptom is severe headache, either of subacute or acute onset, and is present in 90% of patients. In children, seizures, focal neurologic signs, and headache are the most common manifestations. Routine noncontrast and contrast head CT scans and brain MRI scans are often unrevealing, resulting in missed diagnoses, unless CT venogram or MRI venogram are specifically requested.

Approximately 40% of patients with cerebral and sinus vein thrombosis have a hemorrhagic infarct, which is a consequence of the venous occlusion. Currently, no available evidence from randomized controlled trials exists regarding the efficacy or safety of systemic or local thrombolytic therapy in cerebral and sinus vein thrombosis. Based on limited evidence, anticoagulation with heparin appears to be safe, not increasing the risk for intracranial bleeding, but leading to a potentially important reduction in the risk of death or dependency due to neurologic impairment; however, this reduction did not reach statistical significance. Therefore, heparin is often used in acute cerebral and sinus vein thrombosis, even if some parenchymal hemorrhage is present. The 2008 ACCP guidelines do not take any reference to anticoagulant management of patients with sinus vein thrombosis, but the 2006 European Federation of Neurological Societies (EFNS) guidelines recommend LMWH or unfractionated heparin therapy in the acute treatment. The optimal duration of anticoagulant therapy is unknown. Usually, VKAs are given after a first episode of cerebral and sinus vein thrombosis for 3 months if the thrombosis was associated with a transient risk factor, for 6 to 12 months if the event was unexplained and no higher risk thrombophilia has been detected, and for long term if a higher risk thrombophilia is detected or the event is recurrent. In children, use of anticoagulant therapy in cerebral and sinus vein thrombosis has not been well studied in clinical trials, but is not associated with serious hemorrhage in selected patients.

Renal vein thrombosis

In adults, the classical symptom triad of acute renal vein thrombosis, namely acute flank pain, hematuria, and sudden deterioration of renal function, is uncommonly seen. More common is a chronic course with subtle worsening of renal function, progressive proteinuria, and edema, often without pain or hematuria. As many as 30% to 50% of patients with chronic nephrotic syndrome have evidence of renal vein thrombosis, and it is not uncommonly bilateral and often protrudes into the IVC. Nephrotic syndrome leads to hypercoagulability, which may be due to urinary antithrombin loss, free protein S deficiency secondary to an increase in C4b-BP, or unknown causes. Diagnosis is made by Doppler ultrasound or by magnetic resonance venography. Thrombolytic therapy should be considered in case of acute thrombosis, particularly if there is bilateral disease or impending renal failure. Anticoagulation therapy is indicated. The length of anticoagulant therapy depends on whether the thrombotic event was associated with a transient prothrombotic risk factor and whether the patient has permanent risk factors and/or a higher risk thrombophilia. Renal vein thrombosis in children typically presents within the first month of life. In neonates, it may be associated with acute dehydration and perinatal asphyxia. Outside of the neonatal period, nephrotic syndrome is the most common risk factor for thrombosis in children and adults.

Retinal vein thrombosis

Thrombosis can occur as central retinal vein occlusion (CRVO) or as branch retinal vein thrombosis (BRVO). Unfortunately, clinical studies have often grouped CRVO and BRVO together, so that a differential effect of thrombophilia on CRVO and BRVO may have gotten lost in these studies.

CRVO has a prevalence of 1 in 250 to 1000 individuals ≥40 years of age. A number of studies on the association of various thrombophilias and CRVO have shown conflicting results; some have shown associations, but most have not. The presence of cardiovascular risk factors, such as hypertension, hyperlipidemia, and diabetes, has been associated with CRVO. Unfortunately, there is a lack of randomized treatment trials investigating the usefulness of antiplatelet or anticoagulant therapy. The result is a lack of knowledge concerning the appropriate treatment for CRVO in facilitating clot resolution, symptom improvement, or prevention of recurrences.

BRVO is more common than CRVO and is typically due to pressure on the vein from the overlying branch retinal artery, typically due to arteriosclerosis of the retinal artery. BRVO causes a painless sectoral decrease in vision, resulting in misty or distorted vision. Findings are those of intraretinal hemorrhage, retinal exudates, retinal ischemia, and macular edema.

Arterial thromboembolism

General comments

The hematologist typically does not get called upon for input into the management of patients with arteriosclerosis associated ischemic disease. This is more the domain of the cardiologist, neurologist, general internist, and endocrinologist. Therefore, this chapter discusses neither the pathophysiology of arteriosclerosis and its role in arterial occlusive disease nor the management approaches aimed at modifying an individual's arteriosclerosis risk factors, such as weight reduction, cessation of smoking, increased physical activity, and treatment of diabetes mellitus, hypertension, and hyperlipidemia. References to the major treatment guidelines are listed, for the interested reader, in the Bibliography. Because the hematologist may be consulted for some antithrombotic management issues, a few key points on antithrombotic drug use in these disease states are made in the following sections. The more classical reason for consultation about a patient with arterial thromboembolism is when the arterial occlusive event has occurred in a person who is young, has no significant arteriosclerosis risk factors, or has a personal or family history of thrombophilia.

Arterial thrombosis in the absence of arteriosclerosis

Arterial thromboembolic events in the young person (<50 years old) are rare, unless significant arteriosclerosis risk factors are present. No matter which territory the arterial thrombotic event occurs in, a number of risk factors and associated disorders should be investigated to clarify the etiology of the event (Table 7-11). As for specific arterial territories, in the case of upper extremity arterial thromboembolism, thoracic outlet syndrome should be considered; in lower extremity claudication or arterial thromboembolism, popliteal artery entrapment syndrome, cystic adventitial disease of the popliteal artery, fibromuscular dysplasia of the lower extremity arteries, and endofibrosis of the iliac artery should be considered; and in the case of stroke in the young, spontaneous or traumatic cervical artery dissection should be considered.

Relatively little is known about thrombophilias predisposing to arterial thrombosis. Heterozygous FVL and

Table 7-11 Unexplained or nonarteriosclerotic arterial thromboembolism: considerations and workup.

- Arteriosclerotic changes demonstrated on imaging studies (on computed tomography or other vascular imaging studies or pathology specimens)?
- Arteriosclerosis risk factors present?
  - Cigarette smoking
  - Hypertension
  - High level of low-density lipoprotein cholesterol
  - Low level of high-density lipoprotein cholesterol
  - Diabetes mellitus
  - Family history of premature arterial occlusive disease
- Cocaine or anabolic steroid abuse?
- Estrogen use?
- Thromboembolic source ruled out (echocardiography with intravenous normal saline bubble study; evaluation of aorta for plaques)?
- Anatomic abnormalities seen in artery leading to the ischemic area (web, fibromuscular dysplasia, vasculitic changes, external compression)?
- Symptoms suggestive of vasospastic disorder (Raynaud, etc)?
- Evidence for Buerger disease (tobacco or cannabis use)?
- Laboratory workup for vasculitis and immune disorder?
- Thrombophilia workup
  - Hemoglobin and platelet count
  - Antiphospholipid antibodies
    - Anticardiolipin IgG and IgM antibodies
    - Anti–β_2-glycoprotein I IgG and IgM antibodies
    - Lupus anticoagulant
  - Protein C activity
  - Protein S activity and/or free protein S antigen
  - Antithrombin activity
  - Homocysteine
  - Lipoprotein(a)
  - Factor V Leiden and prothrombin 20210 mutation*

*Purpose of testing is to detect the homozygous or double heterozygous state.
IgG = immunoglobulin G; IgM = immunoglobulin M.

heterozygous prothrombin 20210 mutation by themselves do not clearly increase the risk for arterial thromboembolism. Whether the risk is increased in individuals with homozygous FVL or homozygous prothrombin 20210 mutation or in double heterozygous individuals with both FVL and the prothrombin 20210 mutation is not known. Whether such individuals, as well as those with arterial thromboembolic events associated with deficiencies in protein C and S and AT, should be treated with antiplatelet therapy or anticoagulant therapy is also not known.

Peripheral arterial disease

For individuals with symptomatic lower extremity peripheral arterial disease, antiplatelet therapy is indicated, such as aspirin in daily doses of 75 to 100 mg. Clopidogrel (Plavix) is an effective alternative. In patients with moderate to severe claudication, cilostazol (Pletal) at 100 mg every 12 hours is indicated in the absence of heart failure to improve symptoms and walking distance. There is no indication for the use of VKAs. The clinical effectiveness of pentoxifylline (Trental) at 400 mg 3 times per day is marginal and not well established. Thus, the ACCP 2008 guidelines recommend against its use. Patients with an acute ischemic thromboembolic event should be treated with unfractionated heparin. In patients undergoing embolectomy, long-term VKA should be given. For patients with infrainguinal bypass, aspirin, but not routine treatment with VKAs, is indicated. For patients at high risk of bypass occlusion and limb loss, aspirin plus VKA are recommended. Patients undergoing carotid endarterectomy should receive preoperative aspirin at a dose of 75 to 100 mg. Long-term aspirin (75–100 mg/d) should be given to patients after endarterectomy, patients with asymptomatic or recurrent carotid stenosis, and those undergoing extremity balloon angioplasty.

Atrial fibrillation and stroke prevention

Detailed recommendations for anticoagulant and antiplatelet management of patients with atrial fibrillation are available, such as the 2008 ACCP guidelines and the 2006 American College of Cardiology, American Heart Association, and European Society of Cardiology guidelines. Indications for antiplatelet or anticoagulant therapy are based on the $CHADS_2$ score, a clinical prediction rule for estimating the risk of stroke in patients with nonrheumatic atrial fibrillation. The $CHADS_2$ score is made up of the following 5 risk factors for stroke in patients with atrial fibrillation: "C" for congestive heart failure (1 point), "H" for hypertension (1 point), "A" for age >75 years (1 point), "D" for diabetes (1 point), and "S_2" for prior stroke or transient ischemic attack (2 points). The total number of points in an individual patient with atrial fibrillation predicts the risk for stroke and, thus, guides the choice of antithrombotic drug for stroke prevention: for a score of 0, aspirin 81 to 325 mg is indicated; for a sore of 1, aspirin or warfarin with a target INR of 2.0 to 3.0 is indicated; and for a score of ≥2, warfarin with a target INR of 2.0 to 3.0 is indicated.

Neonatal stroke

Neonatal stroke, which is defined as a cerebrovascular event that occurs between 28 weeks of gestation and 7 days of age, occurs in 1 in 250 live births. There is a male predominance. Seizure is the most common clinical presentation. However, many infants do not present for several months until they are noted to have hemiparesis or early hand preference. It is often difficult to determine whether the stroke occurred in utero, at the time of delivery, or within the first week of life. Most neonatal strokes occur in the distribution of the left middle cerebral artery. MRI and magnetic resonance angiography are the best tests to determine extent of disease. There is no standard approach for the evaluation and treatment of perinatal stroke. At the time of diagnosis, though, it is important to determine whether the thrombotic event was related to an underlying disorder such as congenital heart disease; so-called *TORCH infections* (ie, toxoplasmosis, rubella, cytomegalovirus, herpes, and other infections), which are passed in utero from the mother to the developing fetus; systemic bacterial infections; or metabolic diseases. Maternal drugs and medical conditions, placental disorders, perinatal asphyxia, and birth trauma have all been associated with neonatal cerebrovascular events. Several studies have demonstrated an association between inherited prothrombotic conditions and neonatal stroke. The incidence of recurrent stroke is extremely low (<5%); therefore, anticoagulation is not indicated unless there is evidence of embolic heart disease. Children with a cardioembolic cause of stroke should be referred to a pediatric cardiologist for evaluation, management, and correction of the heart defect. Fifty percent of infants with perinatal events will be neurologically normal by 12 to 18 months of age. Long-term sequelae, such as mild hemiparesis, speech or learning problems, behavioral problems, and seizures, are more likely to persist in patients who present outside the newborn period.

Childhood stroke

Stroke affects 1 in 7000 to 35,000 children per year, with a male predominance. As many as 65% of affected children will have lifelong disabilities such as neurologic defects and seizures, and the risk of a second stroke is 20%. Despite therapy, mortality rates as high as 10% have been reported. There are certain comorbid conditions that are highly correlated with stroke, including congenital or acquired cardiac disease that can cause embolic phenomena and sickle cell anemia. Numerous systemic disorders can contribute to stroke, and inherited prothrombotic states are causative as well. A rare cause of stroke in childhood is severe iron deficiency anemia. Fifty percent of children with stroke will have no identifiable disorder. There is limited published information about the etiology and outcome of childhood stroke and little evidence in the literature about appropriate management and prevention approaches. Embolic stroke resulting from cardiac disease or carotid dissection and stroke associated with severe prothrombotic conditions (eg, congenital homozygous protein C deficiency or APLA syndrome) appear to benefit from anticoagulation. Warfarin, unfractionated heparin, and LMWH have been successful in treating and preventing recurrence of acute stroke in children with these underlying disorders. For strokes of other etiologies, anticoagulation does not improve outcome better than treatment with antiplatelet agents. Although the use of thrombolytic agents within 3 hours of initiation of the signs of stroke can be successful in improving outcomes in adults, the safety and efficacy of this strategy in children has not been demonstrated.

Acknowledgment

The authors thank Dr. Keith R. McCrae, Cleveland, OH, for critical review of the manuscript.

Bibliography

Pathophysiology of thrombosis

Furie B, Furie BC. Mechanisms of thrombus formation. *N Engl J Med.* 2008;359:938–949. *Summary of mechanisms of thrombus formation.*

Mackman N. Triggers, targets and treatments for thrombosis. *Nature.* 2008;451:914–918. *Discussion of mechanisms of thrombus formation.*

Thrombophilias
FVL and prothrombin 20210 mutation

Kim RJ, Becker RC. Association between factor V Leiden, prothrombin G20210A, and methylenetetrahydrofolate reductase C677T mutations and events of the arterial circulatory system: a meta–analysis of published studies. *Am Heart J.* 2003;146:948–957. *The role of FVL and prothrombin 20210 mutation in arterial thromboembolism.*

Segal JB, Brotman DJ, Necochea AJ, et al. Predictive value of factor V Leiden and prothrombin G20210A in adults with venous thromboembolism and in family members of those with a mutation: a systematic review. *JAMA.* 2009;301:2472–2485. *Meta-analysis investigating the role of FVL and prothrombin 20210 mutation on recurrent VTE.*

Deficiencies of protein C and S and antithrombin

Goldenberg N, Manco-Johnson M. Protein C deficiency. *Haemophilia.* 2008;14:1214–1221. *Detailed review article about protein C deficiency.*

Mahmoodi BK, Brouwer JLP, Veeger NJ, Van der Meer J. Hereditary deficiency of protein C or protein S confers increased risk of arterial thromboembolic events at a young age. Results from a large family cohort study. *Circulation.* 2008;118:1659–1667. *Study of risk of arterial thromboembolism in individuals with deficiencies of the natural anticoagulants.*

Makris M. Thrombophilia: grading the risk. *Blood.* 2009;113:5038–5039. *Editorial with useful summarizing table about the annual risk of incident and recurrent VTE in various thrombophilias.*

Patnaik MM, Moll S. Inherited antithrombin deficiency: a review. *Haemophilia.* 2008;14:1229–1239. *Detailed review article about AT deficiency.*

ten Kate MK, van der Meer J. Protein S deficiency: a clinical perspective. *Haemophilia.* 2008;14:1222–1228. *Detailed review article about protein S deficiency.*

Antiphospholipid antibodies

Miyakis S, Lockshin MD, Atsumi T, et al. International consensus statement on an update of the classification criteria for definite antiphospholipid syndrome (APS). *J Thromb Haemost.* 2006;4:295–306. *Article describing in detail the Sapporo criteria (ie, classification criteria for APLA syndrome).*

Pierangeli SS, Chen PP, Raschi E, et al. Antiphospholipid antibodies and the antiphospholipid syndrome: pathogenic mechanisms. *Semin Thromb Hemost.* 2008;34:236–235. *Detailed description of various possible mechanisms that may lead to thrombosis in patients with APLA.*

Factor VIII elevation

Koster T, Blann AD, Briet E, Vandenbroucke JP, Rosendaal FR. Role of clotting factor VIII in effect of von Willebrand factor on occurrence of deep-vein thrombosis. *Lancet.* 1995;345:152–155. *Study demonstrating that elevated factor VIII levels are a risk factor for VTE.*

Homocysteine, MTHFR

Den Heijer M, Lewington S, Clarke R. Homocysteine, MTHFR and risk of venous thrombosis: a meta-analysis of published epidemiological studies. *J Thromb Haemost.* 2005;3:292–299. *Meta-analysis showing that MTHFR polymorphisms are not a risk factor for VTE.*

Den Heijer M, Willems HP, Blom HJ, et al. Homocysteine lowering by B vitamins and the secondary prevention of deep vein thrombosis and pulmonary embolism: a randomized, placebo-controlled, double-blind trial. *Blood.* 2007;109:139–144. *Study showing that lowering of elevated homocysteine levels does not change the risk of recurrent VTE.*

Klerk M, Verhoef P, Clarke R, Blom HJ, Kok FJ, Schouten EG. MTHFR 677C–>T polymorphism and risk of coronary heart disease: a meta-analysis. *JAMA.* 2002;288:2023–2031. *Meta-analysis showing that MTHFR polymorphisms are not a risk factor for arterial thromboembolism.*

Rey E, Kahn SR, David M, Shrier I. Thrombophilic disorders and fetal loss: a meta-analysis. *Lancet.* 2003;361:901–908. *Meta-analysis showing that MTHFR polymorphisms are not a risk factor for pregnancy loss and other complications.*

Toole JF, Malinow MR, Chambless LE, et al. Lowering homocysteine in patients with ischemic stroke to prevent recurrent stroke, myocardial infarction, and death: the Vitamin Intervention for Stroke Prevention (VISP) randomized controlled trial. *JAMA.* 2004;291:565–575. *Lowering of elevated homocysteine levels does not change the risk of recurrent arterial thrombotic events.*

Myeloproliferative disorders

Tefferi A, Elliott M. Thrombosis in myeloproliferative disorders: prevalence, prognostic factors, and the role of leukocytes and JAK2V617F. *Semin Thromb Hemost.* 2007;33:313–320. *Patients with myeloproliferative disorders are at increased risk for venous and arterial thromboembolism.*

Paroxysmal nocturnal hemoglobinemia

Parker C, Omine M, Richards S, et al. Diagnosis and management of paroxysmal nocturnal hemoglobinuria. *Blood.* 2005;106:3699–3709. *Study demonstrating the increased risk of thrombosis in patients with PNH.*

Sloand EM, Pfannes L, Scheinberg P, et al. Increased soluble urokinase plasminogen activator receptor (suPAR) is associated with thrombosis and inhibition of plasmin generation in paroxysmal nocturnal hemoglobinuria (PNH) patients. *Exp Hematol.* 2008;36:1616–1624. *Review article discussing the possible mechanisms of thrombosis formation in PNH.*

Abnormalities in fibrinolysis

Mehta R, Shaprio AD. Plasminogen deficiency. *Haemophilia.* 2008;14:1261–1268. *Detailed review article about plasminogen deficiency.*

Meltzer ME, Doggen CJ, de Groot PG, Rosendaal FR, Lisman T. Fibrinolysis and the risk of venous and arterial thrombosis. *Curr Opin Hematol.* 2007;14:242–248. *Detailed review article on the association of various disturbances in fibrinolysis and the risk for thrombosis.*

Lipoprotein(a)

Sofi F, Marcucci R, Abbate RG, Gensini GF, Prisco D. Lipoprotein (a) and venous thromboembolism in adults: a metaanalysis. *Am J Med.* 2007;120:728–733. *Meta-analysis showing that elevated Lp(a) levels are a mild risk factor for VTE in adults.*

Young G, Albisetti M, Bonduel M, et al. Impact of inherited thrombophilia on venous thromboembolism in children: a systematic review and meta-analysis of observational studies. *Circulation.* 2008;118:1373–1382. *Study showing that elevated Lp(a) levels are a risk factor for VTE in children.*

Family history of thromboembolism

Bezemer ID, van der Meer FJ, Eikenboom JC, Rosendaal FR, Doggen CJ. The value of family history as a risk indicator for venous thrombosis. *Arch Intern Med.* 2009;169:610–615. *Study showing that family history of VTE in a first-degree relative is a risk factor for VTE, independent of the absence or presence of an identifiable thrombophilia.*

Thrombophilia testing guidelines

Baglin T, Gray E, Greaves M, et al. Clinical guidelines for testing for heritable thrombophilia. *Br J Haematol.* 2010;149:209–220. *Thrombophilia testing guideline from the British Committee for Standards in Haematology.*

Grody WW, Griffin JH, Taylor AK, Korf BR, Heit JA. American College of Medical Genetics consensus statement on factor V Leiden mutation testing. *Genet Med.* 2001;3:139–148. *Thrombophilia testing guideline from the American College of Medical Geneticists.*

Nicolaides AN, Breddin HK, Carpenter P, et al. Thrombophilia and venous thromboembolism. International consensus statement. Guidelines according to scientific evidence. *Int Angiol.* 2005;24:1–26. *Thrombophilia testing guideline from the European Genetics Foundation.*

Van Cott EM, Laposata M, Prins MH. Laboratory evaluation of hypercoagulability with venous or arterial thrombosis. *Arch Pathol Lab Med.* 2002;126:1281–1295. *Thrombophilia testing guideline from the College of American Pathologists.*

Patient advocacy

Fenninger R. Patient advocacy to promote public awareness about thrombosis and thrombophilia. *Arterioscler Thromb Vasc Biol.* 2008;28:396–397. *Interesting and stimulating editorial about the power of patient advocacy to influence health policies, general education, and health outcomes, with focus on thrombosis and thrombophilia.*

Pediatric studies

Nowak-Göttl U, Strater R, Heinecke A, et al. Lipoprotein (a) and genetic polymorphisms of clotting factor V, prothrombin, and methylenetetrahydrofolate reductase are risk factors of spontaneous ischemic stroke in childhood. *Blood*. 1999;94:3678–3682. *Investigation of association of thrombophilias with ischemic stroke in children.*

Tormene D, Simioni P, Prandoni P, et al. The incidence of venous thromboembolism in thrombophilic children: a prospective cohort study. *Blood*. 2002;100:2403–2405. *Report on the prevalence of VTE in children with thrombophilia.*

Young G, Albisetti M, Bonduel M, et al. Impact of inherited thrombophilia on venous thromboembolism in children: a systematic review and meta-analysis of observational studies. *Circulation*. 2008;118:1373–1382. *Meta-analysis of studies on the risk of first and recurrent VTE with various thrombophilias in children.*

Antithrombotic drugs and therapy

Ansell J, Hirsh J, Hylek E, Jacobson A, Crowther M, Palareti G. Pharmacology and management of the vitamin K antagonists: American College of Chest Physicians Evidence-Based Clinical Practice Guidelines (8th Edition). *Chest*. 2008;133:160S–198S. *Detailed literature review and evidence-based recommendations on diagnostic and therapeutic issues relating to VKAs, including recommendations on management of elevated INRs and bleeding.*

Douketis JD, Berger PB, Dunn AS, et al. The perioperative management of antithrombotic therapy: American College of Chest Physicians Evidence-Based Clinical Practice Guidelines (8th Edition). *Chest*. 2008;133:299S–339S. *Detailed literature review and evidence-based recommendations on perioperative anticoagulation management.*

Hirsh J, Bauer KA, Donati MB, Gould M, Samama MM, Weitz JI. Parenteral anticoagulants: American College of Chest Physicians Evidence-Based Clinical Practice Guidelines (8th Edition). *Chest*. 2008;133:141S–159S. *Detailed literature review and evidence-based recommendations on diagnostic and therapeutic issues relating to heparin, LMWH, fondaparinux, and other parenteral anticoagulants.*

Lo GK, Juhl D, Warkentin TE, Sigouin CS, Eichler P, Greinacher A. Evaluation of pretest clinical score (4 T's) for the diagnosis of heparin-induced thrombocytopenia in two clinical settings. *J Thromb Haemost*. 2006;4:759–765. *Publication introducing the 4T score for the pretest probability assessment of heparin-induced thrombocytopenia (HIT).*

Nutescu EA, Spinler SA, Wittkowsky A, Dager WE. Low-molecular-weight heparins in renal impairment and obesity: available evidence and clinical practice recommendations across medical and surgical settings. *Ann Pharmacother*. 2009;43:1064–1083. *Detailed literature review of LMWH dosing and monitoring, including in obese and renally impaired patients.*

Warkentin TE, Greinacher A, Koster A, Lincoff M. Treatment and prevention of heparin-induced thrombocytopenia: American College of Chest Physicians Evidence-Based Clinical Practice Guidelines (8th Edition). *Chest*. 2008;133:340S–380S. *Detailed literature review and evidence-based recommendations for the diagnosis and management of HIT.*

Venous thromboembolism
Prevention

Geerts WH, Bergqvist D, Pineo GF, et al. Prevention of venous thromboembolism: American College of Chest Physicians Evidence-Based Clinical Practice Guidelines (8th Edition). *Chest*. 2008;133:381S–453S. *Detailed evidence-based recommendations on VTE prevention in various patient populations.*

Diagnosis

Righini M, Perrier A, De Moerloose P, Bounameaux H. D-dimer for venous thromboembolism diagnosis: 20 years later. *J Thromb Haemost*. 2008;6:1059–1071. *Review of the usefulness and limitations of the D-dimer test as a diagnostic tool for the evaluation of VTE.*

Stein PD, Woodard PK, Weg JG, et al. Diagnostic pathways in acute pulmonary embolism: recommendations of the PIOPED II Investigators. *Radiology*. 2007;242:15–21. *Noteworthy study demonstrating the limitations of CT arteriograms in the diagnosis and exclusion of PE.*

Wells PS, Anderson DR, Bormanis J, et al. Value of assessment of pretest probability of deep-vein thrombosis in clinical management. *Lancet*. 1997;350:1795–1798. *Publication of the Wells criteria for the pretest probability assessment of DVT.*

Wells PS, Anderson DR, Rodger M, et al. Excluding pulmonary embolism at the bedside without diagnostic imaging: management of patients with suspected pulmonary embolism presenting to the emergency department by using a simple clinical model and d-dimer. *Ann Intern Med*. 2001;135:98–107. *Publication of the Wells criteria for the pretest probability assessment of PE.*

Treatment

Kahn SR. Frequency and determinants of the postthrombotic syndrome after venous thromboembolism. *Curr Opin Pulm Med*. 2006;12:299–303. *Review article on postthrombotic syndrome.*

Kearon C, Kahn SR, Agnelli G, Goldhaber SZ, Raskob GE, Comerota AJ. Antithrombotic therapy for venous thromboembolic disease: American College of Chest Physicians Evidence-Based Clinical Practice Guidelines (8th Edition). *Chest*. 2008;133:454–545. *Detailed evidence-based recommendations on VTE treatment of various patient populations.*

Khorana AA, Streiff MB, Farge D, et al. Venous thromboembolism prophylaxis and treatment in cancer: a consensus statement of major guidelines panels and call to action. *J Clin Oncol*. 2009;27:4919–4926. *Review of cancer and VTE, including mechanisms, prevalence, and treatment.*

Konstantinides S, Geibel A, Heusel G, Heinrich F, Kasper W. Heparin plus alteplase compared with heparin alone in patients with submassive pulmonary embolism. *N Engl J Med*. 2002;347:1143–1150. *Randomized trial of thrombolytic therapy versus no thrombolytic therapy in patients with submassive PE.*

Unusual thromboses

Darwish Murad S, Plessier A, Hernandez-Guerra M, et al. Etiology, management, and outcome of the Budd-Chiari syndrome. *Ann Intern Med.* 2009;151:167–175. *Review article on hepatic vein thrombosis.*

Einhaupl K, Bousser MG, de Bruijn SF, et al. EFNS guideline on the treatment of cerebral venous and sinus thrombosis. *Eur J Neurol.* 2006;13:553–559. *Management guideline on sinus vein thrombosis.*

Fugate MW, Rotellini-Coltvet L, Freischlag JA. Current management of thoracic outlet syndrome. *Curr Treat Options Cardiovasc Med.* 2009;11:176–183. *Review article on management of thoracic outlet syndrome and upper extremity DVT.*

Arterial thromboembolism

Albers GW, Amarenco P, Easton JD, Sacco RL, Teal P. Antithrombotic and thrombolytic therapy for ischemic stroke: American College of Chest Physicians Evidence-Based Clinical Practice Guidelines (8th Edition). *Chest.* 2008;133:630S–669S. *Detailed literature review and evidence-based recommendations on stroke management.*

Fuster V, Ryden LE, Cannom DS, et al. ACC/AHA/ESC 2006 guidelines for the management of patients with atrial fibrillation: a report of the American College of Cardiology/American Heart Association Task Force on Practice Guidelines and the European Society of Cardiology Committee for Practice Guidelines (Writing Committee to Revise the 2001 Guidelines for the Management of Patients With Atrial Fibrillation): developed in collaboration with the European Heart Rhythm Association and the Heart Rhythm Society. *Circulation.* 2006;114:e257–e354. *Guidelines for anticoagulant management of atrial fibrillation, with details on the CHADS2 score.*

Singer DE, Albers GW, Dalen JE, et al. Antithrombotic therapy in atrial fibrillation: American College of Chest Physicians Evidence-Based Clinical Practice Guidelines (8th Edition). *Chest.* 2008;133:546S–592S. *Detailed literature review and evidence-based recommendations on antithrombotic management of patients with atrial fibrillation.*

Sobel M, Verhaeghe R. Antithrombotic therapy for peripheral artery occlusive disease: American College of Chest Physicians Evidence-Based Clinical Practice Guidelines (8th Edition). *Chest.* 2008;133:815S–843S. *Detailed literature review and evidence-based recommendations on peripheral arterial disease management.*

CHAPTER 08

Bleeding disorders

Guy Young and Amy D. Shapiro

Overview of hemostasis, 217
Approach to the patient with excessive bleeding, 219
Disorders of primary hemostasis, 220
Disorders of secondary hemostasis, 227
Disorders of fibrinolysis, 236
Bibliography, 238

Overview of hemostasis

Hemostasis is the process through which bleeding is controlled at a site of damaged or disrupted endothelium and is a dynamic interplay between the subendothelium, endothelium, circulating cells, and plasma proteins. Immediately after blood vessel injury, plasma and cellular components are recruited and activated to minimize bleeding and begin tissue repair. The hemostatic process is often divided into 3 phases—the vascular, platelet, and plasma phases; although it is helpful to divide coagulation into these phases for purposes of understanding, in vivo, they are intimately linked and occur in a continuum. The vascular phase is mediated by the release of locally active vasoactive agents that result in vasoconstriction at the site of injury and reduced blood flow. Vascular injury exposes the underlying subendothelium and procoagulant proteins, including tissue factor and collagen, that then come into contact with blood. Platelets bind to von Willebrand factor (vWF) incorporated into the subendothelial matrix through their expression of glycoprotein Ib. Platelets bound to vWF form a layer across the exposed subendothelium, a process termed platelet adhesion, and are subsequently activated via receptors such as GPVI and glycoprotein Ia/IIa, resulting in platelet aggregation and thus forming the primary hemostatic platelet plug (Figure 8-1). For a detailed discussion of platelet function, please see Chapter 9.

The plasma phase of coagulation is initiated through the exposure of tissue factor (TF) in the subendothelium and on damaged endothelial cells. TF binds to the small amounts of circulating activated factor VII (FVIIa), resulting in formation of the TF:FVIIa complex, also known as the extrinsic tenase complex, the complex that binds to and activates factor X (FX) to activated FX (FXa). The TF:FVIIa:FXa complex converts a small amount of prothrombin to thrombin, resulting in an initial thrombin burst that is sufficient to cleave factor VIII (FVIII) from vWF and generate an amplification loop through activation of clotting factors such as FVIII, factor IX (FIX), and factor XI (FXI). These reactions include platelet activation resulting in the expression of surface platelet factor V (FV) and activation of FV to FVa, and activated FIX (FIXa) generated though the above reactions binds to the surface of activated platelets. Activated FVIII complexed with FIXa forms the potent intrinsic tenase complex, resulting in conversion of large amounts of FX to FXa, which in association with FVa on the activated platelet surface results in a thrombin burst sufficient to convert fibrinogen to fibrin (Figure 8-2) and subsequent normal clot formation. The clot is then stabilized by the thrombin-mediated activation of factor XIII (FXIII) and thrombin-activatable fibrinolysis inhibitor (TAFI).

Ultimately, the clot undergoes fibrinolysis, resulting in restoration of a blood vessel segment indistinguishable from that prior to injury. The fibrinolytic process is initiated by

---

Conflict-of-interest disclosure: *Dr. Young:* consultancy; Novo Nordisk, Baxter, Bayer; honoraria: Novo Nordisk, Baxter, Bayer; membership on board of directors or advisory committee: Novo Nordisk, Baxter, Bayer. *Dr. Shapiro:* consultancy: Baxter BioScience, Inspiration Biopharmaceuticals, Syntonix; speakers' bureau: Baxter BioScience, Novo Nordisk; membership on board of directors or advisory committee: Baxter BioScience, Novo Nordisk, Bayer Healthcare, Inspiration Biopharmaceuticals, Catalyst Biosciences, American Thrombosis and Hemostasis Network, National Hemophilia Foundation; clinical research protocols: Baxter BioScience, Novo Nordisk, Bayer Healthcare Pharmaceuticals, Wyeth Pharmaceuticals, Inspiration Biopharmaceuticals; NIH/NHLBI: Clinical Trial Review Board, Data Safety Management Board.
Off-label drug use: *Dr. Young:* rFVIIa (Novoseven) for management of bleeding in hemophilia at doses and regimens that are not approved and for other off-label indications; prothrombin complex concentrates (various brand names) for treatment of warfarin overdose, vitamin K deficiency, and liver disease. *Dr. Shapiro:* rFVIIa for high-dose therapy and rare disorders.

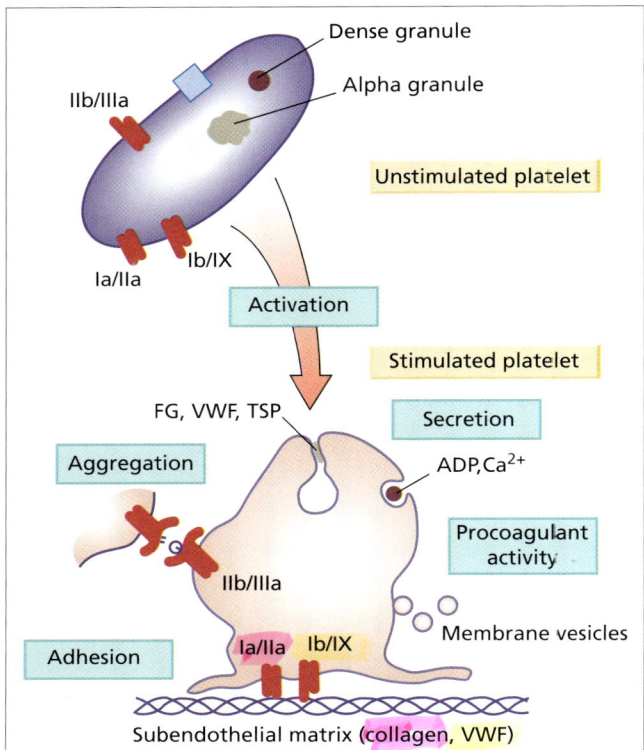

Figure 8-1 Platelet activation. Platelets can undergo activation through stimulation by soluble agonists such as thrombin or by contact (adherence) to the subendothelial matrix. Activation changes the platelet from a disk to a sphere with pseudopods. Activation is followed by secretion of granular contents, aggregation, and rearrangement of membrane phospholipids, resulting in potentiation of phospholipid-dependent procoagulant activity. Reproduced with permission, from George JN, Shattil SJ. The clinical importance of acquired abnormalities of platelet function. *N Engl J Med*. 1991;324:27–39.

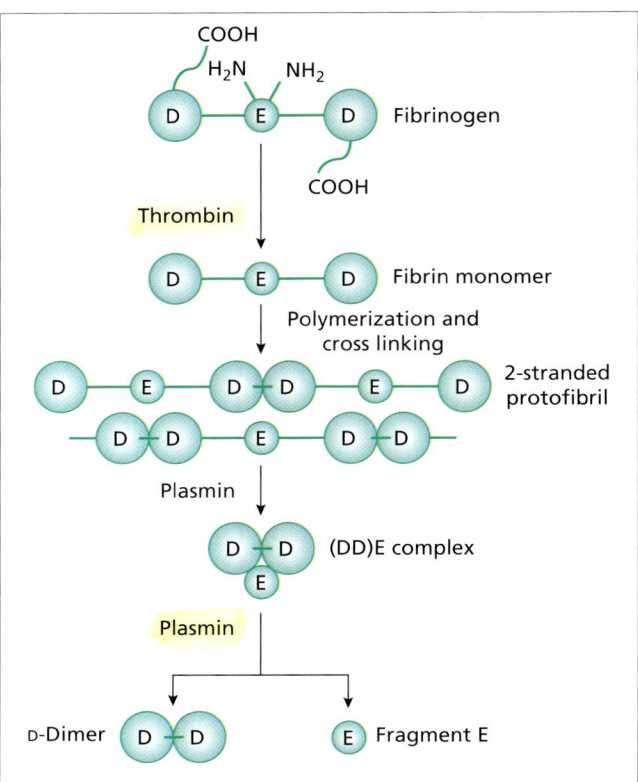

Figure 8-2 Fibrin formation and degradation. Fibrinogen has a trinocular structure with a central E and 2 D domains. Thrombin cleaves fibrinopeptides A and B from the NH2 terminal of the A1 and BJ chains, respectively, located in the E domain. The resultant fibrin monomers polymerize nonenzymatically forming protofibrils. Factor XIIIa cross-links the D domains of adjacent fibrin monomers. Plasmin degrades cross-linked fibrin, thereby generating (DD)E complexes comprised of an E fragment noncovalently bound to D-dimer. With further plasmin attack, the (DD)E complex is degraded into fragment E and D-dimer.

the release of tissue plasminogen activator (tPA) near the site of injury. tPA converts plasminogen to plasmin, which via interactions with lysine and arginine residues on fibrin cleaves fibrin into dissolvable fragments.

Both the hemostatic and fibrinolytic processes are regulated by inhibitors that contain these processes to the site of injury and quench the reactions to prevent systemic activation and pathologic propagation. The hemostatic system has 2 main inhibitory pathways mediated through antithrombin and the protein C/protein S complex. Antithrombin released at the margins of endothelial injury binds in a 1:1 complex with thrombin, inactivating thrombin not bound by the forming clot. Excess free thrombin at the clot margins binds to thrombomodulin, a receptor expressed on the surface of intact endothelial cells that when complexed with thrombin activates protein C; activated protein C complexes with protein S and inactivates activated FV and FVIII. This negative feedback results in reduced subsequent thrombin generation and quenching of fibrin generation. The fibrinolytic system also comprises inhibitors, principally plasminogen activator inhibitor-1 (PAI-1), which as its name implies inhibits tPA, and α_2-antiplasmin (α2AP), which inhibits plasmin.

Key points

1. Hemostasis is a complex and highly regulated process involving the subendothelium, endothelial cells, circulating cells, and plasma proteins that include both positive and negative feedback mechanisms.
2. Defects in primary hemostasis (platelets and vWF) typically result in mucocutaneous bleeding symptoms.
3. Defects in coagulation factors cause variable symptomatology but may result in deep tissue bleeding including intramuscular hematomas, hemarthroses, and retroperitoneal and, occasionally, central nervous system bleeding events.

This chapter is devoted to a discussion of the pathophysiology, clinical presentation, diagnosis, prognosis, and treatment of hemostatic abnormalities hereafter referred to as bleeding disorders. The first section will review the approach to a patient with excessive bleeding followed by a discussion of the specific disorders.

Approach to the patient with excessive bleeding

Excessive bleeding may occur in patients of all ages and ethnicities. Symptoms can begin as early as the immediate newborn period (uncommonly even in utero) or anytime thereafter. The bleeding symptoms experienced are due in large part to the specific factor and level of deficiency; bleeding can be spontaneous, that is, without an identified trigger, or may occur after a hemostatic challenge such as delivery, injury, trauma, surgery, or the onset of menstruation. Furthermore, bleeding symptoms may be confined to specific anatomic sites or may occur in multiple sites. Finally, bleeding symptoms may be present in multiple family members or may occur in the absence of a family history. All of this information is important to arrive at a correct diagnosis rapidly and with minimal yet correctly sequenced laboratory testing. Thus, a detailed patient and family history is a vital part of the approach to each patient with a potential bleeding disorder.

Obtaining a detailed patient and family history is crucial regardless of prior laboratory testing. The history includes a detailed discussion of specific bleeding symptoms or abnormalities. Information regarding bleeding symptoms should include location, frequency and pattern, and duration both in terms of appearance of symptoms and time required for cessation. The location may suggest the part of the hemostatic system affected; patients with disorders of primary hemostasis (platelets and vWF) often experience mucocutaneous bleeding including easy bruising, epistaxis, and menorrhagia in women of childbearing age, whereas patients with disorders of secondary hemostasis (coagulation factor deficiencies) may experience deep tissue bleeding including the joints, muscles, and central nervous system. The bleeding pattern and duration of each episode, particularly for mucus membrane bleeding, assist in determination of the likelihood of an underlying bleeding disorder. For example, a patient with 4 episodes of epistaxis monthly, each lasting <5 minutes, is less likely to have a bleeding disorder than the patient with 4 episodes monthly whose episodes last 10 minutes or longer despite appropriate local interventions. The onset of symptoms can suggest the presence of a congenital versus acquired disorder. Although congenital conditions can present at any age, it is more likely that patients with a long history of symptoms or symptoms that begin during childhood have a congenital condition, whereas patients whose onset occurs at an older age are more likely to have an acquired condition. Congenital clotting factor deficiencies that do not present until later in life do occur and include mild factor deficiencies and coagulation factor deficiencies associated with variable bleeding patterns, most notably FXI deficiency. Additional important information to be collected includes the current use of medications and herbal supplements because these may affect the hemostatic system; the presence or absence of a family history of bleeding; a history of hemostatic challenges including surgery, dental procedures, and trauma; and a menstrual history for females. The goal at the end of the history is to establish the likelihood of a bleeding disorder because this judgment determines the direction of the laboratory investigation. An instrument for the determination of the severity of bleeding symptoms has been published and has been demonstrated to be useful in discriminating patients with and without bleeding disorders.

The laboratory evaluation includes performance of initial screening tests. Specific factor analyses are performed after mixing studies reveal correction of the prolonged coagulation screening test(s) indicative of a deficiency state or in the face of normal screening tests with a positive history. It is important to note that screening tests are not sensitive to all abnormalities associated with a bleeding disorder, including vWF, FXIII, PAI-1, and α2AP deficiencies; therefore, a patient history strongly suggestive of a bleeding disorder may warrant testing for such rare abnormalities regardless of the results of screening tests. The most common screening tests used include the platelet count, prothrombin time (PT), and activated partial thromboplastin time (aPTT). Although some advocate the use of platelet function as screening tests, no strong evidence exists to support this approach, and tests such as the bleeding time or platelet function analyzer (PFA; PFA-100, Platelet Research Laboratory, Barcelona, Spain) should be reserved for individuals in whom the suspicion of a bleeding disorder is high.

Mixing studies are performed via a 1-to-1 mix of patient plasma with known normal standard plasma, thereby increasing any clotting factor deficiency, even those at a level of 0, to at least 50%, the level at which these tests are set to be within the normal range. Correction of these tests indicates a deficiency state, whereas lack of correction indicates an inhibitor, either one directed against a specific factor or a global inhibitor as best exemplified by a lupus anticoagulant.

It is likely that by the time patients are referred to a hematologist that some, if not all, of the previously mentioned tests may have been performed. Abnormalities of screening tests do not necessarily represent the presence of a pathologic process because these tests are sensitive to handling, may vary in reliability based on laboratory, and may be influenced by medications including herbal therapies, among other issues. Repeating laboratory tests is often required; they are optimally performed in the absence of medications known to affect their results.

> ### Key points
> 1. Patients with bleeding disorders may occasionally present for evaluation prior to symptom onset especially in the presence of a known family history and/or abnormal screening laboratory tests.
> 2. Patients with bleeding disorders can present at any age with bleeding in a variety of sites. The more severe disorders tend to present earlier in life and with bleeding symptoms that are often spontaneous or in areas including the joints, muscles, or central nervous system.
> 3. The approach to patients with a potential bleeding disorder requires a detailed personal and family history and involves the use of screening laboratory tests, mixing studies when results are abnormal, and subsequent further specific coagulation factor testing.
> 4. Some patients with a history or physical examination indicative of a bleeding disorder may have a normal laboratory evaluation.

Disorders of primary hemostasis

Platelet function disorders
Pathophysiology

Platelets play a major role in primary hemostasis both by constituting the cellular structure for the primary hemostatic plug and by providing a phospholipid surface upon which plasma coagulation proteins bind and form complexes. Decreases in platelet counts and/or impaired platelet function may result in bleeding symptoms; thrombocytopenic and platelet function defects are reviewed in detail in Chapter 9. A reduced number of platelets may result in reduced platelet adhesion and aggregation. Abnormalities in platelet function can occur in any of the multitude of processes required for normal platelet function including receptor presence and function, signal translation, biochemical pathway, and granule content and secretion. A brief overview of platelet pathophysiology is important to the understanding of described platelet function defects.

It is reasonable to review potential platelet defects in the order in which processes occur during normal platelet function (Figure 8-1). Platelets adhere to a site of bleeding via the binding of vWF through glycoprotein Ib and, to a lesser extent, binding to collagen via glycoprotein Ia/IIa. Defects in glycoprotein Ib result in Bernard-Soulier syndrome, whereas defects in the collagen receptor do not result in an identified bleeding disorder; however, such defects are known to exacerbate coexisting von Willebrand disease (vWD). In addition, a gain of function mutation in glycoprotein Ib results in excess binding of vWF, particularly of the high molecular weight multimers, resulting in platelet-type vWD; although this is technically a platelet defect, it is reviewed in the later section on vWD. After platelet adhesion, platelets become activated through binding of agonists, such as adenosine diphosphate (ADP) or thrombin, and secrete granular contents that enhance vasoconstriction and further platelet aggregation. Defects in the production, storage, and secretion of these vasoactive and hemostatic substances result in excessive bleeding. Such disorders are exemplified by the δ-storage pool defect, resulting in reduced secretion of ADP, and the gray platelet syndrome, a defect in α-granule formation. After granule secretion, platelets aggregate via bridges formed by fibrinogen bound to platelet glycoprotein IIb/IIIa. The absence of, or a defect in, platelet glycoprotein IIb/IIIa results in Glanzmann thrombasthenia, a severe platelet function defect. During activation, the platelet membrane exposes negatively charged phospholipids, the surface upon which the plasma clotting factors bind and form the fibrin meshwork. There are a number of conditions known to disrupt this process through alteration of the composition of the phospholipid surface, most notably dietary substances including vitamin E and omega-3 fatty acids. Although this section briefly encompasses some of the best described defects, a full review of platelet function defects is included in Chapter 9, and a number of excellent review articles that address this topic are available.

Etiology

Platelet function defects may be divided based on congenital or acquired defects and can be conceptualized in terms of the structural components and/or function of the platelets. Congenital disorders of platelet receptors such as glycoprotein Ib and IIb/IIIa result in Bernard-Soulier disease and Glanzmann thrombasthenia, respectively. There are genetic defects resulting in the common ADP secretion defect and the less common absence of dense bodies associated with Hermansky-Pudlak syndrome and α-granule defects such as gray platelet syndrome. Most platelet function defects are diagnosed via standard assays; identification of the specific cause or its presence in multiple family members implies a genetic abnormality.

Acquired platelet defects are most commonly the result of ingestion of medications or herbal supplements, a chronic medical condition such as uremia, or the result of medical interventions such cardiopulmonary bypass. The list of medications resulting in platelet dysfunction is vast. The most commonly used medications that result in platelet dysfunction, many of which are over the counter, include aspirin and other nonsteroidal anti-inflammatory drugs, antihistamines, guaifenesin (the expectorant in many cold remedies), certain anticonvulsants (valproic acid in particular), antibiotics, and antidepressants, including most commonly selective serotonin reuptake inhibitors. The herbal supplements garlic, ginger, omega-3 fatty acids, vitamin E, and gingko biloba are among the most commonly consumed supplements known to affect platelet function. Thus, when taking a history, it is imperative to ask not only about prescribed medications but also over-the-counter and herbal supplements. Although most of these will not lead to a clinically apparent bleeding disorder, they may unmask a mild disorder or confound results of platelet function tests; knowledge of all medications and supplements is critical to interpret laboratory tests.

Clinical presentation

Patients with platelet function disorders present with similar symptoms regardless of the specific defect. The severity of symptoms is dictated by the specific condition or clinical situation. Patients with platelet function defects exhibit mucocutaneous bleeding described in detail in the later section addressing vWD. Central nervous system and retroperitoneal hemorrhage are rare events in patients with platelet function disorders. Patients may present as a result of abnormal bleeding, a known family history of bleeding either with or without a personal history of bleeding, or an abnormal screening test such as a PFA test ordered prior to a planned medical procedure.

Diagnosis

The diagnosis of platelet disorders is covered in Chapter 9. Briefly, the platelet count must be determined; platelet function assays will be abnormal in the setting of significant thrombocytopenia, and the PFA will be abnormal with significant anemia. Thus, a complete blood count (CBC) should be performed prior to obtaining platelet-specific studies. There are 2 commonly available tests to screen for platelet function disorders, both with limitations. The original screening test was the bleeding time, a test that has fallen out of favor due to its limitations, specifically its variability, reproducibility, and inability to predict clinical bleeding. Although the bleeding time was purported to assess platelet adhesion and aggregation, it has significant limitations including interoperator variability, poor reproducibility, and invasiveness especially in children; due to these issues, it is less commonly used than the PFA. Performance of a bleeding time requires a skilled technician and a cooperative patient. There are increasingly fewer laboratories that perform the bleeding time with regularity, and thus, skilled technicians are not commonly available. The need for a cooperative patient renders this assay difficult to perform in children. Importantly, regardless of the result, the bleeding time does not predict for the risk of bleeding during procedures.

The PFA is a widely available laboratory evaluation that may be abnormal in congenital and acquired disorders of platelet function as well as in types 2 and 3 vWD. The usefulness of the PFA in the diagnosis of type 1 vWD is controversial (see discussion in the section on vWD). The PFA will be abnormal if the platelet count is less than approximately 100,000/μL and in patients with anemia because a hemoglobin of <10 g/dL may lead to abnormal results. Patients with severe platelet function defects such as Bernard-Soulier and Glanzmann thrombasthenia will also have abnormal results. The PFA may be abnormal in mild disorders such as common ADP secretion defects; however, its sensitivity for these disorders is insufficient to rule out such defects in the face of a normal result. The PFA is often abnormal in patients on aspirin, clopidogrel, and ticlopidine. The effects of other medications known to affect platelet function such as valproic acid are not clear. The utility of the PFA is limited by insufficient sensitivity, such that it rarely obviates the need for further testing, and its inability to distinguish between the 2 most common bleeding disorders, platelet function defects and vWD. These aspects significantly limit its use as a screening test.

The most specific assay of platelet function is platelet aggregometry. This assay uses platelet-rich plasma and evaluates platelet aggregation via light transmission after addition of a variety of platelet agonists such as ADP, epinephrine, ristocetin, arachidonic acid, collagen, and thrombin-related activation peptide. Patients with a variety of both severe and mild platelet function disorders have abnormal platelet aggregation profiles, and furthermore, the spectrum of abnormalities can be diagnostic of specific disorders. For example, if results demonstrate absent aggregation to all agonists except ristocetin, the pattern is diagnostic of Glanzmann thrombasthenia, whereas the opposite pattern is consistent with Bernard-Soulier syndrome. In addition, a pattern of aggregation followed by disaggregation with ADP is consistent with the common ADP secretion defect. A more detailed discussion of platelet aggregation can be found in reviews of platelet function disorders. Platelet aggregation testing is labor intensive and expensive and often requires a prior appointment. As with the PFA, many medications and supplements affect platelet aggregation studies, and thus if possible, the assay should be performed when patients are no longer receiving these medications or supplements for approximately 10 days. This assay can be performed in anemic and even thrombocytopenic patients (if one suspects a platelet function defect in addition to thrombocytopenia as a cause for bleeding) because it is performed on platelet-rich plasma.

For thrombocytopenic patients, the amount of blood to be drawn may be prohibitive, and consultation with the coagulation laboratory is recommended prior to ordering the assay in this circumstance.

Finally, flow cytometry can be used to quantify the levels of platelet surface receptors and can confirm the diagnosis of Bernard-Soulier and Glanzmann thrombasthenia if the diagnosis is in doubt. In some institutions, these assays are available and have become the method of choice for diagnosis.

Some platelet function defects lead to easily identifiable platelet ultrastructural changes visualized by electron microscopy. In particular, patients with a deficiency or absence of dense bodies (δ-storage pool deficiency) or α-granules (gray platelet syndrome) can be diagnosed by this method. A number of other defects can also be demonstrated by this technique.

Treatment

Congenital platelet function defects may benefit from medical treatment, although ultimately, transfusions may be required because medications or local measures are often ineffective. In acquired conditions, treatment or reversal of the underlying condition will resolve the platelet dysfunction; however, this is not always possible. In such situations, the approach to management of bleeding is similar to that for congenital disorders.

Several medications enhance hemostasis nonspecifically and are useful in the face of platelet dysfunction. These include desmopressin, antifibrinolytic agents, estrogen, and recombinant FVIIa (rFVIIa). Desmopressin may improve platelet function in many congenital disorders, in uremia, and during cardiopulmonary bypass, although the exact mechanism of action is not clear. Desmopressin may be administered intravenously, subcutaneously, and, for home management, intranasally. Intranasal use requires the highly concentrated solution (Stimate; CSL Behring, King of Prussia, PA) because the intranasal formulation used to manage diabetes insipidus or enuresis is ineffective as a hemostatic agent. In some circumstances, it may be useful to perform a desmopressin challenge test prior to its clinical use. The challenge test entails assessment of platelet function before and approximately 90 minutes after administration; however, it is recognized that there is often a poor correlation between the results of platelet function tests and clinical outcomes, and thus, the value of this approach is uncertain. Although desmopressin is a safe agent, its use can lead to vasodilation resulting in facial flushing with rare reductions in blood pressure sufficient to lead to clinical symptoms. Moreover, as an analog of an antidiuretic hormone, desmopressin can result in water retention and hyponatremia. Although this rarely occurs in adults and older children, the risks are increased in children <3 years of age and in individuals receiving intravenous fluids. Therefore, its use should be overseen by an experienced care provider, and its repeated use in close proximity should be limited.

Antifibrinolytic agents (ε-aminocaproic acid [EACA] and tranexamic acid [TXA]) are commonly used adjunctive hemostatic therapies. These agents inhibit plasmin-mediated thrombolysis and exert their effect through clot stabilization and prevention of early dissolution. Thus, these agents may be effective in prevention of rebleeding, a common problem in individuals with bleeding disorders especially in areas with increased fibrinolysis such as the oropharynx. These agents may be administered intravenously, orally, or topically in amenable circumstances. These agents can be used both therapeutically after bleeding has occurred or prophylactically as part of perioperative management. Common practice for treatment of mucosal bleeding includes the use of antifibrinolytic agents in conjunction with desmopressin; the combination is also effective in bleeding from other sites, for example, in the management of menorrhagia. Antifibrinolytic agents have been used widely for many years, have a documented safety profile, and are well tolerated in most patients. Commonly reported symptoms include headaches and abdominal discomfort; however, these symptoms do not preclude its continued use if ameliorated with other agents such as acetaminophen. Antifibrinolytic agents should be used with caution in patients with a history of thrombosis and/or atherosclerosis and are contraindicated when hematuria is present because obstructive uropathy secondary to ureteral clots may develop.

Estrogens have documented effectiveness in the management of bleeding in patients with uremia-induced platelet dysfunction. The mechanism of action is not well elucidated, although their use is associated with an increase in procoagulants including vWF and FVIII and a decrease in naturally occurring inhibitors of coagulation, particularly protein S. Conjugated estrogens are also used for the management of severe menorrhagia with both the previously mentioned hemostatic effects and additional local effect of reduced uterine blood flow. Estrogen in combination with progestins, as in oral contraceptive agents, is useful for home management of menorrhagia in patients with bleeding disorders including platelet function disorders and vWD. The positive effects of these agents are likely similar to conjugated estrogens in conjunction with progestin-induced stabilization of the endometrial lining. The risks associated with estrogens include thrombosis; thus, these agents should be avoided in patients with a history of thrombosis or who are deemed at high risk for thrombosis.

Although rFVIIa has been shown anecdotally to be effective for management of severe bleeding in patients with platelet function defects, its value in this setting has not been clearly defined. This agent is licensed in the European Union for the management of bleeding in patients with Glanzmann thrombasthenia refractory to platelet transfusions. rFVIIa may be associated with adverse events including thrombosis and is costly; therefore, its use should be justified by documentation of efficacy and judicious utilization. Although off-label, the use of rFVIIa in patients with severe bleeding in whom standard therapeutic measures have failed is a reasonable guideline adopted by many institutions.

For severe bleeding unresponsive to the previously mentioned measures, especially in patients with Bernard-Soulier and Glanzmann thrombasthenia, platelet transfusion should be administered to provide normally functioning platelets. The general risks associated with platelet transfusion common to all patients include the risk of transfusion reactions and potential transmission of infectious agents (see Chapter 11 for details on risk of platelet transfusions). An important specific risk associated with Bernard-Soulier and Glanzmann thrombasthenia is alloimmunization due to formation of antibodies against glycoprotein Ib and IIb/IIIa, respectively. Once antibodies develop, future platelet transfusions are likely to be ineffective and may be associated with unusual reactions. Thus, judicious use of platelet transfusions is imperative.

The benefits of local measures cannot be understated in the management of bleeding episodes for which these approaches are amenable. Application of direct pressure is an effective measure for epistaxis and oral and cutaneous bleeding. For accessible bleeding sites including the nose, mouth, and skin, the use of topical adjunctive agents can also be effective and is often safer than systemic therapy.

Prognosis and outcomes

The majority of commonly encountered platelet function disorders are associated with mild intermittent bleeding episodes that do not significantly interfere with a normal life. Among the more serious conditions, Glanzmann thrombasthenia is the most common disorder. In some patients, bleeding has been so severe that bone marrow transplantation was undertaken to correct the defect. This extreme approach is reserved for only the most severe patients for whom an unaffected human leukocyte antigen (HLA)-compatible sibling is available. Patients with platelet function disorders should receive thorough education regarding their condition and its management so that bleeding episodes are recognized early, managed at home, or prevented through appropriate measures or interventions. Importantly, patients should be advised to report their condition to physicians prior to undergoing invasive procedures so that appropriate prophylactic measures are used to avoid adverse events; in addition, all new medications should be checked for their ability to interfere with platelet function.

Gaps in knowledge

The complexity of establishment of a correct diagnosis cannot be underestimated in the appropriate management of patients with platelet function disorders. Although current laboratory assays are helpful, patients may be left without a more specific diagnosis than the broad category of a platelet function defect. The complexity of platelet structure and function makes identification at a molecular or cellular level impractical or impossible in many patients outside of specialized research centers. Therefore, an important area for future research is the development of widely available laboratory assays with increased sophistication, sensitivity, and specificity that are able to unravel platelet function defects into better defined categories. A promising approach is the use of proteomic analysis of platelet proteins. Although this approach is presently used only in the research setting, it is feasible that further research will allow development of a clinically useful assay. In addition, the ongoing development of global hemostatic assays may allow identification of a patient's defects whose previous evaluations were undefined or unrevealing. At present, a number of assays are under evaluation; it is hoped that in the relatively near future, these may become a part of the armamentarium available in the coagulation laboratory.

> **Key points**
>
> 1. Platelet function disorders can be congenital or acquired and typically present with mucocutaneous bleeding symptoms.
> 2. The laboratory evaluation for platelet function disorders involves a variety of tests including platelet aggregation studies and the PFA-100 assay. Neither of these tests, however, is able to predict clinical bleeding episodes.
> 3. Glanzmann thrombasthenia is the most severe platelet function defect and has the potential to result in significant bleeding requiring blood transfusion. Platelet transfusions in this disorder are reserved for life-threatening bleeding due to risk of development of alloantibodies that render further transfusions ineffective.
> 4. The ADP secretion defect is the most common platelet function defect and typically causes mild to moderate mucocutaneous bleeding symptoms that are managed with desmopressin, antifibrinolytic agents, and hormonal therapy for menorrhagia.

von Willebrand disease
Pathophysiology

vWF is the primary plasma protein required for platelet adhesion and also plays an important role in platelet aggregation. The absence or reduced amount of vWF or an abnormal vWF protein results in coagulation defects affecting platelet adhesion and aggregation and resulting in mucocutaneous bleeding. vWF is the carrier protein for FVIII; as a result, patients with vWD may have reduced levels of circulating FVIII that further affect the quality of hemostasis. The effectiveness of vWF as an adhesive protein relies on multimerization of the protein, resulting in large molecules that include high molecular weight multimers required for adequate function.

Etiology

vWD can be either congenital or acquired; the congenital form predominates. Congenital vWD is caused by mutations in the *vWF* gene, and many mutations have been identified that lead to a variety of structural perturbations with either reduced production or secretion of normally structured vWF or to the production of a dysfunctional protein. vWD has been subcategorized into 3 basic types: quantitative defects that may be partial (type 1) or complete (type 3) and qualitative defects (type 2; Table 8-1). Type 1 is a result of reduced amounts of plasma vWF that result from either decreased production/secretion of vWF or increased clearance of circulating vWF (Vicenza type). Type 3 is due to a complete/near-total absence of the plasma protein and is likely due to severe mutations in both vWF genes. There are 4 commonly recognized type 2 defects. Type 2A is due to defects in multimerization and results in an absence of high and medium molecular weight multimers that are required for normal platelet adhesion. Type 2B results from a gain of function mutation (similar to platelet-type vWD) that leads to increased binding of the high molecular weight multimers to circulating platelets that are subsequently removed from the available plasma pool. This type may be associated with thrombocytopenia. Type 2M results from mutations that lead to inability of the vWF to bind to platelets. Type 2N is due to a defect of the vWF to bind and protect FVIII and results in increased proteolysis of FVIII and a resultant reduction in circulating FVIII activity. In general, patients presenting with type 2N are compound heterozygotes for a type 1 defect and the type 2N mutation; these patients may be difficult to distinguish from patients with mild FVIII-deficient hemophilia, and the performance of a specific assay is required (see Diagnosis section).

Acquired von Willebrand syndrome (AvWS) is a rare condition reported in a variety of medical conditions. In children, it has been associated with Wilms tumor, congenital heart disease, and systemic lupus erythematosus, whereas in adults, it may occur in association with a variety of conditions including lymphoproliferative disorders, myeloproliferative disorders, aortic stenosis, hypothyroidism, and after exposure to certain medications. The pathophysiology of AvWS is heterogeneous and depends on the associated condition. Some described mechanisms include antibody formation, decreased production, increased proteolysis, and adsorption of vWF onto malignant cells, among others. AvWS may also occur in association with essential thrombocytosis at high platelet counts due to binding of vWF to the circulating platelets.

Clinical presentation

The clinical presentation of vWD includes mucocutaneous bleeding—specifically easy and excessive bruising and bleeding from mucosal surfaces including the nose, mouth, and

Table 8-1 Classification and diagnosis of von Willebrand disease.

Subtype	Defect	vWF Ag	RCof	FVIII	von Willebrand multimers
1	Partial quantitative	↓	↓	↓	Normal distribution
2A	Multimerization	↓	↓↓	↓	Decreased high and intermediate molecular weight multimers
2B	Increased binding of high molecular weight multimers to platelets	↓	↓↓	↓	Decreased high molecular weight multimers
2M	Decreased binding to platelets	Normal	↓↓	Normal	Normal distribution
2N*	Decreased binding to FVIII	↓	↓	↓↓	Normal distribution
3	Complete deficiency	↓↓↓	↓↓↓	↓↓↓	Absent
Platelet type	Increased binding of high molecular weight multimers to platelets	↓	↓↓	↓	Decreased high molecular weight multimers

*Patients with type 2N are usually compound heterozygotes for a type 1 mutation and therefore have low vWF Ag and RCof.
RCof = Ristocetin Cofactor activity; vWF Ag = von Willebrand factor antigen.

gastrointestinal and genitourinary tract. The extent, location, and nature of bruising are important clinical points. Multiple bruises of various ages in a variety of locations are especially suggestive of a disorder of primary hemostasis. Epistaxis or oral—pharyngeal bleeding that is sufficient to result in anemia also suggests the presence of a hemostatic disorder. Menorrhagia, particularly at the onset of menarche, is also suggestive. Excessive bleeding following procedures involving the mucus membranes may unmask a previously unknown bleeding disorder. The most common of these events include childbirth, oral surgery including dental work, tonsillectomy/adenoidectomy, and sinus surgery. Some patients present as a result of a documented family history of bleeding without an individual specific bleeding event. Less commonly, patients may present due to abnormal screening tests ordered prior to a planned medical procedure.

Clinical manifestations may range from mild to severe. Type 3 vWD may be associated with bleeding events observed in severe hemophilia, likely due to the extremely low FVIII level associated with this syndrome, resulting from the inability to bind and protect FVIII from proteolytic cleavage. Severe menorrhagia resulting in early hysterectomy may also occur in females with a variety of subtypes including types 1, 2, and 3. Because the bleeding manifestations of vWD include common symptoms observed in the normal population such as bruising, epistaxis, and menorrhagia, clinical suspicion is important for accurate diagnosis. The use of agents that inhibit platelet function may unmask vWD; excessive bleeding after the use of a medication such as aspirin or a nonsteroidal agent may trigger an evaluation for a platelet function defect or vWD.

Acquired vWS is less commonly attributable to medication use, although valproic acid has been implicated as a cause of AvWS. Disorders that may lead to AvWS are varied and differ from those associated with platelet function defects. Medications that affect platelet function may contribute to exacerbation of clinical symptoms observed in patients with AvWS as well. Clinical presentation of AvWS is similar to congenital vWD described earlier; however, affected individuals most commonly do not exhibit a lifelong or family history of abnormal bleeding.

Diagnosis

The diagnosis of vWD relies on specific testing because screening tests are insufficient to rule out this disorder. Laboratory testing for vWD includes measurement of the quantity of vWF present and of the 2 presently assayable functions (Table 8-1). Although the PFA may be abnormal in vWD, a normal PFA does not rule out this disorder; therefore, the usefulness of a PFA for detection of vWD is minimal. Assays for vWD include measurement of the amount of vWF (the vWF antigen assay), the platelet binding function (ristocetin cofactor assay, in which the agglutination of fixed platelets in response to patient plasma is measured), and the FVIII binding function (FVIII activity). Recently, a potential role for assays that measure the binding of vWF to collagen has also been described. Based on these results, further testing, which is described in detail later, may be pursued.

Limitations exist with several of these assays. Both vWF and FVIII are acute-phase reactants and will increase to between 2 and 5 times above baseline due to a variety of conditions or circumstances. These increased levels may place previously low values within the normal range when, in fact, the patient being studied is affected with vWD. Therefore, normal levels do not rule out this disorder, especially in the face of a suspicious clinical history, and should be interpreted with caution. Increased estrogen levels, as with the use of oral contraceptive agents, during pregnancy, or at/around the time of ovulation, may also increase vWF levels. The blood type also affects vWF levels; type O is associated with the lowest levels, and type AB is associated with the highest levels.

Performance of the assays to diagnose vWD is not straightforward and requires an experienced coagulation laboratory. The ristocetin cofactor assay has relatively poor inter- and intra-assay variability. It is not unusual for patients who have undergone serial testing to have moderate variations in levels over time. Due to the difficulty in ruling out this disorder with one normal evaluation, it is not uncommon for patients to undergo repeated testing until results appear consistent or congruent with the clinical impression based on history and physical examination. When local laboratory results are inconsistent, a useful strategy is to perform testing in a reference hemostasis laboratory.

Results suggestive of vWD require further evaluation to determine the subtype. This is largely accomplished through the use of vWF multimer analysis (Figure 8-3), as well as other studies such as ristocetin-induced platelet agglutination. These studies and their interpretation are described in Table 8-1. Some cases, such as the diagnosis of vWD Vicenza, may require specialized testing such as determination of the half-life of circulating vWF after desmopressin challenge (see following Treatment section).

Treatment

The principles of management of vWD are to increase or replace vWF to achieve hemostasis. This can be accomplished with either medications that cause the release of endogenous stores of vWF into the circulation (desmopressin) or the use of vWF-containing concentrates derived from human plasma. Mild to moderate bleeding associated with type 1 vWD may be managed with desmopressin, most commonly with the intranasal preparation, and

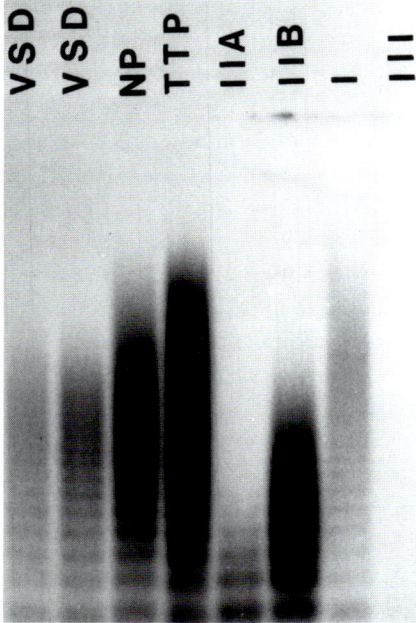

Figure 8-3 Representation of a von Willebrand factor multimer analysis. The third column from the left represents normal plasma as indicated by the NP at the top of the column. In type 2A von Willebrand disease, there is a loss of high and intermediate weight multimers as indicated by the loss of the bands in the gel under the heading. In type 2B von Willebrand disease, there is a loss of high molecular weight multimers. In type 1, all the multimers are present but in reduced amounts as can be seen by the presence of all the bands but with more faint staining than seen in normal plasma. In type 3 disease, there is a complete absence of multimers, and no staining of bands is visible. The labelled columns VSD and TTP stand for ventricular-septal defect, a condition that results in the acquired von Willebrand syndrome with loss of multimers of all sizes, and thrombotic thrombocytopenic purpura where ultra-large multimers can be observed.

antifibrinolytic agents as required. The pathophysiology of the hemostatic response to desmopressin in vWD is well described and results from secretion into the plasma of stored vWF from the Weibel-Palade bodies in endothelial cells. A desmopressin challenge test, as described in the platelet section, should be performed to document a hemostatic response; in vWD, the vWF antigen, ristocetin cofactor, and FVIII activity are performed before and 60 to 90 minutes after dose, depending on the route of administration. Repeat laboratory evaluation at 4 hours after dose may be appropriate if one suspects an altered half-life of the native protein as observed in the Vicenza type. Approximately 90% of patients with type 1 vWD respond with hemostatic levels; however, the response should be measured to determine its adequacy for specific hemostatic challenges. Repeated administration of desmopressin, especially in close proximity, leads to a phenomenon termed tachyphylaxis, with decreased level of the response with repeated use presumably resulting from depletion of the storage pool. Thus, use of desmopressin no more than once daily and on no more than 2 to 3 consecutive days represents acceptable clinical guidelines for home use. There are some reports of the benefits of desmopressin in type 2 vWD, although in general, it is less effective in these subtypes and has been reported to precipitate thrombosis or result in significant thrombocytopenia as a result of in vivo platelet aggregation in type 2B or platelet-type vWD. For these reasons, patients with type 2 vWD are most commonly treated with exogenous normal vWF replacement via a concentrate. Desmopressin is ineffective in type 3 vWD, and treatment is dependent on the use of replacement therapy via concentrate.

There are several products available in the United States that contain intact vWF, including Humate-P (CSL Behring, King of Prussia, PA), Alphanate (Grifols Biologicals, Los Angeles, CA), and Koate DVI (Talecris, Research Triangle Park, NC), with other similar products available in other countries. These concentrates contain vWF and FVIII in varying ratios and with variable amounts of the multimer size or distribution, and all are plasma derived. Both Humate-P and Alphanate are approved by the US Food and Drug Administration (FDA) for the treatment of vWD. Although these products are manufactured via processes that include viral attenuation and inactivation steps, have used donors that have been subjected to rigorous testing, and have been proven to be safe from risk of transmission of blood-borne viral infections, the fact that they are all derived from human plasma suggests that they are associated with a theoretical risk of transmission of infectious agents. As with all human plasma products, there also exists a possibility of allergic reactions; however, these have been infrequently reported with these products. Administration of the first dose in a hospital or clinic setting may be considered.

Antifibrinolytic agents are useful adjunctive therapies and are used in a similar fashion as previously described for platelet defects. Conjugated estrogens and oral contraceptive agents are effective therapies for management of menorrhagia, and topical measures are also useful in some bleeding situations. Case reports exist in the literature regarding the use of rFVIIa in vWD; these are limited to patients with type 3 disease with inhibitors to vWF. The benefits and risks of these agents are identical to those previously described in the section on platelet function disorders.

Management of bleeding in AvWS is similar to congenital vWD. However, treatment of the underlying disorder leading to AvWS often resolves the defect.

Gaps in knowledge

The most challenging aspect in the management of vWD is establishing an accurate diagnosis; this can be especially difficult because vWF levels may appear normal due to associated clinical circumstances despite a clinical history suggestive for this disorder. Recently published data used a Bayesian analysis of laboratory data and personal and family history to help predict the probability of diagnosis of vWD. Future research aimed at development of laboratory assays with improved performance characteristics to decrease these diagnostic dilemmas is needed. It is clear that there exists a wide variation in bleeding symptoms among patients with the same disease subtype, which is likely due to genetic modifiers of the bleeding phenotype. Although currently available therapies overall are effective, it is not completely clear under what circumstances specific therapies are best applied to achieve an optimal outcome. There are few prospective comparative therapy studies to guide physicians in determination of the risks and benefits of available therapies; recently published treatment guidelines published by the National Heart, Lung, and Blood Institute are based on the best available evidence and expert opinion.

Key points

1. vWD is the most common inherited bleeding disorder in the general population.
2. vWD is divided into several subtypes, with type 1 representing a partial quantitative deficiency, the most common.
3. Laboratory diagnosis of vWD may be difficult, especially in type 1.
4. The treatment of vWD is based on the subtype; the most common agents used for treatment include desmopressin, antifibrinolytics, hormonal therapy for menorrhagia, and vWF concentrates for severe bleeding or types 2 and 3.

Disorders of secondary hemostasis

Hemophilia A and B (FVIII and FIX deficiency)
Pathophysiology

The physiology of hemostasis previously reviewed reveals the critical roles played by FVIII and FIX in thrombin generation and ultimately normal fibrin clot formation. The absence or decreased amounts of either FVIII or FIX results in reduced thrombin generation on the surface of activated platelets at injured sites. Inadequate thrombin generation results in a clot with poor structural integrity visualized with electron microscopy; formation of large, coarse fibrin strands as opposed to the normal thinner strands forming a tight network are observed. In addition, reduced thrombin generation results in decreased generation of activated FXIII required for cross-linking of fibrin monomers and decreased TAFI generation, both of which result in a clot less resistant to normal lysis. Therefore, deficiencies of FVIII or FIX result in poorly formed clots that are more susceptible to normal fibrinolysis, which are clinically observed as the bleeding manifestations of hemophilia.

Etiology

Congenital deficiencies of FVIII and FIX occur as a result of genetic mutations on the X chromosome. These deficiencies are observed commonly in males due to their hemizygous state. Heterozygous females may have factor levels observed in the mild hemophilia range as a result of nonrandom X chromosome inactivation. In the past, these women were called symptomatic carriers; they are now more appropriately classified as having mild hemophilia. In addition, females may rarely have levels in the severe or moderate deficiency range due to skewed lyonization or presence of other genetic abnormalities such as Turner syndrome.

There is a wide range of mutations that result in hemophilia, and the mutation type (deletion, inversion, missense, or nonsense) and specific area of the protein affected determine the severity of hemophilia. In approximately 25% of cases, no family history is identified. In such cases, either the disorder was carried silently in females or the pedigree represents a new mutation arising in either the patient's or, more often, the mother's or maternal grandfather's germ cells as demonstrated for a particular FVIII mutation known as the intron 22 inversion.

Rarely, hemophilia can be acquired, due to development of autoantibodies most commonly directed against FVIII. This condition, also known as acquired hemophilia, has been associated with pregnancy, malignancies, and the elderly. In approximately 50% of cases of acquired hemophilia, no known associated disorder can be identified.

These autoantibodies inhibit the functional capability of endogenous FVIII resulting in bleeding symptoms. Although some bleeding symptoms are similar to congenital hemophilia, the incidence of hemarthroses in acquired hemophilia is small, whereas soft tissue, abdominal, and retroperitoneal hemorrhages are more frequent.

Clinical presentation

The clinical presentation of congenital hemophilia is highly variable and is correlated with the level of deficiency. In infants born to known female carriers, the diagnosis can be made shortly after birth by assaying FVIII or FIX from umbilical cord blood. Prenatal testing is also available if the genetic defect has been identified within the family; if the knowledge gained through prenatal testing would not alter the course of pregnancy or the planned mode of delivery, then it is not required. The presentation of symptoms that lead to a diagnosis in patients either without a family history or not tested at birth is quite variable and is dependent on the severity of disease.

Severe hemophilia, defined as a factor activity level <1%, may present in the newborn period with intra- or extracranial bleeding; prolonged bleeding from venipuncture, from heel stick, or after circumcision; or excessive bruising. Infants with severe hemophilia who do not develop symptoms in the newborn period often present during the first year of life with bruising, muscle hematoma with immunization, or bleeding in the joint or muscle due to activity or intercurrent injury. Although the precise prevalence of intracranial hemorrhage is not known, it is likely approximately 1% to 3%.

Moderate hemophilia (factor activity levels between 1% and <5%) has a variable age of presentation; diagnosis may be established due to a known family history, in the newborn period due to bleeding, or later in life, even as an adult, with a bleeding event often associated with intercurrent injury or a procedure. Bleeding symptoms include deep tissue, muscle, or joint bleeding; mucocutaneous bleeding is a common presentation due to the increased fibrinolysis in oropharynx and the inability to form a stable clot.

Mild hemophilia (factor activity levels ≥5%-40%) may be diagnosed at ages similar to moderate hemophilia. For patients without a documented family history, the age of presentation is highly variable; excessive bleeding is always associated with nonincidental injury or surgery. Patients with mild hemophilia typically present later in childhood or during the teenage/adult years.

Joint disease, or hemophilic arthropathy, remains a major morbidity. Although preventive therapy is effective (see Treatment section for details), patients may occasionally present with recurrent hemarthrosis ultimately leading to joint disease. It is not uncommon for patients who have not received optimal treatment, such as those who emigrated from developing nations, to present with hemophilic arthropathy.

Acquired hemophilia usually presents with often dramatic onset of either mucocutaneous or internal bleeding; approximately 50% of patients will have a known associated condition such as pregnancy, autoimmune disorder, or malignancy. Hemarthroses are uncommon in this disorder, and life-threatening bleeding with associated significant morbidity and mortality are observed.

Diagnosis

The laboratory diagnosis of hemophilia begins with screening coagulation studies including PT and aPTT; the aPTT is almost always abnormal, yet it is important to be aware of the instances in which the aPTT may be normal, especially in mild deficiencies (Figure 8-4). After identification of a prolonged aPTT, a mixing study with normal plasma is performed. Correction of the prolongation points to a factor deficiency, and therefore, specific factor analyses are performed including FVIII and FIX. The type and level of severity of the hemophilia are thereby established. As previously discussed, appropriate specimen procurement and handling are critical to obtain accurate results. In newborns where cord blood is tested due to a family history, levels may be altered based on sample procurement or level of deficiency. Therefore, repeat testing may be required based on the results of cord blood testing and the concordance with expected results. In addition, assaying factor activity levels at the lowest range of the curve is technically difficult, and sample analysis at a reference laboratory may help differentiate severe from moderate hemophilia. Finally, because FVIII is an acute-phase reactant, obtaining a true baseline may be difficult in patients with moderate or mild deficiencies based on their clinical circumstances. In addition, mild FIX deficiency may be associated with a normal aPTT in some laboratories or circumstances; therefore, if a clinical suspicion for a bleeding

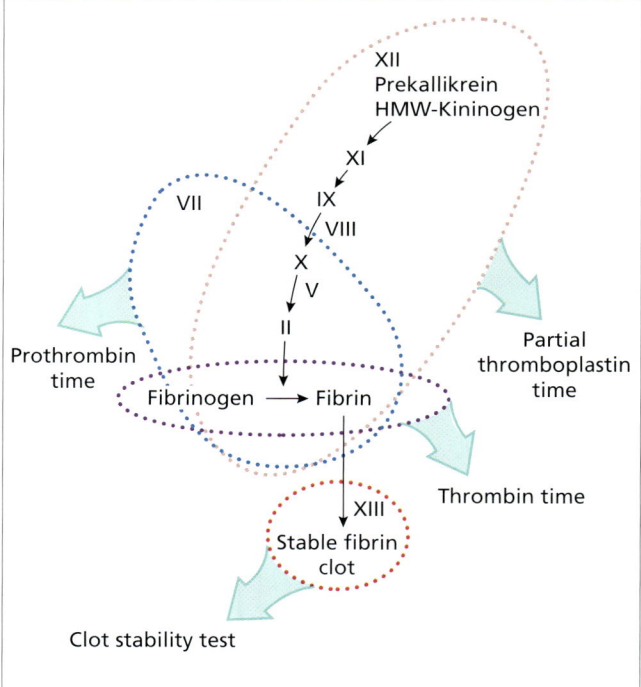

Figure 8-4 Plasma coagulation reactions in in vitro laboratory assays. Note the differences between this diagram and Figure 8-1. Factor XII, prekallikrein, and high molecular weight kininogen are required for a normal partial thromboplastin time but not for normal in vivo hemostasis. Also, plasma factor XI may not always be required for normal in vivo hemostasis. Platelets and tissue factor are required for normal in vivo hemostasis but are supplied by exogenous reagents in the laboratory assays. This diagram outlines the coagulation factors required for each of 4 basic tests.

disorder exists, an FIX activity level should be obtained despite the normal screening test.

Treatment

The mainstay of hemophilia treatment is replacement of the deficient coagulation factor. There are a number of commercially available factor concentrates to treat both FVIII and FIX deficiency (Tables 8-2 and 8-3). The choice of the specific product used includes consideration of availability, cost, method of manufacture, and so on; both recombinant and plasma-derived products are available, and decisions of product used should be made in consultation with the patient and family. Typically, 1 IU/kg of FVIII will increase the FVIII level by 2%; doses can be repeated as needed approximately every 8 to 12 hours. With FIX, dosing depends on the product used—plasma-derived FIX (pdFIX) or recombinant FIX (rFIX). With pdFIX, 1 IU/kg increases the FIX level by 1%, whereas with rFIX, the level increases by 0.6% to 0.8%, with children exhibiting a lower recovery compared with adults. FIX doses can be repeated every 12 to 24 hours as needed.

Treatment approaches are divided into 2 main categories: prophylaxis and on-demand. Prophylaxis is the regular infusion of factor replacement to prevent or suppress bleeding events. Primary prophylaxis is the initiation of replacement therapy prior to or shortly after the first hemarthrosis and has been proven to be the most effective approach to prevent the development of joint disease. Therefore, primary prophylaxis should be considered the optimal therapy for severe hemophilia; however, when it should be instituted and when or if it should be stopped remain controversial. In Sweden, where prophylaxis was pioneered, therapy is initiated prior to the first joint bleed commonly between 9 and 12 months of age. In the United States, a common approach is to wait until 1 or 2 hemarthroses have occurred because some patients even with severe hemophilia may not experience a hemarthrosis until several years of age, thereby limiting invasive therapy until required. Prophylaxis is time and resource intensive and requires adequate venous access often necessitating a central venous catheter; therefore, there may be benefit to institution of therapy after hemarthrosis has occurred to demonstrate its necessity. The negative effect of this approach is that even one significant hemarthrosis may result in joint damage; in addition, this approach allows subclinical bleeding, a potential although as yet not well-defined contributor to joint disease. Once primary prophylaxis has been instituted, it should be continued throughout childhood. The topic of continued prophylaxis into adulthood is an ongoing area of research.

Secondary prophylaxis is the regular infusion of replacement therapy as described earlier but after the onset of significant hemarthroses or joint disease to interrupt a bleeding

Table 8-2 Factor VIII concentrates currently available in the United States.

Brand name	Generation	Plasma derived (Pd) or recombinant (R)	Presence of human proteins	Stability at room temperature
Monoclate	NA	Pd	FVIII (and others)	No
Hemophil M	NA	Pd	FVIII (and others)	No
Recombinate	1st	R	Albumin	No
Kogenate FS	2nd	R	Albumin in processing but not final product	Yes (for 3 months)
Helixate FS	2nd	R	Albumin in processing but not final product	Yes (for 3 months)
Advate	3rd	R	None	Yes (for 6 months)
Xyntha	3rd	R	None	Yes (for 6 months)

There are other FVIII concentrates approved for use in FVIII deficiency, all of which contain vWF as well as FVIII; however, these are not in general use for FVIII deficiency.
NA = not applicable.

Table 8-3 FIX concentrates currently available in the United States.

Brand	Plasma derived (Pd) or recombinant (R)	Presence of human proteins	Stability at room temperature
Mononine	Pd	FIX and others	No
Alphanine	Pd	FIX and others	No
Benefix	R	None	Yes (for 6 months)

The prothrombin complex concentrates were the original FIX concentrates and are still licensed for use in FIX deficiency; however, these products are no longer used in the management of this condition, although they are used to manage rare factor deficiencies (see section on rare factor deficiencies in text).

pattern or prevent further joint damage through suppression of bleeding episodes. Joints with repeated bleeding develop acute and/or chronic synovitis, followed by articular damage; the process of repeated bleeding in a joint is termed target joint. The bleeding pattern in target joints has been documented to be amenable to secondary prophylaxis. Prophylaxis may also be administered for specific patients in circumstances that require adequate hemostatic coverage such as in an adolescent prior to sports. There are other situations where limited prophylactic therapy is reasonable and is reviewed in cited references.

Although primary prophylaxis is used most frequently in patients with severe disease, there are individuals with moderate deficient hemophilia who require this therapy due to their bleeding pattern. Secondary prophylaxis and limited prophylaxis are used in all severities of hemophilia based on circumstances that warrant adequate coverage. Issues related to prophylaxis include adherence, cost, and the need for adequate venous access; prophylaxis and the associated issues have been reviewed. Several prophylactic and general treatment dosing approaches exist and are detailed in Table 8-4. It should be noted that although prophylaxis is very effective in the prevention of the majority of spontaneous bleeding events, patients who experience breakthrough bleeding episodes require immediate treatment according to the recommendations in Table 8-4.

Episodic treatment for bleeding episodes is referred to as on-demand therapy (ie, the use of factor replacement therapy only after bleeding occurs). This treatment approach does not require regular infusions and their associated issues and is less expensive in the short run, but it is ineffective in prevention of joint disease. This mode of therapy is now primarily used for patients with moderate and mild deficient hemophilia because these patients bleed infrequently and the subsequent risk of joint disease is low. On-demand therapy may be used by adults with severe disease who either experience fatigue with prophylaxis or who feel it is not required. The typical dosing for on-demand bleeds can be found in Table 8-4.

Infusion therapy for hemophilia, regardless of the regimen used, is best delivered in the home setting to allow prophylaxis and/or prompt therapy. Family members and patients are trained to administer the factor concentrate at home without need for a medical facility.

Adjunctive therapy for hemophilia is similar to that previously discussed for platelet defects and vWD. Patients with mild FVIII deficiency may be treated with desmopressin after a challenge dose demonstrates an adequate response with an increase in factor levels to hemostatic levels; the level of the response dictates the type of bleeding events that may be treated with this agent. Antifibrinolytic agents are efficacious for mucosal bleeding and are commonly used in conjunction with factor concentrate or desmopressin. For women with hemophilia with menorrhagia, hormonal suppressive therapy previously discussed can be used.

A significant complication of hemophilia after exposure to replacement therapy is development of neutralizing antibodies termed inhibitors. Inhibitors render standard treatment with replacement therapy ineffective and result in hemorrhagic episodes that are prolonged and more difficult to control, resulting in increased risk of morbidity and mortality. The incidence of inhibitors is between 20% and 35% in severe, previously untreated, FVIII-deficient patients and <5% in severe FIX-deficient patients, whereas present inhibitor prevalence is approximately 10% in FVIII deficiency and 3% to 5% in FIX deficiency. Risk factors for inhibitor development include both patient- and environmental-related issues. Among the patient-specific risk factors, the most important is hemophilia severity, with patients with severe disease at highest risk; the specific genetic mutation, ethnicity, and family history of inhibitors have also been shown to impact expression of this complication. Mutations resulting in major disruptions of the gene such as large deletions are associated with increased risk. In addition, patients of African or Hispanic ethnicity have significantly higher rate of inhibitor development. Environmentally related risk factors have been purported to include the source of the factor

Table 8-4 Typical dosing for FVIII and FIX deficiency in different situations.*

Factor	Joint/muscle	Life or limb threatening	Preoperative	Prophylactic
FVIII	25 U/kg (repeat as needed)	50 U/kg (multiple repeated doses required)	50 U/kg	25–40 U/kg 3 times per week or every other day
pdFIX	50 U/kg (repeat as needed)	100 U/kg (multiple repeated doses required)	100 U/kg	50 U/kg twice a week
rFIX	60–70 U/kg (repeat as needed)	120–140 U/kg (multiple repeated doses required)	120–140 U/kg	60–70 U/kg twice a week

*These are general dose recommendations (practice may vary). Due to differences in posttranslational modifications, rFIX doses are approximately 1.2 times higher in adults to 1.4 times higher in children. The duration of therapy for intracranial hemorrhage varies but is at least 2 weeks and in children should prompt consideration for ongoing prophylactic therapy. Prophylaxis regimens vary. These doses are those typically found in the Swedish regimens.

product used (plasma derived vs recombinant); these data remain controversial. A recent systematic review suggests that the rate of inhibitor formation in severe FVIII deficiency is 2-fold higher in patients who received recombinant FVIII versus those who received plasma-derived FVIII. A prospective study is under way to confirm or refute this finding.

Inhibitors are divided into 2 categories: low-titer, low-responding inhibitors and high-titer, high-responding inhibitors. A low-responding inhibitor is characterized as one with a titer, measured in the Bethesda assay, of <5 Bethesda units (BU) despite repeated exposure/stimulation, whereas high-responding inhibitors are those that achieve a titer >5 BU at any time regardless of present titer. Patients with high-responding inhibitors may have a decrease in titer with withdrawal of the stimulation (exposure to the factor for which they are deficient) and may even achieve an undetectable inhibitor level. Despite this, with reexposure, these patients mount a memory response and will demonstrate an increase in inhibitor titer in 7 to 10 days after exposure. Stimulation and increase of inhibitor titer is termed anamnesis. High-responding patients who achieve an undetectable inhibitor titer have not had the inhibitor response ablated and should not be rechallenged unless experiencing life- or limb-threatening bleeding episodes.

Patients with low-responding inhibitors are commonly managed with higher doses of replacement therapy calculated to overcome the inhibitor titer and achieve a hemostatic level; required doses to achieve this are higher than standard doses. A few patients have low-titer inhibitors that resolve without intervention often within a few weeks and are termed transient inhibitors; therefore, ongoing measurement of titers is important to document persistence and for dose calculation. Patients with high-responding inhibitors are not able to achieve a hemostatic level with standard replacement therapy and thus are treated with alternative hemostatic products termed *bypassing agents*.

The 3 important strategies for management of patients with high-responding inhibitors include: (i) management of bleeding episodes, (ii) prevention of bleeding, and (iii) eradication of the inhibitor. Inhibitor eradication, also called *immune tolerance induction* (ITI), requires routine administration of the deficient factor to reset/tolerize the immune system. An international prospective ITI study in good-risk patients has been recently completed, although results are not yet published. This study compared daily high-dose FVIII (200 IU/kg/d) to lower dose FVIII (50 IU/kg/d) 3 times weekly. Typical ITI regimens may include either of these infusion schedules or a regimen of 100 IU/kg given once daily. Retrospective registries have identified several factors impacting ITI success, including the peak inhibitor titer, titer at start of therapy (<10 BU associated with improved outcome), age at initiation, and time from inhibitor development to ITI start. It is best to initiate ITI when the titer is <10 BU, although this must be balanced against the risk of waiting too long. Inhibitor development in FIX deficiency is far less common and has associated unusual complications. Patients with FIX deficiency may develop anaphylactoid reactions to infused FIX concentrate prior to or at the time of inhibitor emergence. For such patients, ITI may not be possible or, if undertaken, requires desensitization to FIX. FIX-deficient patients with inhibitors undergoing ITI are at risk for developing nephrotic syndrome. ITI-associated nephrosis is more likely to occur in patients with a history of an anaphylactoid reaction. The etiology of nephrosis in these patients is unclear, although it is thought to be related to immune complex formation. The overall success rate of ITI in FIX deficiency is 35%, far lower than the 75% achieved in FVIII deficiency. Thus, although fewer FIX inhibitor patients exist, they represent significant treatment challenges.

The management of bleeding episodes in inhibitor patients is challenging, with the majority of hemophilia-related morbidity in the United States occurring in patients with high-responding inhibitors. Bypassing agents are used to treat bleeding episodes in patients with high-responding inhibitors but do not lead to hemostasis as replacement therapy in non-inhibitor patients. There are 2 bypassing agents available for the management of bleeding in inhibitor patients, activated prothrombin complex concentrate (APCC; FEIBA, Baxter, Westlake Village, CA) and rFVIIa (NovoSeven, Novo Nordisk, Bagsvaerd, Denmark). APCC is a plasma-derived concentrate consisting of the vitamin K–dependent clotting factors both in nonactivated and activated forms. The mechanism of action of APCC is largely ascribed to the presence and action of FXa and prothrombin, although FIXa and FVIIa are also contained; small quantities of nonactivated FVIII may be present. rFVIIa contains FVIIa as its sole agent and is genetically engineered. The mechanism of action of rFVIIa is through thrombin generation on the surface of activated platelets through tissue factor–dependent and –independent mechanisms. Both APCC and rFVIIa have been demonstrated to be safe and effective, with variable response rates ranging between 70% and 90%. Two prospective studies compared these products and revealed essentially similar response rates. Both products have considerable data supporting their safety (>30 years for APCC and 10 years for rFVIIa) with few reported thrombotic events in hemophilic inhibitor patients. In addition, APCC as a plasma-derived product has an excellent safety record without documented viral transmission.

The most important consideration when choosing a product in an inhibitor patient is its ability to achieve rapid bleed control and thereby limit morbidity and mortality. Thus product choice is individualized. Note that because APCC is an FIX-based product, its use in FIX inhibitor patients with infusion-associated reactions is contraindicated. Another consideration is that rFVIIa does not stimulate either the FVIII or FIX inhibitor titer and may be preferred if trying to allow the inhibitor to reach a low level prior to starting ITI. APCC may contain small quantities of FVIII and result in continued stimulation of the inhibitor titer in FVIII-deficient patients. Management of acute bleeding is critical; therefore, inhibitor stimulation is not an absolute contraindication to APCC use during this time if any bleeding episode is unresponsive to rFVIIa. Dosing regimens for both products have been established (Table 8-5). Occasionally, patients present with bleeding events refractory to both agents. In such cases, the use of combination APCC and rFVIIa has been reported using an alternative sequential regimen. Although the approach has been demonstrated to be effective and safe in a small number of young children, the reports remain anecdotal. Historically, prevention of bleeding in inhibitor patients was confined to prevention of bleeding during invasive procedures. Due to obvious concern for control of hemostasis during surgery and postoperatively with bypassing agents and concern for thrombotic events with repeated use in a high-risk setting, inhibitor patients were not offered surgery until fairly recently. Few studies demonstrating successful hemostatic strategies for inhibitor patients in the surgical setting have been performed. Over the past decade, several prospective studies have demonstrated the successful use of rFVIIa for both minor and major surgery (see Table 8-5 for dosing recommendations). This has led to an increased availability of required surgical procedures in inhibitor patients, most notably orthopedic procedures for amelioration of hemophilic arthropathy. APCCs have also been used in the surgical setting, but the body of reports supporting their use, dosing, and safety is smaller compared with rFVIIa.

Recently, prophylaxis with bypassing agents to prevent bleeding episodes in inhibitor patients has gained attention as a potentially feasible approach. Several case reports of rFVIIa used prophylactically led to the performance of a prospective study that demonstrated an approximately 50% reduction in bleeding episodes during prophylaxis in patients with a high frequency of bleeding. There are a number of case series and one review (Shapiro et al, 1998) demonstrating the use of APCC for prophylaxis with mixed results; a prospective study is under way. Currently, there are several new agents in development with potential improved hemostatic properties and longer half-lives that may improve overall treatment of inhibitor patients and make prophylaxis more effective and feasible in the future.

The management of bleeding episodes in acquired hemophilia is similar in many respects to that of congenital hemophilia with inhibitors, and the principles outlined earlier largely apply. An exception of note is that patients with acquired hemophilia are often elderly and at increased risk for thrombosis; thus, bypassing agents, although often required for control of bleeding, may have an associated higher rate of thrombotic complications. Inhibitor eradication in acquired hemophilia is quite different than in congenital hemophilia complicated by inhibitors. Because acquired hemophilia is due to development of autoantibodies that result from loss of self-tolerance, they tend to respond to immunosuppressive medications effective in autoimmune disorders in general. Although these patients are too few to allow for well-designed prospective studies, a number of reports have demonstrated the effectiveness of glucocorticoids, cyclophosphamide, and more recently rituximab, with order of use as listed respectively. Although ITI has been reported in acquired hemophilia, it is more cumbersome than immunosuppression alone and is usually not required.

Prognosis and outcomes

Currently, patients with severe hemophilia without inhibitors treated on a prophylactic regimen have an excellent prognosis and lead near-normal lives without hemophilic arthropathy. These outcomes are substantiated by the Swedish cohort followed for nearly 40 years. For patients with inhibitors, the outcome is more variable, and risk of

Table 8-5 Typical dosing for the currently available bypassing agents.

Agent	Joint/muscle	Life or limb threatening	Preoperative	Prophylactic
APCC*	50–75 U/kg (repeat every 8–12 hours as needed)	75–100 U/kg (repeat every 12 hours)	50–75 U/kg	75 U/kg 3 times per week
rFVIIa (low dose)[†]	90–120 μg/kg (repeat every 2–3 hours as needed)	90–120 μg/kg (repeat every 2-3 hours)	90–120 μg/kg	90 μg/kg/d
rFVIIa (high dose)	270 μg/kg (no data available on follow up doses)	270 μg/kg (no data available on follow up doses)	No data	270 μg/kg/d

*Doses >200 U/kg/d are contraindicated per the prescribing information. APCC is only licensed for the treatment of bleeding and not for surgery or prophylaxis.
[†]The licensed dose for rFVIIa in the United States is 90–120 μg/kg, and it is licensed for treatment of bleeding and prevention of bleeding during surgery. It is not approved for prophylaxis.

morbidity is significant. When ITI is successful, the outcome can be converted to that of a noninhibitor patient, yet the morbidity experienced is dependent on the amount of joint disease that occurred prior to ITI success. It is likely that many of these patients will have experienced hemarthroses or muscle or even intracranial hemorrhage and that some will have permanent deficits. For inhibitor patients in whom ITI was not successful or not performed, significant musculoskeletal morbidity is common, resulting in permanent disability and poor quality of life. With improved hemostatic coverage available for surgical interventions, even hemophilic patients with inhibitors may now undergo procedures to reduce pain and increase functionality. Combined with the increased use of prophylaxis, it is possible now to develop treatment strategies to ameliorate the consequences of recurrent bleeding and allow patients to lead more productive lives.

Gaps in knowledge

The greatest challenge with the potential for significant reward lies with gene therapy, a potentially curative approach. Development of improved therapeutic approaches for inhibitor patients who still experience increased morbidity and mortality compared with noninhibitor patients are required. One approach deserving of future work is the prevention of inhibitor formation. An improved understanding of the immunologic pathway involved in inhibitor formation and development of tolerance would open avenues to prevent inhibitor development or increase the rate of tolerance achieved. It is conceivable that an approach could be developed to program the immune system to induce tolerance prior to or in association with exposure to exogenous normal factor concentrate. Future research efforts could also lead to development of replacement products that are less or perhaps not immunogenic. In inhibitor patients, methods to perform ITI in FIX deficiency lag behind those for FVIII deficiency. For patients with anaphylactoid reactions, options for desensitization and subsequent ITI are limited, with an overall outcome that is poor, although rare success has been reported. The FIX-deficient inhibitor population with anaphylactoid reactions represents a small vulnerable population with only 1 therapeutic agent presently available for the management of bleeding episodes; new approaches and treatments are clearly required.

Rare factor deficiencies
Pathophysiology

Deficiencies of other coagulation factors that play a role in thrombin generation, cross-linking, and stabilization of the fibrin clot or down-regulation of fibrinolysis may lead to a bleeding diathesis. Deficiencies of fibrinogen, factor II (FII), FV, FVII, FX, and FXIII result in bleeding disorders where the severity of the bleeding is related to the factor levels, with the exception of FXI deficiency, where even patients with severe deficiencies may exhibit a variable bleeding tendency. Although FVIII and FIX deficiency are defined as rare disorders affecting <200,000 Americans, deficiencies of these other coagulation factors are even less common. Therefore, the clinical presentation related to any specific level and the range of symptoms experienced are less well described than in hemophilia A and B. For detailed discussion of these disorders, the reader is referred to a special issue of the journal *Hemophilia* (Volume 14, Issue 6, November 2008).

Etiology

As with hemophilia, rare factor deficiencies can result from a genetic defect or can be due to an acquired condition. The genes for these coagulation factors are located on somatic chromosomes and are inherited as autosomal recessive conditions with males and females equally affected. Affected individuals may be compound heterozygotes or have a homozygous defect; the resultant coagulation factor activity level and associated phenotypic symptoms are related to the genetic mutations. Because the number of genetic mutations causing each of these rare disorders may be large, the ability to predict a level or phenotypic presentation may be difficult.

Key points

1. Hemophilia is an X-linked disorder due to deficiencies of FVIII or FIX and is categorized as mild, moderate, and severe depending on the factor level.
2. Patients with severe hemophilia are at risk of developing joint disease termed *hemophilic arthropathy* that can be prevented by regular factor infusions (prophylaxis).
3. Factor replacement therapy is available to treat bleeding episodes and is highly effective.
4. Patients with hemophilia, most notably those with severe disease, may develop neutralizing antibodies directed against the deficient/replaced factor termed *inhibitors*; inhibitors are divided into high- and low-responding types, and the presence of inhibitors may render standard substitutive therapy ineffective.
5. Inhibitors can be eradicated through treatment regimens termed *ITI*.
6. Patients with high-responding inhibitors are treated with bypassing agents to manage their bleeding episodes; bypassing products overall are not as effective as factor replacement in noninhibitor patients, and as such, inhibitor patients have an increased risk of hemorrhage-associated morbidity and mortality.

Acquired factor deficiencies may be associated with a wide range of conditions including commonly encountered liver dysfunction and uncommon conditions such as acquired FV deficiency due to thrombin exposure. Acquired disorders may also result in multiple-factor deficiencies, as seen in liver dysfunction and vitamin K deficiency, or in single-factor deficiencies, as in amyloid-associated FX deficiency.

Each acquired clotting factor deficiency may result from a wide range of disorders, and it is beyond the scope of this chapter to review all conditions that may result in any specific coagulation disorder. The more frequently encountered disorders and associated coagulation deficiencies will be highlighted. Hypofibrinogenemia can result from liver disease, use of chemotherapeutic agents such as L-asparaginase, and the Kasabach-Merritt syndrome (hemangioma with consumptive coagulopathy). Other consumptive processes such as disseminated intravascular coagulation lead to multiple coagulation factor deficiencies. FII, FVII, FIX, and FX are vitamin K dependent and synthesized in the liver and thus become abnormal in liver failure, in vitamin K deficiency, and with the use of vitamin K antagonists. A deficiency of FII due to specific factor antibody has been observed as part of the antiphospholipid syndrome; FX deficiency may occur with amyloidosis due to adsorption of the clotting factor onto the abnormal accumulated amyloid. A deficiency of FV may occur due to cross-reacting antibody development after exposure to topical thrombin or use of antimicrobials such as cephalosporins. Acquired specific coagulation factor autoantibodies have been reported for the other coagulation factors outside of FVIII, but these are exceedingly rare.

Two genetic multiple-factor deficiencies occur including combined FV and FVIII and combined vitamin K–dependent coagulation factor deficiency. Combined FV and FVIII deficiency results from mutations in the gene that codes for a protein (endoplasmic reticulum Golgi intermediate compartment [ERGIC]-53) required for assembly and secretion of these 2 similarly structured proteins. The combined vitamin K coagulation factor deficiency is due to a number of mutations in enzymes involved in the vitamin K pathway. Both conditions are very rare and have been reported in consanguineous families or individuals from closed small genetic groups. These combined coagulation factor deficiency states are commonly associated with moderate to severe deficiencies and variable bleeding symptoms.

Clinical presentation

The clinical presentation of the congenital rare factor deficiencies is variable and depends on the specific clotting factor and level of deficiency. These deficiency states may be discovered as a result of a known family history, although this is less common in autosomal recessive disorders unless a sibling has been identified. More commonly, affected individuals present with excessive bleeding ranging from mild mucocutaneous bleeding to catastrophic intracranial hemorrhage. Unique features for each factor deficiency can be found in Table 8-6. Age at presentation is variable and most often is related to the level of deficiency, with severe disorders presenting in childhood, as well as hemostatic challenges that are encountered. Patients with severe FXIII deficiency may present in the newborn period with significant umbilical stump hemorrhage, whereas patients with severe FXI deficiency may present as adults either due to an abnormal aPTT obtained prior to a planned procedure or due to bleeding associated with trauma or major surgery.

Acquired rare factor deficiencies present in the context of selected disorders as described earlier, although these may not always be apparent during the initial presentation of the bleeding disorder. For example, patients with liver disease–associated coagulopathy often have signs and symptoms of liver dysfunction including jaundice, ascites, and caput medusa, among others. Vitamin K deficiency may be seen in newborns who did not receive vitamin K at birth or those with malabsorption conditions. The resultant bleeding symptoms are similar to those seen in congenital factor deficiencies, although hemorrhagic disease of the newborn is associated with a high rate of intracranial hemorrhage.

Diagnosis

Once suspected, the diagnosis of a rare factor deficiency is dependent on the previously discussed principles of clinical history, physical examination, and an ordered systematic approach to laboratory evaluation. The majority of these deficiencies, when present at a severe or moderate level, result in prolongation of the PT and/or aPTT. Exceptions include deficiencies of FXIII, PAI-1, or α2AP, where the PT and aPTT are normal. The section on fibrinolysis addresses PAI-1 and α2AP deficiency. Based on the results of these screening tests and subsequent mixing studies suggesting a factor deficiency, specific factor assays are performed and may result in the establishment of a diagnosis. If the screening tests are not prolonged but the clinical history is suggestive of a bleeding disorder, then specific factor assays should be performed for both deficiencies that are known to be associated with normal screening tests and for others that, when present at a mild level of severity, may not prolong these tests. FXIII deficiency is diagnosed via a qualitative assay (clot solubility assay) or via a quantitative assay. The clot solubility assay is abnormal when the FXIII level is <5% and therefore may not be sensitive to mild deficiencies; it is not well documented at this time that mild FXIII deficiency results in a bleeding diathesis.

Table 8-6 Bleeding sites/symptoms and factor replacement choices for rare factor deficiencies.

Factor deficiency	Bleeding sites	Other symptoms	Factor replacement	Causes for acquired deficiency
Fibrinogen	No typical sites	Splenic rupture Miscarriage Thrombosis	Fibrinogen concentrate (RiaStap) Cryoprecipitate	Liver disease Asparaginase therapy Disseminated intravascular coagulation
Factor II (Prothrombin)	No typical sites	None	PCC	Vitamin K deficiency Liver disease Vitamin K antagonists Antiphospholipid syndrome
Factor V	No typical sites	None	FFP Platelet transfusion	Exposure to topical bovine thrombin
Factor VII	Intracranial	Thrombosis	rFVIIa	Vitamin K deficiency Liver disease Vitamin K antagonists
Factor X	Intracranial	None	PCC	Vitamin K deficiency Liver disease Vitamin K antagonists Amyloidosis
Factor XI	Postoperative or trauma related	None	FFP (FXI concentrates are available in some countries)	Autoantibodies (rare)
Factor XIII	Intracranial Umbilical stump	Poor wound healing Miscarriage	Cryoprecipitate pdFXIII concentrate is available in the United States as part of a clinical trial	Cardiopulmonary bypass Inflammatory bowel disease

RiaStap (fibrinogen concentrate) is only licensed for congenital afibrinogenemia. Recombinant factor VIIa is licensed for the treatment of congenital FVII deficiency. Prothrombin complex concentrates (PCC) are not licensed for the treatment of rare factor deficiencies and contain variable amounts of factors II, VII, and X (the amounts are in the prescribing information). Dosing is based on FIX units.
FFP = fresh frozen plasma.

If suspicion exists that the deficiency is due to an autoantibody, mixing studies will reveal the presence of a time- and/or temperature-dependent inhibitor; if a specific factor inhibitor is subsequently identified, then the coagulation factor against which the inhibitor is directed is identified.

Treatment

For patients with congenital factor deficiencies, the mainstay of therapy is replacement of the deficient coagulation factor either after bleeding occurs or as prophylactic therapy, as previously described for severe hemophilia. Table 8-6 lists presently available therapies for factor replacement in the United States. For the majority of patients with rare disorders, the standard therapy remains treatment when bleeding occurs or prior to procedures or interventions. There are important exceptions to this approach; because severe deficiencies of FX and FXIII frequently result in catastrophic intracranial hemorrhage, these patients receive lifelong prophylaxis. For FX deficiency, this is accomplished through twice-weekly infusions of a prothrombin complex concentrate, whereas for FXIII, this is accomplished via monthly infusions of cryoprecipitate or through a plasma-derived FXIII concentrate available in the United States to patients through an ongoing clinical trial; a recombinant FXIII is in a phase III clinical trial. Severe FVII deficiency may also be associated with intracranial hemorrhage, although this is less consistent than in either FXIII or FX deficiencies; therefore, prophylactic treatment should be considered based on patient and family history.

The approach to management of acquired rare factor deficiencies is 2 pronged and includes both treatment of bleeding and treatment of the associated condition if present. Treatment may be as relatively simple as administration of vitamin K in vitamin K deficiency, or it can be complicated as in some cases of liver failure. For patients in whom an associated condition is not identifiable or when present its treatment is not feasible, the goal of therapy is aimed at intervention for bleeding episodes through either nonspecific therapies, such as fresh frozen plasma, or use of specific factor concentrates as listed in Table 8-6. An individualized approach for each patient's situation and diagnosis is required. Adjuvant therapies including antifibrinolytic and topical agents are used as previously discussed. Desmopressin does not have documented efficacy in these rare deficiencies.

Prognosis and outcomes

Congenital rare factor deficiencies are highly heterogeneous conditions both within and between each disorder. Furthermore, acquired conditions that result in rare factor deficiencies are quite varied; an acquired inhibitor may require specific intervention aimed at ablation or may spontaneously remit as seen with FV antibodies associated with thrombin use, whereas other associated conditions such as liver failure may have significant morbidity and/or mortality. Therefore, prognosis and outcome are very much related to the specific deficiency, its cause, the availability of an adequate replacement product, and the clinical circumstances if bleeding is experienced. In general, mild to moderate congenital rare factor deficiencies often do not result in major sequelae, and the associated bleeding may be manageable. In those with a severe congenital deficiency, particularly if associated with serious bleeding complications, prophylactic therapy may be an effective approach if a replacement product is available; these patients may then experience improved outcomes if permanent sequelae due to bleeding have not yet occurred. For patients with acquired rare factor deficiencies, outcomes may range from excellent to poor. Those who recover from an underlying condition that caused the coagulopathy may have an excellent outcome if a catastrophic bleed has not occurred. For those whose underlying condition is not treatable, prognosis may be poor and often related to consequences of the underlying condition, although bleeding may contribute.

Gaps in knowledge

Large, well-designed prospective studies of congenital rare factor deficiencies are not possible due to the number of affected individuals. Much of current knowledge of these conditions is derived from registry data and small interventional studies. There is a need for both epidemiologic and therapeutic studies in these disorders. Development of international databases is required to establish the natural history and treatment outcomes of these disorders.

A major limitation in some of these conditions is the lack of availability of a specific replacement concentrate for treatment. Presently in the United States, 2 licensed products for rare disorders are available, specifically for afibrinogenemia and FVII deficiency. Globally, and more specifically in the European Union, concentrates also exist for treatment of FXI and FXIII deficiencies. In the United States, off-label use of products continues, including use of prothrombin complex concentrates for deficiencies of FX and FII. In FV and FXI deficiency, fresh frozen plasma remains the mainstay of therapy; in addition, platelet transfusions are sometimes used in FV deficiency because platelets also contain FV. Even when a concentrate is available, its use in these rare disorders is often guided by personal experience or anecdotal reports. For example, determination of appropriate patients for whom prophylaxis is indicated and the appropriate dosing regimen is largely ill defined. Also, the peri- and postoperative care of patients with rare disorders is not founded on evidence-based data. There is a clear and present need for consistent data collection and studies on the clinical management of rare factor deficiencies.

> **Key points**
>
> 1. Rare factor deficiencies occur as a result of congenital mutations and acquired disorders.
> 2. Treatment of an associated underlying acquired disorder may lead to resolution of the acquired deficiency.
> 3. Rare factor deficiencies result in highly variable bleeding symptoms ranging from injury or interventional bleeding (FXI) to severe spontaneous intracranial bleeding (FX and FXIII).
> 4. There are a few specific factor replacement concentrates available for patients with rare factor deficiencies.

Disorders of fibrinolysis

Pathophysiology

The fibrinolytic system is designed to provide orderly clot dissolution. Imbalances in fibrinolysis may lead to excessive fibrinolytic activity through a variety of mechanisms, including increased tPA activity or inadequate inhibition with PAI-1 or α2AP deficiencies, and result in excessive bleeding.

Etiology

Hyperfibrinolysis may result from congenital deficiencies of PAI-1 or α2AP. PAI-1 deficiency is extraordinarily rare, and only in a few cases has the genetic alteration causing this disorder been identified. Defects in α2AP have also been described. Both conditions are inherited as autosomal recessive traits. Additionally, hyperfibrinolysis may occur due to a variety of acquired conditions including liver disease and disseminated intravascular coagulation (DIC); after surgery, particularly cardiac surgery; and some prostatic diseases and cases of acute promyelocytic leukemia. Although these conditions also cause bleeding for other reasons (factor deficiencies due to liver disease, consumption of clotting factors in DIC, and platelet dysfunction in cardiac surgery), the possibility of a contributing hyperfibrinolytic state should be considered as specific therapies are available.

Clinical presentation

The clinical presentation of hyperfibrinolysis is highly variable. Hyperfibrinolytic bleeding may occur in isolation or as a result of a congenital deficiency; most commonly, it occurs as a part of a complex coagulopathy in an acquired disorder. Congenital deficiencies of the fibrinolytic pathway may present with delayed bleeding after injury or intervention and may include mucus membrane, cutaneous, or deep tissue bleeding; however, intracranial hemorrhage has been reported in PAI-1 and α2AP deficiency. Acquired hyperfibrinolysis presents with bleeding in a variety of sites, and in patients with recent surgery, delayed postoperative hemorrhage often occurs at the surgical site.

Diagnosis

Laboratory investigation of the fibrinolytic system is problematic. One screening assay exists, the euglobulin clot lysis time (ELT), that is not currently available in all laboratories, and interpretation of results is not always straightforward. The ELT assesses the capacity of plasma to lyse a clot formed in patient plasma. Under assay conditions, a clot is expected to dissolve within a set period of time, commonly approximately 200 seconds; a shortened ELT suggests hyperfibrinolysis. Several new global hemostatic assays are being evaluated for their ability to more accurately detect hyperfibrinolysis. A currently available global assay is the thromboelastogram and is most commonly used in surgical settings; thromboelastography is a well-established method to assess global hemostasis and can detect hyperfibrinolysis where the use of antifibrinolytic agents may be helpful to control excessive bleeding.

It is possible to measure a few individual components of the fibrinolytic system including α2AP and plasminogen. Although it is possible to measure antigenic levels of PAI-1, the activity assay is problematic because the normal range includes levels of zero, thereby making detection of a dysproteinemic deficiency state impossible. Elevated PAI-1 levels have been associated with atherosclerosis and are not associated with bleeding; PAI-1 levels also exhibit diurnal variation, and any one level may not represent either the highest or lowest physiologic level. A deficiency of α2AP is measurable; however, the correlation of level of deficiency and risk for bleeding is poorly established. It is also possible to measure the fibrinolytic proteins tPA and plasminogen, with a hyperfibrinolytic state expected to result in increased tPA and decreased plasminogen; again, the correlation between specific levels and the degree of hyperfibrinolysis has not been established.

Therefore, laboratory diagnosis of the fibrinolytic system is presently not optimal, requiring the clinician to also rely on clinical suspicion including the presence of delayed bleeding, the clinical context, and at times, response to therapeutic interventions.

Treatment

The treatment of hyperfibrinolytic bleeding is fairly straightforward except when it occurs as a complex coagulopathy when treatment requires careful consideration of thrombotic risk. The control of fibrinolytic bleeding is based on use of antifibrinolytic agents; although several agents are available, 2 are most widely used—EACA and TXA. The mechanism of action of both agents involves competition with negatively charged lysine-rich residues in the kringle domain of plasminogen that render it resistant to activation by tissue or urine plasminogen activators. Thus, these agents are effective in tissues rich in tPA or urine plasminogen activator. Both are available for intravenous and oral administration. Adverse effects and precautions were described previously. When using antifibrinolytic therapy, it is important not to discontinue therapy prematurely due to the risk of delayed bleeding. It is recommended to continue therapy up until the hyperfibrinolysis is felt to have resolved (or possibly on an ongoing basis if a congenital defect is confirmed).

Prognosis and outcomes

Most commonly encountered causes of hyperfibrinolysis are acquired; once the trigger has resolved, the patient's hemostatic system should return to normal, and provided that catastrophic bleeding has not occurred, patients should recover without sequelae. For rare patients with a confirmed congenital disorder, management with antifibrinolytic agents, even as prophylaxis, can minimize or reduce bleeding symptoms. Severe bleeding including intracranial hemorrhage may result in permanent neurologic sequelae.

Gaps in knowledge

The major gap in knowledge in these conditions is the ability to establish an accurate diagnosis; treatment is less difficult than diagnosis. The fibrinolytic pathway remains the most problematic both in terms of diagnosis of a deficiency state and clearly attributable clinical manifestations. Improved and specific laboratory methods are required. A reliable, easily performed, reproducible screening assay would represent an important first step in the diagnosis of these disorders, followed by development of specific factor assays for all components of the fibrinolytic system; levels of deficiency that correlate with clinical bleeding could then be established. An improved understanding of the genetics of congenital fibrinolytic deficiencies and the associated spectrum of clinical manifestations would assist clinicians in the diagnosis of these rare disorders.

Key points

1. Fibrinolytic disorders are the least well-defined hemorrhagic diatheses.
2. Hyperfibrinolytic disorders are most often acquired, although rare congenital defects have been documented.
3. Laboratory diagnosis of fibrinolytic disorders is difficult and not always precise.
4. Treatment of hyperfibrinolytic bleeding is based on the use of antifibrinolytic agents including EACA and TXA.

Bibliography

Almeida AM, Khair K, Hann I, Liesner R. The use of recombinant factor VIIa in children with inherited bleeding disorders. *Br J Haematol*. 2003;121:477–481. *This is a report of the use of rFVIIa in children with congenital bleeding disorders demonstrating positive outcomes in some patients and no response in other patients.*

Astermark J, Donfield SM, Di Michele DM, et al. A randomized comparison of bypassing agents in hemophilia complicated by an inhibitor: the FEIBA NovoSeven Comparative (FENOC) study. *Blood*. 2007;109:546–551. *This was the first study to compare the 2 available bypassing agents currently in use for the management of bleeding in hemophilia patients with inhibitors. Although statistically, equivalence of the 2 products was not demonstrated, the authors concluded that the 2 bypassing agents are equally effective. In addition, this study demonstrated a significant amount of discordance in the responses; that is, some patients responded better to FEIBA, whereas others responded better to rFVIIa.*

Barnett B, Kruse-Jarres R, Leissinger CA. Current management of acquired factor VIII inhibitors. *Curr Opin Hematol*. 2008;15:451–455. *This is a review on the current management of acquired hemophilia.*

Barrowcliffe TW, Cattaneo M, Podda GM, et al. New approaches for measuring coagulation. *Haemophilia*. 2006;12(suppl 3):76–81. *This is an excellent review describing a variety of global hemostatic assays including thrombin generation, thromboelastography, and waveform analysis and the potential clinical applications.*

Bolton-Maggs PH, Chalmers EA, Collins PW, et al. A review of inherited platelet disorders with guidelines for their management on behalf of the UKHCDO. *Br J Haematol*. 2006;135:603–633.

Chitlur M, Warrier I, Rajpurkar M, Lusher JM. Inhibitors in FIX deficiency: a report of the ISTH-SSC international FIX inhibitor registry (1997–2006). *Haemophilia*. 2009;15:1027–1031. *This article updates the data in the largest database of inhibitors in FIX patients.*

Di Michele DM, Hathaway WE. Use of DDAVP in inherited and acquired platelet dysfunction. *Am J Hematol*. 1990;33:39–45. *An early report of DDAVP use for treatment of platelet function defects.*

Di Michele DM, Kroner BL. The North American immune tolerance registry: practices, outcomes, and outcome predictors. *Thromb Haemost*. 2002;87:52–57. *An excellent overall review of immune tolerance for both factor VIII and IX deficiency.*

Di Paola J, Federici AB, Mannucci PM, et al. Low level alpha3beta1 levels in type I von Willebrand disease correlate with impaired platelet function in a high shear stress system. *Blood*. 1999;93:3578–3582. *An early report of genetic modifiers of bleeding in von Willebrand disease.*

Flood VH, Johnson FL, Boshkov LK, et al. Sustained engraftment post bone marrow transplant despite anti-platelet antibodies in Glanzmann thrombasthenia. *Pediatr Blood Cancer*. 2005;45:971–975. *This is a case report on the use of bone marrow transplantation to treat a severe case of Glanzmann thrombasthenia. It should be noted that this is not standard therapy for this condition.*

Franchini M, Lippi G. Acquired von Willebrand syndrome: an update. *Am J Hematol*. 2007;82:368–375. *An excellent review of acquired von Willebrand syndrome.*

Goodeve AC, Peake IR. The molecular basis of hemophilia A; genotype-phenotype relationships and inhibitor development. *Semin Thromb Hemost*. 2003;29:23–30. *An excellent overview of the molecular basis for hemophilia A and inhibitor development.*

Hayward CP, Harrison P, Cattaneo M, Ortel TL, Rao AK. Platelet function analyzer (PFA)-100 closure time in the evaluation of platelet disorders and platelet function. *J Thromb Haemost*. 2006;4:312–319. *This is a report from the Platelet Physiology Subcommittee of the Scientific and Standardization Committee of the International Society on Thrombosis and Haemostasis.*

James P, Lillicrap D. The role of molecular genetics in diagnosing von Willebrand disease. *Semin Thromb Hemost*. 2008;34:502–508. *This is an outstanding overview of the genetics of von Willebrand disease containing very clear and useful figures for identifying the location of the various mutations associated with the different types of von Willebrand disease.*

Kavakli K, Makris M, Zulfikar B, Erhardtsen E, Abrams ZS, Kenet G. Home treatment of haemarthroses using a single dose regimen of recombinant activated factor VII in patients with haemophilia and inhibitors—a multi-centre, randomized, double-blind, cross-over trial. *Thromb Haemost*. 2006;95:600–605. *This is a prospective study randomizing patients to 2 dosing regimens of rFVIIa (same as ter Avest et al [2008]), although this article did not have a FEIBA arm. The results were the same as ter Avest et al (2008) vis-à-vis the comparison of the rFVIIa arms.*

Kitchens CS. To bleed or not to bleed? Is that the question for the PTT? *J Thromb Haemost.* 2005;3:2607–2611. *This is an opinion piece discussing the pros and cons of the PTT.*

Konkle BA, Ebbesen LS, Erhardtsen E, et al. Randomized, prospective clinical trial of recombinant factor VIIa for secondary prophylaxis in hemophilia patients with inhibitors. *J Thromb Haemost.* 2007;5:1904–1913. *This is the first prospective study evaluating any bypassing agent for prophylaxis in inhibitor patients. In this study, patients with a high frequency of bleeding during a preprophylaxis period were randomized to 1 of 2 dosing regimens (270 µg/kg^{-1} and 90 µg/kg^{-1} given once daily). Both arms led to a reduction of bleeding compared with the preprophylaxis period of 50% to 60%.*

Lofqvist T, Nilsson IM, Berntorp E, Pettersson H. Haemophilia prophylaxis in young patients—a long term follow-up. *J Intern Med.* 1997;24:395–400. *This is an update on the initial cohort of patients placed on prophylaxis over 30 years ago describing the effectiveness of this approach at preventing joint disease.*

Macaulay IC, Carr P, Gusnanto A, Ouwehand WH, Fitzgerald D, Watkins NA. Platelet genomics and proteomics in human health and disease. *J Clin Invest.* 2005;115:3370–3377. *A review of platelet genomics and proteomics and the potential clinical applications.*

Manco-Johnson MJ, Abshire TC, Shapiro AD, et al. Prophylaxis versus episodic treatment to prevent joint disease in boys with severe hemophilia. *N Engl J Med.* 2007;357:535–544. *Although prophylaxis had been in wide use by the time this study was published, it is the only randomized study definitively demonstrating the benefits of prophylaxis versus on-demand therapy on joint outcome.*

Mannucci PM. Treatment of von Willebrand's disease. *N Eng J Med.* 2004;351:683–694. *An outstanding review of all aspects of the management of von Willebrand disease including a discussion of desmopressin, antifibrinolytic agents, and replacement therapy.*

Martinowitz U, Livnat T, Zivelin A, Kenet G. Concomitant infusion of low doses of rFVIIa and FEIBA in haemophilia patients with inhibitors. *Haemophilia.* 2009;15:904–10. *This is the first description whereby combination therapy was given simultaneously as opposed to the sequential approach described in Young et al (2008) and Kavakli et al (2006). In this study, lower doses of both bypassing agents given simultaneously demonstrated excellent hemostasis with the clinical results supported by laboratory measurement of thrombin generation.*

McKeown LP, Connaghan G, Wilson O, Hansmann K, Merryman P, Gralnick HR. 1-Desamino-8-arginine-vasopressin corrects the hemostatic defects in type 2B von Willebrand's disease. *Am J Hematol.* 1996;51:158–163. *Although desmopressin is considered contraindicated in patients with type 2B von Willebrand disease, this report describes the successful use in one family.*

Mehta R, Shapiro AD. Plasminogen activator inhibitor type 1 deficiency. *Haemophilia.* 2008;14:1255–1260. *This article reviews this rare bleeding disorder.*

Nichols WL, Hultin MB, James AH, et al. von Willebrand disease (VWD): evidence-based diagnosis and management guidelines. The National Heart, Lung, and Blood Institute (NHLBI) expert panel report (USA). *Haemophilia.* 2008;14:171–232. *This is a comprehensive diagnosis and management guideline that is also available on the NHLBI Web site. There is also a pocket guide (shortened version), which is also available at the NHLBI Web site.*

Nurden P, Nurden AT. Congenital disorders associated with platelet dysfunctions. *Thromb Haemost.* 2008;99:253–263. *An excellent review of congenital platelet disorders.*

O'Connnell KA, Wood JJ, Wise RP, Lozier JN, Braun MM. Thromboembolic adverse events after use of recombinant human coagulation factor VIIa. *JAMA.* 2006;295:293–298. *This is an FDA report discussing the risks for thrombosis in patients receiving off-label use of rFVIIa.*

Owen PS, Golightly LK, MacLaren R, Ferretti KA, Badesch DB. Formulary management of recombinant factor VIIa at an academic medical center. *Ann Pharmacother.* 2008;42:771–776. *This is one center's approach to restricting use of this very expensive and potentially dangerous hemostatic agent.*

Patatanian E, Fugate SE. Hemostatic mouthwashes in anticoagulated patients undergoing dental extraction. *Ann Pharmacother.* 2006;40:2205–2210. *This article discusses the use of tranexamic acid as a topical agent for oral bleeding.*

Pipe SW, Valentino LA. Optimizing outcomes for patients with severe haemophilia A. *Haemophilia.* 2007;13(suppl 4):1–16. *This is an expert panel report discussing the clinical use of prophylaxis in a variety of circumstances including primary, secondary, and limited prophylaxis.*

Poon MC, d'Oiron R. Recombinant activated factor VII (Novoseven) treatment of platelet-related bleeding disorders. International Registry on Recombinant Factor VIIa and Congenital Platelet Disorders Group. *Blood Coag Fibrin.* 2000;11(suppl 1):S55-S68. *This is the first detailed report of the use of rFVIIa in patients with platelet function defects.*

Pruthi RK, Mathew P, Valentino LA, et al. Haemostatic efficacy and safety of bolus and continuous infusion of recombinant factor VIIa are comparable in haemophilia patients with inhibitors undergoing major surgery. Results from an open-label, randomized, multicenter trial *Thromb Haemost.* 2007;98:726–732. *Similar to Shapiro et al (1998), this study demonstrated the efficacy and safety of rFVIIa for surgery in inhibitor patients. This study randomized patients to bolus dosing versus continuous infusion demonstrating no difference between the arms.*

Rodeghiero F, Castaman G, Tosetto A, et al. The discriminant power of bleeding history for the diagnosis of type 1 von Willebrand disease: an international, multicenter study. *J Thromb Haemost.* 2005;3:2619–2626. *The first application of a standardized bleeding score for discriminating patients with and without von Willebrand disease.*

Santagostino E, Mancuso ME, Rocino A, Mancuso G, Scaraggi F, Mannucci PM. A prospective randomized trial of high and standard dosages of recombinant factor VIIa for treatment of hemarthroses in hemophiliacs with inhibitors. *J Thromb Hemost.* 2006;4:367–371. *This is a similar study to the by Kavakli et al (2006) with a different design and different efficacy measures. It essentially demonstrates similar to ter Avest et al (2008) and Chitlur et al (2009) that the standard-dose regimen of rFVIIa*

($90\ \mu g/kg \times 3$ doses) has similar efficacy and safety to the higher single-dose regimen ($270\ \mu g/kg \times 1$ dose).

Schneiderman J, Nugent DJ, Young G. Sequential therapy with activated prothrombin complex concentrates and recombinant factor VIIa in patients with severe haemophilia and inhibitors. Haemophilia. 2004;10:347–351. *This is the first description of the use of combination therapy with rFVIIa and FEIBA, which was previously felt to be contraindicated. This study demonstrates the safety of this approach in children. Similar application of therapy in adults where the risk for thrombotic complications is higher should be approached with a significant degree of caution.*

Schneiderman J, Rubin E, Nugent DJ, Young G. Sequential therapy with activated prothrombin complex concentrates and recombinant factor VIIa in patients with severe haemophilia and inhibitors: update of our previous experience. Haemophilia. 2007;13:244–248. *This is a follow-up to Schneiderman et al (2004) that raised more safety concerns than the original report. Although none of the patients had a thrombotic event, patients on sequential therapy had a steady increase in their D-dimer while on this therapy.*

Seyednejad H, Imani M, Jamieson T, Seifalian AM. Topical haemostatic agents. Br J Surgery. 2008;95:1197–1225. *This review discusses the wide variety of topical hemostatic agents that are available for use. Although much of the use of these agents is in the surgical setting, there are certainly situations where such agents can be used either as adjuncts to systemic hemostatic management or even alone.*

Shapiro AD, Gilchrist GS, Hoots WK, Cooper HA, Gastineau DA. Prospective, randomized trial of two doses of rFVIIa (NovoSeven) in haemophilia patients with inhibitors undergoing surgery. Thromb Haemost. 1998;80:773–778. *This study demonstrated the efficacy and safety of rFVIIa for surgery in patients with inhibitors and has led to less reluctance to perform elective surgery in this group of patients.*

Simion D, Kunicki T, Nugent D. Platelet function defects. Haemophilia. 2008;14:1240–1249. *A review of platelet function defects.*

Spreafico M, Peyvandi F. Combined FV and FVIII deficiency. Haemophilia. 2008;14:1201–1208. *This is a review of an interesting albeit rare condition that illustrates a novel mechanism for factor deficiencies. In this condition, the mutation is in a protein (ERGIC-53) involved in posttranslational protein processing and secretion.*

Sucker C, Scharf RE, Zotz RB. Use of recombinant factor VIIa in inherited and acquired von Willebrand disease. Clin Appl Thromb Hemost. 2009;15:27–31. *This article discusses the use of rFVIIa in patients with selected types of von Willebrand disease.*

Teitel J, Berntorp E, Collins P, et al. A systematic approach to controlling problem bleeds in patients with severe congenital haemophilia A and high-titre inhibitors. Haemophilia. 2007;13:256–263. *This is an expert panel report describing an algorithm to managing bleeds that are refractory to standard therapy.*

ter Avest PC, Fischer K, Mancuso ME, et al. Risk stratification for inhibitor development at first treatment for severe hemophilia A: a tool for clinical practice. J Thromb Haemost. 2008;6:2048–2054. *This article demonstrates a novel approach for attempting to predict the likelihood that a patient will develop an inhibitor.*

Tosetto A, Cataman G, Rodeghiero F. Evidence-based diagnosis of type 1 von Willebrand disease: a Bayes theorem approach. Blood. 2008;111:3998–4003. *This article describes a unique approach to determining whether a patient has von Willebrand disease incorporating the clinical presentation, family history, and laboratory results.*

Valentino LA. The benefits of prophylactic treatment with APCC in patients with haemophilia and high-titre inhibitors: a retrospective case series. Haemophilia. 2009;15:733–742. *This article summarizes all the prior case series of prophylactic therapy with FEIBA for patients with inhibitors.*

Weston BW, Monahan PE. Familial deficiency of vitamin K-dependent clotting factors. Haemophilia. 2008;14:1209–1213. *This is a review of another combined factor deficiency syndrome in which the mutation is not in the genes for the factors themselves. In this case, the mutations occur in enzymes involved in the vitamin K pathway resulting in the abnormal structure of the vitamin K–dependent factors.*

White JG. Use of electron microscope for diagnosis of platelet disorders. Semin Thromb Hemost. 1998;24:163–168. *This is an excellent overview of the ultrastructure of platelets and how abnormalities in the ultrastructure are related to the presence of bleeding disorders.*

Wolberg AS, Allen GA, Monroe DM, Hedner U, Roberts HR, Hoffman M. High dose factor VIIa improves clot structure and stability in a model of haemophilia B. Br J Haematol. 2005;131:645–655. *This is a basic science study that demonstrates how rFVIIa changes clot ultrastructure in a cell-based model of hemophilia.*

Young G. New approaches in the management of inhibitor patients. Acta Haematol. 2006;115:172–179. *This is a review of current therapy for the management of bleeding in inhibitor patients.*

Young G, Shafer FE, Rojas P, Seremetis S. Single $270\ \mu g\ kg^{-1}$-dose rFVIIa vs. standard $90\ \mu g\ kg^{-1}$-dose rFVIIa and APCC for home treatment of joint bleeds in haemophilia patients with inhibitors: a randomized study. Haemophilia. 2008;14:287–294. *This is the only study that randomized patients to 2 doses of rFVIIa and FEIBA in a blinded (for rFVIIa arms) cross-over design. The study confirmed that a single high dose of rFVIIa ($270\ \mu g/kg^{-1}$) is as effective as 3 doses of $90\ \mu g/kg^{-1}$. Chitlur et al (2009) and Astermark et al (2007) had previously demonstrated this. In addition, this study compared the 2 rFVIIa regimens to a standard dose of FEIBA, and although the high rFVIIa dosing regimen appeared to be more effective, this was likely due to the study design. This study essentially confirms the results of the FENOC study demonstrating that both bypassing agents are more or less equally effective.*

CHAPTER 09

Disorders of platelet number and function

Donald M. Arnold and A. Koneti Rao

Platelet biology: structure and function, 241	Immune causes of thrombocytopenia, 243	Disorders of platelet function, 254
Regulation of platelet number, 243	Nonimmune causes of thrombocytopenia, 250	Bibliography, 260

Platelet biology: structure and function

Hemostasis encompasses a series of interrelated and simultaneously occurring events involving the blood vessels, platelets, and coagulation system. Defects affecting any of these major participants may lead to a hemostatic defect and a bleeding disorder. This chapter will focus on the disorders related to platelet number and function.

Platelet structure

Blood platelets are anucleate fragments derived from bone marrow megakaryocytes. The mean diameter of platelets ranges from approximately 1.5 to 3.0 μm, roughly one third to one fourth that of erythrocytes. Platelet volume is approximately 7 fL. Electron microscopy reveals a fuzzy coat (glycocalix) on the platelet surface composed of membrane glycoproteins, glycolipids, mucopolysaccharides, and adsorbed plasma proteins. The plasma membrane is a bilayer of phospholipids in which cholesterol, glycolipids, and glycoproteins are embedded. The phospholipids are asymmetrically organized in the plasma membrane; the negatively charged phospholipids (such as phosphatidylserine) are almost exclusively present in the inner leaflet, whereas the others are more evenly distributed. Platelets have an elaborate channel system, the open canalicular system, which is composed of invaginations of the plasma membrane and that extends throughout the platelet and opens to the surface. The discoid shape of the resting platelet is maintained by a well-defined cytoskeleton consisting of the spectrin membrane skeleton, the marginal microtubule coil, and the actin cytoskeleton. The microtubule coil, present below the platelet membrane, is made up of αβ-tubulin dimers and plays a role in platelet formation from megakaryocytes, in addition to maintaining the discoid platelet shape. In close proximity to the open canalicular system is the dense tubular system, a closed-channel network derived from the smooth endoplasmic reticulum; it is considered the major site of platelet prostaglandin and thromboxane synthesis.

Platelets contain a variety of organelles: mitochondria and glycogen stores, lysosomes, peroxisomes, dense granules, and α granules. The lysosomes contain acid hydrolases; the dense granules contain calcium (which gives them the high electron density), adenosine triphosphate (ATP), adenosine diphosphate (ADP), magnesium, and serotonin (5-hydroxytryptamine). The α granules contain a large number of different proteins, including β-thromboglobulin (βTG) and platelet factor 4 (PF4), which are considered platelet-specific; several coagulation factors (eg, fibrinogen, factor V, factor XIII); von Willebrand factor (vWF); growth factors (eg, platelet-derived growth factor [PDGF], vascular endothelial growth factor [VEGF]); vitronectin; fibronectin; thrombospondin; the factor V binding protein multimerin; and P-selectin.

Conflict-of-interest disclosure: *Dr. Arnold:* consultancy: Amgen Canada; research funding: Hoffmann-La Roche; honoraria: CME lectures accredited by McMaster University, funded by unrestricted educational grant from GlaxoSmithKline. *Dr. Rao* declares no competing financial interest.
Off-label drug use: *Dr. Arnold:* rituximab for ITP. *Dr. Rao:* DDVAP for treatment of platelet disorders.

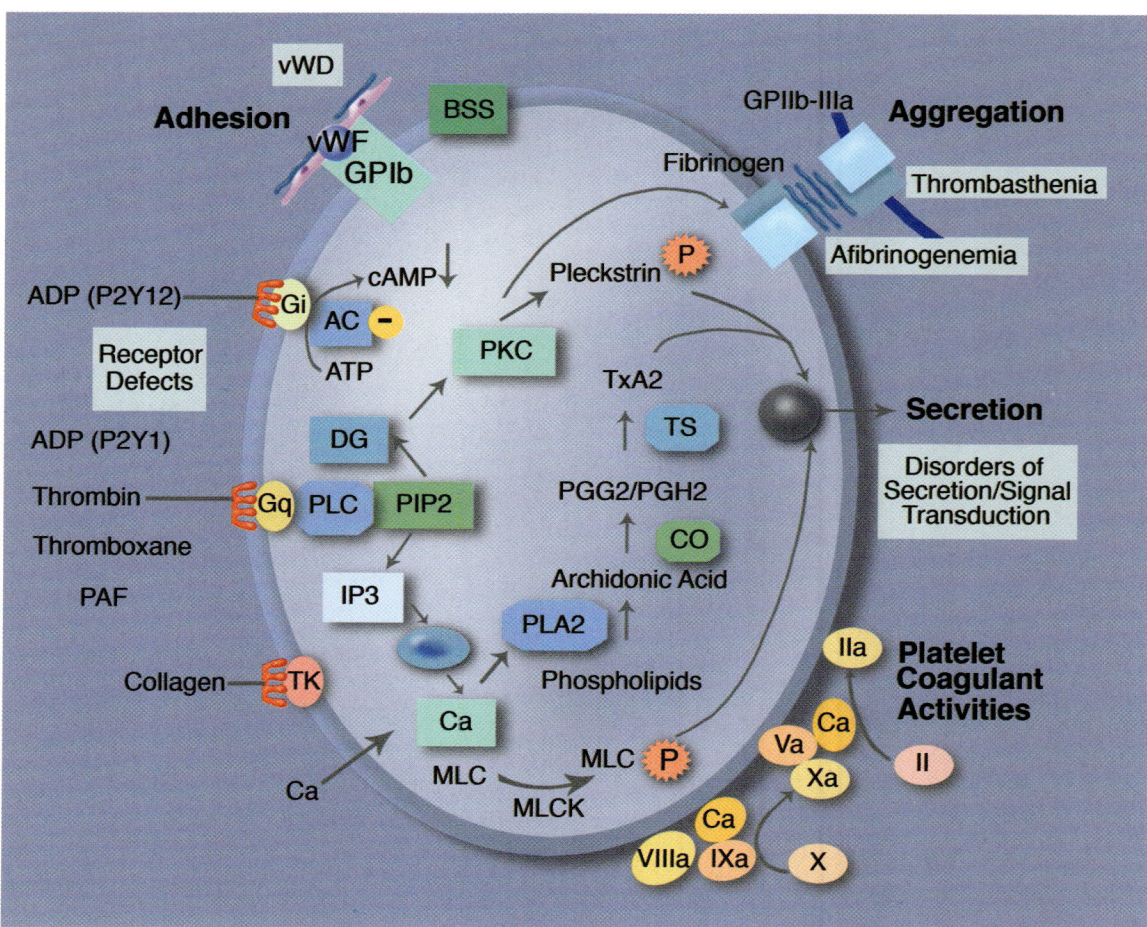

Figure 9-1 Schematic representation of selected platelet responses to activation and inherited disorders of platelet function. AC = adenylyl cyclase; ADP = adenosine diphosphate; BSS = Bernard-Soulier syndrome; CO = cyclooxygenase; DAG = diacylglycerol; G = guanosine triphosphate–binding protein; IP3 = inositol trisphosphate; MLC = myosin light chain; MLCK = myosin light chain kinase; PAF = platelet activating factor; PIP2 = phosphatidylinositol bisphosphate; PKC = protein kinase C; PLC = phospholipase C; PLA2, phospholipase A2; TK = tyrosine kinase; TS = thromboxane synthase; TxA2 = thromboxane A2; vWF = von Willebrand factor; vWD = von Willebrand disease. The Roman numerals in the circles represent coagulation factors. Modified with permission from Rao AK. Congenital disorders of platelet function: disorders of signal transduction and secretion. *Am J Med Sci*. 1998;316:69-76.

Platelet function in hemostasis

Following injury to the blood vessel, platelets adhere to exposed subendothelium by a process (adhesion) that involves, among other events, the interaction of a plasma protein, vWF, and a specific glycoprotein complex on the platelet surface, glycoprotein (GP) Ib-IX-V (GPIb-IX) (Figure 9-1). This interaction is particularly important for platelet adhesion under conditions of high shear stress. Adhesion is followed by recruitment of additional platelets that form clumps, a process called aggregation (cohesion). This involves binding of fibrinogen to specific platelet surface receptors, a complex comprised of GPIIb-IIIa (integrin $\alpha IIb\beta 3$). GPIIb-IIIa is platelet-specific and has the ability to bind vWF as well. Although resting platelets do not bind fibrinogen, platelet activation induces a conformational change in the GPIIb-IIIa complex that leads to fibrinogen binding. Activated platelets release the contents of their granules (secretion), including ADP and serotonin from the dense granules, which causes the recruitment of additional platelets. In addition, platelets play a major role in coagulation mechanisms; several key enzymatic reactions occur on the platelet membrane lipoprotein surface. During platelet activation, the negatively charged phospholipids, especially phosphatidylserine, become exposed on the platelet surface, an essential step for accelerating specific coagulation reactions by promoting the binding of coagulation factors involved in thrombin generation (platelet procoagulant activity).

A number of physiologic agonists interact with specific receptors on the platelet surface to induce responses, including a change in platelet shape from discoid to spherical (shape change), aggregation, secretion, and thromboxane

A_2 (TxA_2) production. Other agonists, such as prostacyclin, inhibit these responses. Binding of agonists to platelet receptors initiates the production or release of several intracellular messenger molecules, including products of hydrolysis of phosphoinositide (PI) by phospholipase C (diacylglycerol and inositol 1,4,5-triphosphate [$InsP_3$]), TxA_2, and cyclic nucleotides (cyclic adenosine monophosphate) (Figure 9-1). These induce or modulate the various platelet responses of Ca^{2+} mobilization, protein phosphorylation, aggregation, secretion, and thromboxane production. The interaction between the platelet surface receptors and the key intracellular enzymes (eg, phospholipases A_2 and C, adenylyl cyclase) is mediated by a group of proteins that bind and are modulated by guanosine triphosphate (G proteins). As in most secretory cells, platelet activation results in an increase in cytoplasmic ionized calcium concentration; $InsP_3$ functions as a messenger to mobilize Ca^{2+} from intracellular stores. Diacylglycerol activates protein kinase C (PKC), and this results in the phosphorylation of several proteins. PKC activation is considered to play a major role in platelet secretion and in the activation of GPI-Ib-IIIa. Numerous other mechanisms, such as activation of tyrosine kinases and phosphatases, are also triggered by platelet activation. Either inherited or acquired defects in the above platelet mechanisms may lead to impaired platelet role in hemostasis.

Regulation of platelet number

Thrombopoietin and the thrombopoietin receptor c-Mpl

In healthy adults, approximately 1×10^{11} platelets are produced each day. The number of circulating platelets is tightly regulated by the hormone thrombopoietin (TPO), which binds to megakaryocytes and hematopoietic stem cells via the TPO receptor, c-Mpl, causing an increase in the production of platelets and megakaryocyte progenitor cells. c-Mpl is also expressed on platelets, which bind TPO and effectively remove it from circulation. TPO is constitutively secreted from the liver, meaning that the amount of TPO released is constant at all times. However, free TPO levels are regulated by the number of circulating platelets and the megakaryocyte mass. Thus, when the platelet count is low, free TPO levels are high, so that more TPO can bind megakaryocytes and increase platelet production; conversely, when the platelet count is high, free TPO levels are low. The role of TPO as the principal physiologic regulator of platelet production has been confirmed in studies of TPO and c-Mpl knockout mice, which have 5% to 15% normal levels of circulating platelets, megakaryocytes, and megakaryocyte progenitor cells.

Normal platelet production

Platelets are produced from bone marrow megakaryocytes. The process of megakaryocyte proliferation and differentiation involves endomitosis and polyploidization, whereby the nucleus divides but the cell does not, and requires the right concentration of interleukins, colony-stimulating factors, and TPO in the bone marrow milieu. In the process of maturation, megakaryocytes form secretory granules and a demarcation membrane system that permeates the cytoplasmic space. This extensive membrane system eventually projects multiple filamentous pseudopod-like structures called proplatelets from which platelets are released into the circulation (shedding). Released platelets circulate for 7 to 10 days and then are cleared by phagocytic cells in the reticuloendothelial system after undergoing a process called senescence, characterized by physiologic changes, loss of membrane integrity, and shedding of antigens including CD42b and GPVI.

Immune causes of thrombocytopenia

Immune thrombocytopenia

> **Clinical case**
>
> A 5-year-old boy is noted by his parents to have multiple large bruises on his arms and legs. The child is brought to the hospital emergency room where the platelet count is found to be 6×10^9/L. No other bleeding signs or symptoms are present. Primary immune thrombocytopenia is suspected, and the hematologist discusses the following management options with the parents: treatment with prednisone, intravenous immunoglobulin, or anti-D, or observation without specific treatment.

Immune thrombocytopenia (ITP) is an autoimmune disease characterized by low platelet counts and a variable risk of bleeding. An international working group has recently proposed standard terminology and definitions for ITP. The term *idiopathic* has been abandoned, and instead, *primary* is used to denote ITP with no precipitating cause. The term *purpura* (as in the old terminology *idiopathic thrombocytopenic purpura*) has also been abandoned because bleeding symptoms, including purpura, are absent or minimal in a large proportion of patients. *Secondary ITP* refers to all forms of immune-mediated thrombocytopenia except primary ITP. In this chapter, we have adopted the new terminology (*primary* and *secondary ITP*).

Primary ITP is a common cause of thrombocytopenia in both adults and children, with an estimated prevalence of 5 to 20 per 100,000 persons and estimated incidence of 1 to 3 per 100,000 persons. In children, the peak age of occurrence is 2 to 4 years, and the frequency is equal in boys and girls.

In adults, the incidence and prevalence of ITP increases with age, and a female predominance is present only in the middle-adult years. Otherwise, the sex distribution is equivalent. In children, ITP is typically self-limited and is often detected after an antecedent viral/infectious illness, whereas adult ITP typically becomes persistent or chronic with no obvious precipitating event. Patients may present with mucocutaneous bleeding, or they may be asymptomatic and identified because of a routine blood count. There is no specific diagnostic test to confirm primary ITP; it is diagnosed by excluding other causes of thrombocytopenia.

Secondary ITP occurs in the setting of drugs such as quinine (see section on drug-induced thrombocytopenia), lymphoproliferative disease, systemic lupus erythematosus, antiphospholipid antibody syndrome, and infections with hepatitis C virus, hepatitis B, human immunodeficiency virus (HIV), and *Helicobacter pylori*. Secondary ITP has also been observed in association with thyroiditis, hemolytic anemia (Evans syndrome), and monoclonal gammopathy of uncertain significance. Nonimmune causes of thrombocytopenia, including hypersplenism, hereditary thrombocytopenias, and von Willebrand disease (vWD) type 2B, are frequently confused with the diagnosis of ITP (Table 9-1).

Table 9-1 Differential diagnosis of immune thrombocytopenia.

Immune
  Primary (no precipitating cause)
  Secondary
    Drug-induced (quinine)
    Posttransfusion purpura
    Human immunodeficiency virus
    Hepatitis C
    Infectious mononucleosis (Epstein-Barr virus)
    Systemic lupus erythematosus
    Crohn disease
    Antiphospholipid antibody syndrome
    Chronic lymphocytic leukemia
    Lymphoma
    Immunoglobulin A deficiency
    Common variable immune deficiency

Nonimmune
  Hypersplenism
  Myelodysplasia
  Acute leukemia
  Drug-induced marrow suppression (valproic acid, alcohol)
  Hereditary thrombocytopenia (*MYH9* mutations and others)
  von Willebrand disease type 2B
  Microangiopathic hemolytic anemia

From Arnold DM, Kelton JG. Current options for the treatment of idiopathic thrombocytopenic purpura. *Semin Hematol*. 2007;44 (Suppl 5):S12–S23, with permission.

Clinical features of primary ITP

By the current definition, a platelet count $<100 \times 10^9$/L is required for the diagnosis of ITP, although it is recognized that some patients may have even milder declines in the platelet count at presentation. Mucocutaneous bleeding is the hallmark of severe primary ITP and manifests as petechiae, purpura, ecchymosis, epistaxis, menorrhagia, oral mucosal bleeding, gastrointestinal bleeding, or rarely, intracranial hemorrhage. Bleeding due to thrombocytopenia is not expected with platelet counts above 30×10^9/L. As the platelet count decreases to below 20 to 30×10^9/L, bleeding symptoms tend to become more severe, yet with significant variability from patient to patient. Primary ITP is rarely life threatening; however, elderly patients with persistent and severe thrombocytopenia (platelets below 20×10^9/L) have the highest rate of fatal bleeding (usually intracranial hemorrhage), which is estimated to occur with a frequency of 0.02 to 0.04 cases per patient-year. Physical examination should focus on typical bleeding sites. Dependent areas and skin underneath tight clothing should be examined for petechiae, and oral mucous membranes should be examined for purpura. The remainder of the physical examination should be normal. The presence of lymphadenopathy or splenomegaly should prompt investigations for underlying infection and/or lymphoproliferative disease. Skeletal, renal, or neurologic abnormalities suggest a familial cause of thrombocytopenia.

Pathophysiology of primary ITP

The prevailing hypothesis to explain the pathophysiology of primary ITP is accelerated platelet destruction by anti–GPIIb-IIIa and anti–GPIb-IX antibodies; however, platelet autoantibodies are detectable only in approximately 60% of patients. Dysregulated T cells in ITP may enable the development of platelet autoantibodies and may have a direct cytotoxic effect on platelets. Another important mechanism of thrombocytopenia in ITP is insufficient platelet production, which was first noted in studies of platelet turnover using autologous radiolabeled platelets and is further supported by the observation that free TPO levels are not consistently elevated (as would be expected). A new and effective class of medications for ITP, called TPO receptor agonists, works by increasing platelet production.

Diagnosis of primary ITP

The diagnosis of ITP rests on a consistent clinical history, physical examination, and the exclusion of other causes. Leukocytes and hemoglobin are normal, unless significant thrombocytopenic bleeding has resulted in anemia. Examination of the peripheral blood film is required to exclude pseudothrombocytopenia (ethylenediaminetetraacetic acid–dependent platelet agglutinating antibodies), microangiopathic hemolytic anemia, or blood cell abnormalities suggestive of other disorders. The mean platelet volume (MPV) is usually increased. Approximately 15% to 25% of ITP patients have detectable antinuclear antibodies or antiphospholipid antibodies, usually in low titers, which have no prognostic significance. Coagulation screen is normal. Thyroid function tests are indicated to uncover occult thyroid dysfunction, especially prior to surgery. Bone marrow examination is not routinely required but should be performed to exclude other causes of thrombocytopenia when atypical features are present such as unexplained anemia, lymphadenopathy, or splenomegaly or when a typical platelet count response to treatment (such as intravenous immunoglobulin [IVIg] or Rh immune globulin [anti-D]) is not observed. Bone marrow examinations may also be warranted in the investigation of elderly patients in whom myelodysplasia is suspected and before splenectomy. Megakaryocyte number is typically normal or increased on bone marrow examination of ITP patients.

Management of children with primary ITP

Because spontaneous recovery is expected in most children with primary ITP, families of children generally need counseling and supportive care, rather than specific drug therapy. Otherwise, a short course of corticosteroids, IVIg, or anti-D (in Rh-positive individuals) generally results in a rapid recovery of the platelet count, although the overall effect of these treatments on bleeding has not been well established. Common adverse effects include behavioral changes from corticosteroids, headache from IVIg, and hemolysis from anti-D. Patients (adults and children) with a positive Coombs test should not receive anti-D due to the risk of severe hemolysis. Severe hemorrhage occurs in approximately 1 in 200 children and intracerebral hemorrhage occurs in approximately 1 in 800 children in the first month after diagnosis.

Recovery of the platelet count ultimately occurs in 80% of children. The remaining 20% have persistent thrombocytopenia, yet even in this group, major bleeding is uncommon. Splenectomy is generally reserved for severe persistent thrombocytopenia and bleeding and results in a complete remission in approximately 75% of children. The risk for overwhelming sepsis after splenectomy is greater in young children, and therefore, splenectomy is generally deferred until after 5 years of age. Immunizing vaccines for *Streptococcus pneumoniae*, *Neisseria meningitides*, and *Haemophilus influenzae* type b should be given before splenectomy, and penicillin prophylaxis is recommended after splenectomy until adulthood.

> **Clinical case (continued)**
>
> With support and reassurance, the parents of the 5-year-old boy with primary ITP described previously accept the hematologist's recommendation for no specific treatment. The boy returns to school the next day. He continues to have new bruises and some petechiae for 1 week, which then resolve. His platelet count gradually increases and returns to a normal level 7 weeks later.

Management of adults with primary ITP

In contrast to children, ITP in adults tends to recur and persist. Nevertheless, asymptomatic patients with mild or moderate thrombocytopenia require no specific treatment. Therefore, deciding which patients do not require treatment is the first important management decision. In general, a period of observation is appropriate when platelet counts are $>30 \times 10^9$/L. Patients with severe thrombocytopenia (usually $<20 \times 10^9$/L) or ITP associated with bleeding symptoms require treatment. Initial treatment is generally with prednisone (staring at 1 mg/kg daily and then tapering over a period of 6 to 8 weeks) or high-dose dexamethasone (in cycles of 40 mg daily for 4 days, repeated monthly for up to 6 cycles or every other week for 4 cycles) with or without IVIg or anti-D. Most patients will achieve an initial platelet count response, which is generally not sustained once treatment is stopped.

For patients who fail to respond durably to initial treatment with corticosteroids, intermittent IVIg or anti-D may be effective. In a prospective study of 28 Rh-positive, nonsplenectomized adults, anti-D, given at a dose of 50 or 75 µg/kg every time the platelet count decreased to $<30 \times 10^9$/L, was an effective maintenance treatment. Rituximab, an anti-CD20 monoclonal antibody that rapidly depletes CD20$^+$ B lymphocytes, has been associated with a platelet count response in ITP, and recent evidence suggests that it may be a reasonable treatment option before splenectomy. In a systematic review of 313 ITP patients, half of whom were nonsplenectomized, 62.5% (95% CI, 52.6%–72.5%) achieved a platelet count response (platelets $>50 \times 10^9$/L), with a median time to response of 5.5 weeks (range, 2–18 weeks) and a median duration of response of 10.5 months (range, 3–20 months). In a single-arm study of 60 nonsplenectomized ITP patients, 40% achieved a platelet count at or above 50×10^9/L with at least a doubling from baseline at 1 year, and in 33.3%, this response was sustained for 2 years. A recent randomized controlled trial in newly diagnosed adults with ITP showed that dexamethasone plus rituximab was associated with a higher rate of response by 6 months compared with a single course of dexamethasone alone.

Adverse effects of rituximab include infusional reactions (eg, hypotension, chills, rash), serum sickness, and cardiac arrhythmia. Neutropenia is rare, and serum immunoglobulin levels rarely fall below the normal threshold. The rate of bacterial infections may be slightly increased, and recent reports have linked rituximab with reactivation of latent JC virus causing progressive multifocal leukoencephalopathy. Reactivation of hepatitis B has been well described in patients with active or remote hepatitis B infection after rituximab.

For patients who relapse or fail to respond to corticosteroids, splenectomy is associated with the highest rate of durable remissions with long-term follow-up. In a systematic review, 1731 (66%) of 2623 adults with ITP achieved a normal platelet count after splenectomy, with responses lasting a median of 7.3 years. Younger age was the only independent predictor of response. Relapses occurred in 15% of patients (range, 0%–51%) after a median of 33 months. Of complete responders, 90% can be expected to attain a normal platelet count from 1 to 6 weeks after splenectomy. Overall mortality with an open or laparoscopic surgical approach is approximately 1% and 0.2%, respectively, and the most common immediate postoperative complications are pneumonia, pleural effusion, bleeding, and thrombosis, occurring in up to 4% of patients. Overwhelming postsplenectomy infection is the most feared late complication, with an estimated lifetime risk of 1% to 2%. Recommendations for immunization before splenectomy are the same as for children; however, penicillin prophylaxis is generally not felt to be necessary.

Persistent primary ITP after splenectomy

Two new TPO receptor agonists, romiplostim (Nplate, previously called AMG 531; given subcutaneously) and eltrombopag (Promacta; given orally), have completed phase III clinical trials and are approved in the United States for patients with primary ITP who have had an insufficient response to corticosteroids, immunoglobulins, or splenectomy. These agents bind and activate the TPO receptor, c-Mpl, and cause an increase in the production of platelets; however, they have no structural similarity to endogenous TPO and thus do not stimulate cross-reactive TPO antibodies. Both drugs are effective in up to 70% of patients with ITP before and after splenectomy (although responses appear to be more pronounced before splenectomy), and platelet count responses are generally maintained as long as the drug is administered. Romiplostim and eltrombopag have been associated with bone marrow reticulin formation and thrombosis, and eltrombopag has been associated with increased liver enzymes. Other treatment options for relapsed ITP or splenectomy failure include rituximab, azathioprine, and immunosuppressant medications; however, evidence from randomized controlled trials is limited in this population.

Emergency treatment of ITP

Hospitalization should be considered for patients with new-onset, severe thrombocytopenia ($<20 \times 10^9$/L) and significant bleeding symptoms. Secondary causes (especially drugs; see next section) should be promptly excluded. Management of major bleeding may require platelet transfusions in combination with high doses of parenteral corticosteroids (methylprednisolone 1 g intravenously daily for 2–3 days) and/or IVIg (1 g/kg for 1–2 days). However, the platelet count typically returns to pretreatment levels 2 to 3 weeks later. Emergency splenectomy may be required for patients with refractory thrombocytopenia and ongoing bleeding.

> **Key points**
>
> - The workup of patients with suspected ITP requires a thorough search for nonimmune causes of thrombocytopenia and underlying (secondary) causes of ITP.
> - Primary ITP in children often resolves spontaneously or with minimal treatment only.
> - Adult-onset primary ITP tends to relapse and often requires ongoing therapy.
> - Splenectomy is associated with a durable response in two-thirds of patients with primary ITP, although relapses occur in approximately 15% of adults.
> - TPO receptor agonists (romiplostim and eltrombopag) work by increasing platelet production and are effective in 60% to 70% of patients with primary ITP.

Drug-induced thrombocytopenia

Unexpected thrombocytopenia is often caused by drugs, and drug-induced thrombocytopenia (DITP) should be suspected in any patient who presents with acute thrombocytopenia. Many drugs have been reported to cause thrombocytopenia, the most common of which are quinine and quinidine (present in tonic water, bitter melon, and certain medications), nonsteroidal anti-inflammatory agents, sulfamethoxazole, vancomycin, anticonvulsants, sedatives, and the platelet GPIIb-IIIa inhibitors tirofiban, eptifibatide, and abciximab. A case-control study of drug use among patients with acute reversible thrombocytopenia compared with nonthrombocytopenic controls showed that trimethoprim/sulfamethoxazole was most frequently implicated, followed by quinine/quinidine, dipyridamole, sulfonylureas, and salicylates. A systematic review of individual patient data also documented that the most commonly reported drugs with a definite or probable causal relation to

Table 9-2 Criteria for assessing reports of drug-induced thrombocytopenia and levels of evidence for a causal relationship between the drug and thrombocytopenia.

Criterion	Description
1	(1) Therapy with the candidate drug preceded thrombocytopenia; and
	(2) recovery from thrombocytopenia was complete and sustained after therapy with the drug was discontinued
2	The candidate drug was the only drug used before the onset of thrombocytopenia; or other drugs were continued or reintroduced after discontinuation of therapy with the candidate drug with a sustained normal platelet count
3	Other causes for thrombocytopenia were excluded
4	Reexposure to the candidate drug resulted in recurrent thrombocytopenia
Level of evidence	
Definite	Criteria 1, 2, 3, and 4 met
Probable	Criteria 1, 2, and 3 met
Possible	Criterion 1 met
Unlikely	Criterion 1 not met

Adapted from George JN, Raskob GE, Shah SR, et al. Drug-induced thrombocytopenia: a systematic review of published case reports. *Ann Intern Med.* 1998;129:886-890, with permission.

thrombocytopenia were quinidine, quinine, rifampin, and trimethoprim/sulfamethoxazole. An online database of implicated drugs has been developed by George and colleagues (Platelets on the Web; available at http://www.ouhsc.edu/platelets). DITP and heparin-induced thrombocytopenia are discussed separately.

Mechanism of DITP

DITP should be suspected when thrombocytopenia occurs approximately 7 days after drug exposure. Notable exceptions are the GPIIb-IIIa antagonists eptifibatide, tirofiban, and abciximab, which may cause acute thrombocytopenia within a few hours of the first exposure. Several mechanisms of DITP have been proposed. Recent data suggest that quinine-type DITP is caused by naturally occurring autoantibodies that acquire strong binding affinity for platelet antigen targets after they have been conformationally altered by the drug. Tight antibody binding stimulates B cells to produce excess antibodies within approximately 7 days. The epitope targets of these antibodies usually reside on GPIIb-IIIa or GPIb-IX. Other drugs such as gold, procainamide, sulfonamide antibiotics, and interferon alfa or beta (but not quinine) can induce platelet autoantibodies causing a syndrome that resembles ITP.

Tirofiban and eptifibatide ("fibans") are small synthetic molecules that bind GPIIb-IIIa and inhibit platelet function. Thrombocytopenia may occur because of preexisting antibodies that recognize structural changes (neoepitopes) induced in GPIIb-IIIa when a fiban binds to it. Abciximab, a chimeric (mouse–human) Fab fragment that is specific for GPIIIa, causes acute profound thrombocytopenia in 0.5% to 1.0% of patients on their first exposure, presumably as a result of preexisting antibodies that recognize the murine portion of abciximab bound to GPIIb-IIIa. Patients with severe thrombocytopenia caused by GPIIb-IIIa antagonists may require platelet transfusions to treat hemorrhagic complications, which are often compounded by the concomitant use of heparin, aspirin, and other antiplatelet agents.

Diagnosis of DITP

Criteria for levels of evidence for DITP have been proposed that may be helpful in the evaluation of patients in whom the condition is suspected (Table 9-2). Clinical criteria used to judge the likelihood of drug being implicated in DITP are temporal association between drug exposure and thrombocytopenia, the exclusion of other causes of thrombocytopenia, and recurrence upon drug rechallenge. The detection of an antibody that binds tightly to normal platelets in the presence of the drug establishes the diagnosis in many cases; however, such testing is not widely available. Furthermore, drug-dependent platelet antibodies cannot be detected when the antibodies recognize a metabolite of the drug instead of the drug itself, such as with nonsteroidal anti-inflammatory drugs and acetaminophen. Thus, DITP remains a clinical diagnosis.

Patients with severe thrombocytopenia (platelets $<10 \times 10^9$/L) are at risk of fatal bleeding. Other symptoms might include faintness, chills, fever, nausea, and hypotension. Treatment is to stop the drug and administer platelet transfusions for patients with severe thrombocytopenia. Bleeding symptoms usually subside after 1 to 2 days, and the platelet count usually returns to normal in 4 to 8 days. Rarely, thrombocytopenia can persist for several weeks.

> **Key points**
>
> - A careful drug history must be taken in any patient presenting with thrombocytopenia.
> - Quinine-induced thrombocytopenia presents after 5 to 7 days and is associated with severe thrombocytopenia and bleeding.
> - Thrombocytopenia induced by quinine is caused by antibodies that bind to platelets only in the presence of the drug.
> - DITP caused by GPIIb-IIIa antagonists may develop within hours of first exposure to the drug and is mediated by preexisting antibodies.

Heparin-induced thrombocytopenia

Heparin-induced thrombocytopenia (HIT) is a drug reaction caused by antibodies against complexes of PF4 and heparin. Binding of HIT antibodies to platelet Fc receptors activates platelets, endothelial cells, and macrophages, resulting in the production of platelet microparticles and an intensely prothrombotic state. HIT is characterized by thrombocytopenia in a patient receiving unfractionated heparin or (less frequently) low molecular weight heparin (LMWH). Despite the occurrence of thrombocytopenia, bleeding is rare, and the risk of thrombosis is high (~50%). HIT is a clinicopathologic syndrome, meaning that the diagnosis relies on a compatible clinical history and supportive laboratory testing. Transient thrombocytopenia following the administration of heparin (previously called type I HIT, or nonimmune HIT) is an innocuous syndrome caused by platelet agglutination because of heparin's strong negative charge. This section will focus on immune-mediated HIT.

Clinical features

HIT occurs more frequently in surgical compared with medical patients, especially following orthopedic and cardiac surgery. Clinical features consistent with HIT include a platelet count decrease of 50% or more (from the highest postoperative platelet count), a platelet count decrease beginning 5 to 10 days after starting heparin (or sooner in patients with recent heparin exposure), the presence of thrombosis, and the exclusion of other causes. These key features (**T**hrombocytopenia, **T**iming, **T**hrombosis and o**T**her) have been incorporated into a clinical scoring system called the 4T score, which can help determine the pretest probability of HIT and aid in the interpretation of functional and quantitative antibody testing (Table 9-3). The scoring system has been shown to have a high negative predictive value (ie, a low score is useful in ruling out HIT); however, a high score has not been consistently predictive, suggesting that patients with HIT cannot be identified reliably based on clinical criteria alone.

Thrombosis occurs in approximately 50% of patients with untreated HIT; thus, the diagnosis should be considered in all patients with acute thrombosis who have been hospitalized within the previous 1 to 2 weeks. Deep vein thrombosis and pulmonary embolism are the most common thrombotic events, but arterial thrombosis including limb artery thrombosis, myocardial infarction, and microvascular thrombosis resembling disseminated intravascular coagulation are well described. Adrenal infarction, skin necrosis at the heparin injection site, and anaphylactoid reactions after an intravenous heparin bolus may also occur as a result of the PF4/heparin antibodies.

Table 9-3 A clinical scoring system (low, 0–3; intermediate, 4–5; high, 6–8) to determine the pretest probability of heparin-induced thrombocytopenia.

4Ts	2 points	1 point	0 point
Thrombocytopenia	Platelet count decrease of >50% and platelet nadir ≥20 × 10⁹/L	Platelet count decrease of 30%–50% or platelet nadir of 10–19 × 10⁹/L	Platelet count decrease of <30% or platelet nadir <10 × 10⁹/L
Timing of platelet count fall	Clear onset of thrombocytopenia 5–10 days after heparin administration; or platelet decrease within 1 day, with prior heparin exposure within 30 days	Consistent with day 5–10 decrease but not clear (eg, missing platelet counts) or onset after day 10; or decrease within 1 day, with prior heparin exposure 30-100 days ago	Platelet count decrease <4 days without recent exposure
Thrombosis or other sequelae	New thrombosis (confirmed); skin necrosis (lesions at heparin injection site); acute systemic reaction after intravenous unfractionated heparin bolus	Progressive or recurrent thrombosis; nonnecrotizing skin lesions; suspected thrombosis (not proven)	None
Other causes for thrombocytopenia	None apparent	Possible	Definite

Adapted from Lo GK, Juhl D, Warkentin TE, et al. Evaluation of pretest clinical score (4 T's) for the diagnosis of heparin-induced thrombocytopenia in two clinical settings. *J Thromb Haemost.* 2006;4:759-765, with permission.

HIT testing

There are 2 types of tests available for the detection of HIT antibodies: quantitative PF4/heparin immunoassays (PF4/heparin enzyme-linked immunosorbent assay [ELISA]) and functional assays demonstrating the platelet-activating potential of these antibodies, such as the serotonin release assay, considered the gold standard for HIT diagnosis.

HIT is caused by anti-PF4/heparin immunoglobulin (Ig) G antibodies that activate platelets; thus, although many susceptible patients form IgG, IgM, and IgA antibodies to PF4/heparin complexes after exposure to heparin, only a few will have platelet-activating IgG antibodies that cause HIT (Figure 9-2).

Treatment of HIT

According to the American College of Chest Physician guidelines, monitoring for HIT should be done with platelet count measurements at least every second day from day 4 of heparin exposure until day 14 (or until heparin is discontinued) for patients at substantial risk of HIT, including medical or surgical patients receiving therapeutic doses of unfractionated heparin, surgical patients receiving postoperative antithrombotic prophylaxis with either unfractionated heparin or LMWH, and medical patients receiving prophylactic unfractionated heparin. When HIT is the likely diagnosis, heparin should be stopped, and therapeutic doses of a rapid-acting, nonheparin anticoagulant should be administered even before the results of HIT testing are known. The use of an alternate anticoagulant such as a direct thrombin inhibitor (argatroban, lepirudin, or bivalirudin) is important even in the absence of thrombosis because the risk of developing a new thrombosis is high. Two other potential agents are the factor Xa inhibitors danaparoid and fondaparinux; however, danaparoid is not available in the United States, and fondaparinux is not approved for this indication. LMWHs should not be used because most heparin-dependent antibodies also react with LMWHs. For patients with strongly suspected or confirmed HIT, ultrasonography of the lower limb veins for investigation of deep venous thrombosis

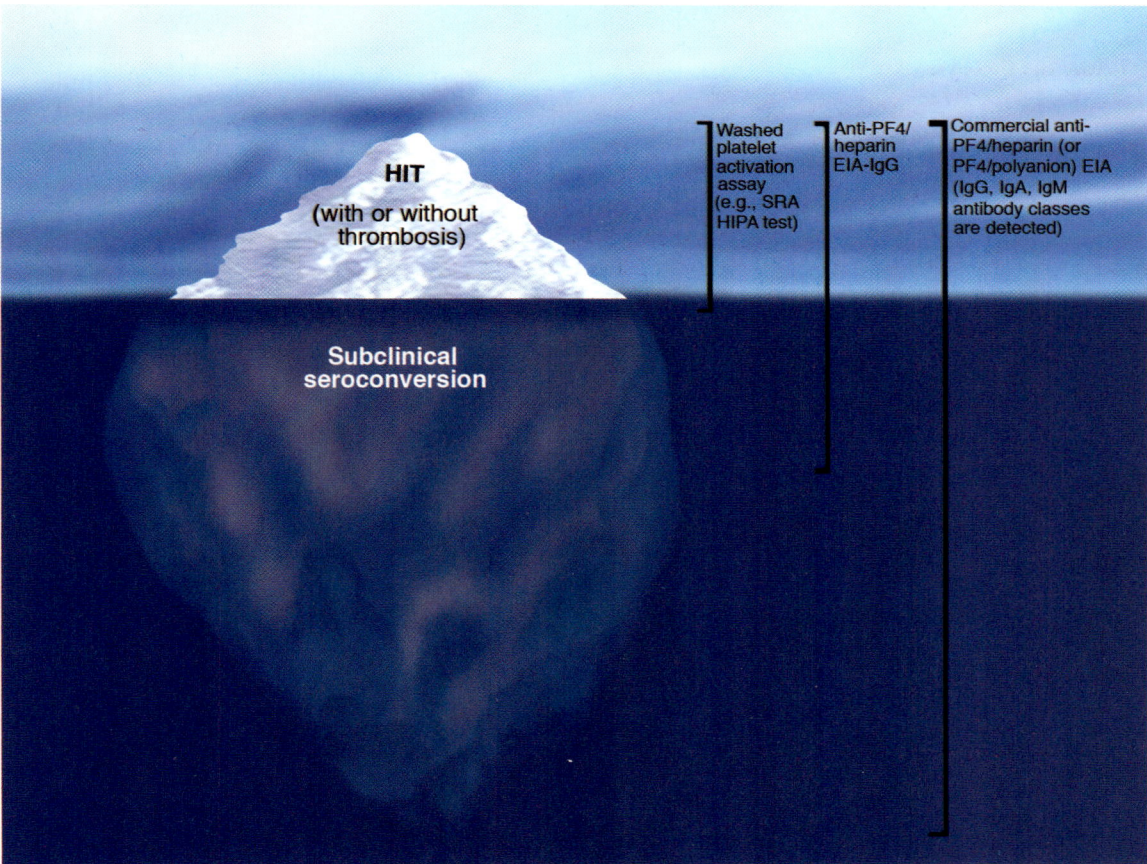

Figure 9-2 Iceberg model of heparin-induced thrombocytopenia (HIT) testing: anti- platelet factor 4 (PF4) immunoglobulin (Ig) G antibodies by enzyme immunoassay (EIA) along with a positive platelet activation assay occur in most HIT patients. Many patients without HIT will have a positive EIA, especially for non-IgG subclasses. HIPA = heparin-induced platelet aggregation; SRA = serotonin release assay. Modified with permission, from Warkentin TE. Heparin-induced thrombocytopenia: pathogenesis and management. *Br J Hematol.* 2003;121:535–555.

should be performed. Vitamin K antagonists (such as warfarin) should not be given to patients with HIT at least until the platelet count has recovered (>100–150 × 10⁹/L). Adequate anticoagulation with a nonheparin anticoagulant is required before warfarin is initiated and should overlap with warfarin to avoid the risk of thrombosis associated with initial reduction in protein C and S levels. Due to the substantial (~50%) frequency of thrombosis, which may occur weeks after thrombocytopenia has resolved, continued treatment with warfarin for 30 days following diagnosis of isolated HIT is advisable.

> **Key points**
>
> - HIT is associated with a high risk of thrombosis.
> - HIT should be suspected in a patient with a 50% decrease in platelet count 5 to 10 days after starting unfractionated heparin or LMWH, or sooner in patients with recent heparin exposure.
> - HIT is caused by platelet-activating IgG antibodies directed against PF4/heparin complexes.
> - Treatment of HIT is to stop heparin and start an alternate, nonheparin anticoagulant in therapeutic doses.

Nonimmune causes of thrombocytopenia

Thrombotic microangiopathies

> **Clinical case**
>
> A 31-year-old woman presents with a 5-day history of progressive headache, fever, and weakness. Laboratory examination reveals a platelet count of 23 × 10⁹/L. Other laboratory abnormalities include anemia with fragmented red blood cells on the blood smear and increased serum creatinine, alanine aminotransferase (ALT), aspartate aminotransferase (AST), and lactate dehydrogenase (LDH). While in the emergency department, she develops left hemiplegia and has a grand mal seizure.

Clinical features

The thrombotic microangiopathies discussed here are thrombotic thrombocytopenic purpura (TTP) and hemolytic uremic syndrome (HUS). Distinguishing between TTP and HUS is sometimes difficult but may be important for prognosis and therapy. For example, neurologic features commonly occur with TTP, which must be treated with plasma exchange, whereas acute renal failure is generally associated with HUS for which plasma therapy may not be required. In addition, contact tracing is important for patients with diarrhea-associated HUS. TTP and HUS are classified here as nonimmune causes of thrombocytopenia, although an immune mechanism is possible.

TTP is classically defined by a pentad of clinical and laboratory features that include thrombocytopenia, microangiopathic hemolytic anemia, neurologic deficits, renal failure, and fever. However, the diagnosis of TTP should be considered in any patient with thrombocytopenia and microangiopathic hemolytic anemia; all 5 features occur in a minority of patients at presentation. Before the therapeutic use of plasma infusions was discovered, TTP was almost always fatal; however, survival rates with plasmapheresis exceed 80%, and most patients can be expected to make a full recovery, even those with neurologic deficits (such as hemiparesis).

HUS is characterized by thrombocytopenia, microangiopathic hemolytic anemia, and acute renal failure. Shiga toxin–producing enterohemorrhagic *Escherichia coli* accounts for the vast majority of childhood HUS in developed countries.

Pathogenesis

Thrombotic microangiopathies are caused by disseminated platelet thrombi, which lead to the shearing of red blood cells inside the blood vessel lumen (intravascular hemolysis). Endothelial cell activation may be an important mediator of the intensely prothrombotic state in HUS caused by Shiga toxin, which is directly toxic to endothelial cells, and in quinine-associated TTP as a result of drug-dependent antibodies that activate endothelial cells. Unusually large vWF multimers are central to the pathogenesis of idiopathic TTP and may be a link between endothelial damage and the development of disseminated platelet thrombi.

Normally, ultralarge multimers of vWF are cleaved by the enzyme ADAMTS13 (**A** **D**isintegrin **A**nd **M**etalloprotease with **T**hrombo**S**pondin-1-like repeats). When ADAMTS13 is deficient, unusually large multimers of vWF are released into the circulation and, under high shear stress, unfold into large strings that bind platelets and form platelet thrombi (Figure 9-3). Inherited or acquired ADAMTS13 deficiency is associated with the development of familial or idiopathic TTP, respectively. In the familial form, genetic mutations cause a quantitative defect of the enzyme. Patients with familial TTP have a lifelong risk for severe neurologic abnormalities and renal failure that is largely preventable by periodic plasma infusions. Many patients with familial TTP are only diagnosed in their adult years. In acquired idiopathic TTP, autoantibodies develop to ADAMTS13 that inhibit its function or accelerate its clearance. However, some patients with what appears to be typical TTP have normal levels of ADAMTS13 and no detectable inhibitors.

Secondary forms of TTP can be caused by drugs including quinine, ticlopidine, clopidogrel, cyclosporine, tacrolimus, mitomycin C, and gemcitabine and may occur in the

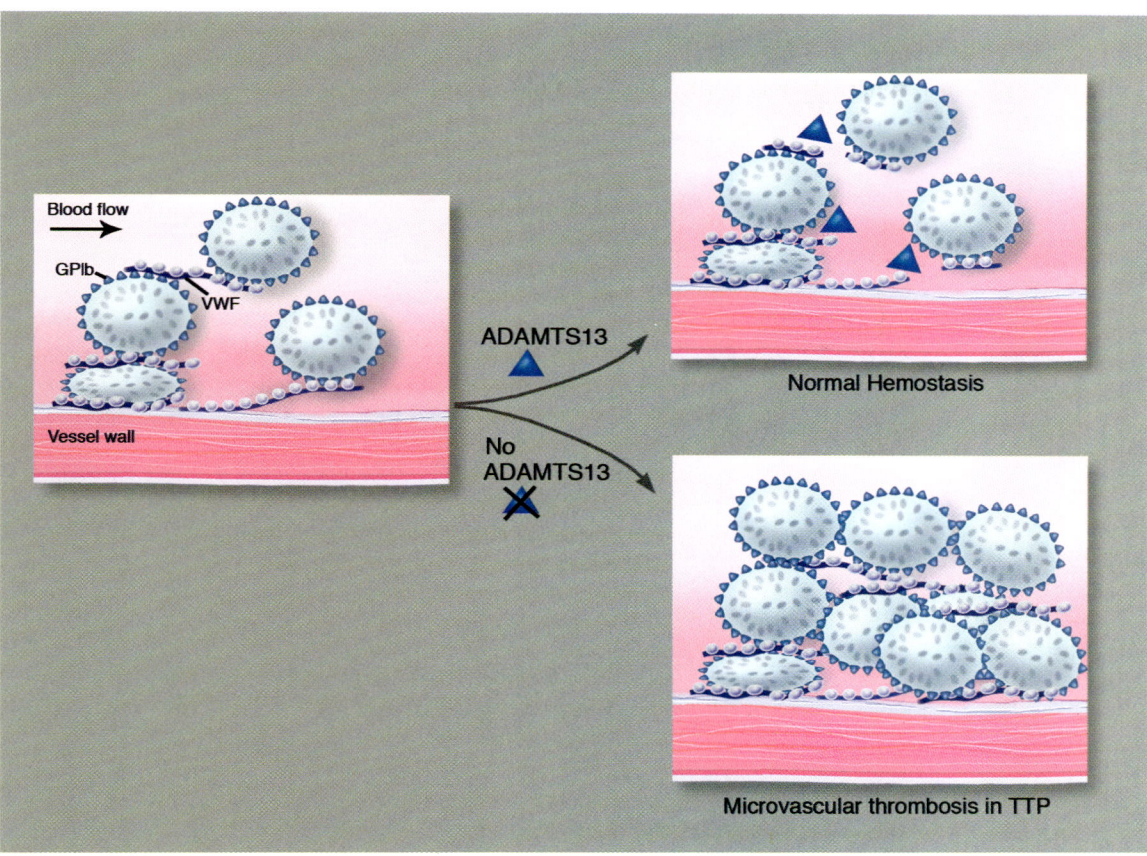

Figure 9-3 A schematic representation of the mechanism of platelet thrombi in thrombotic thrombocytopenic purpura (TTP). ADAMTS13 = a disintegrin and metalloprotease with thrombospondin-1-like repeats; GPIb = glycoprotein Ib; vWF = von Willebrand factor. From Sadler JE. Thrombotic thrombocytopenic purpura: a moving target. *Hematology Am Soc Hematol Educ Program*. 2006:415–420.

setting of pregnancy, bone marrow transplantation, HIV infection, systemic lupus erythematosus, or disseminated malignancy. Secondary forms are often resistant to plasma exchange.

Over 90% of all childhood HUS is caused by Shiga toxin–producing enterohemorrhagic *E coli* or invasive pneumococcal infection. The remainder are mostly associated with disorders of complement regulation, usually due to mutations in complement factor H, factor I, or membrane cofactor protein, or precipitated by other conditions such as pregnancy, HIV, or malignancy. Most patients with acute HUS survive; however, long-term complications include hypertension and chronic renal failure.

Diagnosis

The diagnosis of TTP requires the prompt recognition of clinical symptoms, basic laboratory testing including a complete blood count, and hemolytic indices and examination of the blood film. The presence of acute thrombocytopenia and microangiopathic hemolytic anemia without another clinically apparent etiology is sufficient to assume the diagnosis of TTP. Fever may be present but is often masked by the use of antipyretics. Characteristic laboratory abnormalities include elevated LDH, total and unconjugated hyperbilirubinemia, a negative direct antiglobulin test, and normal coagulation tests. The blood smear must be examined for the presence of red blood cell fragments and large polychromatophilic cells (Figure 9-4). A thorough assessment for secondary causes of TTP is essential and should include a detailed drug history, HIV testing, and a focused search for autoimmune disease and malignancy. Pregnancy should be excluded in females of childbearing potential. The diagnosis of HUS can be made clinically for patients with a diarrheal prodrome and acute renal failure. Specialized testing of complement factors are required to confirm the diagnosis of atypical HUS.

ADAMTS13 testing may be used to support the diagnosis of TTP but should not be used to guide acute management decisions. Two types of testing for ADAMTS13 are available: quantitative and functional tests. Quantitative tests are widely available as commercial ELISA-based kits and provide the concentration of ADAMTS13 antigen or anti-ADAMTS13 antibody in plasma, whereas functional tests are only done in specialized laboratories and provide a measure of antigen or

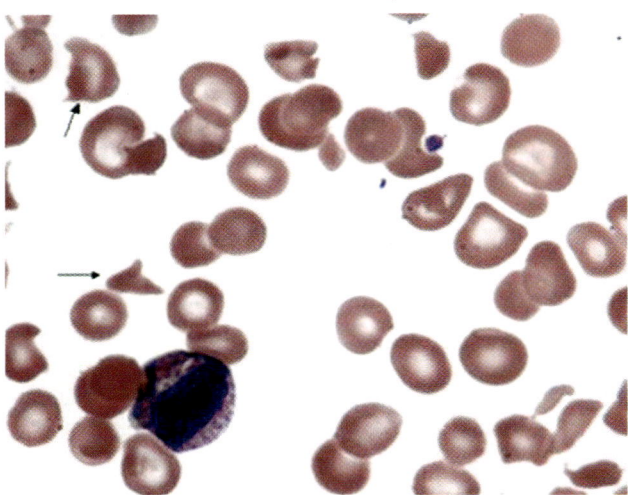

Figure 9-4 Peripheral smear showing red blood cell fragmentation consistent with a microangiopathic hemolytic process in a patient with thrombotic thrombocytopenic purpura.

antibody activity. These tests are not used as diagnostic tests but may be useful for the identification of patients at risk for relapse, which may be associated with severe ADAMTS13 deficiency either at presentation or in remission.

Management

The use of plasma exchange has dramatically changed acute TTP from a disorder with approximately 85% mortality to one with 85% survival. In a randomized trial of 103 adults with TTP, plasma exchange was more effective than plasma infusion. Fresh frozen plasma and cryosupernant plasma (depleted of vWF) are the replacement fluids of choice. The exchange of 1 to 1.5 plasma volumes is standard initial treatment; however, larger volume exchanges may have additional benefit in patients with an inadequate response. Generally, plasma exchange is continued daily until the platelet count reaches normal levels ($>150 \times 10^9/L$), LDH is normal, and symptoms have resolved. Once a response is achieved, plasma exchange may be discontinued or tapered. The role of aspirin and platelet-inhibiting drugs remains to be established. For patients who do not respond to plasma exchange, adjunctive therapies may be required including corticosteroids, immunosuppressive medications, or splenectomy. Promising results of observational studies using rituximab for the treatment of relapsed or refractory TTP are beginning to emerge.

In addition to disease-related morbidities, the procedure of plasma exchange itself is often associated with complications. In a large prospective registry of 249 patients followed from 1996 to 2008, 83 major complications occurred among 64 patients (26%), including catheter-related infection or thrombosis, pneumothorax, pulmonary hemorrhage, severe hypotension, and anaphylaxis. Transfusion-related acute lung injury has also been described in patients undergoing plasma exchange. The transmission of infectious diseases is exceedingly rare with current donor screening even with large volumes of plasma.

Treatment of *E coli*–associated HUS is generally supportive; the use of antibiotics remains controversial and is generally avoided. Plasma therapy is generally not required for HUS caused by *E coli* or pneumococcal infections but may be useful for atypical HUS to replace the deficiencies in complement factors.

> **Key points**
>
> • The presence of thrombocytopenia and microangiopathic hemolytic anemia is sufficient for the diagnosis of TTP and should prompt the initiation of treatment with plasma exchange.
> • HUS in children typically follows a prodrome of bloody diarrhea, is often complicated by acute renal failure, and typically does not require plasma exchange.
> • ADAMTS13 deficiency has been linked to familial and acquired idiopathic TTP as a result of a congenital deficiency or an acquired autoantibody, respectively.
> • Adjuvant rituximab may be effective at inducing a remission in patients with relapsed or refractory TTP.

Splenic sequestration

Splenic enlargement, usually from advanced liver disease or cirrhosis, results in pooling of platelets in the rich splenic vascular network and mild to moderate thrombocytopenia. Other mechanisms of thrombocytopenia in patients with cirrhosis include immune destruction by autoantibodies, the myelosuppressive action of viral agents such as hepatitis C virus, and the toxic effects of excessive alcohol ingestion. Therapy of chronic hepatitis with interferon may also induce thrombocytopenia. Recently, decreased TPO production in the cirrhotic liver has been shown to be an important contributing factor.

Familial thrombocytopenia

Familial thrombocytopenic syndromes are uncommon, and patients are often misdiagnosed as having ITP. Recognition of these disorders is important to avoid unnecessary and potentially harmful treatments including splenectomy. The diagnosis should be considered in any patient with thrombocytopenia (or "chronic ITP") and a family history of thrombocytopenia or in the absence of a platelet count increase after typical ITP treatments. The presence of anatomic defects, including absent radii (thrombocytopenia with absent radii syndrome) or right heart defects (as seen in DiGeorge syndrome), and laboratory features including large platelets and neutrophil inclusions on the blood film (as seen in the *MYH9*-related disorders) support the diagnosis of familial thrombocytopenia.

Autosomal dominant *MYH9*-related macrothrombocytopenic disorders are caused by mutations in the *MYH9* gene, which codes for nonmuscle myosin IIA. These include May-Hegglin, Fetchner, Sebastian, and Epstein syndromes. Associated features include large platelets, leukocyte inclusions called Döhle bodies (Figure 9-5), renal failure, hearing loss, and cataracts. Bernard-Soulier syndrome is an autosomal recessive familial thrombocytopenic disorder characterized by the absence of the platelet GPIb-V-IX complex, associated with giant platelets, lack of platelet aggregation by high-dose ristocetin, and bleeding. Wiskott-Aldrich syndrome is an X-linked disorder characterized by severe immunodeficiency, small platelets, and eczema. Congenital amegakaryocytic thrombocytopenia (CAMT) is a recessive disorder characterized by severe thrombocytopenia and absence of megakaryocytes in the bone marrow and results from mutations in the Mpl receptor. It leads to a trilineage failure. Inherited thrombocytopenias occur also in association with mutations in transcription factors regulating megakaryocytes and platelet production: GATA1 (sex-linked inheritance) and RUNX1 (autosomal dominant). Patients with the Paris-Trousseau/Jacobsen syndrome, an autosomal dominant macrothrombocytopenia, have psychomotor retardation and facial and cardiac abnormalities; this syndrome arises due to deletion of a portion of chromosome 11, 11q23-24, that encompasses transcription factor FLI-1 gene.

Establishing the diagnosis of familial thrombocytopenia is often problematic. Flow cytometry using monoclonal antibodies allows analysis of platelet glycoproteins to diagnose Bernard-Soulier syndrome. The detection of clusters of myosin in granulocytes using an immunofluorescent antibody against nonmuscle myosin heavy chain type IIa may aid in the diagnosis of *MYH9*-related disorders.

Other thrombocytopenic disorders

Thrombocytopenia with infection

Mild and transient thrombocytopenia predictably occurs with many systemic infections. Thrombocytopenia may be caused by a combination of mechanisms, including decreased production, increased destruction, and increased splenic sequestration. In some infections, specific mechanisms may predominate. In viral infections, platelet production may be suppressed; in rickettsial infections, platelets may be consumed in vasculitic lesions; in bacteremia, platelets may be consumed because of disseminated intravascular coagulation (DIC). Thrombocytopenia is commonly associated with HIV infection. Platelet kinetic studies in patients with HIV infection show that decreased platelet production occurs despite the presence of adequate numbers of normal-appearing marrow megakaryocytes. Thrombocytopenia will often improve during treatment with highly active antiretroviral therapy.

Hemophagocytic syndrome

Epstein-Barr virus–associated hemophagocytic syndrome is a rare but important cause of infection-related thrombocytopenia. The diagnosis is supported by hepatosplenomegaly, elevated ferritin, and triglycerides and confirmed by bone marrow or tissue biopsy showing evidence of hemophagocytosis.

Thrombocytopenia in the critically ill

Critically ill patients in the intensive care unit will frequently develop mild to moderate thrombocytopenia. Severe thrombocytopenia (platelet count $<50 \times 10^9$/L) occurs in approximately 5% of patients and may be associated with bleeding. This topic is covered in more detail in Chapter 2. Thrombocytopenia is most often due to a combination of enhanced clearance (eg, in the setting of DIC) and reduced production due to the catabolic state frequently found in such patients. It is likely that platelet transfusion is not needed until the platelet count decreases to $<20 \times 10^9$/L; however, there is no good quality evidence to guide therapy for such patients. Actively bleeding patients or those undergoing invasive procedures such as central venous cannulation should likely receive platelet transfusions, although the optimal threshold for transfusions is not known. In a prospective cohort study, platelet transfusion administered to critically ill patients was associated with an increased risk

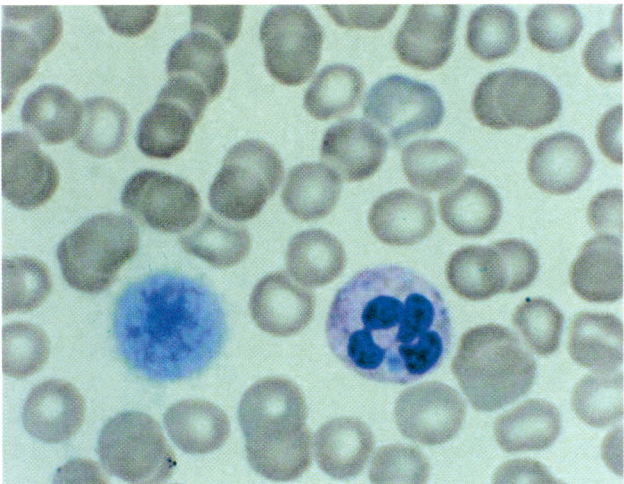

Figure 9-5 Peripheral smear showing a giant platelet (left) and a granulocyte with inclusions called Döhle bodies (right) in a patient with May-Hegglin syndrome.

of deep venous thrombosis. Furthermore, platelets may cause transfusion reactions. Because both of these complications will make management of critically ill patients more complex, such transfusion should be administered after careful consideration.

> **Key points**
>
> • Thrombocytopenia in patients with liver cirrhosis is often multifactorial and may be caused by splenomegaly, hepatitis C virus–induced platelet autoantibodies, or myelosuppression from alcohol.
> • Familial thrombocytopenia should be suspected in patients with presumed ITP who do not respond to treatment.
> • The *MYH9*-related disorders are the most common cause of familial thrombocytopenia and are characterized by large platelets and granulocyte inclusions.

Disorders of platelet function

Disorders of platelet function are characterized by highly variable mucocutaneous bleeding manifestations and excessive hemorrhage following surgical procedures or trauma. Spontaneous hemarthrosis and deep hematomas are unusual in patients with platelet defects. In general, most patients have mild to moderate bleeding manifestations. A majority of patients, but not all, have a prolonged bleeding time. Platelet aggregation and secretion studies provide evidence for the defect but are not always predictive of the severity of clinical manifestations. Defects in platelet function may be inherited or acquired, with the latter being far more commonly encountered. The platelet dysfunction in these patients arises by diverse mechanisms.

Inherited disorders of platelet function

> **Clinical case**
>
> A 9-year-old girl is referred by her pediatrician for evaluation of longstanding easy bruising and recurrent epistaxis. She has not had any surgery. The physical examination reveals scattered bruises on the lower extremities. The platelet count is 190,000/μL, and the hemoglobin is 11 g/dL. The bleeding time is prolonged at 14 minutes (normal range, 3-7 minutes), and plasma levels of factor VIII, vWF antigen, and ristocetin cofactor are within normal range. Previous blood work had also demonstrated normal platelet counts. The hematologist recommends platelet aggregation studies. These studies reveal abnormal platelet aggregation responses upon activation—a primary wave but no secondary wave in response to ADP and epinephrine and decreased aggregation with collagen. The response to ristocetin is normal. The hematologist discusses the diagnosis and management with the parents.

Table 9-4 provides a classification of inherited disorders associated with impaired platelet function, based on the platelet function or responses that are abnormal (Figure 9-1). Of note, not all of them are due to a defect in the platelets per se. Some, such as vWD and afibrinogenemia, result from deficiencies of plasma proteins essential for normal platelet function. Some of these disorders are distinctly rare, but they shed enormous light on platelet physiology. Moreover, in many patients with inherited abnormalities in platelet aggregation responses, the underlying molecular mechanisms remain unknown. In patients with defects in platelet–vessel wall interactions (adhesion disorders), adhesion of platelets to subendothelium is abnormal. The 2 disorders in this group are vWD, due to a deficiency or abnormality in plasma vWF, and the Bernard-Soulier syndrome (BSS), in which platelets are deficient in GPIb (and GPV and GPIX); in both disorders, platelet–vWF interaction is compromised. Binding of fibrinogen to the GPIIb-IIIa complex is a prerequisite for platelet aggregation. Disorders characterized by abnormal platelet–platelet interactions (aggregation disorders) arise because of a severe deficiency of plasma fibrinogen (congenital afibrinogenemia) or because of a quantitative or qualitative abnormality of the platelet membrane GPIIb-IIIa complex, which binds fibrinogen (Glanzmann thrombasthenia). Patients with defects in platelet secretion and signal transduction are a heterogeneous group lumped together for convenience of classification rather than based on an understanding of the specific underlying abnormality. The major common characteristics in these patients, as currently perceived, are abnormal aggregation responses and an inability to release intracellular granule (dense) contents upon activation of platelet-rich plasma with agonists such as ADP, epinephrine, and collagen. In aggregation studies, the second wave of aggregation is blunted or absent. The patient described in the clinical case at the beginning of this section falls in this large group; the platelet dysfunction may arise from a variety of mechanisms. A small proportion of these patients have a deficiency of dense granule stores (storage pool deficiency). In other patients, the impaired secretion results from aberrations in the signal transduction events that govern end responses such as secretion and aggregation. Another group consists of patients who have an abnormality in interactions of platelets with proteins of the coagulation system; the best described is the Scott syndrome, which is characterized by impaired transmembrane migration of procoagulant phosphatidylserine. Defects related to platelet cytoskeleton or structural proteins may also be associated with platelet dysfunction. Recent studies document impaired platelet function associated with mutations in transcription factors (eg, RUNX1, GATA1, FLI-1) that regulate expression of important platelet proteins. In addition to the above groups, there are patients who have abnormal platelet function

Table 9-4 Inherited disorders of platelet function.

1. Defects in platelet–vessel wall interaction (disorders of adhesion)
   a. von Willebrand disease (deficiency or defect in plasma von Willebrand factor)
   b. Bernard-Soulier syndrome (deficiency or defect in GPIb)
2. Defects in platelet–platelet interaction (disorders of aggregation)
   a. Congenital afibrinogenemia (deficiency of plasma fibrinogen)
   b. Glanzmann thrombasthenia (deficiency or defect in GPIIb-IIIa)
3. Disorders of platelet secretion and abnormalities of granules
   a. Storage pool deficiency (δ, α, αδ)
   b. Quebec platelet disorder
4. Disorders of platelet secretion and signal transduction
   a. Defects in platelet-agonist interaction (receptor defects) (ADP, thromboxane A_2, collagen, epinephrine)
   b. Defects in G proteins (Gαq, Gαs, Gαi abnormalities)
   c. Defects in phosphatidylinositol metabolism and protein phosphorylation (phospholipase C-β2 deficiency; PKC-Θ deficiency)
   d. Abnormalities in arachidonic acid pathways and thromboxane A_2 synthesis
      i. Phospholipase A_2 deficiency
      ii. Cyclooxygenase deficiency
      iii. Thromboxane synthase deficiency
5. Disorders of platelet coagulant–protein interaction (Scott syndrome)
6. Defects related to cytoskeletal/structural proteins (Wiskott-Aldrich syndrome protein; β1 tubulin)
7. Abnormalities of transcription factors leading to functional defects
   a. RUNX1 (familial platelet dysfunction with predisposition to acute myelogenous leukemia)
   b. GATA1
   c. FLI-1 (dimorphic dysmorphic platelets with giant α granules and thrombocytopenia; Paris-Trousseau/Jacobsen syndrome)

Modified with permission from Rao AK. Congenital disorders of platelet function: disorders of signal transduction and secretion. *Am J Med Sci.* 1998;316:69–76.
ADP = adenosine diphosphate; PKC = protein kinase C.

associated with systemic disorders, such as Down syndrome and the May-Hegglin anomaly, where the specific aberrant platelet mechanisms are unclear. Overall, the prevalence and relative frequency of the various platelet abnormalities remain unknown.

Disorders of platelet adhesion
Bernard-Soulier Syndrome

BSS is a rare autosomal recessive platelet function disorder resulting from an abnormality in the platelet GPIb-IX complex, which mediates the binding of VWF to platelets and thus plays a major role in platelet adhesion to the subendothelium, especially at the higher shear rates. GPIb exists in platelets as a complex consisting of GPIb, GPIX, and GPV. There are approximately 25,000 copies of GPIb-IX on platelets, and these are reduced or abnormal in the BSS. Although GPV is also decreased in BSS platelets, it is not required for platelet surface GPIb/IX expression. The bleeding time is markedly prolonged, the platelet counts are moderately decreased, and on the peripheral smear, the platelets are markedly increased in size. In platelet aggregation studies, the responses to the commonly used agonists ADP, epinephrine, thrombin, and collagen are normal. Characteristically, the aggregation in platelet-rich plasma in response to ristocetin is decreased or absent, a feature shared with patients with vWD. However, unlike in vWD, plasma vWF and factor VIII are normal in BSS, and addition of exogenous vWF (present in plasma cryoprecipitate fractions) does not restore ristocetin-induced agglutination of platelets because of the GPIb deficiency. Dense granule secretion on activation with thrombin may be decreased.

The blood film from a patient with BSS may resemble that from some patients with ITP in that the platelets tend to be larger than normal, and there is a mild to moderate thrombocytopenia. The diagnosis of BSS is established by demonstrating decreased platelet surface GPIb, which can be performed using flow cytometry.

Von Willebrand disease

See section titled von Willebrand Disease in Chapter 2.

Disorders of platelet aggregation
Glanzmann thrombasthenia

Glanzmann thrombasthenia is a rare autosomal recessive disorder characterized by markedly impaired platelet aggregation, a prolonged bleeding time, and relatively more severe mucocutaneous bleeding manifestations than most platelet function disorders. It has been reported in clusters in populations where consanguinity is common. Normal resting platelets possess approximately 50,000 to 80,000 GPIIb-IIIa complexes on the surface. The primary abnormality in Glanzmann thrombasthenia is a quantitative or qualitative defect in the GPIIb-IIIa complex, a heterodimer consisting of GPIIb and GPIIIa whose synthesis is governed by distinct genes located on chromosome 17. Thus, thrombasthenia may arise due to a mutation in either gene, with decreased platelet expression of the complex. Because of this, fibrinogen binding to platelets on activation and aggregation are impaired. Clot retraction, a function of the interaction of GPIIb-IIIa with the platelet cytoskeleton, is also impaired.

The diagnostic hallmark of thrombasthenia is absence or marked decrease of platelet aggregation in response virtually to all platelet agonists (except ristocetin), with absence of both the primary and secondary wave of aggregation; the shape change response is preserved. Platelet-dense granule secretion may be decreased with weak agonists (eg, ADP) but normal on activation with thrombin. Heterozygotes have approximately half the number of platelet GPIIb-IIIa complexes, but platelet aggregation responses are normal. Although congenital afibrinogenemia is also characterized by a similar absence of platelet aggregation, in this disorder, the prothrombin time, activated partial thromboplastin time, and thrombin time are markedly prolonged, whereas they are normal in thrombasthenia. The diagnosis of thrombasthenia can be established by demonstrating decreased platelet expression of the GPIIb-GPIIIa complex using flow cytometry.

Disorders of platelet secretion and signal transduction

As a unifying theme, patients lumped in this remarkably heterogeneous group are generally characterized by impaired dense granule secretion and absence of the second wave of aggregation upon stimulation of platelet-rich plasma with ADP or epinephrine; responses to collagen, thromboxane analog (U46619), and arachidonic acid may also be impaired. Conceptually, platelet function is abnormal in these patients either when the granule contents are diminished (storage pool deficiency [SPD]) or when the mechanisms leading to aggregation and secretion are impaired (Table 9-4).

Deficiency of granule stores

SPD refers to patients with deficiencies in platelet content of dense granules (δ-SPD), α granules (α-SPD), or both types of granules (αδ-SPD).

Patients with δ-SPD have a mild to moderate bleeding diathesis associated with a prolonged bleeding time. In the platelet studies, the second wave of aggregation in response to ADP and epinephrine is absent or blunted, and the collagen response is markedly impaired. Normal platelets possess 3 to 8 dense granules (each 200-300 nm in diameter). Under the electron microscope, dense granules are decreased in SPD platelets. By direct biochemical measurements, the total platelet and granule ATP and ADP contents are decreased along with other dense granule constituents, calcium, pyrophosphate, and serotonin.

δ-SPD has been reported in association with other inherited disorders such as the Hermansky-Pudlak syndrome (HPS) (oculocutaneous albinism and increased reticuloendothelial ceroid), Chédiak-Higashi syndrome, Wiskott-Aldrich syndrome, thrombocytopenia with absent radii syndrome, and Griscelli syndrome. The simultaneous occurrence of δ-SPD and defects in skin pigment granules, as in the HPS, point to the interrelatedness of the 2 kinds of granules with respect to genetic control.

There is a large group of HPS patients in northwest Puerto Rico where HPS occurs in 1 of every 1800 individuals. There are at least 7 known HPS-causing genes, with most patients having HPS-1 and being from Puerto Rico. These HPS subtypes are autosomal recessive, and the heterozygotes have no clinical findings. In addition to the albinism, most patients have congenital nystagmus and decreased visual acuities. Two additional manifestations in HPS patients are granulomatous colitis and pulmonary fibrosis.

Chédiak-Higashi syndrome is a rare autosomal recessive disorder characterized by SPD, oculocutaneous albinism, immune deficiency, cytotoxic T and natural killer (NK) cell dysfunction, neurologic symptoms, and presence of giant cytoplasmic inclusions in different cells. It arises from mutations in the lysosomal trafficking regulator (*LYST*) gene on chromosome 1.

Patients with the *gray platelet syndrome* have an isolated deficiency of platelet α-granule contents. The name refers to the initial observation that the platelets have a gray appearance with paucity of granules on the peripheral blood smears. These patients have a bleeding diathesis, mild thrombocytopenia, and a prolonged bleeding time. The inheritance pattern has been variable; autosomal recessive, autosomal dominant, and sex-linked patterns have been noted. Under the electron microscope, platelets and megakaryocytes reveal absent or markedly decreased α granules. The platelets are severely and selectively deficient in α-granule proteins including PF4, βTG, vWF, thrombospondin, fibronectin, factor V, and PDGF. In some patients, plasma levels of PF4 and βTG have been found to be raised, suggesting that the defect is not in their synthesis by megakaryocytes but in their packaging into granules. Platelet aggregation responses have been variable. Responses to ADP and epinephrine were normal in most patients; in some patients, aggregation responses to thrombin, collagen, and ADP have been impaired.

The *Quebec platelet disorder*, another disorder affecting the platelet granules, is an autosomal dominant disorder associated with delayed bleeding and abnormal proteolysis of α-granule proteins (including fibrinogen, factor V, vWF, thrombospondin, multimerin, and P-selectin) due to increased amounts of platelet urokinase-type plasminogen activator. These patients are characterized by normal to reduced platelet counts, proteolytic degradation of α-granule proteins, and defective aggregation selectively with epinephrine.

Defects in platelet signal transduction and platelet activation

Signal transduction mechanisms encompass processes that are initiated by the interaction of agonists with specific platelet receptors and include responses such as G protein activation and activation of phospholipase C and phospholipase A_2 (Figure 9-1). If the key components in signal transduction are the surface receptors, the G proteins, and the effector enzymes, evidence now exists for specific platelet abnormalities at each of these levels.

Patients with receptor defects have impaired responses because of an abnormality in the platelet surface receptor for a specific agonist. Such defects have been documented for receptors for ADP, TxA_2, collagen, and epinephrine. Patients with the ADP receptor abnormalities have had a defect in the P2Y12 ADP receptor, which is coupled to inhibition of adenylyl cyclase and is the receptor targeted by thienopyridines (clopidogrel). Because ADP and TxA_2 play a synergistic role in platelet responses to several agonists, these patients with specific receptor defects manifest abnormal aggregation responses to multiple agonists. Patients described with abnormal platelet responses to collagen have had deficiencies in membrane glycoproteins GPIa or GPVI.

G proteins are a link between surface receptors and intracellular effector enzymes, and defects in G protein activation can impair signal transduction. Patients with deficiencies at the level of Gαq, Gαi1, and Gαs have been described.

Patients have been described with impaired signal transduction due to defects in phospholipase C activation, calcium mobilization, and pleckstrin phosphorylation. Specific deficiencies at the level of phospholipase C-β2 and PKC-Θ have been documented.

A major platelet response to activation is liberation of arachidonic acid from phospholipids and its subsequent oxygenation to TxA_2, which plays a synergistic role in the response to several agonists. Patients have been described with impaired thromboxane synthesis due to congenital deficiencies of phospholipase A_2, cyclooxygenase, and thromboxane synthase.

Disorders of platelet procoagulant activities

Platelets play a major role in blood coagulation by providing the surface on which several specific key enzymatic reactions occur. In resting platelets, there is an asymmetry in the distribution of some of the phospholipids such that phosphatidylserine (PS) and phosphatidylethanolamine are located predominantly on the inner leaflet, whereas phosphatidylcholine has the opposite distribution. Platelet activation results in a redistribution with expression of PS on the outer surface, mediated by phospholipid scramblase. The exposure of PS on the outer surface is an important event in the expression of platelet procoagulant activities. A few patients have been described in whom the platelet contribution to blood coagulation is impaired, and this is referred to as Scott syndrome. In these patients, who have a bleeding disorder, the bleeding time and platelet aggregation responses have been normal.

Other abnormalities

Platelet function abnormalities have been described in association with other entities, such as in the *Wiskott-Aldrich syndrome* (WAS), an X-linked inherited disorder affecting T lymphocytes and platelets characterized by thrombocytopenia, immunodeficiency, and eczema. The bleeding manifestations are variable. Several platelet abnormalities including dense granule deficiency and deficiencies of platelet GPIb, GPIIb/IIIa, and GPIa have been reported in WAS. WAS arises from mutations in the gene coding for the WAS protein, which constitutes a link between the cytoskeleton and signaling pathways. Platelet dysfunction occurs also with mutations in tubulin-1, a cytoskeletal protein. More recently, abnormal platelet function has been documented in patients with mutations in transcription factors RUNX1 (also called core-binding factor A2), GATA1, and FLI-1. Patients with RUNX1 mutations have familial thrombocytopenia, platelet dysfunction, and predisposition to acute leukemia.

Therapy of inherited platelet function defects

Because of the wide disparity in bleeding manifestations, management needs to be individualized. Platelet transfusions are indicated in the management of significant bleeding and in preparation for surgical procedures. Platelet transfusions are effective in controlling the bleeding manifestations but come with potential risks associated with blood products including alloimmunization in patients lacking platelet glycoproteins. For example, patients with Glanzmann thrombasthenia and BSS may develop antibodies against GPIIb-IIIa and GPIb, respectively, that compromise the efficacy of subsequent platelet transfusions. An alternative to platelet transfusions is intravenous administration of desmopressin (DDAVP), which shortens the bleeding time in some patients with platelet function defects; this is dependent on the platelet abnormality. Most patients with thrombasthenia do not show a shortening of the bleeding time following DDAVP infusion, whereas responses in patients with signaling or secretory defects have been variable, with a shortening of the bleeding time in some patients. More recently, recombinant factor VIIa has been used in the management of bleeding events in patients with Glanzmann thrombasthenia and some other inherited defects. DDAVP and recombinant factor VIIa are not currently approved by the US Food and Drug Administration for management of patients with inherited platelet defects; however, factor VIIa is indicated to control bleeding in patients with thrombasthenia in Europe.

Key points

- Patients with inherited platelet defects typically have mucocutaneous bleeding manifestations; spontaneous hemarthrosis is rare.
- Patients with the BSS have thrombocytopenia, large platelet size, and a defect in the platelet GPIb-V-IX complex, leading to impaired binding of vWF and adhesion.
- Patients with Glanzmann thrombasthenia have absent or decreased platelet GPIIb-IIIa, leading to impaired binding of fibrinogen and absent aggregation to all of the usual agonists except ristocetin.
- Patients with δ-SPD have decreased dense granule contents; some patients may have associated albinism, nystagmus, and neurologic manifestations.
- Patients with the gray platelet syndrome have decreased α-granule contents.
- In a substantial number of patients with abnormal aggregation responses, the underlying mechanisms are unknown. Some of the patients have defects in platelet activation/signaling mechanisms.

Acquired disorders of platelet function

Alterations in platelet function occur in many acquired disorders of diverse etiologies (Table 9-5). The specific biochemical and pathophysiologic aberrations leading to platelet dysfunction are poorly understood in most of them. In some, such as the myeloproliferative disorders (MPD), there is production of intrinsically abnormal platelets by the bone marrow. In others, the dysfunction results from interaction of platelets with exogenous factors, such as pharmacologic agents, artificial surfaces (cardiopulmonary bypass), compounds that accumulate in plasma due to impaired renal function, and antibodies. In these disorders of platelet dysfunction, the bleeding is usually mucocutaneous with a wide and often unpredictable spectrum of severity. The

Table 9-5 Disorders in which acquired defects in platelet function are recognized.

Uremia
Myeloproliferative disorders
Acute leukemias and myelodysplastic syndromes
Dysproteinemias
Cardiopulmonary bypass
Acquired storage pool deficiency
Antiplatelet antibodies
Drugs and other agents

usual laboratory tests that suggest a platelet dysfunction are a prolonged bleeding time and abnormal results in studies of platelet aggregation or the platelet function analyzer (PFA)-100. The bleeding time and the PFA-100 are not reliable discriminators, because these tests may be variably abnormal or normal, even in individuals with impaired platelet aggregation responses. In patients with acquired platelet dysfunction, the correlation between the abnormalities in platelet aggregation studies and clinical bleeding remains weak.

Myeloproliferative disorders

Bleeding tendency, thromboembolic complications, and qualitative platelet defects are all recognized in MPDs, which include essential thrombocythemia, polycythemia vera, chronic idiopathic myelofibrosis, and chronic myelogenous leukemia. The platelet abnormalities result from their development from an abnormal clone of stem cells, but some of the alterations may be secondary to enhanced platelet activation in vivo. The clinical impact of the in vitro qualitative platelet defects, which occur even in asymptomatic patients, is often unclear.

Numerous studies have examined platelet function and morphology in patients with MPD. Under the electron microscope, the platelet findings include reduction in dense and α granules, alterations in the open canalicular and dense tubular systems, and a reduction of mitochondria. The bleeding time is prolonged in a minority (∼17%) of MPD patients and does not correlate with an increased risk of bleeding. Platelet aggregation responses are highly variable in MPD patients and often vary in the same patient over time. Decreased platelet responses are more common, although some patients demonstrate enhanced responses to agonists. In one analysis, responses to ADP, collagen, and epinephrine were decreased in 39%, 37%, and 57% of patients, respectively. The impairment in aggregation in response to epinephrine is more commonly encountered than with other agonists; however, a diminished response to epinephrine is not pathognomonic of an MPD. Platelet abnormalities described in MPD include decreased platelet α_2-adrenergic receptors, TxA_2 production, and dense granule secretion and abnormalities in platelet surface expression of GPIIb-IIIa complexes, GPIb, and GPIa-IIa.

Platelets from patients with polycythemia vera and idiopathic myelofibrosis, but not essential thrombocythemia or chronic myelogenous leukemia, have been shown to have reduced expression of the TPO receptor (Mpl) and reduced TPO-induced tyrosine phosphorylation of proteins. MPD patients have been reported to have defects in platelet signaling mechanisms.

Acquired abnormalities in plasma vWF have been documented in MPD patients with elevated platelet counts and may contribute to the hemostatic defect. Plasma vWF, particularly the large vWF multimers, is decreased, is inversely related to the platelet counts, and has improved following cytoreduction. These changes in plasma vWF occur in patients with reactive thrombocytosis as well.

Acute leukemias and myelodysplastic syndromes

The major cause of bleeding in these conditions is thrombocytopenia. However, in patients with normal or elevated platelet counts, bleeding complications may be associated with platelet dysfunction and altered platelet and megakaryocyte morphology. Acquired platelet defects associated with clinical bleeding are more common in acute myelogenous leukemia but have been reported in acute lymphoblastic and myelomonoblastic leukemias, hairy cell leukemia, and myelodysplastic syndromes.

Dysproteinemias

Excessive clinical bleeding may occur in patients with dysproteinemias, and this appears to be related to multiple mechanisms including platelet dysfunction, specific coagulation factor abnormalities, hyperviscosity, and alterations in blood vessels due to amyloid deposition. Qualitative platelet defects occur in some of these patients and have been attributed to coating of platelets by the paraprotein.

Uremia

Patients with uremia are at an increased risk for bleeding complications. The pathogenesis of the hemostatic defect in uremia remains unclear, but platelet dysfunction and impaired platelet–vessel wall interaction, comorbid conditions, and the concomitant use of medications that affect hemostasis are major factors. The bleeding time may be prolonged; anemia also contributes to the prolongation, which may shorten following red blood cell transfusion or treatment with erythropoietin.

Multiple platelet function abnormalities are recognized in uremia including impaired adhesion, aggregation, and secretion. These hemostatic defects may be linked to the accumulation of dialyzable and nondialyzable molecules in the plasma. One such compound, guanidinosuccinic acid, accumulates in plasma, inhibits platelets in vitro, and stimulates generation of nitric oxide, which inhibits platelet responses by increasing levels of cellular cyclic guanosine monophosphate.

Aggressive dialysis can ameliorate uremic bleeding diathesis in many patients. Hemodialysis and peritoneal dialysis are equally effective. Platelet transfusions are indicated in the management of acute major bleeds. Other treatments including DDAVP, cryoprecipitate, and conjugated estrogens have also been shown to be beneficial. Elevation of the hematocrit with packed red blood cells or recombinant erythropoietin may shorten bleeding times, improve platelet adhesion, and correct mild bleeding in uremic patients. The beneficial effect of red blood cells has been attributed to rheologic factors whereby the red blood cells exert an outward radial pressure promoting platelet–vessel interactions.

Other factors predisposing to bleeding in patients with renal failure include concomitant administration of antiplatelet agents or anticoagulant medications.

Acquired SPD

Several patients have been reported in whom the dense granule SPD appears to be acquired. This defect probably reflects in vivo release of dense granule contents due to platelet activation or production of abnormal platelets. Acquired SPD has been observed in patients with antiplatelet antibodies, systemic lupus erythematosus, chronic ITP, DIC, HUS, renal transplantation rejection, multiple congenital cavernous hemangioma, MPD, acute and chronic leukemias, and severe valvular disease, and in patients undergoing cardiopulmonary bypass.

Antiplatelet antibodies and platelet function

Binding of antibodies to platelets may produce several effects, including accelerated destruction, platelet activation, cell lysis, aggregation, secretion of granule contents, and outward exposure of PS. Patients with ITP have decreased platelet survival and may have impaired platelet function and prolonged bleeding times even at adequate counts. In many patients, the antibodies are directed against specific platelet surface membrane glycoproteins that play a major role in normal platelet function, including GPIb, GPIIb-IIIa, GPIa-IIa, and GPVI, and glycosphingolipids. These antibodies, in effect, induce acquired forms of BSS and thrombasthenia.

Drugs that inhibit platelet function

Many drugs affect platelet function. For several, the effects on platelets have been studied in vitro, and the relevance of such findings to the drug levels achieved in clinical practice is not well established. Even among those drugs shown to alter platelet responses ex vivo, the impact on hemostasis often remains unclear. Moreover, the impact of concomitant administration of multiple drugs, each with a mild effect on platelet function, is unknown, although this may be clinically relevant. Because of their widespread use, aspirin and nonsteroidal anti-inflammatory agents are an important cause of platelet inhibition in clinical practice. Aspirin ingestion results in inhibition of platelet aggregation and secretion upon stimulation with ADP, epinephrine, and low concentrations of collagen. Aspirin irreversibly acetylates and inactivates the platelet cyclooxygenase, leading to the inhibition of synthesis of endoperoxides (prostaglandin G_2 and H_2) and TxA_2. Typically, it is recommended to wait 5 to 7 days after cessation of aspirin ingestion to perform studies intended to assess platelet function and elective invasive procedures to ensure that the antiplatelet effect is gone. Several other nonsteroidal anti-inflammatory drugs also impair platelet function by inhibiting the cyclooxygenase enzyme and may prolong the bleeding time. Compared with aspirin, the inhibition of cyclooxygenase by these agents is generally short-lived and reversible (1-2 days).

Ticlopidine, clopidogrel, and the recently Food and Drug Administration–approved prasugrel are orally administered thienopyridine derivatives that inhibit platelet function by inhibiting the binding of ADP to the platelet P2Y12 receptor. These drugs prolong the bleeding time and inhibit platelet aggregation responses to several agonists, including ADP, collagen, epinephrine, and thrombin, to various extents depending on agonist concentrations. GPIIb-IIIa receptor antagonists are compounds that inhibit platelet fibrinogen binding and platelet aggregation. These include a monoclonal antibody against the GPIIb-IIIa receptor (abciximab, ReoPro), a synthetic peptide containing the RGD sequence (eptifibatide, Integrilin), and a peptidomimetic (tirofiban, Aggrastat). They are potent inhibitors of aggregation in response to all of the usually used agonists (except ristocetin) and prolong the bleeding time. DITP (secondary to drug-dependent antibodies) occurs in 0.2% to 1.0% of patients on first exposure to GPIIb-III antagonists.

A host of other medications and agents, including oncologic drugs (eg, mithramycin) and food substances, inhibit platelet responses, but the clinical significance for many is unclear. β-Lactam antibiotics, including penicillins and cephalosporins, inhibit platelet aggregation responses and may contribute to a bleeding diathesis at high doses. These include carbenicillin, penicillin G, ticarcillin, ampicillin, nafcillin, azlocillin, cloxacillin, mezlocillin, oxacillin, piperacillin, and apalcillin. The platelet inhibition appears to be dose dependent, taking approximately 2 to 3 days to manifest and 3 to 10 days to abate after drug discontinuation. Cephalosporins may also impair platelet function. Moxalactam has been reported to induce platelet dysfunction associated with prolonged bleeding times and clinical hemorrhage. Other third-generation cephalosporins appear to show little effect on normal platelet function. The clinical significance of the effect of antibiotics on platelet function remains unclear. The general context in which the bleeding events are encountered in patients on antibiotics prevents identification of the precise role played by the antimicrobials because of the presence of concomitant factors (eg, thrombocytopenia, DIC, infection, vitamin K deficiency). Discontinuation of a specifically indicated antibiotic is usually not an option or necessary.

There is growing evidence that selective serotonin reuptake inhibitors (SSRIs) inhibit platelet function, and this has clinical relevance. Serotonin in plasma is taken up by platelets, incorporated into dense granules, and secreted on platelet activation. The SSRIs inhibit the uptake of serotonin and platelet aggregation and secretion responses to activation. In epidemiologic studies, patients on SSRIs have had increased gastrointestinal bleeding and increased bleeding with surgery. Lastly, given the increasing use of herbal medicines and food supplements, their role and interaction with pharmaceutical drugs need to be considered in the evaluation of patients with unexplained bleeding.

Key points

- Alterations in platelet function are described in many disorders of diverse etiologies; the clinical significance in terms of relationship to bleeding manifestations remains unclear in many.
- A careful drug history should be taken in any patient suspected to have platelet dysfunction.
- Aspirin nonsteroidal anti-inflammatory agents and other medications are a major cause of acquired platelet dysfunction.
- Patients with MPD may have altered platelet function that contributes to the bleeding manifestations.
- High platelet counts, as observed in MPD patients, may be associated with a loss of high molecular weight multimers of vWF in plasma.
- Patients with renal failure may have impaired platelet function related to accumulation of substances in plasma that increase platelet cyclic guanosine monophosphate levels.

Bibliography

Regulation of platelet number

de Sauvage FJ, Carver-Moore K, Luoh SM, et al. Physiological regulation of early and late stages of megakaryocytopoiesis by thrombopoietin. *J Exp Med*. 1996;183:651–656.

Italiano JE Jr, Lecine P, Shivdasani RA, Hartwig JH. Blood platelets are assembled principally at the ends of proplatelet processes produced by differentiated megakaryocytes. *J Cell Biol*. 1999;147:1299–1312.

Kaushansky K, Lok S, Holly RD, et al. Promotion of megakaryocyte progenitor expansion and differentiation by the c-Mpl ligand thrombopoietin. *Nature*. 1994;369:568–571.

Kuter DJ, Beeler DL, Rosenberg RD. The purification of megapoietin: a physiological regulator of megakaryocyte growth and platelet production. *Proc Natl Acad Sci U S A*. 1994;91:11104–11108.

Kuter DJ, Begley CG. Recombinant human thrombopoietin: basic biology and evaluation of clinical studies. *Blood*. 2002;100:3457–3469.

Patel SR, Richardson JL, Schulze H, et al. Differential roles of microtubule assembly and sliding in proplatelet formation by megakaryocytes. *Blood*. 2005;106:4076–4085.

Immune thrombocytopenia

Arnold DM, Dentali F, Crowther MA, et al. Systematic review: efficacy and safety of rituximab for adults with idiopathic thrombocytopenic purpura. *Ann Intern Med*. 2007;146:25–33.

Beck CE, Nathan PC, Parkin PC, Blanchette VS, Macarthur C. Corticosteroids versus intravenous immune globulin for the treatment of acute immune thrombocytopenic purpura in children: a systematic review and meta-analysis of randomized controlled trials. *J Pediatr*. 2005;147:521–527.

Bisharat N, Omari H, Lavi I, Raz R. Risk of infection and death among post-splenectomy patients. *J Infect*. 2001;43:182–186.

British Committee for Standards in Haematology Taskforce. Guidelines for the investigation and management of idiopathic thrombocytopenic purpura in adults, children and in pregnancy. *Br J Haematol*. 2003;120:574–596.

Bussel JB, Provan D, Shamsi T, et al. Effect of eltrombopag on platelet counts and bleeding during treatment of chronic idiopathic thrombocytopenic purpura: a randomised, double-blind, placebo-controlled trial. *Lancet*. 2009;373:641–648.

Cines DB, Bussel JB. How I treat idiopathic thrombocytopenic purpura (ITP). *Blood*. 2005;106:2244–2251.

Cines DB, Bussel JB, Liebman HA, Luning Prak ET. The ITP syndrome: pathogenic and clinical diversity. *Blood*. 2009;113:6511–6521.

Cohen YC, Djulbegovic B, Shamai-Lubovitz O, Mozes B. The bleeding risk and natural history of idiopathic thrombocytopenic purpura in patients with persistent low platelet counts. *Arch Intern Med*. 2000;160:1630–1638.

Cooper N, Woloski BM, Fodero EM, et al. Does treatment with intermittent infusions of intravenous anti-D allow a proportion of adults with recently diagnosed immune thrombocytopenic purpura to avoid splenectomy? *Blood*. 2002;99:1922–1927.

George JN, Woolf SH, Raskob GE, et al. Idiopathic thrombocytopenic purpura: a practice guideline developed by explicit methods for the American Society of Hematology. *Blood*. 1996;88:3–40.

Kojouri K, Vesely SK, Terrell DR, George JN. Splenectomy for adult patients with idiopathic thrombocytopenic purpura: a systematic review to assess long-term platelet count responses, prediction of response, and surgical complications. *Blood*. 2004;104:2623–2634.

Kuter DJ, Bussel JB, Lyons RM, et al. Efficacy of romiplostim in patients with chronic immune thrombocytopenic purpura: a double-blind randomised controlled trial. *Lancet*. 2008;371:395–403.

Mazzucconi MG, Fazi P, Bernasconi S, et al; Gruppo Italiano Malattie EMatologiche dell'Adulto (GIMEMA) Thrombocytopenia Working Party. Therapy with high-dose dexamethasone (HD-DXM) in previously untreated patients affected by idiopathic thrombocytopenic purpura: a GIMEMA experience. *Blood*. 2007;109:1401–1407.

Olsson B, Andersson PO, Jacobsson S, Carlsson L, Wadenvik H. Disturbed apoptosis of T-cells in patients with active idiopathic thrombocytopenic purpura. *Thromb Haemost*. 2005;93:139–144.

Provan D, Stasi R, Newland AC, et al. International consensus report on the investigation and management of primary immune thrombocytopenia. *Blood*. 2010;115:168–186.

Rodeghiero F, Stasi R, Gernsheimer T, et al. Standardization of terminology, definitions and outcome criteria in immune thrombocytopenic purpura (ITP) of adults and children: report from an international working group. *Blood*. 2009;113:2386–2393.

Schoonen WM, Kucera G, Coalson J, et al. Epidemiology of immune thrombocytopenic purpura in the General Practice Research Database. *Br J Haematol*. 2009;145:235–244.

Tarantino MD, Young G, Bertolone SJ, et al. Single dose of anti-D immune globulin at 75 microg/kg is as effective as intravenous immune globulin at rapidly raising the platelet count in newly diagnosed immune thrombocytopenic purpura in children. *J Pediatr*. 2006;148:489–494.

Zaja F, Baccarani M, Mazza P, et al. Dexamethasone plus rituximab yields higher sustained response rates than dexamethasone monotherapy in adults with primary immune thrombocytopenia. *Blood*. 2010;115:2755–62.

Drug-induced thrombocytopenia

Aster RH, Bougie DW. Drug-induced immune thrombocytopenia. *N Engl J Med*. 2007;357:580–587.

Aster RH, Curtis BR, McFarland JG, Bougie DW. Drug-induced immune thrombocytopenia: pathogenesis, diagnosis, and management. *J Thromb Haemost*. 2009;7:911–918.

George JN, Raskob GE, Shah SR, et al. Drug-induced thrombocytopenia: a systematic review of published case reports. *Ann Intern Med*. 1998;129:886–890.

Heparin-induced thrombocytopenia

Lo GK, Juhl D, Warkentin TE, et al. Evaluation of pretest clinical score (4 T's) for the diagnosis of heparin-induced thrombocytopenia in two clinical settings. *J Thromb Haemost*. 2006;4:759–765.

Warkentin TE. Heparin-induced thrombocytopenia: pathogenesis and management. *Br J Haematol*. 2003;121:535–555.

Warkentin TE, Greinacher A, Koster A, Lincoff AM. Treatment and prevention of heparin-induced thrombocytopenia: American College of Chest Physicians Evidence-Based Clinical Practice Guidelines (8th Edition). *Chest*. 2008;133 (Suppl 6):340S–380S.

Warkentin TE, Sheppard JA, Moore JC, Cook RJ, Kelton JG. Studies of the immune response in heparin-induced thrombocytopenia. *Blood*. 2009;113:4963–4969.

Thrombotic thrombocytopenic purpura

George JN. Evaluation and management of patients with thrombotic thrombocytopenic purpura. *J Intensive Care Med.* 2007;22:82–91.

Ling HT, Field JJ, Blinder MA. Sustained response with rituximab in patients with thrombotic thrombocytopenic purpura: a report of 13 cases and review of the literature. *Am J Hematol.* 2009;84:418–421.

McCrae KR, Cines DB, Sadler JE. *Derangements in the Complement Cascade Causing HUS.* Hoffman.

McCrae KR, Sadler JE, Cines DB. Thrombotic thrombocytopenic purpura and the hemolytic uremic syndrome. In: Hoffman R, Benz EJ, Shattil SJ, et al. *Hematology: Basic Principles and Practice.* 3rd ed. New York, NY: Churchill Livingstone; 2009:2009–2112.

Nguyen L, Terrell DR, Duvall D, Vesely SK, George JN. Complications of plasma exchange in patients treated for thrombotic thrombocytopenic purpura. IV. An additional study of 43 consecutive patients, 2005 to 2008. *Transfusion.* 2009;49:392–394.

Rock GA, Shumak KH, Buskard NA, et al. Comparison of plasma exchange with plasma infusion in the treatment of thrombotic thrombocytopenic purpura. Canadian Apheresis Study Group. *N Engl J Med.* 1991;325:393–397.

Sadler JE. Von Willebrand factor, ADAMTS13, and thrombotic thrombocytopenic purpura. *Blood.* 2008;112:11–18.

Nonimmune thrombocytopenia

Cines DB, Bussel JB, McMillan RB, Zehnder JL. Congenital and acquired thrombocytopenia. *Hematology Am Soc Hematol Educ Program.* 2004:390–406.

Crowther MA, Cook DJ, Meade MO, et al. Thrombocytopenia in medical-surgical critically ill patients: prevalence, incidence, and risk factors. *J Crit Care.* 2005;20:348–353.

Dong F, Li S, Pujol-Moix N, et al. Genotype-phenotype correlation in MYH9-related thrombocytopenia. *Br J Haematol.* 2005;130:620–627.

Drachman JG. Inherited thrombocytopenia: when a low platelet count does not mean ITP. *Blood.* 2004;103:390–398.

Inherited disorders of platelet function

Coller BS, Mitchell WB, French DL. Hereditary qualitative platelet disorders. In: Lichtman MA, Beutler E, Kipps TJ, Seligsohn U, Kaushansky K, Prchal JT, eds. *Williams Hematology.* 7th ed. New York, NY: McGraw-Hill; 2005:1795–1831.

George JN, Caen JP, Nurden AT. Glanzmann's thrombasthenia: the spectrum of clinical disease. *Blood.* 1990;75:1383–1395.

Huizing M, Helip-Wooley A, Westbroek W, Gunay-Aygun M, Gahl WA. Disorders of lysosome-related organelle biogenesis: clinical and molecular genetics. *Annu Rev Genomics Hum Genet.* 2008;9:359–386.

Lopez JA, Andrews RK, Afshar-Kharghan V, Berndt MC. Bernard-Soulier syndrome. *Blood.* 1998;91:4397–4418.

Mannucci PM, Levi M. Prevention and treatment of major blood loss. *N Engl J Med.* 2007;356:2301–2311.

Michaud J, Wu F, Osato M, et al. In vitro analyses of known and novel RUNX1/AML1 mutations in dominant familial platelet disorder with predisposition to acute myelogenous leukemia: implications for mechanisms of pathogenesis. *Blood.* 2002;99:1364–1372.

Nurden P, Nurden AT. Congenital disorders associated with platelet dysfunctions. *Thromb Haemost.* 2008;99:253–263.

Rao AK. Hereditary disorders of platelet secretion and signal transduction. In: Colman RW, Marder VJ, Clowes AW, George JN, Goldhaber SZ, eds. *Hemostasis and Thrombosis: Basic Principles and Clinical Practice.* 5th ed. Philadelphia, PA: Lippincott Williams & Wilkins; 2006:961–974.

Rao AK, Ghosh S, Sun L, Yang X, Disa J, Polansky M. A randomized double blind trial of 1-desamino-8-D-arginine vasopressin (DDVAP) in congenital platelet defects. *Thromb Haemost.* 1993;69:2316.

Sun L, Mao G, Rao AK. Association of CBFA2 mutation with decreased platelet PKC-theta and impaired receptor-mediated activation of GPIIb-IIIa and pleckstrin phosphorylation: proteins regulated by CBFA2 play a role in GPIIb-IIIa activation. *Blood.* 2004;103:948–954.

Weiss HJ. Impaired platelet procoagulant mechanisms in patients with bleeding disorders. *Semin Thromb Hemost.* 2009;35:233–241.

Acquired disorders of platelet function

Abrams CS, Shattil SJ, Bennett JS. Acquired qualitative platelet disorders. In: Lichtman MA, Beutler E, Kipps TJ, Seligsohn U, Kaushansky K, Prchal JT, eds. *Williams Hematology.* 7th ed. New York, NY: McGraw-Hill; 2005:1833–1856.

Boccardo P, Remuzzi G, Galbusera M. Platelet dysfunction in renal failure. *Semin Thromb Hemost.* 2004;30:579–589.

Budde U, van Genderen PJ. Acquired von Willebrand disease in patients with high platelet counts. *Semin Thromb Hemost.* 1997;23:425–431.

Landolfi R, Marchioli R, Patrono C. Mechanisms of bleeding and thrombosis in myeloproliferative disorders. *Thromb Haemost.* 1997;78:617–621.

Moliterno AR, Hankins WD, Spivak JL. Impaired expression of the thrombopoietin receptor by platelets from patients with polycythemia vera. *N Engl J Med.* 1998;338:572–580.

Noris M, Remuzzi G. Uremic bleeding: closing the circle after 30 years of controversies? *Blood.* 1999;94:2569–2574.

Rao AK. Acquired qualitative platelet disorders. In: Colman RW, Marder VJ, Clowes AW, George JN, Goldhaber SZ, eds. *Hemostasis and Thrombosis: Basic Principles and Clinical Practice.* 5th ed. Philadelphia, PA: Lippincott Williams & Wilkins; 2006:1045–1060.

Schafer AI. Bleeding and thrombosis in myeloproliferative disorders. *Blood.* 1984;64:1–12.

Sohal AS, Gangji AS, Crowther MA, Treleaven D. Uremic bleeding: pathophysiology and clinical risk factors. *Thromb Res.* 2006;118:417–422.

CHAPTER 10

Laboratory hematology

Georgette A. Dent and Charles S. Eby

General concepts, 263
Terminology, 263
Specific laboratory tests, 263
Bibliography, 288

General concepts

Laboratory tests are ordered and interpreted within the context of a specific patient as routine screening during a periodic examination, in the setting of an illness for diagnosis or follow-up, or for preoperative assessment. Clinical judgment is applied in both the selection of tests and in their interpretation, and unexpected results should be considered within the framework of the patient and the disease. Some unexpected results may require confirmation, particularly if the integrity of the specimen cannot be ensured (eg, heparin contamination, wrong collection tube or volume of blood, delayed processing). Additional causes of inaccurate laboratory results include sample mislabeling, analytical mistakes, and reporting errors.

Terminology

Sensitivity is the ability of a test to detect a true abnormality; as the sensitivity of a test increases, the risk of a false-positive result increases (increasing sensitivity comes at the cost of decreasing specificity). Very sensitive tests are helpful for screening, by ruling out a diagnosis or disease when the test is negative (high negative predictive value).

Specificity is the ability of a test to detect a normal result if the abnormality is not present; as the specificity increases, the risk of a false-negative result increases. Specific tests are useful for confirmation, by ruling in a diagnosis or disease when the test is positive (high positive predictive value).

Conflict-of-interest disclosure: *Dr. Dent:* declares no competing financial interest. *Dr. Eby:* consultancy: Barr Pharmaceuticals; research funding: Osmetech, Beckman-Coulter, Stago Diagnostica; honoraria: Genome Quebec.

Precision is reproducibility of a value during repeated testing of a sample.

Accuracy is the ability of a test to obtain the assigned value of an external standard (run as though it were a clinical sample).

Predictive value is the likelihood that an abnormal test indicates a patient with the abnormality (*positive predictive value*) or the likelihood that a normal test indicates a patient without the abnormality (*negative predictive value*). Positive and negative predictive values depend on the frequency of the abnormality being sought in the population as well as the sensitivity and specific of the laboratory methods.

Reference ranges are derived from a sample of a well population, and typically 95% of healthy individuals will have values that fall within the reference range.

Specific laboratory tests

Automated blood cell counting

In addition to complete blood counts (CBCs) and 5-part leukocyte differential counts (LDCs), hematology analyzers now provide quantitative and qualitative information about reticulocytes, nucleated red blood cells, and platelets. Additional information, such as platelet immaturity, extended leukocyte counts, and reticulocyte-specific indices, is only available from selected instrument manufacturers. Due to the large number of cells counted from each blood sample and analysis using multiple physical principles and sophisticated software, hematology analyzers generally produce accurate and precise CBCs and LDCs, with the exception of basophils. They also provide excellent sensitivity to distinguish between normal and abnormal samples via operator alerts prompting microscopic review of a stained peripheral blood smear for selected samples. As a result, approximately 30% of samples require review of a stained blood smear for microscopic review.

Automated blood cell counters use various technologies to enumerate and classify blood cells (Figure 10-1).

Aperture impedance

Cells diluted in a conducting solution are counted, and their volume is determined by measuring change in electrical resistance as they flow through a narrow aperture and interrupt a direct electrical current. Software analysis defines red blood cells, white blood cells (WBCs), and platelets based on volume limits and calculates red blood cell and platelet indices. Coulter (Beckman Coulter, Brea, CA), Sysmex (Mundelein, IL), and some Cell-Dyn instruments (Abbott Diagnostics, Santa Clara, CA) use this technology.

Optical

This method monitors the light-scattering properties of blood cells. Cells pass in single file across the path of a unifocal laser. The amount of light scattered at a low angle from the incident light path is proportional to cell volume. The amount of light scattered at a wide angle depends on factors such as cytoplasmic granules and nuclear shape. All of the major hematology analyzer manufacturers use light-scattering technology.

Erythrocyte analysis

Automated blood cell counters measure the number ($10^6/\mu L$) and volume (10^{-15} L) of red blood cells, and hemoglobin concentration (g/dL) after lysing red blood cells; all other parameters are calculated. Hemoglobin is converted by potassium ferricyanide and potassium cyanide to cyanmethemoglobin, and absorbance is measured by a spectrophotometer at 540 nm. This measurement can be artifactually elevated by increased sample turbidity due to improperly lysed red blood cells, leukocytosis, paraproteinemia, or hyperlipidemia.

The mean corpuscular volume (MCV) is calculated from the distribution of individual red blood cell volumes. This measurement can be artifactually elevated by agglutination of red blood cells, resulting in measurement of more than one cell at a time; hyperglycemia, causing osmotic swelling of the red blood cell; and spherocytes, which have decreased deformity.

Automated hematocrit (%) is calculated by multiplying the MCV by the red blood cell number: hematocrit = MCV (10^{-15} L) × red blood cells (× $10^{12}/L$) × 100.

The mean corpuscular hemoglobin (MCH) is expressed in picograms (10^{-12} g). The MCH is calculated by dividing hemoglobin (g/L) by red blood cell count ($10^{12}/L$). An elevated MCH can be an artifact of increased plasma turbidity.

The mean corpuscular hemoglobin concentration (MCHC) is expressed in grams of hemoglobin per deciliter of packed red blood cells. The MCHC is calculated by dividing the hemoglobin concentration (g/dL) by the hematocrit (%) × 100. Any artifact impacting hematocrit or hemoglobin determinations can alter the MCHC.

The red blood cell distribution width (RDW) is the coefficient of variation of red blood cell size distribution (standard deviation/MCV) and correlates to anisocytosis observed on blood smear review. The RDW is used in the evaluation of

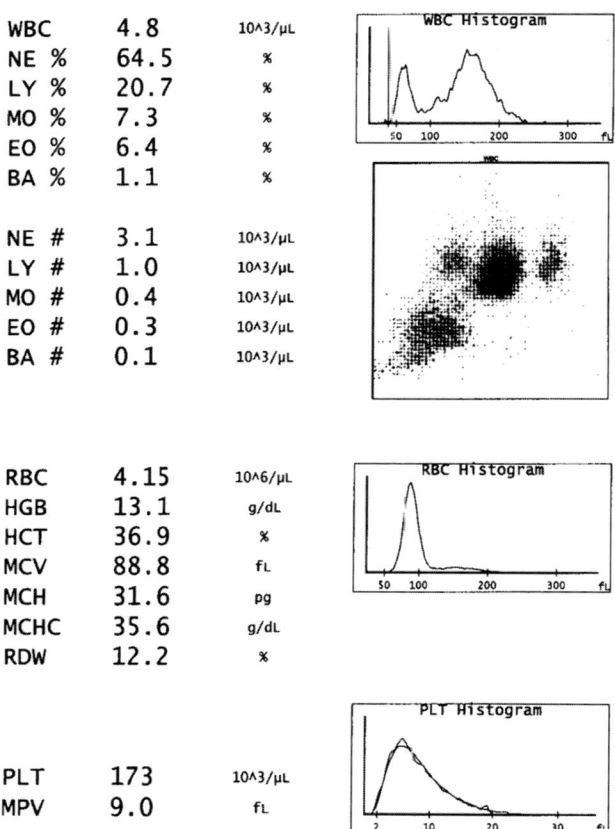

Figure 10-1 Data and histograms performed on a Beckman-Coulter LH 750 automated hematology analyzer from a healthy adult. The white blood cell (WBC), red blood cell (RBC), and platelet (PLT) histograms represent cell volumes determined by impedance. The second histogram from the top displays WBC light scatter in a flow cell; y-axis indicates forward scatter and volume, and x-axis indicates side scatter due to granularity and nuclear features. Basophils (BA) are detected by an alternative physical property not displayed. EO = eosinophil; HCT = hematocrit; HGB = hemoglobin; LY = lymphocyte; MCH = mean corpuscular hemoglobin; MCHC = mean corpuscular hemoglobin concentration; MCV = mean corpuscular volume; MO = monocyte; MPV = mean platelet volume; NE = neutrophil; RDW = red blood cell distribution width.

anemia. The RDW is more frequently elevated with microcytic anemias due to iron deficiency anemia than to thalassemia or anemia of chronic disease and with macrocytic anemias due to vitamin B_{12} or folate deficiency than to liver disease, hypothyroidism, or a reticulocytosis. Myelodysplastic syndromes, such as refractory anemia, or red blood cell transfusions to patients with severe microcytic or macrocytic anemias can produce a dimorphic red blood cell pattern with a very wide RDW.

Reticulocyte counts

Automated hematology analyzers use different dyes to detect residual mRNA in young erythrocytes, and all provide accurate reticulocyte counts expressed as a percentage of red blood cells or as an absolute number. In addition, most instruments sort reticulocytes into 2 or 3 categories based on the quantity of residual mRNA. A relative increase in immature reticulocytes with high mRNA content is a harbinger of erythropoietic recovery from myeloablative therapy, other temporary aplastic states, and nutritional deficiencies, as well as response to erythropoiesis-stimulating agents. An increased immature reticulocyte fraction precedes an increase in reticulocyte number by several days. Some blood cell counters provide reticulocyte indices that are analogous to the standard red blood cell indices, including reticulocyte hemoglobin content (CHr) on Advia analyzers (Siemens, Tarrytown, NY) and reticulocyte MCV (MCVr) on several others. Reductions in CHr and MCVr reflect inadequate hemoglobin synthesis in real time, providing immediate information about functional iron deficiency when other biochemical markers of iron availability may be difficult to interpret due to inflammatory conditions. CHr is particularly useful for assessing response to erythropoiesis-stimulating agents and iron therapy in renal dialysis patients.

Nucleated red blood cells

Circulating erythroblasts occur in newborns; however, beyond this period, the presence of nucleated red blood cells is associated with various hematopoietic stresses including hemolytic anemias, myeloproliferative disorders, metastatic cancer to bone marrow, and hypoxia. All major hematology analyzer brands enumerate nucleated red blood cells and correct WBC and lymphocyte counts for interference from nucleated red blood cells. Accurate enumeration of schistocytes could improve detection and monitoring of microangiopathic hemolytic anemias. Although some analyzers can distinguish small red blood cells from platelets, they cannot determine red blood cell shape, and the fragmented red blood cell counts are not a reportable parameter at this time.

Leukocyte analysis

To differentiate lymphocytes, monocytes, neutrophils, eosinophils, and basophils, most instruments use impedance and or light scattering, plus additional physical properties. Coulter and Sysmex use radiofrequency conductivity, and Advia (Siemens) uses peroxidase staining. Differentials are typically reported as percentages of WBC and as absolute counts. Neither hematology analyzers nor technologists reviewing a blood smear can accurately and precisely count band neutrophils. However, automated blood cell counters do provide sensitive flags and warnings for immature granulocytes and monocytes and abnormal lymphocytes. Quantitative limits, set by the operator, provide further cues for blood smear review. Instrument manufacturers continue to refine technologies to report extended differentials to quantify neutrophil precursors, including metamyelocytes, myelocytes, promyelocytes, and blasts. However, poor sensitivity limits the clinical utility of extended differentials at this time. Some Sysmex analyzers identify a subset of WBCs called hematopoietic progenitor cells, which correlate with CD34 counts and can be used to monitor peripheral stem cell mobilization.

Platelet analysis

Automated blood cell counters enumerate platelets, measure volume, and calculate mean platelet volume (MPV), and some analyzers report platelet distribution width. Associations between MPV and acquired mechanisms of thrombocytopenia suggest that MPV increases with peripheral destruction of platelets due to increased megakaryocyte ploidy and production of larger platelets, whereas MPV decreases when platelet production is suppressed. However, platelets undergo time-dependent shape changes when exposed to ethylenediaminetetraacetic acid (EDTA), leading to ex vivo over- or underestimation of MPV depending on the detection method, thus diminishing its clinical utility. Inaccurate automated platelet counts can result from fragmented red blood cells, congenital (inherited macrothrombocytopenia disorders such as May-Hegglin anomaly) or acquired (myeloproliferative disorders or idiopathic thrombocytopenic purpura) macrothrombocytes, and EDTA-mediated platelet clumping due to IgM autoantibodies. Hematology analyzers provide sensitive warnings for abnormal platelet populations requiring manual smear review to confirm or revise platelet counts. Analogous to reticulocytes, young platelets contain detectable mRNA. Currently, only certain Sysmex analyzers provide an immature platelet count, with a reference range of 1.1% to 6.1%, based on analysis of cell volume and fluorescence intensity of mRNA binding dye. Potential applications include differentiating thrombocytopenia due to megakaryopoiesis failure from peripheral destruction and determining earlier evidence of marrow regeneration following stem cell transplantation. However, wider adoption of immature platelet fraction is hindered by availability from only one manufacturer and limited evidence to support clinical utility.

Examination of peripheral blood smears

The best-quality peripheral blood smears are obtained from fingerstick procedures. Blood smears are stained with either the Wright or the May-Grunwald-Giemsa stains. Microscopic examination of stained blood smears can identify morphologic abnormalities that automated hematology analyzers nonspecifically flag or, rarely, miss. The examination begins at low power (×10), scanning for platelet clumps or abnormal, large, nucleated cells that may be located along the lateral edges of the smear. At higher magnification (×50 and ×100), the optimal area to examine red blood cell, platelet, and leukocyte morphologies and to perform WBC differentials is the transitional area between the thick part of the smear and the feathered edge (Table 10-1), where there are only a few overlapping red blood cells and central pallor of normal red blood cells is evident. Hematologists should review a patient's peripheral smear as part of any consultation potentially involving qualitative or quantitative blood cell abnormalities.

The accuracy of manual WBC differentials suffers from small sample size (typically 100 cells), distributional bias of WBCs on the smear, and variable interobserver agreement regarding cell classification. Advances in digital microscopy and image analysis can improve the accuracy of WBC classification while reducing the required technical time. For example, the CellaVision DM96 (CellaVision, Lund, Sweden)

Table 10-1 Red blood cell abnormalities.*

Abnormality	Description	Cause	Disease association
Acanthocytes (spur cells)	Irregularly spiculated red cell	Altered membrane lipids	Liver disease, abetalipoproteinemia, postsplenectomy
Basophilic stippling	Punctate basophilic inclusions	Precipitated ribosomes	Lead toxicity, thalassemias
Bite cells (degmacyte)	Smooth semicircle taken from one edge	Heinz body pitting by spleen	G6PD deficiency, drug-induced oxidant hemolysis
Burr cells (echinocytes)	Short, evenly spaced spicules	May be related to abnormal membrane lipids	Usually artifactual, uremia, bleeding ulcers, gastric carcinoma
Cabot ring	Circular, blue, threadlike inclusion with dots	Nuclear remnant	Postsplenectomy, hemolytic anemia, megaloblastic anemia
Howell-Jolly bodies	Small, discrete basophilic dense inclusions; usually single	Nuclear remnant	Postsplenectomy, hemolytic anemia, megaloblastic anemia
Pappenheimer bodies	Small dense basophilic granules	Iron-containing siderosomes or mitochondrial remnant	Sideroblastic anemia, postsplenectomy
Schistocytes (helmet cells)	Distorted, fragmented cell, with 2-3 pointed ends	Mechanical distortion in the microvasculature by fibrin strands; damage by mechanical heart valves	Microangiopathic hemolytic anemia, prosthetic heart valves, severe burns
Spherocytes	Spherical cell with dense appearance and absent central pallor; usually decreased diameter	Decreased membrane redundancy	Hereditary spherocytosis, immunohemolytic anemia
Stomatocytes	Mouth- or cuplike deformity	Membrane defect with abnormal cation permeability	Hereditary stomatocytosis, immunohemolytic anemia
Target cell (codocyte)	Targetlike appearance, often hypochromic	Increased redundancy of cell membrane	Liver disease, postsplenectomy, thalassemia, HbC
Teardrop cell (dacryocyte)	Distorted, drop-shaped cell		Myelofibrosis, myelophthisic anemia

*Blood smear abnormalities can be artifacts of poor slide preparation or viewing the wrong part of the smear.
Modified from Kjedsberg C, ed. *Practical Diagnosis of Hematologic Disorders*. 2nd ed. Chicago, IL: ASCP Press; 1995.
G6PD = glucose-6-phosphate dehydrogenase; HbC = hemoglobin C.

scans a stained blood smear, makes digital images of WBCs, classifies them, and presents the sorted WBC images to an operator to confirm or reclassify. When compared with manual differentials, automated morphologic differentials demonstrate excellent routine differential accuracy and sensitivity to detect blasts. In addition, stored images can be reviewed at remote locations such as outpatient clinics.

Supravital stains are used to detect red blood cell inclusions. Crystal violet detects denatured hemoglobin inclusions (Heinz bodies) due to enzymopathies such as glucose-6-phosphate dehydrogenase (G6PD) deficiency; brilliant cresyl blue is used to precipitate and detect unstable hemoglobins (hemoglobin H cells in α thalassemias).

Bone marrow aspirate and biopsy

Bone marrow aspirate and biopsy are commonly performed by collecting specimens from the posterior iliac crests. Bone marrow aspirates can also be obtained from the sternum. In newborns and young infants, marrow aspirates are often obtained from the anterior tibia. Good-quality smears require adequate spicule harvesting because perispicular areas are the most representative areas to examine.

Hemophilia and other coagulation factor deficiencies or anticoagulation are relative contraindications to marrow aspirations and biopsies; thrombocytopenia is not a contraindication. Bleeding disorders are not a contraindication if factor replacement is given.

The bone marrow aspirate and touch prep are stained with either the Wright or May-Grunwald-Giemsa stains; unstained smears should be retained and kept frozen in a dry environment for possible special stains. The bone marrow aspirate is used for cytologic examination of the bone marrow cells and for performing the marrow differential. Bone marrow aspirate clot and core biopsies are fixed in formalin or in a coagulative fixative, and the biopsy specimen is decalcified and embedded in paraffin; 3- to 4-μm sections are then cut and stained with hematoxylin and eosin or Giemsa stains.

Plastic embedding does not require decalcification, and enzymatic activity is better preserved, thereby allowing cytochemical staining of the biopsy; thin cuts of 2 μm can be obtained. Because of the technical expertise required and prolonged processing time, few laboratories process bone marrow specimens using plastic embedding.

When examining pediatric marrows, it is understood that erythroid hyperplasia is present at birth because of high levels of erythropoietin. Lymphocytes may compose 40% of the marrow cellularity in children >4 years of age, and eosinophils are present in higher numbers than in adults.

Perls or Prussian blue reactions are used to identify ferritin and hemosiderin in nucleated red blood cells (sideroblastic iron) and histiocytes (reticuloendothelial iron). Siderocytes containing one or more blue-staining granules account for 20% to 50% of the cells. (See Table 10-2 for other cytochemical stains.)

Ringed sideroblasts are defined as nucleated red cells with blue-staining iron granules surrounding at least two thirds of the nucleus. These iron granules are present in mitochondria surrounding the nuclear membrane.

Iron staining of the biopsy can underestimate the marrow iron stores because of the loss of iron during decalcification.

Table 10-2 Cytochemical stains.

Cytochemical stain	Substrate and staining cells
Myeloperoxidase	Primary granules of neutrophils and secondary granules of eosinophils. Monocytic lysosomal granules stain faintly.
Sudan black B	Stains intracellular phospholipids and other lipids. Pattern of staining is similar to myeloperoxidase.
Naphthol AS-D chloroacetate esterase (specific esterase)	Granulocytes stain; monocytes do not stain. Can be used in biopsies to stain granulocytes and mast cells.
α-Naphthyl butyrate (nonspecific esterase)	Stains monocytes, macrophages, and histiocytes. Does not stain neutrophils.
α-Naphthyl acetate (nonspecific esterase)	Megakaryocytes stain with α-naphthyl acetate but not α-naphthyl butyrate.
Terminal deoxynucleotidyl transferase (TDT)	Intranuclear enzyme. Stains thymocytes and lymphoblasts. Some myeloblasts stain positively.
Tartrate-resistant acid phosphatase (TRAP)	Stains an acid phosphatase isoenzyme. Positive staining in hairy cell leukemia, Gaucher cells, activated T lymphocytes.
Periodic acid-Schiff (PAS)	Detects intracellular glycogen and neutral mucosubstances. Positive staining in acute lymphoblastic leukemia, acute myeloid leukemia, erythroleukemia, and Gaucher cells.
Toluidine blue	Detects acid mucopolysaccharides. Positive in mast cells and basophils.
Tryptase	Positive in mast cells, negative in basophils. Mast cells in systemic mast cell disease frequently have a spindled shape.

Immunohistochemical stains

A large array of specific antibodies detected by enzymatic formation of a colored product linked to the antigen–antibody complex are now available for use on blood smears, marrow aspirates, and bone marrow biopsies or other tissues. Many cytochemical stains, such as tartrate-resistant acid phosphatase (TRAP) and myeloperoxidase, have been converted into immunohistochemical stains.

Immunohistochemical stains are used on marrow aspirates and blood smears when flow cytometry specimens have not been collected or when flow cytometry results are confusing. The advantage of immunohistochemistry is the ability to correlate morphology with phenotype. Immunohistochemistry can be used to phenotype undifferentiated tumors, lymphoproliferative disorders, and atypical lymphoid infiltrates. In patients whose marrow cannot be aspirated ("dry tap"), immunohistochemistry can be performed on the biopsy section. Immunohistochemistry can also be used on sections of lymph nodes or other tissues when there is concern about lymphoma or some other neoplastic disease.

In addition to determining cell lineage—for example, differentiating hematopoietic neoplasms from nonhematopoietic neoplasms or lymphoid processes from myeloid disorders—immunohistochemistry can also be used to help determine prognosis. Immunohistochemical stains can be used to delineate prognostic groups of diffuse large B-cell lymphoma. These different prognostic groups were first detected by gene microarray technology (see Chapter 1). Gene microarray technology has been used to subdivide diffuse large B-cell lymphomas into germinal center B-cell (GCB) and non–germinal center B-cell (NGCB) types. Patients with the GCB phenotype have a better event-free survival and overall survival than patients with the NGCB phenotype. Gene microarray technology is not currently practical for most clinical laboratories, but studies have shown that differentiation of diffuse large B-cell lymphomas into the GCB and NGCB phenotypes can be done by immunohistochemistry using antibodies to CD10, BCL6, and MUM1.

Preparation of bone marrow samples for ancillary studies

Bone marrow collected in EDTA is adequate for both flow cytometry and molecular analysis. Sodium heparin is suitable for flow cytometry but may contaminate DNA preparations and interfere with endonuclease digestion or the polymerase chain reaction (PCR). Bone marrow collected for cytogenetic studies should be collected in a sterile tube containing tissue culture medium such as RPMI (containing fetal bovine serum, l-glutamine, and antibiotics) and anticoagulant.

Bone marrow samples are stable at room temperature for 24 hours for flow cytometry, molecular analysis, and cytogenetics. For cytogenetic studies, shorter storage periods are better. Marrow samples can be frozen in liquid nitrogen for flow cytometry and molecular analysis. However, because flow cytometry requires viable cells, freezing and thawing of samples may yield less than optimal results. Paraffin-embedded tissue can be used for PCR of genomic DNA sequences. Reverse transcriptase PCR (RT-PCR) assays require that RNA preparations be performed as early as possible to prevent digestion by ubiquitous nucleases; alternatively, the RNA can be isolated from cell aliquots stored in frozen nitrogen.

Ancillary testing
Flow cytometry

The most common applications of flow cytometry in hematology include the detection of cell surface proteins using fluorescent-labeled monoclonal antibodies or the assessment of DNA content using DNA-binding dyes.

Flow cytometry is used for phenotyping populations of cells, enumerating early progenitors for stem cell transplantations, detecting minimal residual disease, detecting targets for immunotherapy, and assessing the presence of prognostic markers. See Table 10-3 for a summary of clinical uses of flow cytometry in ancillary studies. When immunophenotyping a cellular population, the panel of antibodies used depends on the cells being analyzed and the question being asked.

Gating is necessary to identify cells of interest in a mixed population of cells. Three major leukocyte populations (lymphocytes, monocytes, and neutrophils) can be defined using light scatter. Forward angle scatter (FS; low angle) measures cell size, and side light scatter (SS) measures internal cellular granularity. Lymphocytes have the lowest FS and SS signals, monocytes have intermediate FS and SS signals, and neutrophils have high SS and slightly lower FS signals.

The most common method for gating different cell populations is by plotting right-angle SS against CD45. Cells can be separated based on the intensity of staining they display with the conjugated antibody that is classified as either bright or dim. Lymphocytes are bright CD45 and have a low SS signal, neutrophils are dim to moderately bright CD45 and have a high SS signal, and monocytes are bright CD45 and have an intermediate SS.

Flow cytometry can also be used to detect populations of natural killer (NK) cells. NK cells express CD2, CD7, CD16, and CD56 and show variable expression of CD57 and CD8. NK cells do not express CD3, and the absence of CD3 expression can be used to differentiate NK cells from T cells.

Table 10-3 Specimen allocation for ancillary studies.

Clinical problem	Ancillary techniques
Pancytopenia	Flow cytometry (LGL, hairy cell leukemia, PNH clone, AML)
	Cytogenetics (AML, MDS)
	Molecular genetics
Myeloid leukemia	Flow cytometry (phenotyping)
	Cytogenetics and FISH
	Molecular genetics (*BCR-ABL, PML/RARA, AML1/ETO*)
Lymphoproliferative disorder	Flow cytometry (phenotyping, prognostic markers such as ZAP-70)
	Cytogenetics: t(l;19) in pre–B-cell ALL, t(14;18) in follicular lymphomas, etc
	FISH
	Molecular genetics (clonality, specific markers such as *BCL2, BCL6*, etc)
	Immunohistochemistry (phenotyping, prognostic markers)
Myeloproliferative disorders	Cytogenetics
	FISH (*BCR-ABL*)
	Molecular genetics (*BCR-ABL, JAK2*)
Plasmaproliferative disorders	Flow cytometry (phenotyping, labeling index)
	Cytogenetics

ALL = acute lymphoblastic leukemia; AML = acute myelogenous leukemia; CLL = chronic lymphocytic leukemia; FISH = fluorescence in situ hybridization; LGL = large granular lymphocyte leukemia; MDS = myelodysplastic syndrome; PNH = paroxysmal nocturnal hemoglobinuria.

In addition to determining cell lineage, flow cytometry can also be used to detect prognostic markers. For example, flow cytometric analysis of the tyrosine kinase ZAP-70 can be used to subdivide chronic lymphocytic leukemia (CLL) into prognostic groups. Positivity for ZAP-70 is highly correlated with unmutated DNA, a feature of CLL arising from pre–germinal center cells, and patients with pre–germinal center CLL have a decreased overall survival when compared with patients with CLL arising from post–germinal center cells. Positivity for CD38 by flow cytometric analysis is also correlated with unmutated DNA, but the correlation is not as strong as it is with ZAP-70.

Flow cytometry can be used to diagnose paroxysmal nocturnal hemoglobinemia (PNH). PNH is associated with the absence of 2 complement regulatory molecules from the cell surface of hematopoietic cells; these are decay-accelerating factor (DAF) and protectin (MIRL). The absence of these proteins from the cell surface of erythrocytes and granulocytes can be detected by flow cytometry using antibodies to CD55 and CD59, respectively.

Normal hematopoiesis

Uncommitted hematopoietic progenitors are CD34+ and CD38−; expression of CD38 is evidence of lineage commitment. In myeloid differentiation, CD33 is one of the earliest antigens to appear. CD33 is followed by CD13, which is then followed by CD15 and CD11b. CD16 and CD10 are seen in late maturation.

Appearance of CD71, loss of CD34 and CD33, and decreased expression of CD45 characterize erythroid maturation. With further differentiation, CD71 expression decreases, glycophorin expression increases, and CD45 disappears.

Megakaryocytic differentiation is indicated by the expression of glycoprotein (GP) IIb (CD41). GPIIb-IIIa (CD61) expression increases as CD34 expression decreases. GPIb (CD42b) is expressed at the promegakaryocyte stage. GPV (CD42d) expression increases with megakaryocyte differentiation.

B- and T-cell precursors express terminal deoxynucleotidyl transferase (TDT), human leukocyte antigen (HLA)-DR, and CD34. B-cell differentiation is indicated by the expression of CD19 followed by CD10. As B cells mature, they lose cell surface expression of CD34 and CD10 and express IgM on the cell surface. Expression of surface IgM is associated with the expression of mature B-lymphocyte markers (CD20, CD21, CD22, and CD79b). Mature B cells express an immunoglobulin heavy chain, such as IgM, and either the κ or a λ light chain. A predominant expression of one type of light chain on the cell surface of a population of B cells is known as light chain restriction and is indicative of a monoclonal process.

T-cell precursors express TDT, HLA-DR, and CD34. Differentiation is indicated by the expression of cytoplasmic CD3 and CD7, followed by the expression of CD2 and CD5. The common thymocyte also expresses CD1, CD4, and CD8. The mature helper/inducer lymphocyte expresses CD2, CD3, CD4, and CD5 and may express CD7. The mature suppressor/cytotoxic T lymphocyte expresses CD2, CD3, CD4, CD5, and CD8 and may express CD7. T-cell neoplasms may be associated with abnormal expression patterns of T-cell antigens, and the abnormal pattern may be detected by flow cytometric analysis. (See Tables 10-4 through 10-10 for useful CD markers.).

Cytogenetics

Cytogenetic analysis can be performed from cultured (indirect) and uncultured (direct) preparations. In the indirect assay, cells are grown so that mitotic forms can be visualized and distinct chromosomal banding patterns can be assessed (conventional cytogenetics). Growing or culturing the cells increases the mitotic rate and improves chromosome morphology. Mitogens may be useful in improving the yield of karyotyping abnormal cells and are particularly useful when analyzing mature B- or T-cell processes.

Cytogenetically, a minimum of 2 mitotic cells with gain of the same chromosome or with the same structural abnormality or 3 mitotic cells with loss of the same chromosome define a clone.

Constitutional chromosome abnormalities, associated with either congenital genetic syndromes or normal variants, are determined on peripheral blood T lymphocytes grown in culture with phytohemagglutinin (PHA), a T-cell mitogen.

Fluorescence in situ hybridization (FISH) is a cytogenetic technique that uses specific fluorescently labeled DNA probes to identify each chromosomal segment. FISH can be performed using either cultured or uncultured preparations. In the uncultured technique, the assay is performed using nuclear DNA from interphase cells that are affixed to a microscope slide. FISH can be performed using bone marrow or peripheral blood smears or fixed and sectioned tissues.

Hybridization of centromere-specific probes is used to detect monosomy, trisomy, and other aneuploidies. Chromosome-specific libraries, which paint the chromosomes, are useful in identifying marker chromosomes or structural rearrangements, such as translocations. Translocations and deletions can also be identified in interphase or metaphase by using genomic probes that are derived from the breakpoints of recurring translocations or within the deleted segment. Multiplex FISH (spectral karyotyping) consists of simultaneously painting all chromosomes in a cell using different colors for each chromosome.

Cytogenetics is particularly useful in the subclassification of acute myeloid leukemias and in confirming the diagnosis and prognosis of B-cell neoplasias. CLL, acute leukemias, B-cell lymphomas, and multiple myeloma all have cytogenetic abnormalities that can be detected using either conventional cytogenetics or FISH.

Molecular diagnostics
Southern blotting

Southern blot analysis begins with the extraction of high molecular weight DNA, followed by its digestion by restriction enzymes. The digested DNA fragments are electrophoresed through a gel to separate the fragments by size. The separated fragments are then blotted onto a piece of filter paper, and the filter is soaked in a solution containing labeled single-stranded DNA probes. The probe hybridizes to the spot on the paper where its complementary strand is found. Unbound DNA is washed away, the filter is exposed to photographic film, and the film reveals the position and size of the electrophoresed fragments.

This technique is slow and has been largely replaced by PCR. Southern blot analysis is used when the genomic fragments being investigated are large and the precise location of the marker sequence is unknown.

Southern blotting has been used on peripheral blood and bone marrow samples to detect immunoglobulin gene rearrangements, T-cell receptor gene rearrangements, and chromosome translocations (eg, *BCR-ABL* and *BCL2*).

Polymerase chain reaction

PCR is designed to permit selective amplification of a specific target DNA sequence within total genomic DNA or a complex complementary DNA (cDNA) population. Partial DNA sequence information from the target sequences is required. Two oligonucleotide primers, which are specific for the target sequence, are used. The primers are added to denatured single-stranded DNA. A heat-stable DNA polymerase and the 4 deoxynucleotide triphosphates are used to initiate the synthesis of new DNA strands. The newly synthesized DNA strands are used as templates for further cycles of amplification. The amplified DNA sequence can be detected by electrophoresis on an agarose gel, and visualization can be accomplished by the use of a DNA dye; alternatively, the amplified DNA can be directly sequenced in an automatic sequencer.

Quantitative real-time PCR is based on detection of a fluorescent signal produced proportionally during the amplification of a PCR product. Forward and reverse primers are extended with *Taq* polymerase as in a traditional PCR reaction. A probe is designed to anneal to the target sequence between the forward and reverse primers. The probe is labeled at the 5′ end with a reporter and a quencher fluorochrome. As long as both fluorochromes are on the probe, the quencher molecule stops all fluorescence from the reporter. As *Taq* polymerase extends the primer, the 5′ to 3′ nuclease activity of *Taq* degrades the probe, releasing the reporter fluorochrome. The amount of fluorescence released during amplification is proportional to the amount of product generated in each cycle.

Table 10-4 Clinically useful CD markers.

Marker	Lineage association
Progenitor cells	
CD34	Progenitor cells, endothelium
CD38	Myeloid progenitors, T, B, NK cells, plasma cells, monocytes, CLL subset
B-cell markers	
CD10	Pre-B lymphocytes, germinal center cells, neutrophils
CD19	B cells (not plasma cells or follicular dendritic cells)
CD20	B cells (not plasma cells)
CD21	Mature B cells, follicular dendritic cells, subset of thymocytes
CD22	Mature B cells, mantle zone cells (not germinal center cells)
CD23	B cells, CLL
CD79b	B cells (not typical CLL)
CD 103	Intraepithelial lymphocytes, hairy cell leukemia, T cells in enteropathic T-cell lymphoma
FMC7	B cells (not typical CLL), hairy cell leukemia
T-cell markers	
CD2	Pro- and pre-T cells, T cells, thymocytes, NK cells, some lymphocytes in CLL and B-ALL
CD3	Thymocytes, mature T cells, cytoplasm of immature T cells
CD5	Thymocytes, T cells, B cells in CLL, B cells in mantle cell lymphoma
CD4	Helper T cells, monocytes, dendritic cells, activated eosinophils, thymocytes
CD7	Pro- and pre-T cells, T cells, thymocytes, NK cells, some myeloblasts
CD8	Suppressor T cells, NK cells, thymocytes
CD25	Activated T and B cells, adult T-cell leukemia/lymphoma
NK/cytotoxic T-cell markers	
CD16	NK cells, monocytes, macrophages, neutrophils
CD56	NK cells, myeloma cells
CD57	NK cells, T-cell subset
Myeloid and monocytic markers	
CD13	Monocytes, neutrophils, eosinophils, and basophils
CD14	Monocytes, macrophages, subset of granulocytes
CD33	Myeloid lineage cells and monocytes
CD117	Immature myeloid cells, AML
Monocytes	
CD11c	Monocytes, macrophages, granulocytes, activated B and T cells, NK cells, hairy cell leukemia
CD15	Myeloid lineage cells and monocytes
CD64	Monocytes, immature myeloid cells, activated neutrophils
Megakaryocytic markers	
CD41	Platelets and megakaryocytes (GPIIb)
CD42	Platelets and megakaryocytes (CD42a: GPI; CD42b: GPIb)
CD61	Platelets, megakaryocytes, endothelial cells (GPIIb-IIIa)
Erythroid markers	
CD71	Transferrin receptor is upregulated upon cell activation
CD235a	Glycophorin A

AML = acute myelogenous leukemia; B-ALL = B-lineage acute lymphoblastic leukemia; CLL = chronic lymphocytic leukemia; GP = glycoprotein; NK = natural killer.

Table 10-5 Acute myeloid leukemia phenotyping.

	HLA-DR	CD34	CD33	CD13	CD11c	CD14	CD41	CD235a
M0	+	+	+	+/–	+/–	–	–	–
M1	+	+	+	+	+/–	+/–	–	–
M2	+/–	+/–	+	+	+/–	+/–	–	–
M3	–	–	+	+	+/–	–	–	–
M4	+	+/–	+	+	+	+	–	–
M5	+	–	+	+	+	+	–	–
M6	+/–	–	–	–	+/–	–	–	+
M7	+/–	+/–	+/–	–	–	–	+	–

Table 10-6 B-lineage acute lymphoblastic leukemia phenotyping.

	TDT	CD19	CD10	CD20	Cyto-μ	Surface Ig
Pro-B	+	+	–	–	–	–
Pre-Pre-B (common ALL)	+	+	+	–	–	–
Pre-B	+	+	+	+/–	+	–
Early B (Burkitt)	–	+	+	+	–	+

Cyto-μ = cytoplasmic μ; Ig = immunoglobulin; TDT = terminal deoxynucleotidyl transferase.

Table 10-7 T-lineage acute lymphoblastic leukemia phenotyping.

Surface	TDT	CD7	CD2	CD5	CD1	CD3	CyCD3	CD4/CD8
Prothymocyte	+	+	+	–	–	–	+	–/–
Immature thymocyte	+	+	+	+	–	–	+	–/–
Common thymocyte	+	+	+	+	+	+/–	+	+/+
Mature thymocyte	–	+	+	+	–	+	+	CD4 or CD8$^+$
Mature T cell	–	+	+	+	–	+	+	CD4 or CD8$^+$

Cy CD3 = cytoplasmic CD3; TDT = terminal deoxynucleotidyl transferase.

Uses of PCR in clinical laboratories include detection of the *BCR-ABL* translocation in chronic myeloid leukemia, detection of *PML-RARA* in acute promyelocytic leukemia, and detection of the *JAK2* mutation in polycythemia vera, essential thrombocythemia, and primary myelofibrosis.

Miscellaneous laboratory hematology methods
Erythrocyte sedimentation rate

The erythrocyte sedimentation rate (ESR) measures a physical phenomenon—the opposing forces of gravity and buoyancy on red blood cells when blood is suspended in an upright tube—and is expressed in millimeters per hour. Elevated plasma proteins, primarily fibrinogen and immunoglobins, neutralize red blood cell membrane negative charge, facilitating rouleaux formation and more rapid sedimentation due to increased mass per surface area. The clinical utility of ESR is generally poor except for selected rheumatologic disorders, and it is not an appropriate screening test in asymptomatic patients. Conditions associated with elevated ESR include malignancies, infections, and inflammatory conditions, particularly polymyalgia rheumatic and temporal arteritis, as well as hematologic conditions such as cold agglutinin disease, cryoglobulinemia, and plasma cell dyscrasia–related M proteins. ESR reference ranges increase with age and are higher for women. Additional variables affect ESR; anemia and macrocytosis can cause faster sedimentation, whereas sickle cells, by impeding rouleaux formation, and microcytosis cause slower sedimentation. The modified Westergren method (EDTA blood diluted 4:1 in sodium citrate and put in a 200-mm vertical glass tube) is the preferred manual method. Automated ESR devices monitor sedimentation for approximately 20 minutes, extrapolate to millimeters per hour, and correlate reasonably well with the Westergren method.

Table 10-8 Common B-cell neoplasms.

	CD20	CD5	CD10	CD23	CD43	CIg	SIg	Cyclin D1	Other
CLL/SLL	+	++	−	++	++	5%+	+	−	
LPL	++	−	−	−	+/−	+	+	−	
PLL	++	+/−		−			++	−	
HCL	++	−	−	−	−	−	+	+/−	CD11c$^+$, CD25$^+$, CD103$^+$
MCL	++	++	−	−	++	−	++	++	
MZL	++	−	−	−	+/−	+/−	++	−	
FCL	++	−	60% +	−	−	−	++	−	BCL2$^+$
LCL	++	10%+	25%-50% +	+	+/−	+/−	+/−	−	BCL2$^+$ in 30%-40%
Burkitt	++	−	+	−	−	+	+	−	
Myeloma	−	−	Occ +	−	+	++	−	15%-20% +	CD56$^+$, CD38$^+$, CD138$^+$

CIg = cytoplasmic immunoglobulin; CLL = chronic lymphocytic leukemia; FCL = follicular center cell lymphoma; HCL = hairy cell leukemia; LCL = large-cell lymphoma; LPL = lymphoplasmacytic lymphoma; MCL = mantle cell lymphoma; MZL = marginal zone lymphoma; PLL = B-cell prolymphocytic leukemia; SIg = surface immunoglobulin; SLL = small lymphocytic lymphoma.

Screening and diagnosis of hemoglobinopathies
Solubility testing for hemoglobin S

Manual qualitative methods to detect hemoglobin S (Hgb S) rely on visual detection of a turbid solution when blood containing Hgb S is added to a solution containing a reducing agent, detergent to lyse red blood cells, and high-concentration salt buffer. Deoxygenated Hgb S forms tactoids that defract and reflect light, whereas nonsickling hemoglobins remain soluble, allowing the detection of lines or letters when viewed through the hemolysis solution. A positive solubility test cannot discriminate between Hgb S trait, Hgb S homozygous, and Hgb S β thalassemia. False-positive results can occur due to paraprotein or cryoglobulin precipitation, and false-negative results can occur in anemic (hemoglobin <7.0 g/dL) sickle trait individuals or when Hgb S concentration is <2.6 g/dL. Due to the low concentration of Hgb S in affected newborns, sickle solubility testing should not be performed on infants <6 months old due to the risk of false-negative results. If used as a screening test, a positive solubility test requires evaluation by an alternative method to confirm and quantify Hgb S and to identify coexisting nonsickling hemoglobinopathies or thalassemias. There are other rare hemoglobinopathies that produce a positive solubility test, including hemoglobin C Harlem, and if coinherited with Hgb S, they will produce a sickle cell disease phenotype.

Table 10-9 Common mature T-cell and NK-cell neoplasms.

	CD3S	CD3C	CD5	CD7	CD4	CD8	CD30	CD16	CD56	EBV
T-PLL	+	+	−	+	4>8	4>8	−	−	+	−
T-LGL	+	+	−	+	−	+	−	+	−	−
NK-leukemia	−	−	−	+/−	−	+/−	−	−	+	+
EN-NK/T	−	+	−	+/−	−	−	−	+	+	+
HS-γδ lym	+	+	−	+	−	−	−	+	+/−	−
Ent-T lym	+	+	+	+	−	+/−	+/−	−	−	−
SC pannic T lym	+	+	+	+	−	+	+/−	−	−	−
PTCL-NOS	+	−	+/−	+/−	+/−	+/−	+/−	−	+	+/−
AILD	+	+	+	+	+/−	−	−	−	+	+/−
ALCL	+	−	+/−	+/−	+/−	+/−	+	−	−	−

AILD = angioimmunoblastic lymphadenopathy; ALCL = anaplastic large-cell lymphoma; CD3C = cytoplasmic CD3; CD3S = surface CD3; EBV = Epstein-Barr virus; Ent-T lym = enteropathic T-cell lymphoma; EN-NK/T = extranodal natural killer/T-cell lymphoma; HS-γδ lym = hepatosplenic γδ lymphoma; NK-leukemia = natural killer cell leukemia; PTCL-NOS = peripheral T-cell lymphoma, not otherwise specified; SC pannic T lym = subcutaneous panniculitis T-cell lymphoma; T-LGL = T-large granular lymphocyte leukemia; T-PLL = T-prolymphocytic leukemia.

Table 10-10 Immunohistochemical diagnosis of Hodgkin disease.

	CD45	CD30	CD15	CD20	CD3
Hodgkin (R-S cells)	−	+	+	LPHD(+)	−
B lymphoma	+	+/−	−	+	−
T lymphoma	+	+/−	+/−	−	+

LPHD = lymphocyte-predominant Hodgkin disease; R-S = Reed-Sternberg.

If an abnormal hemoglobin consistent with Hgb S is first detected by screening electrophoresis or high-performance liquid chromatography (HPLC), a positive solubility result is an acceptable confirmatory test. A negative solubility result, if abnormal Hgb concentration is >2.6 g/dL, supports less common hemoglobinopathies that can comigrate or coelute with Hgb S.

Methods to separate normal (hemoglobins A, A_2, and F) and abnormal hemoglobins, primarily based on differences in charge, include alkaline and acid gel electrophoresis, isoelectric focusing, HPLC, and capillary electrophoresis (Figure 10-2). No method can definitively identify and quantify all hemoglobin variants, and any abnormal hemoglobin identified by the method chosen for screening must be confirmed by an alternative method (including solubility test for presumed Hgb S). HPLC and capillary electrophoresis instruments are fully automated, provide precise measurements of normal and variant hemoglobins, and are well suited for laboratories performing many analyses to diagnosis hemoglobins S, C, and E and other uncommon hemoglobinopathies and β thalassemia trait. For optimal counseling, DNA analysis may be appropriate to completely characterize α and β thalassemias and some hemoglobinopathies.

G6PD testing

Evaluation for inherited red blood cell enzymopathies is appropriate in patients with nonspherocytic, non–immune-mediated hemolytic anemia. X-linked inheritance of G6PD deficiency is the most common red blood cell enzyme defect and is associated with hemolysis during oxidative stresses due to acute illness, medications, or, rarely, ingestion of fava beans. Decreased G6PD activity diminishes nicotinamide adenine dinucleotide phosphate (NADPH) production and prevents reduction of methemoglobin by reduced glutathione, leading to Heinz body formation and shortened red blood cell survival. Sensitive qualitative screening tests for G6PD deficiency include dye decolorization and fluorescent spot tests, which monitor NADPH-dependent chemical reactions. However, false-negative results may occur if testing is performed during or shortly after a hemolytic event in individuals (typically African and African American males) with the A− mutation because enzyme activity is near normal in reticulocytes. Pyruvate kinase deficiency is the second most common red blood cell enzyme defect, presenting with chronic hemolysis of variable severity and an autosomal recessive inheritance pattern. In patients with hemolysis, a suspicion for a red blood cell enzymopathy, and normal G6PD screening, blood should be sent to a reference laboratory that offers a panel of additional red blood cell enzyme tests.

Hemostasis and thrombosis

Hemostasis is a complex process, involving multiple molecular and cellular interactions to initiate and regulate platelet aggregation (primary hemostasis) and coagulation (secondary hemostasis) at the site of vascular injury to produce a durable "patch" without occluding blood flow. Laboratory evaluation

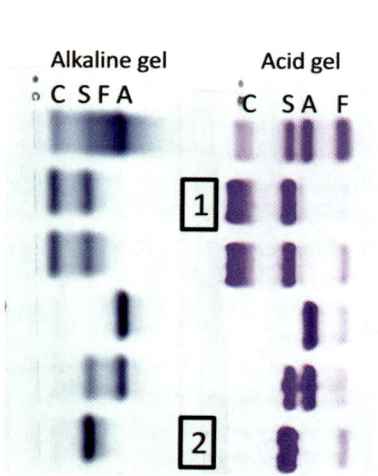
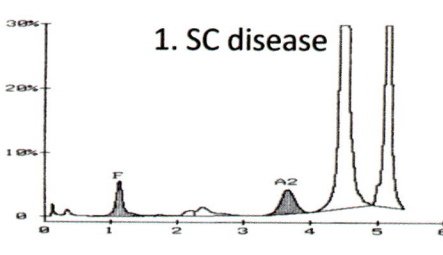
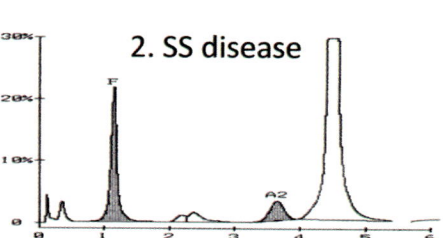

Figure 10-2 Examples of alkaline and acid gel electrophoresis and high-performance liquid chromatography patterns for a patient with hemoglobin SC disease (1) and a patient with homozygous SS sickle cell disease (2).

of hemostasis is performed in several clinical settings, including screening of asymptomatic patients prior to selective invasive procedures and of patients with underlying disorders associated with bleeding complications, evaluation of patients with personal or family histories of abnormal bleeding or bruising, assessment for inherited and acquired thrombosis risk factors, and antithrombotic drug monitoring.

Hemostasis screening typically consists of a prothrombin time (PT), activated partial thromboplastin time (aPTT), and platelet count, with assessment of platelet function reserved for procedures that cannot tolerate excessive bleeding. Abnormal screening test results require additional laboratory investigation to determine the etiologies. History, medication lists, and physical examination findings guide test selection in patients with signs and symptoms of hemostasis defects. Mucosal bleeding, menorrhagia, petechiae, and ecchymoses suggest primary hemostasis disorders such as von Willebrand disease (vWD) and qualitative platelet disorders, whereas hematomas, hemarthroses, and delayed bleeding suggest a coagulation defect.

Testing for thrombophilia is usually performed when a patient has a venous thromboembolic event (VTE) in the absence of compelling acquired risk factors such as major surgery or trauma, cancer and its treatment, and immobility. The decision to test for a predisposition to VTE also depends on the patient's age, history of thrombosis, family history of thrombosis, and anticipated use of the results in future management decisions. Laboratory testing for inherited deficiencies of coagulation regulatory proteins should be done after a patient has completed treatment for a VTE and is in stable health. The levels of protein C, protein S, and antithrombin can decrease during the acute phase of a VTE. Protein C and S levels are reduced by anticoagulation with warfarin. Antithrombin will decrease during anticoagulation with unfractionated heparin. Lupus anticoagulant testing ideally should be done before anticoagulation is begun, in conjunction with serologic assays (anticardiolipin and β_2-GPI antibodies), and abnormal results should be repeated at least 12 weeks later to determine if they are persistent to fulfill the laboratory criteria for antiphospholipid antibody syndrome. Genetic thrombophilia testing can be ordered at any time and is not affected by clinical status or medications. Heparin-induced thrombocytopenia (HIT) and thrombotic thrombocytopenia (TTP) are unique acquired thrombocytopenia disorders with potential for thrombotic complications. Laboratory test results can provide subsequent support for these diagnoses, but immediate therapeutic interventions should be based on clinical assessment alone.

Two major forms of anticoagulation therapy, coumarin antagonism of vitamin K–dependent gamma carboxylation of coagulation factors X, IX, VII, and II, represented by warfarin in this chapter, and unfractionated heparin, require therapeutic drug monitoring due to unpredictable anticoagulant activities and risks of bleeding. Efforts to harmonize interlaboratory monitoring of warfarin with the PT and heparin with the aPTT have led to the international normalized ratio (INR) and heparin activity assays, respectively.

It is important to be aware of the differences in hemostasis factor reference ranges between infants and older children and adults to avoid mislabeling newborns with inherited defects, particularly for coagulation factors and natural inhibitors (see Chapter 2 for details).

The following sections will provide specific information regarding hemostasis laboratory methods as they apply to the aforementioned clinical situations.

Screening coagulation testing

Our current understanding indicates that most coagulation reactions are initiated by exposure of tissue factor and that important interactions occur between the extrinsic and intrinsic pathways. Although the division into 2 separate pathways, as shown in Figure 10-3, does not reflect these extrinsic–intrinsic pathway interactions, it does provide a useful way to interpret screening coagulation test results when evaluating a clinical problem.

Preanalytical variables

The aPTT and, to a lesser degree, the PT are sensitive to changes in the ratio of sodium citrate solution in the collection tube and added plasma. Filling a tube with less than the recommended volume to obtain a sodium citrate-to-blood ratio of 1:9 or collecting blood in the proper proportions from a polycythemic patient increases the concentration of citrate in the plasma compartment, leading to incomplete recalcification when a fixed volume of $CaCl_2$ is added and artifactual prolongation of the aPTT. Heparin contamination due to blood collection from central lines can cause a prolonged aPTT even after discarding the initially removed blood. A direct peripheral venipuncture is required in these cases to exclude heparin as a cause of the prolonged aPTT. A prolonged thrombin time that corrects when repeated after treatment of plasma with a heparin-neutralizing agent or enzymatic digestion (Hepzyme; Siemens) confirms heparin contamination. Alternatively, a prolonged thrombin time and a normal reptilase time, which uses a snake venom not neutralized by heparin-accelerated antithrombin, will confirm the presence of heparin. Most PT reagents contain heparin-neutralizing agents, making this screening clotting test insensitive to heparin contamination.

Mixing studies

The purpose of a mixing study is to determine whether a prolonged aPTT or, occasionally, a prolonged PT is more likely

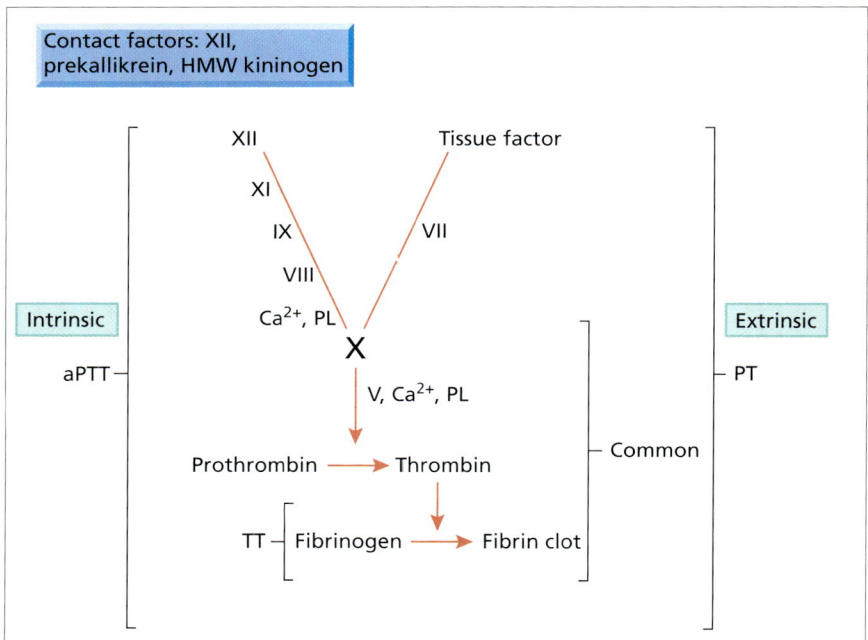

Figure 10-3 Simplified coagulation cascade indicating the intrinsic pathway measured by the activated partial thromboplastin time (aPTT), the extrinsic pathway measured by the prothrombin time (PT), the common pathway (factor X, factor V, prothrombin, and fibrinogen) measured by PT and aPTT, and the conversion of fibrinogen to fibrin measured by the thrombin time (TT). HMW = high molecular weight.

due to a deficiency of one or more coagulation factors or to an inhibitory antibody. The first step is to rule out preanalytical artifacts and then contamination with heparin or direct thrombin inhibitors by performing a thrombin time; if the thrombin time is prolonged, the cause must be determined before proceeding. Next, the aPTT or PT is repeated on a 1:1 mixture of patient plasma and pooled normal plasma (PNP), which should provide at least 50% activity for all coagulation factors and substantial correction if deficiency is the cause. Because factor VIII inhibitors and some lupus anticoagulants produce a delayed aPTT prolongation, 1:1 mixtures are incubated at 37°C for 1 to 2 hours followed by repeating the aPTT. There is no consensus for interpretation of mixing study results, and inflexible requirements such as correction to within the laboratory's PT or aPTT reference ranges to rule out inhibitor activity can be misleading. One must consider the clinical context (bleeding or thrombosis events) and the initial extent of PT and aPTT prolongation when assessing the 1:1 mix results. Sometimes mixing studies will not be definitive, especially when an aPTT is mildly prolonged and "corrects" with mixing, in which case performing both selected factor activity assays and lupus anticoagulant screening will be necessary.

Coagulation factor activity assays

Determination of a coagulation factor activity in a patient's plasma requires 2 additional reagents: PNP and plasma completely deficient in the factor of interest. Combining equal volumes of plasma from a large number of healthy adults averages the interindividual variability for coagulation factors, which typically ranges from approximately 50% to 150%, to produce PNP with 100% activity for all factors. Mixing PNP and factor-deficient plasma in different ratios produces calibrators of known factor activities. PTs are performed on the calibration samples for factors VII, X, V, and II, and aPTTs are performed for the intrinsic pathway factors. When the factor activities of the calibrators are plotted against the corresponding PT or aPTT results on logarithmic axes, a line or curve is generated. Then, a PT or aPTT is performed on patient plasma mixed with factor-deficient plasma, and the corresponding activity is determined from the calibration curve.

Additionally, factor activities are done on serial dilutions of a patient's plasma, and the results, corrected for the dilution factor, are compared. If an inhibitor is present, the factor activity appears to increase with dilution. To determine whether the inhibitor interference is specific for one factor, such as factor VIII, or nonspecific like a lupus anticoagulant may require performance of additional factor activities.

The end point for most coagulation tests is detection of a fibrin clot based on changes in light transmission, decreased motion of a magnetic bead, or other measurable physical properties. The advantages of clot-based assays include low costs, simplicity, and wealth of clinical experience to interpret the results. A factor VIII chromogenic activity assay exists but is not widely used. The end point is cleavage of a small chromogenic substrate by an activated coagulation factor that generates a change in color (optical density) proportional to the activity of the factor. Chromogenic assays can be more precise than clotting assays, but they may not detect some defects in a factor that disrupt the binding of the factor to its natural (larger) substrate.

Prothrombin time

The PT measures the time to form a fibrin clot after adding thromboplastin (tissue factor combined with phospholipid) and $CaCl_2$ to citrated plasma and assesses 3 of the 4 vitamin K–dependent factors (factors II, VII, and X) plus factor V and fibrinogen. Commercial thromboplastins contain either recombinant human tissue factor combined with phospholipid or thromboplastins derived from rabbit or bovine tissues. Almost all PT reagents contain a heparin-neutralizing additive to allow monitoring of vitamin K antagonist anticoagulation during concurrent heparin therapy.

Isolated prolongation of the PT most often reflects a deficiency of vitamin K–dependent factors due to poor nutrition, inadequate absorption of vitamin K, antagonism of γ carboxylation of the vitamin K–dependent factors by coumarins (warfarin in North America, phenprocoumon and acenocoumarol in other countries), or decreased hepatic synthesis. Congenital deficiencies of factors X, V, and II and fibrinogen are rare (1 in 1-2 million people), whereas the estimated incidence of factor VII deficiency is 1 in 300,000 people. Some factor VII mutations produce greater PT prolongations with rabbit/bovine tissue factor than with human tissue factor. Therefore, it is important to confirm a suspected congenital factor VII deficiency by measuring factor VII activity with recombinant human thromboplastin. Dysfibrinogenemia occasionally causes a prolongation of the PT without a prolongation of the aPTT, and factor VII inhibitory autoantibodies are extremely rare (Figure 10-4).

Warfarin and other coumarins cause prolonged PTs (and, variably, prolonged aPTTs depending on the degree of factor IX, X, and II suppression). Therapeutic monitoring of warfarin depends on the PT. However, thromboplastins have different sensitivities to the effects of warfarin on the vitamin K–dependent proteins. To account for this variability, manufacturers compare PTs obtained with commercial thromboplastin lots to a World Health Organization reference thromboplastin, with the behavior of human tissue factor, performed on plasma samples from healthy controls and stable anticoagulated patients to obtain an international sensitivity index (ISI). A sensitive thromboplastin with an ISI of 1.0 is equivalent to human tissue, whereas a thromboplastin with an ISI of 2 is relatively insensitive to depletion of vitamin K–dependent clotting factors. The INR is a calculation that represents the ratio of the patient's PT to the laboratory's mean normal PT raised to the exponent of the thromboplastin ISI.

$$INR = \left[\frac{PT \text{ of patient}}{\text{Mean normal PT of lab}}\right]^{ISI}$$

Normal subjects have an INR of 1.0 ± 0.2. The INR is designed to accurately monitor patients who have been stabilized on warfarin regardless of the sensitivity of the thromboplastin used to perform the PT. Instrument variables can add imprecision to the ISI calculation, which can be minimized by calibration of specific reagent/instrument combinations by manufacturers.

The INR is a mathematical conversion based on chronic effects of warfarin and is *not* intended for assessing coagulopathies due to congenital deficiencies or liver disease because the ISI is not validated for these conditions.

> **Key points**
>
> Isolated prolonged PT:
> - Poor nutrition (decreased dietary vitamin K)
> - Malabsorption of vitamin K
> - Liver disease (decreased synthesis of vitamin K–dependent factors)
> - Warfarin therapy
> - Rare congenital deficiency or inhibitor (factor VII)

Activated partial thromboplastin time

The aPTT is a 2-step assay to measure the time to form a fibrin clot after incubation of citrated plasma with phospholipid and negatively charged particles followed by addition of $CaCl_2$. The negative surface and the phospholipid activate the contact factors (factor XII, prekallikrein [PK], and high molecular weight kininogen [HMWK]) and factor XI. The addition of $CaCl_2$ permits activation of factor IX and the remaining reactions to proceed to form a fibrin clot.

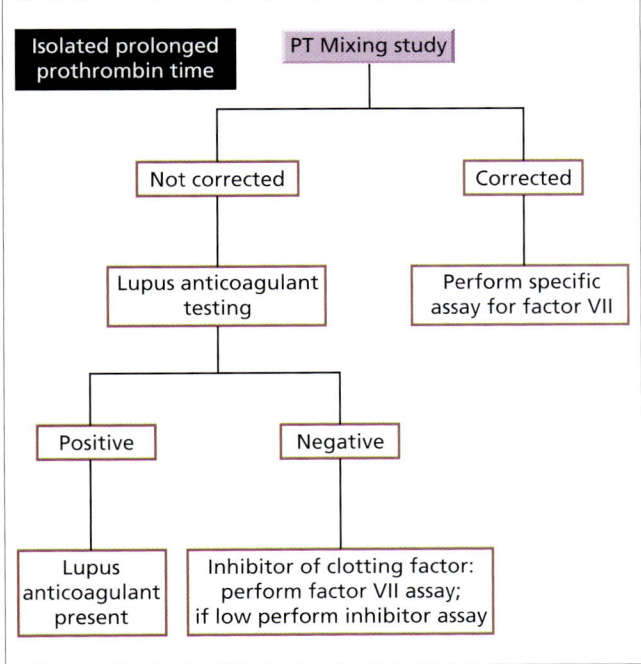

Figure 10-4 Algorithm for evaluation of an isolated prolonged prothrombin time.

Causes of an isolated prolonged aPTT include preanalytical artifacts, congenital factor deficiencies, acquired inhibitors, and anticoagulation therapies (Figure 10-5).

Deficiency of factors VIII, IX, XI, XII, PK, and HMWK prolong the aPTT. Severe deficiencies of factor XII, PK, and HMWK are rare, typically produce aPTTs >100 seconds, and do not cause a bleeding disorder. Depending on the coagulation reagents and instrument in use, in order for an isolated intrinsic factor deficiency to prolong the aPTT, activity is usually <30% to 40%.

Factors VIII and IX deficiencies, or hemophilia A and B, respectively, are X-linked inherited disorders that are often diagnosed early in life due to spontaneous bleeding or a positive maternal family history of hemophilia. Occasionally, diagnosis is delayed until adulthood if it is a mild deficiency (5%-40%).

A patient with type 1 vWD may have a slightly prolonged aPTT if the factor VIII level is below the threshold of detection.

Factor XI deficiency should be investigated when a prolonged aPTT is encountered in a person of Ashkenazi ancestry. Bleeding risk is variable and does not correlate particularly well with the severity of factor XI deficiency.

Lupus anticoagulants can cause a prolonged aPTT (see section on thrombophilia testing). If a prolonged aPTT does not substantially shorten when repeated on a 1:1 mix with PNP, perform lupus anticoagulant testing and/or specific factor activities depending on the clinical context.

Inhibitors to factor VIII are detected in 25% to 30% of males with severe hemophilia A due to development of alloantibodies to infusions of "foreign" factor VIII. Alloantibody formation to factor IX in males with severe hemophilia B occurs less often. Acquired hemophilia caused by autoantibodies to factor VIII is the most common acquired specific factor inhibitor. A factor VIII antibody is suspected in patient with a prolonged aPTT that fails to fully correct immediately after 1:1 mixing and subsequently prolongs after a 1- to 2-hour incubation of the 1:1 mixture at 37°C. The inhibitor may be apparent only after prolonged incubation because it may be directed against a protected site in factor VIII. A very low or undetectable factor VIII activity and mild inhibitor patterns for factors IX and XI due to partial inhibition of factor VIII in these aPTT-based activity assays confirm the presence of a specific factor VIII inhibitor. The Bethesda assay determines the potency of a factor VIII inhibitor by incubating dilutions of patient plasma combined 1:1 with PNP at 37°C for 2 hours, followed by determination of residual factor VIII activity. The antibody titer is expressed in Bethesda units (BU) equal to the reciprocal of the patient plasma dilution required to obtain recovery of 50% of the expected factor VIII activity in the incubated 1:1 mixture. A BU of 0.5 to 5.0 is a low titer and may be overwhelmed with larger infusions of factor VIII, whereas a BU >10 will require treatment of bleeding episodes with a factor VIII bypass product such as recombinant factor VIIa. The Nijmegen modification of the 1:1 mix conditions improves accuracy and precision of the Bethesda assay for low titer inhibitors.

Most hospitals use aPTT-based nomograms to guide therapeutic anticoagulation with unfractionated heparin. A therapeutic aPTT range is typically determined by collecting plasma samples from patients on heparin infusions and comparing aPTTs to heparin activity using the anti-Xa chromogenic assay. The aPTT therapeutic range in seconds will correspond to an anti-Xa range of 0.3 to 0.7 IU/mL. The aPTT is also used to monitor the direct thrombin inhibitors lepirudin and argatroban, and the therapeutic targets recommended by the manufacturers are 1.5 to 2.5 and 1.5 to 3.0 times the baseline aPTT, respectively. Therapeutic infusions of direct thrombin inhibitors also prolong the PT/INR, and the intensity depends on the specific direct thrombin inhibitor and the thromboplastin reagent.

The anti-Xa assay is a variation of a chromogenic antithrombin assay (see section on thrombophilia testing) comparing an unknown concentration of heparin in the patient plasma to a calibration curve prepared with an unfractionated heparin standard. Activated factor Xa is added to the test

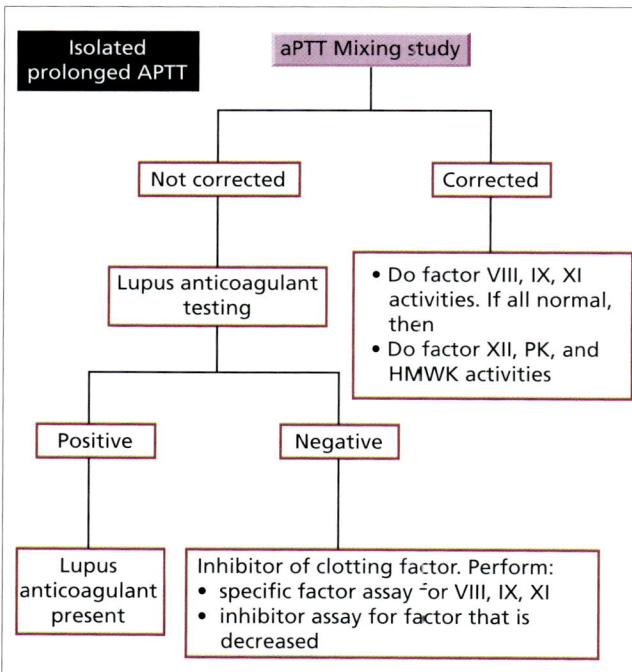

Figure 10-5 Algorithm for evaluation of an isolated prolonged activated partial thromboplastin time (aPTT). HMWK = high molecular weight kininogen; PK = prekallikrein.

plasma, and the rate of factor Xa neutralization by antithrombin is positively correlated with the heparin concentration, and the rate of chromogenic substrate cleavage by factor Xa is inversely correlated with the heparin concentration. Directly monitoring heparin anticoagulation with the anti-Xa assay is the preferred approach in some hospitals and is an alternative to the aPTT when unusually high rates of heparin infusion are required or when a patient's baseline aPTT is prolonged due to a lupus anticoagulant or deficiency of a contact activator (factor XII, PK, or HMWK). Low molecular weight heparins (LWMHs) will minimally prolong the aPTT at therapeutic concentrations. LMWHs typically do not require monitoring. However, under certain situations, including patients of extremely low and high weights, pregnant patients, and patients with impaired renal function, monitoring plasma LMWH activity approximately 4 hours after a subcutaneous injection using a chromogenic anti-Xa assay calibrated against an LMWH standard with a therapeutic target of 0.6 to 1.0 IU/mL is recommended.

Key points

Isolated prolonged aPTT:
- Factor VIII, IX, or XI deficiency
- Lupus anticoagulant
- Factor VIII inhibitor
- vWD (if factor VIII is <30%-40%)
- Factor XII, PK, or HMWK deficiency
- Heparin therapy or contamination of sample
- Direct thrombin inhibitor

Combined abnormalities of PT and aPTT

Deficiency or inhibition of a factor in the common pathway (factors X, V, II, and fibrinogen), hypofibrinogenemia, dysfibrinogenemia DIC, and lupus can cause combined prolongation of the PT and aPTT. Advanced liver disease can cause decreased hepatic synthesis of all coagulation factors, except for factor VIII, and acquired dysfibrinogenemia, which is suggested by a low fibrinogen level in a functional assay combined with a normal or high level of immunologic fibrinogen (see section on fibrinogen assays). See Figure 10-6 for evaluation of a prolonged PT and aPTT.

Symptomatic inhibitors to factor V rarely occur after patient exposure to bovine thrombin (which also contains bovine factor V) is combined with fibrinogen to produce "fibrin glue" during cardiothoracic, neurosurgery, and other surgical procedures to control bleeding. Bovine factor V antibodies may cross-react with human factor V to cause bleeding. Low factor V activity and specific in vitro inhibition of factor V confirm the diagnosis. Fortunately, fibrin glue therapeutics containing either plasma-derived or recombinant human thrombin are now available, making it possible to avoid iatrogenic development of acquired factor V inhibitors.

Acquired prothrombin deficiency rarely accompanies lupus anticoagulants and can cause abnormal bleeding. The autoantibodies do not produce an inhibitor pattern in mixing studies because they are not directed against the active site of the molecule. Rather, they form immune complexes, increasing the clearance rate and lowering prothrombin activity.

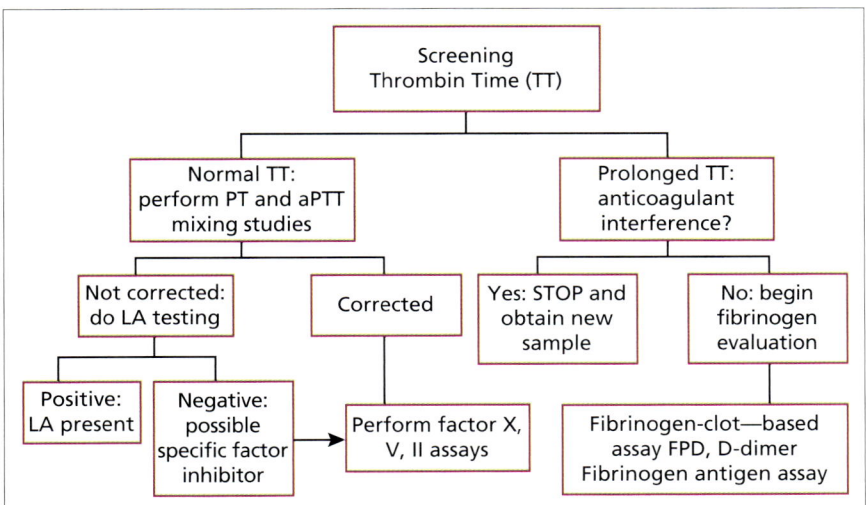

Figure 10-6 Algorithm for evaluation of a prolonged prothrombin time (PT) and activated partial thromboplastin time (aPTT). FDP = fibrin degradation product.

> **Key points**
>
> Prolonged PT and aPTT:
> - Prolonged thrombin time
> - Factors X, V, or prothrombin deficiency
> - Hypofibrinogenemia or dysfibrinogenemia
> - Liver disease
> - Excessive warfarin anticoagulation or vitamin K deficiency
> - Factor V or prothrombin autoantibodies

Thrombin time

The thrombin time (TT) measures the time required to convert fibrinogen to a fibrin clot, bypassing the intrinsic, extrinsic, and common pathways. TT requires sufficient amounts of normal fibrinogen and absence of thrombin inhibitors and substances that impede fibrin polymerization. The only reagent is bovine or human thrombin, and the test sample is undiluted citrated plasma.

- *Unfractionated heparin, LMWH, lepirudin, argatroban, bivalirudin, and oral thrombin inhibitors* inhibit thrombin and prolong the TT.
- *Dysfibrinogenemias* usually prolong the TT and are suspected if the functional test (clottable fibrinogen) is disproportionately low compared with an immunologic measurement of fibrinogen.
- *Hypofibrinogenemia* usually prolongs the TT when levels of fibrinogen are below approximately 90 mg/dL. L-Asparaginase can cause hypofibrinogenemia by inhibiting synthesis.
- *Neutralizing thrombin autoantibodies* are rare, but antibodies to bovine thrombin can occur after the use of fibrin glue. The antibodies to bovine thrombin usually do not cross-react with human thrombin. The TT will be prolonged when the activator is bovine thrombin.
- *Fibrin degradation products* in very high concentrations and M proteins can inhibit fibrin polymerization and prolong the TT.
- Heparin-like anticoagulants (heparan sulfates) have occurred in patients with multiple myeloma and other tumors. They prolong the TT by interacting with antithrombin in a manner similar to heparin. The reptilase time will be normal in these patients.

> **Key points**
>
> Prolonged TT:
> - Heparin and direct thrombin inhibitors in plasma sample
> - Hypofibrinogenemia or dysfibrinogenemia
> - Thrombin autoantibodies
> - Heparin-like anticoagulants
> - Elevated fibrin degradation products

Fibrinogen assays

The most commonly performed fibrinogen assay is a modified TT where fibrinogen rather than the thrombin is limiting. The time to clot formation is proportional to fibrinogen activity calibrated against a standard of known concentration and expressed as milligrams per deciliter. The thrombin concentration is high enough to not be affected by therapeutic concentrations of heparin and direct thrombin inhibitors. Fibrinogen can also be measured in immunologic tests (radial immunodiffusion) to evaluate for possible dysfibrinogenemia.

Reptilase time

Reptilase is a snake venom that cleaves fibrinopeptide A from fibrinogen and results in fibrin clot formation. This assay is prolonged by hypofibrinogenemia and most dysfibrinogenemias but is not prolonged by heparin because the reptilase enzyme is not inactivated by antithrombin.

Global hemostasis tests

Two different approaches to assessing a patient's hemostatic capacity are gaining more attention lately, although the underlying methods date back decades. Thromboelastography involves monitoring the viscoelasticity properties of whole blood during clot initiation, contraction, and lysis. The thromboelastograph (TEG; Haemoscope, Niles, IL) is the most commonly used instrument in the United States, employing a plastic cup, containing a whole blood specimen, that rotates back and forth and a pin immersed into the blood that is connected to a mechanical-electrical transducer. As fibrin forms and platelets aggregate, the pin begins to turn, producing a tracing of clot firmness over time. Certain patterns correlate with coagulopathies, fibrinogen deficiency, thrombocytopenia, and hyperfibrinolysis. Most experience with thromboelastography has been in the liver transplantation and cardiopulmonary bypass surgery settings, where rapid point-of-care hemostasis information is used to select blood component replacement products. The test conditions can be modified in several ways, including to specifically assess residual platelet responsiveness in patients prescribed aspirin. Modest clinical research has been done with this technology in other medical settings to evaluate patients' bleeding or thrombotic risk, but thromboelastography is not ready for general use as a diagnostic test.

The clotting end point for PT and aPTT tests requires approximately 5% of the total thrombin-generating capacity of plasma. Investigators have developed new reagents and software to enable continuous monitoring of thrombin generation based on hydrolysis of a fluorogenic thrombin-specific substrate. Several properties can be quantified including lag time, maximum rate of thrombin generation, and area under the curve or endogenous thrombin generation. Conditions can be modified to measure thrombin generation with different activators in plasma or platelet-rich plasma and with activation of the protein C pathway to monitor endogenous anticoagulant activity. Although ongoing clinical research suggests thrombin-generation assays could have diagnostic utility for some hemostasis disorders, they are not ready for routine clinical use.

von Willebrand factor assays

Endothelial cells and megakaryocytes synthesize von Willebrand factor (vWF) molecules, which undergo dimerization and subsequent linkage of dimers to form a wide range of vWF multimers prior to secretion into blood. Once released, very large multimers undergo remodeling to smaller molecules via cleavage by the protease ADAMTS13. There are multiple domains in vWF with specific functions to support its 2 activities: adhesion to connective tissue and platelets and binding factor VIII. Deficiencies of vWF (vWD) can be congenital or acquired, associated most often with lymphoproliferative disorders, particularly monoclonal gammopathy of unknown significance, hypothyroidism, and severe aortic stenosis. Laboratory testing for suspected vWD is challenging due to the variability of personal and family bleeding histories, multiple types of vWF defects, physiologic variables affecting vWF levels, and analytical imprecision of certain vWF test methods. Repeated testing is frequently indicated to confirm abnormal results before diagnosing a patient with vWD. See Chapter 9 for additional information regarding clinical presentation, classification, and management of vWD.

Initial testing for vWD

Global tests of primary hemostasis, including bleeding time and PFA-100 (Siemens) closure times, lack both sensitivity and specificity for vWD, and aPTT is an indirect and potentially insensitive screening test for low factor VIII activity. vWF antigen concentration (vWF:Ag), vWF adhesion to platelets and/or collagen, and factor VIII activity measurements are sufficient initial screening tests. Reference intervals for these analytes vary based on blood type, and type O individuals have mean values approximately 25% lower than non–type O controls. Some laboratories provide blood type–specific reference intervals, whereas other laboratories provide a single reference range (with lower limits of approximately 50%) and note that asymptomatic type O individuals may have vWF antigen, activity, and factor VIII levels as low as 35% to 40%. It is reasonable to consider vWF levels in the range of 30% to 50% as biomarkers for mild bleeding tendency rather than an inheritable disease, and this is supported by weak and inconsistent bleeding histories and lack of plausible genetic mutations for most patients with values in this range. The variable levels of vWF in patients during physiologic alterations associated with acute-phase reactions, the menstrual cycle, or pregnancy can also make the interpretation of theses analytes problematic, and patients may require repeat testing after an interval of several weeks. There are several equivalent and accurate methods to quantify vWF:Ag, including enzyme-linked immunosorbent assay (ELISA) and automated immunoassays that monitor agglutination of latex particles coated with vWF antibodies. Measuring vWF adhesion activity is another matter. The most widely used method to assess vWF binding to platelet GPIb/IX/V complex is the ristocetin cofactor assay (vWF:RCo) performed on a platelet aggregometry instrument. Ristocetin, an antibiotic, binds to vWF, causing a change in conformation that mimics the affect of high shear stress in vivo to expose the platelet binding domain. Control platelets adhere to the modified vWF multimers, causing agglutination and increased light transmission. The vWF:RCo activity is sensitive both to quantitative deficiencies of vWF (type 1 deficiency) and to mutations causing reductions in large and medium vWF multimers or defects in platelet binding (types 2A, 2B, and 2M vWD). A vWF:RCo/vWF:Ag ratio of <0.7 supports a qualitative, or type 2, vWF defect and warrants specialized confirmatory testing (Tables 10-11 and 10-12). The vWF:RCo assay is technically demanding, labor intensive, and imprecise, leading to the development of alternative methods to assess adhesive activity including binding to immobilized collagen, immobilized platelet GPIb to capture vWF, and automated immunoturbidity assays using lyophilized platelets and ristocetin. The collagen binding assay is not widely used due to variable performance of commercial collagen binding ELISA assays, which is attributed to different types of collagen, and the possibility of not detecting type 2M vWD. An automated immunoturbidity assay using latex particles coated with monoclonal antibodies to the vWF GPIb binding domain compares favorably with vWF:RCo activity for detection of vWD.

Specialized testing to classify vWD

Dismissing a possible diagnosis of vWD or confirming a diagnosis of type 1 or type 3 vWD can usually be accomplished by reviewing vWF:Ag, vWF activity, and factor VIII activity results, although repetition of this test panel may be necessary due to biologic variability and analytical imprecision. However, vWF activity or factor VIII activity much lower than vWF:Ag is an indication for more specific testing. vWD multimer analysis provides qualitative information by identifying structural abnormalities that correlate with qualitative defects in vWF adhesion (Figure 10-7). Electrophoresis of plasma through low-concentration agarose gel

Table 10-11 vWF assays.

Name	Function	Assay
vWF activity	Activity of vWF that causes binding of vWF to platelet GPIb in the presence of ristocetin with consequent agglutination	Ristocetin cofactor activity: quantitates platelet agglutination after addition of ristocetin and vWF
	Ability of vWF to bind to collagen	Collagen binding activity: quantitates binding of vWF to collagen-coated plates
vWF antigen	vWF protein as measured by protein assays; does not measure functional ability	Immunologic assays such as ELISA
vWF multimers	Size distribution of vWF multimers as assessed by agarose gel electrophoresis	vWF multimer assay: electrophoresis of plasma in low-concentration agarose gel and visualization by monospecific antibody to vWF
RIPA	Measures the ability of patient vWF to bind to patient platelet receptor GPIb in the presence of variable concentrations of ristocetin	RIPA: aggregation of patient platelet-rich plasma with decreasing concentrations of ristocetin

ELISA = enzyme-linked immunosorbent assay; RIA = radioimmunoassay; RIPA = ristocetin-induced platelet aggregation; vWD = von Willebrand disease; vWF = von Willebrand factor.

separates vWF multimer bands by size, which are detected with radiolabeled, enzyme-linked, or fluorescent vWF antibodies. Analysis of the band patterns can distinguish normal or subtly abnormal patterns (consistent with type 1, 2M, and 2N vWD) from major losses of large and intermediate-size bands (consistent with type 2A, type 2B, and platelet-type vWD). The ristocetin-induced platelet aggregation assay is a variation on the vWF:RCo activity to investigate platelet adhesion defects. Several ristocetin concentrations (ranging from 0.6-1.5 mg/mL) are added to separate aliquots of a patient's platelet-rich plasma, while change in light transmission is monitored as platelets bind to vWF and aggregate (Figure 10-8). Normal and mild type 1 vWD platelet-rich plasma typically produces no or minimal aggregation at low ristocetin concentrations and increasing aggregation at higher concentrations. Platelet-rich plasma from severe type 1 and types 2A and 2M vWD patients produces attenuated aggregation at high ristocetin concentrations, whereas platelet-rich plasma from type 2B or platelet-type vWD patients shows an enhanced aggregation response to low ristocetin concentrations. Estimates of the relative frequency of type 2B vWD to platelet-type vWD range from 8-10 to 1. Although the disorders have similar clinical presentations and inheritance is autosomal dominant, they require different types of hemostasis replacement products (vWF concentrate vs platelets, respectively). Mixing studies using normal washed platelets plus patient plasma, or vice versa, can distinguish whether the patient's vWF or platelet receptor is abnormal. Genotyping to detect known mutations associated with each disorder is offered by a few reference laboratories. Rarely, men and women with mild or moderate factor VIII deficiencies lacking inheritance patterns consistent with hemophilia A may be homozygous for type 2N vWD (decreased vWF binding affinity for factor VIII) or compound heterozygous (type 1/2N). Decreased binding of control factor VIII to the patient's immobilized vWF in an ELISA assay and equivalent vWF:Ag and vWF activity results are consistent with type 2N vWD. Genotyping specific for type 2N mutations is offered by a few reference laboratories.

Bleeding disorders with normal screening hemostasis tests

Abnormal, typically delayed bleeding due to severe factor XIII deficiency and fibrinolytic pathway defects is rare, yet should be considered when evaluations for coagulopathies and primary hemostasis defects are negative. Thrombin activates factor XIII, and factor XIIIa cross-links fibrin monomers to produce a durable clot. The urea clot lysis test is a

Table 10-12 Assays for vWD classification.

vWD type	vWF Activity	vWF Antigen	RIPA	FVIII	Multimers
Type 1	↓	↓	↓	↓	Uniform ↓
Type 2A	↓↓	↓	↓↓	↓	↓ Large and intermediate
Type 2B	↓↓	↓	↑	↓	↓ Large
Type 2M	↓↓	↓	↓↓	↓	Normal
Type 2N*	Normal	Normal	Normal	↓	Normal
Type 3	↓↓↓	↓↓↓	↓↓↓	↓↓↓	Undetectable

* FVIII low;
RIPA = ristocetin-induced platelet aggregation;
vWD = von Willebrand disease.

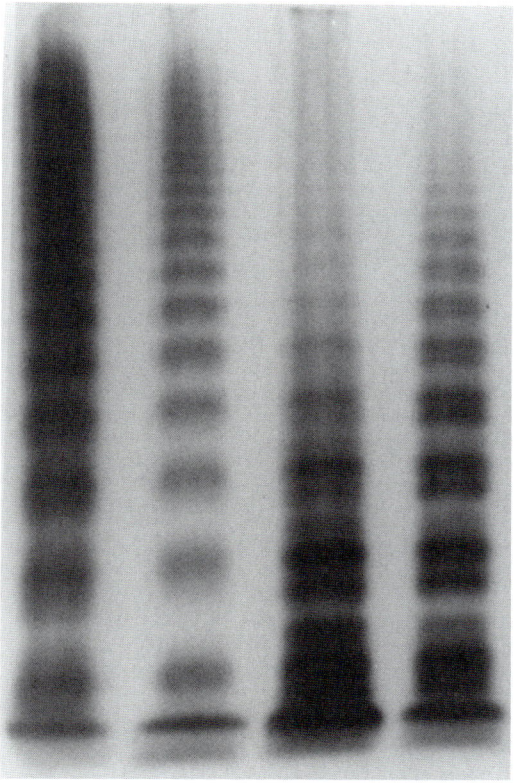

Figure 10-7 von Willebrand multimer patterns. 1 = type 1 von Willebrand disease (vWD) with normal bands but decreased staining intensity; 2A = type 2A vWD with loss of large and intermediate multimers; 2B = type 2B vWD with loss of large multimers; NP = normal plasma.

qualitative screening test for severe factor XIII deficiency. Thrombin is added to plasma, and the clotted fibrin is added to a high-molar solution of urea that will disrupt the clot if fibrin has not been cross-linked by factor XIIIa. Alternative quantitative assays are available to directly measure factor XIII concentration and activity. Global screening tests of the fibrinolytic system include the euglobulin clot lysis time (ECLT), which measures the time to lyse a fibrin clot in the absence of plasmin inhibitors, and the whole blood clot lysis time, which is measured by changes in the viscoelasticity. Few laboratories perform ECLT, and thromboelastometry instruments are typically used during liver transplantation and cardiac surgeries to monitor for acquired hyperfibrinolysis. Congenital hyperfibrinolysis is due to deficiencies of tissue plasminogen activator (tPA) or plasmin natural inhibitors, and laboratory evaluation requires a panel of analytes, including plasminogen activator inhibitor 1 (PAI-1) activity and antigen, tPA antigen, and α_2-antiplasmin activity.

Causes of acquired hyperfibrinolysis resulting in circulating plasmin overwhelming α_2-antiplasmin inhibition include decreased hepatic clearance of tPA due to advanced cirrhosis or during liver transplantation, increased release of tPA from endothelial cells during cardiopulmonary bypass, amyloidosis, envenomization from several species of snakes, and as a component of the disseminated intravascular coagulation (DIC) process associated with acute promyelocytic leukemia. Laboratory support for primary fibrinolysis includes reduced fibrinogen levels due to cleavage by plasmin, elevated fibrin(ogen) degradation products, and no significant elevation of D-dimer levels because lysis of cross-linked fibrin clot is not the dominant process. DIC is the result of a primary disease process that leads to release of tissue factor or other coagulation-activating factors into the blood (see Chapter 2 for more details). Due to variations in the amount and rate of procoagulant material released determined by the underlying disease, there are no diagnostic patterns of laboratory results. In acute, overwhelming DIC, initial platelet counts and fibrinogen levels are low, or serial testing shows a downward trend. PT, aPTT, and TT may be prolonged depending on the severity of consumption, and D-dimer levels are markedly elevated, indicating unregulated thrombin activity and secondary fibrinolysis.

Vessel wall defects, such as collagen diseases (eg, Ehlers-Danlos and Marfan syndromes), can also cause abnormal bleeding. In addition to physical examination and imaging information, genetic testing is becoming more readily available for some of these syndromes.

> **Key points**
>
> Bleeding disorders with normal screening tests:
> - Factor XIII deficiency
> - α_2-Antiplasmin deficiency
> - PAI-1 deficiency
> - Vessel wall defects (eg, inherited collagen disorders)

Platelet function tests

In vitro assessment of platelet activation and aggregation in response to selected platelet agonists should be reserved for patients with convincing bleeding histories in whom evaluations for coagulopathies, vWD, and moderate to severe thrombocytopenia are negative. In addition, prescribed and over-the-counter medications that can inhibit platelet function must be discontinued prior to testing. Many disease processes can produce acquired qualitative platelet defects, including uremia, liver failure, and myeloproliferative and myelodysplastic disorders, but formal aggregation studies testing usually are not very informative in these cases. Platelet

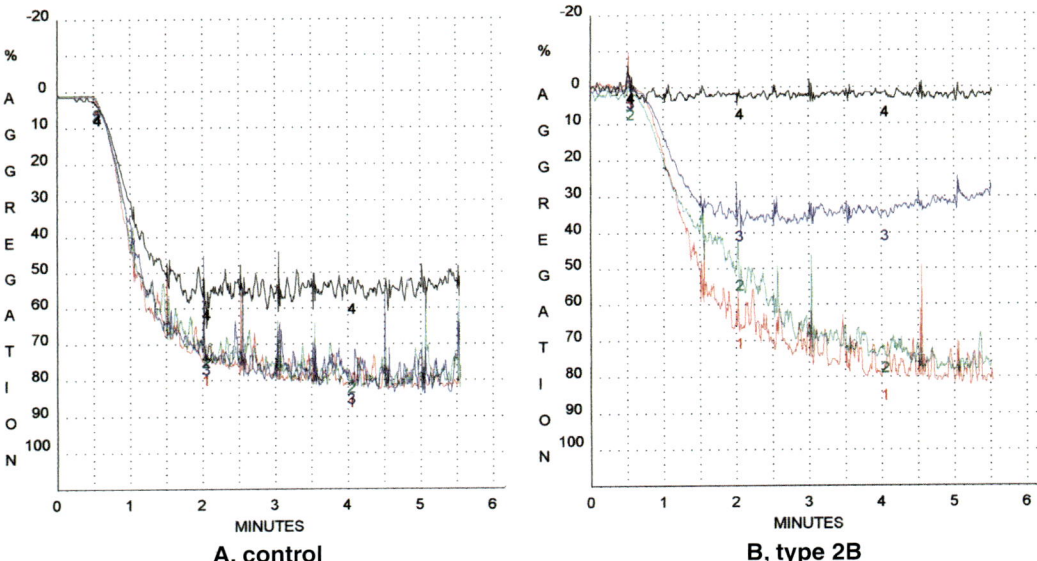

Figure 10-8 Examples of platelet-rich plasma aggregation responses to a range of ristocetin concentrations [1 = 1.5, 2 = 1.2, 3 = 0.9, 4 = 0.6 (µg/mL)]. A, Normal control demonstrating concentration-dependent aggregation. B, Type 2B vWD patient showing >50% aggregation with all ristocetin concentrations.

function testing is technically demanding, time consuming, and poorly standardized, although efforts are under way to develop guidelines for performing and interpreting these studies. Testing is performed on aliquots of citrated blood or platelet-rich plasma with different concentrations of agonists such as adenosine diphosphate (ADP), epinephrine, and collagen; arachidonic acid, which platelets metabolize to the agonist thromboxane A_2 via the cyclooxygenase pathway; and ristocetin to screen for platelet GPIb/IX/V deficiency. Formation of platelet aggregates causes an increase in light transmission over time. Figure 10-9 shows a normal, dose-dependent aggregation response of platelet-rich plasma to

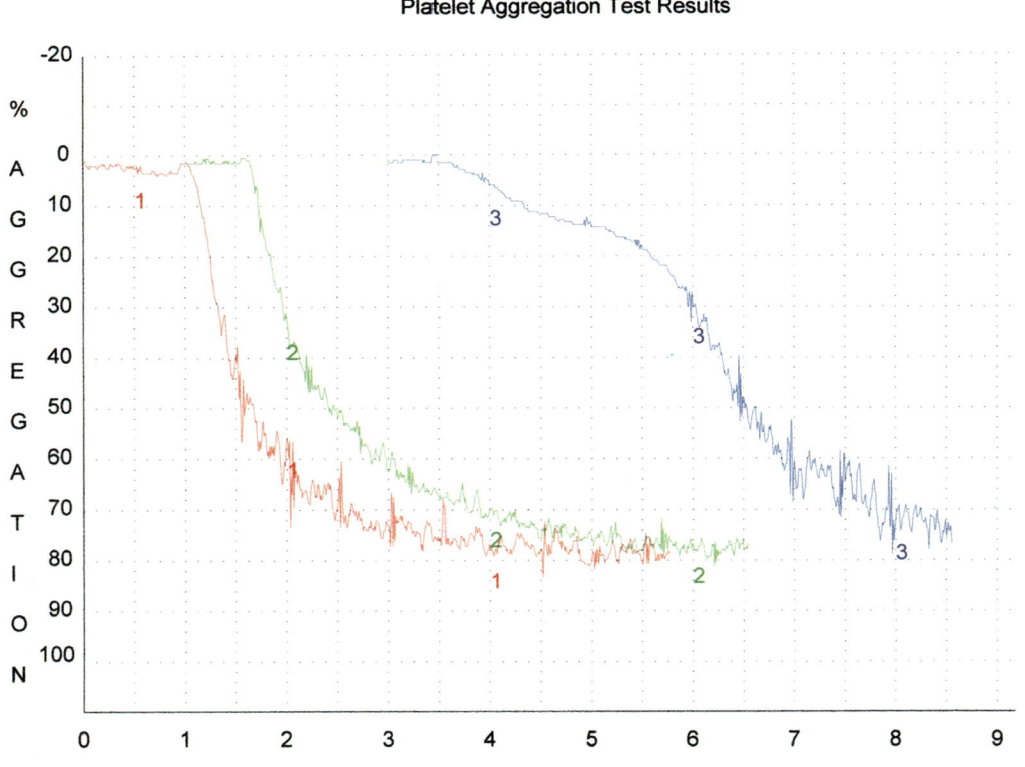

Figure 10-9 Representative platelet aggregation curves performed on normal platelet-rich plasma: 1 = collagen 5µg/mL, 2 = ADP 5µM/mL, 3 = epinephrine 5µM/mL.

collagen and ADP, including a clear first and second wave at the lowest ADP concentration indicating initial aggregation in response to exogenous ADP followed by additional, irreversible aggregation due to release of ADP from platelet-dense granules. The platelet release reaction can be assessed in a lumi-aggregometer, which simultaneously monitors change in electrical impedance through whole blood as platelets aggregate and platelet activation when released adenosine triphosphate combines with luciferin-luciferase enzyme releasing light. Certain patterns of platelet aggregation responses to a panel of agonists are sensitive for specific inherited and rare qualitative platelet disorders including Glanzmann thrombocythemia, Bernard-Soulier disease, and collagen receptor defects. Platelet secretion defects due to abnormal signal transduction and qualitative and quantitative granule disorders are more common, produce variable aggregation patterns, and require additional diagnostic tests that are not readily available.

Global primary hemostasis screening tests

The template bleeding time is an invasive test, fraught with difficult-to-control technical and patient variables, that lacks specificity and sensitivity for detection of primary hemostasis disorders. Prolonged bleeding times performed on asymptomatic patients do not predict risk of abnormal bleeding during surgery or other invasive procedures. The test is performed by making a standard incision in the forearm using a spring-loaded blade while maintaining a blood pressure cuff at 40 mm Hg. Blood oozing from the incision is wicked away with filter paper every 30 seconds until bleeding stops. The typical reference range in adults is approximately 5 to 10 minutes.

Most laboratories have discontinued bleeding times and substituted automated in vitro screening methods, which are more convenient and precise yet have similar limitations. The PFA-100 instrument monitors vWF-dependent platelet adhesion and aggregation under conditions that mimic the shear forces in the arterial circulation. Citrated blood is aspirated through a minute hole in a membrane coated with collagen and ADP (COLL/ADP) or collagen and epinephrine (COLL/EPI). vWF multimers bind to collagen, and platelets adhere to vWF, are activated by COLL/ADP or COLL/EPI, aggregate, and occlude the aperture, which is recorded as closure time in seconds. Reference intervals must be determined by each laboratory, although typical ranges are approximately 55 to 137 seconds and 78 to 199 seconds for COLL/ADP and COLL/EPI cartridges, respectively. Prolonged PFA-100 closure time is not sufficiently sensitive for all congenital qualitative platelet disorders and types of vWD to be used as a general screening test. In addition, as anemia and thrombocytopenia worsen, closure times increase, and these variables should be considered when interpreting prolonged closure times in the setting of hematocrit <25% to 30% and platelet count <$100 \times 10^6/\mu L$. Prolonged COLL/EPI closure time is a sensitive test for aspirin inhibition of platelets, but the COLL/ADP closure time is insensitive to blockade of the platelet P2Y12 ADP receptor by thienopyridines. One prospective preoperative assessment study, combining bleeding history, PFA-100 testing, and selective prophylactic treatment with desmopressin, showed a reduction in blood transfusions. However, the results do not validate using PFA-100 closure times to predict bleeding or direct platelet transfusions or other hemostasis therapies in unselected patients.

Specialized testing for acquired thrombocytopenia
Assays for platelet antibodies

Immune-mediated thrombocytopenia remains a clinical diagnosis of exclusion due to the general poor performance of laboratory methods to detect platelet-specific antibodies. Assays detecting total or surface bound platelet immunoglobulins are nonspecific and are not recommended. More specific direct tests have been adapted for immunoassays (monoclonal antibody immobilization of platelet antigen [MAIPA]) and flow cytometry analysis. Platelet lysates provide immune complexes that are captured by platelet-specific antibodies to GPIIb/IIIa, GPIb, and GPIa/Ia attached to beads or immobilized in microtiter wells and detected with labeled antihuman immunoglobulin antibodies. These methods have similar excellent specificity but sensitivities of only 50% to 70%, and they require large blood samples in severely thrombocytopenic patients. Indirect methods for detection of platelet-specific autoantibodies in patient serum following incubation with normal platelets are even less sensitive.

Assays for HIT

Heparin induced thrombocytopenia (HIT) is a clinical diagnosis supported by serologic and functional assays. In vitro functional assays monitor activation of normal control platelets by patient serum in the presence of therapeutic concentrations of heparin and at high heparin concentrations. Activation with a low heparin concentration and no activation at high heparin concentration are considered to be both specific and sensitive for detection of platelet factor-4–heparin immune complexes capable of causing in vivo platelet activation, thrombocytopenia, and thrombosis. In North America, selective laboratories perform the serotonin release assay to monitor carbon-14–labeled serotonin secretion from control platelets. In Europe, heparin-induced platelet aggregation performed in microtiter wells with visual detection of platelet aggregation is the preferred method. Both assays are technically difficult, labor intensive, and not readily available.

Commercial ELISA assays detect antibodies recognizing immobilized platelet factor-4 (PF4) bound to heparin or polyvinylsulfonate complex. Although very sensitive, HIT ELISA results are nonspecific, detecting antibodies incapable of activating platelets in vitro or causing thrombocytopenia and thrombosis in vivo. The positive predictive value of a positive PF4 ELISA result alone to confirm a diagnosis of HIT is a low as 28%, and if used as the only criterion, a positive PF4 ELISA result is estimated to overdiagnosis HIT by 100%. Growing evidence supports 3 approaches toward improving the specificity of PF4 ELISA testing. First, clinicians can improve the pretest likelihood that thrombocytopenia is due to HIT by applying a validated clinical scoring system called the *4Ts* (*T*hrombocytopenia, *T*iming, *T*hrombosis, and o*T*her more likely causes of thrombocytopenia). Patients with low 4T scores are unlikely to have HIT, even with a positive PF4 ELISA, removing the need for testing. Second, identifying only IgG instead of a combination of IgG/IgM/IgA PF4 antibodies improves the specificity of a positive PF4 ELISA with little impact on sensitivity. Finally, the cutoff for a PF4 ELISA result is based on optical density (OD) ranges derived from control groups not exposed to heparin, and many patients exposed to heparin with normal platelet counts have ODs above these cutoff values. In addition, there is ample evidence that the higher a PF4 ELISA OD is, the more likely a functional HIT assay will be positive and the clinical presentation and course will be consistent with HIT. However, no cutoff point will completely segregate all platelet-activating antibodies from nonactivating antibodies. Conversion from viewing PF4 ELISA results as simply positive or negative to considering OD as a continuous variable with increasing probability for HIT as OD increases is still evolving as clinical research continues.

Assays for TTP and vWF cleaving protease (ADAMTS13)

In sporadic cases of TTP, ultra-large forms of vWF initiate the formation of platelet aggregates and lead to thrombi and thrombocytopenia. In these cases, the activity of the vWF cleaving protease, ADAMTS13, is typically <5%, and in many cases, in vitro evidence of an inhibitory autoantibody is present. In hereditary forms of TTP, there are mutations in the gene encoding the enzyme, and the activity of ADAMTS13 is absent or markedly decreased; however, no inhibitor is present.

Initial techniques to detect ADAMTS13 function and neutralizing antibodies were slow and labor intensive. A patient's ADAMTS13 activity is determined by prolonged incubation of plasma with partially denatured plasma-derived vWF multimers, and enzyme activity is determined by direct visualization of intact and degraded multimers or indirectly by measuring residual vWF binding activity. Development of a recombinant 73–amino acid peptide from the A2 domain of vWF containing the Y1605-M1606 bond recognized by ADAMTS13 has led to rapid commercial assays to detect substrate cleavage by either ELISA or fluorescence resonance energy transfer (FRET) methods. Two amino acids in the peptide substrate are modified in the FRET assay; one fluoresces when exited, and the other absorbs or quenches the released energy. When ADAMTS13 cleaves the substrate and separates the modified amino acids, emitted energy is detected in a fluorescent plate reader. The method for ADAMTS13 neutralizing antibody detection is similar to the Bethesda assay for factor VIII inhibitors; dilutions of patient serum/plasma are mixed with PNP followed by measurement of residual enzyme activity using the synthetic substrate. Typical reference values are ADAMTS13 activity ≥67% and inhibitor titer <0.4. Measuring ADAMTS13 antigen is not necessary when evaluating a patient for sporadic/idiopathic TTP.

The decision to initiate plasma exchange is based on clinical assessment and should not be delayed until ADAMTS13 activity and inhibitor results return because they improve diagnostic specificity at the expense of sensitivity. Although persistently low ADAMST13 activity and positive inhibitor titer are predictors of relapse during remission, the clinical utility of monitoring ADAMTS13 during the acute management phase of TTP is unclear at this time.

Assays for thrombophilia

Inherited deficiency of one or more of the identified natural inhibitors of coagulation (antithrombin, protein C, and protein S) is a risk factor for venous thrombosis, and functional and immunologic assays are available to measure these inhibitors. The use of these assays is generally restricted to patients who present with spontaneous thrombosis not temporally related to recent surgery, trauma, immobilization, cancer, or other acquired risk factors. The likelihood of identifying a deficiency is increased if thrombosis is recurrent or in an unusual location, the patient is young (<45 years old), or the patient has a positive family history of thrombosis. To avoid misleading low results due to temporary conditions related to acute illness, thrombosis, and anticoagulation therapy, testing ideally should be delayed until several weeks after completion of treatment when a patient has returned to baseline. The biologic and analytical variability associated with phenotypic diagnoses of these deficiencies requires verification of an abnormal test result on a new sample. Due to the large number of mutations associated with deficiencies of antithrombin, protein C, and protein S, genotyping is not routinely performed.

Antithrombin deficiency

The most sensitive screening tests for antithrombin deficiency are chromogenic activity assays designed to quantify antithrombin inhibition of factor Xa or IIa in the presence of unfractionated heparin. Abnormal low antithrombin activity results require measurement of antithrombin antigen to classify the deficiency as type I (activity = antigen) or type II (activity < antigen). Type I antithrombin deficiency is more common than type II deficiency in symptomatic kindreds. Subclassification of type II deficiency requires performance of the chromogenic activity assay without heparin to differentiate type IIa due to reactive site defects and IIb due to antithrombin heparin-binding defects. Although type IIb is associated with a low risk of thrombosis, progressive antithrombin activity assays are not readily available and are not typically performed.

Protein C deficiency

The preferred screening tests for protein C (PC) deficiency are chromogenic assays. PC is activated with a snake venom. PC activity correlates with hydrolysis of a synthetic peptide and change in OD. Clot-based PC activity assays are an alternative, but potentially inaccurate results may occur due to variations in factor VIII and protein S levels, factor V Leiden, inhibitory antibodies, and anticoagulants. An abnormal low PC activity result requires measurement of PC antigen to classify the deficiency as type I (activity = antigen) or type II (activity < antigen).

Protein S deficiency

Protein S (PS) assays are challenging due to the unique biology of PS. Total plasma PS is partitioned between the nonfunctional state when bound to C4B binging protein and the free state, which is capable of being a cofactor for activated PC (aPC). The typical PS bound-to-free ratio of 60:40 varies under different physiologic and pathologic conditions. Clot-based PS activity assays are the most sensitive screening tests for PS deficiency but suffer from potential inaccuracy due to the same variables that can affect PC activity testing. An alternative screening assay is free PS antigen concentration to avoid confounding variables. However, free PS testing is insensitive to type II PS deficiency (activity < free antigen). Some laboratories screen with PS activity, some screen with free PS antigen, and other laboratories use both assays. Total PS measurement is reserved for classification of type III PS deficiency (total PS normal, free PS and PS activity low).

Factor V Leiden and prothrombin gene mutation

Two autosomal inherited coagulation factor mutations increase the risk for VTEs; these are factor V G1691A (factor V Leiden) and prothrombin G20210A. Several sensitive commercial clot-based screening assays for factor V Leiden mutation demonstrate a resistance of factor Va cleavage by aPC in the presence of factor V Leiden mutation. Coagulation testing, activated with aPTT, PT, or Russell viper venom reagents, is performed with or without added aPC, and the clotting times are expressed as a ratio (seconds + aPC/seconds + buffer). Abnormally low ratios represent aPC resistance (APCr). Specificity is improved by repeat testing of positive plasmas after dilution with factor V–depleted plasma to minimize impact of inhibitors, anticoagulants, and high factor VIII levels. Genotyping should be performed on all APCr-positive patients to determine whether they are heterozygous or homozygous for factor V Leiden. Although prothrombin G20210A mutation is associated with elevated prothrombin levels, measuring factor II activity is not a sensitive screening test, and genetic testing is the primary method.

Antiphospholipid syndrome

The antiphospholipid antibody syndrome (APS) is an important acquired thrombotic condition. APS requires certain clinical conditions (unexplained venous or arterial thromboembolic events, pregnancy complications), and persistent laboratory evidence of autoantibodies that recognize epitopes on selected proteins associated with phospholipids and identified by coagulation-based (lupus anticoagulants) and/or serologic-based (cardiolipin and β_2-GPI antibodies) testing. Lupus anticoagulants (LACs) are heterogeneous antibodies that interfere with in vitro clotting assays. Indirect evidence for the presence of a LAC requires (i) prolongation of a screening clotting assay designed to be sensitive to the phospholipid-dependent behavior of LAC; (ii) ruling out prolongation due to a coagulopathy by showing incomplete correction in a 1:1 mix of patient and normal pooled plasma; and (iii) confirming phospholipid dependence by shortening the clotting time with the addition of more phospholipid. Although some LACs are discovered when a routine aPTT is prolonged, a normal aPTT is not a sensitive LAC screening test and should not prevent performance of more sensitive LAC testing based on the clinical circumstances. There is no "gold standard" LAC method. Recent updated consensus expert guidelines from the International Society of Thrombosis and Hemostasis Scientific Subcommittee on Lupus Anticoagulant/Phospholipid Antibodies recommend performing 2 sensitive LAC tests in parallel—one aPTT-based test and one Russell viper venom (activation of factor Xa)–based test—and accepting a positive result from either or both as evidence of an LAC. Preanalytical variables requiring attention include platelet contamination (>5000/μL) due to inadequate centrifugation, which can produce false-negative LAC results due to the neutralizing effect of platelet-derived phospholipid, and concurrent anticoagulation therapy. Presence of a direct thrombin inhibitor or factor Xa inhibitor in the test plasma nullifies performance of LAC testing. Heparin can be neutralized by additives in the LAC test reagents or in a separate step before testing, and the mixing step can compensate for mild to moderate coagulopathies due to liver disease or vitamin K antagonists like warfarin. However, the preferred time for LAC testing is before or after anticoagulation treatment. Rarely, a specific factor inhibitor can cause a false-positive LAC result, typically with an aPTT-based LAC test due to a factor VIII inhibitor. Abnormal bleeding would likely be present, and specific factor assays would confirm an isolated factor deficiency. LAC tests are either positive or negative, and there is insufficient evidence to support reporting gradations of positive. Due to differences in test methods, reagents, instrumentation, preanalytical variables, and approaches to analyzing and reporting results, there is substantial interlaboratory variability of LAC results based on external proficiency testing surveys.

LAC can cause reagent-dependent prolongations of PT results. Although this is usually mild, occasionally LAC-positive patients will have elevated INRs prior to starting warfarin. Chromogenic factor X activity is an alternative to the INR for therapeutic anticoagulation monitoring (target 20%); however, availability of the test is limited. Another option is to measure PT-based factor II, VII, and X activities and observe whether the LAC produces an "inhibitor pattern" on the serial dilutions of plasma. If one or more factor assays appear unaffected by the LAC, then suppression of a specific clotting factor can serve as the therapeutic target for warfarin anticoagulation. A markedly prolonged PT in the setting of LAC may be a result of acquired factor II deficiency due to a nonneutralizing prothrombin autoantibody that increases clearance rate. These patients are at risk for spontaneous bleeding. To recognize this rare condition, a factor II activity level should be obtained in a LAC-positive patient with a prolonged PT/INR.

Performance of ELISA testing for anticardiolipin (aCL) and anti–β_2-GPI (aβ2GPI) antibodies should accompany LAC testing to maximize sensitivity because persistently positive (arbitrarily defined as ≥12 weeks apart) results from serologic tests or LAC, or both, fulfill the laboratory criteria for APS. Commercial ELISA kits for aCL and aβ2GPI lack standardization, and interlaboratory agreement is poor for weakly positive sera. To improve specificity, only medium and high titer positive IgG and IgM aCL and aβ2GPI results are considered clinically important by some experts.

> **Key points**
>
> Thrombophilic states:
> - Deficiency of PC, PS, and antithrombin
> - Coagulation factor polymorphisms: factor V Leiden, prothrombin 20210 mutation
> - High levels of factors VIII, IX, and XI and fibrinogen
> - LAC

Bibliography

Automated hematology reviews

Briggs C. Quality counts: new parameters in blood cell counting. *Int J Lab Hematol*. 2009;31:277–297.

Buttarello M, Plebani M. Automated blood cell counts. *Am J Clin Pathol*. 2008;130:104–116.

Fernandes B, Hamaguchi Y. Automated enumeration of immature granulocytes. *Am J Clin Pathol*. 2007;128:454–463.

Kartz A, Bengtsson H-I, Casey JE, et al. Performance evaluation of the CellaVision Dm96 system. *Am J Clin Pathol*. 2005;124:770–781.

Padmanabhan A, Reich-Slotky R, Jhang JS, et al. Use of the haematopoetic progenitor cell parameter in optimizing timing of peripheral blood stem cell harvest. *Vox Sang*. 2009;97:153–159.

Thomas C, Kirschbaum A, Boehm D, Thomas L. The diagnostic plot: a concept for identifying different states of iron deficiency and monitoring the response to epoetin therapy. *Med Oncol*. 2006;23:23–36.

van der Meer W, van Gelder W, de Keijzer R, Wilems H. Does the band cell survive the 21st century? *Eur J Haematol*. 2006;76:251–254.

Miscellaneous laboratory hematology tests

Cappellini MD, Fiorelli G. Glucose-6-phosphate dehydrogenase deficiency. *Lancet*. 2008;371:64–74.

Keren DF, Hedstrom D, Gulbranson R, Ou C-N, Bak R. Comparison of Sebia Capillarys capillary electrophoresis with the Primus high-pressure liquid chromatography in the evaluation of hemoglobinopathies. *Am J Clin Pathol*. 2008;130:824–831.

Old JM. Screening and genetic diagnosis of haemoglobinopathies. *Scand J Clin Lab Invest*. 2007;67:71–86.

Perovic E, Bakovic L, Valcic A. Evaluation of Ves-Matic Cube 200—an automated system for the measurement of the erythrocyte sedimentation rate. *Int J Lab Hematol*. 2010;32:88–94.

Schmidt RM, Wilson SM. Standardization in detection of abnormal hemoglobins. Solubility test for hemoglobin S. *JAMA*. 1973;225:1225–1230.

Sox HC, Liang MH. The erythrocyte sedimentation rate: guidelines for rational use. *Ann Intern Med*. 1986;104:515–523.

Bone marrow aspiration review

Bain BJ. Bone marrow aspiration. *J Clin Pathol*. 2001;54:657–663. *Review article describing the clinical usefulness of the aspirate as well as the technical aspects of obtaining and staining an aspirate.*

Flow cytometry reviews

Gudgin EJ, Erber WN. Immunophenotyping of lymphoproliferative disorders: state of the art. *Pathology*. 2005;37:457–478.

Marti GE, Stetler-Stevenson M, Blessing JH, et al. Introduction to flow cytometry. *Semin Hematol*. 2001;38:93–99.

Stetler-Stevenson M, Braylan RC. Flow cytometric analysis of lymphomas and lymphoproliferative disorders. *Semin Hematol*. 2001;38:111–123.

Weir EG, Borowitz MJ. Flow cytometry in the diagnosis of acute leukemia. *Semin Hematol*. 2001;38:124–128.

Lymphoma immunohistochemistry

Hans CP, Weisenburger DD, Greiner TC, et al. Confirmation of the molecular classification of diffuse large B-cell lymphoma by immunohistochemistry using a tissue microarray. *Blood*. 2004;103:275–282.

Hsi ED, Yegappan S. Lymphoma immunophenotyping: a new era in paraffin section immunohistochemistry. *Adv Anat Pathol*. 2001;8:219–239.

Molecular diagnostic reviews

Alizadeh AA, Ross DT, Perou CM, et al. Towards a novel classification of human malignancies based on gene expression patterns. *J Pathol*. 2001;195:41–52.

Burmeister T, Thiel E. Molecular genetics in acute and chronic leukemias. *J Cancer Res Clin Oncol*. 2001;27:80–90.

Campbell L. Cytogenetics of lymphoma. *Pathology*. 2005;37:493–507.

Dunphy CH. Gene expression profiling data in lymphoma and leukemia. *Arch Pathol Lab Med*. 2006;130:483–520.

Kearney L. Molecular cytogenetics. *Best Pract Res Clin Hematol*. 2001;14:645–668.

General hemostasis testing

Ansell J, Hirsh J, Hylek E, et al. The pharmacology and management of the vitamin K antagonists. *Chest*. 2008;133:160S–198S.

Berntorp E, Salvagno GL. Standardization and clinical utility of thrombin-generation assays. *Semin Thromb Hemost*. 2008;34:670–682.

Bolton-Maggs PHB, Perry DJ, Chalmers EA, et al. The rare coagulation disorders: review with guidelines for management from the United Kingdom Hemophilia Centre Doctors' Organization. *Hemophilia*. 2004;10:593–628.

Kamal AH, Tefferi A, Pruthi RK. How to interpret and pursue an abnormal prothrombin time, activated partial thromboplastin time, and bleeding time in adults. *Mayo Clin Proc*. 2007;82:864–873.

Wagenman BL, Townsend KT, Crookston KP. The laboratory approach to inherited and acquired coagulation factor deficiencies. *Clin Lab Med*. 2009;29:229–252.

von Willebrand disease

Favaloro EJ. Laboratory identification of von Willebrand disease: technical and scientific perspectives. *J Thromb Haemost*. 2006;32:456–471.

Sadler JE, Budde U, Eikenboom CJ, et al. Update on the pathophysiology and classification of von Willebrand disease: a report of the Subcommittee on von Willebrand factor. *J Thromb Haemost*. 2006;4:2103–2114.

Assays for qualitative and quantitative platelet disorders

Bakchoul T, Giptner A, Najaoui A, et al. Prospective evaluation of PF4/heparin immunoassays for the diagnosis of heparin-induced thrombocytopenia. *J Thromb Haemost*. 2009;7:1260–1265.

Chen A, Teruya J. Global hemostasis testing thromboelastography: old technology, new applications. *Clin Lab Med*. 2009;29:391–407.

Doldan-Silvero A, Acevedo-Gadea C, Habib C, et al. ADAMTS13 activity and inhibitor. *Am J Hematol*. 2008;83:811–814.

Harrison P, Mumford A. Screening tests of platelet function: update on their appropriate uses for diagnostic testing. *Semin Thromb Hemost*. 2009;35:150–157.

Hayward PM, Pai M, Liu Y, et al. Diagnostic utility of light transmission platelet aggregometry: results from a prospective study of individuals referred for bleeding disorder assessments. *J Thromb Haemost*. 2009;7:676–684.

Lo GK, Sigouin CS, Warkentin TE. What is the potential for over diagnosis of heparin-induced thrombocytopenia? *Am J Hematol*. 2007;82:1037–1043.

McGlasson DL, Fritsma GA. Whole blood platelet aggregometry and platelet function testing. *Semin Thromb Hemost*. 2009;35:168–180.

Warkentin TE, Greinacher A, Koster A. Treatment and prevention of heparin-induced thrombocytopenia. *Chest*. 2008;133:340S–380S.

Warkentin TE, Sheppard JI, Moore JC, et al. Quantitative interpretation of optical density measurements using PF4-dependent enzyme-immunoassays. *J Thromb Haemost*. 2008;6:1304–1312.

Thrombophilia testing

Herskovits AZ, Lemire SJ, Longtine J, et al. Comparison of Russell viper venom-based and activated partial thromboplastin time-based screening assays for resistance to activated protein C. *Am J Clin Pathol*. 2008;130:796–804.

Khor B, Van Cott EM. Laboratory evaluation of hypercoagulability. *Clin Lab Med*. 2009;29:339–366.

Miyakis S, Lockshin MD, Atsumi T, et al. International consensus statement on an update of the classification criteria for definite antiphospholipid syndrome (APS). *J Thromb Haemost*. 2006;4:295–306.

Patnaik MM, Moll S. Inherited antithrombin deficiency: a review. *Haemophilia*. 2008;14:1229–1239.

Pengo V, Tripodi A, Reber JH, et al. Update of the guidelines for lupus anticoagulant detection. *J Thromb Haemost*. 2009;7:1737–1740.

CHAPTER 11

Transfusion medicine

Don L. Siegel and Karen Quillen

Red blood cell transfusion, 291
Platelet transfusion, 297
Granulocyte transfusion, 303
Transfusion of plasma products, 304
Pretransfusion testing, 306
Apheresis, 308
Transfusion support in special clinical settings, 312
Transfusion risks, 321
Bibliography, 327

Red blood cell transfusion

ABO system

The ABO system is a group of carbohydrate antigens in which the individual alleles are defined by the terminal saccharide moiety. Specifically, addition of N-acetylgalactosamine or galactose to the subterminal galactose yields red blood cells (RBCs) of group A or group B, respectively. Individuals who express neither of these sugars on the subterminal galactose are group O, and individuals who express both sugars are group AB. The subterminal galactose, in association with a constitutively expressed fucose moiety, defines the so-called H antigen. As such, some authors refer to the ABO antigen system as the ABH system. For reasons that are still not clear, healthy persons past infancy nearly always produce circulating immunoglobulin (Ig) M anti-A and/or anti-B antibodies, also known as isohemagglutinins, directed against the respective ABO antigen(s) that are not present on their own cells. Thus, group O individuals have circulating anti-A and anti-B antibodies, group A individuals have anti-B antibodies, group B individuals have anti-A antibodies, and group AB individuals have neither. The expression of A and B antigens is the most important factor in determining whether blood from a specific donor can be transfused into a specific recipient because preformed recipient-derived isohemagglutinins predictably induce acute hemolysis in individuals who receive ABO-incompatible RBCs. Because anti-A and anti-B isohemagglutinins are predominantly of the IgM isotype and thus very efficient at fixing complement, the ensuing hemolysis is intravascular in nature and can be severe, leading to shock, renal failure, disseminated intravascular coagulation, and death. It should be noted that in blood group O individuals, levels of anti-A and anti-B of the IgG isotype can be prevalent. Because IgG antibodies readily cross the placenta, whereas IgM antibodies cannot, the presence of IgG isohemagglutinins in blood group O individuals explains the higher frequency of ABO hemolytic disease of the newborn in blood group O mothers carrying non–blood group O fetuses and newborns.

The ABO gene locus is on chromosome 9. The A and B genes encode specific transferases that covalently attach the specific terminal saccharide moiety to the subterminal galactose. These genes have been cloned, and numerous genetic variants accounting for group O and unusual A and B subgroup phenotypes have been defined. In most cases, the gene underlying the group O phenotype is identical to the A transferase gene except for a single base pair deletion that leads to premature termination of translation. The large number of A and B transferase polymorphisms has precluded the development of reliable genotyping methods for the determination of ABO blood group.

Variations in the strength of ABO antigen expression are occasionally clinically significant. For example, so-called type A_2 individuals manifest substantially weaker A antigen expression and can occasionally develop antibodies directed against the common type A RBCs (referred to as "A_1") despite the presence of detectable A carbohydrate. The differences in A antigen expression among RBCs of differing A subgroups are qualitative as well. Consequently, the anti-A_1 antibodies made by non–A_1-expressing individuals are not self-reactive. Furthermore, anti-A_1 antibodies typically bind only to A_1-positive RBCs at nonphysiologic temperatures. However, when reactive at 37°C, only A_2 or O RBCs should be used for transfusion. Subgroups of B antigen exist as well but are much less frequently encountered.

Conflict-of-interest disclosure: *Dr. Siegel* declares no competing financial interest. *Dr. Quillen* declares no competing financial interest.
Off-label drug use: *Dr. Siegel*: use of recombinant factor VIIa for bleeding. *Dr. Quillen*: use of recombinant activated factor VII in refractory bleeding.

Recent work has explored the conversion of group A blood or group B blood into group O blood. This can be accomplished using an N-acetylgalactosaminidase or a galactosidase, respectively. Preliminary studies of transfusion of type B blood modified by galactosidase have suggested that the procedure is probably safe but are limited by the relatively small supply of type B blood, present in 11% of white donors in the United States. Attempts are underway to enzymatically modify group A blood, present in 40% of white donors in the United States, to produce group O blood from A, although the cost of doing so may be economically impractical.

Rh system

Clinically, the Rh blood group system is second in importance to the ABO system. Unlike the ABO system, which comprises carbohydrate antigens, Rh antigens are proteins. Also unlike the ABO system, antibodies to Rh antigens are rarely present unless a person has been previously immunized by transfusion or pregnancy or has undergone an allogeneic hematopoietic stem cell transplantation (HSCT) using an Rh-alloimmunized donor or an Rh-mismatched donor.

The Rh system is a collection of >50 different antigens encoded by 2 genes, designated *RHD* and *RHCE*. *RHD* and *RHCE* are 97% identical, comprise 10 exons, and evolved from a gene duplication event on chromosome 1p34-36. Individuals who are referred to as Rh positive express both genes (ie, D and CE proteins are present on their RBCs). Individuals who are referred to as Rh negative express CE but not D, either because they have a complete deletion of the *RHD* gene (individuals of European descent) or have nonfunctioning *RHD* resulting from premature stop codons, gene insertions, or other causes (individuals of Asian and African descent). The fact that some individuals whose RBCs are phenotypically D negative have genomes that may contain the bulk of the *RHD* gene has complicated the development and interpretation of polymerase chain reaction (PCR)-based methods to predict the D status of the fetus in the evaluation of possible hemolytic disease of the newborn as well as the general use of genotyping for predicting donor or patient RBC phenotype.

On a protein level, D and CE are 417-amino acid, nonglycosylated transmembrane proteins that are predicted to span the membrane bilayer 12 times. Whereas one protein carries the D antigen and identifies an individual as Rh positive or Rh negative, the other protein carries various combinations of the CE antigens (eg, ce, cE, Ce, or CE). D differs from CE by 32 to 35 amino acids, depending on which of the 4 possible forms of CE protein is present. This magnitude of difference between the 2 Rh proteins may explain the relatively high degree of immunogenicity of the D antigen to the Rh-negative individual when compared with the immunogenicity of other blood group antigens in which single amino acid changes distinguish between their polymorphic alleles.

Inheritance of the Rh_{null} phenotype, in which none of the previously listed Rh antigens are expressed on the cell surface, is associated with stomatocytic erythrocytes and low-grade hemolytic anemia. Many physiologic defects have been described in Rh_{null} cells, but the function of the Rh proteins themselves is only now becoming appreciated. Initial clues to the putative function of Rh proteins came from amino acid sequence analysis that linked them to the family of ammonium (NH_4^+) transporters present in bacteria, fungi, and plants. Recent experiments in which Rh-related proteins were expressed in frog oocytes and yeast have established their function as an NH_4^+–H^+ exchanger.

Blood is routinely typed and matched for the presence of the D antigen for 2 primary reasons. First, as noted previously, the D antigen is highly immunogenic, and approximately 80% of D-negative individuals exposed to D become alloimmunized to D. Second, before the advent of prophylaxis with Rh(D)-immune globulin (for example, RhoGAM; Ortho-Clinical Diagnostics, Raritan, NJ), anti-D commonly caused hemolytic disease of the newborn. Prevention of immunization to the D antigen in women of childbearing potential continues to be extremely important, and failure of prophylaxis continues to account for a significant percentage of cases of hemolytic disease of the newborn. When a dose of Rh(D)-immune globulin (typically 300 μg) is administered at 28 weeks of pregnancy and again at delivery (if the newborn turns out to be Rh positive), the drug is >99.9% effective in preventing maternal alloimmunization to D. The mechanism by which Rh(D)-immune globulin prevents sensitization in the Rh-negative individual when exposed to Rh-positive RBCs remains unknown. It has been proposed that Rh-positive fetal RBCs coated with Rh(D)-immune globulin in the maternal circulation serve to cross-link surface immunoglobulin to inhibitory Fc receptors on maternal naive B cells to render them anergic, although this mechanism has yet to be proven experimentally.

The other major antigens of the Rh system—C, c, E, and e—are also relatively potent immunogens and can also cause severe hemolytic disease of the newborn, albeit at lower frequencies than D. There are no immune globulin preparations available for the prevention of alloimmunization to Rh antigens other than D.

As is the case with the ABO system, variations in the strength of expression of Rh antigens can be clinically significant. In the case of D, clinical significance depends on the etiology of its reduced expression. Two types of scenarios are worthy of discussion. The first is one that is strictly quantitative in nature, that is, RBCs express a structurally "normal" D protein, but in reduced amounts. Historically, this phenotype was referred to as D^u, although "weak D" is now the preferred term. Individuals with this phenotype can be considered Rh positive for all intents and purposes; that is, they are immunologically tolerant to D and thus can receive "wild-type" Rh-positive RBCs. Likewise, if pregnant with an Rh-positive fetus, they would not need to receive Rh(D)-immune globulin to prevent D sensitization. The second scenario is one in which an individual's D antigen is qualitatively different than wild-type D, which, in turn, can lead to a quantitative reduction in the level of cell surface expression. In many of these cases, the qualitative alteration is the result of the replacement by homologous recombination of one or more exons of the *RHD* gene by the corresponding exon(s) of the nearby *RHCE* gene. As a consequence, the RBCs of such individuals, referred to as *partial D cells*, express D proteins that are chimeric in nature and comprise pieces of CE. The immunologic ramification of this genetic alteration is that such individuals may type as Rh positive (depending on the particular formulation of anti-D typing reagent used) but, after being transfused with true Rh-positive RBCs, may make anti-D alloantibodies to the D epitopes they lack. Such antibodies may be clinically significant in terms of their ability to cause hemolysis and/or hemolytic disease of the newborn. Therefore, such individuals should ideally be transfused with Rh-negative RBCs and should be given Rh(D)-immune globulin if pregnant. The important point here is that with routine serologic testing, it is difficult to distinguish a weak D from a partial D phenotype. As a result, this has led to the practice in some centers of using different reagents for performing D typing depending on whether one is typing a patient or a donor. For a patient, reagents that do not pick up weakened D phenotypes would be used so that such individuals would be labeled as Rh negative and receive only Rh-negative blood products. For blood donors, reagents with the ability to detect all forms of weakened D expression (whether due to weak D or partial D phenotypes) would be used so that such units would be labeled Rh positive and would not be inadvertently transfused to those who are truly Rh negative. The use of genotyping using automated microarray technologies is gaining popularity in large blood centers and some hospital transfusion services as a means to sort out true "partial D" individuals from "weak D" individuals.

Other protein antigen systems

Outside the ABO and Rh systems, most clinically significant blood group alloantibodies are directed against protein-based antigens, particularly antigens in the Kell, Kidd, Duffy, and MNSs systems (Table 11-1). As is the case with the Rh system, and unlike the ABO system, these systems are defined by protein (as opposed to carbohydrate) antigenic

Table 11-1 Commonly occurring red blood cell (RBC) antigens of clinical significance.

RBC antigen system	Molecule expressing antigen	Function of molecule	Antibody immune/naturally occurring	Hemolytic transfusion reaction from antibody	Hemolytic disease of the newborn from antibody
ABO	Glycoprotein or glycolipid	Unknown	Naturally occurring	Yes, acute	Yes, mild (IgG form of anti-A,B generally present in blood group O mothers)
Rh	Protein	Ammonium ion transport	Immune	Yes, delayed	Yes, can be severe
Kell	Glycoprotein	Member of neprilysin (M13) family of zinc metalloproteases	Immune	Yes, delayed	Yes, often severe; hypoproliferative component
Kidd	Glycoprotein	Urea transport	Immune	Yes, delayed	Yes
Duffy	Glycoprotein	Chemokine receptor DARC (Duffy antigen receptor for chemokines)	Immune	Yes, delayed	Yes
MNSs	Glycoprotein	Structural role in RBC membrane (glycophorins A and B)	Naturally occurring (anti-M/N); immune (S/s)	Rare (anti-M/N); yes (anti-S/s)	Rare (anti-M/N); yes (anti-S/s)
P	Glycolipid	Unknown	Immune (anti-P); naturally occurring (anti-P_1)	Yes (anti-P); rare (anti-P_1)	Variable

determinants. In general, antibodies to these antigens are acquired only after exposure to blood products or fetal blood during pregnancy, or via HSCT. Some patients appear predisposed to develop antibodies and can form several antibodies simultaneously, which can limit the availability of donor blood.

Antibodies to certain blood group antigens are seen in patients more commonly than others. It should be appreciated that this is not simply a function of the inherent antigenicity of the antigen but is also a consequence of the relative frequency of the antigen in blood donor and patient populations because that will define the proportion of individuals who are capable of mounting an immune response to that antigen. For example, the K1 antigen of the Kell blood group system (often referred to as just "K") is expressed on the RBCs of approximately 10% of blood donors and patients. Therefore, there is a sizable proportion of individuals capable of mounting an immune response to K1 (90%) and a reasonable chance of one of these individuals receiving a unit of K1-positive cells during a transfusion. Consequently, anti-K1 antibodies are the most commonly identified antibodies and can cause accelerated clearance of transfused cells as well as significant hemolytic disease of the newborn. In contradistinction to the hemolytic disease of the fetus/newborn due to anti-Rh blood group antibodies, the anemia seen in fetuses and newborns of anti-K1–associated hemolytic disease appears to have a hypoproliferative component as well, due to the expression of Kell antigens on fetal hematopoietic progenitor cells. From a clinical management standpoint, the apparent dual effects of maternal anti-K1 on the fetus whose cells express K1 have rendered the use of the maternal anti-K1 titer less reliable as an indicator of fetal status as in Rh antibody–associated disease, and more invasive monitoring is often used (eg, amniotic fluid analysis, percutaneous umbilical blood sampling, etc). The Kell blood group system is interesting for several other reasons as well. The protein bearing the Kell system antigens is structurally related to a number of metalloproteases, including CALLA (common acute lymphoblastic leukemia antigen, or enkephalinase) and endothelin-converting enzyme. In addition, weakened expression of inherited Kell antigens may be associated with a rare phenotype, called the McLeod phenotype, due to deficiency of a protein called Kx. Unlike Kell, Kx is encoded by the *XK* gene on the X chromosome, near the locus affected in the X-linked form of chronic granulomatous disease (CGD); therefore, the McLeod phenotype is associated with CGD in some families. McLeod phenotype cells are classified as *spur cells* (acanthocytes) because they contain sharp, irregular cytoplasmic projections. Absence of the Kx protein is responsible for most instances of congenital acanthocytosis associated with neurologic dysfunction.

Another important protein antigen system is the Kidd system, which is located on the erythrocyte urea transporter. Antibodies directed against antigens in the Kidd system are notorious for their involvement in delayed hemolytic transfusion reactions (DHTRs). The pathophysiology of DHTRs is as follows: (i) An individual acquires antibodies directed against one or more nonself blood group antigens via transfusion, pregnancy, or HSCT. (ii) The antibody titer decays over time, such that the antibody becomes undetectable by standard serologic techniques at the time that the individual is screened as a candidate for a subsequent RBC transfusion. (iii) The recipient develops a rapid anamnestic antibody response, which results in clinically significant hemolysis several days after the transfusion. Although antibodies to other blood group antigens can cause DHTRs, the severity of DHTRs due to antibodies of the Kidd blood group system is compounded by the fact that Kidd antibodies, although IgG, are excellent at fixing complement so that the rapid anamnestic response leads to the more clinically significant intravascular form of hemolysis.

Alloantibodies that develop to antigens in the Duffy blood group system may cause hemolytic transfusion reactions, which are acute or delayed, and cause hemolytic disease of the fetus/newborn. Their clinical significance in both scenarios can vary from mild to severe. The Duffy glycoprotein itself is structurally related to chemokine receptors that bind interleukin (IL)-8, monocyte chemotactic protein-1 (MCP-1), and other chemokines, although its function on RBCs is not clear. It may impart RBCs with the ability to scavenge excess chemokines from the circulation. The Duffy glycoprotein also serves as a receptor for the malarial parasite *Plasmodium vivax*.

The MNSs blood group system is highly complex, comprising >46 antigens in large part created from the recombination of closely linked homologous genes. They reside on one or both of the major RBC membrane glycoproteins—glycophorin A (GPA) and glycophorin B (GPB). GPA is critical to invasion of RBCs by *Plasmodium falciparum*. Alloantibodies to the M and N antigens are generally not reactive at 37°C and rarely clinically significant. Alloantibodies to the S and s alloantigens are clinically significant and can cause hemolytic transfusion reactions and hemolytic disease of the fetus and newborn.

As is the case with antibodies directed against antigens of the Rh blood group system, antibodies directed against other protein antigen systems are typically of the IgG isotype when discovered in patient serum during pretransfusion testing. However, in the acute phase of alloimmunization to nonself protein antigens, T-cell–independent IgM antibodies may appear first, which subsequently isotype switch to IgG.

Other carbohydrate antigen systems

Carbohydrate antigen systems other than the ABO system are rarely significant in clinical transfusion practice, but some issues of pathophysiologic importance are of interest. The Lewis antigens (Le^a and Le^b) and the P$_1$ antigen are common targets of cold-reacting IgM alloantibodies. Lewis antigens are technically not blood group antigens because they are not intrinsic to RBCs but are passively acquired by absorption from the plasma. Lewis antigens expressed on gastric mucosa serve as receptors for *Helicobacter pylori*. Persons who lack all P system antigens (Tj[a$^-$]) may produce a clinically significant antibody directed against the P antigen. These individuals are also resistant to parvovirus B19 infection because the P antigen on RBCs acts as the receptor for this virus. Interestingly, recent studies have suggested that the presence or absence of certain members of the P/P1/P^k blood group system on mononuclear cells may modulate susceptibility to human immunodeficiency virus (HIV) infection. Individuals with infectious mononucleosis sometimes develop cold agglutinins directed against the i antigen, whereas persons with *Mycoplasma pneumoniae* infections sometimes develop cold agglutinins directed against the I antigen. The I antigen is also the predominant specificity for RBC autoantibodies responsible for IgM-mediated autoimmune hemolytic anemia (AIHA). The expression of the Ii antigen system is age dependent. In newborns, the predominant allele is the i antigen, which comprises linear repeats of *N*-acetylglucosamine and galactose (*N*-acetyllactosamine). In older individuals, the predominant allele is the I antigen, which comprises the same polysaccharides but arrayed in a branched configuration rather than a linear configuration. Activity of the "branching enzyme" that forms the branched structure is absent in fetal erythrocytes but appears at about 6 months of age. Fetal and cord blood cells thus express strong i and weak I antigens, whereas adult erythrocytes express i weakly and I strongly.

As is the case with antibodies directed against ABO antigens, antibodies directed against other carbohydrate antigens tend to be of the IgM isotype. One exception to this rule is found in the syndrome of paroxysmal cold hemoglobinuria (PCH), in which so-called Donath-Landsteiner antibodies—that is, cold-reacting IgG autoantibodies directed against the P antigen—appear, sometimes in the setting of secondary or tertiary syphilis. Of historical interest, PCH is considered the first example of an autoimmune disease and was referred to by Ehrlich as *horror autoxicus*.

Collection and storage of RBCs

Most RBCs collected in the United States are obtained from healthy volunteer donors, although collection of autologous RBCs and RBCs obtained from so-called *directed donors* also occur. Most units of whole blood collected from volunteer donors are fractioned into one or more transfusable components, including packed RBCs, platelets, fresh frozen plasma (FFP), and others.

Largely due to advances in storage techniques, RBCs have the longest shelf life of any of the 3 major transfusable cell types (RBCs, platelets, and granulocytes). RBCs are routinely stored for up to 6 weeks at 4°C in currently available storage media, and techniques for freezing RBCs impart essentially indefinite shelf life in special situations such as storage of rare blood types, autologous blood donation, and so on; although strictly speaking, the American Association of Blood Banks (AABB) standards limit storage to 10 years. RBCs can be stored in plasma or in a variety of additive solutions (ASs). One commonly used AS for RBC storage is AS-1. AS-1 contains glucose, adenine, and mannitol.

Clinical transfusion of RBCs

> **Clinical case**
>
> A 29-year-old man with chronic renal failure has a peripheral blood hemoglobin of 6.7 g/dL and is seen in the emergency department for flu-like symptoms and cough. The attending physician orders a blood transfusion, but the patient states that he usually has this degree of anemia and that his nephrologist is considering starting him on recombinant erythropoietin. He has been able to conduct his normal office duties without difficulty and routinely drives himself to the outpatient dialysis unit.

From the perspective of the clinician, the most important consideration for ensuring the safe administration of RBCs is definitive identification of the patient. Specifically, it is imperative that the labeling of the type and crossmatch specimen as well as the definitive identification of the unit to be transfused occur at the bedside, not outside the patient's room, as unfortunately occurs with some frequency.

Table 11-2 summarizes the major available RBC products and their respective indications. Because the primary function of erythrocytes is the delivery of oxygen to tissues, the primary goal of erythrocyte transfusion is to improve the oxygen-carrying capacity of the blood in patients with anemia. In addition, in patients with intravascular volume depletion due to acute blood loss, hypoalbuminemia, systemic inflammatory syndrome with third spacing, or other etiologies, erythrocyte transfusion can provide one component of the overall management of hypovolemia.

Numerous compensatory mechanisms exist to maintain oxygen delivery in the face of reduced erythrocyte mass, that is, anemia. These mechanisms include increased pulse rate and cardiac contractility, peripheral vasodilatation, increased

Table 11-2 Characteristics and indications for various red blood cell and platelet products.

Product	Characteristics	Indication(s)
Whole blood	450 mL; coagulation factors adequate; platelets low in number; not widely available	To provide increased oxygen-carrying capacity and blood volume
Packed red blood cells	250–300 mL; can be stored up to 42 days	To provide increased oxygen-carrying capacity
Leukocyte-reduced packed red blood cells	Contain $<10^7$ leukocytes per unit	To reduce the incidence of febrile reactions, CMV transmission, HLA alloimmunization, and platelet transfusion refractoriness
Leukocyte-reduced, γ-irradiated packed red blood cells	Leukoreduced and γ-irradiated	To reduce the incidence of febrile reactions, CMV transmission, HLA alloimmunization, platelet transfusion refractoriness, and transfusion-associated graft-versus-host disease
Deglycerolized frozen red blood cells	200 mL	To support patients with rare blood group phenotypes; to prevent allergic reactions in patients with IgA deficiency
Washed red cells	Saline-suspended red cells 200–250 mL	To support patients with severe or recurrent allergic reactions
Pooled platelets*	300–325 mL, 4–8 donors	Prophylaxis of bleeding: platelet count $<10,000$–$15,000/\mu L$; treatment of bleeding: platelet count $<100,000/\mu L$
Single-donor platelets*	150–350 mL, 1 donor	Similar to pooled platelets; limits donor exposure, eg, in aplastic anemia
HLA-matched single-donor platelets*	150–350 mL, 1 donor	Platelet transfusion refractoriness in association with a documented anti-HLA (lymphocytotoxic) antibody

* Platelet products should be subjected to leukoreduction and/or γ-irradiation for the same indications as discussed for red blood cells.
CMV = cytomegalovirus; HLA = human leukocyte antigen; IgA = immunoglobulin A.

oxygen delivery to tissues resulting from decreased hemoglobin–oxygen affinity due to increased erythrocyte 2,3-diphosphoglycerate (2,3-DPG) concentration and decreased plasma pH, and altered oxygen consumption and utilization within the tissues themselves. Studies relating hemoglobin level to anaerobic threshold indicate that, in healthy persons, a shift to anaerobic metabolism occurs at hemoglobin levels of approximately 7.5 g/dL or lower when the blood hemoglobin concentration is reduced rapidly. Below this level, compensatory mechanisms to enhance oxygen transport are likely to be inadequate in patients with relatively rapid-onset anemia. When cardiopulmonary disease or other disorders affecting oxygen availability or consumption exist, the hemoglobin level at which anaerobic metabolism begins to occur may be increased.

As a result of the previous factors, there is no fixed hemoglobin target for the transfusion of RBCs. For example, a relatively young, otherwise healthy individual involved in a sedentary occupation may tolerate a blood hemoglobin concentration of 6.0 g/dL or less without particular difficulty, as long as the anemia was gradual in onset. In contrast, an older individual with a severe cardiac or pulmonary disorder or an individual with acute-onset anemia due to traumatic blood loss may require a blood hemoglobin concentration of 10.0 g/dL or greater to maintain clinical stability. The efficacy of a low or high transfusion threshold in acutely ill patients in the intensive care unit (ICU) is discussed in detail in Chapter 2.

Another factor that may influence the patient's target hemoglobin level is concurrent thrombocytopenia. Both clinical and laboratory evidence suggests that the hemorrhagic defect associated with thrombocytopenia may be exacerbated by moderate to severe anemia. Therefore, many clinicians attempt to maintain a hemoglobin level of 8.0 g/dL or higher in patients with severe concurrent thrombocytopenia, for example, in patients undergoing acute leukemia induction or HSCT.

Finally, there is some evidence to suggest that patients with acute coronary syndromes may have a better outcome when the hemoglobin level is maintained above 10 g/dL. However, the data are conflicting, and randomized trials will be required to clarify exactly which subsets of patients may benefit.

Whole blood is not widely available in most regions of the United States, and therefore, packed RBCs are the most frequently used form of RBCs. For acute blood loss, packed erythrocytes are used either alone or in combination with crystalloid solutions or FFP. Washed erythrocytes are indicated for patients who have had severe allergic or anaphylactic reactions to blood transfusion. Patients with IgA deficiency often have antibody to IgA, which may cause anaphylaxis with transfusion. Although washed erythrocytes have been recommended to reduce complement levels in patients with paroxysmal nocturnal hemoglobinuria (PNH), it is not known to what degree this practice is necessary. Cryopreserved erythrocytes are used for autologous transfusion when the interval between donation and use exceeds the usual upper limit for erythrocyte storage time (approximately 6 weeks) and for multiply alloimmunized patients who require inventoried units of rare blood type.

All cellular blood products, including both RBCs and platelets, are contaminated with small numbers of leukocytes sometimes referred to as *passenger leukocytes*. Several lines of evidence suggest that passenger leukocytes play an important role in alloimmunization to human leukocyte antigens (HLAs), transmission of cytomegalovirus (CMV) infection, cytokine-mediated febrile transfusion reactions, transfusion-induced graft-versus-host disease (t-GVHD), and other adverse events. Reduction in the number of passenger leukocytes has therefore been a major focus of research in recent years. Randomized trials have suggested that significant reductions in the number of passenger leukocytes, achievable with commercially available leukocyte reduction filters, result in clinically important reductions in the incidence of platelet transfusion refractoriness, alloimmunization to HLA antigens, and transfusion-transmitted CMV infection. As a result, there has been a strong trend toward the use of universal prestorage or poststorage leukoreduction of both RBCs and platelets, particularly in patients who are likely to require prolonged transfusion support. Leukoreduction techniques, however, are not thought to provide adequate protection against t-GVHD (see discussion later in the chapter), so γ-irradiation of all cellular blood products, in addition to leukodepletion, continues to be used in immunosuppressed recipients.

After the clinician's decision to request RBCs for a particular patient, the next important step in the clinical transfusion of RBCs is the transfusion medicine department's selection of the appropriate unit(s). The steps involved in the selection of an RBC unit comprise A-, B-, and D-antigen typing of the patient's RBCs; screening of the patient's serum for preformed antibodies to clinically significant RBC antigens; and performing a crossmatch, in which immunologic compatibility between the patient and the prospective RBC unit is assessed. Details of this process are presented in the section on pretransfusion testing.

In the clinical case described previously, the attending physician's initial decision to administer RBCs was incorrect because it failed to consider the fact that young, otherwise healthy individuals with gradual-onset anemia often tolerate strikingly low hemoglobin levels without difficulty. Therefore, the case illustrates the importance of using bedside clinical judgment in making transfusion decisions rather than relying on arbitrary hemoglobin cutoffs.

As the previous case illustrates, individuals with a propensity to develop antibodies are best managed by attempting autologous blood donation whenever possible. However, in many situations—for example, patients with chronic sickle cell anemia or patients who are candidates for HSCT—autologous blood donation is not feasible. In these cases, adequate time for the acquisition of crossmatch-compatible units must be planned, and accessing rare blood types through major regional or national blood centers that maintain collections of frozen erythrocytes may be required.

Key points

- The ABO system is the most important determinant of transfusion compatibility.
- Rh compatibility is also necessary because of its high immunogenicity and potential role in hemolytic disease of the fetus and newborn.
- Other frequently relevant antigen systems include Kell, Kidd, Duffy, and MNSs.
- There is no fixed threshold for transfusion of RBCs.

Platelet transfusion

The HLA system

Alloimmunization to HLAs is the major cause of immune-mediated refractoriness to platelet transfusion in patients undergoing chronic platelet transfusion therapy. Of the HLA antigens, only the class I antigen systems at the HLA-A and HLA-B loci have been shown to be important in causing immune-mediated refractoriness to platelet transfusion. The relative insignificance of HLA class II antigens, that is, the HLA-DR, HLA-DP, and HLA-DQ antigen systems, in clinical platelet transfusion practice stands in contrast to the major importance of these systems, particularly HLA-DR, in the selection of donors for HSCT. Given the high degree of polymorphism in the HLA system, large numbers of HLA-typed donors need to be available to blood centers to provide HLA-compatible platelets to individual patients. Antibodies directed against HLA antigens can be categorized into cross-reactive groups (CREGs; Table 11-3). In the common situation in which an exact HLA-identical platelet donor is not available, blood centers often use CREGs to locate platelet donors in whom the risk of cross-reactivity between the recipient's antibodies and the donor's antigens may be minimized. For example, if a particular recipient has an

Clinical case

A 44-year-old multiparous female requires orthopedic surgery. Pretransfusion compatibility testing reveals antibodies to 3 separate RBC antigens, K1 (Kell system), Fy^a (Duffy system), and E (Rh system). Crossmatch-compatible blood is transfused, and the patient does well. A second operation is needed, and at this time, repeat screening of the patient's plasma detects an additional antibody directed against C (Rh system). Because of the multiple antibodies, a large number of donor units must be screened to find the required number of antigen-negative units. The hematologist advises that the patient undergo autologous blood donation prior to the procedure.

Table 11-3 Class I HLA cross-reactive groups (CREGs).

Cross-reactive group	HLA antigens within group
A1C	1, 3, 9, 10, 11, W19, 28
A2C	2, 9, 10, 17, 28, 33
B5C	5, 15, 17, 18, 35, 49, 53, 70
B7C	7, 13, 22, 27, 40, 41, 42, 47, 48
B8C	8, 13, 14, 16, 22, 40, 41, 42, 47, 48
B12C	12, 13, 21, 40, 41

HLA = human leukocyte antigen.

anti–HLA-A3 antibody, a donor whose platelets express HLA-A9 would be less desirable than a donor whose platelets express, for example, HLA-A17, because the recipient's anti–HLA-A3 is likely to cross-react with the HLA-A9 antigen on donor platelets as a result of the fact that HLA-A9 is in the same CREG as HLA-A3.

Human platelet antigens

In addition to anti-HLA antibodies, antibodies to platelet-specific antigens may also cause platelet transfusion refractoriness. The human platelet antigens (HPAs) arise as a result of polymorphisms involving various platelet membrane glycoproteins. There are a number of well-characterized HPA antigen systems, but alloimmunization is most commonly due to polymorphisms involving the PLA1 system, also known as the HPA-1a/1b system. The HPA-1a/1b system is attributable to a polymorphism on the β_3 subunit of the platelet fibrinogen receptor, GPIIb/IIIa, also known as integrin $\alpha_{2b}\beta_3$ or CD41/CD61. Alloimmunization to HPAs can cause neonatal alloimmune thrombocytopenia (NAIT) and posttransfusion purpura (PTP) and accounts for approximately 8% of platelet transfusion refractoriness in multiply transfused platelet transfusion recipients. In addition, there are case reports of alloimmune thrombocytopenia after HPA-mismatched allogeneic HSCT. HPA antigens typically arise as a result of single nucleotide substitutions; thus, a particular patient's HPA type may be readily determined using DNA-based methods. There appear to be important differences in the various HPA allelic frequencies in different ethnic populations. These differences may partially account for differences in the rates of alloimmunization to HPA antigens reported by different investigators. In addition to ethnic differences in allelic frequencies, alloimmunization to the most prevalent HPA-1 allele (HPA-1a) is strongly associated with expression of HLA-DRB3*0101 and HLA-DQB1*0201 in the recipient.

PTP is a fascinating syndrome in which transfused platelets are destroyed by HPA alloantibodies through a process loosely analogous to a DHTR, as discussed previously. However, what then follows is the apparent destruction of the patient's own antigen-negative platelets as though an immune thrombocytopenic purpura (ITP)-like syndrome had manifested. Therefore, a more appropriate analogy to the RBC transfusion reaction may be the development of AIHA that can follow DHTRs in the sickle cell patient. The mechanism by which autologous platelets are destroyed in PTP is unclear, although a process involving cross-reactivity of HPA alloantibodies to patient platelets is a favored explanation. However, the presence of self-reactive platelet antibody reactivity has yet to be demonstrated in PTP plasma. From a transfusion perspective, for the patient with a history of PTP, RBC units should be washed to remove any contaminating potentially alloreactive platelets that could incite an additional episode of PTP. For platelet transfusions, alloantigen-negative platelets should be selected.

Collection and storage of platelets

There are 2 basic types of platelet products available for clinical use: pooled products and single-donor products. Pooled products are obtained by pooling individual platelet concentrates derived from whole blood units obtained from approximately 4 to 8 volunteer whole blood donors. The platelet content of pooled platelet products varies significantly depending on the number of units in the pool and various technical factors. However, a pooled product derived from 6 units of whole blood (commonly known as a *6-pack*) typically contains at least 3×10^{11} platelets, which is sufficient to raise the peripheral blood platelet count by at least 10,000 to 20,000/μL in the average-sized adult recipient.

The second basic category of platelet products is single-donor platelets (SDPs). Unlike pooled platelet concentrates, which are derived from multiple volunteer donors' whole blood, SDPs are collected from single donors using continuous centrifugation plateletpheresis techniques in which most of the RBCs and plasma are returned to the donor at the time of collection. Plateletpheresis donors must undergo insertion of a relatively large-bore intravenous catheter to allow processing of the large volumes of blood that are needed to collect an adequate number of platelets. Plateletpheresis collection techniques have been refined such that approximately 3×10^{11} platelets—that is, approximately the same number of platelets contained in a 6-pack of pooled-donor platelets—can usually be collected from a single donor in a single session. Modern apheresis devices are equipped with software that can predict the platelet yield based on the donor's size, platelet count, and hematocrit.

The passenger leukocyte content of a pooled-donor platelet 6-pack is approximately 6×10^8 leukocytes when the 6-pack has been prepared using the so-called platelet-rich plasma method of platelet separation commonly used in the United States, versus approximately 6×10^6 leukocytes per 6-pack for platelets prepared using the so-called buffy coat method of platelet separation commonly used in Europe. The relatively lower leukocyte content in platelets prepared by the buffy coat method reduces the incidence of alloimmunization and febrile transfusion reactions. However, the increasingly widespread use of prestorage or poststorage leukofiltration techniques lessens this relative advantage. The leukocyte content of SDPs depends on the technology used, but most devices currently in use yield units that contain $<10^6$ leukocytes, that is, approximately equivalent to the European pooled buffy coat products.

Unlike RBCs, which can be stored for up to 6 weeks in the refrigerator, bacteriologic considerations limit the storage of platelets to 5 days. Platelets must be stored at room temperature to maintain viability, which increases the risk of bacterial overgrowth with prolonged storage. With regard to preservation of platelet function, clinical studies indicate that there is relatively little loss of platelet function and viability as long as storage is limited to approximately 5 days. Functionally, storage of platelets is limited to this comparatively short period because of the so-called storage lesion. The storage lesion primarily involves platelet activation. Currently available collection and storage systems initiate platelet activation, which can become self-perpetuating as more platelets are recruited into the activated state. These activation changes may be reflected in platelet shape change, adhesion, aggregation, secretion of platelet granular contents, and the expression of activation antigens. An ongoing challenge of preparing platelets for transfusion has been to minimize the damaging effects of preparation and storage.

Cryopreservation of platelets has been investigated as a potential method for enhancing long-term platelet storage and allowing the use of autologous platelet donation in patients who are alloimmunized to HLA antigens or who are at high risk of developing alloimmunization, such as multiparous females. For example, in patients with acute leukemia, platelets could be collected during remission, frozen, and used during subsequent courses of treatment. Extensive research has examined the utility of using either dimethylsulfoxide (DMSO) or glycerol as platelet cryopreservation agents. The average posttransfusion recovery of cryopreserved platelets appears to be approximately 50%, but hemostatic efficacy seems to be preserved. Despite promising early results using cryopreserved platelets, these methods have not yet been successfully adapted for widespread clinical practice, in part due to logistical problems involving the storage and retrieval of cryopreserved platelets.

The long-held belief that storage of platelets in the cold compromised their use as viable hemostatic agents due to cold-induced functional alterations has been recently challenged by several investigators. Although cold-induced changes in platelet shape and other properties of the cells are undeniable, it has been hypothesized that it is really a change in particular platelet membrane receptors induced by the cold temperature that results in a more rapid platelet clearance upon transfusion rather than in an alteration in platelet function per se. The mechanism underlying this proposed clearance mechanism relates to murine studies that revealed a cold-induced clustering of von Willebrand factor (vWF) receptor complexes [(glycoprotein $Ib_{\alpha\beta}IX)_2V$] on the platelet surface that are subsequently recognized by $\alpha_M\beta_2$ integrin receptors present on hepatic macrophages. This interaction, which leads to rapid clearance of the transfused platelets in the murine model, apparently requires recognition of a β-N-acetylglucosamine (β-GlcNAc) residue on the clustered platelet glycoprotein. Experiments have shown that these β-GlcNAc residues can be modified in vitro with galactose by simply incubating platelet-rich plasma with the substrate uridine diphosphate (UDP) galactose and allowing the platelets' endogenous galactosyltransferase enzyme to attach galactose covalently to β-GlcNAc. Such sugar-coated platelets were found to circulate normally in mice, whether stored in the cold or at room temperature. These findings suggested that if both mice and humans share this same cold-induced clearance mechanism, the routine carbohydrate modification of human platelets by collection facilities may provide a practical means for refrigerated storage of platelets. Unfortunately, a phase I clinical trial conducted with human autologous platelets glycosylated in a manner similar to those in the murine model did not demonstrate that galactosylation prevented accelerated platelet clearance after a 48-hour period of storage in the cold. A subsequent murine study conducted in the same way (ie, 48 hours of storage in the cold) showed that UDP-galactose treatment of murine platelets also did not prevent rapid platelet clearance, suggesting that different mechanisms of clearance may exist for short- and long-term cold-stored platelets.

Clinical case

A 56-year-old multiparous female develops acute myeloid leukemia and is admitted to the hospital for intensive induction therapy. The platelet count rapidly decreases to <10,000/μL, and she responds well initially to prophylactic transfusion with pooled platelet concentrates. However, during the second week of hospitalization, her postinfusion platelet count increments are persistently <5000/μL. Having obtained HLA typing on the patient prior to initiating the induction therapy, the attending physician asks the blood bank director to obtain HLA-matched platelets from the regional blood center.

Clinical transfusion of platelets
Prophylactic platelet transfusion

Prior to the advent of effective platelet transfusion support, hemorrhage accounted for >50% of deaths in patients with acute leukemia. With the advent of effective platelet transfusion support, death due to hemorrhage has been reduced to <5%. In an effort to identify a "hemorrhagic threshold" related to the degree of thrombocytopenia, Gaydos et al (1962) reviewed hemorrhagic episodes in 92 consecutive patients treated for acute leukemia between 1956 and 1959 at the National Cancer Institute. Platelet counts <100,000/μL were associated with a slight but demonstrable increased risk of bleeding, whereas patients with platelet counts of ≤5000/μL manifested gross hemorrhage on approximately one third of days at risk. The authors could not identify a discrete platelet count threshold for bleeding. Rather, the risk of hemorrhage increased progressively as the platelet count decreased. In examining patients with fatal hemorrhage, the authors noted that patients in "blast crisis" sometimes manifested hemorrhage despite adequate platelet counts. Excluding such patients, 8 of the 92 patients developed fatal hemorrhage. Of these 8 cases, 1 patient with fatal hemorrhage had a platelet count >5000/μL, and none exceeded 10,000/μL.

In recent years, evidence has accumulated that the appropriate prophylactic transfusion threshold in the nonbleeding patient may be lower than the time-honored threshold of 20,000/μL. Rebulla et al (1997) conducted a randomized study of prophylactic platelet transfusion in patients undergoing therapy for acute leukemia, which demonstrated that giving prophylactic transfusions only when the platelet count decreased below 10,000/μL significantly decreased platelet utilization. However, trends were observed toward increased incidences of both major and minor bleeding within the group transfused at a threshold of 10,000/μL, and the statistical power of the study to detect these trends at a statistically significant level was extremely limited due to the low number of actual bleeding episodes observed during the course of the study. In addition, the only fatal intracerebral hemorrhage observed during the course of the study occurred in the group being transfused at a threshold of 10,000/μL. Similar trends were observed in at least one other randomized trial of similar design. Nevertheless, some centers now administer prophylactic platelet transfusions only if the count decreases below 5000/μL, whereas other centers have maintained thresholds in the 10,000 to 20,000/μL range. Ongoing trials in Europe are exploring the possibility of transfusing platelets only when therapeutically necessary and not prophylactically. Common indications for raising the prophylactic platelet transfusion target include blast crisis or acute promyelocytic leukemia during induction; recent or upcoming invasive procedures; qualitative platelet dysfunction due to uremia, drugs, or other causes; concurrent coagulopathy; anemia; fever; hypertension; and acute pulmonary processes, all of which are thought to increase the risk of spontaneous bleeding. In patients with active bleeding, most clinicians target the platelet count to 50,000 to 100,000/μL, especially in patients with definite or suspected central nervous system bleeding.

The survival of endogenously produced platelets in healthy individuals is in the range of 7 to 9 days. However, the half-life of platelets in individuals undergoing induction chemotherapy for acute leukemia, HSCT, or other acute medical situations is typically 1 to 3 days or less. Most centers check the platelet count in patients receiving platelet transfusion support at least every 24 hours. However, checking an immediate postinfusion platelet count is often extremely helpful in monitoring the platelet response and half-life. In addition, as detailed later, poor immediate postinfusion counts appear to be predictive of the presence of alloantibodies to HLA antigens, which is an indication for requesting HLA-matched products. Table 11-2 summarizes the major platelet preparations and their respective indications.

Choice of platelet product

Several arguments have been proposed for the superiority of apheresis platelets over pooled platelets, including reduced rates of alloimmunization and transfusion reactions. However, the bulk of the currently available data does not clearly support these advantages. For example, the Trial for the Reduction of Alloimmunization to Platelets (TRAP; see Bibliography) suggests that leukocyte-reduced apheresis platelets provide no additional reduction in alloimmunization compared with leukocyte-reduced pooled platelet concentrates. Another argument that has been proposed for the superiority of apheresis platelets over pooled platelets is the theoretical reduction in the incidence of transfusion-transmitted infections. However, because of the very low absolute magnitude of the infectious risk associated with transfusion of blood products (Table 11-4) in comparison with the magnitude of the other treatment-related and disease-related risks to which most platelet transfusion recipients are subject, the cost effectiveness of requiring single-donor transfusions for all platelet transfusion recipients has been seriously questioned. In addition, all platelet products, whether pooled whole blood–derived or apheresis-derived, must now undergo some procedure for the detection of bacterial contamination.

In contrast to the availability of universal-donor (O-negative) RBCs and universal-donor (AB-positive) plasma, universal-donor platelets do not exist because platelet products contain substantial quantities of both plasma (typically 200-400 mL) and cells. For example, group O platelets contain

Table 11-4 Infectious complications of transfusion.

Infectious agent	Approximate risk per transfused unit
Hepatitis B	1:220,000
Hepatitis C	1:1,800,000
HIV-1, HIV-2	1:2,300,000
HTLV-1, HTLV-2	1:2,993,000
Bacterial sepsis	1:75,000 (platelet transfusions); 1:250,000 to 1:10,000,000 (red blood cell transfusions)
Babesia	1:1800 in endemic areas
Malaria (*Plasmodium* spp.)	1:4,000,000

HIV = human immunodeficiency virus; HTLV = human T-cell lymphotrophic virus.

anti-A and anti-B isohemagglutinins that would react against the RBCs of all but type O recipients, whereas group AB platelets are likely to yield a decreased platelet count increment when transfused into all but type AB recipients. However, recent data suggest that platelets obtained from group A_2 donors—that is, individuals who are blood type A but have substantially weaker than average A antigen expression on their RBCs—can be administered to group O recipients without the reduction in platelet count increment that would ordinarily be expected in the A-into-O platelet transfusion setting. In addition, because platelets from many group A_2 donors lack anti-A_1 isohemagglutinin (ie, alloantibody to the more common A antigen structure), such platelets may represent a near universal-donor product except in type B or type AB recipients.

Platelet transfusion dose

The dose of platelets that one administers to a thrombocytopenic patient depends on the therapeutic goal. If one administers prophylactic platelet transfusions to a myelosuppressed patient, the primary goal is to administer a sufficient number of platelets to prevent bleeding, that is, to keep the trough peripheral blood platelet count above approximately 10,000/μL. To select the appropriate platelet dose, one must take into consideration factors that affect the response to individual transfusions including the size of the patient and the presence of splenomegaly, active bleeding, disseminated intravascular coagulation, platelet antibodies, and other factors. In addition, it appears that thrombocytopenia itself decreases platelet survival such that more severely thrombocytopenic patients may require higher doses and/or more frequent transfusions to maintain a particular peripheral blood platelet level.

Knowing the number of platelets in a particular platelet product or the average content of platelets in products supplied by a particular blood center, one can calculate the approximate volume of platelets that should be transfused. US Food and Drug Administration (FDA) guidelines dictate that SDPs must contain at least 3×10^{11} platelets and that individual platelet concentrates prepared from single units of whole blood must contain at least 5.5×10^{10} platelets, that is, the equivalent of approximately 3×10^{11} platelets per 6-pack. In an average-sized patient in the absence of any of the risk factors for poor platelet transfusion response as listed previously, approximately 3×10^{11} platelets is considered an appropriate starting dose. On average, this dose can be supplied by a single apheresis unit of SDP or a pooled-donor 6-pack. If a patient is being managed as an outpatient, larger doses of platelets may extend the interval between transfusions. Many centers calculate pooled platelet dose based on the weight of the recipient; the appropriate prophylactic pooled platelet dose in a nonbleeding, thrombocytopenic patient is approximately 1 unit per 10 kg body weight. For example, an 8-pack would be an appropriate starting dose in an 80-kg patient. A multicenter randomized trial comparing low, average, and high platelet dosing transfused prophylactically for a platelet count of <10,000/μL in patients undergoing chemotherapy or HSCT (where average is equivalent to 4-6 pooled platelet concentrates or 1 apheresis unit of SDP) found that the low-dose group did not experience increased bleeding and received significantly fewer platelets, albeit over more transfusion episodes.

Diagnosis and management of platelet transfusion refractoriness

A commonly used bedside definition of platelet transfusion refractoriness is 2 consecutive postinfusion platelet count increments <10,000/μL. A more formal definition of refractoriness, which adjusts for both the size of the patient and the number of platelets actually infused, uses the so-called *corrected count increment* (commonly referred to as the CCI), which is calculated as follows:

$$CCI = \frac{\left(\begin{array}{c}\text{postinfusion} \\ \text{platelet} \\ \text{count}\end{array} - \begin{array}{c}\text{preinfusion} \\ \text{platelet} \\ \text{count}\end{array}\right) \times \begin{array}{c}\text{body} \\ \text{surface} \\ \text{area}\end{array}}{(\text{number of platelets infused}) \times 10^{11}}.$$

In the peer-reviewed transfusion medicine literature, platelet transfusion refractoriness is often defined as 2 or more consecutive postinfusion CCIs of <5000/μL.

As noted previously, alloimmunization to HLA antigens accounts for a large fraction of cases of platelet transfusion refractoriness, although the fraction appears to be decreasing due to the increasing use of prestorage blood product leukodepletion and other factors. In the absence of obvious nonimmune causes of platelet transfusion refractoriness, such as marked splenomegaly, disseminated intravascular coagulation, or the use of relatively small platelet doses in relatively large patients, the clinician should request a serum anti-HLA antibody assay. In larger patients, simply increasing the platelet dose is often sufficient to achieve adequate postinfusion increments; a trial of fresh ABO-matched platelets is often worthwhile also. To facilitate the acquisition of HLA-matched platelets in case immune-mediated refractoriness occurs, clinicians should request pretreatment HLA typing in patients who are anticipated to require extended platelet transfusion support, for example, patients undergoing induction therapy for acute leukemia or HSCT.

Anti-HLA antibodies are typically detected by means of a so-called lymphocytotoxic antibody screen, also commonly referred to as a plasma reactive antibody or percent reactive antibody (PRA) screen. In this assay, patients' plasma samples are incubated with complement and a panel of normal donor lymphocytes is chosen to represent a cross-section of HLA types. Increasingly, HLA antibody testing is being performed on high-throughput platforms such as Luminex microbeads coated with HLA class I and II antigens. When properly performed, this assay allows both the detection of anti-HLA antibodies as well as the determination of the serologic HLA specificities of the antibodies. In patients whose PRA screen is positive, one should select platelets based on HLA matching, avoiding the antibody specificities found in the patient, and/or platelet crossmatching, although these methods do not always guarantee improved platelet responses. There is no evidence that the use of single-donor and/or HLA-matched platelets enhances response to platelets in the absence of documented alloimmunization to HLA antigens. It should also be noted that alloimmunization sometimes appears to resolve spontaneously; thus, the requirement for HLA-matched products may not persist indefinitely.

Normally, platelets express HLA-A and HLA-B antigens, but not HLA-C, -DR, -DQ, or -DP antigens. Therefore, most blood centers attempt to optimize matching at the HLA-A and HLA-B loci only, as noted earlier. Depending on the HLA type of an individual, one may have little difficulty in locating platelets that are HLA identical, or at least within the same CREG as the patient, as detailed in Table 11-3. An "A, B, C, D" grading system has been developed to semiquantitatively define the degree to which the platelet donor and the platelet recipient are matched at these loci, although the predictive value of this system is modest.

It is important to note that the relatively low-stringency, serologic, 4-loci, HLA-matching protocols that transfusion medicine specialists typically use to select platelet products is quite different from the relatively high-stringency, molecular-level, 10- to 12-loci, HLA-matching schemas that bone marrow transplantation (BMT) specialists typically use to select HSCT donors. Nevertheless, for some patients with unusual HLA types, such as patients who are members of certain ethnic groups, locating an appropriate HLA-matched platelet donor may still be difficult. The blood center will attempt to locate platelet donors whose HLA-A and HLA-B types are within the same serologic CREG(s) as the recipient's leukocytes and/or whose HLA-A and HLA-B types are not within same the CREG(s) as antibodies that have been defined in the recipient's serum using the PRA assay (Table 11-3).

Relying solely on HLA matching has certain shortcomings. In some cases, it is overly restrictive because some HLA-B locus antigens are not present on platelets. In addition, there is only a modest correlation between the degree of HLA match and the observed postinfusion platelet count increment. For these reasons, there has been a great deal of interest in adopting a "platelet crossmatching" approach similar to that used in RBC compatibility testing. In the latter approach, a sample of the patient's serum is incubated with 2 or more small aliquots of platelets from candidate donor units, and those units that manifest the least cross-reactivity are selected for transfusion. At present, it is not clear which method (HLA matching or platelet crossmatching) is superior, and some centers use a combination of both methods.

A variety of approaches have been taken when no compatible platelets can be found for a patient who is alloimmunized to HLA antigens. Therapeutic modalities used have included splenectomy, corticosteroids, plasmapheresis, administration of intravenous γ-globulin, frequent platelet transfusion, continuous-infusion platelet transfusion, and ε-aminocaproic acid. There are little randomized clinical data to support any one of these modalities over the others. Platelet transfusion refractoriness in HSCT recipients can often be overcome by obtaining platelets from the original stem cell donor.

Prevention of alloimmunization to HLA antigens

Results of early animal studies showed that the depletion of passenger leukocytes from donor blood components was effective in prevention of alloantibody response to major histocompatibility complex (MHC) antigens (HLA antigens are the MHC antigens in humans). The study of other approaches, including inactivating passenger leukocytes by ultraviolet irradiation, provided further evidence of the important role of passenger leukocytes in eliciting immune responses to class I MHC antigens. With the development of highly efficient methods to remove leukocytes from blood products, a number of clinical trials were instituted. In general, it was shown that if $<10^6$ contaminating leukocytes remained in each transfused unit, alloimmunization could be reduced by 30% to 50%. Several studies in thrombocytopenic patients have demonstrated success in using leukocyte-reduced blood components to prevent HLA alloimmunization and resultant platelet transfusion refractoriness. A large multicenter randomized trial, the TRAP study, tested the efficacy of transfusing patients with platelets that were modified by leukocyte reduction or ultraviolet irradiation or transfusing patients with leukocyte-depleted SDPs. The effect of using these platelet products was compared with the effect of using conventional, unmodified pooled platelet concentrates. Patients in the study who required RBC transfusion received leukocyte-depleted RBCs. A total of 534 patients were studied for the development of alloantibodies during an 8-week period. Forty-five percent of patients in the control group developed HLA antibodies, compared with 22% in the ultraviolet-irradiated group, 18% in the filtered pooled platelet group, and 17% in the filtered SDP group. All of the differences were statistically significant compared with the control group. Importantly, none of the treatment maneuvers reduced the rate of alloimmunization to human platelet alloantigens as opposed to alloimmunization to HLAs per se. In summary, this large study documented the usefulness of either leukocyte removal or leukocyte inactivation by ultraviolet irradiation in patients undergoing repetitive prophylactic platelet transfusion.

It is important to point out that most of the data documenting the ability of leukoreduction to reduce alloimmunization to HLA antigens have been obtained in the setting of the immunosuppressed/myelosuppressed patient. There is some evidence to suggest that similar improvements may not be observed in the setting of RBC transfusions to immunologically normal recipients; further study is required to clarify these issues.

> **Key points**
>
> - Antibodies directed against HLAs commonly develop following blood transfusion or pregnancy and are the most important cause of platelet transfusion refractoriness.
> - Human platelet alloantigens are polymorphisms on platelet surface glycoproteins that may also mediate platelet transfusion refractoriness, as well as NAIT, PTP, and alloimmune thrombocytopenia following HSCT.
> - Prophylactic platelet transfusion should be considered when the peripheral blood platelet count decreases below approximately 10,000/μL, but the platelet count target should be increased in the presence of specific risk factors for bleeding, including recent or upcoming invasive procedures, coagulopathy, fever, hypertension, or acute pulmonary processes.

Granulocyte transfusion

Granulocyte antigen systems

As is the case with RBC antigens and platelet antigens, antigen systems on neutrophils can be classified as shared or restricted. Shared antigens, which are also found on other hematopoietic cells, include the ABO, HLA, and Ii systems. The biallelic NA-1/NA-2 antigen system, now called HNA-1a/HNA-1b, appears to be the most antigenic, and donor–recipient or fetal–maternal mismatches involving the NA-1/NA-2 system appear to be responsible for a significant percentage of reported cases of neonatal alloimmune neutropenia (NAIN), granulocyte transfusion refractoriness, transfusion-related acute lung injury (TRALI; see discussion later in the chapter), and delayed neutrophil recovery or secondary graft failure following HSCT.

The molecular characterization of neutrophil-restricted antigens is incomplete, although some of the more important antigen systems, such as the NA-1/NA-2 system, have now been characterized at the molecular level. Common properties of neutrophil-specific alloantigen systems include their absence on early myeloid precursors and the acquisition of expression during neutrophil differentiation. NA antigens reside on a neutrophil IgG Fc receptor called FcγRIII, also known as CD16. FcγRIII is linked to the outer leaflet of the cell membrane bilayer by a glycosylphosphatidylinositol (GPI) anchor. As a result, NA antigens are poorly expressed on neutrophils in patients with PNH as well as in a proportion of patients with a variety of other clonal myeloid disorders, including some patients with myeloid leukemia, in which the expression of GPI-linked proteins has been reported to be absent or reduced. Antibody to the FcγRIII receptor has been identified as a cause of neonatal granulocytopenia in cases where the mother was congenitally deficient in this protein, whereas the fetus expressed the protein through paternally derived genes.

Alloantibodies to neutrophil-specific antigens appear to play an important role in some cases of febrile transfusion reaction and TRALI. In addition, a recently published prospective study has demonstrated that over one third of patients undergoing HSCT acquire antibodies directed against neutrophils in the posttransplantation period and that the presence of such antibodies is independently correlated with both delayed neutrophil engraftment and postengraftment neutropenia—that is, secondary graft failure. The latter observation is important because such patients often respond to steroids and/or granulocyte colony-stimulating factor (G-CSF) and thus may be able to avoid retransplantation, which is far more dangerous. In some patients alloimmunized to neutrophil-specific antigens, transfused granulocytes do not migrate to sites of infection, which suggests that some neutrophil-specific antibodies can interfere with qualitative neutrophil function.

Collection and storage of granulocytes

Approximately 10^{10} granulocytes can be harvested from a healthy donor during a single leukapheresis session not dissimilar to the SDP apheresis procedure described previously. Pretreatment with corticosteroids has been used to induce neutrophilia in donors, and this slightly increases the granulocyte yield. Some experimental evidence suggests that pretreatment of granulocyte donors with small doses of G-CSF significantly increases the granulocyte yield. Several studies suggest that administering G-CSF to healthy donors does not lead to an increased incidence of hematologic disorders, but the duration of the follow-up period in such studies is somewhat limited. Because of the very short natural half-life of granulocytes and a 24-hour expiration period imposed by accrediting organizations, granulocytes should be harvested, transported, and infused into the intended recipient within a matter of hours. Ironically, this is often confounded by current constraints related to the time required for infectious disease screening of the donor, particularly with the introduction of the more time-consuming viral nucleic acid testing (NAT), which can take 24 to 48 hours to complete. Because of these issues, some institutions have procedures in place by which the physician of the intended granulocyte recipient can transfuse the product before infectious disease testing has been completed. In these situations, the physician is given the opportunity to weigh the potential benefit of granulocyte transfusions with the putative risk of infectious disease transmission by the blood product.

Clinical transfusion of granulocytes

Most cases of prolonged marrow aplasia can be adequately treated without the transfusion of granulocytes. However, several studies indicate that certain subsets of patients appear to benefit from granulocyte transfusions, including patients with sepsis caused by organisms resistant to antibiotics and patients in whom fungal infection progresses despite the administration of appropriate antifungal agents. Currently, it appears that the initial treatment of patients with neutropenic fever should consist of broad-spectrum antibiotics and recombinant growth factors and that granulocyte transfusions should be considered only in patients with ongoing neutropenia in whom bacterial or fungal infections persist or progress despite the administration of appropriate antibiotics. A randomized controlled trial is ongoing in the United States comparing conventional therapy with the addition of G-CSF–mobilized granulocytes (see "Transfusion support after HSCT") in HSCT patients.

Once the decision to use granulocyte transfusions has been made, an adequate dose should be given. A minimum dose of 2 to 3×10^{10} neutrophils should be given to adults. Achieving this dose requires transfusing multiple units from unstimulated donors or using a collection method that increases the granulocyte yield from a single donor, such as pretreatment of the donor with corticosteroids or G-CSF. ABO-compatible donors should be used unless effective RBC sedimentation is performed. Daily granulocyte transfusions are continued until the infection is controlled; until the patient's neutrophil count has increased to $>500/\mu L$; or until significant toxicity, particularly pulmonary toxicity, intervenes. Patients with alloantibodies to granulocyte-specific antigens may not achieve a satisfactory therapeutic response to granulocyte transfusions and are at higher risk of pulmonary toxicity. Granulocyte transfusions should be temporally separated from amphotericin administration by a few hours because anecdotal evidence suggests that pulmonary toxicity is increased otherwise. Serologic testing for antineutrophil antibodies is not routinely performed, but it is indicated if significant transfusion reactions develop. If antibodies are found, leukocytes from compatible donors should probably be used, particularly the peripheral blood stem cell (PBSC) donor if applicable. Leukocyte reduction filters should obviously not be used with granulocytes. Unlike stem cells and donor lymphocyte infusions (DLIs), however, granulocytes should undergo γ-irradiation. In addition, if the potential for CMV transmission is a concern, then granulocytes collected from CMV-seronegative donors should be used because leukoreduction filters cannot be used.

> **Key points**
>
> - The neutrophil alloantigen system known as NA-1/NA-2 (HNA-1a/HNA-1b) is in some respects analogous to the ABO system on RBCs.
> - Antibodies directed against NA-1/NA-2 and other neutrophil antigen systems may mediate TRALI, refractoriness to granulocyte transfusions, NAIN, alloimmune neutropenia following HSCT, and qualitative neutrophil dysfunction.
> - Transfusion of granulocytes should be considered in patients with severe prolonged neutropenia and antibiotic-refractory infections.

Transfusion of plasma products

Fresh frozen plasma

As is the case with packed RBCs, units of FFP are most commonly obtained from units of whole blood donated by volunteer blood donors. New viral inactivation methods to sterilize plasma exist that are not yet universally used. The most commonly used technique to sterilize plasma uses detergents that disrupt lipid-containing viruses. It has been shown that a 5-log reduction of virus is achievable in plasma derivatives such as factor VIII, antithrombin III concentrate, and prothrombin concentrates. Recovery of clotting factors is generally well preserved with these methods. For a relatively short time period, a solvent detergent-treated form of FFP was available; the use of solvent detergent-treated plasma and plasma fractions would eliminate the risk of transmission of hepatitis B, hepatitis C, and retrovirus to patients receiving FFP. Methylene blue is another method of pathogen inactivation, commonly used in Europe, in addition to the use of ultraviolet-activated psoralen derivatives.

In theory, FFP can be used to treat acquired or congenital deficiencies of virtually any circulating procoagulant or anticoagulant. However, it is standard practice to use relatively purified preparations of appropriate coagulation-related proteins in situations in which specific preparations of the required factor are available, including hemophilia A, hemophilia B, factor VII deficiency, and protein C deficiency. Thus, the most common indications for FFP include situations in which multiple factor deficiencies are present simultaneously, such as patients with liver disease, with disseminated intravascular coagulation, on warfarin, with vitamin K deficiency requiring urgent therapy, with massive transfusion secondary to acute blood loss, or requiring plasma exchange for such indications as thrombotic thrombocytopenic purpura (TTP). After thawing, FFP expires within 24 hours. At many institutions, FFP that has been thawed and relabeled as "thawed plasma" is used instead of thawed FFP that retains its designation as "FFP." Thawed plasma has a shelf-life of 5 days instead of 24 hours; a standing inventory of thawed plasma can be made available much more quickly in emergency bleeding situations. ADAMTS13 metalloprotease activity is stable up to 5 days of storage and such thawed plasma can be used for plasma exchange in TTP. However, thawed plasma should not be used for hemophilia A or factor V deficiency due to the lability of factors VIII and V. For hemophilia A management where factor VIII concentrate is not available or factor V deficiency, FFP should be used.

More plasma is transfused relative to RBCs in the United States. Most prophylactic plasma transfusions to "correct" mild prolongations of coagulation values prior to an invasive procedure do not actually correct the result. Randomized controlled trials to determine the appropriate indications and dosing of plasma therapy are sorely needed. In emergency situations involving life-threatening bleeding in patients with hemophilia A or B where factor concentrates are not readily available, it is theoretically possible to initiate replacement therapy with FFP (for factor IX) or cryoprecipitate (for factor VIII, see "Cryoprecipitate," below), but adequate factor correction (from 0% to 50% normal, for instance) precludes the exclusive use of plasma due to volume limitations. Second-generation prothrombin complex concentrates are increasingly being used to reverse warfarin-related bleeding, although these newer concentrates are not yet licensed for use in the United States.

Cryoprecipitate

Cryoprecipitate is a concentrated preparation of procoagulant factors including fibrinogen, factor VIII, vWF, factor XIII, and fibronectin. Thus, cryoprecipitate contains almost exclusively procoagulants and, unlike FFP, does not contain appreciable quantities of physiologic anticoagulants such as protein C, proteins S, and others. Therefore, cryoprecipitate alone may not be the optimal replacement strategy in patients with disease processes that deplete both procoagulants and anticoagulants such as disseminated intravascular coagulation or severe hepatic failure. The most common clinical indication for the transfusion of cryoprecipitate is congenital or acquired hypofibrinogenemia. In theory, cryoprecipitate can be used to treat von Willebrand disease or hemophilia, but other blood products are now considered preferable. Cryoprecipitate has also been used to treat qualitative platelet dysfunction due to uremia.

Cryoprecipitate is prepared by thawing FFP at 4°C and then removing the supernatant from the cryoprecipitable proteins following centrifugation at 1°C to 6°C. Use of the supernatant plasma (sometimes referred to as *cryosupernatant*) has been explored in the treatment of TTP because it lacks the high molecular weight multimers of vWF that are involved in the pathogenesis of most cases of TTP. However, unequivocal clinical data supporting this concept are not yet available. Unlike intravenous immunoglobulin (see following section), factor concentrates, and albumin, cryoprecipitate is not pathogen inactivated, and a pool of 8 to 10 units of cryoprecipitate needed to correct hypofibrinogenemia in a adult would carry a multiplicative donor exposure risk compared with a single unit of RBC transfusion.

Immunoglobulin

Commercially available intravenous immunoglobulin (IVIg) products are typically prepared by cold ethanol fractionation of large pools of human plasma followed by viral inactivation procedures such as solvent detergent treatment or heat pasteurization. As is the case with virally inactivated FFP, the risk of transmission of hepatitis B, hepatitis C, or HIV appears to be negligible, although concerns remain regarding the potential transmission of certain difficult-to-inactivate pathogens such as parvovirus B19 and the agent responsible for transmitting Creutzfeldt-Jakob disease. There have been reports of acute renal failure occurring in association with the administration of IVIg, particularly in patients with pre-existing renal failure, hypovolemia, diabetes, or other risk factors. Most of the immunoglobulin in commercially available preparations of IVIg is IgG itself, and the IgG immunoglobulin subtype distribution (ie, IgG_1 through IgG_4) appears similar to that found in normal human plasma. Relatively small amounts of IgA and IgM are also present. IVIg has been used to treat a variety of hematologic disorders including congenital immunodeficiency syndromes, ITP, AIHA, autoimmune neutropenia (AIN), and recurrent bacterial infections occurring in association with chronic lymphocytic leukemia or multiple myeloma. In autoimmune cytopenias such as AIHA and ITP, IVIg is often considered the best "emergency" intervention when a rapid, albeit often transient, response is required. A large randomized trial published in the early 1990s suggested that prophylactic administration of IVIg is associated with a variety of beneficial effects in patients undergoing allogeneic HSCT. Two more recently published trials do not appear to have confirmed these findings. However, these more recent trials must be interpreted with caution because their statistical power was limited as result of enrolling smaller patient numbers and administering lower doses of IVIg.

The mechanism by which IVIg ameliorates autoantibody destruction of blood cells is unknown. Historically, it has been assumed that the infused IgG blocked Fc receptors on phagocytic cells of the reticuloendothelial system. Numerous other theories have been proposed including autoantibody neutralization by anti-idiotypic antibodies, saturation of FcRn receptors causing increased autoantibody catabolism, cytokine modulation, and complement neutralization. Unfortunately, none of these theories appears to hold up when tested by well-designed and controlled experimental studies. However, recent studies have provided experimental evidence that IVIg may serve to create soluble immune complexes that interact with activating FcγR on dendritic cells, which leads to inhibition of macrophage phagocytic activity.

A significant proportion of patients receiving IVIg develop a positive direct antiglobulin test (DAT, also known as a direct Coombs test) due to the presence of anti-A or anti-B derived from type O individuals in the donor pools, and there are occasional case reports of overt acute alloimmune hemolytic anemia developing. Fever is a relatively common sequela of IVIg administration and does not necessarily preclude the administration of additional IVIg.

> **Key points**
>
> - The most common indications for the transfusion of FFP include rapid reversal of anticoagulant effects; treatment of deficiencies of coagulation factors for which specific coagulation replacement products are not available; treatment of multiple coagulation factor deficiencies in conditions such as disseminated intravascular coagulation or vitamin K deficiency; and plasma exchange in patients with TTP.
> - The most common indication for transfusion of cryoprecipitate is hypofibrinogenemia.

Pretransfusion testing

The preceding sections discussed the importance of providing immunologically compatible blood products to patients. The term *pretransfusion testing* refers to the series of laboratory tests that blood banks and transfusion services perform to ensure this compatibility. Although a detailed description of such testing is beyond the scope of this chapter and, in any case, not necessarily relevant to the practicing hematologist, it is nevertheless important for such individuals to have a general working knowledge of what takes place behind the scenes in the blood bank between the time when blood is ordered and when it is received. Such an understanding can help the hematologist better understand and anticipate delays in finding compatible blood for his or her patient as well as appreciate any potential additional immune-related risks or consequences of transfusing blood to a given patient. For more in-depth reading, clinicians are encouraged to consult several excellent transfusion medicine texts listed at the end of this chapter, particularly the *Technical Manual* published by the AABB.

ABO/Rh(D) typing

Determining a patient's ABO blood group actually comprises 2 independent sets of tests that should yield complementary results (Table 11-5). In the *forward typing* reaction, patient RBCs are mixed with either IgM anti-A typing sera or IgM anti-B typing sera. Agglutination of cells with either reagent indicates the presence of the A or B antigen, respectively. Because of the medical importance of determining a patient's ABO blood type with absolute certainty, a second test known as *reverse typing* is performed in which drops of the patient's serum are mixed with reagent RBCs that are known to be either blood group A or B and agglutination is assessed. This second test exploits the phenomenon noted earlier in which individuals naturally produce the isohemagglutinins to the A and/or B antigens that their RBCs lack. Table 11-5 illustrates the expected forward and reverse typing results for the 4 possible ABO blood types.

It should be appreciated that discrepancies between the forward and reverse typing reactions occur and can usually be explained by examining the patient's recent transfusion

Table 11-5 ABO blood group typing reaction results.

Patient's ABO type	Forward typing		Reverse typing	
	Reaction of patient's RBCs with:		Reaction of patient's serum with:	
	Anti-A	Anti-B	A RBCs	B RBCs
O	0	0	+	+
A	+	0	0	+
B	0	+	+	0
AB	+	+	0	0

RBC = red blood cell.

history. For example, a blood group B individual who received a number of units of blood group O platelets (a not uncommon scenario in times of platelet shortage or when additional constraints such as HLA matching of platelets is required) would have a forward typing reaction indicating a reaction with only anti-B typing reagent (interpretation: blood group B individual) due to the B antigen on his or her cells but could have a reverse typing reaction in which the patient's serum agglutinates both A and B reagent RBCs (interpretation: blood group O individual) due to passively transferred anti-A and anti-B contained in the plasma in which the platelets were suspended. Conversely, a blood group B individual given a small amount of O RBCs in an emergency situation could continue to demonstrate only the appropriate anti-A isohemagglutinin by reverse typing but show a "mixed field" of RBCs, that is, both agglutinated (the patient's blood group B cells) and unagglutinated RBCs (the transfused blood group O cells) upon forward typing with anti-B.

In the case of newborns, forward and reverse typing discrepancies can be expected to occur because the production of the appropriate isohemagglutinins are delayed for several months while their immune systems are maturing (ie, the ABO type for all newborns would be interpreted as blood group AB based solely on their reverse typing reactions). For this reason, only forward typing is performed on newborns. Less trivial settings for forward and reverse typing discrepancies would be in some patients who have undergone ABO-mismatched BMTs who are tested during their transition from one ABO blood type to another. Whatever the cause, it is important to resolve the etiology for the ABO typing discrepancy to select the appropriate ABO type for transfusion.

Typing for the presence or absence of the Rh(D) antigen on RBCs is a one-step or multistep process, depending on the particular kind of typing reagent used at a given institution. Historically, anti-D typing reagent was manufactured from pooled human sera containing high titers of IgG anti-D antibodies [the same material from which Rh(D)-immune globulin is prepared]. Although bivalent, such molecules were not generally capable of forming visible RBC agglutinates when added to D-positive RBCs. As a result, Rh(D) typing consisted of incubating RBCs with the IgG anti-D, washing away unbound reagent, and then adding antihuman IgG (Coombs reagent) to induce agglutination by bridging between anti-D–coated cells. However, with recent advances in the production of human monoclonal anti-D typing reagents by tissue culture, directly agglutinating, decavalent IgM anti-D is now readily available, and typing for D is accomplished in the same manner as for the blood group A and B antigens.

It should be noted that the affinity of such IgM anti-D reagents is not as high as for the conventional serum-derived polyclonal anti-D and may mistype patients with the weak D phenotype as D negative. As a result, the less prevalent Rh-negative blood products that need to be reserved for the true Rh-negative patient would be unnecessarily consumed by such mistyped patients. For this reason, most blood banks use anti-D reagents that consist of a blend of monoclonal IgM and polyclonal IgG. All reactions that are negative by direct agglutination are washed and then incubated with Coombs reagent to allow the IgG anti-D component of the blend to agglutinate RBCs with weaker forms of D, thus avoiding false-negative results. The issue of weak D versus partial D phenotypes and their clinical significance has been discussed previously in the section on Rh antigens.

Regardless of the anti-D reagent used, typing for D does not involve a reverse typing as for the ABO typing process because anti-D is not constitutively expressed in the sera of Rh-negative individuals, as noted previously.

Antibody screen and specificity identification

In general, a patient who has never been transfused or pregnant in the past would be expected to have only the appropriate "naturally occurring" isohemagglutinins based on his or her ABO type. For such patients, transfusion with blood products that are selected solely on the basis of ABO compatibility should, in theory, be well tolerated. However, because patient transfusion and pregnancy histories can be unreliable or not readily obtained, and possible exposure and hence sensitization to non-ABO blood group antigens cannot be ruled out with absolute certainty, it is the standard of care to test all patient sera for the possible presence of such serum alloantibodies. If any clinically significant alloantibodies are detected, then ABO-compatible RBCs lacking the corresponding antigen(s) must be selected for transfusion.

Alloantibody identification is perhaps the most time-consuming series of all pretransfusion tests. Testing consists of performing agglutination reactions between patient sera and 2 (or 3) reagent RBCs whose extended phenotype (ie, antigenic composition across many blood groups) is known. Initially, patient serum is tested against a pair of reagent RBCs that, between them, express all common, clinically significant alloantigens. If the patient's serum does not react with either screening cell, then the patient is said to have a *negative screen* and ABO-compatible units can be selected for crossmatch, as described in the following section.

If the patient's antibody screen is positive, then further testing is required to determine the precise antigen specificity or specificities (in the case of multiple alloantibodies). To accomplish this, the patient serum is run against a larger set of reagent cells (typically ~11–16, referred to as an *RBC panel*). The set of panel cells provided by the reagent supplier is chosen so that by comparing the resulting pattern of reactivity (ie, which cells agglutinate and which do not) with the phenotype of each of the reacting and nonreacting cells, the alloantibody specificity(ies) can be identified to an acceptable degree of certainty. Note that all reagent RBCs used as screening cells and panel cells are purposely selected to be blood group O so that the presence of anti-A and/or anti-B isohemagglutinins will not affect the results.

Based on the results of the antibody identification panel, units of ABO/Rh-compatible RBCs are selected from inventory, and aliquots of RBCs from each of the units are tested with preparations of reagent antisera to identify antigen-negative units.

Crossmatching

There are 2 basic types of crossmatch procedures, and the one used depends on the results of the patient's antibody screen. If the screen is negative and the blood bank has no historical records indicating a presence of alloantibodies in the patient, then an immediate spin crossmatch may be carried out in which the patient's serum is mixed at room temperature with an aliquot of RBCs from the prospective ABO-compatible unit and the absence of agglutination is verified. The purpose of this type of crossmatch is to serve as a final check for ABO compatibility. However, it is now acceptable practice for blood banks to perform an electronic or computer crossmatch, in which the laboratory information system runs through an algorithm to ensure that both patient and prospective RBC unit have been properly typed for the ABO antigens. This type of crossmatch is thus a *virtual crossmatch* because no physical mixing of cells and sera takes place.

The other type of crossmatch procedure is known as a full or Coombs crossmatch. This type of crossmatch is required for cases in which the patient has a historical and/or currently positive antibody screening result. A full crossmatch consists of incubating patient serum with aliquots of cells from prospective ABO/Rh-compatible units as in the immediate spin type, but the reactions are carried to the Coombs phase (ie, cell/serum samples are washed and resuspended in Coombs reagent) to ensure that the selected units are not only ABO compatible, but also lack the additional antigens to which the patient's serum contains preformed alloantibodies.

Patients with AIHA present a special challenge to transfusion services by virtue of the presence of pan-reactive serum antibodies (ie, anti-RBC antibodies that not only bind to their own RBCs, but to all RBCs, including reagent screening and panel cells). As a result, the presence of additional alloantibodies to specific blood group alloantigens may be masked by the autoantibodies. Time-consuming methods known as absorption techniques must be used in these cases and are discussed later in the section on AIHA.

Key points

- For blood products to be issued to a patient, the patient's ABO/Rh blood type must be determined and the patient's serum must be screened for the presence of RBC alloantibodies that may have formed following a previous transfusion or through pregnancy.
- If a patient's serum lacks clinically significant RBC alloantibodies, then an immediate spin or computer crossmatch is performed with prospective RBC units to ensure ABO blood group compatibility.
- If a patient's serum demonstrates the presence of clinically significant RBC alloantibodies, then ABO/Rh-compatible RBCs must be identified that lack the corresponding antigen(s). These prospective units must undergo a full or Coombs crossmatch to ensure that the selected units are not only ABO compatible, but also lack the additional antigens to which the patient's serum contains preformed alloantibodies.

Apheresis

Plasma exchange and plasmapheresis

A number of the more common indications for therapeutic apheresis are given in Table 11-6. For a more comprehensive list and discussion using an evidence-based medicine approach, a recent special issue of the *Journal of Clinical Apheresis* is cited at the end of this chapter. Plasma exchange has traditionally involved centrifugation of whole blood removed from the patient. Typically, one plasma volume of patient plasma is removed and replaced with 5% albumin (or FFP, in the case of TTP), which is combined with the patient's cellular blood elements in the extracorporeal circuit, and returned to the patient. Centrifugal apheresis is typically performed in a continuous-flow fashion, so that the patient remains euvolemic throughout the procedure. An alternative technology, namely, hemofiltration, has more recently been introduced and involves the extraction of selected plasma constituents by passing the patient's blood over specially designed membranes. With this form of ultrafiltration, greater selectivity is possible so that clotting factors and albumin may be retained by the patient. This technology is designed primarily to remove high molecular weight immune complexes. Other large materials such as low-density lipoprotein (LDL) can also be removed. This technology is especially useful in the management of patients with hyperviscosity due to hypergammaglobulinemia. Nevertheless, conventional plasma exchange continues to be used far more frequently than hemofiltration for the previously listed indications in the United States.

Immunoaffinity columns can also be used to remove various substances from the patient's plasma. Adsorbents that have been tested include staphylococcal protein A (SpA) to extract IgG and immune complexes, synthetic blood group substances to remove isohemagglutinins, and factor VIII

Table 11-6 Abbreviated list of therapeutic apheresis procedures grouped by ASFA indication category.

Disease/disorder	Procedure
Category 1. Standard and acceptable therapy, including primary therapy	
Chronic inflammatory demyelinating polyradiculoneuropathy (CIDP)	Plasmapheresis
Cryoglobulinemia	Plasmapheresis
Cutaneous T-cell lymphoma; mycosis fungoides (erythrodermic)	Extracorporeal photopheresis
Familial hypercholesterolemia (homozygotes)	Selective absorption
Goodpasture syndrome	Plasmapheresis
Guillain-Barré syndrome	Plasmapheresis
Hyperleukocytosis/leukostasis	Leukopheresis
Hyperviscosity in monoclonal gammopathies	Plasmapheresis
Myasthenia gravis	Plasmapheresis
Sickle cell disease (life and organ threatening)	Red blood cell exchange
TTP	Plasmapheresis
Category 2. Sufficient evidence to suggest efficacy; acceptable therapy on an adjunctive basis	
ABO-incompatible hemopoietic progenitor cell transplantation	Plasmapheresis
Babesiosis	Red blood cell exchange
Familial hypercholesterolemia	Plasmapheresis
Familial hypercholesterolemia (heterozygotes)	Selective absorption
Graft-versus-host disease (skin)	Extracorporeal photopheresis
ITP (refractory)	Immunoadsorption
Malaria	Red blood cell exchange
Renal allograft rejection (antibody-mediated)	Plasmapheresis
Rheumatoid arthritis	Immunoadsorption
Sickle cell disease (prevention of iron overload)	Red blood cell exchange
Sickle cell disease (stroke prophylaxis)	Red blood cell exchange
Wegener granulomatosis	Plasmapheresis
Category 3. Insufficient evidence for efficacy; uncertain benefit-to-risk ratio. Conditions that may fall into this category might be an exception effort for an individual patient.	
Aplastic anemia; pure red blood cell aplasia	Plasmapheresis
Catastrophic antiphospholipid disorder	Plasmapheresis
Coagulation factor inhibitors	Plasmapheresis/immunoadsorption
Graft-versus-host disease (nonskin)	Extracorporeal photopheresis
Hyperleukocytosis/leukostasis (prophylaxis)	Leukopheresis
Idiopathic HUS	Plasmapheresis
Myeloma and acute renal failure	Plasmapheresis
Posttransfusion purpura	Plasmapheresis
Rapidly progressive glomerulonephritis	Plasmapheresis
Warm- and cold-type autoimmune hemolytic anemia	Plasmapheresis
Category 4. Disorders for which controlled trials have not shown benefit or anecdotal reports have been discouraging	
Cutaneous T-cell lymphoma (nonerythrodermic)	Extracorporeal photopheresis
Dermatomyositis/polymyositis	Plasmapheresis
ITP (refractory)	Plasmapheresis
Rheumatoid arthritis	Plasmapheresis
SLE nephritis	Plasmapheresis

ASFA = American Society for Apheresis; HUS = hemolytic-uremic syndrome; ITP = immune thrombocytopenic purpura; SLE = systemic lupus erythematosus; TTP = thrombotic thrombocytopenic purpura.

coupled to Sepharose to remove factor VIII antibodies. The only immunoaffinity system that has received FDA approval for the treatment of ITP and rheumatoid arthritis (RA) in the United States is the ProSorba SpA/silica-based column. However, due to the apparent more effective use of B-cell–depleting agents for the treatment of these disorders, the ProSorba system is no longer commercially available. Although the mechanism by which these SpA columns exerted their therapeutic effect had been assumed to be by the adsorption of pathogenic autoantibodies, recent experimental data have demonstrated that soluble SpA, upon infusion, can induce apoptosis of specific B-cell populations, notably those implicated in autoantibody production. It is now considered likely that it was the leaching off of microgram quantities of SpA from the columns and subsequent intravenous infusion of this material that may have been responsible for the clinical improvement often seen in ITP and RA patients treated with the ProSorba system. Other brands of SpA-based immunoaffinity devices are still in use outside of the United States. Regardless of mechanism of action, the use of immobilized SpA immunoaffinity columns has been associated with fever, chills, hypotensive episodes, and (rarely) death. Pretreatment with corticosteroids appears to decrease the severity and frequency of these reactions. SpA treatment is contraindicated in patients receiving angiotensin-converting enzyme (ACE) inhibitors because severe hypotensive reactions can occur if these drugs have been administered within 24 to 48 hours of the procedure depending on drug half-life. ACE inhibitor–associated hypotensive reactions have been reported in patients undergoing other types of plasmapheresis as well.

Extracorporeal photochemotherapy (ECP or photopheresis) involves collecting peripheral blood mononuclear cells by apheresis (processing about one third of the blood volume), adding a photoactivating agent (8-methoxypsoralen) into the mononuclear cell suspension, irradiating the mononuclear cells with ultraviolet A irradiation, and returning the irradiated mononuclear cells to the patient; the whole process takes about 2.5 hours. ECP is an adjunctive therapy for erythrodermic cutaneous T-cell lymphoma; patients are typically treated on 2 consecutive days every 4 weeks; the median response time is 4 to 6 months. Response correlates with the presence of circulating clonal tumor cells and a CD8-mediated antitumor response. ECP is also used to treat chronic graft-versus-host disease (GVHD) after allogeneic stem cell transplantation and has a 70% response rate when used as second-line therapy.

LDL apheresis selectively removes LDL from plasma and is used to treat homozygous familial hypercholesterolemia or the heterozygous carrier refractory to maximal lipid-lowering drug therapy. The most common method used in the United States uses a dextran sulfate column to bind LDL and very low–density lipoprotein (but sparing high-density lipoprotein [HDL]). Heparinized blood separated into plasma by hollow fiber filters perfuses twin columns alternately, each column being automatically regenerated between successive adsorption cycles. A typical procedure reduces LDL by 50% to 75%, and is performed every 2 weeks; fibrinogen is lowered by 20% to 40%, although bleeding or other complications are rare. Some authorities believe that homozygous children should start LDL apheresis around age 7 years to prevent premature atherosclerosis. Vascular access may necessitate an arteriovenous fistula, and iron deficiency anemia may occur; otherwise the procedure is well tolerated and avoids the nonspecific removal of immunoglobulins as well as HDL cholesterol in standard plasmapheresis.

Exchange transfusion

RBC exchange transfusion therapy is most often performed in patients with sickle cell disease to treat acute complications of the disease such as central nervous system infarction or hemorrhage and acute chest syndrome. Preoperative exchange transfusion is always indicated when the surgeon intends to create a dry field using a vaso-occlusion tourniquet (common in orthopedic procedures) or if the procedure requires an especially long anesthesia time. In addition, exchange transfusion is indicated to prevent strokes in sickle cell patients who have had an ischemic stroke in the past, or in children at high risk for development of stroke, and may be indicated in the treatment of priapism. In such circumstances, patients should be transfused with blood that is known to contain only hemoglobin A; using directed-donor or family-donor blood that has not been subjected to hemoglobin electrophoresis may impart a significant risk of infusing additional hemoglobin S, thus decreasing the potential therapeutic benefit. Most clinicians attempt to achieve a final concentration of hemoglobin S of <30%. In many centers, a hemapheresis apparatus is used to perform RBC exchange; the patient's erythrocytes are removed and replaced with donor erythrocytes while the patient's own plasma is being continually returned, thus inducing little perturbation of hemodynamic and coagulation parameters. Developments in these apparatuses now allow the use of hemapheresis in relatively young children. In other centers, incremental phlebotomy followed by infusion of donor RBCs is performed without the use of hemapheresis. When manual exchange is done, careful attention should be paid to the potential for volume depletion. The goal of exchange transfusion in most situations such as acute chest syndrome and stroke, whether performed manually or via automated RBC apheresis, is to achieve a hematocrit of 30% with a hemoglobin S of <30%.

PBSC harvesting

Mobilization refers to the technique of increasing the number of circulating progenitor cells in the peripheral blood. It was noted in the 1970s that progenitor cells in peripheral blood increased up to 20-fold after chemotherapy for ovarian cancer. The introduction of hematopoietic growth factors in the late 1980s shortened the period of neutropenia after chemotherapy and was noted to increase circulating hematopoietic progenitors up to 1000-fold. G-CSF downregulates the expression of, and/or cleaves, adhesion molecules on the surface of hematopoietic stem cells (HSCs), progenitor cells, and precursor cells, and mobilizes clinically significant numbers of HSCs and progenitor cells into the peripheral blood. There are many mobilization regimens that combine chemotherapy with growth factors. Although earlier studies suggested that leukapheresis should commence when the white blood cell count reached 1×10^9/L, more recent data suggest that a more optimal time to start collecting is when the white blood cell count exceeds 10×10^9/L or the peripheral blood CD34$^+$ cell count exceeds 20×10^6/L. Cyclophosphamide (at 2.5–4 g/m^2) followed by G-CSF (at 5–10 μg/kg/d) is among the more commonly used protocols. The white blood cell count reaches 1 to 10×10^9/L around days 11 to 13 after chemotherapy. Leukapheresis is usually scheduled for days 10 to 12 after chemotherapy. A mobilization regimen that has a predictable rebound phase allows for more efficient use of apheresis and stem cell processing staff. The use of growth factor alone for mobilization avoids the risk of febrile neutropenia with chemotherapy and can be used in allogeneic donors. G-CSF at 10 μg/kg/d has been the mobilization regimen of choice for allogeneic PBSC donors. With this regimen, leukapheresis begins on day 5, when the white blood cell count is 20 to 50×10^9/L. There is an excellent correlation between the number of CD34$^+$ cells in the peripheral blood on the day of leukapheresis (or the preceding day) and the number of CD34$^+$ cells that can be collected by apheresis. For instance, for a target collection of 2.0×10^6/kg CD34$^+$ cells, the preceding day CD34$^+$ cell count in the peripheral blood should exceed 20×10^6/L. If collections are planned to take place over a number of consecutive days, many centers begin collections when the peripheral CD34$^+$ cell count is lower (eg, 10×10^6/L).

Although the administration of mobilizing doses of G-CSF can induce seemingly worrisome degrees of leukocytosis— transient peripheral blood leukocyte counts of 80,000/μL or higher are not uncommon—follow-up studies reported to date suggest that administration of short courses of G-CSF to healthy donors is not associated with any adverse long-term consequences. A rare complication of G-CSF for PBSC mobilization is splenic rupture; at least 4 cases of splenic rupture have been reported in healthy adult PBSC donors, most commonly after 5 days of daily G-CSF administration.

Large-volume leukapheresis (LVL) refers to the processing of large volumes of blood (15–30 L over 5 hours) made possible by current automated cell separators; data suggest that committed progenitor cells are recruited into the circulation during LVL. Although the magnitude of recruitment from LVL is small relative to the effects of chemotherapy/growth factor mobilization, the 2 techniques can be combined for maximal benefit. The principles of LVL involve establishing good venous access that would permit flow rates on the order of 80 to 110 mL/min. This may necessitate the insertion of an apheresis catheter in a central vein. To minimize the risks of citrate toxicity, heparin may be added to the citrate; calcium supplementation is an alternative to heparin use. Platelet depletion is another predictable consequence of LVL. Newer cell separators may be able to collect PBSCs with less platelet loss.

Use of PBSCs instead of bone marrow for hematopoietic rescue after high-dose chemoradiotherapy has been shown to increase the rapidity of neutrophil recovery following transplantation and, in some diseases, appears to reduce the risk that the harvested stem cell product will be contaminated with tumor cells. PBSC is clearly the optimal autograft source. The optimal graft choice in allogeneic transplantation is less clear; the benefits of rapid neutrophil and platelet engraftment come at the cost of an increased incidence of GVHD. The increased incidence of GVHD is most likely due to the approximately 10-fold increase in the number of CD3$^+$ cells administered with blood-derived, as opposed to marrow-derived, HSCs.

A relatively common problem with PBSC harvesting is inadequate collection. Although multiple definitions of inadequate collection have been used, it is clear that the incidence of inadequate collection is much higher in heavily pretreated patients than in healthy donors. In healthy PBSC donors, age, white ethnicity, and female sex were associated with lower post–G-CSF peripheral blood CD34$^+$ counts, which correlate with CD34$^+$ yields from collection. Risk factors for an inadequate autologous collection include multiple prior chemotherapeutic regimens, extensive prior radiation therapy, or administration of certain chemotherapeutic agents such as fludarabine, lenalidomide, melphalan, chlorambucil, and nitrosoureas. Plerixafor is a small-molecule reversible inhibitor of the chemokine receptor CXCR4 on stem cells; this inhibition facilitates HSC egress from the bone marrow and is synergistic with the mobilizing effects of G-CSF. One dose of plerixafor given with G-CSF has been shown to successfully mobilize CD34$^+$ cells in patients with multiple myeloma, Hodgkin disease, and non-Hodgkin lymphoma who failed previous mobilization attempts; plerixafor as a

Key points

- The most common hematologic conditions for which therapeutic apheresis is indicated include cryoglobulinemia/cold agglutinin disease, paraproteins causing hyperviscosity syndromes, TTP, severe symptomatic leukocytosis or thrombocytosis, and exchange transfusion in patients with sickle cell disease in whom acute complications develop or prolonged surgery is anticipated.
- Harvesting HSCs from the peripheral blood has increased the rapidity of neutrophil engraftment and abrogated the need to subject stem cell donors to general anesthesia and surgical bone marrow harvesting.
- A variety of nonhematologic disorders can be successfully treated with apheresis, including Goodpasture syndrome, Guillain-Barré syndrome, and myasthenia gravis.

single agent is being studied in healthy PBSC donors. The adverse effect profile of plerixafor (mostly gastrointestinal) does not appear to overlap with that of G-CSF.

Transfusion support in special clinical settings

Patients with aplastic anemia and other candidates for HSCT

As autologous and nonmyeloablative HSCTs are becoming offered to a wider population of patients with hematologic malignancies, the clinician must take into account the possibility that many patients newly diagnosed with hematopoietic malignancies are likely to become potential candidates for HSCT at some point in their clinical course. Therefore, it is important to avoid administering transfusion products obtained from family members because they may increase the risk of graft rejection via alloimmunization to minor histocompatibility antigens. For newly diagnosed patients with acute leukemia, it is useful to perform HLA typing earlier in the course of induction therapy and to anticipate problems in platelet support in patients who are at risk of HLA alloimmunization such as multiparous females; HLA typing results will, of course, be useful for potential allogeneic HSCT.

Transfusion support in patients with aplastic anemia merits discussion because several studies have supported a strong association between the number of blood product exposures prior to allogeneic HSCT and the risk of the often-fatal complication of graft rejection in such patients. It is believed that recipient-derived T cells directed against a variety of hematopoietic targets contribute to the genesis of the aplastic anemia itself and may also be responsible for the particularly high incidence of graft rejection that has been observed among patients undergoing HSCT for aplastic anemia. Administration of irradiated, leukoreduced blood products in such patients may reduce the risk of subsequent graft rejection. Serious attention must be paid to minimizing the number of blood product exposures in patients with aplastic anemia because older patients are often eligible for HSCT with nonmyeloablative conditioning. Menstrual suppression in young women can be helpful. RBCs should be transfused only for significantly symptomatic anemia. Single-donor (apheresis-derived) platelet products should be used in preference to pooled random-donor platelets whenever possible; antifibrinolytics are a useful adjunct to a lower platelet transfusion threshold.

Hematopoietic stem cell infusion

In the setting of allogeneic HSCT, PBSCs are typically infused "fresh," without cryopreservation. RBC or plasma depletion of the PBSC component may be required if the donor is major or minor ABO incompatible, respectively. Autologous PBSCs are nearly always cryopreserved prior to use because most transplantation preparative regimens require at least several days to administer before the stem cells can be infused. Optimal viability is obtained by automated controlled-rate freezing, using DMSO as the cryopreservative. PBSCs are typically stored in the vapor phase of liquid nitrogen; they are frozen in aliquots of 50 to 75 mL and thawed sequentially during the infusion, at the bedside, or in the laboratory. This approach allows the maintenance of a relatively slow infusion rate while simultaneously maximizing PBSC viability by minimizing the interval between the thawing and the infusion of each aliquot. DMSO toxicity commonly manifests as flushing, nausea, vomiting, and blood pressure fluctuations; to minimize toxicity, the volume of DMSO infused should be limited to 1 mL/kg at one sitting (which translates to 10 mL/kg of PBSCs for components that were cryopreserved with 10% DMSO).

> **Key points**
>
> - As is the case with transfusion of any other blood product, the most important issue with regard to the safe infusion of HSCs is definitive bedside identification of the patient.
> - To obtain optimal cell viability, frozen aliquots of HSCs must be rapidly thawed and infused into the patient without delay.

> **Clinical case**
>
> A 56-year-old woman is being evaluated for matched HSCT from her brother for high-risk acute myeloid leukemia in first remission. She is A positive, and he is O negative. She is enrolled on a nonmyeloablative conditioning protocol. On day 0, the PBSC is plasma-depleted and infused without incident. On day +8, she is noted to have a hemoglobin of 6 g/dL (down from 9 g/dL the day before). She is asymptomatic without any evidence of bleeding.

Transfusion support after HSCT

The intensity of transfusion support varies widely for different conditioning regimens; typically, the transfusion needs are much less in autologous transplantation and nonmyeloablative allogeneic conditioning regimens compared with allogeneic myeloablative regimens. The optimal transfusion threshold in HSCT patients for RBCs and platelets is not well studied. In a hemodynamically stable patient without underlying cardiovascular disease, it is common practice to transfuse RBCs for a hemoglobin of 8 g/dL. A recent multicenter pilot study was reported to support the concept of maintaining a higher hemoglobin (12 g/dL) in patients undergoing leukemia induction or HSCT, the rationale being that a higher hematocrit facilitates platelet–vessel wall interaction and may decrease thrombocytopenic bleeding. The landmark studies that support a platelet transfusion threshold of 10×10^9/L were conducted in patients undergoing leukemia induction. However, a recent multicenter randomized trial comparing different platelet transfusion doses (see Platelet Transfusion Dose section earlier in chapter) did include both autologous and allogeneic HSCT recipients, who were transfused prophylactically at the 10×10^9/L threshold. Risk factors for platelet refractoriness such as fever, infection, bleeding, amphotericin, and vancomycin are common occurrences in HSCT patients. Veno-occlusive disease increases platelet consumption from cytokine-induced endothelial damage and activation of vWF; portal hypertension with hypersplenism further increases platelet transfusion requirements. The availability of the original PBSC donor in related matched HSCTs can be a useful option in platelet-refractory patients.

There has been renewed interest in granulocyte transfusions since the mid-1990s when it became possible to collect adequate doses of granulocytes in donors who are willing to undergo stimulation with G-CSF with or without corticosteroids. Despite new antifungal agents, fungal infections in patients who have prolonged neutropenia remain problematic. There are case series of patients who received granulocyte transfusions as adjunctive therapy for refractory fungal (and bacterial) infections after HSCT and as secondary prophylaxis during HSCT after a prior episode of fungal infection, typically during leukemia induction or consolidation. The use of granulocyte transfusions as primary prophylaxis after allogeneic HSCT produced a modest decrease in febrile days and antibiotic usage but no difference in treatment-related mortality in one study and is not warranted given the potential risks, however slight, of subjecting healthy individuals to G-CSF and corticosteroids. Patients known to be HLA alloimmunized are at risk of greater pulmonary toxicity from granulocyte transfusions compared with patients without HLA antibodies, although routine screening for HLA antibodies before granulocyte transfusions is not universal. A randomized controlled trial is under way to study the incremental benefits of granulocyte transfusions in HSCT-related neutropenic infections.

All cellular blood components—RBCs, platelets, and granulocytes—must be γ-irradiated prior to transfusion in HSCT recipients to prevent t-GVHD. Some institutions with high-volume oncology and HSCT caseloads have elected to irradiate all platelets and RBCs to avoid the disastrous consequence of omitting this step; γ-irradiated components are safe for patients who are not at risk of t-GVHD. Gamma-irradiation shortens the shelf-life of RBCs (but not platelets), necessitating attention to inventory management. Most centers recommend that HSCT survivors receive irradiated blood components indefinitely, in the absence of data that show the safety of nonirradiated components in long-term HSCT survivors.

Prevention of CMV infection is an important part of transfusion management in CMV-seronegative HSCT recipients. Leukoreduction filters achieve a 3- to 4-log reduction of contaminating leukocytes in blood products. A landmark randomized comparison of leukoreduced/filtered versus CMV-seronegative blood components in CMV-seronegative HSCT recipients (with seronegative donors) found no significant difference in the incidence of CMV infection; others have argued that the study was not powered to detect differences in CMV disease, which was 2.4% in the filtered group and 0% in the seronegative group. With the improvement in CMV surveillance followed by pre-emptive antiviral therapy, which has further reduced the incidence of CMV disease after HSCT, this question will never be answered definitively. A subsequent cohort study reported from the same center, where CMV-seronegative components were preferentially used when available, found that the number of filtered RBC units from CMV-positive donors is the primary predictor of transfusion-transmitted CMV infection, which occurred in 3% of the CMV-seronegative HSCT recipients. Pre-emptive therapy with ganciclovir after detection of antigenemia prevented all but one case of CMV disease, which was successfully treated, prior to day 100. Most transplantation centers not closely related to regional blood suppliers or centers in regions of the world where CMV prevalence is very high will, in practice, use filtered blood components for CMV prevention; prestorage leukoreduction at the blood supplier (with adequate quality control) is preferred to bedside filtration.

ABO incompatible HSCTs

Allogeneic HSCTs do not require ABO matching because ABO antigens are not expressed on pluripotent stem cells. Because the genes for HLA are encoded on chromosome 6 and the genes for ABO are on chromosome 9, 2 siblings can have an identical HLA type but different ABO types. A recent report compiled from multicenter data reported to the International Blood and Marrow Transplant Research group included >3000 patients with early-stage leukemia who underwent transplantation between 1990 and 1998 with bone marrow from an HLA-identical sibling donor. In this large homogeneous group, there was no difference in overall survival, transplantation-related mortality, and grades 2 to 4 acute GVHD in the ABO-identical or ABO-mismatched groups. However, a single-institution study that focused exclusively on nonmyeloablative regimens found that ABO incompatibility was associated with increased nonrelapse mortality within the first year after HSCT. Similarly, the Japanese Marrow Donor Program has reported increased acute

GVHD in ABO-mismatched unrelated donor transplantations and increased transplantation-related mortality in the subset that received nonmyeloablative conditioning. In the unrelated donor setting, there may be multiple potential HLA matches for any given patient, and in light of these findings, ABO compatibility is a secondary consideration (in addition to other factors such as donor sex, age, CMV status, etc) that ultimately dictates donor choice.

A major ABO mismatch occurs when the recipient's plasma contains antibodies against the donor's RBCs. An example would be a group O recipient/group A donor pair. Early investigators used large-volume plasma exchange followed by infusion of incompatible RBCs to lower the isohemagglutinin titer before infusing the donor marrow; subsequent groups depleted RBCs from the donor marrow in lieu of recipient antibody depletion. Either of these approaches can effectively prevent immediate hemolytic transfusion reactions during marrow infusion. ABO-mismatched HSCT recipients have a slightly slower neutrophil recovery. Mature erythroid progenitors do express ABO antigens, and immune-mediated delayed erythropoiesis with reticulocytopenia can occur, leading to prolonged transfusion dependence up to 1 year after transplantation. The incidence is approximately 10%, and there is an inverse correlation between ABO hemagglutinin titers and reticulocyte counts, although attempts to lower hemagglutinin titers by plasma exchange have not been effective in treating RBC aplasia in this setting; extracorporeal immunoadsorption columns, cyclosporine withdrawal, erythropoietin, DLIs, and rituximab have also been used. One retrospective analysis found that pretransplantation reduction of recipient hemagglutinins helped to prevent pure RBC aplasia, although the majority of patients underwent isoagglutinin reduction by transfusion of ABO-incompatible, donor-type RBCs without plasmapheresis, which carries substantial risk of acute hemolysis.

A minor ABO mismatch occurs when the donor's plasma contains antibodies against the patient's RBCs (group A recipient/group O donor, such as in the illustrative case). Plasma depletion of the HSC product is performed by some centers, but acute hemolysis from donor plasma is uncommon. A more important concern is the phenomenon of immune hemolysis from mature, competent passenger lymphocytes transfused with the HSC component, especially with T-cell–depleted marrows, PBSCs versus marrow, the use of cyclosporine alone (without methotrexate) for GVHD prophylaxis, and reduced-intensity conditioning regimens. The hemolysis can occur abruptly, from days 7 to 14 after HSCT, and can be very severe or even fatal. A positive DAT distinguishes passenger lymphocyte hemolysis from thrombotic microangiopathy after transplantation; some centers perform periodic DAT screening in minor ABO–mismatched HSCT recipients, although the effectiveness of this strategy is not clear. It is prudent to maintain a higher transfusion threshold in minor mismatch recipients during the at-risk period after transplantation. Massive hemolysis may be treated by erythrocyte exchange transfusion using donor-type RBCs.

HSCT recipients with non-ABO RBC antibodies such as anti-D have undergone transplantation with antigen-positive grafts using the same principle of RBC depletion if marrow is the HSC component. An Rh(D)-positive recipient who undergoes HSCT from an Rh-negative donor may develop anti-D as the donor lymphocytes respond to the residual Rh-positive RBCs. Sickle cell patients undergoing HSCT may present a challenge if they have developed

Recipient blood type	Donor blood type	RBC transfusion	Platelet/plasma transfusion
O	A	O	A
O	B	O	B
O	AB	O	AB
A	B	O	AB
B	A	O	AB
A	O	O	A
B	O	O	B
A	AB	A	AB
B	AB	B	AB
AB	O	O	AB
AB	A	A	AB
AB	B	B	AB
Rh neg	Rh pos	Rh neg	Rh pos or Rh neg
Rh pos	Rh neg	Rh neg	Rh pos or Rh neg

Table 11-7 Guidelines for blood component selection in ABO-incompatible HSCT.

HSCT = hematopoietic stem cell transplantation; neg = negative; pos = positive; RBC = red blood cell.

multiple RBC alloantibodies or antibody to a high-incidence antigen. The optimal time to discontinue antigen-negative blood is not known, but one strategy is to wait until lymphocyte type is 100% donor because residual recipient lymphocytes may resume production of RBC alloantibodies with antidonor specificity.

It is important to consider alloimmune hemolysis in the differential diagnosis of hyperbilirubinemia in the posttransplantation patient because veno-occlusive disease and liver GVHD are likely to be more common occurrences. Finally, HSCT patients whose disease relapses may revert to the recipient ABO/Rh type. The transfusion service must be alert to subtle changes in mixed-field agglutination in ABO blood grouping during these situations. Table 11-7 provides useful guidelines for the selection of the appropriate blood group type for RBCs, platelets, and plasma for various scenarios of donor/recipient ABO-HSCT incompatibility.

Autoimmune cytopenia after HSCT

Autoimmune cytopenias occasionally develop in HSCT recipients. ITP appears to respond to standard therapy for de novo ITP. AIHA has been reported after myeloablative and nonmyeloablative conditioning regimens. One report suggests that cold-reactive (IgM) autoantibodies are more common earlier in the posttransplantation course (2–8 months) and warm autoantibodies occur later (after 6 months). AIHA occurs in 4% to 6% of allogeneic HSCT, and unrelated donor graft is a risk factor. In one pediatric series, almost all cases occurred in patients <10 years of age, and patients who underwent transplantation for nonmalignant disease had a higher incidence of AIHA compared with patients who underwent transplantation for malignancies. Mortality is high after the onset of AIHA; in the pediatric series, the majority of deaths occurred from the hemolytic anemia or from infection while on immunosuppressive therapy to treat hemolysis. The pathogenesis is presumed to be immune dysregulation during the period of immune constitution, and there appears to be an association with chronic GVHD.

> **Key points**
>
> - All cellular blood products administered to recipients of HSCT must be γ-irradiated and leukoreduced to minimize the risk of potentially fatal complications of t-GVHD, CMV transmission, and alloimmunization to HLA antigens.
> - Donor–recipient mismatches involving the ABO system are usually well tolerated but can occasionally cause delayed alloimmune hemolytic anemia, pure RBC aplasia, or other adverse effects.

Pediatric transfusion issues
In utero transfusion

Intrauterine transfusion (IUT) is much less commonly needed today compared with a decade or 2 ago, and technical expertise should be concentrated in centers that specialize in high-risk obstetrics and perform IUT regularly. In a sensitized pregnancy, Doppler ultrasound and amniotic fluid studies guide the need for fetal blood sampling, which is performed after 20 weeks of gestation. Blood is prepared for IUT if the fetal hematocrit is <25% to 30%. Group O, D-negative RBCs lacking the implicated RBC antigen are selected; some centers match the extended maternal RBC phenotype beyond the implicated antigen. Maternal serum/plasma is used for crossmatch. A fresh unit (<5 days old) is used, either CPD-A unit (without additive solution) or an additive solution unit with the supernatant removed. The unit must be γ-irradiated to prevent t-GVHD because the fetal immune system is immature; leukoreduction or a CMV-seronegative donor is used to provide a "CMV-safe" component. The unit should also be negative for sickle hemoglobin. Once IUT is initiated, it is repeated every 3 to 4 weeks until 35 weeks to maintain fetal hematocrit at approximately 25%. Neonates who have undergone IUT will type as O negative; such neonates may have suppressed erythropoiesis, which necessitates postnatal transfusion support for up to 3 months. Complications of IUT are related to the technical complexity of vascular access.

Neonatal exchange transfusion

Advances in phototherapy and use of IVIg have made exchange transfusion for hemolytic disease of the newborn or for hyperbilirubinemia a rare occurrence. Appropriate unit selection follows the same principles for IUT described previously (ie, fresh O-negative unit, negative for any offending antigen, crossmatched against maternal serum, leukoreduced, irradiated, hemoglobin S negative). In addition, the RBCs are concentrated and reconstituted with group AB FFP, typically in a 1:1 ratio to produce a unit of reconstituted whole blood (hematocrit 50%) for the exchange. A double volume exchange removes approximately 85% of the neonate's antigen-positive RBCs but is much less efficient in lowering plasma bilirubin. Complications of exchange transfusion include hypocalcemia, dilutional thrombocytopenia, and catheter-related thrombosis, infection, or bleeding.

Neonatal transfusion

The physiologic anemia of infancy occurs at 10 to 12 weeks, and the nadir hemoglobin is rarely <9 g/dL. Among preterm infants, this decline occurs at an earlier age, and the nadir is 7 to 8 g/dL; the physiologic nadir is compounded by phlebotomy blood loss. The blood loss through cumulative phlebotomy in a preterm infant's first weeks of life commonly exceeds the entire blood volume. Delaying umbilical cord clamping for 30 to 60 seconds for infants who do not require immediate resuscitation has been advocated by some to be the first step in counteracting the anemia of prematurity. Limiting phlebotomy blood loss is a crucial part of minimizing transfusion in a preterm infant. Pretransfusion specimens for crossmatching are not necessary as long as a cord blood sample is available to determine the infant's ABO/Rh type and DAT. Erythropoietin has limited efficacy at best and appears to increase the risk of retinopathy of prematurity. There should be a program to limit donor exposure in neonatal transfusions. Typically, a fresh additive-solution O-negative unit (<7 days old) is dedicated to 1 or 2 preterm infants and used exclusively for all transfusions for those 1 or 2 infants for up to 6 weeks of allowable storage. Two randomized clinical trials of restrictive versus liberal transfusion criteria used transfusion thresholds that varied with patients' respiratory and other status and postnatal age. A stable older infant in the restrictive arm, for instance, would be transfused at a hemoglobin level of approximately 7.5 g/dL; a younger mechanically ventilated preterm infant would be transfused at a hemoglobin level of approximately 11.5 g/dL. Significantly, in both trials, the number of donor exposures from RBC transfusions alone was not reduced by restrictive transfusion criteria, presumably reflecting the efficacy of using dedicated donor units; only 1 of the 2 trials demonstrated that a restrictive transfusion threshold increased the percentage of infants who avoided transfusion altogether (from 5% to 11%). However, infants in the restrictive transfusion group in the smaller trial had a higher incidence of apnea, severe brain injury, and mortality. Long-term follow-up of these infants would be important.

The fact remains that 90% of preterm neonates require a transfusion. Most US centers routinely irradiate all cellular components for neonates for a variable period of time after birth (typically 4–6 months). Other centers base irradiation criteria on gestational age and birth weight. In addition, leukoreduced cellular components are used to reduce the risk of CMV transmission. Some centers may use CMV-seronegative components for specific subgroups such as neonates weighing <1200 g. The quantity of additives in stored RBCs such as citrate, adenine, and mannitol is far less than levels believed to be toxic. Plasma potassium in stored RBCs approximates 50 mEq/L, but the volume of plasma infused with a small-volume "top-up" neonatal transfusion is so small that the dose of potassium infused with a 15 mL/kg RBC transfusion to a 1-kg infant is only 0.4 mEq. Although 2,3-DPG is depleted in stored RBCs, it is rapidly regenerated after transfusion; infants given stored RBCs had stable 2,3-DPG levels after small-volume RBC transfusions.

Component therapy in neonates

Newborns may require FFP, most commonly for disseminated intravascular coagulation secondary to sepsis; 10 to 15 mL/kg produces a 15% to 20% increase in factor level, assuming ideal recovery. If cryoprecipitate is required for persistent hypofibrinogenemia despite FFP, a dose of 1 unit should produce a 100 mg/dL increase in fibrinogen (in older infants, the cryoprecipitate dose is 1 unit per 5 to 10 kg of body weight).

Neonatal thrombocytopenia is not uncommon in preterm neonates, occurring in 22% of infants in one series. It is frequently a sign of sepsis or severe inflammation and often precedes other signs of sepsis. Prophylactic transfusions are often recommended in neonates with platelet counts <20,000 to 30,000/μL if otherwise stable; in unstable neonates or those requiring invasive procedures, platelets are transfused to maintain a count >50,000/μL. The usual platelet dose in neonates is 10 to 15 mL/kg, which is one platelet concentrate (allowing for tubing volume). Platelets should be ABO identical to avoid the transfusion of minor incompatible plasma into the small blood volume of a neonate. If ABO-identical (or group AB) platelets are not available, platelets should be washed to remove incompatible plasma. Routine volume reduction of platelets is not necessary or recommended because the procedure can jeopardize platelet quality.

Extracorporeal membrane oxygenation and congenital heart surgery

Extracorporeal membrane oxygenation is used to treat respiratory and cardiac failure in neonates secondary to diverse conditions such as persistent pulmonary hypertension, congenital diaphragmatic hernia, and meconium aspiration syndrome. The membrane oxygenator consumes platelets, and RBCs are needed to prime the circuit and maintain a hematocrit typically >40%. A program to limit donor exposure that includes using dedicated RBC units and aliquots of single-donor apheresis platelets can significantly decrease donor exposure, although the duration of extracorporeal

Key points

- The immune system in the fetus and in neonates up to the age of 4 months is immature and probably not capable of generating antibody responses to transfusions. Thus, the most crucial compatibility issues involve the passive transfer of antibodies from the mother to the fetus, as well as maintaining ABO compatibility between the donor and the fetus or neonate.
- Current blood banking practice attempts to limit the number of donor exposures to fetal and neonatal patients by using modern technology to retrieve multiple transfusion aliquots from single blood products.

membrane oxygenation drives the transfusion demands. Similarly, bypass cardiac surgery is frequently performed on small infants with congenital heart disease. Although smaller infants are more likely to require transfusion, transfusion-free procedures have been safely performed for infants as small as 5 kg using miniaturized bypass systems and a variety of blood-conservation techniques.

Pediatric transfusion beyond the neonatal period

The posttransfusion long-term survival rate in pediatric transfusion recipients is much higher than in adults, so the principle of minimizing donor exposure, which carries risks of transfusion-transmitted disease (involving known and unknown infectious agents), continues beyond the neonatal period. A multicenter trial of restrictive versus liberal transfusion thresholds (7 g/dL vs 9.5 g/dL) in pediatric intensive care units found that a restrictive transfusion strategy was noninferior in the primary outcomes (28-day mortality and new or progressive multiorgan dysfunction) and successfully avoided transfusion in 54% of patients (compared with 2% in the liberal transfusion group). Cardiac, craniofacial, and scoliosis surgery account for many cases of perioperative transfusion in older children; the older child or adolescent undergoing elective scoliosis surgery benefits from judicious use of autologous blood donation and intraoperative cell salvage in an integrated blood-conservation approach. Large-volume transfusion in the perioperative setting dictates careful monitoring of electrolytes and coagulation status. Hematologic or oncologic disease accounts for the remaining cases of pediatric transfusion. Pediatric patients with sickle cell disease and thalassemia benefit from leukoreduced blood transfusion to reduce HLA alloimmunization (and febrile nonhemolytic transfusion reactions); there is some evidence to suggest that development of HLA antibodies is associated with the development of RBC antibodies in the sickle cell patient. They also benefit from the use of extended RBC phenotypic matching to reduce alloimmunization; DHTRs from RBC alloantibodies can precipitate vaso-occlusive crises, hyperhemolysis, or autoantibody development.

Pediatric immune disorders

Hemolytic disease of the newborn (HDN; or erythroblastosis fetalis) is most commonly due to maternal–fetal mismatches involving Rh or ABO antigens, which can cause an antigen-negative mother to mount an IgG antibody response against the antigen-positive fetal RBCs. These antibodies can be transported across the placenta and cause passively acquired immune-mediated hemolytic anemia in the fetus, leading to profound anemia and hydrops fetalis. Fetal demise may be seen in severe cases. The incidence of this disorder has been dramatically reduced with the use of antenatal and peripartum administration of anti-D to Rh(D)-negative mothers, which abrogates the maternal immune response to primary exposure to the D antigen. As a result, most cases of HDN today are attributed to Rh antigens other than D, as well as K1 (Kell blood group system), and ABO. ABO HDN is characterized by hyperbilirubinemia with mild anemia (if any); the mother is typically group O with IgG anti-A,B alloantibodies (an antibody with cross-reactivity to both A and B antigens), and the infant is typically group A; HDN responds well to phototherapy. Cord blood should be ABO and Rh typed and a DAT performed for all infants born to group O mothers, all infants born to Rh-negative mothers (mother of an Rh-negative infant does not require anti-D prophylaxis), and all infants born to mothers with known (non-D) alloimmunization.

In an analogous fashion, maternal–fetal mismatches involving platelet-specific or neutrophil-specific alloantigen systems may result in NAIT or NAIN, respectively. The target antigens are quite diverse but often consist of membrane glycoproteins that are specific to the cell implicated in the immune cytopenia. The most common antibody specificity in NAIT in whites is anti-HPA-1a (PL^{A1}), which resides on the platelet fibrinogen receptor GPIIb/IIIa, although numerous other polymorphisms and specificities on this and other membrane constituents are documented in the literature. NAIN is often due to fetal–maternal mismatches involving the neutrophil-specific NA-1/NA-2 system. No prophylactic therapies are currently available for NAIT or NAIN.

Management of these disorders often includes antenatal maternal IVIg to reduce antibody levels, decrease placental transfer of antibodies, and reduce cellular destruction in the fetus. Transfusion support of NAIT is most often with washed irradiated maternal platelets, usually prepared through apheresis. Maternal platelets are essentially always negative for the target antigen in question; their use abrogates the need to wait for the often lengthy serologic determinations that are required to identify platelet alloantibody specificity. Some blood centers have registries of specific platelet antigen–negative donors available for emergency apheresis if the mother is unable to donate.

Maternal ITP or NAIN can cause passively acquired immune thrombocytopenia or immune neutropenia in the fetus, respectively. It is important to rule out the latter disorders by checking a complete blood count, bone marrow biopsy, and/or appropriate antibody assays in the mother prior to using the mother as a source for platelets or neutrophils. It is important to keep in mind that the currently available assays for antiplatelet antibodies and antineutrophil antibodies are not always highly sensitive or specific and that the diagnosis or exclusion of AIN or ITP should thus not be based solely on the results of assays for antibodies.

In addition to alloimmune cytopenias caused by passively transferred maternal alloantibody and autoimmune cytopenias caused by passively transferred maternal autoantibody, cytopenias in the pediatric population can also be due to the production of autoantibodies by the child's own immune system. Typically, these syndromes present at a later age than the passively acquired cytopenias discussed previously. Nevertheless, children can present with serologic and clinical features that are similar to adult ITP, AIN, AIHA, or PCH. Unlike their adult counterparts, however, ITP, AIHA, and PCH are often acute and self-limited when they present during childhood, in which setting they are frequently manifestations of a postviral syndrome. Fewer data are available regarding the typical course of childhood AIN. The latter disorder is probably underdiagnosed in both adults and children, in part as a result of the paucity of laboratories that are able to carry out antineutrophil antibody assays. As in adults, immune cytopenias can complicate a variety of rheumatologic or immunologic disorders in childhood. Evan syndrome (concurrent AIHA and ITP) has also been reported in childhood.

Autoimmune hemolytic anemia

> **Clinical case**
>
> An elderly woman presents with a hemoglobin of 6.0 g/dL and a positive DAT that reveals IgG, but not complement, on the surface of her RBCs. Her reticulocyte count is <1%. She has never been previously transfused and has never been pregnant. She is started on prednisone for the treatment of presumed warm-type (IgG-mediated) AIHA. Because of shortness of breath and a previous history of heart disease, RBC transfusions are ordered. Multiple RBC crossmatches are incompatible. Three units of leukocyte-depleted RBCs are transfused. The peripheral blood hemoglobin concentration increases to 9.0 g/dL, and she experiences no untoward reactions.

Autoantibodies to RBCs can result in multiple incompatible RBC crossmatches, which may lead blood banks to advise clinicians that no compatible RBC units are available. FDA regulations require the patient's physician to provide written consent to release incompatible units, which makes many clinicians uncomfortable. However, in instances in which the patient has not previously been transfused or pregnant, alloantibodies to non-ABO antigens are unlikely to be present and patients can usually be safely transfused with ABO-compatible blood. Even in patients who have previously been transfused or pregnant, withholding transfusions because the crossmatches are incompatible may preclude the administration of lifesaving transfusions. Techniques are available to minimize the risk of transfusion in such situations; these techniques are important because failure to identify underlying alloantibodies in patients with AIHA not only leads to the destruction of the transfused donor cells, but also can cause serious exacerbation of the concomitant autohemolytic process. Some transfusion services routinely perform extended RBC phenotyping; that is, the patient's RBCs are typed with regard to antigen systems in addition to ABO and Rh(D), at the time that a diagnosis of AIHA is first rendered, to facilitate the identification of alloantibodies that may appear subsequently.

Several studies have examined the incidence of clinically significant alloantibodies in multiply transfused patients with AIHA and found that up to 30% to 35% of such patients develop alloantibodies. Thus, if a patient has previously received a transfusion or been pregnant, the transfusion service must perform specific testing to determine whether alloantibodies are present concurrently with the panagglutinating autoantibodies that are typically associated with AIHA. The term *panagglutinating* refers to the fact that most autoantibodies that cause AIHA will agglutinate most units of RBCs because the antigenic target is typically a "public" antigen, that is, an antigen present on the RBCs of a large fraction of the population as a whole. The public antigen is often a common epitope on the Rh protein that is distinct from the common alloantigenic Rh epitopes. The most definitive technique for detecting alloantibodies in the presence of autoantibodies is called *autoadsorption*. With the autoadsorption technique, an aliquot of the patient's serum is repeatedly adsorbed with the patient's own erythrocytes and then tested for alloreactivity with panel or donor erythrocytes in a standard antibody screen.

However, if the patient has undergone transfusion recently, autoadsorption can be used only if sufficient quantities of recipient-derived reticulocytes can be harvested by a special density gradient centrifugation procedure that is not widely available. Otherwise, autoadsorption cannot be reliably interpreted because the transfused RBCs present in the prospective recipient's blood could adsorb the very same alloantibodies that the laboratory is attempting to detect. In this situation, a method called *differential adsorption* is used. Differential adsorption involves adsorbing different aliquots of patient serum against RBCs of different defined phenotypes to produce several adsorbed sera that give differential reactivity in standard antibody screens. The differential reactivity results from the fact that alloantibodies are left behind in the serum following the adsorption if the adsorbing cells are negative for the antigen in question. Because most warm-reacting autoantibodies react with erythrocyte-surface determinants that do not vary among patients (ie, public antigens), adsorption with erythrocytes of different phenotypes removes the autoantibody but, depending on the phenotype, either removes or fails to remove alloantibody. For example, if the patient's serum contains an anti-Jk^a antibody along with an autoantibody, both the autoantibody and the anti-Jk^a antibody will be adsorbed by Jk^a-positive adsorbing cells, but only the autoantibody will be adsorbed by Jk^a-negative adsorbing cells. The presence of the anti-Jk^a in the patient's serum can then be deduced by demonstrating that the aliquot of the serum that was adsorbed by Jk^a-positive cells is nonreactive in a standard antibody screen, whereas the aliquot of serum that was adsorbed by Jk^a-negative cells reacts only with Jk^a-positive cells in a standard antibody screen.

Warm-reacting autoantibodies occasionally demonstrate preferential reactivity against certain alloantigens, even though the patient is positive for the alloantigen in question. This preferential reactivity can be striking, such that if the autoantibody has relative specificity for a particular alloantigen, the antibody may demonstrate much stronger reactions against alloantigen-positive RBCs in comparison with alloantigen-negative RBCs. The preferential reactivity may be so strong that autoantibody reactivity against RBCs negative for the alloantigen in question cannot be detected. These antibodies are referred to as *mimicking* antibodies. In these situations, donor RBCs that do not express the target antigen may survive longer following transfusion.

In patients with cold-reacting autoantibodies such as anti-I, blood lacking the antigen in question is generally unavailable. In this situation, blood transfused through a blood warmer will usually survive adequately if the patient is kept warm while other forms of treatment, such as cytotoxic chemotherapy or plasmapheresis, are instituted. If requested, a blood bank workup of the cold-reacting autoantibodies can include the performance of a "thermal amplitude" determination in which RBC binding in vitro to the patient's autoantibodies is assessed as a function of temperature (eg, at 4°C, 22°C, 30°C, and 37°C). The results of such tests can give the clinician a sense of the potential clinical significance of the autoantibodies in vivo at body temperature.

In the clinical case described previously, note that the patient's reticulocyte count was relatively low. A substantial minority of patients will manifest at least transient reticulocytopenia early in the course of AIHA, a phenomenon that may be due to the fact that autoantibody titers may increase more quickly than the bone marrow can generate a reticulocyte response and/or due to rapid destruction of reticulocytes by the autoantibody itself.

> **Key points**
>
> - RBC transfusions in patients with life-threatening AIHA should not be withheld simply because all available units are crossmatch incompatible.
> - Special blood bank techniques are available to minimize the risk of transfusion in patients with AIHA.

Autoimmune and consumptive thrombocytopenias

Transfusion of platelets in patients with autoimmune thrombocytopenia (commonly known as ITP) is problematic because the efficacy of platelet transfusions in such patients is unpredictable due to the potential destruction of transfused platelets by the autoantibody. (As is the case with AIHA, the autoantibody in ITP often reacts with public antigens.) Transfusion of platelets in patients with ITP is usually attempted only in patients with life-threatening hemorrhage; in a small retrospective series, 40% of platelet transfusions did result in immediate posttransfusion increments of at least 20,000/μL. Administration of IVIg may improve the survival of transfused platelets in patients with ITP, and the administration of IVIg and/or continuous infusions of platelets have been tried in patients with life-threatening hemorrhage and patients undergoing major surgery. Elective splenectomy is typically managed with preoperative IVIg or a pulse of corticosteroids. Intravenous Rh(D) IgG can be administered more quickly than IVIg, but its use is limited to Rh(D)-positive, nonsplenectomized patients. Recent introduction of 2 thrombopoietin mimetics (eltrombopag and romiplostim) has further expanded the therapeutic armamentarium for ITP.

Except in life-threatening bleeding situations such as intracranial hemorrhage, platelet transfusions should be avoided in consumptive thrombocytopenias such as TTP and heparin-induced thrombocytopenia because they could exacerbate the thrombotic process that characterizes both of these disorders.

Sickle cell disease

Patients receiving long-term transfusion therapy often become alloimmunized to multiple blood components, including RBC antigens, leukocyte antigens, and plasma proteins. For reasons that are not entirely clear, this is especially true in patients with sickle cell disease, of whom 3.5% to 35% become alloimmunized to non-ABO RBC antigens. Leukocyte-depleted or saline-washed blood products may minimize febrile and allergic reactions and are useful once alloimmunization to leukocyte and plasma antigens occurs. Patients with sickle cell disease, however, are particularly prone to alloimmunization against RBC alloantigens and account for more than half of the requests for rare-phenotype blood received by the American Red Cross Rare Donor Registry, which collects and distributes blood from donors with unusual phenotypes. The reasons for the high rate of alloimmunization to RBC antigens among patients with sickle cell disease are poorly understood. Likely factors include repeated exposure to RBC antigens in combination with differences in the frequencies of certain RBC antigens between the predominantly white donor population and the predominantly black patient population. However, patients with sickle cell disease may also have a higher intrinsic immune responsivity to blood group antigens.

Indications for transfusion in sickle cell disease include stroke, acute chest syndrome, aplastic crisis, and preoperative preparation to reduce the risk of postoperative respiratory complications. Sickle cell patients who require chronic transfusion therapy accumulate iron much less rapidly if the transfusion occurs in the form of exchange procedures rather than simple transfusions, although exchange carries the risk of additional donor exposures and requires adequate vascular access. Techniques for preventing and managing alloimmunization in patients with sickle cell disease are controversial. In many institutions, RBCs from patients with sickle cell disease are subjected to extended antigen typing for the most important antigen systems in addition to ABO and Rh(D), including Kell, Kidd, Duffy, MNSs, Rh(C), Rh(E), and others, before transfusion therapy is initiated. Extended RBC phenotyping facilitates future identification of antibody specificities and the transfusion of at least partially extended antigen–matched units, which may reduce the incidence of subsequent alloimmunization. Most commonly, matching is performed for the extended Rh antigens (C, c, E, and e) and the major Kell antigen (K), in part because providing RBC units that are matched for these antigens does not require use of phenotypically rare blood units. It is usually not possible to match routinely for all antigens for which the patient has been typed because most blood centers that identify and store phenotypically rare blood provide these units only to patients with demonstrated alloantibodies due to limited supplies of rare-phenotype blood.

The development of alloantibodies is occasionally associated with autoantibody formation, which complicates transfusion therapy. The prevalence was 8% in a pediatric series of sickle cell patients; about half the patients with detectable autoantibody had evidence of hemolysis, often associated with a positive DAT for complement. Hyperhemolysis is another transfusion-related complication observed in sickle cell disease, often presenting with severe anemia and reticulocytopenia 7 to 10 days after an index transfusion. The hematocrit is typically lower than the pretransfusion value, indicating the destruction of autologous RBCs. The DAT is often negative, and new alloantibodies may or may not be detectable. It is important to recognize this syndrome because the management consists of the judicious avoidance of additional transfusions in the face of severe anemia, corticosteroids, IVIg, and erythropoietin. Many centers that treat patients with sickle cell disease have observed an apparent association between DHTRs, the onset of sickle cell crises, and the occurrence of other complications of sickle cell disease. Thus, although DHTRs cause relatively little morbidity in other populations, they may cause significant morbidity in patients with sickle cell anemia.

> **Key points**
>
> - Patients with sickle cell disease on a chronic transfusion program should receive extended-match RBCs to prevent alloimmunization to non-ABO RBC antigens.
> - DHTRs caused by alloimmunization to non-ABO RBC antigens represent a significant problem in chronically transfused patients with sickle cell disease.
> - Simple transfusion to a hemoglobin of 10 g/dL is indicated in patients with sickle cell disease who are undergoing surgical procedures in which the operative time is expected to be approximately >30 minutes, and exchange transfusion is indicated in patients with major complications such as cerebral infarction or acute chest syndrome.

Massive transfusion

Massive transfusion is defined as the replacement of one blood volume within 24 hours, typically 4 to 6 hours after severe trauma or major surgery. Coagulopathy of massive transfusion is multifactorial: hypothermia, acidosis, the dilutional effect of blood loss and inadequate coagulation factor replacement, reduced hepatic synthesis of coagulation factors in massive hepatic injury, disseminated intravascular coagulopathy from hypotension and tissue injury, and consumption of coagulation factors/platelets. Unfortunately, neither laboratory tests nor transfusion volume correlates well with the severity of bleeding. In the absence of hypovolemic shock and significant liver dysfunction, the exchange of one circulating plasma volume does not reduce the clotting factor activities below levels necessary to maintain hemostasis, that is, approximately 50% of the normal levels. Thrombocytopenia is the most frequent abnormality associated with massive transfusion. When transfusions of 1.5 to 2.0 blood volumes are administered over 4 to 8 hours, the mean reduction in the peripheral blood platelet count is approximately 50%. Ideally, it is preferable to obtain appropriate coagulation tests, including prothrombin time (PT), international normalized ratio (INR), activated partial thromboplastin time (aPTT), and plasma fibrinogen level, to guide plasma replacement therapy. In practice, many trauma centers have adopted an empiric pre-emptive approach to prevent coagulopathy based on military experience using early aggressive plasma transfusion. Some institutional massive transfusion protocols also incorporate the off-label use of recombinant factor VIIa, typically at a lower dose than that used in hemophilia patients with inhibitors, although there is no consensus on this use and thromboembolism is a potential adverse effect. Patients undergoing massive transfusion need to be monitored for electrolyte disturbances such as hypocalcemia (citrate in the anticoagulant used for all blood components binds free calcium), hyperkalemia or hypokalemia, and metabolic alkalosis (from citrate metabolism).

Cardiopulmonary bypass

Alterations in the laboratory parameters of hemostasis are observed in virtually all patients undergoing open-heart surgery and extracorporeal circulation. However, <10% of these patients experience severe bleeding, and during the history of cardiopulmonary bypass procedures, blood usage for surgery involving extracorporeal circulation has markedly decreased. Platelet abnormalities account for most cases of correctable nonsurgical bleeding following such procedures. Platelet dysfunction and aggregation may result from platelet contact with the foreign surfaces of extracorporeal circuits, including pumps and aortic assist devices. Preoperative therapy with antiplatelet agents such as clopidogrel and GPIIb/IIIa inhibitors exacerbates platelet dysfunction. Dilution by priming the extracorporeal circuit with nonblood solutions may reduce the platelet count by as much as 50%. Changes in platelet function due to exposure to the extracorporeal circuit may persist for several hours after discontinuation of bypass. Although plasma coagulation factor levels are diluted by nonblood priming solutions, coagulation factor levels ordinarily remain above the minimal level needed for hemostasis, that is, approximately 50% of the normal factor levels. The extracorporeal circuit is not thought to consume clotting factors directly. As a result of these issues, platelet transfusion to correct quantitative and/or qualitative platelet defects is the mainstay of treatment of nonsurgical bleeding associated with cardiopulmonary bypass procedures. Even if routine blood testing reveals significant coagulation abnormalities, it is important to keep in mind that such testing will not detect qualitative defects in platelet function. In addition, because platelet products themselves contain significant quantities of plasma, platelet transfusion alone may still be the treatment of choice even when the primary laboratory abnormalities appear to be coagulation factor related. Routine transfusion of platelets to patients who are not bleeding and not severely thrombocytopenic does not appear to be justified.

Aplastic anemia

Transfusion support in patients with aplastic anemia merits discussion because, as mentioned previously, several studies have supported a strong association between the number of blood product exposures prior to allogeneic HSCT and the risk of the often-fatal complication of graft rejection in such patients. It is believed that recipient-derived T cells directed against a variety of hematopoietic targets contribute to the genesis of the aplastic anemia itself and may also be responsible for the particularly high incidence of graft rejection that has been observed among patients undergoing HSCT for aplastic anemia. For both of the previous reasons, serious attention must be paid to minimizing the number of blood product exposures in patients with aplastic anemia who may be potential candidates for HSCT. With the advent of reduced dose-intensity conditioning regimens and other methods for preventing and treating GVHD and other complications of transplantation, this may now include patients up to the age of 70 with moderate or severe aplastic anemia, particularly because such patients frequently fail to respond to nontransplantation interventions or manifest progression and transformation of the aplastic anemia to more immediately life-threatening conditions such as acute myelogenous leukemia.

In addition to transfusing RBCs only for significantly symptomatic anemia, some authors have proposed that ε-aminocaproic acid be used in lieu of routine prophylactic platelet transfusions and that single-donor, leukoreduced platelet products be used in conjunction with a lower than usual platelet count target. As noted previously, most HSCT teams strongly discourage or prohibit the use of directed-donor transfusions obtained from family members for fear that the patient may become alloimmunized to minor (ie, non-HLA) histocompatibility antigens expressed on HSCs obtained from HLA-matched family donors, thus further increasing the risk of graft rejection.

Transfusion risks

Clinical case

Shortly after the initiation of an RBC transfusion, a 33-year-old patient with sickle cell anemia develops pain at the infusion site followed by dyspnea, fever, chills, and low back pain. His urine is noted to be red, and his plasma demonstrates free hemoglobin. Repeat testing of both the RBC product and the patient reveals that the product is type A, the patient is type O, and the crossmatch is incompatible.

Acute hemolytic reactions

The patient in the previous clinical case illustrates the typical presentation of an acute hemolytic transfusion reaction: pain at the administration site, fever, chills, back pain, dark urine, and laboratory evidence of intravascular hemolysis. As noted previously, ABO isohemagglutinins are complement fixing and lead to the intravascular destruction of the transfused RBCs, as manifested in the previous patient by hemoglobinemia and hemoglobinuria. Activation of complement leads to the release of cytokines, including tumor necrosis factor, accounting for fever and chills. The serologic hallmark of an acute hemolytic reaction is a DAT that demonstrates both IgG and complement on the surface of the recipient's RBCs. Disseminated intravascular coagulation also occurs, and bleeding may result. ABO incompatibility accounts for more deaths from transfusion than HIV transmission and hepatitis transmission combined. Most ABO-related hemolytic episodes are caused by clerical errors, particularly mislabeling of the pretransfusion type and crossmatch sample. An important but often overlooked technique for reducing the risk of this type of incident is to label the samples to be used in the crossmatch at the patient's bedside. Treatment of acute intravascular hemolytic reactions is supportive and includes fluids and vasopressors if hypotension occurs. Intravenous mannitol is also given to prevent renal shut down.

Delayed hemolytic reactions

As mentioned previously, DHTRs occur when a patient acquires an alloantibody to an RBC antigen following pregnancy, transfusion, or HSCT, but the titer of the antibody falls to below the detectable limit prior to a subsequent RBC transfusion. Following the subsequent transfusion, the patient develops an anamnestic immune response to the mismatched antigen, leading to delayed destruction of the transfused RBCs. Clinical symptoms of hemolysis may include fever, anemia, and jaundice, which may not become evident until approximately 5 to 10 days after the transfusion. Hemolysis is usually IgG mediated and thus extravascular, although IgG alloantibodies to Kidd blood group antigens may fix complement and cause intravascular hemolysis, as noted earlier. Hemoglobinuria may occur, and occasional instances of severe complications such as acute renal failure or disseminated intravascular coagulation have been reported. The antibodies most often implicated in DHTR are directed against antigens in the Rh (34%), Kidd (30%), Duffy (14%), Kell (13%), and MNSs (4%) antigen systems.

Febrile reactions

Multiparous women and multiply transfused patients commonly develop leukoreactive antibodies that cause nonhemolytic febrile reactions to RBC or platelet transfusions. In addition, during the storage of blood, clinically significant quantities of cytokines are sometimes liberated from donor-derived passenger leukocytes present in platelet and RBC products, as discussed previously. These cytokines include IL-2, IL-6, IL-8, and tumor necrosis factor. Occasional cases of severe hypotensive and/or hypoxic reactions that appear to have been caused by preformed cytokines have been observed. Prestorage leukocyte depletion, as opposed to poststorage bedside leukofiltration, may reduce the accumulation of these biomediators and the probability of febrile, hypotensive, or hypoxic transfusion reactions. Most transfusion services have adopted universal leukocyte depletion, and in some parts of the world, including Canada, regulatory agencies dictate universal leukocyte depletion. Regardless of the exact pathophysiology in a particular instance, mild febrile transfusion reactions are usually self-limited, and in most cases, the clinician can administer subsequent transfusions without undue risk. It should be appreciated that the main issue regarding the limiting and prevention of such febrile reactions is not concern about morbidity or mortality associated with this type of transfusion reaction. Rather, the main concern is that an elevation in temperature during a transfusion, although most likely the result of this innocuous febrile transfusion reaction, cannot be distinguished from the sole sign of a developing life-threatening acute hemolytic transfusion reaction in which fever can be the only clue. Consequently, the repeated occurrence of true febrile transfusion reactions in a given patient can lead to the otherwise unnecessary termination of transfusions, blood unit wastage, and time-consuming blood bank hemolytic transfusion reaction workups that will invariably be negative for hemolysis. Of interest, a recently published consecutive cohort study from Johns Hopkins University suggested that the switchover to universal leukoreduction was associated with a significant reduction in febrile nonhemolytic transfusion reactions but no change in the incidence of allergic reactions.

Allergic reactions

Minor allergic reactions manifested by urticaria are frequent in multiply transfused patients. These reactions can usually be prevented by the administration of prophylactic antihistamines. Many urticarial reactions are donor specific and thus do not recur with subsequent transfusions. If a recipient experiences multiple urticarial reactions, the clinician should consider premedication with antihistamines and/or washed products resuspended in albumin and saline. However, the clinician must take into consideration the possibility that washing platelets may impair platelet function.

IgA-deficient patients may make anti-IgA antibodies that can cause anaphylactic reactions. However, this is a rare occurrence considering the number of patients at risk. When such a patient is encountered, extensively washed RBCs must be given, and plasma products from IgA-deficient donors must be transfused. Platelets should also be derived from IgA-deficient donors to avoid platelet washing procedures, as noted previously. In addition to the well-known propensity of IgA-deficient patients to develop anaphylactic reactions to blood products, there are also reports of patients with deficiencies of haptoglobin and various complement components, such as C4a (Rogers antigen) or C4b (Chido antigen), developing anaphylactic reactions to platelets.

Transfusion-related acute lung injury

TRALI is a potentially life-threatening reaction that in many cases appears to be caused by passive transfusion of antigranulocyte antibodies (in particular, anti-HLA antibodies), ILs, biologically active lipids, or other substances. The resulting clinical picture is thus referred to as *noncardiac pulmonary edema*. Signs and symptoms include dyspnea, hypoxemia, hypotension, fever, and a chest x-ray showing bilateral infiltrates with pulmonary edema. Aggressive pulmonary support, including intubation and mechanical ventilation, is frequently needed. Approximately 80% of patients improve within 48 to 96 hours, 20% have a protracted course of fatal outcome, and 100% of patients require oxygen support with approximately 70% requiring mechanical ventilation. Infrequently, antibodies in the recipient may react with donor granulocytes that are introduced by units of RBCs or platelets. Prestorage leukodepletion of blood products may diminish this less frequent initiator of TRALI. In some cases of TRALI, neither patient-derived nor donor-derived antibodies can be identified, and other mechanisms have been advanced such as the priming of neutrophils by bioactive lipids that accumulate during blood storage.

Much attention has been recently focused on improving the recognition and prevention of TRALI given that in 2006, TRALI represented approximately 50% of all transfusion-related fatalities reported to the US FDA. Although the true incidence rate of TRALI is unknown, it may occur in as many as 1 in 5000 transfusions of any plasma-containing blood product (ie, packed RBCs, platelet concentrates, and FFP) with a 5% to 10% fatality rate. One of the difficulties in recognizing TRALI when it is occurring is that it can be difficult to distinguish from the manifestations of a patient's underlying medical problems, particularly those of cardiac origin such as congestive heart failure and fluid overload brought on by the transfusion. To deal with this problem better, a recent consensus conference provided a working definition of TRALI: acute lung injury (ALI) occurring during a transfusion or within 6 hours of completion with no other temporally associated causes of ALI. ALI was defined as a syndrome of (i) acute onset; (ii) hypoxemia (PAO_2/FIO_2 <300 mm Hg, O_2 saturation <90% on room air, or other clinical evidence); (iii) bilateral pulmonary infiltrates, as noted previously; and (iv) no evidence of circulatory overload.

Clinical management is supportive with the goal of reversing progressive hypoxemia. At the present time, there does not appear to be any universally satisfying means by which to prevent TRALI. Once blood from a particular donor is implicated in a case of TRALI, that donor is excluded from the donor pool. However, preventing those first cases of TRALI by those donors would require the elimination of all blood donors whose plasmas contain anti-HLA and/or neutrophil antibodies. Because screening donors for such antibodies would be extraordinarily expensive and time consuming, an approach has been investigated in which FFP is simply not prepared from female donors whose plasmas have a greater chance of containing anti-HLA antibodies due to pregnancy. When this approach was adopted in the United Kingdom in late 2003 where 60% of TRALI cases had previously been caused by FFP transfusions, no reports of TRALI deaths due to plasma occurred after 2004 (6 deaths occurred in 2005, none from plasma). Recent studies investigating the relationship of HLA antibodies in blood donors to pregnancy and transfusion history have shown that the incidence of class I and class II HLA antibodies is about the same in nontransfused males, transfused males, and females who have never been pregnant (0.9%, 1.2%, and 1.5%, respectively). However, the incidence of HLA antibodies dramatically increased with increasing number of pregnancies (11.2%, 23.1%, and 28.1% with 1, 2, and ≥3 pregnancies, respectively). This, in part, has led some major blood suppliers in the United States to limit the use of female plasma for the production of FFP in an attempt to decrease the incidence of TRALI. Even with these precautions in place, cases of TRALI in which HLA or other granulocyte-specific antibodies do not appear to be responsible will not be eliminated. Therefore, strict transfusion criteria for FFP, early recognition, and proper clinical management are currently the best options available to deal with this potentially fatal form of transfusion reaction.

Infectious complications
Bacterial and protozoal transmission by transfusion

Fatal transfusion reactions from bacterially contaminated RBCs are rare, although occasional cases of acute hypotensive and febrile reactions due to gross bacterial contamination have been observed. However, bacterial contamination of platelet products is recognized as a more significant issue given that platelets are stored at room temperature. Before the recent introduction of specific precautions to reduce bacterial contamination of platelet products, as many as 1 in 1000 to 1 in 2000 platelet units were contaminated with bacteria, resulting in clinical sepsis after 1 in 4000 platelet transfusions and a risk of death that was estimated to be between 1 in 7500 and 1 in 100,000. Because bacterial contamination of platelets became recognized as the most common cause of transfusion-associated morbidity and mortality due to an infectious source (greater than hepatitis, HIV, and other viral sources combined), laboratory accreditation agencies in the

United States recently mandated that organizations that collect or prepare platelets for transfusion have methods in place to limit and detect the presence of bacteria in platelet components. Since the introduction of bacterial screening, the risk of septic transfusion reactions for apheresis platelets has declined to approximately 1 in 75,000, and the risk of a fatal septic reaction has declined to approximately 1 in 500,000. These new requirements have been addressed in various ways; for example, efforts to limit the introduction of bacteria into platelets have involved the diversion of the first aliquot of donor blood from the collection bag as a means of removing the bacteria-ridden skin core that would otherwise be introduced by the phlebotomy needle. Efforts to detect the presence of bacteria in platelet units prior to dispensing to a patient include culturing an aliquot of the unit as though one were performing a blood culture or, for more rapid albeit less sensitive detection, using a surrogate marker for evidence of bacterial metabolism such as a low pH (eg, pH <6.5) in an aliquot of the platelet suspension.

In recent years, several fatal reactions to RBCs caused by contamination with *Yersinia enterocolitica* have been reported. This gram-negative organism can survive during refrigerated storage and lead to bacteremia or septic shock in the transfusion recipient. With the immigration of individuals from South America to the United States, there is concern that Chagas disease may emerge as a common transfusion-transmitted infection. *Trypanosoma cruzi* parasites can survive several weeks of storage in blood, and contamination of blood products with this organism is already a significant problem in parts of South America. Transfusion-transmitted babesiosis has been reported in New England and has been identified in patients receiving platelets, refrigerated RBCs, and even frozen-thawed RBCs. *Borrelia burgdorferi*, the etiologic agent of Lyme disease, has yet to be confirmed as having been transmitted by blood transfusions.

Hepatitis

Despite the elimination of commercial blood donors and screening of donor blood for hepatitis B and hepatitis C, posttransfusion hepatitis still occasionally develops. Although transmitted in a similar fashion to hepatitis B, acute transfusion-related hepatitis C infection is subclinical and anicteric in most cases. However, hepatitis C infection frequently becomes chronic and often results in clinically significant liver dysfunction. Recent data suggest that patients who have undergone HSCT are at much increased risk for late-onset cirrhosis after hepatitis C exposure. Prior to the availability of anti–hepatitis C virus (anti-HCV) testing, assays for serum alanine aminotransferase (ALT) levels and antibodies to hepatitis B core antigen testing were performed as surrogate tests. In the early 1990s, routine screening of all donors with a first-generation assay to detect antibody to a nonstructural antigen of hepatitis C was adopted in the United States. However, not all donors who transmitted hepatitis C were found to be positive by this assay. Therefore, in 1992, a second-generation assay that tests for antibodies to additional gene products (core and putative protease epitopes) was introduced. With such second-generation tests and now NAT, it is estimated that the risk of posttransfusion hepatitis C is <1 per 1,800,000 units transfused. Table 11-4 summarizes the estimated risks of various transfusion-associated infections. A number of recent studies have examined the utility of photochemical treatment of platelets with amotosalen and ultraviolet A to inactivate HIV, hepatitis viruses, and other viral pathogens. To date, this approach appears both efficacious and relatively sparing in terms of qualitative platelet function, although decreases in quantitative platelet recovery have been observed in some studies. Concern with the use of these viral inactivation methods focuses more on the potential untoward systemic effects of residual pathogen-inactivation agents introduced during transfusion.

Acquired immunodeficiency syndrome–related retroviruses

The risk of acquiring HIV-1 or HIV-2 infection as a result of transfusion is currently estimated to be 1 in 2,300,000. Nucleic acid amplification testing for HIV has reduced the window of serologic conversion from 16 days to 8 days. Because the HIV-1 RNA response detected by nucleic amplification testing occurs before or simultaneously with p24 antigen and because HIV-1 RNA is detected after p24 disappearance, p24 testing has been replaced by this newer technology. The availability of heat-treated concentrates, solvent detergent-treated products, and recombinant DNA-synthesized products has eliminated acquired immunodeficiency syndrome (AIDS) as a risk for hemophiliacs.

Human T-cell lymphotrophic viruses

Human T-cell lymphotrophic virus 1 (HTLV-1) is a retrovirus associated with adult T-cell leukemia/lymphoma and tropical spastic paraparesis. Because asymptomatic blood donors can transmit this virus, resulting in seroconversion and possible illness in transfusion recipients, screening for HTLV-1 in blood donors was initiated in 1989. Several cases of neuropathy had been reported in transfusion recipients prior to the availability of testing. HTLV-2, a related virus with antigenic cross-reactivity to HTLV-1, is endemic in certain Native American populations and is associated with an increase in common infections suggesting immune suppression. A high fraction of users of injectable drugs are infected with HTLV-2.

West Nile virus

Recently there have been a number of well-documented reports indicating that transfusion can transmit West Nile virus (WNV) and that recipients can develop fever, confusion, and encephalitis characteristic of WNV infection within days to weeks of transfusion. During the 2002 West Nile virus epidemic in the United States, 23 individuals acquired WNV after blood transfusion. As a result, blood centers have implemented nucleic acid–based testing to screen all donations for WNV. In a survey of 2.5 million donations in 2003, 601 donations (0.02%) were found to contain WNV. A subsequent follow-up study detected no cases of transfusion-transmitted WNV infection among recipients of tested blood; however, rare breakthrough transmissions have been reported.

Parvovirus B19

A recent study documented persistence of low levels of parvovirus B19 DNA in a high percentage of multitransfused patients. The long-term clinical implications of this finding are currently unknown.

Cytomegalovirus

Passenger leukocytes that inevitably contaminate RBC and platelet products, albeit in relatively small numbers, are capable of transmitting CMV infection. Transfusion-transmitted CMV infection is an important issue in transfusion of cellular blood products to neonates, HSC transplantation recipients, and other highly immunosuppressed patients. For example, there is a high risk of mortality among patients who acquire CMV infection within the first few months after transplantation. The risk of acquiring CMV from transfusions is particularly high when pretransplantation serologic testing reveals that neither the donor nor the recipient has been previously exposed to CMV. In addition, transplantation recipients are at increased risk for transplantation-associated CMV reactivation when either the donor or the recipient is seropositive for CMV prior to transplantation. The latter consideration often affects the choice of HSC donors. Another at-risk group for CMV infection is neonates, particularly low birth weight infants born to seronegative mothers.

For the previous reasons, many teams use blood products obtained exclusively from CMV-negative donors when providing blood products to neonatal recipients or recipients of HSC transplantations. Other teams simply use leukoreduced blood products in all such recipients, regardless of CMV status. The latter strategy has the additional advantage of reducing the risk of alloimmunization to HLA antigens and thus of developing refractoriness to platelet transfusions. However, none of the previous strategies to reduce the risk of CMV transmission eliminate the necessity of γ-irradiating blood products administered to the same subsets of patients. For reasons discussed previously, γ-irradiation of blood products must also be performed to prevent the development of t-GVHD. There is evidence that the use of CMV-seronegative leukoreduced blood products may be superior to the use of leukoreduced products alone. Therefore, some centers advocate the use of CMV-seronegative products in highly immunosuppressed patients such as patients receiving HSC from unrelated donors.

Transfusion-associated graft-versus-host disease

t-GVHD is an important risk in patients undergoing treatment of hematologic malignancies, patients undergoing HSCT, and patients with certain congenital immunodeficiency syndromes. The pathophysiology of t-GVHD is thought to involve engraftment of small numbers of donor-derived passenger leukocytes in a host whose immune system is unable to eliminate the passenger leukocytes. Unlike *transplantation*-associated GVHD, in which the hematopoietic organ is donor derived and thus relatively protected from immune assault by donor-derived T cells, in *transfusion*-associated GVHD, the hematopoietic organ is recipient derived. Therefore, when t-GVHD develops, mortality approaches 100% as a result of the severe pancytopenia that usually develops. Patients may also develop signs and symptoms of classic transplantation-associated GVHD, including skin rash, diarrhea, liver function test abnormalities, and other symptoms. The infusion of any cellular blood product can theoretically cause t-GVHD, and the conventional leukoreduction techniques discussed earlier in this chapter have not been proven adequate to eliminate the risk of this usually fatal complication. In contrast, γ-irradiation of all cellular blood products prior to transfusion virtually eliminates the risk of t-GVHD. Many hospitals that have HSCT programs and/or treat large numbers of patients with hematologic malignancies and congenital immunodeficiency states have acquired their own in-house blood irradiators. It is important to note that γ-irradiation of cellular blood products has not been proven to be adequate to reduce the risk of alloimmunization to HLA antigens or the risk of CMV transmission. Therefore, most centers subject blood products to be administered to at-risk patients to both γ-irradiation and leukoreduction.

Until relatively recently, t-GVHD had not been described in immunocompetent patients. However, recent data suggest that transfusion within relatively inbred populations, such as in Israel or Japan, appears to increase the risk of t-GVHD because of the increased prevalence of donors who are homozygous at an HLA locus at which the recipient is heterozygous but who share one allele. This appears to set up a unidirectional HLA mismatch in which the recipient immune system is unable to recognize the donor-derived passenger leukocytes as being foreign and is thus unable to eliminate the passenger leukocytes, whereas the passenger leukocytes appear to recognize the nonshared HLA allele on the recipient's cells and thereby initiate a graft-versus-host reaction. For similar reasons, directed-donor transfusions between closely related family members may also theoretically increase the risk of t-GVHD.

Strategies to reduce transfusion risks in general

Clinicians can reduce virtually all of the previously listed risks by following a few basic principles. First, patients should receive the minimum necessary number of blood components specifically required to correct the deficiency at hand without supplying unnecessary cells or plasma products. Second, clinicians must keep in mind that it is unnecessary to correct a cytopenia or a clotting protein deficiency to normal levels; transfusion should be directed toward restoring only functionally adequate levels. For example, many patients with chronic anemia or thrombocytopenia tolerate much lower blood counts than patients with acute cytopenias involving the same lineages, and most patients tolerate clotting factor levels of 50% without difficulty. Third, patient misidentification due to clerical error remains the most common cause of acute hemolytic transfusion reactions; therefore, the importance of definitive bedside patient identification, both at the time that type and crossmatch specimens are obtained and at the time that the product is ready to be administered, cannot be overemphasized. Various high-technology methodologies to assure correct patient identification have been shown to reduce the risk of mistransfusion.

Autologous blood donation is an important technique that is available to reduce the risks associated with RBC transfusion among patients scheduled for elective surgical procedures. However, it is important to appreciate that although the use of autologous blood may eliminate transfusion risks due to immunologic incompatibility or transfusion-transmitted infection (although not bacterial contamination of the unit), the etiology for the most common cause of transfusion-related mortality still exists—that is, the transfusion of ABO-incompatible blood due to a clerical error (ie, the inadvertent transfusion of the wrong patient's autologous blood). Likewise, transfusion-associated complications such as those related to fluid overload in a patient with cardiac disease can occur whether the patient is receiving autologous or allogeneic blood. Therefore, many of the same principles regarding the judicious use of allogeneic blood components apply to the use of autologous blood. Unless the clinical condition of the patient actually warrants transfusion, autologous units of blood should not be used "because they couldn't hurt," a philosophy that must be discouraged among clinicians.

Blood substitutes and "bloodless" medicine

Currently, there are no licensed blood substitutes available for clinical use in the United States, although some formulations are available for clinical trials. The 2 types of blood substitutes that are being investigated are hemoglobin solutions and perfluorochemical-based compounds. With regard to the former, stroma-free hemoglobin or recombinant hemoglobin solutions that have been modified to increase intravascular dwell time are being evaluated. Because free hemoglobin is rapidly cleared, polymerization or linking to a macromolecule appears to be required. Compassionate use of hemoglobin-based blood substitutes has been reported in patients who either declined transfusion or were impossible to transfuse by virtue of multiple high-frequency antibodies or severe AIHA. However, a recent meta-analysis of hemoglobin-based blood substitutes found excess myocardial infarction and mortality in surgical patients who received the blood substitute compared with controls; patient groups included trauma, cardiac surgery, vascular surgery, and elective orthopedic surgery.

Perfluorochemical solutions have been licensed to supplement oxygen delivery to the heart during coronary artery balloon angioplasty. However, perfluorochemical formulations have not yet proved clinically valuable as general-use blood substitutes because of their insolubility in water, brief intravascular dwell time, reticuloendothelial and granulocyte blockade, and high inspired oxygen requirement. Newer formulations may circumvent the need for high concentrations of inspired oxygen. Because of the insolubility of perfluorochemical compounds, egg phospholipids are required as emulsifying agents. Some of these agents are antigenic and may lead to allergic reactions. Most perfluorochemical compounds are excreted within days of administration, but some remain in the tissues for months.

The use of recombinant erythropoietin (epoetin alfa) for patients with chronic renal failure who require dialysis has virtually eliminated the need for transfusion in these patients. Erythropoietin may also be used to treat patients with earlier stages of chronic kidney disease, who typically have less severe anemia that is not transfusion dependent. A recent study showed that the hemoglobin level in these patients should be maintained no higher than 11 to 12 g/dL because the incidence of cardiovascular events was increased when this threshold level was exceeded. Erythropoietin is also useful in Jehovah's Witness patients, who decline transfusion, either therapeutically to treat anemia or prophylactically before elective surgery.

In patients scheduled to undergo elective surgery with significant blood loss, allogeneic transfusion can be minimized by optimizing preoperative hemoglobin levels and using autologous blood donations. Achieving optimal hemoglobin levels, including correction of iron deficiency (if present), is often overlooked; >30% of patients scheduled for orthopedic surgery were anemic in several series. Preoperative autologous blood donation has been used for many years to reduce the risks associated with allogeneic transfusion. However, autologous blood transfusion is not risk free because clerical errors, volume overload, and bacterial contamination can and do occur. In addition, patients who donate autologous blood have an increased risk of developing perioperative anemia and an increased need for additional blood transfusions, particularly if the interval between donation and surgery is short. Directed donations from relatives or friends selected by the patient have not been shown to be any safer in terms of transmitting infectious agents. In addition, blood from first-degree relatives must be irradiated to prevent t-GVHD.

The management of Jehovah's Witness patients who require chemotherapy for hematologic malignancies can present a challenge. Autologous PBSC transplantation and reduced-intensity allogeneic transplantation have been performed in these patients. A comprehensive approach is required, including minimizing phlebotomy and gastrointestinal blood loss; optimizing pretransplantation blood counts using erythropoietic-stimulating agents, iron and folate repletion, and possibly the newer thrombopoietic growth factors; prophylactic use of antifibrinolytic agents during the period of thrombocytopenia; and use of desmopressin and recombinant factor VIIa for active bleeding.

Key points

- Life-threatening acute hemolytic reactions due to patient misidentification are significantly more common than transfusion-transmitted HIV or hepatitis.
- A number of strategies are available for reducing transfusion risks, including reducing the number of units transfused, γ-irradiating blood products, leukoreduction of blood products, and the use of autologous blood donation.

Bibliography

Ackerman SJ, Klumpp TR, Guzman GI, et al. Economic consequences of alterations in platelet transfusion dose: analysis of a prospective, randomized, double-blind trial. *Transfusion.* 2000;40:1457-1462. *This economic analysis of a prospective, randomized trial of platelet transfusion dose demonstrated that efforts to decrease costs by reducing the mean platelet dose are likely to result in a disproportionate increase in the number of transfusions per patient, resulting in a corresponding increase in overall hospital transfusion costs.*

American Association of Blood Banks. *Technical Manual.* 16th ed. Bethesda, MD: AABB Press; 2008. *Despite the rather dry-sounding title, this text provides an outstanding overview of essentially all topics in transfusion medicine from blood collection and transfusion to serology and apheresis.*

Bell EF. When to transfuse preterm babies. *Arch Dis Child Fetal Neonatal Ed.* 2008;93:F469-F473. *A succinct review of transfusions in the neonatal intensive care unit, from the Iowa group that conducted 1 of the 2 randomized controlled trials comparing liberal versus restrictive transfusion thresholds in preterm babies.*

Blanchette VS, Rand ML, Carcao MD, et al. Platelet transfusion therapy in infants and children. In: Kickler TS, Herman JH, eds. *Current Issues in Platelet Transfusion Therapy and Platelet Alloimmunity.* Bethesda, MD: AABB Press; 1999:177–222. *A comprehensive review of pediatric platelet transfusion practice.*

Busch MP, Glynn SA, Stramer S, et al. A new strategy for estimating risks of transfusion-transmitted viral infections based on rates of detection of recently infected donors. *Transfusion.* 2005;45:254–264. *Provides a method by which the risks of transfusion-transmitted viral infection can be estimated given the effectiveness of NAT of donors.*

Centers for Disease Control and Prevention. Update: detection of West Nile virus in blood donations – United States, 2003. *JAMA.* 2003;290:2248–2250. *A clearly written review, including representative case reports, of the current status of the US blood supply with regard to the transmission and prevention of WNV infections.*

Cooling LWW, Kelly K, Barton J, et al. Determinants of ABH expression on human blood platelets. *Blood.* 2005;105:3356–3364. *This study indicates that platelets obtained from type A2 blood donors may represent a universal platelet product for all except type B and type AB recipients, in the sense that A antigen is not expressed on the platelets, whereas anti-A is not present in the supernatant plasma.*

Crow AR, Lazarus AH. The mechanisms of action of intravenous immunoglobulin and polyclonal anti-D immunoglobulin in the amelioration of immune thrombocytopenic purpura; what do we really know? Transfus Med Rev. 2008;22:103–116. *This excellent paper reviews and critiques the numerous theories proposed for the mechanism(s) of action of intravenous immune globulins in the treatment of autoimmune disorders with particular focus on their use in ITP.*

Dacie SJ. The immune hemolytic anemias. *Br J Haematol.* 2001;114:770–785. *An authoritative review on the diagnosis and treatment of AIHA.*

Denomme GA. The structure and function of the molecules that carry human red blood cell and platelet antigens. *Transf Med Rev.* 2004;18:203–231. *An updated review of the structure–function relationship of RBC and platelet antigens, such as the Duffy glycoprotein as a chemokine receptor, and the transporter functions for the Rh proteins, band 3 glycoprotein (Diego blood group), and aquaporin-I (Colton blood group).*

Dodd RY. Current viral risks of blood and blood products. *Ann Med*. 2000;32:469–474. *An overview of current strategies for preventing viral transmission of disease by blood transfusion.*

Gaydos LA, Freireich EI, Mantel N. The quantitative relationship between platelet count and hemorrhage in patients with acute leukemia. *N Engl J Med*. 1962;266:905–909. *One of the few studies to address the relationship between the degree of thrombocytopenia and the risk of hemorrhage.*

Hébert PC, Wells G, Blajchman MA, et al. A multicenter, randomized, controlled clinical trial of transfusion requirements in critical care. *N Engl J Med*. 1999;340:409–417. *An excellent multicenter clinical trial showing that a conservative transfusion protocol for the administration of RBCs to critically ill patients did not significantly change morbidity or mortality.*

Heddle NM, Klama L, Singer J, et al. The role of the plasma from platelet concentrates in transfusion reactions. *N Engl J Med*. 1994;331:625–628. *One of the first reports documenting the role of cytokines in transfusion reactions.*

Hume H, Bard H. Small volume red blood cell transfusions for neonatal patients. *Transfus Med Rev*. 1995;9:187–199. *A practical review of transfusion strategies in neonates.*

Klein HG. The prospects for red-cell substitutes. *N Engl J Med*. 2000;342:1666–1668. *Summarizes 3 decades of work toward the development of an RBC substitute.*

Klein HG, Spahn DR, Carson JL. Red blood cell transfusion in clinical practice. *Lancet*. 2007;370:415–426. *A review of RBC transfusion, balancing the principles of oxygen transport with the uncertainties of the transfusion trigger, and the practical aspects of component modification and transfusion reactions.*

Kleinman S, Caulfield T, Chan P, et al. Toward an understanding of transfusion-related acute lung injury. Statement of a consensus panel. *Transfusion*. 2004;44:1774–1789. *A seminal paper in the field that provides a much-needed set of criteria for defining this potentially fatal complication of transfusion.*

Klumpp TR, Herman JH, Schnell MK, et al. Association between antibodies reactive with neutrophils, rate of neutrophil engraftment, and incidence of post-engraftment neutropenia following BMT. *Bone Marrow Transplant*. 1996;18:559–564. *The only prospective study documenting the high incidence of antibodies reactive with neutrophils following BMT and the independent statistical correlation of such antibodies with both delayed neutrophil engraftment and secondary graft failure.*

Kruskall MS, Aubuchon JP, Anthony K, et al. Transfusion to blood group A and O patients of group B RBCs that have been enzymatically converted to group O. *Transfusion*. 2000;40:1290–1298. *This article describes early efforts in the area of ABO blood group conversion for therapeutic use.*

Luban NLC, Strauss RG, Hume HA. Commentary on the safety of red blood cells preserved in extended storage media for neonatal transfusions. *Transfusion*. 1991;31:229–235. *This paper discusses the safety of using RBC preservative solutions in neonates.*

Lund N, Olsson ML, Ramkumar S, et al. The human P^k histo-blood group antigen provides protection against HIV-1 infection. *Blood*. 2009;113:4980–4991. *Fascinating study that demonstrated that the presence of the Pk antigen on mononuclear cells confers resistance to HIV-1 infection whereas cells completely lacking Pk (blood group "p" phenotype) were 10 to 1000 times more susceptible to HIV-1 infection.*

McCullough J. Current issues with platelet transfusion in patients with cancer. *Semin Hematol*. 2000;37:3-10. *Despite recent advances, alloimmunization to HLA antigens is still a significant issue. This paper discusses approaches to reducing the incidence of this problem.*

McCullough J, Vesole DH, Benjamin RJ, et al. Therapeutic efficacy and safety of platelets treated with a photochemical process for pathogen inactivation: the SPRINT Trial. *Blood*. 2004;104:1534–1541. *This randomized trial compared photochemically treated platelets and conventionally prepared platelets and demonstrated an equivalent incidence of grade 2 bleeding along with a reduced incidence of transfusion reactions. The posttransfusion platelet increments were somewhat reduced.*

McFarland JG. Platelet and neutrophil alloantigen genotyping in clinical practice. *Transfus Clin Biol*. 1998;5:13–21. *This paper describes the clinically relevant antigens on platelets and neutrophils.*

Nichols WG, Price TH, Gooley T, et al. Transfusion-transmitted cytomegalovirus infection after receipt of leukoreduced blood products. *Blood*. 2003;101:4195–4200. *This paper compares the incidence of transfusion-transmitted CMV infection using 2 different commonly used prevention strategies.*

Read MS, Reddick RL, Bode AP, et al. Preservation of hemostatic properties of rehydrated lyophilized platelets. *Proc Natl Acad Sci USA*. 1995;92:397–401. *Describes efforts to move toward the use of lyophilized platelets, the potential advantages of which are detailed in the text.*

Rebulla P, Finazzi G, Marangoni F, et al. The threshold for prophylactic platelet transfusions in adults with acute myeloid leukemia. *N Engl J Med*. 1997;337:1870–1875. *A randomized clinical trial examining the consequences of using a prophylactic platelet transfusion threshold of 10,000/μL versus 20,000/μL. The use of the lower threshold appeared to be associated with minimal increased risk, but the statistical power of the study to detect clinically meaningful increases in the risk of major hemorrhage was limited.*

Rock G, Neurath D, Toye B, et al. The use of a bacteria detection system to evaluate bacterial contamination in PLT concentrates. *Transfusion*. 2004;44:337–342. *Demonstrated that the use of a commercially available bacterial detection system can identify culture-negative platelets that could be stored for up to 7 days and function appropriately.*

Schiffer CA, Anderson KC, Bennett CL, et al. Platelet transfusion for patients with cancer: clinical practice guidelines of the American Society of Clinical Oncology. *J Clin Oncol*. 2001;19:1519–1538. *Evidence-based clinical practice guidelines based on an extensive review of the literature.*

Seftel MD, Growe GH, Petraszko T, et al. Universal prestorage leukoreduction in Canada decreases platelet alloimmunization and refractoriness. *Blood*. 2004;103:333–339. *A large study documenting that prestorage leukodepletion of blood products markedly reduces the incidence of platelet transfusion refractoriness.*

Sensebe L, Giraudeau B, Bardiaux L, et al. The efficiency of transfusing high doses of platelets in hematologic patients with thrombocytopenia: results of a prospective, randomized, open, blinded end point (PROBE) study. *Blood*. 2005;105:862–864. *A small trial that randomized leukemia and HSCT patients to low-dose versus high-dose platelet transfusion; the high-dose group underwent fewer transfusion episodes but a similar number of transfused platelets, compared with the low-dose group.*

Silliman CC, Boshkov LK, Mehdizadehkashi Z, et al. Transfusion-related acute lung injury: epidemiology and a prospective analysis of etiologic factors. *Blood*. 2003;101:454–462. *A large prospective study documenting both the incidence of TRALI and the apparent contribution of granulocyte antibodies, cytokines, and biologically active lipids.*

Silverman GJ, Goodyear CS, Siegel DL. On the mechanism of staphylococcal protein A immunomodulation. *Transfusion*. 2005;45:274–280. *This paper describes the "superantigen" properties of bacterial SpA and demonstrates how it is the leaching off of small quantities of this substance from the SpA columns and the subsequent intravenous infusion into the patient during apheresis procedures that imparts this molecule's B-cell–suppressive effects.*

Slichter S, Davis K, Enright H, et al. Factors affecting posttransfusion platelet increments, platelet refractoriness, and platelet transfusion intervals in thrombocytopenic patients. *Blood*. 2005;105:4106–4114. *A follow-up analysis from the TRAP trial to explore patient and component factors that influence platelet transfusion response; higher doses of platelets transfused and filtered apheresis platelets decreased platelet refractoriness.*

Slichter SJ, Kaufman RM, Assmann SF, et al. Dose of prophylactic platelet transfusions and prevention of hemorrhage. *New Engl J Med*. 2010;362:600–613. *Recent multicenter RCT showing no difference in bleeding episodes when patients were randomized to prophylactic transfusions at low, medium, or high doses. The low-dose arm received fewer platelets but more transfusion episodes.*

Snyder EL, Haley NR. *Cellular Therapy: A Physician's Handbook*. Bethesda, MD: AABB Press; 2000. *A good review of HSC mobilization and harvesting.*

Stanworth SJ, Brunskill SJ, Hyde CJ, McClelland DBL, Murphy MF. Is fresh frozen plasma clinically effective? A systematic review of randomized controlled trials. *Br J Haematol*. 2004;126:139–152. *A review that shows how little evidence there is to support the widespread use of FFP and the dire need for clinical trials in this area.*

Stramer SL, Fang CT, Foster GA, et al. West Nile virus among blood donors in the United States, 2003 and 2004. *N Engl J Med*. 2005;353:451–459. *This study suggests that the introduction of nucleic acid amplification testing for WNV appears to have essentially eliminated transfusion-transmitted infection with this pathogen.*

Stramer SL, Glynn SA, Kleinman SH, et al; for the National Heart, Lung, and Blood Institute Nucleic Acid Test Study Group. Detection of HIV-1 and HCV infections among antibody-negative blood donors by nucleic acid amplification testing *N Engl J Med*. 2004;351:760–768. *Reports on the effectiveness of NAT to detect individuals infected with HIV-1 and HCV who are in the seronegative window period of infection.*

Stroncek DF, Rebulla P. Platelet transfusions. *Lancet*. 2007;370:427–438. *An excellent review of platelet transfusion practice including the transfusion trigger and platelet refractoriness.*

Szczepiorkowski ZM, Bandarenko N, Kim HC, et al. Guidelines on the use of therapeutic apheresis in clinical practice—evidence-based approach from the apheresis applications committee of the American Society for Apheresis. *J Clin Apheresis* 2007;22:106–175. *Comprehensive analysis of the indications for apheresis using a rigorous evidence-based approach.*

Trial to Reduce Alloimmunization to Platelets Study Group. Leukocyte reduction and ultraviolet B irradiation of platelets to prevent alloimmunization and refractoriness to platelet transfusions. *N Engl J Med*. 1997;337:1861–1869. *A landmark study comparing 4 major options for the reduction of alloimmunization to HLA antigens with consequent reduction in the incidence of platelet transfusion refractoriness.*

Vamvakas EC, Blajchman MA. Transfusion-related mortality: the ongoing risks of allogeneic blood transfusion and the available strategies for their prevention. *Blood*. 2009;113:3406–3417. *An up-to-date review of transfusion-related morbidity including hemolysis, bacterial contamination, and TRALI but also immunomodulation and the benefits of leukoreduction.*

Vaughn JI, Manning M, Warwick RM, et al. Inhibition of erythroid progenitor cells by anti-Kell antibodies in fetal alloimmune anemia. *N Engl J Med*. 1998;338:798–803. *This paper was the first to describe the hypoproliferative effect of anti-Kell alloantibodies on fetal erythroid progenitor cells, thus explaining how the anemia in anti-Kell–induced hemolytic disease of the newborn results from a combination of decreased production as well as increased destruction.*

Vichinsky EP. Current issues with blood transfusions in sickle cell disease. *Semin Hematol*. 2001;38:14–22. *Transfusion practices in sickle cell disease are important if one treats this group of patients. This paper gives a comprehensive overview.*

Westhoff CM, Burd C, Siegel DL, et al. Evidence that the erythrocyte Rh-blood group glycoprotein functions as an NH_4^+/H^+ exchanger. *J Biol Chem*. 2004;279:17443–17448. *Using strains of yeast transfected with the human Rh-associated glycoprotein, the authors were the first to demonstrate an ammonium ion/proton ion exchange transport function for Rh.*

CHAPTER 12

Cellular basis of hematopoiesis and stem cell transplantation

Alan B. Cantor, Hillard M. Lazarus, and Ginna G. Laport

Introduction and historical perspective, 331	Transplantation for specific diseases, 354	Bibliography, 367
Hematopoietic stem cell concepts, 331	Late effects and long-term follow-up after transplantation, 365	
Ontogeny of hematopoiesis, 334		
Stem cell enrichment strategies, 335	Summary, 367	

Introduction and historical perspective

Most terminally differentiated blood cells have a relatively short life span and must be continually replenished through the lifetime of an individual. In 1961, a series of seminal experiments by Till and McCulloch showed that the transfer of bone marrow cells from donor mice into lethally irradiated host mice resulted in the formation of macroscopic colonies of myeloid, erythroid, and megakaryocytic cells in the spleens of the recipients 7 to 14 days after transplantation (Till and McCulloch, 1961) (Figure 12-1). These colonies were shown to arise from a single implanted cell, were capable of extensive proliferation, and could be retransplanted into secondary recipients. Although later work showed that these cells (called spleen colony-forming unit [CFU-S] cells) likely represent short-term, rather than long-term, hematopoietic repopulating cells, these studies laid the foundation for concepts of hematopoietic (and nonhematopoietic) stem cell biology.

Hematopoietic stem cell concepts

Hematopoietic stem cell properties

The remarkable ability of hematopoietic stem cells (HSCs), at the single-cell level, to reconstitute and maintain a functional hematopoietic system over extended periods of time in vivo is related to 3 intrinsic properties: extensive proliferative capacity, pluripotency (the ability to differentiate into all blood cell types), and self-renewal capacity (the ability to replace the cells that became progressively committed to differentiation).

Stem cell assays
Colony-forming assays

The identification of a cell capable of clonal differentiation in vivo by Till and McCulloch (1961) prompted other groups to develop a simple quantitative assay for the growth and differentiation of single-cell suspensions of mouse bone marrow in vitro. When hematopoietic cells were cultured in a semi-solid soft agar medium, discrete colonies were formed and included cells in multiple stages of differentiation (Figure 12-2). In line with the properties observed for CFU-S, it was subsequently established that colonies generated in vitro could be initiated by the proliferation of a single colony-forming cell/unit (CFC or CFU). However, contrasting with the self-renewal potential of most CFU-S, colonies grown in vitro showed no or limited ability to proliferate in secondary cultures. This limitation implied that the most primitive stem cells failed to survive or proliferate in this assay, and therefore, CFCs were suggested to define a population of committed progenitors, fed from an earlier, more immature compartment of HSCs.

Long-term bone marrow culture

Attempts to develop procedures that mimic the normal bone marrow microenvironment resulted in the development

---

Conflict-of-interest disclosure: *Dr. Cantor* declares no competing financial interest. *Dr. Lazarus:* honoraria: Genentech/Biogen IDEC; speakers' bureau: Genentech/Biogen IDEC. *Dr. Laport:* honoraria: Genzyme.

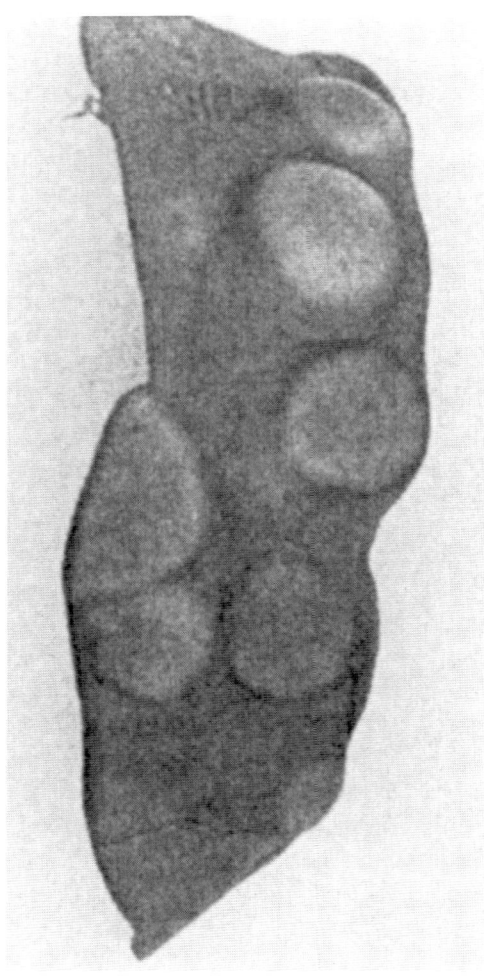

Figure 12-1 Spleen colony-forming unit (CFU-S) assay. Macroscopic splenic hematopoietic colonies arising from the CFU-S stem/progenitor cell 14 days after injection of murine bone marrow into lethally irradiated mice. Reproduced with permission from Williams DA. Stem cell model of hematopoiesis. In: Hoffman R, Benz EJ Jr, Shattil SJ, Furie B, Cohen HJ, eds. *Hematology: Basic Principles and Practice*. New York, NY: Churchill Livingstone, 1995.

of long-term bone marrow cultures. In this assay, formation of an adherent stromal cell layer, which produces and deposits an extracellular matrix meshwork, is a prerequisite for the development of hematopoietic cells. In association with the feeder layer, hematopoietic cells proliferate and differentiate over several months in culture releasing clonogenic and mature cells. The ongoing production of these cells is the result of differentiation and proliferation of very primitive cells. In recognition of their method of detection, these cells have been called long-term culture-initiating cells (LTC-ICs). They represent the most primitive immature cells that can be assayed in vitro. The presence of LTC-ICs can be detected by assaying for the presence of CFU in cultures maintained for a minimum of 5 weeks. Beyond this point, any CFCs initially present in the culture should have disappeared through differentiation or death, and those detected will be the result of differentiation by LTC-IC. However, several lines of evidence suggest that LTC-ICs are not true HSCs and, therefore, are incapable of definitive long-term reconstitution and maintenance of hematopoiesis in vivo.

Transplantation assays

The definitive assay for mouse HSC activity is the ability to provide long-term (>4 months) repopulation of all blood lineages of myeloablated host mice. For studies of human HSCs, xenograft models involving transplantation of primitive human hematopoietic cells have been developed. Primitive human hematopoietic cells will engraft fetal sheep at low levels, and at least 50% will have long-term persistence of human cells, with secondary or tertiary transplantation into additional fetal sheep possible. Unfortunately, this model is technically challenging and not practical for most research groups. Murine xenotransplant models have been developed using several alternative immunodeficient mouse strains. The strain NOD-SCID IL-2R$_\gamma^{-/-}$ is severely immunodeficient, and a number of groups have shown it to be a best host for human hematopoietic cells. This model has been used to identify a pluripotent stem cell, termed severe combined immune-deficient mouse (SCID)-repopulating cells (SRCs), that is more primitive and clearly distinct from prior multipotent primitive human hematopoietic cell populations identified using in vitro methodology.

HSC number

The most primitive HSCs are rare, representing approximately 1 in 10^4 bone marrow cells. It is estimated that in healthy persons, there are approximately 50 million self-renewing HSCs, which can give rise to approximately 10^{13} mature blood cells over a normal life span. During normal steady-state hematopoiesis, adult HSCs cycle slowly. When they are recruited into active hematopoiesis, they exit the G0 phase of the cell cycle and undergo a series of maturational cell divisions that culminate in the generation of progenitor cells with progressively limited self-renewal, proliferative, and differentiative potentials.

HSC niche

Hematopoietic cells develop in vivo in intimate association with a heterogeneous population of stromal cells and extracellular matrix molecules that constitute the microenvironment of the bone marrow. Fibroblasts, smooth muscle cells, adipocytes, osteogenic cells, and macrophages compose the stromal cell compartment. Extracellular matrix molecules

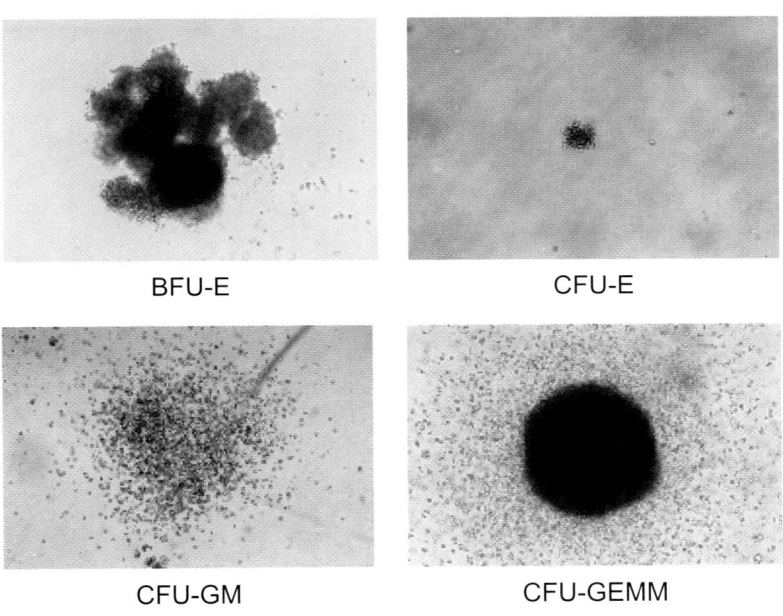

Figure 12-2 Examples of colony-forming assays of human hematopoietic progenitors, including colony-forming unit (CFU) erythroid (CFU-E), burst-forming unit erythroid (BFU-E), CFU granulocyte/macrophage (CFU-GM), and CFU granulocyte/erythroid/macrophage/megakaryocyte (CFU-GEMM). From Stem Cell Technologies, Inc; reprinted with permission.

of 7 distinct families have been identified, including collagens, proteoglycans, fibronectin, tenascin, thrombospondin, laminin, and hemonectin. Unique locales within the marrow, termed *niches*, exist that favor HSC self-renewal versus differentiation. HSCs are thought to occupy 1 of 2 niches within the bone marrow: an osteoblastic niche, which is located in the periosteal region of the bone cavity; and a vascular niche, which involves vascular sinusoids within the bone marrow. The relationship between these 2 niches remains under investigation, but it is possible that they represent similar locales due to intermingling of vascular sinusoids with the osteoblastic regions of the bone marrow. Various experimental systems have served to provide evidence that intimate contacts between HSCs and other cells and extracellular matrix molecules in these areas are involved in the maintaining of HSC properties. In addition, there is increasing evidence for a role of Wnt and angiopoietin 1/Tie-2 signaling in these processes.

HSC circulation, homing, and mobilization

Stem cells migrate from one site of blood cell production, circulate, home, and enter other supportive sites. Experiments using parabiotic mice, in which the circulations of 2 separate mice were joined surgically, have indicated that murine HSCs exit the bone marrow and transit the peripheral blood system at surprisingly high flux rates (estimated to be $\sim 10^4–10^5$ long-term repopulating HSCs [LT-HSCs] per day in a mouse). What controls the rate, timing, and destination of the HSCs is not currently well understood but appears to involve lectins, integrin adhesion molecules, chemokines and their receptors (especially stromal-derived factor-1 [SDF-1] and its receptor CXCR4), and members of the RhoGTPase family. The ability to alter these interactions with agents such as granulocyte colony-stimulating factor (G-CSF) or CXCR4 antagonists allows for "mobilization" of HSCs into the peripheral blood system and their collection by apheresis for HSC transplantation.

Hierarchal differentiation of HSCs

A complex network of transcription factor and growth factor signaling pathways tightly regulates HSC recruitment, lineage commitment, and differentiation. The advent of flow cytometric techniques has allowed cell surface markers to be used to prospectively isolate cell populations with selective potentials. These studies, in combination with classical CFC assays, have led to a hierarchal map of hematopoiesis shown in Figure 12-3. Although it was initially thought that these cell populations were irreversibly committed to their downstream lineages, more recent studies show that they retain some degree of potential lineage plasticity.

Summary

The fundamental concept uncovered by these studies can be summarized as follows: hematopoietic reconstitution during bone marrow transplantation is mediated by a succession of cells at various stages of development. Immediately following transplantation, the most mature cells contribute to

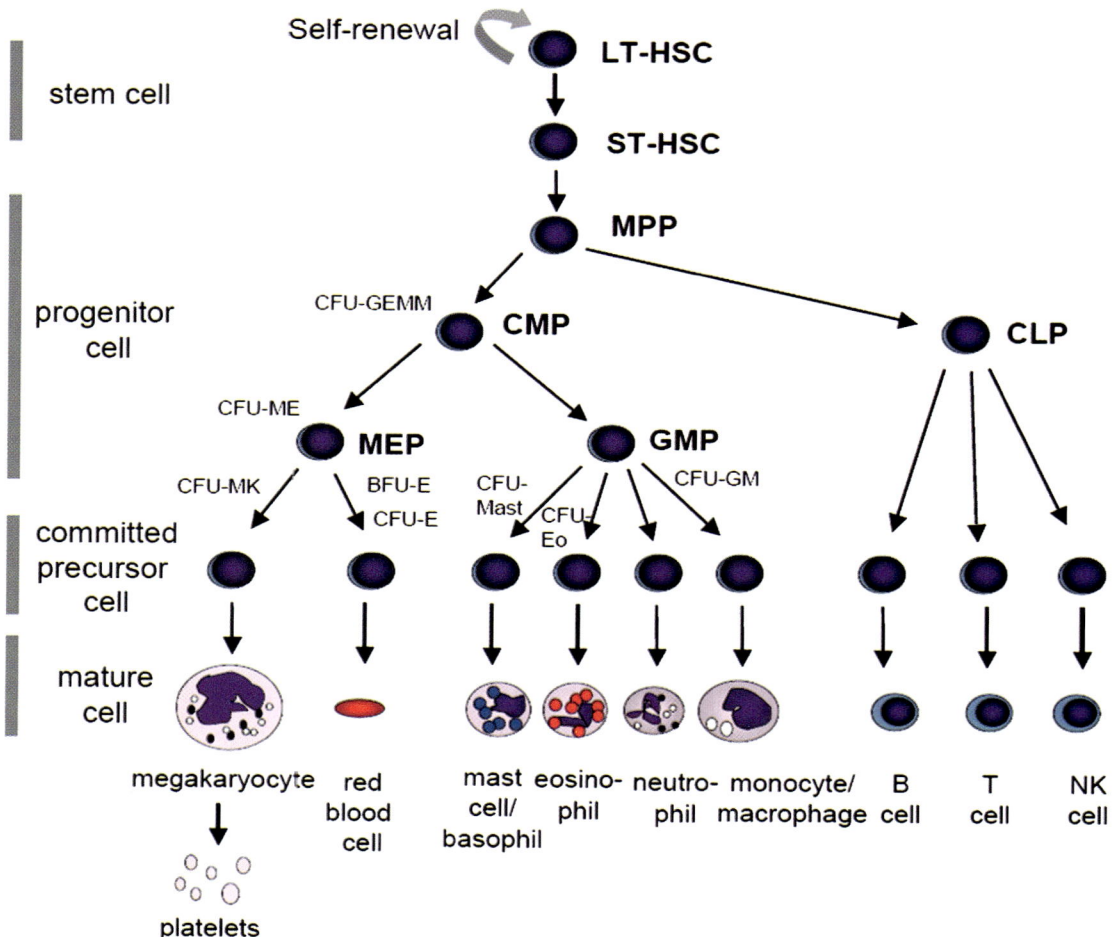

Figure 12-3 Classical hierarchal map of hematopoietic development. Schematic diagram depicting hierarchal relationships between immunophenotypically and functionally defined hematopoietic cell populations. CLP = common lymphoid progenitor; CMP = common myeloid progenitor; GMP = granulocyte-macrophage progenitor; LT-HSC = long-term repopulating hematopoietic stem cell; MEP = megakaryocyte-erythroid progenitor; MPP = multipotential progenitor cell; NK = natural killer; ST-HSC = short-term repopulating hematopoietic stem cell. Corresponding CFCs are indicated.

repopulation. With time, cells at progressively earlier stages of development contribute, with the final stable repopulation being provided by long-lived, multipotential stem cells. Long-term hematopoiesis is sustained by a relatively small number of HSCs, some of which can remain active for >2 years in primary, as well as secondary and tertiary, hosts. Consequently, durable, long-term reconstitution of the hematopoietic system of a recipient animal after transplantation remains the only definitive means of identifying and characterizing HSCs.

Ontogeny of hematopoiesis

The primary sites of hematopoiesis change in a temporally and spatially ordered fashion during development in most vertebrates. In humans, the yolk sac serves as the initial site of erythropoiesis from weeks 3 to 6 of gestation. The primary

> **Key points**
>
> - Key features of HSCs are as follows:
>   - Ability, at the single-cell level, to reconstitute and maintain a functional hematopoietic system over extended periods of time in vivo
>   - Extensive proliferative capacity
>   - Self-renewal capacity
>   - Pluripotency
>   - Quiescence
> - In vivo transplantation models are currently the only reliable assays of HSC activity.
> - Key features of progenitor cells are as follows:
>   - Inability to maintain long-term hematopoiesis in vivo
>   - Limited proliferative capacity
>   - Diminished or no self-renewal capacity
>   - Lineage commitment
>   - More actively cycling

site of hematopoiesis then shifts to the fetal liver from 6 to 22 weeks, and finally to the bone marrow, which becomes the predominant and lifelong site of blood cell production. Erythroid development during the yolk sac phase has been termed *primitive erythropoiesis*, whereas development during fetal liver and adult bone marrow stages is referred to as *definitive* or *adult erythropoiesis*. Primitive erythrocytes differ from definitive erythrocytes in a number of ways, but most notably in the expression of specific embryonic globin genes. There is some evidence that a distinct "primitive" stage of megakaryopoiesis also exists during yolk sac stages of embryogenesis, but further investigation is needed to confirm this.

The sequential development of hematopoietic sites led to the belief that the complete prenatal and postnatal blood system is ultimately generated from yolk sac–derived stem cells. However, subsequent experimental data indicate that definitive hematopoiesis arises from an independent intraembryonic source of stem cells. These HSCs develop during a brief developmental window at approximately 4 to 5 weeks of gestation in the vicinity of the developing aorta termed the *aorto-gonadal-mesonephros* (AGM) region. Several new studies in mice indicate that the HSCs develop directly from specialized "hemogenic" endothelial cells lining the ventral aspect of the dorsal aorta. HSCs also arise in the umbilical arteries and allantois at about the same time. It is believed that these HSCs then seed the developing fetal liver, where they expand and differentiate into committed progenitor cells. It is not clear whether AGM/umbilical artery–derived HSCs also directly seed the developing bone marrow or whether they first must reside in the fetal liver before seeding the bone marrow. Recently, a large transient pool of HSCs has also been identified in the placenta of mice around the time of AGM HSC development. It remains to be determined whether an equivalent population of HSCs exists in developing human placenta.

HSCs isolated from different locations (eg, bone marrow, fetal liver, placenta) and from organisms of different ages have been shown to have distinct gene expression patterns and other features. These differences may have implications regarding choice of stem sources for human transplantation therapies.

> **Key points**
> - Hematopoiesis develops in distinct waves during development.
> - Definitive HSCs first develop within the embryo in specialized regions of the dorsal aorta and umbilical arteries and then seed the fetal liver and bone marrow.
> - HSC characteristics differ based on their site of development and age of the organism.

Stem cell enrichment strategies

Attempts to purify stem cell populations have used a combination of approaches based on the physical and biologic properties of HSCs.

Physical properties

Early work on murine bone marrow revealed that the transplantable HSCs co-purified with lymphocytes and led to the idea that HSCs are morphologically indistinguishable from lymphocytes. Density gradient separation, such as Ficoll and Percoll gradient, are commonly used as a pre-enrichment step in stem cell purification protocols.

Biologic properties

As discussed earlier, progenitor cells cycle actively, whereas HSCs are relatively quiescent. This difference has been exploited in techniques for HSC enrichment in mouse systems. Treatment of mice with the antimetabolite agent fluorouracil markedly reduces progenitor cells, while relatively sparing populations enriched in HSC activity.

HSCs, but not later progenitor cells, express high levels of the verapamil-sensitive multidrug resistance membrane efflux pump (P-glycoprotein), which confers resistance to multiple chemotherapeutic agents. This pump also excludes certain fluorescent dyes such as rhodamine-123 or Hoechst-33342. Using these dyes in combination with flow cytometry, it has been possible to identify a population of hematopoietic cells with low dye retention (so-called *side population cells*). Although this population is enriched for HSCs, it nonetheless represents a heterogeneous mix and is not equivalent to pure HSCs.

Immunophenotype

Combinations of cell surface markers have been used to enrich for HSC populations. In mice, the immunophenotype of c-Kit$^+$, Thy-1$^+$, Lin$^-$ (a cocktail of surface markers found on mature cells of distinct lineages), and Sca-1$^+$ (so-called *KTLS cells*) enriches for cells with HSC activity. Flk2 expression can be used to distinguish LT-HSCs (Flk2$^-$) from short-term repopulating HSCs (ST-HSCs; Flk2$^+$).

Other protocols have used CD105 (endoglin) and the SLAM receptor CD150 as additional markers to enrich for LT-HSCs.

In humans, the most primitive stem cells are CD34$^+$/CD38$^-$, human leukocyte antigen (HLA)-DR$^{-/low}$, CD45 RA$^{-/low}$, CD71$^{-/low}$, and c-kit$^{-/low}$. Approximately 5% to 25% of CD34$^+$ cells also express low to moderate levels of Thy-1 antigen. As in the mouse, Thy-1 expression by human hematopoietic cells decreases with differentiation, and most lineage-restricted progenitors are CD34$^+$ Thy-1^{low} cells. The clinical transplantation potential of CD34$^+$ cells was first shown by engraftment of lethally irradiated baboons with autologous or allogeneic immunoaffinity-selected marrow cells. To date, several groups have shown human CD34$^+$ cells to contain stem cells capable of fully reconstituting the lymphohematopoietic system in humans after myeloablative chemotherapy and radiation therapy. However, recent studies suggest that some human stem cell activity can also be found in the CD34$^-$ population of cells.

Ex vivo expansion of HSCs

Due to the limited number of HSCs available from some sources, there has been great interest over the years to define conditions allowing ex vivo expansion of HSCs. Such systems require the ability to increase the number of HSCs without sacrificing any of the properties of HSCs, such as self-renewal, proliferative capacity, and pluripotency. Combinations of hematopoietic cytokines such as interleukin (IL) 11, SCF, Flt-ligand, and thrombopoietin, with or without stromal support cells, have led to modest expansion of HSCs in culture (~6-fold). Recently, a family of angiopoietin-like molecules has been shown to markedly expand bona fide HSCs cultured from mice. Whether similar findings will be applicable to human HSCs has yet to be determined.

The isolation of human embryonic stem cells and induced pluripotent stem cells has raised the possibility of in vitro differentiation of HSCs, including patient-specific HSCs. Unfortunately, this remains a significantly inefficient process using current techniques. Enforced expression of transcription factors such as HoxB4 and Cdx4 expands HSC populations. However, concerns about potential effects of transcription factor manipulation on transforming potential and/or long-term repopulating activity, even if induced transiently, may undermine the clinical utility of this approach in humans. This area remains an active field of research.

Key points

- HSCs can be enriched using their known biologic, physical, and immunophenotypic properties.
- The consensus human stem cell phenotype is CD34$^+$, CD38$^-$, Thy-1^{low}, HLA-DR$^{-/low}$, CD45 RA$^{-/low}$, CD71$^{-/low}$, c-kit$^{-/low}$, and rhodamine-123 dull.
- Limited ex vivo expansion of HSCs has been reported in experimental systems but is not at the stage of clinical utility as of yet.
- In vitro generation of HSCs from embryonic stem cells remains a very inefficient process.

Number of stem cells required for engraftment

Normal hematopoiesis in cats and humans is characterized by many simultaneously active stem cells, each contributing a small proportion of the blood cells present at any given time. In contrast, the hematopoietic system regenerated in animals that have undergone transplantation is, after an initial period of clonal disequilibrium, characterized by the contribution of a relatively few stem cells. Monoclonal hematopoiesis has also been documented in humans after allogeneic stem cell transplantation (SCT). However, experiments in which mice were injected with varying numbers of unseparated marrow cells or purified stem cells have shown that the number of clones contributing to hematopoiesis increases in proportion to the number of stem cells injected. Limiting numbers of repopulating stem cells in a graft may force such cells to exhibit a larger proliferative response than stem cells in a transplantation that exceeds minimal requirements. Although it may be possible to regenerate a functioning immunohematopoietic system after transplantation of relatively few stem cells, it is less likely that these cells are capable of sustaining hematopoiesis for the life span of the patient without periodic replacement. Therefore, although in clinical transplantation the adage appears to be "the more stem cells, the better," the practical questions are: "How many stem cells are enough?" and "How are such cells measured?" In practice, mobilization of stem cells can be monitored by the total number of nucleated cells, CFU-granulocyte macrophages (CFU-GMs), or CD34$^+$ cells to optimize harvesting time and achieve maximum yield. Successful engraftment in the clinical setting is predicted by a minimal dose of 2 to 5×10^5 CFU-GMs or 2×10^6 CD34$^+$ cells/kg of recipient body weight. Estimates of CD34$^+$ cells have been shown to correlate with CFU-GM numbers and have the significant advantage of providing an essentially immediate measure of the composition of a graft, which can be used to guide apheresis timing.

Key points

- CD34$^+$ cell counts correlate with CFU-GM numbers.
- In transplantation, CD34$^+$ cell counts can guide timing of apheresis for stem cell collection.
- Successful engraftment is predicted by a minimal CD34$^+$ dose of 2×10^6/kg of recipient body weight.

HSC transplantation (HSCT) is an accepted curative treatment modality for patients with selected malignant and nonmalignant diseases. Allogeneic and autologous HSCT have been used with great success in the management of diseases that otherwise were incurable. With the advent of improved supportive care, reduced-intensity conditioning regimens, and alternative sources of stem cells, the role of HSCT continues to evolve and to become more available to more patients in need.

Allogeneic transplantation

Stem cell sources

Bone marrow harvest was the original method for harvesting HSCs for clinical transplantation, but mobilized peripheral blood stem cells and umbilical cord blood cells are now commonly used. The term *hematopoietic stem cell transplantation* (HSCT), instead of the term *bone marrow transplantation* (BMT), is now more often used to encompass these various sources of stem cells. However, the basic goal of each of these methods is to replace host marrow cells (creating complete chimerism) or to supplement them (resulting in mixed chimerism). Donors can be related or unrelated and can be matched or mismatched at the major histocompatibility complex (MHC).

Histocompatibility and HLA typing

The MHC refers to the entire genetic region containing the genes encoding tissue antigens. In humans, the MHC region lies on the short arm of chromosome 6 and is designated the HLA region. The HLA region is a relatively large section of chromosome 6 with many genes, not all of which are involved in immune responses. The HLA region has been divided into class I, class II, and class III regions, each containing numerous gene loci that may encode a large number of polymorphic alleles. Antigens from class III are not thought to play a significant role in transplantation tolerance and are not used to identify donor/recipient pairs at this time.

Class I

Class I antigens are composed of 2 chains: a heavy chain containing the polymorphic region that combines with the nonpolymorphic light chain, β_2-microglobulin (from chromosome 15), to form the final molecule (Figure 12-1). The class I HLA antigens include HLA-A, -B, and -C antigens and are expressed on almost all cells of the body at varying densities. Other class I HLA antigens have also been identified, but these genes generally have quite restricted expression and uncertain functional significance.

Class II

Class II antigens are composed of 2 polymorphic chains: an α chain and a β chain (both encoded on chromosome 6; Figure 12-4). Both chains of class II antigens are encoded in the MHC. The class II antigens are further divided into DR, DQ, and DP antigens. Class II antigens are expressed on B cells and

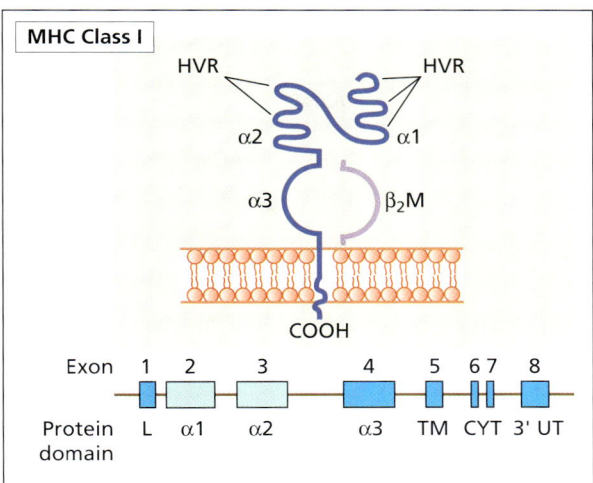

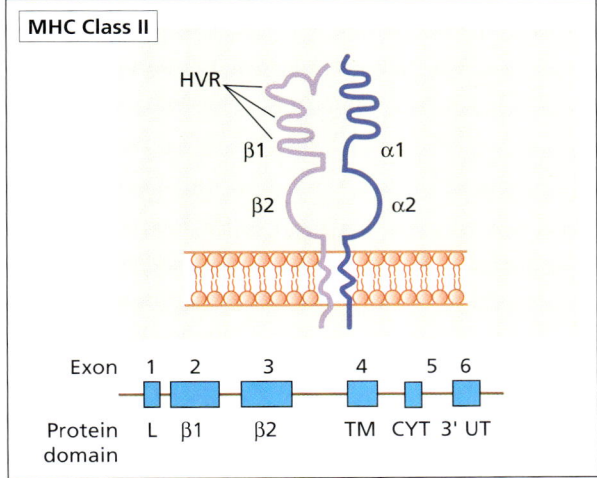

Figure 12-4 Molecular structure of human leukocyte antigen (HLA) class I and II antigens.

monocytes and can be induced on many other cell types following inflammation or injury. The DQ and DP antigens each have polymorphic α and β chains, which can dimerize in various combinations. DR dimers all share an essentially invariant α chain, whereas the β chain is extremely polymorphic.

Typing

HLA-A, -B, and -C antigens all have approximately equivalent importance in determining transplantation outcome. Matching of the DR β chain is also extremely important in determining transplantation outcome. The importance of matching in DQ and particularly in DP is less well established. (Until the late 1990s, HLA-C typing was not thought to be important, and routine typing was limited to HLA-A, -B, and -DR, hence the common terminology of 6/6 matching.)

Determination of HLA types has become much more accurate as typing has become molecularly based, replacing the earlier serologic or cellular techniques. The naming of antigens used in typing reflects the methodology used, resulting in confusing nomenclature and potential pitfalls for those reviewing HLA typing. All typing should be reviewed by an expert to ensure correct interpretation and accuracy. Seemingly disparate typing may in fact be identical, with the differences accounted for by the typing nomenclature or by previously large serologic groups being "split" into new groups by more refined typing. Optimal typing relies on molecular techniques such as polymerase chain reaction (PCR) amplification of the test DNA, followed by probing with labeled short sequence-specific oligonucleotide probes or, more recently, sequencing of the MHC class I and class II alleles. An increasing number of unique polymorphisms have been identified by molecular typing (Figure 12-5). By convention, differences recognized by serologic typing are called antigen mismatches, and differences recognized only by molecular techniques are called allele mismatches.

Inheritance of HLA antigens is determined by Mendelian genetics with coexpression of the maternal and paternal alleles; the likelihood of siblings sharing both HLA haplotypes (ie, a particular sequence of HLA-A, -B, -C, -DR, -DQ, and -DP on chromosome 6) is approximately 25%. Parents share one HLA haplotype with their offspring and are considered haploidentical. Within the United States, the current family size makes the identification of more than one HLA-identical sibling an uncommon event. However, the high degree of polymorphisms of each of the individual HLA alleles results in an enormous range of possible HLA recombination in the general population.

Certain HLA antigens commonly occur in association with one another, a phenomenon called *linkage disequilibrium*. This accounts for identification of certain haplotypes far more commonly than would be expected by chance alone. Also, certain haplotypes occur with high frequency within certain racial groups and are nearly absent in others. For example, Japan was isolated from much of the rest of the world until the 20th century. Because of their island location, the genetic diversity within Japan is much lower than in many other racial groups. But certain haplotypes that are common in Japan will be extremely rare in other ethnic groups. Contrasting with Japan is Africa, where there is a great deal more polymorphism than in other parts of the world. Even with equal numbers of donors available, patients of African descent will have greater difficulty finding an unrelated donor (Figure 12-6). In patients with mixed heritage, the mixing of the genetic material decreases the chances of identifying a donor.

Class I A, B, and C and class II DR antigens are the major determinants for risk of graft-versus-host disease (GVHD) and graft rejection. But even when a patient and donor are completely identical for HLA, there is a substantial risk of GVHD. The antigens responsible for GVHD in this setting have been called minor histocompatibility antigens. It

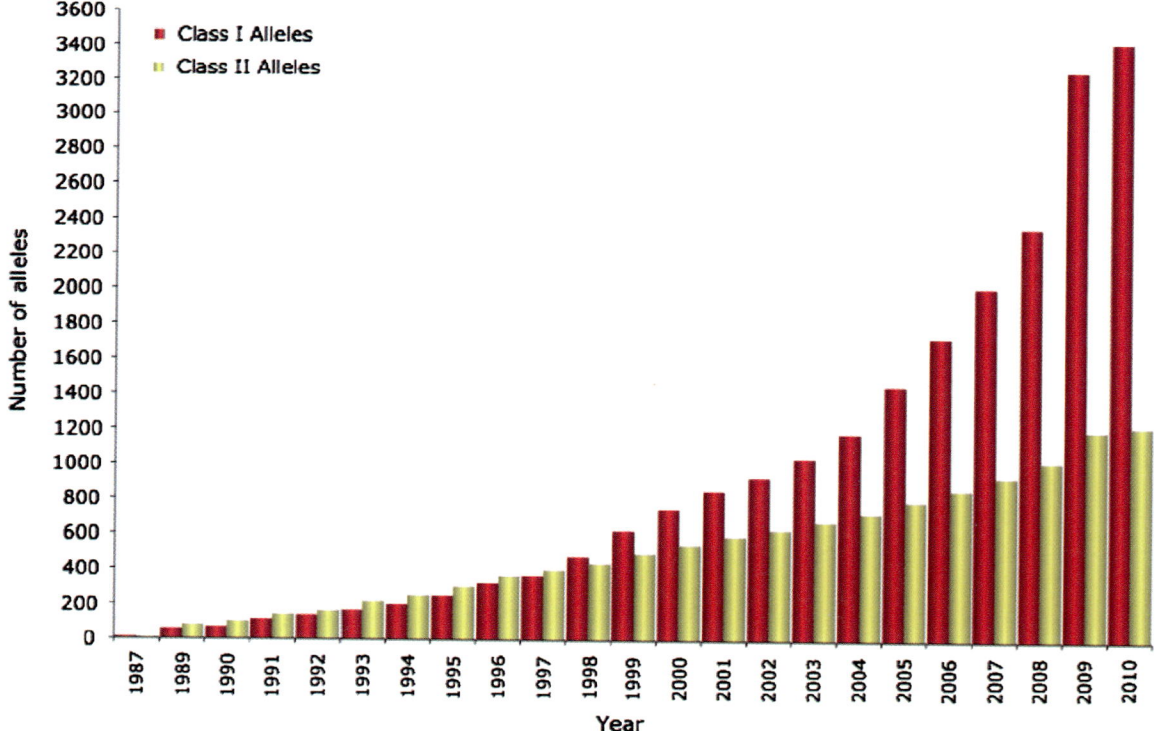

Figure 12-5 Number of class I and class II polymorphisms identified. Kindly provided by Professor Steven Marsh, Anthony Nolan Research Institute, London, United Kingdom (www.hla.alleles.org).

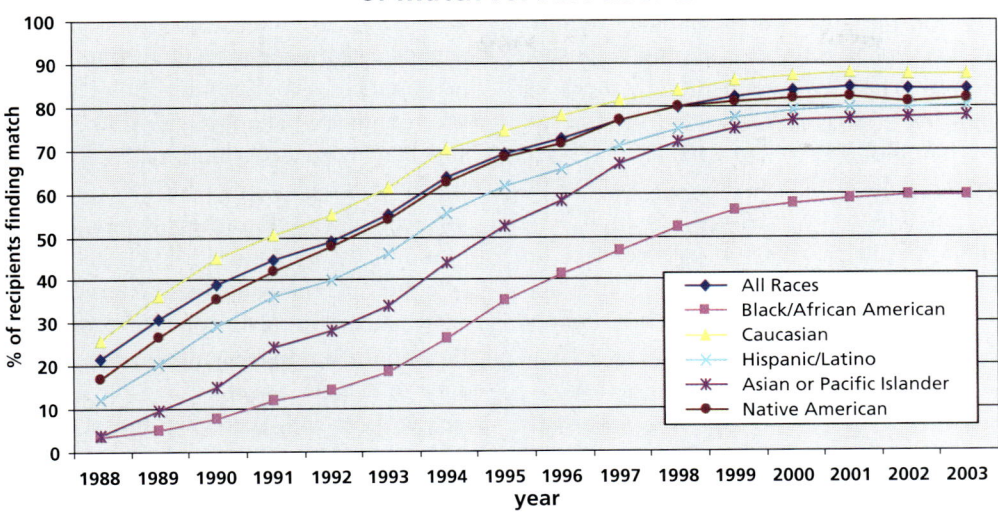

Figure 12-6 Likelihood of finding an unrelated adult donor. Used with permission from the National Marrow Donor Program.

appears that most minor antigens are a consequence of polymorphisms of endogenous proteins (ie, variants with subtle variations in the amino acid sequence) that distinguish the donor and recipient. Peptide products of the cellular metabolism of such proteins presented on the cell surface by HLA molecules are recognized by donor T lymphocytes and result in their activation. Although further elucidation of these minor antigens is a fascinating problem, they currently have minimal implications for donor selection because not all are known and few can be routinely identified. Minor histocompatibility antigens encoded for on the Y chromosome and absent in females explain the increased incidence of GVHD when a male recipient receives cells from a female donor. An HLA-identical unrelated donor is likely to have more differences in minor histocompatibility antigens with the recipient than an HLA-identical sibling. Therefore, there is a higher incidence of GVHD in patients receiving unrelated-donor transplantation, even when the donor is perfectly HLA identical. Syngeneic transplantation, that is, transplantation between identical twins, is a situation of complete matching in HLA and in minor histocompatibility antigens and therefore has a very low incidence of either GVHD or graft-versus-leukemia/lymphoma (GVL) effect.

Clinical case

A 15-year-old boy has recently relapsed with acute lymphoblastic leukemia (ALL) while still in the intensive part of his therapy and is referred with his parents to the nearest transplantation center to discuss treatment options. The patient has one sibling who is described as healthy. His mother has just learned that she is pregnant.

Graft-versus-tumor effects/donor leukocyte infusions

In contrast to autologous HSCT, which relies solely on chemotherapy and/or total-body irradiation to eradicate disease, allogeneic HSCT is associated with a graft-versus-tumor (GVT) effect mediated by alloreactive donor T and B cells. The importance of GVT was initially studied by comparing relapse rates between syngeneic and allogeneic transplantation recipients, by considering the relation between GVHD and relapse, and by examining the effect of T-cell depletion of the graft on risk of disease recurrence. Patients with acute myelogenous leukemia (AML) in first complete remission (CR1) and chronic myelogenous leukemia (CML) in chronic phase had an increased rate of recurrence after syngeneic transplantation. However, relapse rates after syngeneic transplantation for lymphoma or for ALL in CR1 are not increased compared with those after allogeneic transplantation. Definitive evidence for a GVT effect comes from the use of donor leukocyte infusions (DLIs). DLI confers a direct graft-versus-malignancy effect by infusion of alloreactive donor lymphocytes. Purposes of DLI include conversion of mixed donor chimerism to full donor chimerism after HSCT as preemptive therapy to prevent relapse or for the treatment of relapse. The use of DLI was first reported in 1990; 3 patients with relapsed CML achieved long-term remissions with the use of interferon and donor buffy coat cells. Since then, numerous reports using related and unrelated donors have confirmed the efficacy of DLI in reinducing remissions in patients with hematologic malignancies, with the highest responses observed in patients with CML. Disease status at the time of DLI and disease type (acute vs chronic leukemia) appear to be the most important predictors of response. The incidence of durable molecular remissions after DLI in CML patients with cytogenetic relapse approaches 70%. However, remission rates for CML patients with accelerated or blast phase are much lower, and responses are transient. In contrast to the notable positive response rates for early-phase CML relapse, DLI is much less successful for patients with relapsed acute leukemia and myelodysplastic syndromes (MDS). For patients with AML, the response rates range from 15% to 45%, but most of the responses are not durable. DLI has limited activity in ALL, and long-term responses in patients with relapsed ALL are uncommon. DLI for relapsed multiple myeloma after allogeneic HSCT has yielded response rates ranging from 30% to 50%. However, despite these moderate response rates, long-term survival has been the exception rather than the rule.

The application of DLI, however, is not without toxicity and carries a mortality rate of 3% to 10%, with acute GVHD and marrow aplasia being the leading causes of death. The incidence of both acute and chronic GVHD after DLI is approximately 40% to 60%, with more than half of the patients who develop chronic GVHD having extensive disease. The onset of acute GVHD typically occurs 32 to 42 days after DLI. The incidence of marrow aplasia has ranged from 18% to 50%, although sustained pancytopenia occurs in <5% of patients. Marrow aplasia is thought to occur when donor lymphocytes ablate recipient cells but donor hematopoietic cells are unable to maintain adequate hematopoiesis, especially when there is little or no donor-derived hematopoiesis at the time of DLI. Therefore, the use of DLI is cautioned in patients who relapse and have mostly recipient-type hematopoiesis.

Donor types
Related donors

Using strict Mendelian laws of inheritance, the likelihood that a sibling pair is HLA identical would be exactly 25%. Crossover phenomena during meiosis explain unusual cases of aberrant recombination of HLA antigens. For this reason, the chance that 2 siblings are HLA matched is slightly <25%. Parents usually are only haploidentical, but parental donors can be more closely matched with their offspring if by chance the parents share certain HLA alleles or even a complete haplotype.

Unrelated donors

For the majority of patients who lack a matched related donor, an HLA-identical unrelated donor usually represents the next best option. One of the major advances in unrelated SCT has been the establishment of donor marrow registries. Millions of potential donors have been HLA typed and are listed with national and international registries. The utility of these registries has been greatest for patients with common haplotypes where, because of linkage disequilibrium, the haplotype is found frequently within the registry. Thus, for patients with common HLA types, it is now possible to find donors on a routine basis. However, it is still difficult to find a donor for patients with infrequent haplotypes or for patients with very polymorphic HLA backgrounds such as African Americans.

Searching donor registries often requires a minimum of 3 to 4 months of search time because potential donors must be contacted and their willingness to serve as donors confirmed. Confirmatory typing must be performed, a mutually agreeable date for the transplantation must be selected, and the donor undergoes a history and physical examination. For many patients with aggressive disease, the time required to find the donor is prohibitive.

Outcomes of unrelated-donor transplantation are greatly influenced by the degree of donor matching. The continued refinement of molecular typing has resulted in more precise identification of the best donor, resulting in lower rates of GVHD and graft failure in patients highly matched to their donors. There is now agreement that outcomes are optimal when a donor and recipient are completely matched at the allele level (ie, as determined by molecular typing) in HLA-A, -B, -C, and -DR (8/8 molecular match). With each additional mismatch in A, B, C, or DR, the risks of transplantation increase, and few centers are willing to accept more than one antigen mismatch between an adult unrelated donor and recipient. The importance of matching for DQ and DP is less well established. Because of differences in minor histocompatibility antigens between donors and recipients, transplantation with unrelated donors is still associated with a higher incidence of GVHD and graft failure even when donor and recipient are perfectly matched.

Cord blood

Because of the inability to identify a fully matched related or unrelated donor in a timely fashion, additional sources of stem cells have been explored. It is estimated that only one third of patients in need of an unrelated donor will be able to find a match. Therefore, umbilical cord blood (UCB) cells harvested from the umbilical cord of newborns represent a rapidly growing source of HSCs. UCB contains hematopoietic progenitors capable of hematopoietic reconstitution, can be obtained within a short time span (available on average in 13.5 days in contrast to a matched unrelated donor search of 3–4 months), and demonstrates less allogeneic reactivity responsible for GVHD compared with marrow or peripheral blood grafts.

The initial UCB transplantations were performed in young children using HLA-identical siblings and resulted in rapid engraftment and a low incidence of GVHD. Mismatched related cord transplantations have a low incidence of GVHD as well, with 2- and 3-antigen mismatches well tolerated in children. Subsequently, unrelated donor cord blood was established as a source of stem cells with low rates of acute and chronic GVHD. As a result, both private and public cord banks have been established, allowing for the successful collection, typing, freezing, and dispensing of cord blood units. Because HLA mismatching between cord blood and recipients is better tolerated compared with marrow and peripheral blood grafts, there is a greater likelihood of finding a suitable donor for each patient.

The greatest limitations of UCB transplantation are the slow rate of engraftment, prolonged myelosuppression, and delayed immune reconstitution, which results in higher rates of death from infection; all of these limitations are related to the relatively low progenitor cell dose in cord blood. This low progenitor cell dose has hampered the ability to obtain rapid engraftment in patients >50 kg.

A number of trials have been performed to determine the feasibility of UCB transplantation for adults. In a review by Laughlin et al (2001) of 68 adult patients transplanted using UCB, the median weight of the recipients was 69.2 kg, and the median cell dose was 2.1×10^7 total nucleated cells/kg. Engraftment was slow, with a median time to neutrophil engraftment of 27 days (range, 13–59 days), and 10% of patients failed to engraft. A more recent analysis from the International Bone Marrow Transplant Registry (IBMTR) showed that the results with UCB transplantation were equivalent to those of mismatched unrelated donor transplantation but inferior to matched unrelated-donor transplantation. Attempts to speed engraftment have included the use of 2 cord products in a single patient, supplementation with $CD34^+$ selected cells from a related donor, and the use of ex vivo partially expanded UCB products.

Routine cord blood banking for newborns as a precaution for potential treatment of illness later in life is advertised by private companies. Currently, the American Academy of Pediatrics recommends that private banking be used only in families where there is an affected child of a disease known to be cured by allogeneic transplantation. Others should be encouraged to donate the cord blood to public banks.

Haploidentical-related donors

Haploidentical-related donors share one haplotype with the recipient, and their use is considered investigational. Parents are always haploidentical with their children, and siblings have a 50% chance of being haploidentical. It is estimated that approximately 90% of patients will have an available haploidentical donor.

The major challenges associated with haploidentical transplantation are the high rate of severe acute GVHD and delayed immune reconstitution. Strategies to ameliorate GVHD include T-cell depletion both through in vivo and ex vivo means, novel immunosuppressive combinations, and posttransplantation chemotherapy. Graft failure has been reduced with the use of large doses of stem cells and intensified conditioning regimens. Encouraging results have been reported, particularly in myeloid malignancies and in patients in remission at the time of HSCT.

> **Clinical case (continued)**
>
> Children and adolescents with ALL who relapse while receiving chemotherapy and, in particular, <18 months after obtaining a remission should be referred for SCT. This young man and his sibling and parents should undergo HLA typing. If his sister is not genotypically identical or a 7/8 match and his parents are not at least a 7/8 match, an unrelated donor search should be initiated as soon as possible. The length of subsequent remissions is generally shorter than previous ones. Therefore, delaying transplantation until his new sibling is born is not advised. You recommend proceeding to transplantation once a donor is identified and the leukemia is in remission. A haploidentical donor can be used if there is an ongoing trial and a delay in time to transplantation to locate an alternative donor is not acceptable.

Peripheral blood stem cells (PBSCs) predominate over bone marrow as the major source of stem cells. PBSCs result in more rapid engraftment (due to more committed progenitors being collected) and therefore less early complications. Recent trials have suggested that there may be a survival benefit for PBSCs, especially in adult patients with high-risk disease such as leukemia that is not in remission. For example, one relatively large study conducted at the Fred Hutchinson Cancer Research Center found that overall survival (OS) was modestly improved in patients receiving PBSCs (66%) compared with BMT (54%), potentially due to the slightly higher rates of acute GVHD (64% vs 57%) and chronic GVHD (46% vs 35%), resulting in a greater GVT effect. An analysis by Champlin et al (2000) of the IBMTR of 288 patients receiving PBSC transplantation compared with 536 patients receiving BMT demonstrated that both the transplantation-related mortality (TRM) and the relapse rates were lower for patients who received PBSCs for advanced leukemia (acute leukemia in second remission or CML in accelerated phase). However, the relative risk (1.66) of chronic GVHD is increased in patients receiving allogeneic PBSC transplantation; thus, there may be more late morbidity and mortality.

In a similar retrospective study of children of the IBMTR, poorer outcome was seen in all groups of patients receiving PBSC grafts. Prospective studies to evaluate this issue in children are urgently needed. In addition, in the pediatric population, the donor is frequently a minor, for whom the risks of G-CSF and leukapheresis (the smaller the size of the patient, the more technically difficult the collection due to the fluid shifts involved) must be weighed against the risk of a marrow harvest. A recent report found no major untoward events for the healthy sibling donors evaluated following PBSC mobilization. The Pediatric Bone Marrow Transplant Consortium is currently investigating the ability to decrease the time to engraftment of marrow grafts through the use of G-CSF mobilization prior to donor harvest.

In adult and pediatric patients receiving transplantations for nonmalignant conditions and/or where rapid engraftment is not a critical issue, bone marrow may be a superior source of stem cells due to the lower rates of acute and chronic GVHD.

Conditioning regimens

Prior to HSCT, recipients receive a course of intensive chemotherapy or combined chemotherapy and total-body irradiation (TBI; Table 12-1). The purpose of this conditioning regimen is usually 2-fold. First, it serves to suppress the host immune system, resulting in an inability for the host to reject the transplanted stem cells. The more immunosuppressive the conditioning regimen is, the better the chance for engraftment. The other purpose is to eradicate malignant cells. Many newer conditioning regimens are minimally myelosuppressive (ie, nonmyeloablative or reduced intensity) but remain immunosuppressive.

Myeloablative regimens

The first conditioning regimen that achieved widespread application consisted of the combination of cyclophosphamide and TBI (CyTBI). High doses of cyclophosphamide, typically 120 to 200 mg/kg (the higher doses are used more frequently in children) are combined with radiation in a dose of 8 to 12 Gy (depending on the fractionation). This regimen is considered myeloablative, meaning that without transfusion of donor cells, the patient would almost invariably die of marrow failure. It is also profoundly immunosuppressive. Graft rejection is slightly more common after unrelated donor transplantation compared with matched sibling donor transplantation. Disease relapse, however, remains the most common cause of treatment failure. More intensive variants of this conditioning regimen have been developed, none of which have been proven superior.

High-dose busulfan and cyclophosphamide (BuCy) conditioning was developed as an alternative to CyTBI. Several randomized studies and a meta-analysis have been conducted to compare BuCy with CyTBI. Both regimens are equally efficacious for treatment of AML and CML. For treatment of patients with ALL, TBI-containing regimens may be slightly superior. Treatment-related morbidity and mortality rates are also similar after both regimens, although the patterns of toxicity are slightly different. TBI is associated with more pulmonary toxicity, cataract formation, and thyroid dysfunction. BuCy is associated with a higher incidence of veno-occlusive disease (VOD) and irreversible alopecia. The long-term effects of TBI on development in very young children have resulted in an increased use of busulfan-based protocols over TBI when possible.

Table 12-1 Commonly used conditioning regimens.

Allogeneic stem cell transplantation	
Myeloablative conditioning	
CyTBI	Cyclophosphamide 120 mg/kg + TBI 8–12 Gy*
BuCy	Cyclophosphamide 120 mg/kg + busulfan 16 mg/kg PO or 12.8 mg/kg IV
Nonmyeloablative conditioning	
Flu TBI	Fludarabine + TBI 2 Gy
Flu Mel	Fludarabine + melphalan 140 mg/m^2
Flu Cy	Fludarabine + cyclophosphamide 60 mg/kg
Flu Bu	Fludarabine + busulfan 8 mg/kg PO
Cy ATG	Cyclophosphamide 4 gm/m^2 + ATG†
Predominantly autologous stem cell transplantation	
Lymphoma	
BEAM	BCNU + etoposide + cytarabine + melphalan
BEAC	BCNU + etoposide + cytarabine + cyclophosphamide
CBV	Cyclophosphamide + BCNU + etoposide
Myeloma	
High-dose melphalan	Melphalan 200 mg/m^2

*Various fractionation schedules in use.
†Mainly for conditioning in severe aplastic anemia.
ATG = antithymocyte globulin; BCNU = Carmustine; IV = intravenously; PO = per os; TBI = total-body irradiation.

Nonmyeloablative/reduced-intensity conditioning

Myeloablative conditioning regimens were long considered necessary for engraftment of allografts, but their considerable extramedullary toxicity typically limited their use to patients under the age of 50 to 60 years who had a good performance status and no comorbidities. The demonstration that engraftment can be achieved without myeloablation led to the investigation of so-called *nonmyeloablative* or *reduced-intensity conditioning* (RIC) regimens (also called minitransplantation regimens). These regimens often use lower doses of busulfan or TBI (typically 2 Gy) or reduced doses of cyclophosphamide, often combined with fludarabine, an immunosuppressive drug with limited extramedullary adverse effects. Nonmyeloablative regimens have more frequently been used in older patients and in patients with comorbidities. These regimens rely more heavily on immunologic (GVL) effects to induce tumor regression and contain lower doses of drugs with cytoreductive activity. GVHD and infections remain the major causes of nonrelapse mortality (NRM), so these transplantations should not be considered reduced risk.

The definitive role of RIC transplantation remains a matter of debate. There is relative agreement that it might be most useful in situations where patients are at high risk for toxicity from conventional conditioning. However, because this type of regimen confers little to moderate cytoreduction, patients must be in a minimal disease state prior to HSCT because the GVL effect requires a minimum of 2 to 3 months to confer a maximal immunotherapeutic effect.

Conditioning for benign hematologic disorders

Patients with aplastic anemia, metabolic disorders, or hemoglobinopathies represent a special category. There is no underlying malignancy that requires eradication. There is a higher risk of graft rejection, in part because of the nature of the underlying disease, the lack of previous immunosuppressive chemotherapy, and, in many cases, exposure to prior transfusions with HLA sensitization. The conditioning regimens for such patients have thus traditionally emphasized more immunosuppression and less myelosuppression. A combination of high-dose cyclophosphamide with antithymocyte globulin (ATG) has emerged as the standard conditioning regimen for aplastic anemia, although it may need modification in patients with underlying Fanconi syndrome (discussed later in this chapter).

Influence of genomic variation in allogeneic HSCT

Advances in DNA sequencing technology have enabled large-scale single nucleotide polymorphism (SNP) genotyping, which greatly facilitates detailed genetic analysis between patient and donor. Although information obtained from HLA typing helps predict the alloreactivity between donor–antihost response, recent reports have suggested that the genetic information obtained from SNPs may help identify individual susceptibility to transplantation-related toxicities. Polymorphisms in the innate immune genes (non-HLA) alter the inflammatory response and thus can affect the incidence of GVHD.

The nucleotide oligomerization domain 2 (*NOD2*) gene encodes a protein involved in the immune response to intracellular bacterial lipopolysaccharides, and polymorphisms within this gene may lead to a deregulated immune response contributing to the pathogenesis of acute GVHD. SNPs in the *NOD2* gene have been shown to have significant impact on treatment-related mortality, acute GVHD, and disease relapse in HLA-matched sibling pairs. Additionally, several cytokine gene polymorphisms have been studied in the context of HSCT especially related to IL-10 and tumor necrosis factor (TNF), both key components of the GVHD inflammatory response. One large study of nearly 1000 recipient–donor pairs found that the presence of an SNP in the promoter region of the recipient's IL-10 gene was significantly associated with severe acute GVHD and death. One weakness of this study, however, was the lack of understanding of the true biologic significance of the findings because IL-10 levels were not directly measured. The effects of polymorphisms have also been studied in drug metabolism genes, which can interfere with metabolism of agents used in conditioning regimens. In one particular study, polymorphisms in the candidate gene *CYP2B6* of the P450 cytochrome family caused interference with cyclophosphamide metabolism, resulting in worse oral mucositis, hemorrhagic cystitis, and VOD. Thus, these observations represent only a few of the clinical examples of the impact of genetic heterogeneity on the outcomes after HSCT. The variation in the human genome contributes to host–donor antigen disparity and provides functional polymorphisms leading to individual patient responses. Once the biologic and clinical implications of genetic polymorphisms are clearly elucidated, non-HLA genetic typing of potential donors may eventually allow optimization of donor selection and lead to more individualized patient treatment.

Complications of allogeneic transplantation (Table 12-2)

GVHD: features, risk factors, prophylaxis, and treatment

Acute and chronic GVHD traditionally were defined by the time of onset. Acute GVHD was defined as any GVHD occurring before day 100 after transplantation, and chronic GVHD was defined as any GVHD occurring after day 100. It is now recognized that typical features of chronic GVHD can occur

Table 12-2 Infections and complications in allogeneic transplantations.

Complication/infection	Aplasia	Day 100	Late (on immunosuppression)
Bacterial	Gram negative ——————————————————————————→		
	Gram positive ——————————————————————————→		
			Encapsulated organisms
Viral	Herpes simplex ————————————————————————→		
	RSV ——————————————————————————————————→		
	Adenovirus ——————————————————————————→		
		CMV ————————————————→	
		Varicella ————————————→	
	BK/JC ——————————————————————————————→		
Fungal	Candida		
	Aspergillus ——————————————————————————→		
Parasitic		*Pneumocystis jiroveci* ————→	
		Toxoplasma ——————————→	
VOD	VOD		
GVHD	Acute ——————————————————————————————→		
		Chronic ————————————→	
TM	TM →		

BK = virus; CMV = cytomegalovirus; GVHD = graft-versus-host disease; JC = virus; RSV = respiratory syncytial virus; TM = thrombotic microangiopathy; VOD = veno-occlusive disease.

before day 100 and that typical features of acute GVHD can occur after day 100. Acute and chronic GVHD are no longer defined by their time of onset but by their clinical features. Two subcategories of acute (classic and persistent/late onset or recurrent) and 2 subcategories of chronic GVHD (classic and overlap acute/chronic) are recognized.

Acute GVHD

Acute GVHD is characterized in its mildest forms by skin rash. As the disease worsens, the confluent rash may progress to blistering of the skin similar to a severe burn, profound diarrhea with crampy abdominal pain, and hepatic dysfunction with marked hyperbilirubinemia. Patients with acute GVHD lack, by definition, any diagnostic or distinctive features of chronic GVHD.

Acute GVHD is graded by the extent of skin rash, the amount of diarrhea, and the bilirubin elevation. There are several methods of grading GVHD, but all rely on the same features, and most continue to use the original Glucksberg criteria or the modified Keystone criteria. Patients with stage I disease have skin disease and a mild course. Those with stage II to IV disease have multiorgan disease, and patients with stage III or IV disease have a grave prognosis, with mortality rates >90%.

Acute GVHD was first considered a "pure" T-cell–mediated disease with cellular injury thought to be due to infiltration of T-effector cells into target tissues. However, recent immunohistochemical studies demonstrate that some infiltrating cells are natural killer (NK) cells rather than mature T cells. This observation has led many investigators to consider acute GVHD as a "cytokine storm." This model accounts for many of the observations made in GVHD. It proposes that damage to host tissues during chemotherapy and infection results in the release of inflammatory cytokines such as TNF and IL-1. These cytokines provoke increased MHC expression and upregulate other adhesion molecules that, in turn, amplify recognition of allogeneic minor HLA differences by T cells in the donor graft. The reactive donor T cells proliferate and secrete more cytokines that further activate additional donor T cells and other inflammatory cells, including macrophages induced to secrete more IL-1 and TNF. A powerful inflammatory response occurs that involves multiple cytokines recruiting more cells into the response and damaging more tissues. This cascade eventually produces the clinical manifestations of GVHD. Factors such as gut decontamination, sterile environment, intravenous immunoglobulin, lower dose preparative regimens, and ex vivo lymphocyte depletion of a marrow graft may decrease GVHD by interrupting this cascade. Of particular interest will be the further elucidation of the role of CD4$^+$ subpopulations in GVHD because in experimental models, the T-helper cell type 2 (T$_H$2) subpopulation that produces IL-4 and IL-10 (in contrast to T$_H$1 cells, which secrete IL-2 and interferon) inhibits GVHD. Recent data have shown that allogeneic PBSC transplantation is relatively enriched for the T$_H$2 population, which may account for the relatively moderate rate of acute GVHD seen after the large T-cell load given with the peripheral blood.

Prophylaxis of GVHD has been more successful than treatment. The most commonly used prophylaxis regimens use a calcineurin inhibitor (cyclosporine or tacrolimus) plus methotrexate. These regimens carry toxicity, with renal compromise from cyclosporine/tacrolimus and with significant mucositis from methotrexate-containing regimens. Sirolimus and mycophenolate mofetil are now commonly used as alternatives to methotrexate to decrease the toxicity of GVHD prophylaxis.

Other methods to prevent GVHD include depleting the graft of donor T cells either by an in vitro procedure after procurement of the stem cells or by exposure to T-cell–depleting antibodies such as ATG or alemtuzumab. These strategies result in a significant reduction in acute GVHD but can result in higher infection rates due to delayed immune reconstitution. Additionally, T-cell depletion compromises the graft-versus-malignancy effect and can potentially increase relapse rates.

Therapy for acute GVHD consists of high-dose steroids, typically 2 mg/kg/d, which are tapered upon obtaining a response. Calcineurin inhibitors will be continued or restarted. Patients not responding to or experiencing recurrence on high doses of steroids (considered steroid refractory) have a very poor prognosis from continued acute GVHD, infection, and chronic GVHD. Other agents added in the steroid-refractory setting include mycophenolate mofetil, pentostatin, ATG, and monoclonal antibodies such as infliximab, etanercept, and rituximab. However, the responses are low, and patients typically succumb to opportunistic infection in the setting of profound immunosuppression.

Chronic GVHD

Chronic GVHD affects from 40% to 80% of long-term survivors of allogeneic HSCT. Although chronic GVHD was once arbitrarily designated as any GVHD occurring after day 100, it is now recognized as a distinct disorder in which the manifestations often resemble those seen in spontaneously occurring autoimmune disorders. The diversity of the manifestations has proven a great hindrance to clinical study of chronic GVHD. A recent National Institutes of Health consensus conference produced working definitions for clinical and pathologic diagnosis, staging, and response criteria, as well as suggestions for supportive care, clinical trial design, and biomarkers.

Many of the features of acute GVHD can also be found in patients with chronic GVHD. But patients with chronic GVHD always have, in addition, other diagnostic or distinctive features. Diagnostic features of chronic GVHD are features that are sufficient to establish the diagnosis. They are summarized in Table 12-3. Diagnostic features of chronic GVHD typically involve the skin and mucosa. They include poikiloderma, lichen planus–like features, sclerotic features, and morphea-like features of the skin. Lichen-type features and hyperkeratotic plaques of the mouth are also diagnostic, as is vaginal scarring. Other diagnostic features of chronic GVHD are the development of an esophageal web and strictures, fasciitis, and joint contractures. Finally, bronchiolitis obliterans is a diagnostic feature of chronic GVHD if confirmed by biopsy.

Distinctive signs are also typical for chronic GVHD but are not by themselves considered sufficient for a diagnosis. They include depigmentation, nail loss, alopecia, xerostomia, and myositis. Features such as thrombocytopenia, eosinophilia, lymphopenia, hypo- or hypergammaglobulinemia, exocrine pancreatic insufficiency, myasthenia gravis, cardiac conduction abnormalities, and nephrotic syndrome can occur in chronic GVHD but are not sufficient for diagnosis.

Chronic GVHD used to be scored as limited or extensive based on the need for treatment. In the new proposal, chronic GVHD is classified as mild, moderate, or severe based on the number of organs involved and the extent of involvement within each organ.

The incidence of chronic GVHD is increasing due to the older age of patients being transplanted, the predominant use of PBSCs, and the use of mismatched and unrelated donors. The greatest risk factor for development of chronic GVHD is prior acute GVHD. Chronic GVHD has been poorly studied compared with acute GVHD because most patients have returned to their home institutions at the time this complication develops. These same factors have also hindered studies of the pathophysiology of this disorder. An additional problem has been the lack of a good animal model. There are 2 basic theories regarding the mechanism of chronic GVHD. Some believe that chronic GVHD is simply late allogeneic reactivity. That is, chronic GVHD represents old acute GVHD. Others believe that chronic GVHD may be poor/dysfunctional immunologic recovery akin to autologous GVHD (discussed elsewhere). This model may account for the marked similarities between chronic GVHD and spontaneously occurring human autoimmune disorders, especially scleroderma. This hypothesis has been supported by the demonstration of class II–specific T cells in humans and mice with chronic GVHD.

Therapy in patients with chronic GVHD has relied on steroids after a report by the Seattle transplantation group that steroids are more effective than steroids plus azathioprine. A study comparing cyclosporine plus prednisone therapy with prednisone was unable to show a benefit to combination therapy other than a steroid-sparing effect and less bone damage compared with the prednisone-alone group. Other therapies currently under evaluation include psoralen plus ultraviolet A, extracorporeal photopheresis, pentostatin, imatinib, and rituximab.

Table 12-3 Signs and symptoms of chronic graft-versus-host disease (GVHD).

Organ of site	Diagnostic (sufficient to establish the diagnosis of chronic GVHD)	Distinctive (seen in chronic GVHD, but insufficient alone to establish a diagnosis of chronic GVHD)	Other features*	Common (seen with both acute and chronic GVHD)
Skin	Poikiloderma Lichen planus-like features Sclerotic features Morphea-like features Lichen scleroses-like features	Depigmentation	Sweat impairment Ichthyosis Keratosis pilaris Hypopigmentation Hyperpigmentation	Erythema Maculopapular rash Pruritus
Nails		Dystrophy Longitudinal ridging, splitting, or brittle features Onycholysis Pterygium unguis Nail loss (usually symmetric; affects most nails)[†]		
Scalp and body hair		New onset of scarring or nonscarring scalp alopecia (after recovery from chemoradiotherapy) Scaling, papulosquamous lesions	Thinning scalp hair, typically patchy, scarce, or dull (not explained by endocrine or other causes) Premature gray hair	
Mouth	Lichen-type features Hyperkeratotic plaques Restriction of mouth opening from sclerosis	Xerostomia Mucocele Mucosal atrophy Pseudomembranes[†] Ulcers[†]		Gingivitis Mucositis Erythema Pain
Eyes		New onset dry, gritty, or painful eyes[†] Cicatricial conjunctivitis Keratoconjunctivitis sicca[†] Confluent areas of punctate keratopathy	Photophobia Periorbital hyperpigmentation Blepharitis (erythema of the eyelids with edema)	
Genitalia	Lichen planus-like features Vaginal scarring or stenosis	Erosions[†] Fissures[†] Ulcers[†]		
GI tract	Esophageal web Strictures or stenosis in the upper to mid third of the esophagus[†]		Excrine pancreatic insufficiency	Anorexia Nausea Vomiting Diarrhea Weight loss Failure to thrive (infants and children)

(Continued)

Table 12-3 Signs and symptoms of chronic graft-versus-host disease (GVHD) (continued).

Organ of site	Diagnostic (sufficient to establish the diagnosis of chronic GVHD)	Distinctive (seen in chronic GVHD, but insufficient alone to establish a diagnosis of chronic GVHD)	Other features*	Common (seen with both acute and chronic GVHD)
Liver				Total bilirubin, alkaline phosphatase >2 × upper limit of normal† ALT or AST >2 × upper limit of normal† BOOP
Lung	BO diagnosed with lung biopsy‡	BO diagnosed with PFTs and radiology†		
Muscles, fascia, joints	Fasciitis Joints stiffness or contractures secondary to sclerosis	Myositis or polymyositis†	Edema Muscle cramps Arthralgia or arthritis	
Hematopoietic and immune			Thrombocytopenia Eosinophilia Lymphopenia Hypo- or hypergammaglobulinemia Autoantibodies (AIHA and ITP)	
Other			Pericardial or pleural effusions Ascites Peripheral neuropathy Nephrotic syndrome Myasthenia gravis Cardiac conduction abnormality or cardiomyopathy	

*Can be acknowledged as part of the chronic GVHD symptomatology if the diagnosis is confirmed.
†In all cases, infection, drug effects, malignancy, or other causes must be excluded.
‡Diagnosis of chronic GVHD requires biopsy or radiology confirmation (or Schirmer test for eyes).
From Filipovich AH, Weisdorf D, Pavletic S, et al. National Institutes of Health consensus development project on criteria for clinical trials in chronic graft-versus-host disease: I. Diagnosis and staging working group report. Biol Blood Marrow Transplant. 2005;11:945–956.
AIHA = autoimmune hemolytic anemia; ALT = alanine aminotransferase; AST = aspartate aminotransferase; BO = bronchiolitis obliterans; BOOP = bronchiolitis obliterans organizing pneumonia; GI = gastrointestinal; ITP = idiopathic thrombocytopenic purpura; PFT = pulmonary function test.

The major cause of death in patients with chronic GVHD is infection from the profound immunodeficiency associated with chronic GVHD and its therapy. Careful monitoring with antibiotic prophylaxis for encapsulated organisms is warranted in all patients. Patients with frequent infections and low immunoglobulin levels may benefit from intravenous immunoglobulin replacement. Patients should remain on prophylaxis for viruses, *Pneumocystis jiroveci* pneumonia (formerly known *as Pneumocystis carinii*), and fungal infections (yeast and mold).

Graft failure

Graft failure is an unusual but often fatal complication of allogeneic HSCT. Mechanisms include immunologic rejection, abnormalities in the marrow microenvironment/

stroma, inadequate dose or composition of the graft, viral infections (in particular cytomegalovirus [CMV]), or drug-induced myelosuppression. It is often impossible to determine the exact cause of graft failure in an individual patient, but the risk for graft failure is increased with increasing disparity of the graft, with T-cell depletion of the graft, and in transplantation for certain diseases such as severe aplastic anemia or hemoglobinopathies. The risk for graft rejection can be decreased by infusing larger numbers of HSCs and by increasing the intensity of the conditioning regimen.

Infections

Infections are another major source of life-threatening complications in allogeneic HSCT. Their prevention, diagnosis, and treatment are important components of the care of the allogeneic HSCT patient. Major advances in this area have decreased TRM. Although this is an ever-changing field, the Centers for Disease Control and Prevention (CDC) recommendations published in 2000 provide a framework. Some modifications for the pediatric patient are required. We briefly discuss bacterial, parasitic, fungal, and viral infections.

Bacterial infections occur with high frequency during the neutropenic period after transplantation, and guidelines for their prevention and management are similar to those in other neutropenic patients. Many centers use prophylactic quinolone therapy for gut decontamination in patients older than 12 years of age during the neutropenic period. Their use in younger children is controversial secondary to older safety data in an animal model that restricted the use of quinolones in this age group. The American Academy of Pediatrics currently recommends that quinolones be limited in children to a number of circumstances that include gram-negative bacteremia in the immunocompromised host in which an oral agent is desired. As the experience with quinolones in young children grows, there is likely to be an analysis of their benefit in this age group. Patients with chronic GVHD are immunosuppressed by their therapy. They are at particular risk for fulminant infections with encapsulated gram-positive organisms, particularly *Pneumococcus*. They should receive prophylaxis with penicillin V potassium or trimethoprim-sulfamethoxazole.

Allogeneic transplantation patients are also at high risk for *P jiroveci*, and prophylaxis is recommended. For those allergic to trimethoprim-sulfamethoxazole, alternatives such as pentamidine or dapsone are routine. Trimethoprim-sulfamethoxazole prophylaxis may also prevent toxoplasmosis, which has occasionally been reported in recipients of allogeneic transplantation.

Fungal infections remain a major problem in allogeneic transplantation patients and are associated with prolonged neutropenia and also with immunosuppression and GVHD. Yeast (*Candida*) infections are rare with fluconazole prophylaxis. When such infections occur, they are frequently caused by fluconazole-resistant organisms. Airborne molds, particularly *Aspergillus*, remain a major hazard for patients undergoing allogeneic transplantation, despite the use of high-efficiency particulate air filtration. The azoles (voriconazole and posaconazole) and echinocandins (caspofungin, micafungin, and anidulafungin) with potent activity against molds have improved the outcome for such patients. Concerns with new azoles include their toxicity profile (neurologic and hepatic toxicity), which can be life threatening. Interactions with the metabolism of calcineurin inhibitors warrant the need for careful monitoring and often dose reduction of tacrolimus and cyclosporine. Also, as *Aspergillus* is treated more successfully, cases of mucormycosis are increasingly reported and necessitate treatment with amphotericin derivatives or posaconazole.

Viral infections are also common after allogeneic transplantation. The herpesvirus family and, in particular, CMV represent the major threat to transplantation patients. Herpesviruses are DNA viruses that are commonly acquired during childhood and adolescence and remain quiescent in the immunocompetent host because of immunosurveillance. Each of these viruses can reactivate after transplantation with serious and possibly fatal consequences. It is customary to test the donor and recipient for CMV, varicella-zoster virus (VZV), Epstein-Barr virus (EBV), and herpes simplex virus (HSV) by determining antibody levels prior to transplantation.

Approximately 80% of adult donors and recipients have been exposed to CMV, as indicated by positive antibody titers (although there are considerable variations in incidence depending on geographic region). Those who have been exposed (commonly called CMV$^+$) prior to transplantation are likely to experience virus reactivation in the first 100 days after transplantation. The incidence of reactivation ranges from 40% to 60% depending on the technology used for screening, the target tissue evaluated (eg, blood, urine, bronchoalveolar lavage [BAL]), the conditioning regimen, and the method of GVHD prophylaxis. Detection of CMV in the blood (CMV viremia), either by PCR or rapid antigen screening, indicates a high risk for CMV disease, usually CMV pneumonia but occasionally (especially at later time points after transplantation) CMV hepatitis, retinitis, or gastroenteritis. Patients who have not been exposed prior to transplantation (CMV$^-$) are still at risk for CMV infection either by transmission from a CMV$^+$ stem cell donor or via transfusion of blood products from a CMV$^+$ blood donor. To avoid risk of CMV infection in CMV$^{-/-}$ donor/recipient pairs, CMV$^-$ blood products were formerly recommended but are often not readily available. Fortunately, filtration of blood products efficiently reduces the risk of CMV transmission, and most centers no longer require use of CMV⁻ blood products.

Frequent screening for CMV viremia is mandatory in the first 3 months after transplantation including for CMV⁻ recipients (unless receiving CMV⁻ blood products). Ganciclovir, oral valganciclovir, high-dose acyclovir, or valacyclovir have all been used for prophylaxis of CMV reactivation in patients at high risk. Each of these approaches has potential problems including cost, inconvenience, and adverse effects. Myelosuppression, especially neutropenia, is the most serious and common toxicity associated with ganciclovir and valganciclovir. Maribavir, a member of a new class of drugs called benzimidazole ribosides, is currently under investigation and carries a much more favorable toxicity profile compared with ganciclovir and valganciclovir. It is an oral agent that does not induce myelosuppression or nephrotoxicity associated with the other anti-CMV agents. For patients who develop CMV viremia, preemptive treatment with ganciclovir or valganciclovir is immediately initiated. This strategy of preemptive treatment has significantly decreased the occurrence of CMV disease in the early months after transplantation. Oral valganciclovir (but not oral ganciclovir) is a convenient and effective oral alternative for preemptive and prophylactic treatment. Alternative medications for preemptive treatment include foscarnet (equally efficacious but more nephrotoxic) and cidofovir (requires only once-weekly administration but is less extensively tested and much more nephrotoxic and myelosuppressive). Acyclovir and valacyclovir, although moderately active for CMV prevention, have no role in preemptive treatment.

CMV disease tends to occur in the early months after transplantation and usually presents as interstitial pneumonia. This is a highly fatal disease that can be controlled only occasionally with a combination of antivirals such as ganciclovir and intravenous immunoglobulin. CMV disease can also occur late after transplantation in patients who are chronically immunosuppressed because of GVHD. Such patients may present with retinitis, hepatitis, or gastroenteritis. Guidelines for screening and treatment of late CMV disease are less well established. With the use of preemptive ganciclovir, the incidence of CMV disease after day 100 may increase because patients may not have developed an adequate T-cell response against the previously suppressed virus.

Other important herpesviruses include HSV, VZV, EBV, and human herpesvirus 6 (HHV-6). HSV used to be a major cause of mucositis and pneumonia occurring during the neutropenic phase after transplantation and is prevented by acyclovir. VZV can cause zoster, a frequent problem after transplantation with patients at risk for dissemination when profoundly immunosuppressed. In a single-institution double-blind controlled trial, patients after an allogeneic transplantation who were at risk for VZV reactivation were randomized to acyclovir 800 mg twice daily or placebo given from 1 to 2 months until 1 year after transplantation. Acyclovir significantly reduced VZV infections at 1 year after transplantation (hazard ratio, 0.16; $P = .006$). EBV can cause posttransplantation lymphoproliferative disease, particularly in patients who are extremely immunosuppressed because of mismatched or T-cell–depleted transplantation. Treatment with rituximab is typically first-line therapy. HHV-6 is a cause of posttransplantation encephalitis and aplasia. Others have postulated a link with interstitial pneumonia.

The exact roles of other viruses are not as well defined. Adenovirus has been the cause of fatal hepatitis, gastroenteritis, and pneumonitis in transplantation patients. The epidemiology and value of screening remains a matter of ongoing study. There is no established treatment; however, there is a growing experience in some transplantation centers with antivirals such as cidofovir. Respiratory viruses such as respiratory syncytial virus (RSV) and influenza can lead to fatal pneumonias. Some centers have recommended screening of all patients during RSV season and treatment with ribavirin and immunoglobulin in patients who become infected. This is, however, a very controversial issue. BK virus and adenovirus have been associated with severe hemorrhagic cystitis. The frequency of infection, treatment, and value of screening are not determined. Finally, JK virus is a rare cause of encephalitis.

Because there is evidence for loss of immunity against common childhood infections, revaccination is routinely recommended after HSCT.

VOD/sinusoidal obstruction syndrome

> **Clinical case**
>
> A 16-year-old girl from New Jersey with AML in third complete remission is admitted to the transplantation unit for an allogeneic transplantation from an unrelated donor. The patient has been heavily treated and transfused prior to transplantation, with a liver function test 3 times normal on admission. Her transplantation is complicated by a busulfan level that is near the high range of the target dose. She starts to develop a distended abdomen on day 4 and 5% weight gain with increasing right upper quadrant pain. Her total bilirubin on day 4 is 4 mg/dL. An abdominal ultrasound and Doppler studies show ascites, hepatomegaly, and reversal of flow through the portal system.

VOD/sinusoidal obstruction syndrome (SOS) is one of the most common and lethal toxicities of SCT; it occurs in 10% to 60% of patients receiving transplantations, depending on both the risk factors for the patients and the vigor with which the diagnosis is pursued. VOD is caused by preparative regimen toxicity and is thought to be caused by damage to endothelial cells, sinusoids, and hepatocytes in the area surrounding terminal hepatic venules. Endothelial cells are directly sensitive to chemotherapy and radiation therapy, and cytokines released during endothelial injury may also be implicated. For instance, elevated levels of TNFα predict development of VOD.

There are several risk factors for the development of VOD. VOD is more common in patients with evidence of prior hepatocellular damage at the time of transplantation, heavy pretreatment prior to SCT, prolonged and elevated busulfan levels, and/or >10 to 12 Gy TBI. Other drugs such as nitrosoureas (carmustine) have also been implicated in VOD/SOS. Studies suggest that prior exposure to gemtuzumab significantly increases the risk of VOD, especially in those who receive the drug shortly before the transplantation. Patients entering SCT with significantly impaired hepatic function from hepatitis also have a higher rate of VOD.

Most centers now define a clinical diagnosis of VOD with the following triad: weight gain and/or ascites, tender hepatomegaly, and jaundice. Ideally, the diagnosis should be confirmed by liver biopsy, but liver biopsy is not always possible because of the risks in critically ill patients. VOD tends to occur 8 to 10 days after the start of the preparative regimen and has a worse prognosis the earlier the presentation.

> **Clinical case (continued)**
>
> Based on these radiographic findings, the patient in this case is felt to have VOD. The patient develops worsening ascites and renal failure. This is a classic case of VOD—a heavily pretreated patient with abnormal liver function entering transplantation. The early onset, tender hepatomegaly, weight gain, radiographic findings, and rapid decline clinically are consistent with severe disease. Her platelets become difficult to support, and she develops worsening respiratory disease resulting in the need for mechanical ventilation. She experiences a pulmonary hemorrhage and care is withdrawn.

Until recently, the treatment of VOD has been largely supportive. Several studies have evaluated the use of recombinant tissue-type plasminogen activator (tPA) and heparin in the treatment of VOD. In general, a response rate of approximately 30% to 40% was seen in association with a significant risk of hemorrhage. Studies using defibrotide, a polydeoxyribonucleotide, have shown encouraging response rates. Defibrotide is an adenosine receptor agonist that increases levels of endogenous prostaglandins (PGI_2 and PGE_2), reduces levels of leukotriene B_4, stimulates expression of thrombomodulin in endothelial cells, modulates platelet activity, and stimulates fibrinolysis by increasing endogenous tPA function and decreasing the activity of plasminogen activator inhibitor 1 (PAI-1). Defibrotide has little systemic anticoagulant activity, which is an advantage in patients with multiorgan failure. In the latest published update, 88 patients with severe VOD were treated with defibrotide. At treatment, median bilirubin was 12.6 mg/dL, and multiorgan failure was present in 97%. No severe hemorrhage or other serious toxicity was reported. Complete resolution of VOD was seen in 36%. Younger patients, those receiving autologous SCT, and those with abnormal portal flow had the highest response rates. Defibrotide is not approved by the US Food and Drug Administration (FDA), although the results of a recently completed phase III trial are eagerly awaited. Low-dose heparin and ursodiol have been used for prevention of VOD/SOS but remain controversial.

Cardiac and pulmonary toxicity

Pulmonary complications occur frequently after HSCT and are associated with a high mortality. In an attempt to stratify transplantation patients into different risk categories, pretransplantation evaluation often includes a detailed pulmonary function test (PFT) and two-dimensional echocardiogram or radionuclide ventriculography. The utility of these tests, however, is doubtful. In a retrospective study from the Fred Hutchinson Cancer Research Center that included 1297 patients, decreased diffusing capacity of the lung for carbon monoxide and elevated alveolar-arterial partial pressure of oxygen were predictors for increased mortality. However, most transplantation centers will not exclude a patient from transplantation based solely on an abnormal pre-SCT PFT. Similarly, baseline reduced left ventricular ejection fraction predicted for cardiac toxicity after HSCT but failed to predict life-threatening events.

During the early posttransplantation period (days 0–30), regimen-related toxicity and infectious etiologies account for most of the pulmonary events. Although most focal infiltrates are infectious in origin, diffuse infiltrates related to regimen-related toxicity should also be considered. The differential diagnosis of diffuse infiltrates during early post-SCT includes iatrogenic fluid overload, pulmonary edema (cardiogenic and noncardiogenic), idiopathic pneumonia syndrome (IPS), adult respiratory distress syndrome from chemoradiotherapy injury or sepsis, and diffuse alveolar hemorrhage (DAH). Cardiogenic pulmonary edema and septicemia in particular need to be excluded. After engraftment, the risk of fungal/viral infection increases. Historically, CMV pneumonitis was the most common cause of diffuse infiltrates during days 30 to 150, but its incidence has dramatically decreased with the use of preemptive treatment strategies for prevention of CMV disease. During this period, opportunistic and idiopathic pneumonias dominate the pulmonary complications. It takes approximately 3 to 6 months for the immune function of patients undergoing HSCT to return to normal and longer for patients who suffer from chronic GVHD. Infectious etiologies during this phase include bacteria, fungi, viruses, *Nocardia*, mycobacteria, and *P jiroveci*. Furthermore, approximately 10% of patients with chronic GVHD develop bronchiolitis obliterans, a severe obstructive airflow disease.

Idiopathic pneumonia syndrome

IPS is a condition characterized by diffuse alveolar injury with fever, cough, dyspnea, hypoxemia, and restrictive physiology. Chest x-ray usually demonstrates multilobar pulmonary infiltrates. This is a diagnosis of exclusion. BAL must be negative for infectious etiologies including bacteria, fungi, CMV, and other viral infections. The incidence of IPS is approximately 7%, with a median time to onset of 21 days and hospital mortality of >70%. The risk factors for IPS include the use of TBI or carmustine-based conditioning regimens and previous exposure to bleomycin. Treatment of IPS is mostly supportive, but high-dose steroids are often given. They may be beneficial in patients in whom pulmonary damage is due to carmustine or in those with the closely related syndrome of DAH.

Diffuse alveolar hemorrhage

DAH occurs most commonly in the first weeks after SCT and presents as idiopathic pneumonia with or without hemoptysis. The classic finding on BAL is increasingly bloody returns during BAL washings. Analysis of BAL fluid usually demonstrates red blood cells, hemosiderin-laden macrophages if blood has been present for more than 2 to 3 days, and negative microbiologic studies. Treatment of DAH is largely supportive, but retrospective studies suggest that high-dose steroids with a starting dose in the range of 1 g/d are often beneficial.

Transplantation-related obstructive airway disease

Approximately 6% to 10% patients with chronic GVHD develop chronic airway obstruction. The most common histologic finding is constrictive bronchiolitis obliterans. Bronchiolitis obliterans typically presents 3 to 12 months after an allogeneic SCT with gradual onset of dyspnea, dry cough associated with occasional wheezing, and inspiratory crackles. PFTs demonstrate an obstructive pattern that does not respond to bronchodilator therapy and reduced diffusing capacity of the lung for carbon monoxide. Thin-section computed tomography scans reveal bronchial dilation, mosaic pattern attenuation, and evidence of air trapping on expiration. The diagnosis is often based on clinical, imaging, and spirometric findings without a tissue biopsy. There is no effective treatment of patients with bronchiolitis obliterans, and current treatment is mostly directed at the underlying chronic GVHD with immunosuppressive therapy. Lung transplantation offers some promise.

Thrombotic microangiopathy

Posttransplantation thrombotic microangiopathy (TMA) presents as a spectrum of disease ranging from mild microangiopathic anemia to thrombocytopenic purpura (TTP) or hemolytic uremic syndrome and occurs more commonly after allogeneic and unrelated donor SCT. TTP frequently presents with fever, neurologic symptoms, microangiopathic hemolytic anemia, thrombocytopenia, and renal impairment. In children, TMA more closely resembles hemolytic uremic syndrome. In some patients, TMA appears to be related to cyclosporine nephrotoxicity and responds to discontinuing the cyclosporine. But other patients have a fulminant course and a very high mortality rate. Autopsy findings include arteriolar thrombosis in the kidneys. In many patients, fungal infection, sepsis, and/or severe acute GVHD appear to be underlying the microangiopathic processes. Unlike patients with idiopathic TTP, patients with transplantation-related TTP do not respond to plasma exchange. TTP outside the transplantation setting has been associated with immunoglobulin G (IgG) antibodies that inhibit the cleaving protease of von Willebrand factor in the plasma. No such mechanism was found in cases of posttransplantation TTP, pointing to another as yet unidentified cause for this syndrome.

Bleeding

Although all patients with thrombocytopenia are at risk for bleeding, there are several hemorrhagic syndromes that are peculiar to transplantation. Hemorrhagic cystitis early after transplantation is usually attributed to toxicity to the bladder from cyclophosphamide metabolites. Late-onset hemorrhagic cystitis is often associated with viral infection with BK virus and occasionally with adenovirus. Hemorrhagic cystitis can be severe and can require continuous bladder irrigation, diverting nephrostomy tubes, and occasionally formalin instillation until the bladder heals. As mentioned previously, pulmonary hemorrhage can be a serious complication of transplantation and is most often attributed to preparative regimen toxicity.

Iron overload

Iron overload has been identified to be an adverse prognostic factor for children with thalassemia undergoing HSCT, and there is an increasing evidence that iron overload also may have deleterious effects for patients with hematologic malignancies who undergo HSCT. This particular patient population often is heavily transfused prior to HSCT and continues to require transfusions in the peritransplantation period. One red blood cell unit contains 200 to 250 mg of iron, and significant iron accumulation can occur after 10 to 20 red blood cell transfusions. Iron overload increases the risk of infections, VOD, and hepatic dysfunction. Although the serum ferritin level is commonly used to estimate body iron stores, it is not specific enough to accurately assess body iron burden and can be elevated from infectious and inflammatory conditions. However, serum ferritin may serve as an initial screening test. Liver biopsy with estimation of liver iron concentration (LIC) is considered the most accurate method to measure hepatic iron. Hepatic magnetic resonance imaging is a less invasive method to measure LIC and has been shown to be a reproducible, sensitive, and specific method. A retrospective study of 590 patients from the Dana-Farber Cancer Institute found that an elevated pretransplantation serum ferritin level was an adverse risk factor for OS and disease-free survival (DFS) for patients with MDS and AML. The inferior survival rates were attributed to a significant increase in NRM with a trend toward an increased risk of VOD. There are no published guidelines on the management of iron overload in HSCT patients, but phlebotomy or iron chelation therapy should be considered in HSCT patients with an LIC of >7 mg/g or in patients with iron-related hepatic or cardiac dysfunction. The natural history of post-HSCT iron overload has not been extensively studied and further investigation is warranted.

Key points

- Current sources of HSCs include matched sibling donors, unrelated donors, UCB, and related haploidentical donors.
- Choice of the stem cell source depends on the disease, disease status, prior treatment, patient age, patient size, frequency of HLA type, and comorbid medical conditions.
- Nonmyeloablative preparative regimens are increasingly being offered, particularly in diseases with a demonstrated GVT effect and older patients.
- The results of unrelated donor transplantation have improved due to more refined HLA typing. HLA typing should be reviewed by an expert.
- The outcome of transplantation is determined to a large extent by the prevention and treatment of complications such as GVHD, infections, and VOD/SOS.
- Acute and chronic GVHD are currently defined by their clinical and pathologic features, not by their time of occurrence.
- The long-term care of the transplantation survivor requires the careful evaluation of the patient over time with at least an annual follow-up visit.

Syngeneic transplantation: syngeneic autologous GVHD

Syngeneic transplantation (ie, transplantation between identical twins) provides a unique opportunity to evaluate the clinical effects of GVL in allogeneic transplantation and the role of graft contamination in autologous transplantation. The donor and recipient are genetically identical; therefore, GVHD occurring through mismatching for major or minor histocompatibility antigens is thought not to occur. The rare cases of GVHD after syngeneic transplantation have occurred more frequently when the donors were parous females and may be due to passenger fetal lymphocytes remaining from prior pregnancies. Still, these are unusual cases, and one can consider a syngeneic transplantation the equivalent of an allogeneic transplantation without GVHD or GVL. When such transplantations are used for CML or AML, relapse rates tend to be considerably higher than after allogeneic transplantation. This observation has long served as a strong argument for the importance of GVL effects in allogeneic transplantation. By contrast, when outcomes in ALL or lymphoma were compared, no excess risk of disease recurrence was documented. This observation does not rule out the existence of GVL effects in lymphoma or ALL but suggests that the GVL effect may be outweighed by the risks of GVHD and the need for immunosuppressive agents.

Syngeneic transplantation can also be considered the equivalent of an autologous transplantation in which the graft is not contaminated with lymphoma cells. In this regard, it is of interest that in lymphoma patients, the risk of relapse after syngeneic transplantation is much lower than that after autologous transplantation.

Autologous GVHD is a phenomenon that is observed in approximately 5% of autologous transplantation recipients and is clinically indistinguishable from acute GVHD. A number of models for its development have been proposed. It may be related to microchimerism from residual fetal cells, a hypothesis supported by a higher rate of occurrence in females. An alternative hypothesis is self-recognition of the CLIP molecule in the MHC molecule, resulting in recognition of self and GVHD. This hypothesis is currently being tested in an autologous transplantation setting in the Children's Oncology Group in patients with relapsed Hodgkin disease.

Autologous transplantation
HSC collection and manipulation

Autologous transplantation was developed as a salvage treatment for patients diagnosed with hematologic malignancies with primary refractory disease after frontline treatments or with relapsed disease after initially obtaining a complete remission or as frontline therapy in disorders such as multiple myeloma. The dose escalation of chemotherapeutic agents made possible by use of HSC rescue allows for eradication of microscopic residual disease that contributes to relapse after conventional treatment. Initially developed in the 1980s, the complication rates of autologous transplantation have declined precipitously, and NRM now ranges from 0% to 3%. The decreased early NRM is likely due to multiple factors, including better patient selection, improved supportive care, hematopoietic growth factors, and use of PBSCs as the stem cell source.

Peripheral blood progenitor cells have almost completely replaced bone marrow as the HSC source for patients undergoing autologous HSCT because of the less invasive collection method and more rapid blood count recovery. Under steady-state conditions, most HSCs reside in the marrow, and various strategies have been developed to mobilize them. This includes single-agent cytokine, cytokine combinations, and combinations of chemotherapy with cytokines followed by leukapheresis. HSC concentration in the blood stream usually peaks 4 to 6 days after initiation of therapy with cytokines alone. When chemotherapy with cytokines is given, maximum recovery of stem cells in the blood occurs at the time of marrow recovery. Collection is usually initiated when the white blood cell (WBC) count recovers to >1 to 5×10^9L WBC/L. In an attempt to improve the accuracy and efficacy of stem cell collections, daily measurement of peripheral blood $CD34^+$ content has been used, and many centers initiate HSC collection when $CD34^+$ cell count exceeds 5 to 10 cells/mL.

Historically, the number of mononuclear cells per kilogram and/or granulocyte-macrophage CFUs per kilogram was used to predict the quality of the graft and engraftment kinetics. Currently, most transplantation centers use peripheral blood CD34 counts as surrogate markers for rapid and sustained engraftment. A minimum of 1×10^6 is considered necessary, and ideally at least 3×10^6 $CD34^+$ cells/kg body weight are collected. So far, no single mobilization regimen has been shown to be superior. In general, mobilization with a combination of chemotherapy and cytokines achieves a better yield of $CD34^+$ cells when compared with cytokine mobilization alone, but this fails to translate into a shorter time to engraftment.

Despite the use of chemotherapy–cytokine combination regimens, mobilization failure still occurs in some patients. Prior treatment is the single most important factor affecting stem cells yields. Prior treatment with stem cell toxins, short interval since last chemotherapy, previous radiation, hypocellular marrow, malignancies involving the bone marrow, and refractory disease have been associated with poor mobilization. This underscores the importance of referring a potential transplantation candidate early for transplantation evaluation before repeated salvage attempts that may adversely affect stem cell collections.

A novel chemokine, plerixafor (Mozobil; Genzyme, Cambridge, MA), was approved in 2009 as a mobilization agent in combination with G-CSF. Plerixafor, formerly known as AMD3100, a bicyclam derivative, is a specific antagonist of CXCR4, a coreceptor for the entry of human immunodeficiency virus (HIV) into host cells, and was initially developed as a potential therapeutic agent for HIV. In a phase I study, it induced modest leukocytosis when administered intravenously to HIV-1–infected patients. Based on this observation, plerixafor was tested for its ability to mobilize $CD34^+$ and hematopoietic progenitor cells from marrow to peripheral blood. In a pilot study that included patients with myeloma or lymphoma, plerixafor caused a rapid and statistically significant increase in the total WBC and peripheral blood $CD34^+$ counts at 4 and 6 hours after a single injection. The results of 2 phase III randomized studies, one involving lymphoma patients and the other for myeloma patients, were recently reported. Patients were randomized to receive G-CSF alone or G-CSF in combination with plerixafor. The primary end point was the percentage of patients who collected $\geq 6 \times 10^6$ $CD34^+$ cells/kg. In both studies, there was a significantly higher proportion of patients in the G-CSF plus plerixafor arm who reached the primary end point compared with the G-CSF–alone arm. Plerixafor was a well-tolerated agent, and the most common adverse events were gastrointestinal disorders and injection site reactions. These results led to FDA approval of this agent in 2009.

One of the major disadvantages of autologous SCT is the potential contamination of the graft by the tumor cells. Tumor cell contamination is associated with disease recurrence, particularly in autologous transplantation for lymphoma. To decrease the risk of contamination of the graft, various "purging" techniques have been explored, including pharmacologic and immunologic methods. Multiple autologous transplantation series including patients with acute leukemia and non-Hodgkin lymphoma (NHL) have suggested potential benefits of purging, but results are not conclusive. Relapse after autologous SCT usually occurs at sites of prior bulky disease, which then questions the benefit of purging. In vivo purging with chemoimmunotherapy before stem cell collection is also used, which may improve the quality of the collection with less contamination. Examples include using rituximab-containing chemotherapy mobilization and high-dose cytarabine mobilization regimens for patients with B-cell lymphoma and AML, respectively.

Alternatively, many centers have used methods to enrich for HSCs (a process called positive selection). Currently, the most common method is the use of $CD34^+$ selection of the product prior to cryopreservation. The advantage of this system is the lack of a need for a different purging agent for each disease type. However, immune reconstitution following the transplantation is delayed. As with purging, CD34$^+$ selection continues to be performed but is of unproven benefit.

Conditioning regimens for autologous transplantation

The rationale for high-dose cytotoxic chemotherapy stems from the steep dose–response curve of alkylating agents and radiotherapy and tumor cell response in human tumors. Doubling the dose of alkylating agents increases tumor cell kill by a log or more, and increasing the dose of alkylating agents by 5- to 10-fold overcomes the resistance of tumor cells against lower doses. High-dose chemotherapy also aims to destroy the tumor cells in an expediently timely manner to prevent the emergence of resistant clones. In 1978, investigators from the National Cancer Institute were the first to report the use of high-dose chemotherapy followed by autologous BMT for patients with relapsed lymphoma. These encouraging results were the initial clinical evidence that led to the widespread application of autologous HSCT.

Commonly used regimens are often based on regimens initially developed for allogeneic transplantation. Such regimens include high-dose busulfan for acute leukemia. Other regimens are used nearly exclusively for autologous transplantation; they include carmustine-based regimens such as carmustine, etoposide, cytarabine, and melphalan or cyclophosphamide, carmustine, and etoposide for large-cell lymphoma; the high-dose melphalan regimens used for myeloma; and the ifosfamide, etoposide, and carboplatin (ICE) regimens for lymphoma and germ cell tumors (GCTs).

Complications of autologous transplantation

Some of the complications of autologous transplantation, including infections and regimen-related complications, are similar to those occurring after allogeneic transplantation (Table 12-4). Patients are not required to take immunosuppressive medications to maintain their grafts, and if there has not been a large amount of manipulation of the cells, immune recovery is much more rapid than in the allogeneic setting. CMV infections are rare, and there is no role for routine CMV screening. *Aspergillus* infections are also distinctly less common after autologous transplantation. Prophylaxis with quinolone antibiotics, an antifungal with activity against yeast such as fluconazole, and acyclovir (for HSV and VZV prophylaxis) is recommended. Many centers also recommend routine prophylaxis for *P jiroveci*. Because there is evidence for loss of immunity against common childhood infections, revaccination is recommended by the CDC.

Conditioning-related complications such as VOD/SOS can occur after autologous transplantation. Their incidence is lower than after allogeneic transplantation, possibly because patients undergoing autologous transplantation tend to be less heavily pretreated or because of the absence of agents used for GVHD prophylaxis. Carmustine-based conditioning can be associated with pulmonary (interstitial pneumonitis) and hepatic toxicity.

> **Key points**
>
> - PBSCs are the most commonly used stem cell course in adults.
> - NRM ranges from 1% to 3% for autologous HSCT.
> - HSCs can be collected after mobilization with cytokines or a combination of chemotherapy and cytokines.
> - There is no definitive evidence that ex vivo purging of autologous stem cell grafts affects relapse rates or outcomes.
> - Treatment-related myelodysplasia and leukemia represent significant late complications of autologous SCT.

Transplantation for specific diseases

Non-Hodgkin lymphoma
Aggressive lymphomas

Many patients with NHL can be cured today with frontline combination chemotherapy and/or radiotherapy. However,

Table 12-4 Infections and complications in autologous transplantations.

Infection/complication	Aplasia	Day 100	Late (to 6 months)
Bacterial	Gram negative Gram positive		
Viral	Herpes simplex RSV		
		Varicella ⟶	
	BK/JC		
Fungal	Candida		
Parasitic		*Pneumocystis jiroveci* ⟶	
VOD	VOD		

RSV = respiratory syncytial virus; VOD = veno-occlusive disease.

for patients with suboptimal responses to initial therapy or for patients with relapsed or refractory disease, salvage therapy alone is typically inadequate to achieve long-term survival. High-dose chemotherapy with autologous HSCT offers curative potential. Dose-intensive treatment has unequivocally been shown to be the treatment of choice for patients with relapsed, chemotherapy-sensitive intermediate-grade lymphomas.

Autologous HSCT is the standard of care for most patients with chemotherapy-sensitive relapsed or refractory diffuse large-cell lymphoma. The international, multicenter, prospective PARMA trial was the pivotal study that established the role of autologous HSCT for patients with relapsed, chemotherapy-sensitive, diffuse large B-cell NHL. In this trial, 109 of 215 patients who had relapsed diffuse large B-cell NHL and who responded to platinum-based salvage chemotherapy were randomly assigned to 4 more courses of conventional chemotherapy or autologous HSCT. The 5-year event-free survival (EFS) and OS were 46% and 53%, respectively, for the transplantation arm and 12% and 32%, respectively, for the chemotherapy arm. An important prognostic indicator was response to salvage chemotherapy. Patients with relapsed diffuse large B-cell NHL who were chemotherapy sensitive unequivocally fared better compared with patients with chemotherapy-resistant disease.

Patients with diffuse large B-cell NHL who demonstrate primary refractory disease or relapsed disease that is not responsive to salvage chemotherapy have poor outcomes even after autologous HSCT. However, autologous HSCT is indicated for patients who respond to salvage therapy after demonstrating resistant disease to frontline therapy. There is no consensus on the optimal salvage regimen, but platinum-containing regimens are the most commonly used. Such regimens include ICE; dexamethasone, high-dose cytarabine, and cisplatin (DHAP); and etoposide, methylprednisolone, high-dose cytarabine, and cisplatin (ESHAP). Ifosfamide-based regimens are also used, such as ICE and mesna, ifosfamide, mitoxantrone, and etoposide (MINE), and rituximab is usually added to all of these regimens.

The introduction of rituximab has improved the prognosis of aggressive B-cell lymphoma, and rituximab has a growing role in the peritransplantation management of patients with aggressive lymphoma. Rituximab is now commonly added to salvage regimens (eg, R-ICE, R-DHAP) for added cytoreduction and because it also confers an in vivo purging effect and reduces the incidence of tumor contamination in the autograft. It is also given after transplantation as maintenance therapy to eradicate minimal residual disease in an effort to reduce recurrence. However, transient neutropenia has been observed in patients given rituximab before or after transplantation, but the mechanism for this is poorly understood.

Investigators have studied various prognostic factors at relapse that help predict outcome after autologous HSCT. The International Prognostic Index (IPI) is the validated scoring system designed to predict survival of patients with newly diagnosed aggressive NHL. However, the IPI at relapse (second-line IPI) also has been shown to correlate with prognosis after autologous HSCT. Positron emission tomography (PET) scanning also appears to have predictive value; several studies have shown that patients who demonstrate PET positivity after salvage therapy have an inferior failure-free survival compared with patients who are PET negative, and these results are independent of second-line age-adjusted IPI. Other poor prognostic features include relapse within 12 months of diagnosis, advanced stage, poor performance status, and failure to achieve only a partial response and not a complete response (CR) after transplantation.

The use of autologous HSCT for patients with aggressive lymphoma as frontline therapy has been explored, but several phase II and III trials have failed to show a benefit. Early autologous HSCT confers higher CR rates but does not appear to improve EFS or OS compared with conventional therapy in both good-risk and high-risk patients, as detailed in a recent systematic review and meta-analysis of 15 randomized controlled trials comparing autologous HSCT as frontline therapy with conventional therapy in patients with aggressive NHL. The use of autologous HSCT for patients with high-risk disease, however, is still the subject of active investigation.

Allogeneic HSCT is not routinely offered to patients with aggressive lymphoma. Exceptions include young patients with advanced disease, patients who failed to mobilize an adequate number of autologous peripheral blood progenitor cells, or patients who failed a previous autologous HSCT. Although relapse rates are lower compared with autologous HSCT, the higher NRM associated with myeloablative conditioning regimens abrogates any benefit in OS. However, there is renewed interest in the role of allogeneic HSCT with the advent of RIC regimens. This type of transplantation relies primary on the donor T-cell–mediated GVL effect to confer a response rather than high-dose cytoreductive chemotherapy. RIC allogeneic HSCT is not standard therapy as of yet but is more commonly offered to patients with aggressive NHL who have failed a prior autologous HSCT. Chemotherapy sensitivity is a strong predictor of outcome in this setting.

Mantle cell lymphoma

Mantle cell lymphoma accounts for 5% to 10% of lymphoid malignancies and is characterized by the t(11;14) translocation. Most patients present with advanced disease and experience an aggressive course with a median OS of 3 to 5 years. For patients in first remission, the role of autologous or allogeneic HSCT is not well defined. Most patients currently receive a high-dose cytarabine-containing regimen such as hyperfractionated fractionated cyclophosphamide, vincristine, doxorubicin, and dexamethasone combined with rituximab and obtain response rates >90% and failure free survival rates of approximately 50%. Patients more often receive autologous HSCT as consolidation with promising results, although it is not clear whether autologous HSCT significantly increases cure rates. For patients with relapsed or refractory disease, autologous HSCT does not confer durable remissions, and these patients should either be guided toward a clinical trial or consideration of allogeneic HSCT because this modality remains the only possible option for cure. Myeloablative allogeneic HSCT can induce durable remissions in mantle cell lymphoma even in heavily pretreated patients, but it is associated with high up-front mortality. Therefore, reduced-intensity regimens are increasingly being offered to this subgroup and yielding EFS rates ranging from 50% to 85% even in patients who failed a prior autologous HSCT. As seen with most other NHL subtypes, the existence of a GVL effect in mantle cell lymphoma stems from findings of lower relapse rates after allogeneic HSCT compared with autologous HSCT.

As discussed in Chapter 18, children usually present with aggressive NHL and only rarely with low-grade lymphoma. Children with refractory disease or relapsed disease require SCT for long-term survival. Research is ongoing to determine whether there is a pediatric population at high risk for relapse who would warrant a transplantation in first remission. Children and adults with HIV-associated NHL have undergone successful autologous SCT while on antiretroviral therapy.

Indolent lymphoma

Although most patients with follicular lymphoma (FL) typically experience a relatively indolent disease course, FL is typically incurable with conventional chemotherapy. However, the addition of rituximab to frontline, salvage, and maintenance therapy has resulted in prolonged survivals. There currently are no uniform guidelines as to the optimal time of HSCT for patients with this disease. Autologous HSCT in first remission is not recommended. In the prerituximab area, the results of 3 large randomized trials from Europe suggested improved DFS but no benefit in OS for patients randomized to the transplantation arm versus the conventional chemotherapy arm. Additionally, the incidence of therapy-related MDS ranged from 3.5% to 12% in the transplantation arm, which was a significantly higher incidence compared with the conventional chemotherapy arm.

For patients with relapsed disease, only one randomized trial from Europe, known as the CUP (Conventional Chemotherapy, Unpurged Autograft, Purged Autograft) trial, has been conducted but closed early due to slow accrual. A total of 89 patients with relapsed disease were randomized to either 3 cycles of salvage chemotherapy versus autologous HSCT with ex vivo purged marrow versus autologous HSCT with unpurged marrow. After a median follow-up of 69 months, the hazard ratio for PFS favored the HSCT arms compared with the salvage chemotherapy arms, and there was a trend for a superior OS favoring the high-dose therapy arms. The samples sizes were not large enough to detect the effect of ex vivo purging of the graft. Conditioning regimens incorporating radioimmunoconjugates such as yttrium-90 ibritumomab have also been used in the autologous setting with the intent of delivering therapeutic radiation doses without the toxicity of TBI, and but this is currently investigational.

Myeloablative allogeneic HSCT has been offered to patients with relapsed FL to harness the GVL effect and to circumvent the tumor cell contamination associated with autologous HSCT. Although no randomized trials have been completed, several studies have consistently reported a lower relapse rate compared with autologous HSCT. However, the benefit of the lower relapse rates has been invariably offset by the NRM associated with myeloablative allogeneic HSCT, and thus, this modality if not routine offered to FL patients. However, the results with allogeneic HSCT using RIC appear very promising even in patients who have failed a prior autologous HSCT. Two prospective studies, one from M.D. Anderson Cancer Center and one from the Cancer and Leukemia Group B (CALGB), used fludarabine-based conditioning regimens. The M.D. Anderson trial reported 6-year PFS and OS rates of 83% and 85%, respectively, with a TRM of 15%. The CALGB trial reported 2-year PFS and OS rates of 71% and 76%, respectively, with a TRM of only 7%. Patients with chemotherapy-sensitive disease prior to transplantation fared better than patients with chemotherapy-resistant disease. Thus, FL patients with recurrent disease may be salvaged after RIC allogeneic HSCT with a lower TRM compared with myeloablative regimens.

Hodgkin lymphoma

For patients with relapsed or refractory disease, autologous HSCT is the standard of care and confers cure rates of 40% to 60% in patients with relapsed, chemotherapy-sensitive disease and 25% to 40% in patients with chemotherapy-refractory disease. Prior to proceeding to autologous HSCT, patients should receive salvage therapy for maximum cytoreduction, with the platinum-based regimens being the most commonly used regimens.

However, the role of allogeneic HSCT in patients with Hodgkin lymphoma is controversial because the existence of a robust GVL effect in Hodgkin lymphoma is under debate. As seen in aggressive B-cell NHL, allogeneic HSCT has historically been only offered to Hodgkin lymphoma patients who have marrow involvement, refractory disease, or relapsed disease after autologous HSCT. The literature now contains several reports detailing the outcomes of Hodgkin lymphoma patients who have undergone allogeneic HSCT with RIC regimens, with the majority of these patients having failed a prior autologous HCT. Thus far, results demonstrate that 30% to 50% of these patients may be cured with RIC allogeneic HSCT; further trials are ongoing.

The focus of first-line therapy for pediatric patients has been to decrease the toxicity of the current therapy while still achieving high cure rates. For children and adolescents who fail conventional chemotherapy, autologous HSCT is offered as a curative option. The Children's Oncology Group is investigating the role of immune modulation in an attempt to induce autologous GVHD in the immediate posttransplantation period. For those with bone marrow involvement or with relapse following an autologous transplantation, allogeneic transplantation has been performed and appears to be better tolerated than in the adult population.

Plasma cell dyscrasia

Over the last 20 years, autologous HSCT has been generally recommended to myeloma patients who are relatively young and who do not have serious comorbid conditions. The results of randomized trials in the 1990s demonstrated a survival advantage for autologous HSCT compared with conventional therapy and formed the basis of this approach. When autologous HSCT is given as part of the planned frontline treatment, approximately 22% to 44% patients achieve CR, with median time to progression and OS time of 18 to 24 months and 4 to 6 years, respectively. High-dose melphalan alone at a dose of 200 mg/m^2 is the most commonly used preparative regimen for patients with multiple myeloma undergoing HSCT. TBI-based regimens have been compared with single-agent high-dose melphalan, and results demonstrated that the TBI-based regimens produced inferior outcomes due to increased toxicity compared with single-agent melphalan. The procedure is well tolerated, with a TRM of <2% in most recent series. Because of the potential tumor contamination during stem cell collection that may contribute to subsequent relapse, stem cell purging and positive selection have both been tested. No significant benefit has been demonstrated. It is also possible for patients with severe renal insufficiency to undergo transplantation, but the experience of performing transplantation in this group of patients is small, and the benefits remain unclear.

However, the advent of the immunomodulators, such as lenalidomide and thalidomide, and proteasome inhibitors, such as bortezomib, as frontline treatment for myeloma has changed the treatment paradigm. The newer agents result in more patients attaining CR, near CR, and very good partial response with frontline therapy and provide the platform toward improving results with autologous HSCT. Current guidelines state that high-dose chemotherapy with autologous HSCT should be offered as initial therapy in patients with newly diagnosed myeloma who are under 65 years old and have a good performance status. However, it appears that patients with adverse prognostic features at diagnosis such a high serum β_2-microglobulin or an unfavorable karyotype such del(13) still have a poor outcome even after tandem (double) autologous HSCT.

Because of concerns over the potential toxicities associated with SCT, a strategy of delayed transplantation has also been tested. In a French randomized study, up-front transplantation was compared with transplantation at relapse with stem cells collected at diagnosis. Early transplantation significantly improved PFS, but there was no difference in OS. Early transplantation, however, was associated with a shorter period of chemotherapy and hence improved quality of life (QOL). Currently, the utility of planned double or tandem transplantation as the primary treatment remains controversial. In a randomized study from the French group, both response rates and survival favored tandem transplantation, in particular for patients with significant residual disease after their first transplantations. A recently published meta-analysis of 6 randomized trials with >1000 patients concluded that tandem autologous HSCT confers higher response rates compared with single autologous HSCT, but it did not find conclusive evidence for improvement in PFS or OS. However, a registry analysis from the European BMT group demonstrated that when a second transplantation is performed within 3 to 6 months after the first transplantation, survival is improved. Thus, the evidence is mixed regarding the utility of tandem autologous HSCT compared with single autologous HSCT. Based on the results of the previously mentioned French study, patients who have residual disease after the first HSCT may benefit from the aggressive cytoreduction of a second autologous HSCT.

The role of maintenance therapy after autologous SCT is unclear and is currently not standard therapy. Trials incorporating thalidomide maintenance have consistently shown improvement in PFS but with variable results in OS. However, thalidomide is usually not well tolerated at full doses for lengthy durations due to sedation and neuropathy. We await the results of a US intergroup trial that recently completed accrual and evaluated the role of lenalidomide as maintenance therapy after single autologous HSCT and the results of another cooperative group trial that studied the role of thalidomide and dexamethasone after double autograft.

Allogeneic HSCT has been tested in younger patients with multiple myeloma. The advantages of an allogeneic HSCT include an uncontaminated graft and the well-documented graft-versus-myeloma immunologic effect that may reduce the relapse rate. Unfortunately, this approach is associated with high TRM (20%–50% by day 100). In addition, a pattern of continuous relapse was observed after allogeneic transplantation of approximately 7% per year with long-term follow-up. This raises the question of the curative potential of allogeneic transplantation. Nonmyeloablative transplantation approaches have also been extensively studied in myeloma, but relapse remains the major cause of treatment failure.

AL (light-chain amyloid) amyloidosis is a clonal plasma cell disorder similar to multiple myeloma and characterized by widespread disposition of amorphous extracellular materials composed in part of immunoglobulin light- or heavy-chain fragments in many vital organs such as the heart, lung, kidney, liver, and central nervous system (CNS). This infiltrative process ultimately leads to organ failure and death. The prognosis of patients with AL amyloidosis is poor, with median survival of approximately 1 to 2 years. Although conventional chemotherapy has limited utility in patients with AL, autologous SCT using high-dose chemotherapy, mostly melphalan, to eradicate the clonal plasma cells can reverse the disease process for selected patients with AL and possibly prolong survival. It is critical to establish an accurate diagnosis of AL amyloidosis because patients with nonimmunoglobulin forms of amyloidosis will not benefit from cytotoxic therapy, including transplantation. Because of the preexisting organ dysfunction in patients with AL amyloidosis, despite careful patient selection, the TRM is still 4 to 8 times ($\sim$25%) higher compared with that of autologous transplantation for multiple myeloma (<5%). The causes of TRM include gastrointestinal bleeding, cardiac arrhythmias, and the development of intractable hypotension and multiorgan failure.

In a single-institution study from the Boston Medical Center that included 205 patients, 115 patients (56%) survived for at least 1 year after SCT. Nearly half of the patients achieved complete hematologic responses, and the amyloid-related organ disease improved in three quarters of the complete responders. Although the median survival of patients with cardiac involvement was 2 years, patients with other dominant organ involvement had a median survival of >4 years. In a study from the Mayo Clinic, 66 patients with AL amyloidosis underwent autologous SCT; the 30-month actuarial survival was 72%, but survival for patients with involvement of >2 organs was <20%. It is clear from these studies that patients with advanced cardiomyopathy or involvement of >2 organs rarely benefit and are not suitable candidates for HSCT. However, a phase III trial was recently published in which AL amyloid patients were randomized to receive autologous HSCT with high-dose melphalan versus oral melphalan and high-dose dexamethasone. After a median follow-up of 3 years, the OS was significantly longer in the conventional-dose group (57 vs 22 months; $P = .04$). When the groups were stratified by risk, there was no difference in OS between the 2 treatment arms in the low-risk group, but in the high-risk group, there was a nonsignificant survival difference favoring the conventional treatment arm. The TRM was 24%. Based on these results, AL amyloid patients should be carefully selected for HSCT, and patients must be fully informed of the up-front TRM.

POEMS syndrome is characterized by polyneuropathy, organomegaly, endocrinopathy, monoclonal gammopathy, skin changes, and a clonal plasma cell disorder. Investigators from the Mayo Clinic performed transplantation in 16 patients with POEMS syndrome; 15 patients had a severe, rapidly progressive sensorimotor polyneuropathy, and 9 patients were wheelchair dependent. All 14 evaluable patients achieved neurologic improvement or stabilization. Other symptoms also improved substantially. Because POEMS syndrome is a very rare disease, it would be difficult to perform any prospective study to define the exact role of SCT. Nevertheless, HSCT results in significant clinical improvement in a majority of patients and should be considered a therapeutic option in these patients.

Acute myelogenous leukemia

Allogeneic HSCT is a treatment option for selected AML patients in CR1 and the only curative option for patients with primary refractory or relapsed AML. In adults, allogeneic transplantation in CR1 is usually reserved for those with high-risk features of AML such as patients with unfavorable cytogenetic abnormalities at diagnosis. For patients with favorable features, the treatment-related mortality associated with transplantation in CR1 exceeds the benefits.

Approximately 40% to 50% of adult AML patients present with a normal karyotype at the time of diagnosis and thus fall into the intermediate-risk category. The optimal postremission therapy for this subgroup remains controversial, but molecular risk stratification can aid in determining prognoses. Patients with the *FLT3-ITD* and *MLL* mutations demonstrate relapse rates approaching 90% after conventional chemotherapy and should be offered allogeneic HSCT in CR1 if a matched sibling donor is available. The presence of the *NPM1* or *CEBPα* mutation confers a favorable prognosis, and thus, HSCT in CR1 is usually not indicated if these mutations do not appear concurrently with any of the poor-risk mutations such as *FLT-ITD*.

Patients with recurrent AML have very low cure rates with conventional chemotherapy. Allogeneic and occasionally autologous transplantation represents their only realistic chance for cure. Patients in second complete remission (CR2) have a survival rate of approximately 25% to 30% after allogeneic transplantation. Most patients with refractory disease (primary treatment failures or refractory relapse) have very low rates of long-term DFS (5%–15%) and should be considered for novel transplantation strategies or investigational therapies. However, DFS approaching 30% has been reported in a subset of primary refractory patients who receive related donor grafts and who do not have an unfavorable karyotype at diagnosis.

Most of the data with allogeneic HSCT transplantation are derived from experience in patients with HLA-identical sibling donors, but it is generally accepted that the outcomes of patients with HLA-identical unrelated donors approach those of HLA-identical sibling transplantation recipients. For patients who lack an available matched sibling donor or unrelated donor, alternative donors include UCB donors or related haploidentical donors. UCB transplantation was initially offered to pediatric patients because the number of hematopoietic progenitor cells in a cord blood graft is adequate enough to rapidly engraft a patient <50 kg. However, for adults, UCB transplantation is now being performed with double cord blood units, which increases the number of stem cells infused, aids in faster engraftment, and is associated with lower relapse rates compared with single UCB transplantation thought due to the synergistic alloreactivity of the 2 grafts. Allogeneic HSCT using related haploidentical donors is highly investigational, with success mostly limited to patients with myeloid malignancies in remission at the time of HSCT. When cord blood units or haploidentical donors are used, opportunistic infections stemming from delayed immune reconstitution represent a major cause of NRM.

Randomized clinical trials in children show that allogeneic SCT provides superior DFS for patients in CR1 compared with either chemotherapy or autologous SCT as consolidation. Thus, children with AML lacking favorable features [eg, t(8;21), inv(16), or AML M7 associated with Down syndrome] who have an HLA-matched sibling often receive allogeneic transplantations after induction therapy.

Busulfan- and TBI-based regimens are generally considered equivalent. The newer RIC and nonmyeloablative conditioning regimens have been tested mainly in older or more infirm patients. Their precise role remains to be determined, but in at least one study, reduction of dose-intensity was associated with increased rates of recurrence.

Autologous transplantation for AML has been explored as consolidation for patients in CR1 or CR2. Patients undergoing autologous transplantation in CR1 have a decreased rate of recurrence compared with those receiving conventional chemotherapy but a higher recurrence rate than those undergoing allogeneic transplantation. Overall long-term outcome is generally considered comparable to that of patients receiving intensive consolidation therapy, and in the United States, autologous transplantation is not commonly offered in CR1. Occult AML cells contaminating the marrow graft are responsible for recurrence in a fraction of patients undergoing autologous transplantation, and stem cell purging by in vitro exposure to chemotherapeutic agents may be important for long-term outcome. Enthusiasm in the United States for this approach has been limited due to lack of availability of purging agents. Appropriate consolidation therapy prior to harvest and transplantation has been investigated as a method to improve cure rates and optimize autologous (and even allogeneic) transplantation.

Autologous transplantation has also been investigated as consolidation of CR2. Excellent results have been reported in patients with recurrent acute promyelocytic leukemia [t(15;17)]. Results in other AML subtypes are less encouraging, and allogeneic transplantation is usually preferred in the United States.

Acute lymphoblastic leukemia

Allogeneic SCT is a treatment option for selected patients in CR1 of ALL and the only curative option for all patients with Philadelphia chromosome–positive ALL and most patients with primary refractory or relapsed ALL. In adults, allogeneic transplantation in CR1 is usually reserved for those with high-risk features of ALL. High risk is often defined by the following characteristics: poor-risk cytogenetics such as t(9;22), t(4;11), t(1;19), and t(8;14); complex karyotype (ie, >5 abnormalities); WBC >30,000/μL with the B-cell phenotype; WBC >100,000/μL with the T-cell phenotype; requiring >4 weeks to achieve CR; or age >30 to 35 years. Approximately 30% to 65% of patients who receive transplantation in first remission become long-term survivors.

For patients with standard-risk ALL, the benefit of allogeneic transplantation in CR1 continues to be debated. The largest prospective trial to date addressing this question is the MRCUKALLXII-ECOG2993 trial, which accrued nearly 2000 newly diagnosed ALL patients from 1993 to 2006. Of the 1031 Philadelphia chromosome–negative patients who obtained a CR with frontline therapy, the 5-year OS among patients who had a donor versus patients without a donor (and who received autologous HSCT or chemotherapy) was 53% versus 45%, respectively ($P = .01$). However, in contrast to other studies, the standard-risk patients with a donor had a superior OS compared with patients without a donor. Despite the significantly reduced relapse rates among all patients who had a donor, there was no survival benefit for HSCT in the high-risk group due to the high TRM of 39% in patients >35 years old. A meta-analysis of >1200 ALL patients in 7 studies showed a higher survival in the patients with a donor compared with the no-donor group. In contrast to the Medical Research Council Eastern Cooperative Oncology Group trial, the meta-analysis demonstrated that the survival advantage was even more pronounced in the high-risk group.

Survival of adult patients with ALL who receive transplantation in relapse is dismal, with long-term survival rates of 5% to 10%. Unfortunately, despite better patient selection, the long-term DFS for adult patients who receive transplantation beyond CR1 is still, at best, between 20% and 25%. The GVL effect appears less potent in patients with ALL because there is no statistical difference in relapse rate between allogeneic and syngeneic transplantations for ALL.

The prognosis of pediatric patients with ALL is very good with standard therapy. SCT in first remission using a matched related donor is limited to a small, very high-risk population including children with t(9;22), those whose blasts are hypodiploid, those who have an *MLL* rearrangement [t(4;11)] with a slow response to therapy, and/or those who fail to obtain a remission after induction therapy. In a recent retrospective study, children with t(9;22) translocation achieved a 65% long-term EFS after SCT from an HLA-identical sibling compared with an approximately 25% EFS for patients treated with standard chemotherapy regimens. Several reports of infants with *MLL* rearrangements treated with SCT in first remission have documented EFS ranging between 64% and 76%. This compares favorably to an EFS of approximately 33% attained with the most aggressive chemotherapy regimens in this setting. However, all of these studies need to be interpreted cautiously due to their nonrandomized nature and the relatively small numbers of patients studied.

The prognosis of patients with relapsed childhood ALL depends on the site and timing of relapse. Among patients with early marrow relapse (during chemotherapy or within 6 months of stopping), only 10% achieve long-term EFS with standard chemotherapy. A retrospective review found that children with relapsed ALL had better EFS with allogeneic SCT than with chemotherapy alone for early relapse and that, in this population, a TBI-based regimen was superior. The role of SCT in later relapses is debatable due to relatively good results with standard chemotherapy alone. Extramedullary relapse in children is quite different from adult ALL. Pediatric patients with early CNS relapse (<18 months from diagnosis) have a 40% EFS using chemotherapy and irradiation. Patients with late CNS relapse can achieve up to 80% EFS using chemotherapy plus irradiation. Similar results have been achieved with late testicular relapse. The role of allogeneic SCT in this setting remains controversial. The bias of each transplantation center influences these retrospective analyses, demonstrating the need for a case–control prospective study.

Chronic myelogenous leukemia

Prior to the introduction of the tyrosine kinase inhibitors (TKIs) such as imatinib, dasatinib, and nilotinib, allogeneic HSCT was part of standard therapy for patients with CML since the early 1980s. Earlier retrospective analyses data showed that patients who underwent allogeneic HSCT within 1 year of diagnosis experienced better outcomes compared with patients who underwent transplantation later in their disease course. In the preimatinib era, for patients with chronic-phase CML undergoing myeloablative allogeneic HSCT, the 10-year OS rate was between 40% and 80%, with TRM ranging from 5% to 30%. The DFS rates with matched related donor allogeneic SCT were 40% to 80% in chronic phase, 15% to 40% in accelerated phase, and 5% to 10% in blastic phase CML. Similar results have been obtained from patients receiving a transplantation from HLA-identical unrelated donors.

However, TKIs, especially imatinib, have unequivocally emerged as standard frontline therapy for all newly diagnosed CML patients. The 5-year update of the International Randomized Study of Interferon Versus STI571 (IRIS) trial demonstrated that for the imatinib-treated patients, the cumulative best complete hematologic response rates and complete cytogenetic response rates were 98% and 87%, respectively, and that treatment response improved with ongoing therapy. Additionally, there is no clear evidence that pretransplantation imatinib will negatively influence outcome of patients undergoing future transplantation. A retrospective analysis of >400 patients who underwent HSCT in first chronic phase or beyond first chronic phase clearly showed no negative impact of pre-HSCT imatinib, and pre-HSCT imatinib was associated with a higher OS with a trend toward lower NRM. Interestingly, however, higher hematologic relapse rates were seen.

So which CML patients should be considered for allogeneic HSCT? During imatinib therapy, it is of utmost importance to observe for therapeutic milestones, especially during the first 12 to 18 months of therapy. It is universally accepted that the lack of a complete hematologic response at 3 months, a lack of major cytogenetic response (CyR) at 12 months, or a lack of a complete cytogenetic response by 18 months is consistent with imatinib failure. Despite the high response rates achieved with imatinib, a few patients will not achieve a complete hematologic response, and 20% to 25% will not achieve a complete cytogenetic response. These patients are considered to have primary resistance to imatinib and should be considered for allogeneic HSCT. Approximately 25% of patients will acquire secondary resistance, which is defined as loss of complete hematologic response, loss of complete cytogenetic response, or an increase in 30% of Philadelphia chromosome–positive metaphases, and these patients should also be directed toward allogeneic HSCT. Patients who are diagnosed with resistance should be screened for the T315I mutation and advised to receive transplantation because none of the current first- and second-generation TKIs can overcome this mutation. Patients without the mutation are often given another TKI, such as nilotinib or dasatinib, for temporary disease control, but durable remissions are unlikely, and allogeneic HSCT should be planned accordingly. A recent study found that the majority of patients who develop imatinib resistance have a high likelihood of developing resistance to second- and third-generation TKIs.

In summary, for patients with CML, the role of allogeneic HSCT has considerably shifted in the imatinib era, but this modality is still of value in the treatment of selected patients who have failed TKI therapy. For CML patients in accelerated phase or blast crisis, TKIs can induce transient responses, and a search for a donor should commence as soon as possible. However, it has been reported that in other countries where the cost considerations of taking imatinib or another TKI for a lifetime weigh heavily on medical decision making, the rate of allogeneic HSCT for CML patients has not fallen since TKIs were introduced.

The care of the pediatric patient with CML is also evolving with the development of imatinib. Related and unrelated HSCT in pediatric patients with this disease results in EFS rates of 60% to 75%. The lack of long-term data for new agents makes a definitive recommendation difficult. Most centers will begin the child or adolescent on imatinib while initiating HLA typing and donor search. If there is a good match, the child may proceed to HSCT. As the data on imatinib and other similar agents mature, the role in the treatment of childhood CML should be investigated within clinical trials including close observation for late effects of this novel therapy.

Chronic lymphocytic leukemia

Chronic lymphocytic leukemia (CLL) is the most common adult leukemia in North America and Europe. Although this disease usually follows an indolent course, it remains incurable with standard therapy, and once patients become fludarabine-refractory, the median survival is <12 months. Allogeneic HSCT is the only curative modality, but historically, many CLL patients were not offered this treatment because most patients were elderly and could not tolerate high-dose chemotherapy.

High-dose chemotherapy with autologous HSCT confers high response rates in CLL and reported remission durations lasting up to 5 tro 6 years. However, the enthusiasm for autologous HSCT has significantly waned due to the significant incidence of late toxicities (mainly posttransplantation MDS/AML, with an incidence as high as 12% reported in one series), the comparable outcomes after combination chemotherapy or chemoimmunotherapy, and the fact that autologous HSCT does not appear to overcome adverse prognostic factors.

The advantages of allogeneic HSCT include the GVL effect associated with the donor's immune system and the elimination of potential tumor contamination associated with an autologous graft. Studies involving myeloablative conditioning regimens have reported plateaus in survival curves, with DFS ranging from 39% to 78%. Chemotherapy-sensitive and less heavily pretreated patients fare better than the chemotherapy-refractory patients. However, myeloablative conditioning is not commonly offered due to the high TRM, which approaches 50% to 60% in published studies, and the increasing use of nonmyeloablative/RIC regimens, which appear to be better tolerated.

RIC regimens allow transplantation in older patients and patients with comorbid conditions. The outcomes of CLL patients, including heavily pretreated patients and patients with adverse prognostic factors, look very promising after RIC allogeneic HSCT. A study from the M.D. Anderson Cancer Center of 39 patients who received the fludarabine, cyclophosphamide, and rituximab (FCR) regimen reported 4-year PFS and OS rates of 44% and 48%, respectively, with chemotherapy sensitivity being a major prognosticator for diseases progression. The risk of progression for chemotherapy-sensitive versus chemotherapy-refractory patients was 22% versus 73%, respectively, and interestingly, ZAP-70 status had no impact on outcomes, suggesting that the GVL effect was able to overcome this adverse prognostic factor. Investigators from Seattle reported the outcomes of 82 CLL patients who received an RIC regimen of low-dose TBI with or without fludarabine. The 5-year OS and DFS rates were 50% and 39%, respectively, which was notable considering that nearly 90% of patients were fludarabine refractory. The NRM was 23%.

In summary, allogeneic HSCT has a selected role in CLL, with RIC regimens offering the most promising results to date. Patients who should be considered earlier for HSCT include young patients who do not achieve a CR, patients who experience progression with a fludarabine-based regimen within 24 months of therapy, patients with the 17p deletion, patients with Richter transformation, and patients who have relapsed after a prior autologous HSCT. Ongoing prospective clinical trials are currently studying the merit of early HSCT in patients who have other high-risk factors such as unmutated *IgVH* and deletion of 11q.

Aplastic anemia and other autoimmune diseases

For patients with aplastic anemia, allogeneic HSCT is an established therapy. Fortunately, in aplastic anemia, several strategies provide long-term survival for the majority of patients. The pathophysiology and results of treatment using immunosuppression and transplantation are discussed in other chapters in this book.

For young patients with newly diagnosed idiopathic severe aplastic anemia and an HLA-identical sibling, many centers recommend immediate transplantation to minimize the sensitization with transfusions, which historically has resulted in an increased risk for graft rejection. Although the use of cyclosporine, as well as the use of leukodepleted blood products, has reduced the problem of rejection, sensitization should be minimized; directed family donations of blood products should be avoided. Transplantation remains the treatment of choice for patients up to the age of 40 years. Typically, a combination of high-dose cyclophosphamide and ATG is used for conditioning. Excellent results have been reported with related and unrelated donor transplantation alike, with cure rates approaching 80%. For older patients (age >40 years), results with SCT drop off considerably. Even for patients with HLA-identical siblings, many centers reserve SCT for those failing immunosuppression in this age group.

It is important to rule out Fanconi anemia in potential transplantation recipients. Patients with Fanconi anemia frequently do not have all of the stigmata of the disease, and the diagnosis is easily overlooked. The sensitivity of patients with Fanconi anemia to alkylating agents is well known, and transplantation can be done successfully using only reduced-intensity regimens. Recent trials have focused on reducing radiation exposure in addition to reducing doses of alkylating agents in these patients. Patients with Fanconi anemia are also at high risk for solid tumors, especially following radiation exposure. Much like for other inherited disorders, siblings should be screened for both HLA compatibility and to rule out the presence of the disease itself.

There has been increasing interest in autologous transplantation as a method of treating life-threatening autoimmune disorders. Autologous transplantations have been used in multiple sclerosis, systemic sclerosis (usually for lung disease), rheumatoid arthritis, juvenile idiopathic arthritis, systemic lupus, dermatomyositis/polymyositis, and autoimmune cytopenias. The therapeutic rationale for these transplantations is that high-dose chemotherapy may eradicate/modulate clones of autoreactive T cells. Although the integration of this approach into treatment of each disease will depend on the results of ongoing trials, some general observations are now possible. First, ASCT has considerable treatment-related morbidity and even mortality. This has been particularly true in patients with advanced multiple sclerosis. Second, the underlying organ dysfunction often progresses acutely through the transplantation, even if there is stability to improvement later. Third, durability of response and the need for continued therapy remain to be defined. The waxing and waning course of autoimmune disorders makes it difficult to define end points in these diseases. Results that have been considered encouraging in the transplantation literature have been considered disappointing (both regarding the rates of response and toxicity) in the rheumatology literature. Nonetheless, patients with aggressive autoimmune disorders should consider clinical trials and examine this approach as one of their treatment options.

Hemoglobinopathies

Thalassemia major

The Pesaro team has pioneered transplantation for thalassemia and has reported high cure rates. Three factors predict adverse transplantation outcomes: hepatomegaly (>2 cm below the costal margin), hepatic fibrosis, and irregular chelation. Quality chelation therapy is defined as deferoxamine therapy initiated not later than 18 months after the first transfusion and given for at least 5 days each week. Class I patients have none of these factors, class II patients have 1 or 2 factors, and class III patients have all 3 factors. For class I patients <17 years of age, the rates of survival, thalassemia-free survival, TRM, and recurrence of thalassemia were 94%, 87%, 6%, and 7%, respectively. The rates of survival, thalassemia-free survival, TRM, and recurrence of thalassemia were 84%, 81%, 15%, and 4%, respectively, for class II patients. Patients with class III disease have more complications and a higher rate of graft rejection. The probability of thalassemia-free survival for young patients who are in class III is 62%, and the risk of dying is 35%. RIC regimens have been investigated in these patients. Class III adults receiving reduced-dose conditioning appear to have a lower rate of rejection. The Pesaro team notes a 24% chance of rejection if the individual has received >100 transfusions, compared with a 53% chance in patients who have received fewer transfusions.

The optimal source of stem cells for patients with hemoglobinopathies is still under investigation. To avoid chronic GVHD, the use of bone marrow rather than PBSCs has been advocated. For those lacking sibling donors, unrelated and cord blood donor transplantations have shown promising results in both pediatric and adult patients, provided donor compatibility is stringent.

The 2-year probability of survival after cord blood transplantation for children with thalassemia was 79% in 33 patients who received transplantation. Unfortunately, 7 of the children rejected the graft. Additional work to improve engraftment is needed before this method can be universally applied.

Patients with thalassemia major not infrequently develop mixed chimerism following transplantation, which usually leads to marked improvement in their transfusion requirements. However, the patients remain at risk for graft rejection, especially those whose percentage of host cells remains >25%. Attempts to reduce the conditioning regimen intensity may lead to a higher incidence of stable mixed chimerism.

Sickle cell disease

Although supportive therapy, including prophylactic antibiotics, hydroxyurea, and chronic transfusion, have improved the survival of individuals with sickle cell disease and its variants, life expectancy and QOL for sickle cell patients is much reduced. By contrast, results from the 150 children who have received transplantation from HLA-identical siblings indicate a >90% survival rate and that 85% are disease free. Of particular interest is that successful SCT so far has prevented further sickle cell complications. Chronic transfusion reduces the rate of complications but does not prevent them. A study from Belgium demonstrated that patients who received transplantation early in the course of their disease (<4 blood transfusions) had a 100% survival rate and 93% DFS rate compared with an 88% survival rate and 80% DFS rate in patients who received transplantation later in the course of their disease.

Despite these successes, many recommend reserving transplantation for children at high risk from their sickle cell disease because of the toxicities and risks. Frequently, however, children at significant risk are not identified until they have suffered end-organ damage including stroke and/or severe lung injury. In addition, the clinical course for a patient may vary over time. Attempts to identify risk factors of severe disease have suggested high WBC count, severe anemia, and early dactylitis as surrogate markers. But the ability to predict the clinical course for each individual remains elusive. In addition, finding suitable, unaffected sibling donors has been difficult. In one study, only 14% of patients with siblings had a suitable HLA-matched donor.

Similar to thalassemia major, stable mixed chimerism has developed in a subset of patients. Studies of various nonmyeloablative regimens are ongoing. The degree of chimerism (in particular red blood cell chimerism) to ensure stable engraftment while consistently eliminating end-organ damage in these patients is not known.

Immune deficiency disorders

Many immune deficiency disorders become evident in infancy secondary to an increased rate of infections and/or the presence of opportunistic infections. In such cases, the possibility of HIV infection must be ruled out. For patients suspected of having a primary immune deficiency, definitive diagnosis of the exact molecular defect is important to predict the course of the disease and to be able to tailor therapy appropriately. The most common diseases for which transplantation is indicated include severe combined immunodeficiency syndrome (SCIDS), adenosine deaminase deficiency, Wiskott-Aldrich syndrome, Nezelof syndrome, Omenn syndrome, MHC antigen deficiency, leukocyte adhesion defect, Chédiak-Higashi syndrome, chronic granulomatous syndrome, and DiGeorge anomaly.

Newborns known to have or to be at high risk for severe SCIDS should be isolated at birth because infection increases the risk for complications of SCT. Evaluation of early complete blood counts may suggest a neutrophil (neutrophil adhesion disorder or Kostmann syndrome) or lymphocyte disorder, such as SCIDS. Cord blood, when available, should be studied for lymphocyte numbers and in vitro function.

HLA typing should be undertaken as soon as a diagnosis of SCIDS or other combined deficiency potentially correctable by SCT is established. SCT approaches are modified based on the exact diagnosis. The need for a preparative regimen and its intensity are determined in part by the function of the lymphocytes and NK cells.

SCT is undertaken in these disorders to provide a stable source of immunologically competent cells. The major complications are host-versus-graft reactions (ie, rejection of the marrow graft) and GVHD. Graft rejection occurs when sufficient immune function remains for the recipient to mount a cellular immune response against donor HLA molecules. Although this may be prevented by a preparative regimen, the preparative regimen also exposes the recipient to potentially toxic effects. In some forms of SCIDS with absent T-cell function, such as X-linked SCIDS, Jak3 deficiency, and complete RAG-1 and RAG-2 deficiencies, the patient is unable to reject the stem cells. In these patients, simple infusion of stem cells is usually all that is required. However, many of the recipients who received stem cells without a preparative regimen failed to develop normal B-cell function and required ongoing IgG replacement. This has led many centers to tailor the preparative regimen to include some chemotherapy, most recently fludarabine, to attempt to ensure full immune reconstitution. Patients with adenosine deaminase deficiency, the largest subset of this group, require a preparative regimen despite the absence of detectable T-cell function because the donor lymphocytes may rescue the host cell function, thus allowing for ultimate graft rejection. Patients with normal NK cell activity (including some X-linked, Jak3, and RAG defects) also often require preparative regimens, again emphasizing the need for determining the exact defect before initiating therapy.

Results of transplantation are best for children receiving HLA-identical sibling transplantations, with survival ranging from 70% to 100%. For patients lacking a sibling donor, results have ranged from 30% to 50%. In the past, many patients lacking a sibling donor have received haploidentical grafts from a parent. The use of this option provides the ability to proceed with transplantation rapidly, which improves the chances for success. The older the infant is, the greater the likelihood of TRM secondary to opportunistic infection becomes. The increasing availability of cord blood stem cells provides another option, and the optimal choice of stem cell source is far from clear. Cord blood stem cells are particularly appealing because they can be accessed readily and are not infection carriers, decreasing the risk of CMV disease and EBV lymphoproliferative disorders after transplantation.

Inherited metabolic disorders

A number of inborn errors of metabolism have been corrected with SCT. One of the most important steps is the early identification of the disorder prior to the development of end-organ damage. Unfortunately, this is frequently done following the diagnosis in a severely affected older sibling. The role of transplantation varies according to the disorder identified. For instance, certain storage disorders such as Niemann-Pick type IA are not treatable by transplantation. Other disorders such as globoid cell leukodystrophy; metachromatic leukodystrophy; adrenoleukodystrophy; mannosidosis; fucosidosis; aspartylglucosaminuria; Hurler, Hunter, Maroteaux-Lamy, and Sly syndromes; and Gaucher disease type III have been successfully treated with SCT. Siblings and parents should be typed as soon as possible, and the genetic status of the donor should be identified. In a number of these disorders, transplantation using marrow from a donor heterozygous for the trait will not cure the disease. For those lacking a suitable related donor, the best donor source is unclear. The pace of the disease may make the time required for the typical search for a matched unrelated donor unrealistic. The use of cord blood for SCT may require a more intensive preparative regimen to prevent rejection in these immunocompetent patients. GVHD in some of these disorders (ie, adrenal leukodystrophy) may accelerate their disease process and increase the risk of rapid decline. The timing of the transplantation may also be difficult because not all patients with the same apparent diagnosis have the same course of disease. In adrenal leukodystrophy, some patients have rapid neurologic decline at an early age, whereas others may not manifest symptoms until later in childhood, adolescence, or adulthood, if at all. In a number of these disorders, SCT will halt the disease progression, but the patient may not regain lost milestones or function. Decisions regarding the need for a transplantation require the team effort of a metabolic geneticist as well as the transplant physician.

Recently, it has become possible to perform in vitro fertilization using embryos selected for not having the genetic defect and being HLA identical. Although this raises numerous ethical issues, many families may wish to explore this possibility for finding a donor for a sibling patient with these disorders as well as other inherited diseases such as the hemoglobinopathies and Fanconi anemia.

SCT for solid tumors
Germ cell cancer

Germ cell cancer is highly curable, even in patients with disseminated disease. Although conventional-dose cisplatin-based chemotherapy cures the majority of patients, patients presenting with very advanced disease have a somewhat higher rate of recurrence. Some patients at first relapse can achieve a durable remission with salvage chemotherapy, but most of the patients who failed salvage chemotherapy or had cisplatin-refractory disease ultimately died of the disease. Approximately 15% to 20% of patients with multiply relapsed or overtly cisplatin-refractory germ cell cancer, however, can be cured with high-dose carboplatin and etoposide followed by HSCT. In a large retrospective study, progressive disease before transplantation, primary mediastinal tumor, refractoriness to conventional-dose cisplatin, and human chorionic gonadotropin levels >1000 IU/L before transplantation predicted for transplantation failure. The estimated 2-year survival rates were 51% and 5% for patients with no risk factors and multiple risk factors, respectively.

Transplantation has also been investigated as consolidation therapy after initial treatment of patients with advanced disease. In a European Bone Marrow Transplantation Group prospective study, patients were randomized between 4 cycles of etoposide, ifosfamide, and cisplatin (VIP) versus 3 cycles of VIP plus a single cycle of high-dose therapy followed by ASCT. The 3-year EFS for patients who received VIP only was 35% versus 42% for patients randomized to transplantation, with no difference in OS. A recently completed US intergroup phase III randomized study failed to demonstrate any benefits in high-dose therapy for patients with newly diagnosed intermediate- or poor-risk germ cell cancer.

Pediatric solid tumors

Many pediatric solid tumors demonstrate exquisite chemosensitivity, leading to the exploration of SCT as a method of dose intensification for children presenting with high-risk or recurrent disease.

Neuroblastoma

In 1999, the Children's Cancer Group reported a study of 539 patients with high-risk neuroblastoma defined as age >1 year, metastatic disease, amplification of *MYCN* oncogene, and/or histologic findings. All patients were treated with the same initial regimen of chemotherapy, and those with progression of disease were then randomly assigned to continued chemotherapy or SCT using purged autologous bone marrow. Patients still without disease progression were then randomized to differentiation therapy with 13-*cis*-retinoic acid or no further therapy. The EFS was superior for the SCT group (34% vs 22% at 3 years). Among patients assigned to receive *cis*-retinoic acid and SCT, EFS was 55% versus 18% in those assigned to chemotherapy and no *cis*-retinoic acid. Although neuroblastoma may have late relapses that may decrease this apparent effect, this large study established the benefit of SCT for these high-risk patients. More recently, the use of purged mobilized PBSCs has replaced purged bone marrow at many centers and is associated with decreased SCT-related mortality. Ongoing studies are investigating additional SCT-related strategies for further improving the outcome of high-risk patients, such as the use of sequential autologous transplantations (tandem transplantations), combination therapies with high-dose radiopharmaceutical agents such as iodine-131 meta-iodobenzylguanidine, and allogeneic SCT. There have been a few reports of a possible GVT effect in neuroblastoma, but this will require further study.

Ewing sarcoma

Like neuroblastoma, the Ewing sarcoma and primitive neuroectodermal tumor family is chemotherapy-sensitive and radiotherapy-sensitive tumors. High-risk features of Ewing sarcoma include a large primary tumor >8 cm in diameter, pelvic location of the primary, and presence of overt metastatic disease at diagnosis. Patients with metastatic Ewing tumors have a DFS rate of 20% when treated with conventional therapy. Dose intensification with stem cell support has been tried in Ewing sarcoma patients. Results from several large retrospective studies covering patients who received transplantation in the 1980s to 2000 showed no clear benefit from SCT compared with conventional therapies. The prognosis still remains very poor for those receiving transplantation in the setting of residual disease. In a study from the National Cancer Institute, 91 patients were enrolled on a series of 3 protocols consisting of induction chemotherapy, radiation to the primary site, consolidation with TBI (8 Gy), and autologous BMT. In this group, 79% of the patients achieved a CR with surgery, local radiation, and chemotherapy; 90% of eligible patients proceeded to transplantation; and 30% survived long term without progression of disease. Although this proportion is higher than expected for a poor-prognosis group of patients, this may represent selection of a chemotherapy-sensitive better risk group because only patients who did not progress after chemotherapy were eligible for SCT. Current recommendations for the use of SCT in this patient population are mixed.

Late effects and long-term follow-up after transplantation

As the number of long-term survivors following a transplantation increases and many of these individuals have returned to their referring physicians, the need for understanding and continued follow-up is essential both for the care of the survivors themselves and to anticipate the needs of the group as a whole. The joint recommendations of the European Bone Marrow Transplantation Group, the Center for International Blood and Marrow Transplant Research, and the American Society of Blood and Marrow Transplantation were recently published. These recommendations are based in part on published data and in part on common practice. Careful evaluation on an annual basis is recommended with close monitoring and preventive screening, especially for the problems discussed in this chapter. Many of the late complications seen after SCT are especially profound for younger patients.

Endocrine adverse effects

Endocrine sequelae of myeloablative transplantation have been well documented but may be underappreciated. Children should be followed to assure that adequate growth is obtained through adolescence. After conditioning with CyTBI, 20% to 70% of children develop growth hormone deficiency. Some children have benefited from growth hormone therapy. In addition, many patients have thyroid dysfunction, often compounded by the effects of therapy prior to the transplantation.

The prevalence of damage to the gonadal tissue is high and may result in delay or absence of development of secondary sexual characteristics and the need for hormonal replacement. The risk for gonadal damage appears to be dependent on multiple factors including age, sex, type of transplantation, previous therapy, and conditioning regimen. For many young adults, the high risk of infertility after SCT is a major issue, and counseling for sperm or egg banking should be considered for such young patients before SCT. Recent evaluation of 39 male patients 2 years following SCT at a single institution demonstrated spermatogenesis in 28% of the patients. Those more likely to have sperm included men <25 years of age at transplantation, men with a longer interval from transplantation, and men who had not had chronic GVHD. Unfortunately, although sperm banking is readily available, currently, only fertilized eggs are readily stored. Research is ongoing into the cryopreservation of unfertilized eggs or ovaries. For many patients, the course of their disease does not allow this luxury; however, counseling with fertility specialists after the procedure may, in the future, allow new options.

Musculoskeletal complications

Patients receiving high-dose steroids for their disease or for GVHD have an increased risk of developing avascular joint necrosis and myopathies. In addition, loss of range of motion may be seen in patients with a history of chronic GVHD even if the disease is controlled. Osteoporosis due to steroid use and therapy-induced menopause is common. All patients should obtain a bone densitometry at 1 year after transplantation.

Psychosocial considerations

The long-term cognitive effects of prior therapy and SCT continue to be evaluated. Significant CNS toxicity has been seen, especially in young patients receiving intensive intrathecal chemotherapy and/or CNS radiotherapy prior to transplantation. Previous evaluations involving QOL assessments completed by parents appear to underestimate the child's QOL and functioning. Newer methods of neuropsychiatric testing have begun to reveal subtle problems that greatly affect school performance. Identification of these deficiencies and adaptive measures help to improve school functioning. Use of neuropsychiatric testing should be considered on a regular basis for children as well as adults who are finding tasks at home and work more difficult after transplantation. The loss of executive function after therapy has not been evaluated. For patients who receive transplantation as adults, changes in executive function, attention, and memory have been reported and may affect the ability to return to a particular job or to continue the previous role of the individual in his or her family life.

Second malignancies and posttransplantation lymphoproliferative disorders

Survivors of allogeneic transplantation are at increased risk for a variety of second malignancies including a 2- to 3-fold increased risk of solid tumors compared with their age-matched controls. The risk increases over time after transplantation, with the greater risk among younger patients. In a retrospective multicenter study that included approximately 20,000 patients who had received either allogeneic or syngeneic transplantations, the cumulative incidence rates for the development of a new solid cancer were 2.2% and 6.7% at 10 and 15 years, respectively. The risk was significantly elevated for cancers of the buccal cavity, liver, brain, bone, and connective tissue as well as malignant melanoma. Higher doses of TBI were associated with a higher risk of solid cancers. Chronic GVHD and male sex were also associated with increased risk of squamous cell cancers of the buccal cavity and skin. Melanoma and basal cell carcinoma are common in patients, especially those with chronic GVHD. Patients should be instructed to avoid ultraviolet exposures and to use sunscreens and protective clothing.

Posttransplantation lymphoproliferative disorders after allogeneic transplantation are usually related to EBV. They occur more commonly after T-cell–depleted transplantation or in other profoundly immunosuppressed states. Treatment consists of decreasing immunosuppression, monoclonal antibody therapy (in particular rituximab), DLIs (see earlier section on DLIs), and sometimes chemotherapy.

Long-term survivors of autologous transplantation are at considerable risk for therapy-related leukemia. In some series, the cumulative incidence exceeds 10%. The risk is increased with high-dose TBI used for conditioning, is related to the type and intensity of chemotherapy received prior to transplantation, and possibly is related to the chemotherapy agents used for stem cell mobilization (high-dose etoposide is thought to confer an increased risk). In some cases, cytogenetic abnormalities were detected in the marrow or stem cell product of patients destined to develop therapy-related MDS, further implicating pretransplantation chemotherapy. Donor cell leukemia is a rare complication of allogeneic transplantation.

> **Key points**
>
> - Autologous transplantation is the standard of care for relapsed aggressive lymphoma and Hodgkin disease.
> - Autologous HSCT for indolent lymphoma induces high remission rates, but to date, most trials have not shown improved survival compared with conventional therapy. Reduced-intensity allogeneic HSCT shows promising results for patients with relapsed/refractory FL and carries decreased NRM compared with myeloablative regimens.
> - Early autologous transplantation for multiple myeloma increases survival but does not cure. The use of immunomodulators and proteasome inhibitors confers improved remission rates as frontline therapy. Longer follow-up is necessary to determine the long-term impact of the newer agents and their influence on HSCT outcomes.
> - In acute leukemia, generally, second remission or high-risk first remission patients are offered allogeneic transplantations. In all but the youngest adults with chronic-phase CML, allogeneic transplantation has been replaced by imatinib as first-line therapy. All adults should still be HLA typed for potential HSCT in case of TKI failure or intolerance. Allogeneic HSCT remains the treatment of choice for children with CML.
> - HSCT is being studied in selected solid tumors and in autoimmune diseases.
> - HSCT is the treatment of choice for certain congenital immunodeficiencies and inborn errors of metabolism.
> - HSCT should be considered in young patients with severe aplastic anemia. Fanconi anemia should be ruled out.
> - HSCT is a curative treatment of hemoglobinopathies in children. It is also being investigated in young adults.

Summary

HSCT is a rapidly evolving field. Results have improved over the past decade, and indications have changed. Transplantation is more widely applicable due to improvements in supportive care and donor selection and the advent of RIC regimens. For patients with malignant diseases, especially the lymphoid malignancies, the chance for a better outcome is significantly improved if patients are referred when their disease still demonstrates chemotherapy sensitivity. For most of the other indications, it is important to identify high-risk features or poor prognostic factors at the time of diagnosis to help determine the optimal time for HSCT.

Bibliography

Cellular basis of hematopoiesis

Bryder D, Rossi DJ, Weissman IL. Hematopoietic stem cells: the paradigmatic tissue-specific stem cell. *Am J Pathol*. 2006;169:338–346. *A nice review on hematopoietic stem cell properties.*

Lengerke C, McKinney-Freeman S, Naveiras O, et al. The cdx-hox pathway in hematopoietic stem cell formation from embryonic stem cells. *Ann N Y Acad Sci*. 2007;1106:197–208. *A description of the challenges of deriving HSCs by in vitro differentiation of embryonic stem cells and the role of cdx-hox gene pathways in enhancing efficiency.*

Orkin SH, Zon LI. Hematopoiesis: an evolving paradigm of stem cell biology. *Cell*. 2008;132:631–644. *An up-to-date review of concepts in hematopoiesis.*

Raaijmakers MH, Scadden DT. Evolving concepts on the microenvironmental niche for hematopoietic stem cells. *Curr Opin Hematol*. 2008;15:301–306. *A current perspective article incorporating recent new findings in the field of hematopoietic niche biology. This includes a summary of current knowledge about key components of the niche, as well as discussion regarding the potential role of the niche in hematologic disease and as a therapeutic target.*

Rossi DJ, Bryder D, Zahn JM, et al. Cell intrinsic alterations underlie hematopoietic stem cell aging. *Proc Natl Acad Sci USA*. 2005;102:9194–9199. *Provides data regarding age-related differences in HSCs.*

Tavian M, Peault B. Embryonic development of the human hematopoietic system. *Int J Dev Biol*. 2005;49:243–250. *A comprehensive review of the ontogeny of blood cell development in humans, including comparison to murine and avian models.*

Till JE, McCulloch EA. A direct measurement of the radiation sensitivity of normal mouse bone marrow cells. *Radiat Res*. 1961;14:213–222. *The first example of a quantitative assay for hematopoietic stem cells; beginning of stem cell research.*

Unrelated donor transplantation and HLA

Flomenberg N, Baxter-Lowe LA, Confer D, et al. Impact of HLA class I and class II high-resolution matching on outcomes of unrelated donor bone marrow transplantation: HLA-C mismatching is associated with a strong adverse effect on transplantation outcome. *Blood*. 2004;104:1923–1930.

Petersdorf EW, Malkki M. Human leukocyte antigen matching in unrelated-donor hematopoietic cell transplantation [review]. *Semin Hematol*. 2005;42:76–84.

Sasazuki T, Juji T, Morishima Y, et al. Effect of matching of class I HLA alleles on clinical outcome after transplantation of hematopoietic stem cells from an unrelated donor. Japan Marrow Donor Program [published correction appears in *N Engl J Med*. 1999;340:402]. *N Engl J Med*. 1998;339:1177–1185.

Cord blood

Armson BA. Umbilical cord blood banking: implications for perinatal care providers. *J Obstet Gynaecol Can*. 2005;27:263–290.

Barker JN, Rocha V, Scaradavou A. Optimizing unrelated donor cord blood transplantation. *Biol Blood Marrow Transplant*. 2008;15(1 Suppl):154–161.

Kurtzberg J. Update on umbilical cord blood transplantation. *Curr Opin Pediatr*. 2009;21:22–29.

Laughlin MJ, Barker J, Bambach B, et al. Hematopoietic engraftment and survival in adult recipients of umbilical-cord blood from unrelated donors. *N Engl J Med*. 2001;344:1815–1822.

Laughlin MJ, Eapen M, Rubinstein P, et al. Outcomes after transplantation of cord blood or bone marrow from unrelated donors in adults with leukemia. *N Engl J Med*. 2004;351:2265–2275.

Rocha V, Labopin M, Sanz G, et al. Acute Leukemia Working Party of European Blood and Marrow Transplant Group; Eurocord-Netcord Registry. Transplants of umbilical-cord blood or bone marrow from unrelated donors in adults with acute leukemia. *N Engl J Med*. 2004;351:2276–2285.

Schoemans H, Theunissen K, Maertens J, et al. Adult umbilical cord blood transplantation: a comprehensive review. *Bone Marrow Transplant*. 2006;38:83–93.

Yu LC, Wall DA, Sandler E, et al. Unrelated cord blood transplant experience by the pediatric blood and marrow transplant consortium. *Pediatr Hematol Oncol*. 2001;18:235–245.

Haploidentical transplantation

Koh LP, Chao N. Haploidentical hematopoietic cell transplantation. *Bone Marrow Transplant*. 2008;42(Suppl 1):S60–S63.

Peripheral blood versus marrow

Bensinger WI, Martin PJ, Storer B, et al. Transplantation of bone marrow as compared with peripheral-blood cells from HLA-identical relatives in patients with hematologic cancers. *N Engl J Med*. 2001;344:175–181.

Champlin RE, Schmitz N, Horowitz MM, et al. Blood stem cells compared with bone marrow as a source of hematopoietic cells for allogeneic transplantation. IBMTR Histocompatibility and Stem Cell Sources Working Committee and the European

Group for Blood and Marrow Transplantation (EBMT). *Blood.* 2000;95:3702–3709.

Eapen M, Horowitz MM, Klein JP, et al. Higher mortality after allogeneic peripheral-blood transplantation compared with bone marrow in children and adolescents: the Histocompatibility and Alternate Stem Cell Source Working Committee of the International Bone Marrow Transplant Registry. *J Clin Oncol.* 2004;22:4872–4880.

Eapen M, Logan BR, Confer DL, et al. Peripheral blood grafts from unrelated donors are associated with increased acute and chronic graft-versus-host disease without improved survival. *Biol Blood Marrow Transplant.* 2007;13:1461–1468.

Grupp SA, Frangoul H, Wall D, et al. Use of G-CSF in matched sibling donor pediatric allogeneic transplantation: a consensus statement from the Children's Oncology Group (COG) Transplant Discipline Committee and Pediatric Blood and Marrow Transplant Consortium (PBMTC) Executive Committee. *Pediatr Blood Cancer.* 2006;46:414–421.

National Marrow Donor Program (NMDP). Homepage. http://www.marrow.org. Accessed April 30, 2010.

Pulsipher MA, Levine JE, Hayashi RJ, et al. Safety and efficacy of allogeneic PBSC collection in normal pediatric donors: the pediatric blood and marrow transplant consortium experience (PBMTC) 1996–2003. *Bone Marrow Transplant.* 2005;35:361–367.

Ringden O, Remberger M, Runde V, et al. Peripheral blood stem cell transplantation from unrelated donors: a comparison with marrow transplantation. *Blood.* 1999;94:455–464.

Schmitz N, Eapen M, Horowitz MM, et al. Long-term outcome of patients transplanted with mobilized blood or bone marrow: a report from the International Bone Marrow Transplant Registry and the European Group for Blood and Marrow Transplantation. *Blood.* 2006;108:4288–4290.

Conditioning regimens

Craddock CF. Full-intensity and reduced-intensity allogeneic stem cell transplantation in AML. *Bone Marrow Transplant.* 2008;41:415–423.

Kim I, Yoon SS, Lee KH, et al. Comparative outcomes of reduced intensity and myeloablative allogeneic hematopoietic stem cell transplantation in patients under 50 with hematologic malignancies. *Clin Transplant.* 2006;20:496–503.

Schattenberg AV, Levenga TH. Differences between the different conditioning regimens for allogeneic stem cell transplantation. *Curr Opin Oncol.* 2006;18:667–670.

Complications

Graft-versus-host disease

Deeg HJ, Antin JH. The clinical spectrum of acute graft-versus-host disease. *Semin Hematol.* 2006;43:24–31.

Ferrara JL, Levine JE, Reddy P, Holler E. Graft-vs-host-disease. *Lancet.* 2009;373:1550–1561.

Filipovich AH. Diagnosis and manifestations of chronic graft-versus-host disease. *Best Pract Res Clin Haematol.* 2008;21:251–257.

Joseph RW, Couriel DR, Komanduri KV. Chronic graft-versus-host disease after allogeneic stem cell transplantation: challenges in prevention, science, and supportive care. *J Support Oncol.* 2008;6:361–372.

Martin PJ, Weisdorf D, Przepiorka D, et al. National Institutes of Health Consensus Development Project on Criteria for Clinical Trials in Chronic Graft-Versus-Host Disease: VI. Design of Clinical Trials Working Group report. *Biol Blood Marrow Transplant.* 2006;12:491–505.

Pavletic SZ, Martin P, Lee SJ, et al. Measuring therapeutic response in chronic graft-versus-host disease: National Institutes of Health Consensus Development Project on Criteria for Clinical Trials in Chronic Graft-Versus-Host Disease: IV. Response Criteria Working Group report. *Biol Blood Marrow Transplant.* 2006;12:252–266.

Schultz KR, Miklos DB, Fowler D, et al. Toward biomarkers for chronic graft-versus-host disease: National Institutes of Health Consensus Development Project on Criteria for Clinical Trials in Chronic Graft-Versus-Host Disease: III. Biomarker Working Group report. *Biol Blood Marrow Transplant.* 2006;12:126–137.

Infections

Boeckh M, Kim HW, Flowers ME, et al. Long-term acyclovir for prevention of varicella zoster virus disease after allogeneic hematopoietic cell transplantation—a randomized double-blind placebo-controlled study. *Blood.* 2006;107:1800–1805.

Centers for Disease Control and Prevention; Infectious Disease Society of America; American Society of Blood and Marrow Transplantation. Infection guidelines for preventing opportunistic infections among hematopoietic stem cell transplant recipients. *MMWR Recomm Rep.* 2000;49:1–125. *Important consensus statement.*

Hiemenz JW. Management of infections complicating allogeneic hematopoietic stem cell transplantation. *Semin Hematol.* 2009;46:289–312.

Ison MG. Respiratory syncytial virus and other respiratory viruses in the setting of bone marrow transplantation. *Curr Opin Oncol.* 2009;21:171–176.

Leung TF, Chik KW, Li CK, et al. Incidence, risk factors and outcome of varicella-zoster virus infection in children after haematopoietic stem cell transplantation. *Bone Marrow Transplant.* 2000;25:167–172.

Veno-occlusive disease

Ho V, Momtaz P, Didas C, et al. Post-transplant hepatic venoocclusive disease: pathogenesis, diagnosis and treatment. *Rev Clin Exp Hematol.* 2004;8:E3.

Ho VT, Revta C, Richardson PG. Hepatic veno-occlusive disease after hematopoietic stem cell transplantation: update on defibrotide and other current investigational therapies. *Bone Marrow Transplant.* 2008;41:229–237.

Thrombotic microangiopathy

Hale GA, Bowman LC, Rochester RJ, et al. Hemolytic uremic syndrome after bone marrow transplantation: clinical characteristics and outcome in children. *Biol Blood Marrow Transplant.* 2005;11:912–920.

Ho VT, Cutler C, Carter S, et al. Blood and marrow transplant clinical trials network toxicity committee consensus summary: thrombotic microangiopathy after hematopoietic stem cell transplantation. *Biol Blood Marrow Transplant.* 2005;11:571–575.

Hemorrhagic complications

Gorczynska E, Turkiewicz D, Rybka K, et al. Incidence, clinical outcome, and management of virus-induced hemorrhagic cystitis in children and adolescents after allogeneic hematopoietic cell transplantation. *Biol Blood Marrow Transplant.* 2005;11:797–804.

Hale GA, Rochester RJ, Heslop HE, et al. Hemorrhagic cystitis after allogeneic bone marrow transplantation in children: clinical characteristics and outcome. *Biol Blood Marrow Transplant.* 2003;9:698–705.

Pihusch M. Bleeding complications after hematopoietic stem cell transplantation [review]. *Semin Hematol.* 2004;41(Suppl 1): 93–100.

Pulmonary complications

Dudek AZ, Mahaseth H. Hematopoietic stem cell transplant-related airflow obstruction [review]. *Curr Opin Oncol.* 2006;18:115–119.

Kurland G, Michelson P. Bronchiolitis obliterans in children [review]. *Pediatr Pulmonol.* 2005;39:193–208.

Tichelli A, Rovó A, Gratwohl A. Late pulmonary, cardiovascular, and renal complications after hematopoietic stem cell transplantation and recommended screening practices. *Hematology Am Soc Hematol Educ Program.* 2008:125–133.

Watkins TR, Chien JW, Crawford SW. Graft versus host-associated pulmonary disease and other idiopathic pulmonary complications after hematopoietic stem cell transplant [review]. *Semin Respir Crit Care Med.* 2005;26: 482–489.

Yanik G, Cooke KR. The lung as a target organ of graft-versus-host disease [review]. *Semin Hematol.* 2006;43:42–52.

Genomic variation and iron overload

Armand P, Kim HT, Cutler CS, et al. Prognostic impact of elevated pretransplantation serum ferritin in patients undergoing myeloablative stem cell transplantation. *Blood.* 2007;109:4586–4588.

Holler E, Rogler G, Herfarth H, et al. Both donor and recipient NOD2/CARD15 mutations associate with transplant-related mortality and GvHD following allogeneic stem cell transplantation. *Blood.* 2004;104:889–894.

Majhail NS, Lazarus HM, Burns LJ. Iron overload in hematopoietic cell transplantation. *Bone Marrow Transplant.* 2008;41:997–1003.

Mullaly A, Ritz J. Beyond HLA: the significance of genomic variation for allogeneic hematopoietic stem cell transplantation. *Blood.* 2007;109:1355–1362.

Autologous stem cell sources and mobilization

Bensinger W, DiPersio JF, McCarty JM. Improving stem cell mobilization strategies: future directions. *Bone Marrow Transplant.* 2009;43:181–195.

DiPersio JF, Stadtmauer EA, Nademanee A, et al. Plerixafor and G-CSF versus placebo and G-CSF to mobilize hematopoietic stem cells for autologous stem cell transplantation in patients with multiple myeloma. *Blood.* 2009;113:5720–5726.

Pulsipher MA, Nagler A, Iannone R, et al. Weighing the risks of G-CSF administration, leukopheresis, and standard marrow harvest: ethical and safety considerations for normal pediatric hematopoietic cell donors [review]. *Pediatr Blood Cancer.* 2006;46:422–433.

Yaniv I, Cohen IJ, Stein J, et al. Tumor cells are present in stem cell harvests of Ewings sarcoma patients and their persistence following transplantation is associated with relapse. *Pediatr Blood Cancer.* 2004;42:404–409.

Graft-versus-leukemia effect and donor lymphocyte infusions

Horowitz MM, Gale RP, Sondel PM, et al. Graft-versus-leukemia reactions after bone marrow transplantation. *Blood.* 1990;75:555–562.

Porter D, Levine JE. Graft-versus-host disease and graft-versus-leukemia after donor leukocyte infusion [review]. *Semin Hematol.* 2006;43:53–61.

Schmid C, Labopin M, Nagler A, et al. Donor lymphocyte infusion in the treatment of first hematological relapse after allogeneic stem-cell transplantation in adults with acute myeloid leukemia: a retrospective risk factors analysis and comparison with other strategies by the EBMT Acute Leukemia Working Party. *J Clin Oncol.* 2007;25:4938–4945.

Syngeneic and autologous GVHD

Adams KM, Holmberg LA, Leisenring W, et al. Risk factors for syngeneic graft-versus-host disease after adult hematopoietic cell transplantation. *Blood.* 2004;104:1894–1897.

Bierman PJ, Sweetenham JW, Loberiza FR Jr, et al. Lymphoma Working Committee of the International Bone Marrow Transplant Registry and the European Group for Blood and Marrow Transplantation. Syngeneic hematopoietic stem-cell transplantation for non-Hodgkin's lymphoma: a comparison with allogeneic and autologous transplantation. *J Clin Oncol.* 2003;21:3744–3753.

Holmberg L, Kikuchi K, Gooley TA, et al. Gastrointestinal graft-versus-host disease in recipients of autologous hematopoietic stem cells: incidence, risk factors, and outcome. *Biol Blood Marrow Transplant.* 2006;12:226–234.

Late effects and long-term follow-up

Burns LJ. Late effects after autologous hematopoietic cell transplantation. *Biol Blood Marrow Transplant.* 2008;15 (Suppl 1):21–24.

Deeg HJ, Socie G. Malignancies after hematopoietic stem cell transplantation: many questions, some answers. *Blood.* 1998;91:1833–1844.

Rizzo JD, Wingard JR, Tichelli A, et al. Recommended screening and preventive practices for long-term survivors after hematopoietic cell transplantation: joint recommendations of the European Group for Blood and Marrow Transplantation, the Center for International Blood and Marrow Transplant Research, and the American Society of Blood and Marrow Transplantation. *Biol Blood Marrow Transplant.* 2006;12:138–151.

Tichelli A, Rovó A, Gratwohl A. Late pulmonary, cardiovascular, and renal complications after hematopoietic stem cell transplantation and recommended screening practices. *Hematology Am Soc Hematol Educ Program.* 2008:125–133.

Transplantation for specific diseases

Non-Hodgkin lymphoma

Barr PM, Lazarus HM. Follicular non-Hodgkin lymphoma: long-term results of stem-cell transplantation. *Curr Opin Oncol.* 2008;20:502–508.

Ghielmini M, Zucca E. How I treat mantle cell lymphoma. *Blood.* 2009;114:1469–1476.

Sandlund JT, Bowman L, Heslop HE, et al. Intensive chemotherapy with hematopoietic stem-cell support for children with recurrent or refractory NHL. *Cytotherapy.* 2002;4:253–258.

Schouten HC, Qian W, Kvaloy S, et al. High-dose therapy improves progression-free survival and survival in relapsed follicular non-Hodgkin's lymphoma: results from the randomized European CUP trial. *J Clin Oncol.* 2003;21:3918–3927.

Seshadri T, Kuruvilla J, Crump M, Keating A. Salvage therapy for relapsed/refractory diffuse large B cell lymphoma. *Biol Blood Marrow Transplant.* 2008;14:259–267.

Tam CS, Khouri IF. Autologous and allogeneic stem cell transplantation: rising therapeutic promise for mantle cell lymphoma. *Leuk Lymphoma.* 2009;26:1–10.

Hodgkin disease

Brice P. Managing relapsed and refractory Hodgkin lymphoma. *Br J Haematol.* 2008;141:3–13.

Laport GG. Allogeneic hematopoietic cell transplantation for Hodgkin lymphoma: a concise review. *Leuk Lymphoma.* 2008;49:1854–1859.

Lieskovsky YE, Donaldson SS, Torres MA, et al. High-dose therapy and autologous hematopoietic stem-cell transplantation for recurrent or refractory pediatric Hodgkin's disease: results and prognostic indices. *J Clin Oncol.* 2004;22:4532–4540.

Plasma cell dyscrasias

Dispenzieri A. POEMS syndrome. *Hematology Am Soc Hematol Educ Program.* 2005:360–367.

Harousseau JL, Moreau P. Autologous hematopoietic stem cell transplantation for multiple myeloma. *N Engl J Med.* 2009;360:2645–2654.

Kumar SK, Rajkumar SV, Dispenzieri A, et al. Improved survival in multiple myeloma and the impact of novel therapies. *Blood.* 2008;111:2516–2520.

Mhaskar R, Kumar A, Behera M, Kharfan-Dabaja MA, Djulbegovic B. Role of high-dose chemotherapy and autologous hematopoietic cell transplantation in primary systemic amyloidosis: a systematic review. *Biol Blood Marrow Transplant.* 2009;15:893–902.

Acute myelogenous leukemia

Hamadani M, Awan FT, Copelan EA. Hematopoietic stem cell transplantation in adults with acute myeloid leukemia. *Biol Blood Marrow Transplant.* 2008;14:556–567.

Schlenk RF, Döhner K, Krauter J, et al. Mutations and treatment outcome in cytogenetically normal acute myeloid leukemia. *N Engl J Med.* 2008;358:1909–1918.

Shenoy S, Smith FO. Hematopoietic stem cell transplantation for childhood malignancies of myeloid origin. *Bone Marrow Transplant.* 2008;41:141–148.

Tallman MS, Pérez WS, Lazarus HM, et al. Pretransplantation consolidation chemotherapy decreases leukemia relapse after autologous blood and bone marrow transplants for acute myelogenous leukemia in first remission. *Biol Blood Marrow Transplant.* 2006;12:204–216.

Woods WG, Neudorf S, Gold S, et al. A comparison of allogeneic bone marrow transplantation, autologous bone marrow transplantation, and aggressive chemotherapy in children with acute myeloid leukemia in remission. *Blood.* 2001;97:56–62.

Acute lymphoblastic leukemia

Eapen M, Raetz E, Zhang MJ, et al. Outcomes after HLA-matched sibling transplantation or chemotherapy in children with B-precursor acute lymphoblastic leukemia in a second remission: a collaborative study of the Children's Oncology Group and the Center for International Blood and Marrow Transplant Research. *Blood.* 2006;107:4961–4967.

Gaynon PS, Harris RE, Altman AJ, et al. Bone marrow transplantation versus prolonged intensive chemotherapy for children with acute lymphoblastic leukemia and an initial bone marrow relapse within 12 months of the completion of primary therapy: Children's Oncology Group Study CCG-1941. *J Clin Oncol.* 2006;24:3150–3156.

Goldstone AH, Richards SM, Lazarus HM, et al. In adults with standard-risk acute lymphoblastic leukemia, the greatest benefit is achieved from a matched sibling allogeneic transplantation in first complete remission, and an autologous transplantation is less effective than conventional consolidation/maintenance chemotherapy in all patients: final results of the International ALL Trial (MRC UKALL XII/ECOG E2993). *Blood.* 2008;111:1827–1833.

Hahn T, Wall D, Camitta B, et al. The role of cytotoxic therapy with hematopoietic stem cell transplantation in the therapy of acute lymphoblastic leukemia in adults: an evidence-based review [review]. *Biol Blood Marrow Transplant.* 2006;12:1–30.

Krance RA. Transplantation for children with acute lymphoblastic leukemia. *Bone Marrow Transplantation.* 2008;42:S25–S27.

Moorman AV, Harrison CJ, Buck GA, et al. Karyotype is an independent prognostic factor in adult acute lymphoblastic leukemia (ALL): analysis of cytogenetic data from patients treated on the Medical Research Council (MRC) UKALLXII/Eastern Cooperative Oncology Group (ECOG) 2993 trial. *Blood.* 2007;109:3189–3197.

Rowe JM. Optimal management of adults with ALL. *Br J Haematol.* 2009;144:468–483.

Chronic myelogenous leukemia and chronic lymphocytic leukemia

Goldman JM. How I treat chronic myeloid leukemia in the imatinib era. *Blood.* 2007;110:2828–2837.

Gribben JG. Stem cell transplantation in chronic lymphocytic leukemia. *Biol Bone Marrow Transplant.* 2009;15:53–58.

Lee SJ, Kukreja M, Wang T, et al. Impact of prior imatinib mesylate on the outcome of hematopoietic cell transplantation for chronic myeloid leukemia. *Blood.* 2008;112:3500–3507.

Maziarz RT. Who with chronic myelogenous leukemia to transplant in the era of tyrosine kinase inhibitors? *Curr Opin Hematol.* 2008;15:127–133.

Milojkovic D, Apperly J. State of the art in the treatment of chronic myelogenous leukemia. *Curr Opin Hematol.* 2008;20:112–121.

Sorror ML, Storer BE, Sandmaier BM, et al. Five-year follow-up of patients with advanced chronic lymphocytic leukemia treated with allogeneic hematopoietic cell transplantation after nonmyeloablative conditioning. *J Clin Oncol.* 2008;26:4912–4920.

Autoimmune diseases and aplastic anemia

Brodsky RA, Jones RJ. Aplastic anaemia. *Lancet.* 2005;365:1647–1656.

Griffith LM, Pavletic SZ, Tyndall A, et al. Feasibility of allogeneic hematopoietic stem cell transplantation for autoimmune disease: position statement from a National Institute of Allergy and Infectious Diseases and National Cancer Institute-Sponsored International Workshop, Bethesda, MD, March 12 and 13, 2005. *Biol Blood Marrow Transplant.* 2005;11:862–870.

Kurre P, Johnson FL, Deeg HJ. Diagnosis and treatment of children with aplastic anemia. *Pediatr Blood Cancer.* 2005;45:770–780.

Hemoglobinopathies/thalassemia

Bolanos-Meade J, Brodsky RA. Blood and marrow transplantation for sickle cell disease: overcoming barriers to success. *Curr Opin Oncol.* 2009;21:158–161.

Gaziev J, Lucarelli G. Stem cell transplantation and gene therapy for hemoglobinopathies. *Curr Hematol Rep.* 2005;4:126–131.

Gaziev J, Sodani P, Polchi P, et al. Bone marrow transplantation in adults with thalassemia: treatment and long-term follow-up. *Ann NY Acad Sci.* 2005;1054:196–205.

Immune deficiencies

Bielorai B, Trakhtenbrot L, Amariglio N, et al. Multilineage hematopoietic engraftment after allogeneic peripheral blood stem cell transplantation without conditioning in SCID patients. *Bone Marrow Transplant.* 2004;34:317–320.

Buckley RH, Schiff SE, Schiff RI, et al. Hematopoietic stem-cell transplantation for the treatment of severe combined immunodeficiency. *N Engl J Med.* 1999;340:508–516.

Grunebaum E, Mazzolari E, Porta F, et al. Bone marrow transplantation for severe combined immune deficiency. *JAMA.* 2006;295:508–518.

Veys P, Rao K, Amrolia P. Stem cell transplantation for congenital immunodeficiencies using reduced-intensity conditioning. *Bone Marrow Transplant.* 2005;35(Suppl 1):S45–S47.

Metabolic disorders

Peters C, Steward CG. Hematopoietic cell transplantation for inherited metabolic diseases: an overview of outcomes and practice guidelines. *Bone Marrow Transplant.* 2003;31:229–239.

Adult solid tumors

Einhorn LH, Williams SD, Chamness A, et al. High-dose chemotherapy and stem-cell rescue for metastatic germ-cell tumors. *N Engl J Med.* 2007;357:340–348.

Pediatric solid tumors

Fish JD, Grupp SA. Stem cell transplantation for neuroblastoma. *Bone Marrow Transplant.* 2008;41:159–165.

Hale GA. Autologous hematopoietic stem cell transplantation for pediatric solid tumors. *Expert Rev Anticancer Ther.* 2005;5:835–846.

Gardner SL, Carreras J, Boudreau C, et al. Myeloablative therapy with autologous stem cell rescue for patients with Ewing sarcoma. *Bone Marrow Transplant.* 2008;41:867–872.

Ladenstein R, Potschgr U, Hartman O, et al. 28 years of high-dose therapy and SCT for neuroblastoma in Europe: lessons from more than 4000 procedures. *Bone Marrow Transplant.* 2008;41:S118–S127.

Matthay KK, Villablanca JG, Seeger RC, et al. Treatment of high-risk neuroblastoma with intensive chemotherapy, radiotherapy, autologous bone marrow transplantation, and 13-cos-retinoic acid. Children's Cancer Group. *N Engl J Med.* 1999;341:1165–1173.

CHAPTER 13

Myeloid disorders

Daniel C. Link and Geoffrey L. Uy

Granulocytes: neutrophils, eosinophils, and basophils, 373
Monocytes and tissue histiocytes, 375
Dendritic cells, 376
Neutrophilia, 376
Neutropenia, 378
Disorders of neutrophil function, 385
Monocytosis, 388
Monocytopenia, 388
Disorders of histiocytes and DCs, 388
Lysosomal storage diseases, 392
Bibliography, 394

The term "myeloid" derives from the Greek *myelos*, meaning "marrow." Sometimes the term "myeloid" is used to describe hematologic conditions or diseases not involving the lymphoid tissues or lymphocytes. "Myeloid" is also used to describe disorders primarily involving granulocytes (neutrophils, eosinophils, or basophils) and monocytes. Tissue macrophages (histiocytes), Langerhans cells, and interdigitating dendritic cells also arise from monocytic progenitors or precursors. Other important immunoregulatory dendritic cell types and mast cells derive from marrow progenitors that are distinct from myeloid and monocytic progenitors. This chapter covers disorders of granulocytes, monocytes, histiocytes, and dendritic cells. The myeloproliferative disorders (ie, the clonal disorders of myeloid origin), including polycythemia vera, essential thrombocytosis, idiopathic myelofibrosis/myeloid metaplasia, systemic mastocytosis, and chronic myelogenous leukemia, are described in Chapter 14.

Granulocytes: neutrophils, eosinophils, and basophils

The term *granulocytes* refers to circulating neutrophils, eosinophils, and basophils, although because of their predominance in the blood, the terms *neutrophil* and *granulocyte* are sometimes used synonymously. The names for these cells originated with the work of a medical student, Paul Ehrlich. In 1877, he developed the system of aniline dyes that allowed the clear definition of the nucleus, cytoplasm, and other features of white blood cells, as examined on dried films on glass slides. Counting and carefully examining white blood cells on stained blood films remain cornerstones for diagnosing many infectious, inflammatory, and malignant diseases. Normal values for the differential count for leukocytes in the blood are shown in Table 13-1.

Neutrophils are a critical component of the innate immune response, and persistent neutropenia is associated with a marked susceptibility to infection. Conversely, there is increasing evidence that neutrophils may be a major contributor to tissue damage in inflammatory diseases. Thus, regulation of the level of blood neutrophils may be important in controlling both infectious and inflammatory diseases. Neutrophil homeostasis in the blood is regulated at 3 levels: neutrophil production in the bone marrow (granulopoiesis), neutrophil release from the bone marrow to blood, and neutrophil clearance from the blood (Figure 13-1).

Granulopoiesis

Under normal conditions, neutrophils are produced exclusively in the bone marrow, where it is estimated that 10^{12} are generated on a daily basis. Granulocytic differentiation of hematopoietic stem cells is regulated by the coordinated expression of a number of key myeloid transcription factors, including PU.1, CCAAT enhancer binding protein α (C/EBPα), C/EBPε, and GFI-1. A number of hematopoietic growth factors provide extrinsic signals that regulate granulopoiesis (see Chapter 3). The most important of these is granulocyte colony-stimulating factor (G-CSF), which stimulates the proliferation of granulocytic precursors, reduces the average transit time through the granulocytic

Conflict-of-interest disclosure: *Dr. Link* declares no competing financial interest. *Dr. Uy:* consultancy: Genzyme; research funding: Genzyme, Novartis Oncology; honoraria: Novartis Oncology; speakers' bureau: Genzyme.

Table 13-1 Normal leukocyte values in peripheral blood.

A, Adults

Cell type	Cells/μL*	
	Median	Range
All leukocytes (white blood cells)	7000	4300–10,000
Total neutrophils	4000	1800–7200
Band neutrophils	500	100–2000
Segmented neutrophils	3500	1000–6000
Lymphocytes	2500	1500–4000
Monocytes	450	200–900
Eosinophils	150	0–700
Basophils	30	0–150

*To calculate the number of cells per liter, multiply by 10^6.

B, Children

Age	All leukocytes (cells/μL)	Neutrophils	Lymphocytes	Monocytes	Eosinophils
Neonate	9000–38,000 (range)	5000–28,000	2000–11,500	1100–1200	400–500
1 week to 1 month	5000–21,000	1000–10,000	2000–17,000	700–1100	300–500
6 months to 2 years	6000–17,500	1000–8500	3000–13,500	500–600	300
4 to 8 years	4500–15,500	1500–8500	1500–8000	400–500	200–300
10 to 16 years	4500–13,500	1800–8000	1200–6500	400	200

Adult data: Copyright 2001 WebMD Corp. All rights reserved. From Scientific American Medicine, WebMD Corp., 2002. Pediatric data: Adapted from Geaghan SM. Normal blood values: selected reference values of neonatal, pediatric, and adult populations. In: Hoffman R, Benz EJ, Shattil SJ, et al, eds. *Hematology Basic Principles and Practice*. 3rd ed. Philadelphia, PA: Churchill Livingstone; 1999.

compartment, and stimulates neutrophil release from the bone marrow. As discussed later, disruption of normal granulopoiesis is a common cause of congenital and acquired neutropenia.

Neutrophil release

Neutrophils, under normal conditions, are produced solely in the bone marrow and are released into the blood in a regulated fashion to maintain homeostatic levels of circulating neutrophils. The bone marrow provides a large reservoir of mature neutrophils that can be readily mobilized in response to infection. A broad range of substances has been shown to induce neutrophil release from the bone marrow, including chemokines, cytokines, microbial products, and various other inflammatory mediators (eg, C5a). Recent evidence suggests that the chemokine stromal derived factor-1 (SDF1, CXCL12) plays a key role in regulating neutrophil trafficking in the bone marrow; this issue will be discussed in detail in the section on WHIM syndrome.

Neutrophil clearance

Neutrophil homeostasis in the blood is determined, in part, by the rate of clearance from the circulation. Once released into the circulation, neutrophils are rapidly cleared with a half-life of only 6 to 8 hours. Neutrophils are cleared primarily in the liver, spleen, or bone marrow, where apoptotic or aged neutrophils are thought to be phagocytosed by macrophages. Recent studies suggest that CXCR4 may play a role in the clearance of aged, senescent neutrophils, particularly at bone marrow sites.

Neutrophil extravasation

Neutrophils in the circulation loosely attach and subsequently adhere to vascular endothelium in response to the local production of inflammatory cytokines and chemokines (Figure 13-1). Selectins mediate neutrophil rolling and β_2-integrins mediate firm adherence and vascular transmigration. Indeed, deficiency of selectin ligands or β_2-integrins causes leukocyte adhesion deficiency, a rare syndrome manifested by normal neutrophil production but impaired emigration to sites of inflammation.

Once emigrated to the inflammatory site, neutrophils function primarily as tissue phagocytes. These vital functions depend on several critical features of these cells. Surface receptors for immunoglobulins and complement enhance ingestion and killing of microorganisms. Within the cell, the reduced nicotinamide adenine dinucleotide phosphate (NADPH) oxidase system, enzymes found in the cell's primary and secondary granules, and cytoplasmic glycogen are involved in the intracellular oxidative burst that accompanies phagocytosis and in the killing

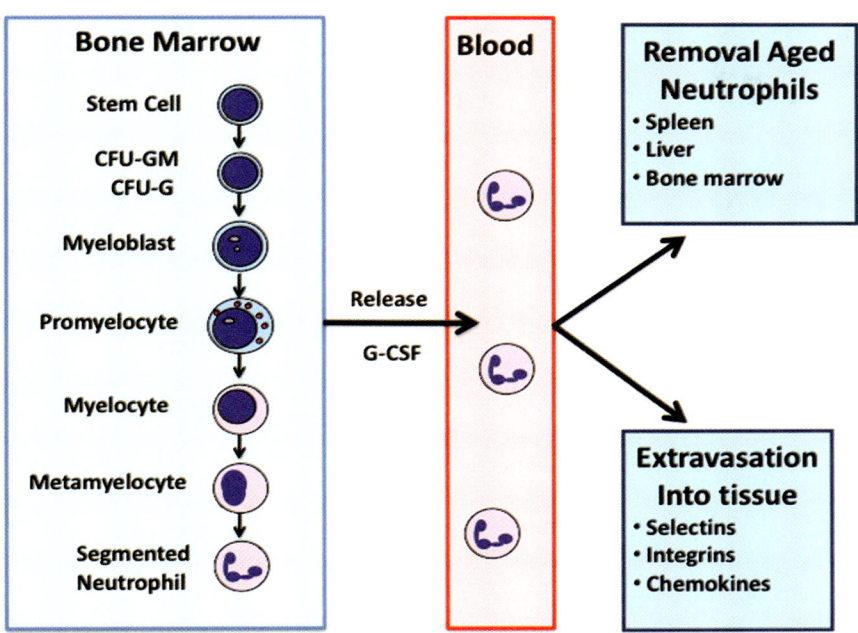

Figure 13-1 Neutrophil homeostasis. The bone marrow is the primary site of granulopoiesis in humans. Under basal conditions, the bone marrow contains a large reservoir of mature neutrophil. Neutrophils are released into the circulation in a regulated fashion. The principal cytokine regulating both granulopoiesis and neutrophil release into the blood is granulocyte colony-stimulating factor (G-CSF). Neutrophils in the circulation have 2 general fates. In response to local infection or inflammation, neutrophils can emigrate into tissue. Neutrophil emigration is a highly orchestrated process that includes sensing of chemokine gradients, selectin-mediated rolling on inflamed endothelium, and integrin-mediated adhesion and diapedesis through the endothelium. Alternatively, senescent (aged) neutrophils are cleared from the circulation primarily by the macrophages in the spleen, liver, and bone marrow. CFU-G = colony-forming unit–granulocyte; CFU-GM = colony-forming unit–granulocyte macrophage.

and digesting of microorganisms. Maintenance of both the supply of cells and the integrity of all of these functions is critical for normal host defense mechanisms. Diseases affecting each of these features and functions of neutrophils result in enhanced susceptibility to infection (see discussion later in chapter).

Normally, the marrow contains a very small proportion of eosinophils and basophils. The granules of eosinophils contain histamine and proteins important for the killing of parasites. Eosinophil production is increased and eosinophilia (ie, $>0.7 \times 10^9$/L) occurs in many allergic disorders (ie, asthma, allergic rhinitis, dermatitis), parasitic infections, collagen vascular diseases, and drug reactions. Eosinophilia also frequently occurs with myeloproliferative disorders and is the hallmark feature of the hypereosinophilic syndrome, a disorder characterized by autonomous eosinophil production with end-organ or tissue complications (see Chapter 14). Basophils are the least numerous blood leukocytes. Basophilic granules contain histamine, glycosaminoglycans, major basic protein, proteases, and a variety of other vasoactive inflammatory mediators. Basophils primarily function to activate the immediate (type 1) hypersensitivity responses. Increases in basophils are associated with hypersensitivity reactions including drug and food allergies. Basophilia has been reported with some chronic inflammatory diseases, such as tuberculosis, ulcerative colitis, and rheumatoid arthritis, but these reactions are quite rare. The most important association of basophilia is with myeloproliferative disorders, particularly chronic myeloid leukemia.

Monocytes and tissue histiocytes

Monocytes share their origin and functions with neutrophils. They are phagocytes, ingesting and killing microorganisms. Monocytes also may become the fixed phagocytic cells that line portions of the circulation, particularly in the spleen and liver. In these tissues, their role is to clear particulate matter, including microorganisms, and aged or damaged blood cells from the circulation. They are also an important source of inflammatory cytokines (eg, tumor necrosis factor, interleukin 1, interferon-γ) that cause fever and many of the symptoms associated with infectious and inflammatory diseases. Monocytes can differentiate to tissue histiocytes, and these cells may then fuse to form giant cells, as occurs in tuberculosis and sarcoidosis. Alveolar macrophages in the lung, Kupffer cells in the liver, and osteoclasts and phagocytic cells in reticuloendothelial tissue are all forms of tissue histiocytes that are thought to derive from blood monocytes or, in some cases, from circulating monocyte progenitors. These phagocytic cells not only serve antimicrobial, scavenger, and secretory functions, but they also participate in wound repair and antigen processing and presentation. Chronic inflammatory states may increase monocytes in the blood and the tissues. Transient monocytopenia occurs with stress and infections. In aplastic anemia and hairy cell leukemia, monocyte numbers are suppressed, but circulating monocyte counts and function are maintained in many other conditions that cause neutropenia. Inappropriate overstimulation of tissue macrophages, usually in the setting of infectious stimuli with or without underlying acquired or congenital immune dysregulation, may contribute to the sepsis-associated systemic inflammatory response syndrome and/or can lead to a severe pathologic disorder called hemophagocytic syndrome (see later discussion).

Dendritic cells

Dendritic cells (DCs) are a heterogeneous group of hematopoietic-derived cells that are critical participants in innate and adaptive immune responses. These cells are widely distributed throughout virtually all tissue types and, in particular, lymphoid organs and organs with barrier function such as the skin and mucosal surfaces. A major function of DCs is to process and present antigen to the immune system. Immature DCs in the peripheral tissue express a number of surface receptors, which allow them to recognize and take up extracellular antigens in their environment via mechanisms including phagocytosis, pinocytosis, and receptor-mediated endocytosis. Upon encountering antigen, immature DCs undergo activation and maturation and migrate to secondary lymphoid organs where they bind and present antigen in the context of major histocompatibility complex (MHC) class I and II molecules to stimulate naive T cells. Mature DCs also produce a number of cytokines, which can prime T cells toward either a T_H1 versus T_H2 response. In addition, DCs possess a number of other immunomodulatory functions including the activation of other lymphocyte subsets and induction of immune tolerance. Specific DC subsets have been identified and characterized based on their location, cell surface phenotype, function, or developmental stage. The ability of DCs to present tumor antigens has led to their use in vaccine immunotherapy trials. An important pathologic condition of DCs is Langerhans cell histiocytosis, an acquired clonal disorder that can lead to local or systemic tissue infiltration and organ failure.

Neutrophilia

> **Clinical case**
>
> A 50-year-old businessman is seen because of knee and foot pain of 2 weeks in duration. Physical examination is normal, except for tenderness of the proximal metatarsal joint of the right first toe and swelling of the right knee. On further questioning, the knee swelling may be due to a recent injury playing handball. Laboratory examination shows a white blood cell count of 18×10^9/L, with an absolute neutrophil count (ANC) of 16×10^9/L. Blood counts on previous annual physical examinations were normal.

Neutrophilia is defined as an ANC >2 standard deviations above the mean or, in adults, >7700 neutrophils/μL. Neutrophilia is associated with many different types of stress, including recent exercise, infection, and inflammatory diseases (Table 13-2). A prompt increase in the blood neutrophil count, as well as the circulating levels of other leukocytes, occurs with acute stress, exercise, anxiety (including visits to a physician), and epinephrine administration. Only rarely does this response more than double the count. It is attributable to demargination of cells, not to the release of cells from the marrow reserve. Normally, approximately one half of the neutrophils in the circulation are loosely adherent to blood vessels and not counted in a routine blood count. These cells are described as being in the marginal pool. The other half of the neutrophils are circulating freely with the red cells and platelets. They are described as being in the circulating pool.

Neutrophilia associated with infections and inflammatory disorders occurs by 2 general mechanisms. First, during infection, a number of inflammatory cytokines are released into the circulation that induce the release of mature neutrophils from the bone marrow. Second, the sustained cytokine response associated with infections may stimulate neutrophil production in the bone marrow. In contrast to neutrophil demargination, neutrophilia associated with infections and inflammatory disorders is marked by the presence of an increase in immature granulocytes in the blood, mostly comprising band forms but also including metamyelocytes and occasionally early granulocytic precursors. In addition, there often is a change in the morphology of neutrophils with the appearance of vacuoles and "toxic granulation," due to more intense staining of the primary granules of neutrophils. Cells released prematurely also may contain bits of endoplasmic reticulum that stain as blue bodies in the cytoplasm, called *Döhle bodies* (Figure 13-2). In patients with neutrophilia, it is helpful to examine a blood smear to look for these changes.

Table 13-4 Genetic causes of congenital neutropenia.

Syndrome	Genetics
Severe congenital neutropenia (AD)	*ELA2* (sporadic and AD), *GFI*, *CSF3R*
Autosomal recessive	*HAX1*; *G6PC3*
X-linked recessive	WAS
Cyclic neutropenia	*ELA2*
WHIM syndrome/myelokathexis	*CXCR4*
Shwachman-Diamond syndrome	*SBDS*
Barth syndrome	*TAZ*
Glycogen storage disease type Ib	*G6PT1*
Cartilage-hair hypoplasia	*RMRP*
Pearson syndrome	Variable mitochondrial DNA deletions
Dyskeratosis congenita	*DKC1* (XL), *TERC* (AD)
Neutropenia associated with impaired vesicular transport	
Chédiak-Higashi syndrome	*LYST*
Griscelli syndrome, type II	*RAB27A*
Hermansky-Pudlak syndrome, type II	*AP3B1*
p14 deficiency	*MAPBPIP*
Cohen syndrome	*VPS13B*
Neutropenia associated with primary immunodeficiency	
Hyper IgM syndrome	*HIGM1*, *IKBKG* (XL), *AICDA* (AR)
X-linked agammaglobulinemia	*BTK* (XL)
Reticular dysgenesis	*AK2*

AD = autosomal dominant; AR = autosomal recessive; XL = X-linked.

Severe congenital neutropenia (SCN) is a heterogeneous group of disorders first described in an extended consanguineous family by the Swedish physician Rolf Kostmann. Thus, the disease has also been known as Kostmann syndrome, although this eponym has since been used to define a subset of patients with autosomal recessively inherited SCN. SCN is characterized by severe neutropenia present at birth with ANCs generally <200 cells/μL. The bone marrow typically shows an arrest in myeloid maturation with an accumulation of promyelocytes or myelocytes. Other hematologic parameters are generally normal, although peripheral monocytosis and increase in bone marrow eosinophils are often observed.

SCN demonstrates multiple modes of inheritance, including autosomal recessive, autosomal dominant, X-linked, and sporadic patterns. Accordingly, recent genetic studies have identified multiple gene mutations in SCN, including *ELA2*, *GFI1*, *CSF3R*, *WASP*, *HAX1*, and *G6PC3*. A recent study of patients with SCN enrolled in the North American Severe Chronic Neutropenia International Registry (SCNIR) reported that 90 (56%) of 162 patients had mutations of *ELA2* (all in autosomal dominant or sporadic SCN). Collectively, mutations of *GFI1*, *CSF3R*, *WASP*, *HAX1*, and *G6PC3* were detected in only 5% of patients. Thus, in nearly 40% of cases, the genetic basis of SCN remains unknown. Based on these data, it is recommended that *ELA2* genotyping be performed in all patients with suspected SCN. For SCN patients with an autosomal recessive pattern of inheritance, *HAX1* and *G6PC3* genotyping also should be considered.

As noted earlier, by far the most common mutations affect the *ELA2* gene encoding neutrophil elastase. To date, 73 different, mostly missense, *ELA2* mutations have been identified in patients with SCN. Recent studies suggest that these *ELA2* mutations may disrupt granulopoiesis through induction of the unfolded protein response. In this model, the shared feature of the *ELA2* mutations is the production of misfolded neutrophil elastase protein that induces endoplasmic reticulum stress, activation of the unfolded protein response, and ultimately induction of apoptosis of neutrophil precursors.

Historically, affected patients had a poor prognosis and often succumbed in the first or second decade of life with recurrent severe bacterial infections. The use of G-CSF has changed the natural history of this disease; the results of a randomized phase III trial comparing G-CSF with no treatment in patients with SCN demonstrated that the majority (>90%) of patients had a significant increase in circulating levels of neutrophils and reduction in the incidence and severity of bacterial infections. There is substantial patient-to-patient variability in the dose of G-CSF that is required to achieve an acceptable neutrophil count, with some children requiring only 1 to 2 μg/kg on alternate days and others only responding to doses of

25 to 50 μg/kg/d. Recognized adverse effects of chronic G-CSF therapy include splenomegaly, bone pain, vasculitis, and osteoporosis.

With longer survival and close observation, it has become clear that congenital neutropenia is a preleukemic disorder. A recent update of the SCNIR showed that the cumulative incidence of myelodysplastic syndrome (MDS) or acute myeloid leukemia (AML) was 21%. The hazard rate for AML/MDS increases with time, reaching 8% per year in patients on G-CSF therapy for 12 years. Patients less responsive to G-CSF (defined as an ANC of <2188/μL after 6 months of treatment) are at the highest risk of developing AMD/MDS, with a cumulative risk at 10 years of 40%. It should be emphasized that there is no definitive proof that G-CSF directly contributes to leukemic transformation. Indeed, reports of AML/MDS in SCN predate the use of G-CSF. Moreover, myeloid malignancies are rare in children and adults with cyclic neutropenia despite many years of G-CSF treatment (see later discussion on cyclic neutropenia). Thus, the contribution of G-CSF to the development of AML/MDS in patients with SCN remains controversial, and therapy with G-CSF should not be withheld from newly diagnosed patients on this basis. Additional studies have addressed the molecular lesions that are associated with transformation to MDS/AML in patients with SCN. The most fascinating of these is the acquisition of somatic mutations in the G-CSF receptor, which truncate the carboxyl terminus. Monosomy 7 is also common in the bone marrows of patients with MDS and AML, and some cases also show *RAS* mutations. Based on the risk of leukemic transformation in SCN, patients should receive the lowest dose of G-CSF that is required to maintain an acceptable neutrophil count and should undergo yearly bone marrow examinations with cytogenetic analysis.

Hematopoietic stem cell transplantation (HSCT) from a human leukocyte antigen (HLA)-identical sibling is potentially curative for patients with SCN who are refractory to G-CSF treatment. A more difficult question involves when to perform transplantation in SCN patients who are doing well on G-CSF and have an HLA-matched sibling donor. The limited published data indicate that transplantation cures a high percentage of patients with neutropenia only but is usually ineffective in children who have progressed to MDS/AML. Patients who acquire a G-CSF receptor mutation or are less responsive to G-CSF (see previous discussion) appear to have an elevated risk of developing MDS or AML, and this may prove useful for identifying children who should receive transplantation. However, no prospective data exist that address this question. HSCT from unrelated donors is not recommended for patients with SCN who are doing well on G-CSF treatment.

Cyclic neutropenia

> ### Clinical case
>
> A 2½-year-old boy is seen because of frequent fevers, mouth sores, and treatment for recurrent pharyngitis and otitis. The symptoms occur approximately every 3 weeks. The patient's mother had similar problems as a child, which seemed to get better in her late teenage years. The patient has a temperature of 38.7°C with inflamed gingivae and a large ulcer on the tip of his tongue. Cervical lymph nodes are enlarged; the abdomen is slightly tender. The rest of the examination is normal. The white blood cell count is 3.5×10^9/L, and the ANC is 0.

Cyclic neutropenia (CN) is a disorder of granulopoiesis characterized by 21-day oscillations in the number of circulating neutrophils. In CN patients, neutrophil counts often fluctuate between normal or near-normal levels and <200/μL. The diagnosis of CN should be considered in patients with recurrent fever, mouth sores, and upper respiratory infections. Usually these symptoms recur at regular, 3-week intervals. CN is diagnosed by serial blood counts. The "up" time of neutrophils is usually much shorter than the "down" time. Therefore, counts 2 or 3 times a week for at least 6 weeks are required to be sure of the diagnosis. CN is usually diagnosed as a sporadic or (in approximately one third of cases) an autosomal dominantly inherited disorder in young children who are healthy at birth but soon thereafter begin to have recurrent respiratory illnesses. These children may be treated as having recurrent viral or bacterial infections before serial blood counts are performed. The differential diagnosis in this case includes CN, SCN, autoimmune neutropenia, and idiopathic neutropenia. Rare acquired cases of adult-onset CN (or cyclic hematopoiesis) have been reported in association with clonal T-lymphocyte disorders, Crohn disease, pregnancy, and exposure to radiation or certain drugs.

Although not required to make the diagnosis, serial marrow examinations in CN show periodic interruptions of cell production, with arrest of development at the promyelocyte stage during the first days of severe neutropenia with each cycle. Over the next few days, hematopoietic recovery occurs with appearance of a complete complement of cells of the neutrophil lineage.

Recent genetic studies have identified mutations of the *ELA2* gene in nearly all patients with CN. Consequently, genetic testing for *ELA2* mutations is a valuable diagnostic tool. As noted earlier, *ELA2* mutations also are found in the majority of patients with SCN, suggesting that CN and SCN are related and fall along a continuum of disorders of granulopoiesis. Interestingly, the amino acid substitutions

Table 13-2 Causes of neutrophilia.

Acute neutrophilia	Chronic neutrophilia
Infections	*Infections*
Many localized and systemic, acute bacterial, mycotic, rickettsial, spirochetal, and certain viral infections	Persistence of many infections associated with acute neutrophilia
Inflammation or tissue necrosis	*Inflammation*
Burns, electric shock, trauma, infarction, gout, vasculitis, antigen–antibody complexes, complement activation	Continuation of most acute inflammatory reactions, such as rheumatoid arthritis, gout, chronic vasculitis, myositis, nephritis, colitis, pancreatitis, dermatitis, thyroiditis, drug-sensitivity reactions, periodontitis, Sweet syndrome, familial periodic fever syndromes
Physical or emotional stimuli	*Tumors*
Cold, heat, exercise, convulsions, pain, labor, anesthesia, surgery, panic, rage, severe stress, depression	Gastric, bronchogenic, breast, renal, hepatic, pancreatic, uterine, and squamous cell cancers; rarely, Hodgkin disease, lymphoma, brain tumors, melanoma, and multiple myeloma
Drugs, hormones, and toxins	*Drugs, hormones, and toxins*
Epinephrine, etiocholanolone, endotoxin, glucocorticoids, venoms, vaccines, colony-stimulating factors	Continued exposure to many substances that produce acute neutrophilia; lithium; rarely, as a reaction to other drugs
Hereditary and congenital disorders	*Metabolic and endocrinologic disorders*
Down syndrome, familial Mediterranean fever, leukocyte adhesion deficiency	Eclampsia, thyroid storm, overproduction of adrenocorticotropic hormone or glucocorticoids
	Hematologic disorders
	Rebound from agranulocytosis or therapy of megaloblastic anemia, chronic hemolysis or hemorrhage, asplenia, myeloproliferative disorders, chronic neutrophilic leukemia

Adapted from Dale DC. Neutropenia and neutrophilia. In: Williams WJ, et al, eds. *Hematology*. 6th ed. New York, NY: McGraw-Hill; 2001:823–834.

Neutrophilia is also a feature of the myeloproliferative syndromes, particularly chronic myeloid leukemia (CML) and chronic neutrophilic leukemia. Other than molecular testing (Chapter 14), there are no diagnostic tests that will definitively distinguish reactive neutrophilia from a myeloproliferative disorder, but there are certain clinical features that are highly suggestive. Most importantly, in most cases of reactive neutrophilia, the inciting infection (or other stress) is usually clinically obvious, and the neutrophilia is self-limited. In addition, the presence of splenomegaly, leukoerythroblastic features on the blood smear (tear drop and nucleated red blood cells), basophilia, or circulating promyelocytes or blasts is suggestive of a myeloproliferative disorder and may merit further evaluation. Finally, although molecular testing for the *BCR-ABL* fusion gene is the test of choice, measurement of leukocyte alkaline phosphatase, which is high in reactive neutrophilia but usually low in CML, may be helpful in some cases. In the patient described earlier in the clinical case, the uric acid level was high, leading to the

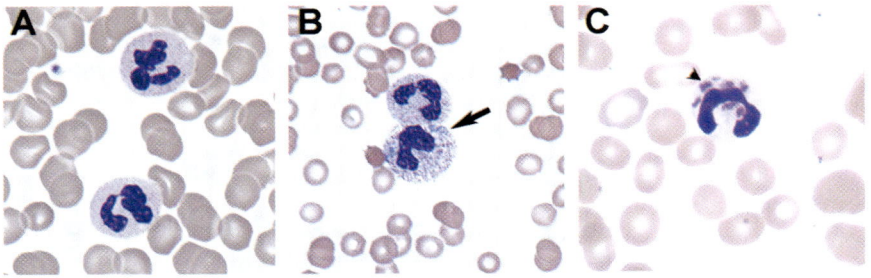

Figure 13-2 Photomicrographs of blood smears showing typical neutrophil morphology from A, a healthy individual; B, a patient with sepsis showing Döhle bodies (*arrow*) and toxic granulations; and C, a patient with Chédiak-Higashi syndrome showing large cytoplasmic inclusions (*arrowhead*). Images from the American Society of Hematology Image Bank.

diagnosis of gout as the cause of neutrophilia. This finding plus the neutrophilia initially raised concern about an underlying myeloproliferative disease. However, the neutrophilia rapidly resolved after institution of anti-inflammatory medications, essentially eliminating myeloproliferative disorders from consideration.

In rare cases, neutrophilia may be due to intrinsic defects of neutrophil function. Leukocyte adhesion deficiency and familial Mediterranean fever are associated with neutrophilia; they are discussed in detail in the section on disorders of neutrophil function.

Neutropenia

Neutropenia is defined as an ANC of <1500 cells/μL. Of note, neutrophil levels are lower in some ethnic and racial groups (eg, Africans, African Americans, and Yemenite Jews). For example, in adult African Americans, the 95% confidence limits for the ANC are 1300 to 7400 cells/μL. A survey of 25,222 participants in the National Health and Nutrition Examination Survey showed that 4.5% of black participants had an ANC of <1500/μL, compared with 0.79% and 0.35% of whites and Mexican Americans, respectively.

Neutropenia is classified based on the ANC as severe (<500/μL), moderate (500–1000/μL), or mild (1000–1500/μL). The risk of infection begins to increase with an ANC <1000/μL. Patients with neutropenia are prone to develop bacterial infections, typically caused by endogenous flora and involving mucous membranes, including gingivitis, stomatitis, perirectal abscesses, cellulitis, and pneumonia. Fungal infections are less common, and there is no increase in susceptibility to viral or parasitic infections. The differential diagnosis of neutropenia is wide (Table 13-3). In this section, congenital syndromes associated with neutropenia and other common acquired causes of neutropenia are discussed. Neutropenia is a frequent manifestation of myelodysplastic syndromes (Chapter 15), acute leukemia (Chapters 16 and 17), and marrow-infiltrative processes such as myelofibrosis (Chapter 14) or metastatic carcinoma; these disorders are discussed in detail in the indicated chapter. Recent studies have identified many of the genetic lesions responsible for congenital neutropenia (Table 13-4). Accordingly, genetic testing is now becoming an important diagnostic tool in the evaluation of patients with congenital neutropenia. The discussion of congenital neutropenia is focused on those syndromes in which neutropenia is the sole or major clinical feature. The bibliography contains several excellent reviews that include the congenital neutropenic syndromes shown in Table 13-4 that are not covered in this chapter.

Table 13-3 Causes of neutropenia.

I. Congenital neutropenia syndromes
   Severe congenital neutropenia (Kostmann syndrome)
   Cyclic neutropenia
   Shwachman-Diamond syndrome
   WHIM syndrome (myelokathexis)
   Disorders of vesicular transport
      Chédiak-Higashi syndrome
      Griscelli syndrome, type II
      Hermansky-Pudlak syndrome, type II
      p14 deficiency
      Cohen syndrome
   Barth syndrome
   Cartilage-hair hypoplasia syndrome
   Pearson syndrome
   Glycogen storage disease type Ib
   Dyskeratosis congenita
   Neutropenia associated with immunodeficiency syndromes

II. Acquired neutropenia
   Neonatal alloimmune neutropenia
   Primary autoimmune neutropenia
   Secondary autoimmune neutropenia
      Systemic lupus erythematosus
      Felty syndrome
   Nutritional deficiencies
      Vitamin B_{12}, folic acid, copper
   Myelodysplastic syndrome
   Acute leukemia
   Myelophthisis (bone marrow infiltration)
      Tumor, fibrosis, granulomas
   Large granular lymphocytic leukemia
   Neutropenia associated with infectious disease
      Sepsis
      Rickettsial: human granulocytic ehrlichiosis
      Viral: mononucleosis, HIV
   Drug-induced neutropenia
   Hypersplenism

HIV = human immunodeficiency virus.

Severe congenital neutropenia (Kostmann syndrome)

> **Clinical case**
>
> A 2½-week-old infant has had persistent neutropenia since birth. Because of fever during the first week of life, he had several blood counts. One ANC was 0.9×10^9/L, but all other counts were 0.0 to 0.2×10^9/L. He now has neutropenia, monocytosis, and thrombocytosis but is doing well without infection. On marrow examination, there is "maturation arrest" at the myelocyte stage. There are almost no metamyelocytes, bands, or mature neutrophils in the marrow. The appearance of the erythroid cells, lymphocytes, and megakaryocytes is normal.

identified in patients with CN are, for the most part, distinctive from those found in patients with SCN.

CN is now treated with daily or alternate-day G-CSF, which largely eliminates the periodic fevers, mouth ulcers, and most of the other inflammatory complications associated with this disease. In contrast to SCN, there is no evidence of an increased risk of MDS or AML in patients with CN. In many children, the cyclic pattern evolves to a state of chronic, persistent neutropenia.

Shwachman-Diamond syndrome

Shwachman-Diamond syndrome (SDS; also known as Shwachman-Bodian-Diamond syndrome) is a rare multisystem disorder characterized by exocrine pancreatic insufficiency, bone marrow dysfunction, and skeletal abnormalities. Bone marrow dysfunction is present in nearly all patients with SDS. In the largest series, 86 of 88 patients with SDS displayed chronic or intermittent neutropenia. Moreover, defects in neutrophil function, most notably impaired chemotaxis and motility, have been reported. Anemia and thrombocytopenia, although less common, are present in more than a third of patients. Defects in B- and/or T-lymphocyte function also have been described. Similar to SCN, patients with SDS have a marked propensity to develop MDS or AML. SDS is the second most common cause of congenital exocrine pancreatic insufficiency (behind cystic fibrosis). Maldigestion caused by pancreatic insufficiency is present in nearly all patients in early life but improves with increasing age in most patients. Bony abnormalities are common, with rib cage abnormalities and metaphyseal dysostosis being the most common features. Growth retardation also is common in SDS patients, but it is not thought to be secondary to malnutrition.

SDS is inherited in an autosomal recessive fashion. Recent studies have identified compound heterozygous mutations of the *SBDS* gene in approximately 90% of patients with SDS. Thus, genetic testing for *SBDS* mutations is a valuable diagnostic tool for SDS. Recent studies suggest that the *SBDS* gene encodes for a protein involved in ribosome biogenesis and microtubule stability.

Treatment of SDS includes pancreatic enzyme replacement and fat-soluble vitamins for pancreatic insufficiency. Neutropenia is usually treated with G-CSF. Stem cell transplantation is generally reserved for patients with bone marrow failure or who have transformed to AML/MDS. A recent study reported a 5-year event-free survival rate of 60% in patients with SDS following stem cell transplantation.

WHIM syndrome

WHIM (warts, hypogammaglobulinemia, infections, and myelokathexis) syndrome is a rare inherited disorder characterized by neutropenia, hypogammaglobulinemia, and extensive human papillomavirus (HPV) infection. Affected individuals typically present with recurrent bacterial infections from birth with ANCs of <1000/μL. Despite the peripheral neutropenia, the bone marrow of affected patients is generally hypercellular with increased numbers of mature neutrophils (a condition termed myelokathexis). Patients commonly have lymphopenia or T-cell dysfunction, yet immunity to most viral pathogens is normal. The major exception is HPV, which is the cause of warts in patients with WHIM syndrome. Although some patients have few, if any, warts, the majority of patients suffer from extensive verrucosis. They typically appear in the first or second decades of life and can involve any mucocutaneous surface. Hypogammaglobulinemia is variable, ranging from normal to modestly decreased serum immunoglobulin (Ig) G, IgM, and IgA. Treatment with G-CSF or granulocyte-macrophage colony-stimulating factor (GM-CSF) is effective in correcting the neutropenia.

The majority of patients with WHIM syndrome have heterozygous mutations of the *CXCR4* gene. CXCR4 is a G protein–coupled heptahelical receptor that is the major receptor for SDF1 (CXCL12). There is convincing evidence that SDF1/CXCR4 signaling is a key regulator of neutrophil release from the bone marrow. Specifically, SDF1/CXCR4 provides a signal to retain neutrophils in the bone marrow. The mutations of *CXCR4* in WHIM syndrome truncate the carboxyl-terminal (cytoplasmic) tail, resulting in enhanced CXCR4 signaling. These observations support the current model in which enhanced signaling by the *CXCR4* mutants in WHIM syndrome leads to abnormal neutrophil retention in the bone marrow.

Chédiak-Higashi syndrome

Chédiak-Higashi syndrome (CHS) is a rare inherited syndrome characterized by partial albinism, a mild bleeding diathesis, severe immunodeficiency, and progressive neurologic defects. The pathognomonic feature of CHS is the presence of giant inclusion bodies in virtually all granulated cells, particularly neutrophils (Figure 13-2). Neutropenia is common, and the residual neutrophils display functional defects. Approximately 85% of patients will progress to an accelerated phase characterized by a nonclonal lymphohistiocytic infiltration of multiple organs, leading to multiorgan system failure. CHS is inherited in an autosomal recessive fashion and is due to mutations of the *LYST* gene. The loss of LYST protein disrupts vesicular trafficking, leading to impaired formation of secretory lysozymes and resulting in hypopigmentation and dysregulated immune cell function. Of note, there are several other rare neutropenic disorders in which impaired vesicular trafficking appears to be the primary mechanisms of disease pathogenesis (Tables 13-3 and 13-4). Other than allogeneic bone marrow transplantation, treatment of CHS and related syndromes is largely supportive.

Neonatal alloimmune neutropenia

Physiologic and acquired neutropenia in premature infants, including neutropenia as a result of idiopathic or immune causes, is much more common than inherited/congenital neutropenia. In alloimmune neonatal neutropenia, there is transplacental transfer of maternal IgG directed against paternal antigens expressed on neonatal neutrophils. It is analogous to neonatal erythroblastosis secondary to Rh incompatibility. Rarely, the maternal antibody is secondary to autoimmune neutropenia in the mother. The incidence has been estimated at 2 per 1000 live births. The bone marrow usually shows normal cellularity with a late myeloid arrest. Maternal alloimmunization probably occurs during the first trimester of pregnancy. Only some of the antigens provoking this response are known. Two antigens known to be responsible for this syndrome, NA1 and NA2, originally described by Lalazari, are now known to be isotypes of CD16 or FCγRIII. These children may develop omphalitis or skin infections; however, they are also at risk of severe, life-threatening infections. Aggressive antibiotic therapy must be given for documented infection, and recombinant G-CSF should be considered, although the response is variable and unpredictable. With supportive care, the neutropenia usually spontaneously resolves within 3 to 28 weeks (average of 11 weeks). Overall, the prognosis for infants with alloimmune neutropenia syndrome is generally quite favorable.

Primary autoimmune neutropenia

Primary autoimmune neutropenia (also termed chronic benign neutropenia of infancy and childhood) typically occurs in children between the ages of 5 and 15 months but can be present from 1 month through adulthood. The ANC is typically between 500 and 1000/μL. Serious infections are infrequent and may reflect the ability of patients to increase their neutrophil counts during acute illnesses. Bone marrow examination is rarely indicated. When performed, it reveals minimal abnormalities or only a deficit of mature neutrophils. Spontaneous remission occurs in most patients. In the largest series, 95% of 240 patients with autoimmune neutropenia had a spontaneous remission, usually within 24 months of diagnosis. The pathogenesis is thought to be immune-mediated neutrophil clearance. Indeed, in the great majority of published cases, antibodies to neutrophil antigens can be detected, although multiple blood samples may need to be analyzed. Antibodies directed against FCγRIII or CD11b/CD18 (also termed the type 3 complement receptor) are the most common antibodies detected. Many patients remain free of infections, and no specific therapy is required. For patients with recurrent infections, prophylactic antibiotics or intermittent treatment with G-CSF may be indicated. Although rarely needed, high-dose intravenous immunoglobulin and/or corticosteroid therapy have been reported to be effective.

Secondary autoimmune neutropenia

Neutropenia is occasionally associated with autoimmune disease, most commonly rheumatoid arthritis (RA), systemic lupus erythematosus (SLE), and Sjögren syndrome. Moreover, there is a strong association of neutropenia with large granular lymphocytic leukemia (LGL) often in association with RA. LGL is discussed separately in the following section. In SLE, neutropenia occurs in approximately 50% of patients. The neutropenia is generally mild, has little impact on disease, and requires no specific treatment. The pathogenesis of neutropenia in SLE is unclear. Neutrophil antibodies have been implicated but are present in some SLE patients without neutropenia; thus, the clinical utility of measuring antineutrophil antibodies in SLE is questionable. Of note, sera samples from a portion of neutropenic patients with SLE contain anti-SSA/Ro or anti-SSB/La antibodies with potent binding and functional activity against neutrophils; however, the clinical relevance and applicability of these findings await further confirmatory studies. As with SLE, the differential diagnosis for neutropenia in RA is wide, and drug-induced neutropenia must be considered. Felty syndrome is defined as the triad of unexplained neutropenia, long-standing RA, and variable splenomegaly. There is an increased risk of infections in these patients. Treatment is usually directed at the underlying RA.

Large granular lymphocyte leukemia

> **Clinical case**
>
> A 60-year-old female presents with fatigue and arthralgias. She has recurrent fevers and complains of upper respiratory infections but has not had documented bacterial infections. On examination, there is no lymphadenopathy or splenomegaly. A complete blood cell count shows hematocrit 35%, platelets $225 \times 10^9/L$, white blood cells $3.5 \times 10^9/L$, and ANC $0.2 \times 10^9/L$. Peripheral blood smear shows frequent large lymphocytes with azurophilic granules.

The previous clinical case is suggestive of LGL, a clonal disorder of cytotoxic T lymphocytes or natural killer cells. Discussion here is limited to T-cell LGL (TLGL) because it is most strongly associated with severe chronic neutropenia. TLGL is a disease of older patients (median age, 60 years) that is associated with RA in 25% of cases. Neutropenia is seen in approximately 85% of cases. Increased numbers of large lymphocytes with abundant cytoplasm and azurophilic granules are often, but not always, apparent on examination of the blood smear. Splenomegaly is present in 25% to 50% of patients. The diagnosis is based on the finding of an elevated number of LGL cells ($CD3^+/CD16^+/CD28^-/CD57^+$) by flow cytometry in blood or bone marrow concurrent with evidence of T-cell clonality. Neutropenia is present in 85% of patients and is often severe (50% with an ANC of $<500/\mu L$). The pathogenesis of neutropenia in TLGL is the subject of intense study. Current models suggest that increased peripheral destruction of neutrophils secondary to immune complexes and bone marrow suppression of granulopoiesis via Fas ligand secretion contribute to the neutropenia. TLGL typically has an indolent but chronic course with median survival of >10 years. In the absence of symptomatic cytopenia, no treatment is required. The most common indication for therapy is recurrent infection secondary to neutropenia. A wide variety of therapeutic interventions have been used in TLGL, and standard therapy remains undefined. It is most commonly managed with immunosuppressive agents including methotrexate, cyclosporine, glucocorticoids, or G-CSF.

Nonimmune chronic idiopathic neutropenia

In a subset of patients with chronic neutropenia, there is no evidence of immune-mediated disease. The diagnosis of nonimmune chronic idiopathic neutropenia in adults (NI-CINA) is based on the presence of chronic acquired neutropenia in the absence of underlying autoimmune disease, cytogenetic abnormality, antineutrophil antibodies, or other obvious explanation for neutropenia. In addition to neutropenia, lymphopenia, monocytopenia, anemia, and thrombocytopenia are occasionally seen. Bone marrow findings are highly variable, with both hyperplastic and hypoplastic bone marrow cellularity reported. The pathogenesis of NI-CINA is poorly understood, although it has been suggested that chronic low-grade inflammation may contribute. Fortunately, the clinical course is usually benign, infections are infrequent, and specific treatment is not required.

Neutropenia due to idiosyncratic drug reactions

Clinical case

A 50-year-old teacher with a history of ulcerative colitis for 1 year presents to the emergency room with fever, chills, and sore throat for 24 hours. On examination, the temperature is 39.6°C, blood pressure is 90/60 mm Hg, pulse is 105 beats/min, and respiratory rate is 28. The patient is confused and reports that her throat is very sore. The abdomen is slightly tender, and bowel sounds are absent. Based on the patient's presentation, therapeutic measures for septic shock are initiated. Within a few minutes, a complete blood cell count reveals a white blood cell count of $1.5 \times 10^9/L$ with an ANC of 0. On questioning of the patient's husband, you learn that she had been in her usual state of health until a few days ago. She has had long-standing complaints of chronic diarrhea with intermittent blood and mucous in the stool. Her only medication is sulfasalazine begun about 3 months ago.

Drug-induced neutropenia and agranulocytosis are serious medical problems, with an estimated frequency of 1 per 1.6 to 7 million and a case fatality rate of approximately 5%. Agranulocytosis refers to the complete absence of neutrophils in the blood. Although certain medications carry a higher risk of neutropenia (Table 13-5), it is probably wise to consider most medications as potential offenders, thus emphasizing the need for a careful drug history in all patients who present with acquired neutropenia. A recent systematic review of the literature identified 10 drugs that accounted for $>50\%$ of cases of definite or probable reports of drug-induced neutropenia: carbimazole, clozapine, dapsone, dipyrone, methimazole, penicillin G, procainamide, propylthiouracil, rituximab, sulfasalazine, and ticlopidine. In most cases, agranulocytosis presents within 6 months, and usually within 3 months, after starting the offending drug. The clinical presentation of drug-induced agranulocytosis is often less dramatic than in this case, but patients often have fever and pharyngitis as their first symptoms. Sepsis and/or pneumonia may occur in 10% to 30% of patients. Usually the prognosis is good because neutrophil counts recover within approximately a week if the offending medication is withdrawn. The disease mechanism is often unclear. In some well-studied cases, the offending drug serves as a hapten in association with an endogenous protein, probably an antigen expressed on the neutrophil surface. The immune response to this complex results in neutrophil destruction, severe neutropenia, and susceptibility to infection. Other drugs may impair production of neutrophils by a direct, toxic effect on myeloid precursors.

Table 13-5 Selected drugs associated with neutropenia.

Anti-inflammatory agents	Antimicrobial agents
Aminopyrine*	Ampicillin*
Diclofenac*	Cefotaxime*
Diflunisal*	Cefuroxime*
Dipyrone*	Flucytosine*
Ibuprofen*	
Gold salts	Fusidic acid*
Penicillamine	Imipenem-cilastatin*
Phenylbutazone	Nafcillin*
Sulfasalazine	Oxacillin*
	Quinine*
Cardiovascular agents	Ticarcillin*
Clopidogrel*	Chloramphenicol
Disopyramide*	Sulfonamides
Methyldopa*	Amodiaquine
Procainamide*	Dapsone
Quinidine*	Terbinafine
Ramipril*	Vancomycin
Spironolactone*	
Dipyridamole	Antithyroid agents
Captopril	Propylthiouracil*
Ticlopidine	Carbimazole
	Methimazole
Anticonvulsants	
Phenytoin*	Other agents
Carbamazepine	Amygdalin*
	Calcium dobesilate*
Psychotropic agents	Cimetidine*
Chlorpromazine*	Infliximab*
Clozapine*	Levamisole*
Fluoxetine*	Metoclopramide*
Mianserin	Mebhydrolin*
	Rituximab
Hypoglycemic agents	Ranitidine
Chlorpropamide	Famotidine
Tolbutamide	Metiamide
Glyburide*	

* Level I evidence based on Andersohn F, Konzen C, Garbe E. Systematic review: agranulocytosis induced by nonchemotherapy drugs. Ann Intern Med. 2007;146:657–665.
NOTE: Documentation of the role of specific drugs in the causation of neutropenia is dependent on (i) the frequency of the occurrence among patients; (ii) the timing of the event in relationship to drug use; (iii) the absence of alternative explanations; and (iv) the inadvertent or intentional reuse of the drug (rechallenges) with a similar response.

Drug-induced agranulocytosis is difficult to anticipate. Serial blood counts are now recommended for patients on some drugs (ie, sulfasalazine, clozapine, phenothiazines, and antithyroid drugs) because of the relatively high frequency of drug-induced neutropenia associated with these agents.

Practices are not standardized, however, and the benefit of frequent blood counts is not established.

Management includes prompt withdrawal of all potentially offending drugs and administration of broad-spectrum antibiotics, usually with inpatient management. The mean time to recovery is approximately 10 days, but the duration of neutropenia is highly variable. Therapy with hematopoietic growth factors, particularly G-CSF, is controversial. A number of nonrandomized trials have reported a shortened duration of neutropenia, less antibiotic use, and reduced hospital stay with the use of G-CSF. Bone marrow examination is usually not necessary in cases with otherwise normal hematocrit, platelet count, and red blood cell morphology. The time to hematologic recovery may be proportional to the severity of the marrow defect; that is, if no cells at the myelocyte stage are seen on an aspirate sample, it will probably be several days before recovery occurs. Overall survival is approximately 95%. A neutrophil count $<0.1 \times 10^9$/L and the presence of sepsis or severe infection are associated with delayed neutrophil recovery and increased mortality.

Chemotherapy-induced neutropenia

Clinical case

A 65-year-old woman with stage III multiple myeloma is treated with vincristine, doxorubicin, and dexamethasone using a tunneled central venous catheter. Approximately 9 days after the initial course of therapy, she develops fever, chills, and rigors and is admitted to the hospital with presumed sepsis. The hematocrit is 32%, platelet count is 25×10^9/L, and ANC is 300/μL. She is initially treated with broad-spectrum antibiotics. Blood cultures are positive for Staphylococcus aureus.

Chemotherapy-induced neutropenia is a common complication of the treatment of cancer. Risk of infection increases with the severity and duration of neutropenia, increasing age, and coexistence of other severe illnesses. In this case, the presence of an intravenous catheter provided a route for serious infection to occur. Chemotherapy-induced neutropenia occurs with a wide range of myelotoxic drugs and treatment regimens. In current practice, the occurrence of fever in a patient with severe, chemotherapy-induced neutropenia is an indication for hospitalization with immediate initiation of broad-spectrum antibiotics pending culture results. Evidence-based guidelines for the indications and use of antibacterial, antifungal, and antiviral agents in patients with neutropenia and cancer were published by the Infectious Diseases Society of America (Hughes et al, 2002). The reader is referred to this report for specifics regarding prophylaxis and treatment of neutropenic patients. Chapter 3 contains an excellent review of the use of hematopoietic growth factors in the prevention and treatment of neutropenia after chemotherapy.

> **Key points**
>
> - Transient neutropenia is not uncommon in infants and children and may be due to infection, auto- or alloimmune mechanisms, unidentified causes (ie, idiopathic), or, less commonly, genetic disorders of granulopoiesis.
> - The genetic basis for many congenital neutropenia syndromes has been identified, and genetic testing is becoming an important diagnostic tool in the evaluation of patients with chronic neutropenia.
> - CN and many cases of congenital neutropenia are associated with mutations of *ELA2*, the gene encoding for neutrophil elastase. Treatment with G-CSF improves neutrophil counts and prevents clinical infections; however, patients with congenital neutropenia must be monitored for evolution to MDS or AML.
> - Neutropenia in adults is frequently due to drugs, both as a predictable response to myelotoxic agents and as an idiosyncratic reaction to almost any drug. Less commonly, neutropenia is due to infection, acquired hematopoietic disease, autoimmune disorder, or a clonal proliferation of large granular lymphocytes.

Disorders of neutrophil function

> **Clinical case**
>
> A 2-year-old boy has had recurrent furuncles and deep abscesses since the first few months of life. On examination, there is no active infection, but there are scars from drainage of previous abscesses. Complete blood cell count shows a hematocrit of 32%, white blood cell count of 12×10^9/L, and platelet count of 400×10^9/L. The differential count is normal, and the morphology of the leukocytes is normal. The IgG level is increased; the levels of IgM and IgA are normal.

Recurrent fevers, otitis media, and sinopulmonary infections are common in young children, and it may be difficult to assess when a child has had "too many" infections and requires a careful workup. However, there are certain conditions that should raise concern for an underlying immunodeficiency syndrome, including neutrophil function disorders, and that may merit further evaluation. These include the following: (i) recurrent systemic bacterial infections (eg, sepsis, osteomyelitis, meningitis); (ii) infections at unusual sites (eg, hepatic or brain abscess); (iii) recurrent bacterial infections (eg, pneumonia, sinusitis, cellulitis, lymphadenitis, draining otitis media); (iv) infections caused by unusual pathogens (eg, *Aspergillus* pneumonia, disseminated candidiasis, *Serratia marcescens*, *Nocardia* species, *Burkholderia cepacia*); and (v) chronic gingivitis or recurrent aphthous ulcers (Boxer, 2003). In the previous clinical case, the history of recurrent abscesses in the face of a normal ANC would merit further evaluation for a neutrophil function disorder. The most widely known disorders with abnormalities of neutrophil function are described in the following sections.

Myeloperoxidase deficiency

Myeloperoxidase (MPO) deficiency is the most common disorder of phagocytes, with 1 in 4000 individuals having a complete deficiency of MPO. It is inherited in an autosomal recessive fashion and is due to mutations of the *MPO* gene. MPO is a primary granule enzyme that catalyzes the conversion of H_2O_2 to hypochlorous acid and other toxic intermediates that greatly enhance polymorphonuclear neutrophil microbicidal activity. The diagnosis can be made with histochemical assays for MPO on neutrophils. Of note, most patients (95%) with MPO deficiency are asymptomatic. An increase in mucocutaneous infections with *Candida* strains has been reported, particularly in patients with concurrent diabetes mellitus. There is no specific treatment.

Leukocyte adhesion deficiency

Leukocyte adhesion deficiency (LAD) is a rare disorder manifested by delayed wound healing, recurrent bacterial infections, and neutrophilia. There are 3 distinct forms of LAD. In LAD-I, mutations of *ITGB2*, encoding the β_2-integrin (CD18) chain, disrupt β_2-integrin function. In LAD-II, mutations of *FUCT2*, encoding GDP-fucose transporter-1, disrupt the generation of ligands on neutrophils required for selectin binding. Patients with LAD-II also display short stature, abnormal facies, and severe cognitive impairment. Finally, in LAD-III, mutations of *FERMT3* (KINDLIN3) or *RASGRP2* lead to impaired β-integrin function. In addition to immunodeficiency, patients with LAD-III also have a bleeding diathesis due to a defect in β_3-integrin function on platelets. All mutations result in severely impaired neutrophil chemotaxis and emigration from the blood to sites of infection. A history of consanguinity may be an important clue in evaluating children for LAD. Definitive treatment of LAD requires allogeneic HSCT, with a recent study reporting a 5-year survival of 75%.

Hyperimmunoglobulin E syndrome

Hyperimmunoglobulin E syndrome (previously known as Job syndrome) is manifested by defective neutrophil chemotaxis, recurrent bacterial infections (typically involving the skin, sinuses, or lung), mucocutaneous infections with *Candida albicans*, and elevated serum IgE levels. Patients may also present with a pruritic dermatitis in the first few weeks of life. Associated features that might aid in the diagnosis include coarse facial features, recurrent fractures, and short stature. Recent studies have identified mutations of *STAT3* in the majority (60%–70%) of cases of hyperimmunoglobulin E syndrome. In addition, mutations of *DOCK8* (encoding dedicator of cytokinesis 8) are present in many cases of the autosomal recessive form of hyperimmunoglobulin E syndrome. Finally, homozygous mutations of *TYK2* have been identified in a single patient with this syndrome.

Neutrophil-specific granule deficiency

Neutrophil-specific granule deficiency is a rare disorder also associated with recurrent severe skin and lung infections caused by *S aureus*, *Staphylococcus epidermidis*, and gram-negative bacteria. These patients' neutrophils are morphologically abnormal; they are devoid of secondary and tertiary granules but contain normal azurophilic granules, and they do not migrate normally in response to chemotactic stimuli. This syndrome is associated with loss-of-function mutations of C/EBPϵ.

Chronic granulomatous disease

The most frequent manifestations of chronic granulomatous disease (CGD) are cutaneous and pulmonary infections. In the lymph nodes and other tissues, granulomatous inflammatory responses develop. The 5 main groups or microorganisms responsible for infections in CGD include *Aspergillus* species, *Burkholderia* species, *S aureus*, *Nocardia* species, and *Mycobacteria* species. The incidence is approximately 1 in 200,000 live births. This disorder is due to mutations in one of the components of the NADPH oxidase system that results in a failure to generate the oxidative burst that normally produces reactive oxygen species and the bactericidal agent, hypochlorous acid, within the neutrophil (Figure 13-3). Approximately two thirds of CGD cases are due to mutations affecting the X-linked gene *CYBB*, which encodes the gp91^{phox} component of the membrane cytochrome b$_{558}$ protein complex. Rare X-linked cases have also implicated defects in glucose-6-phosphate dehydrogenase (G6PD). For this reason, most patients with CGD are boys. The other cases involve mutations of autosomal genes, including *CYBA*, which encodes p22^{phox} (the second membrane component of cytochrome b$_{558}$; 5% of CGD cases); *NCF-1*, which encodes p47^{phox} (20% of cases); and *NCF-2*, which encodes p67^{phox} (6% of cases) (Figure 13-2). Diagnosis is usually made by a typical clinical history and a laboratory test demonstrating abnormal neutrophil oxidative burst. The quantitative dihydrorhodamine 123 flow cytometry assay is the most accurate and commonly used test. However, the older burst nitroblue tetrazolium (NBT) test also is still in use. Patients with CGD benefit from prophylactic treatment with antibiotics and antifungal agents and prompt antibiotic administration for specific infections. Chronic treatment with interferon-γ reduces the incidence of bacterial and fungal infections by approximately 70%. HSCT is curative and should be performed in patients in whom the clinical course or specific mutation portends a poor outcome and who have an HLA-matched donor.

Autoinflammatory diseases

Autoinflammatory diseases, also called periodic fever syndromes, refer to a group of rare hereditary disorders characterized by recurrent episodes of unprovoked inflammation in the absence of infection. The most common and prototypical autoinflammatory disease is familial Mediterranean fever (FMF). FMF is characterized by sporadic paroxysmal attacks of fever, serosal inflammation, and neutrophilia. The most common presentation is recurrent attacks of acute peritonitis, although pleuritis and synovitis also are frequent. It is an autosomal recessive disorder that mainly occurs in populations from the Mediterranean basin, such as Sephardic Jews, Arabs, Turks, and Armenians. However, sporadic cases have been reported in individuals of French, Italian, Greek, Belgian, and Northern European heritage. Mutations in the *MEFV* gene, which encodes a myeloid-specific protein of unclear function, appear to cause dysregulation of inflammation control that leads to unpredictable episodes of neutrophil overactivity and tissue infiltration by activated neutrophils. Because the chronic, recurrent inflammatory attacks also cause persistent elevations of serum amyloid A protein, patients with FMF are at high risk of developing complications of AA amyloidosis, especially in the kidneys. In this regard, FMF is the leading cause of secondary amyloidosis in Turkey. The diagnosis of FMF is usually made based on clinical criteria, including unexplained episodes that persist over many months to years in the absence of other etiologies of inflammation. Most of the common *MEFV* mutations are well characterized. Thus, the diagnosis can now be confirmed and family studies carried out using molecular studies done by a reference research laboratory. Colchicine prevents clinical attacks and tissue amyloid deposition in most patients with FMF. Rare patients with exceptional, refractory disease have undergone successful HSCT.

Hyper-IgD syndrome is another rare autosomal recessive autoinflammatory disease found in Dutch and French families that is associated with mutations in the mevalonate kinase gene *MVK*. The tumor necrosis factor (TNF) receptor–associated periodic syndrome (TRAPS; previously known as familial Hibernian fever) is an autosomal dominant disorder affecting Scottish and Irish individuals and associated with mutations in the gene encoding TNF

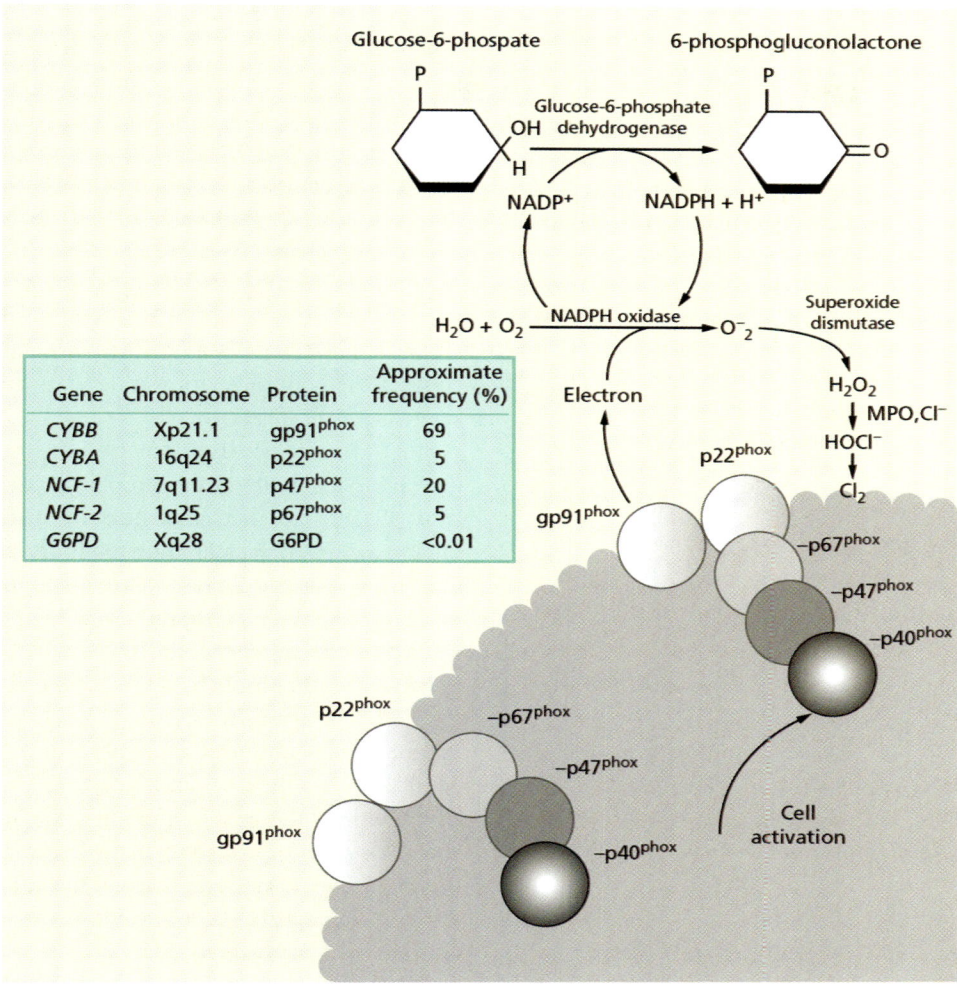

Figure 13-3 Relation among the components of nicotinamide adenine dinucleotide phosphate (NADPH) oxidase that are affected in patients with chronic granulomatous disease. The membrane-bound phagocyte oxidase components, the 91-kd glycoprotein (gp91^{phox}) and the 22-kd protein (p22^{phox}), interact with the cytoplasmic components, the 47-kd protein (p47^{phox}) and 67-kd protein (p67^{phox}). Glucose-6-phosphate dehydrogenase (G6PD) converts glucose-6-phosphate to 6-phosphogluconolactone, generating NADPH and a hydrogen ion from NADP$^+$. NADPH oxidase catalyzes the monovalent reduction of O_2 to superoxide anion (O_2^{-1}), with the subsequent conversion to hydrogen peroxide (H_2O_2) by superoxide dismutase. Neutrophil-derived myeloperoxidase (MPO) converts hydrogen peroxide to hypochlorous acid (HOCL$^-$, bleach), which is converted to chlorine (Cl_2). The genes for the components of NADPH oxidase, their chromosomal locations, and the frequency of mutations as a cause of chronic granulomatous disease are indicated in the box. From Leckstrom-Himes JA, Gallin JI. Immunodeficiency diseases caused by defects in phagocytes. *N Engl J Med*. 2000;343:1703–1714.

receptor 1, *TNFRSF1A*. Cryopyrin-associated periodic syndromes (CAPS) are a group of autosomal dominant inherited disorders that are caused by mutations of a pyrin-like protein called NALP3, encoded by the *CIAS1* gene. The type of *CIAS1* mutation determines the clinical severity. Familial cold autoinflammatory syndrome is the most severe form of CAPS, followed by Muckle-Wells syndrome and familial cold autoinflammatory syndrome. Although neutrophils are not the primary mediators of pathogenesis in these non-FMF disorders, they share many clinical features with FMF and should be considered in the differential diagnosis of unexplained recurrent fever with noninfectious autoinflammation.

> **Key points**
>
> - Genetic disorders affecting neutrophil function are possible but uncommon causes of recurrent infections, unexplained fever, and inflammation.
> - Disorders affecting neutrophil adhesion, chemotaxis, and killing are usually diagnosed in young children with recurrent infections.
> - CGD is characterized by recurrent bacterial and fungal infections and is due to mutations that impair the ability of phagocytes to generate reactive oxygen intermediates.
> - FMF should be considered in children or adults with unexplained recurrent fever and inflammation and the appropriate ethnic background.

Monocytosis

Monocytes normally account for approximately 1% to 9% of peripheral blood leukocytes, with absolute monocyte counts ranging from 0.3 to 0.7×10^9/L. An increase in circulating monocytes may be observed in chronic inflammatory conditions and infectious diseases such as tuberculosis, endocarditis, and syphilis. Monocytosis is a hallmark of chronic and juvenile myelomonocytic leukemias and may also be observed in other malignancies including lymphomas and acute monocytic leukemias. In the inflammatory conditions, monocytosis is a reactive process resulting from the peripheral production of cytokines, which stimulate monocyte production. Malignant monocytosis is presumed to be due to specific molecular defects affecting monocyte proliferation, differentiation, and survival.

Monocytopenia

A decreased absolute monocyte count can be encountered in bone marrow failure states such as aplastic anemia and, less commonly, MDS. Monocytopenia, along with neutropenia, is characteristic of hairy cell leukemia. Low monocyte counts are also encountered with overwhelming sepsis and as the result of cytotoxic chemotherapy.

Disorders of histiocytes and DCs

Hemophagocytic lymphohistiocytosis

> **Clinical case**
>
> A 9-month-old girl is admitted to the hospital after presenting with a fever of 40.5°C, sore throat, and lethargy. Over the course of the next 48 hours, the child continues to have high fevers despite broad-spectrum antibiotics and develops progressive splenomegaly and pancytopenia. Laboratory data are also notable for a markedly elevated ferritin of 24,000 ng/mL (normal, 4–76 ng/mL) and hypofibrinogenemia of 68 mg/dL (normal, 150–450 mg/dL). A bone marrow biopsy reveals marked histiocyte hyperplasia with hemophagocytosis. The patient begins treatment with dexamethasone, cyclosporine, and etoposide. Mutational testing reveals the presence of a homozygous mutation in the *PRF1* gene.

Hemophagocytosis is the histologic finding of activated macrophages engulfing leukocytes, erythrocytes, platelets, and their precursor cells. Although hemophagocytosis may be observed in a variety of conditions including hemolytic anemias, infections, and malignancies, it is also a principal feature of hemophagocytic lymphohistiocytosis (HLH), a clinical syndrome characterized by fever, pancytopenia, and splenomegaly that results from the abnormal activation and proliferation of cytotoxic T lymphocytes and tissue macrophages (Figure 13-4).

The major pathophysiologic abnormality in HLH is cytokine dysfunction. Cytokines found at high levels in the plasma of patients with HLH include interferon-γ; TNFα; interleukin (IL) 6, IL-10, and IL-12; and soluble IL-2 receptor (CD25). Elevated IL-16 levels may be important for a T_H1-type response that recruits macrophages and other cells pertinent to HLH. Severe impairment in natural killer (NK) cell activity and cytotoxic T-cell function are also characteristic of the disease.

HLH may occur either as an inherited or acquired disorder (Table 13-6). Familial hemophagocytic lymphohistiocytosis (FHL) is an autosomal recessive disease that typically presents in infancy and early childhood with an estimated incidence of approximately 1 in 50,000. Mutations involving the *PRF1* gene, encoding perforin, have been found in up to 50% of patients with FHL. Perforin is a critical component of the granule exocytosis pathway, which enables NK cells and cytotoxic T lymphocytes to induce apoptosis in target cells. Additional mutations in the Munc13-4 gene (*UNC13D*), resulting in defective granule exocytosis, and in *STX11*, a t-SNARE involved in intracellular trafficking, have also been described in FHL. In addition to FHL, HLH also occurs in the context of inherited immune deficiency syndromes including CHS, Griscelli syndrome, and X-linked proliferative syndromes.

Acquired HLH syndrome, also known as reactive hemophagocytic syndrome or secondary HLH (SHLH), can affect both adults and children and is usually associated with an underlying infection or other immunocompromised state. Predisposing conditions associated with SHLH include infections, autoimmune/rheumatologic disorders, hematologic and (less commonly) nonhematologic malignancies, acquired immunodeficiency syndrome (AIDS; with or without opportunistic infections), and posttransplantation immunosuppression. The pathophysiology of SHLH appears to be similar to that described for FLH, except that in these patients, the underlying predisposing disorder, and not a congenital defect, is responsible for the secondary dysregulation of T cells and NK cells that leads to histiocyte activation. A form of SHLH, known as macrophage activation syndrome, occurs in individuals with autoimmune disorders, most frequently systemic-onset juvenile RA or adult-onset Still disease. The clinical manifestations are similar, although cytopenias have been reported to be less pronounced in macrophage activation syndrome.

The clinical presentation, laboratory features, and tissue histopathology of inherited and acquired HLH are similar. HLH should be considered in the differential diagnosis in patients who develop sepsis and/or multiorgan dysfunction

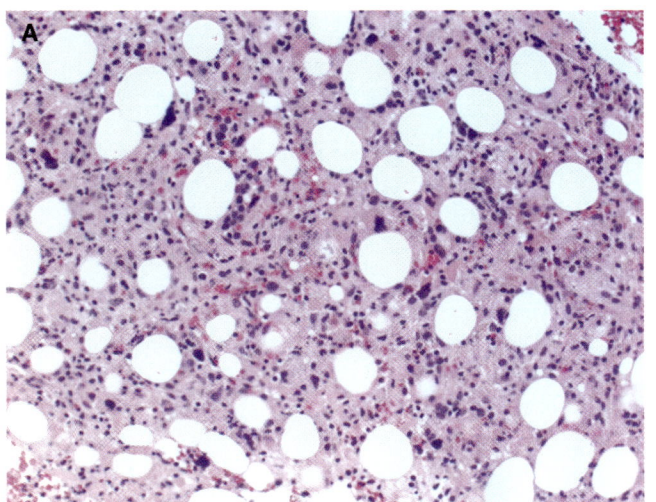
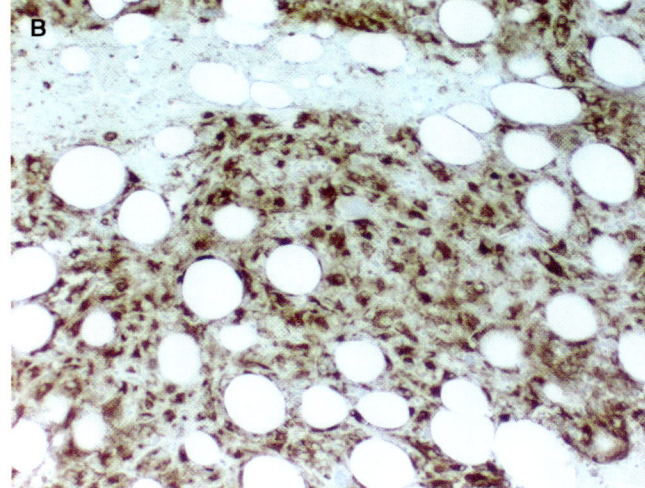
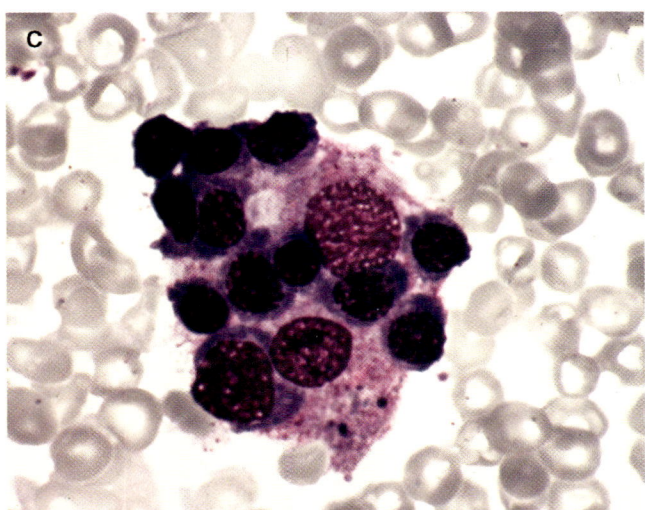

Figure 13-4 Marrow findings in hemophagocytic lymphohistiocytosis. A, Marrow biopsy reveals increased numbers of macrophages scattered among the normal hematopoietic precursors (hematoxylin-eosin stain; original magnification, ×85). B, Immunohistochemical staining for CD68 reveals the macrophages (×85). C, Cytophagic histiocytes are more easily identified in the marrow aspirate (Wright-Giemsa stain). Photos courtesy of Steven J. Kussick, MD, PhD, Associate Director of Hematopathology, Assistant Professor, Department of Laboratory Medicine, University of Washington.

in the setting of fever, unexplained progressive pancytopenia, and hepatosplenomegaly. Laboratory findings include elevated ferritin and triglycerides with low fibrinogen. Central nervous system (CNS) involvement may range from irritability, bulging fontanel, and neck stiffness to seizures, cranial nerve palsies, ataxia, or coma. Lymphadenopathy, rash, and liver disease may also be present. A bone marrow biopsy is crucial to identify histiocytic hyperplasia and hemophagocytosis, although hemophagocytosis may not be observed early in the clinical course. Lumbar puncture and magnetic resonance imaging of the brain should be performed in those with suspected CNS involvement.

Although evaluation for an underlying infection should be performed, both familial and secondary forms of HLH are frequently triggered by an infection. Diagnostic criteria for HLH have been established by the Histiocyte Society (Table 13-7). In addition to the original criteria proposed in 1991 of fever, splenomegaly, cytopenias, hypertriglyceridemia and/or hypofibrinogenemia, and hemophagocytosis, 3 additional criteria were introduced in 2004; these are low or absent NK-cell activity, hyperferritinemia, and high levels of sIL-2r. At least 5 of 8 clinical criteria or the presence of either familial disease or one of the known genetic abnormalities is required for diagnosis of HLH.

Although secondary HLH may resolve after treatment of the underlying condition or with a short course of immunosuppression, untreated FHL is uniformly fatal within 1 to 2 months. Treatment of FHL consists of chemoimmunotherapy followed by allogeneic stem cell transplantation. The HLH-94 protocol of the Histiocyte Society for FHL consists of an initial 8 weeks of dexamethasone and etoposide followed by maintenance cyclosporine with pulses of etoposide and dexamethasone. Intrathecal therapy with methotrexate and corticosteroids is administered in individuals with evidence of CNS involvement. Results of HLH-94 demonstrate a 3-year survival rate of 51%. The subsequent protocol, HLH-2004, is similar to the HLH-94 protocol and includes etoposide, dexamethasone, and cyclosporine with an earlier introduction of cyclosporine

Table 13-6 Hereditary and acquired causes of HLH.

Primary HLH
  Familial HLH
  Chédiak-Higashi syndrome
  Griscelli syndrome
  X-linked lymphoproliferative disease
  Wiskott-Aldrich syndrome

Secondary HLH
Infections
  Herpes virus infection (EBV, CMV, HHV-6, HHV-8, VZV, HSV)
  HIV
  Parvovirus, adenovirus, hepatitis virus
  Bacteria, rickettsial, fungal, spirochete-associated infections
Malignancy
  AML, MDS, lymphomas, multiple myeloma
  Metastatic carcinoma
Autoimmune diseases (macrophage activation syndrome)
Other immunodeficiency states
  Posttransplantation
  Cytotoxic and/or immunosuppressive therapy
  Postsplenectomy

AML = acute myeloid leukemia; CMV = cytomegalovirus; EBV = Ebstein-Barr virus; HHV = human herpesvirus; HIV = human immunodeficiency virus; HLH = hemophagocytic lymphohistiocytosis; HSV = herpes simplex virus; MDS = myelodysplastic syndrome; VZV = varicella zoster virus.

Table 13-7 2004 revised diagnostic criteria for hemophagocytic lymphohistiocytosis.

The diagnosis HLH can be established if one criterion from either 1 or 2 below is fulfilled
1. A molecular diagnosis consistent with HLH
2. Diagnostic criteria for HLH fulfilled (5 out of the 8 criteria below)
   A. Initial diagnostic criteria (to be evaluated in all patients with HLH)
      Fever
      Splenomegaly
      Cytopenias (affecting ≥2 of 3 lineages in the peripheral blood):
         Hemoglobin <90 g/L (in infants <4 weeks: hemoglobin <100 g/L)
         Platelets <100 × 10^9/L
         Neutrophils <1.0 × 10^9/L
      Hypertriglyceridemia and/or hypofibrinogenemia:
         Fasting triglycerides ≥3.0 mmol/L (ie, ≥265 mg/dL)
         Fibrinogen ≤1.5 g/L
      Hemophagocytosis in bone marrow or spleen or lymph nodes
      No evidence of malignancy
   B. New diagnostic criteria
      Low or absent NK-cell activity (according to local laboratory reference)
      Ferritin ≥500 μg/L
      Soluble CD25 (ie, soluble IL-2 receptor) ≥2400 U/mL

NOTE: (1) If hemophagocytic activity is not proven at the time of presentation, further search for hemophagocytic activity is encouraged. If the bone marrow specimen is not conclusive, material may be obtained from other organs. Serial marrow aspirates over time may also be helpful. (2) The following findings may provide strong supportive evidence for the diagnosis: (a) spinal fluid pleocytosis (mononuclear cells) and/or elevated spinal fluid protein; or (b) histologic picture in the liver resembling chronic persistent hepatitis (biopsy). (3) Other abnormal clinical and laboratory findings consistent with the diagnosis are cerebromeningeal symptoms, lymph node enlargement, jaundice, edema, skin rash, hepatic enzyme abnormalities, hypoproteinemia, hyponatremia, decreased very low-density lipoprotein, and high-density lipoprotein.
HLH = hemophagocytic lymphohistiocytosis; IL-2 = interleukin 2; NK = natural killer.

to reduce the risk of relapse while corticosteroids are being tapered. Allogeneic HSCT is recommended in patients with FHL and in patients with relapsed or refractory secondary HLH.

Langerhans cell histiocytosis

Langerhans cells are specialized DCs that are found in the skin and mucosa. Langerhans cell histiocytosis (LCH), a clonal disorder of Langerhans DCs, is associated with polymorphic cellular infiltration and damage at either unifocal tissue sites or in multiple organs and tissues. Historically, localized LCH was referred to as eosinophilic granuloma, whereas clinical variants of multisystem disease were referred to as histiocytosis X, Letter-Siwe disease, and Hand-Schüller-Christian syndrome.

Patients with LCH are categorized as having either uni- or multifocal involvement of a single organ system (SS-LCH) or multisystem LCH (MS-LCH). SS-LCH most commonly involves the bone (particularly the skull, femur, pelvis, and ribs) and less commonly involves the skin, lymph nodes, and lung. Usual presentations of limited disease include persistent or recurrent/progressive bony pain and/or swelling, chronic skin rash, chronic ear drainage, dyspnea, cough, and/or pneumothorax (isolated bony involvement resulting in ear drainage is more common in children, and pulmonary disease occurs predominantly in adults). MS-LCH most commonly occurs in young children and may present with various combinations of bony and/or soft tissue masses with symptoms including fever, eczematoid rash, gingival swelling, cough/dyspnea, tooth loss, hepatosplenomegaly, lymphadenopathy, abnormal chest x-ray, and/or cytopenias. Diabetes insipidus may result from intracranial extension of craniofacial bone lesions and is the most common CNS manifestation, occurring in up to 30% of patients. LCH is rare, with an annual incidence of approximately 5 per million. The etiology of LCH is unknown, although LCH of the lungs in adults is frequently associated with smoking.

Tissue biopsy is required to confirm the diagnosis of LCH. Histologically, the lesions contain a mix of characteristic

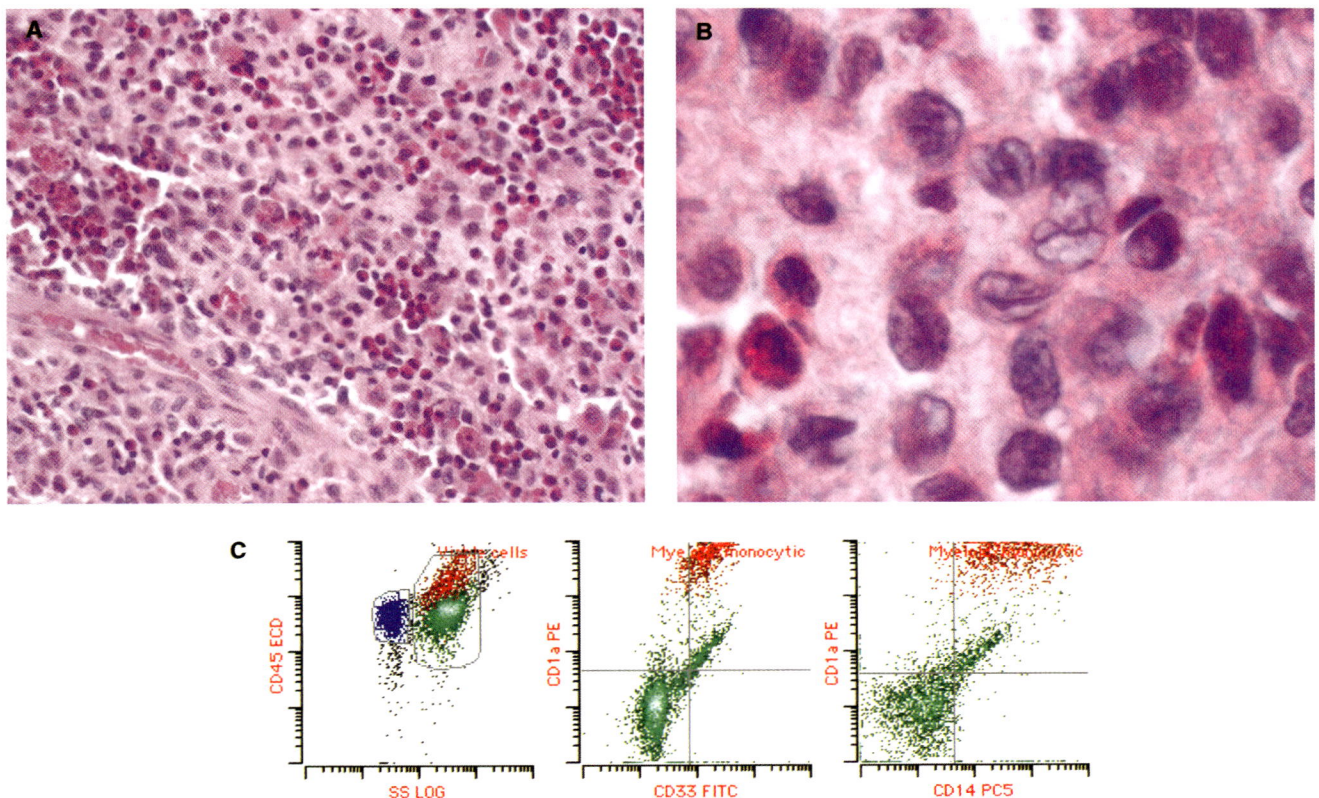

Figure 13-5 Histopathology of Langerhans cell histiocytosis (LCH). A, LCH lesions typically consist of benign-appearing histiocytes frequently admixed with scattered eosinophils, neutrophils, and/or lymphocytes (hematoxylin-eosin stain; original magnification, ×85). B, Langerhans cells frequently have a cleaved or indented nucleus (reticulin stain; ×850). C, Flow cytometry analysis of side scatter (SS) and CD45 expression patterns reveals lymphocytes (blue), eosinophils (green), and monocyte/macrophage cells (red) within the LCH lesion (left panel). The monocyte/macrophage cells are identified as Langerhans cells by their coexpression of CD33, CD1a, and CD14 (middle and right panels). Photos courtesy of Steven J. Kussick, MD, PhD, Associate Director of Hematopathology, Assistant Professor, Department of Laboratory Medicine, University of Washington.

Langerhans cells in a background of eosinophils, neutrophils, and lymphocytes. Langerhans cells are positive for CD1a and S-100, and by ultrastructural examination, they contain the hallmark Birbeck granules (Figure 13-5). Birbeck granules are tennis racket–shaped cytoplasmic granules approximately 200 to 400 nm in length and 33 nm in width with a zipper-like appearance. Because expression of langerin (CD207) confirms the presence of Birbeck granules, electron microscopy is now rarely done for diagnosis. Some tumors contain an abundance of eosinophils and neutrophils with central necrosis, whereas fibrosis and foamy macrophages are found in more long-standing lesions. A full staging workup including chest x-ray, skeletal survey, and measurement of urine osmolality is required to categorize the extent and activity of disease and to guide treatment decisions. Pulmonary function testing and high-resolution computed tomography scanning of the chest should be performed in individuals with suspected lung disease, whereas magnetic resonance imaging of the brain should be performed if there is evidence of CNS or endocrine dysfunction.

Treatment of LCH is based on the extent and activity of the disease. SS-LCH generally confers a good prognosis and frequently requires minimal or no treatment. Bony or soft tissue SS-LCH can be treated with surgical resection or bony curettage, local irradiation (usually 4–8 Gy), and/or injection of steroids. Limited skin disease often responds to topical steroids, nitrogen mustard, or psoralen and ultraviolet A (PUVA) light therapy. Management of lung disease includes discontinuation of smoking and judicious use of prednisone, vinblastine, methotrexate, and/or immunosuppressive agents. Disease-free survival with limited/local LCH exceeds 95%; however, recurrences are common, and some patients require multiple courses of treatment to be cured. Therefore, patients must be monitored closely for evolution to multisystem disease, secondary malignancies, and in the case of lung involvement, progressive pulmonary compromise.

MS-LCH and SS-LCH with progressive multifocal involvement or involvement of critical anatomic sites are treated with systemic therapy. Although initial therapy with vinblastine and prednisone or etoposide and prednisone results in equivalent response rates, vinblastine is currently favored due to the leukemogenic risk of etoposide. Various combinations and schedules of vinblastine, methotrexate, prednisone, and mercaptopurine have been used as additional therapy based on disease risk and initial response. Involvement of the hematopoietic system, spleen, liver, and lung is considered high risk, with a mortality of approximately 20% compared with <5% for patients without high-risk features. Recurrences and progression are most common in patients with extensive visceral disease and suboptimal initial response to therapy. Persistent organ and endocrine dysfunction are common long-term sequelae of even successful therapy. Salvage and palliative therapies include 2-chlorodeoxyadenosine, cyclosporin A, pamidronate (for bony lesions), thalidomide, interferon-γ, etanercept, liver transplantation, and HSCT.

Non–Langerhans cell histiocytoses

A number of other rare histiocytic disorders that are phenotypically distinct from Langerhans cells have been characterized. Juvenile xanthogranuloma, the most common of these disorders, is a proliferative disorder of young children that generally appears as a solitary or multiple red, yellow, or brown papular skin lesions. The condition generally follows a benign clinical course and usually resolves spontaneously, although extracutaneous lesions do rarely occur.

Sinus histiocytosis with massive lymphadenopathy, also known as Rosai-Dorfman disease, is a nonmalignant proliferation of histiocytes within lymph node sinuses and lymphatics in extranodal sites. The condition most commonly occurs in children and young adults and presents as massive, painless, bilateral lymph node enlargement in the neck with fever. Other nodal and extranodal sites may sometimes be involved. Although spontaneous resolution is observed in most cases, relapses can occur, and the condition can be fatal in a small proportion of patients.

Lysosomal storage diseases

Lysosomal storage diseases are a collection of approximately 50 genetically inherited disorders characterized by a deficiency or defect in 1 or more specific lysosomal enzymes. These disorders lead to an accumulation of undigested material inside the lysosome, leading to cell degeneration and accumulation of macromolecules in various tissues and organs of the body and resulting in organ dysfunction. Gaucher disease and Niemann-Pick disease are 2 lysosomal storage diseases, also known as sphingolipidoses or lipid storage disorders, in which undigested lipids accumulate in the lysosome-rich cells of the monocyte/macrophage system and are of particular importance to hematologists because they frequently present with cytopenias and hepatosplenomegaly.

Gaucher disease

> **Clinical case**
>
> A 23-year-old male from the Ukraine presents with a several-month history of easy bruising, worsening fatigue, and hip pain. On physical examination, the patient is noted to be pancytopenic, with a hemoglobin of 8.0 and platelet count of 40×10^9/L, and has marked hepatosplenomegaly with a spleen measuring 12 cm below the costal margin. A bone marrow biopsy reveals the presence of lipid-laden macrophages consistent with Gaucher cells infiltrating the marrow. Measurement of leukocyte glucocerebrosidase is markedly reduced, measuring at <10% of normal levels.

Gaucher disease is a lipid storage disease that results from the deficiency of glucocerebrosidase (acid β-glucosidase), which hydrolyzes glucocerebroside to glucose and ceramide. Deficiency of the enzyme causes glucocerebroside accumulation in the cytoplasm of tissue macrophages, known as Gaucher cells, resulting in a characteristic wrinkled-paper appearance (Figure 13-6).

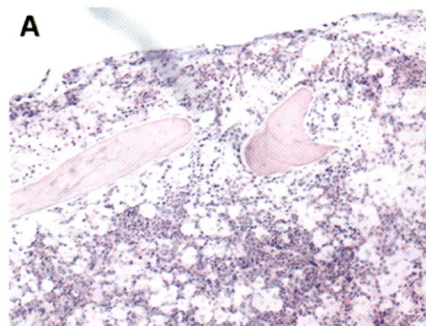
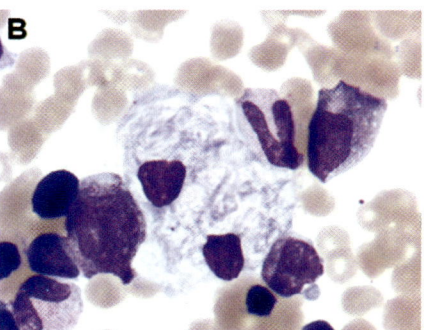

Figure 13-6 Gaucher disease. A, Proliferation of benign-appearing macrophages with interspersed normal hematopoietic elements are easily identified. B, High-power view of bone marrow aspirate demonstrating a Gaucher cell, an abnormal macrophage with the characteristic "wrinkled paper" cytoplasm.

Gaucher disease is the most common lysosomal storage disease, with an incidence of approximately 1 in 75,000 births, and is more common in Ashkenazi Jewish populations, with an incidence of 1 in 1000. Gaucher disease is inherited as an autosomal recessive disorder, with >300 mutations having been described. The disease is divided into 3 clinical subtypes based on pattern and severity of neurologic involvement. Type I (nonneuropathic) is most common (90% of all patients), has the most variable clinical presentation, and is associated with the highest residual enzyme activity. Symptoms consist of hepatosplenomegaly, cytopenias, and bone disease. Skeletal manifestations include osteopenia, pain crises, and osteolytic lesions, with radiographs showing flaring of the ends of the long bones (Erlenmeyer flask deformity) and cortical thinning. Although the clinical severity may not be predicted by the genotype, early onset is associated with more rapidly progressive and severe disease. Type II (acute neuronopathic) is rarest, with the lowest enzyme activity. Disease onset occurs during infancy and results in progressive neurologic deterioration that includes generalized seizures, hypertonia, profound mental retardation, and death during infancy. Type III (subacute neuronopathic) falls between types I and II in incidence, enzyme activity, and clinical severity. Onset occurs at any time during childhood, and manifestations include progressive dementia and ataxia, bone and visceral involvement, and supranuclear palsies.

The diagnosis of Gaucher disease can be established by enzyme assay for glucocerebrosidase activity in leukocytes, fibroblasts, or urine, which is between 0% and 30% of normal values. In addition, mutational analysis of the 4 most common mutations of the glucocerebrosidase gene (N370S, IVS2+1G>A, L444P, and 1035insG [84G>GG]) can detect 90% to 95% of the mutations associated with Gaucher disease in the Ashkenazi Jewish population and 50% to 75% of the associated mutations in the general population. The onset of symptoms ranges from 2 years of age to late adulthood, and it has been estimated that up to 60% of individuals harboring the most common N370S mutation never present to medical attention.

Enzyme replacement therapy (ERT) is the mainstay of treatment of individuals with nonneuropathic manifestations of Gaucher disease. Imiglucerase (Cerezyme) is a recombinant modified placental glucocerebrosidase in which the glycosylation sites of the enzyme are processed to terminate in mannose sugars to improve uptake and trafficking to the lysozymes of macrophages via the mannose receptor. In clinical studies, ERT at 30 to 60 U/kg administered every 2 weeks results in normalization of cytopenias and reduction in organomegaly within 6 to 12 months, whereas skeletal symptoms improve more slowly. Studies using low-dose ERT at 15 to 30 U/kg/month administered more frequently at 3 times a week have shown that this regimen appears to produces similar effects on cytopenias and organomegaly at significantly reduced cost. Given the high cost of ERT, published guidelines advocate treatment only for symptomatic children and adults with severe disease (eg, platelet counts <60,000/μL, marked splenomegaly, skeletal disease). In addition, because imiglucerase does not cross the blood–brain barrier, it has limited utility in neuropathic forms of the disease. An alternative therapy, miglustat (Zavesca) acts by reducing substrate accumulation in Gaucher disease by inhibiting glucosylceramide synthase, a key enzyme in glycosphingolipid synthesis. Miglustat is available for use in the United States for patients unable to receive ERT and in Europe for adult patients with mild to moderate disease. In clinical studies, miglustat decreased liver and spleen volumes by 12% and 19%, respectively, with modest improvements in hemoglobin and platelet counts.

Niemann-Pick disease

Type A and type B Niemann-Pick disease (NPD) are caused by mutations in the sphingomyelin phosphodiesterase-1 (*SMPD1*) gene, which result in deficient sphingomyelinase activity and accumulation of sphingomyelin (ceramide phosphorylcholine). Type C NPD is an unrelated defect caused by mutations of the *NPC1* and *NPC2* genes, which result in impaired cellular processing and transport of low-density lipoprotein cholesterol.

NPD is inherited as an autosomal recessive disorder. Type A patients have <5% of normal sphingomyelinase activity, and the disease is characterized by hepatosplenomegaly, failure to thrive, and rapidly progressive neurodegeneration, with death occurring by age 2 to 4 years. Examination reveals cherry-red maculae in approximately half of affected infants. Type B patients have sphingomyelinase activity within 5% to 10% of normal, often have minimal to no neurologic involvement, and can survive into adulthood. Cytopenias and hepatosplenomegaly are typical, and patients can also develop progressive pulmonary infiltrates.

The histologic hallmark of NPD is the pathologic foam cell or Niemann-Pick cell; these cells are histiocytes filled with lipid droplets or particles that are uniform in size, giving the cells a "mulberry-like" or "honeycomb-like" appearance, and are found in involved organs. Type A and B NPD may be readily diagnosed by assays for sphingomyelinase in leukocytes or cultured fibroblasts, which demonstrate reduced activity (1%–10%) in the disease. Genetic testing can detect the most common mutations in type A, which account for approximately 90% of the mutant alleles in the Ashkenazi Jewish population. Currently, no specific treatment exists for NPD.

> **Key points**
>
> - HLH is a pathologic activation and proliferation of tissue histiocytes leading to severe multisystem clinical consequences. HLH may present in young children with an inherited predisposition (eg, due to perforin gene mutations) or in children and adults with acquired disorders of immune regulation due to infection, autoimmune disorder, malignancy, and/or acquired immunodeficiency state.
> - LCH is a clonal DC disorder that can present with involvement of a single tissue (usually the bone) or multiple tissues and organs, including the pituitary and hypothalamus (with diabetes insipidus). The clinical course may be variable, with periods of disease inactivity and/or chronic progression, and treatment must be individualized.
> - Gaucher disease is a lysosomal storage disorder caused by mutations in glucocerebrosidase, leading to abnormal accumulation of glucocerebroside in tissue macrophages and resulting in hepatosplenomegaly, cytopenias, and skeletal disorders. ERT can reverse both nonhematologic and hematologic manifestations.

Bibliography

General

Christopher MJ, Link DC. Regulation of neutrophil homeostasis. *Curr Opin Hematol.* 2007;14:3–8. *Current review of neutrophil homeostasis and emigration.*

Friedman AD. Transcriptional control of granulocyte and monocyte development. *Oncogene.* 2007;26:6816–6828. *Review of transcription factors that control neutrophil and monocyte development.*

Hsieh MM, Everhart JE, Byrd-Holt DD, Tisdale JF, Rodgers GP. Prevalence of neutropenia in the U.S. population: age, sex, smoking status, and ethnic differences. *Ann Intern Med.* 2007;146:486–492. *Recent population-based study of ethnic differences in blood neutrophil counts.*

Sullivan BM, Locksley RM. Basophils: a nonredundant contributor to host immunity. *Immunity.* 2009;30:12–20. *Recent review of basophil biology.*

von Vietinghoff S, Ley K. Homeostatic regulation of blood neutrophil counts. *J Immunol.* 2008;181:5183–5188.

Zarbock A, Ley K. Mechanisms and consequences of neutrophil interaction with the endothelium. *Am J Pathol.* 2008;172:1–7.

Neutrophilia

Reding MT, Hibbs JR, Morrison VA, Swaim WR, Filice GA. Diagnosis and outcome of 100 consecutive patients with extreme granulocytic leukocytosis. *Am J Med.* 1998;104:12–16. *Classic paper on neutrophilia.*

Seebach JD, Morant R, Ruegg R, et al. The diagnostic value of the neutrophil left shift in predicting inflammatory and infectious disease. *Am J Clin Pathol.* 1997;107:582–591. *Classic paper on neutrophilia.*

Congenital neutropenia

Boocock GR, Morrison JA, Popovic M, et al. Mutations in SBDS are associated with Shwachman-Diamond syndrome. *Nat Genet.* 2003;33(1):97–10. *Original report of SBDS mutations in SDS.*

Boxer LA, Newburger PE. A molecular classification of congenital neutropenia syndromes. *Pediatr Blood Cancer.* 2007;49:609–614. *Nice review of congenital neutropenia from leaders in the field.*

Boztug K, Appaswamy G, Ashikov A, et al. A syndrome with congenital neutropenia and mutations in G6PC3. *N Engl J Med.* 2009;360:32–43. *Original report of mutations in G6PC3 in congenital neutropenia.*

Dale DC, Bonilla MA, Davis MW, et al. A randomized controlled phase III trial of recombinant human G-CSF for treatment of severe chronic neutropenia. *Blood.* 1993;181:2496–2502. *Randomized trial showing efficacy of chronic G-CSF treatment in patients with SCN.*

Dale DC, Person RE, Bolyard AA, et al. Mutations in the gene encoding neutrophil elastase in congenital and cyclic neutropenia. *Blood.* 2000;96:2317–2322. *Original report of mutations of ELA2 in congenital neutropenia.*

Ginzberg H, Shin J, Ellis L, et al. Shwachman syndrome: phenotypic manifestations of sibling sets and isolated cases in a large patient cohort are similar. *J Pediatr.* 1999;135:81–88. *Review of clinical features of SDS.*

Gorlin RJ, Gelb B, Diaz GA, et al. WHIM syndrome, an autosomal dominant disorder: clinical, hematological, and molecular studies. *Am J Med Genet.* 2000;91:368–376. *Summary of the clinical features of WHIM syndrome.*

Hernandez PA, Gorlin RJ, Lukens JN, et al. Mutations in the chemokine receptor gene CXCR4 are associated with WHIM syndrome, a combined immunodeficiency disease. *Nat Genet.* 2003;34:70–74. *Original report of CXCR4 mutations in WHIM syndrome.*

Horwitz M, Benson KF, Person RE, Aprikyan AG, Dale DC. Neutrophil elastase mutations define a 21-day biological clock in cyclic hematopoiesis. *Nat Genet.* 1999;23:433–436. *Original report of mutations of ELA2 in congenital neutropenia.*

Klein C, Grudzien M, Appaswamy G, et al. HAX1 deficiency causes autosomal recessive severe congenital neutropenia (Kostmann disease). *Nat Genet.* 2007;39:86–92. *Original report of mutations of HAX1 in congenital neutropenia.*

Rosenberg PS, Alter BP, Bolyard AA, et al. The incidence of leukemia and mortality from sepsis in patients with severe congenital neutropenia receiving long-term G-CSF therapy. *Blood.* 2006;107:4628–4635. *Update from the Severe Chronic Neutropenia International Registry on the incidence of leukemia in severe congenital neutropenia.*

Ward DM, Shiflett SL, Kaplan J. Chédiak-Higashi syndrome: a clinical and molecular view of a rare lysosomal storage disorder. *Curr Mol Med.* 2002;2:469–477. *Review of the clinical features and genetics of Chédiak-Higashi syndrome.*

Immune neutropenia and neutropenia associated with autoimmunity

Berliner N, Horwitz M, Loughran TP. Congenital and acquired neutropenia. *Hematology Am Soc Hematol Educ Program.* 2004:63–69.

Bux J, Behrens G, Jaeger G, Welte K. Diagnosis and clinical course of autoimmune neutropenia in infancy: analysis of 240 cases. *Blood.* 1998;91:181–186. *Classic paper on autoimmune neutropenia in infants and young children.*

Gramatges MM, Fani P, Nadeau K, Pereira S, Jeng MR. Neonatal alloimmune thrombocytopenia and neutropenia associated with maternal human leukocyte antigen antibodies. *Pediatr Blood Cancer.* 2009;53:97–99. *Recent review of neonatal alloimmune neutropenia.*

O'Malley DP. T-cell large granular leukemia and related proliferations. *Am J Clin Pathol.* 2007;127:850–859. *Excellent review of neutropenia, particularly LGL and Felty's syndrome.*

Papadaki HA, Palmblad J, Eliopoulos GD. Non-immune chronic idiopathic neutropenia of adult: an overview. *Eur J Haematol.* 2001;67:35–44. *A review of nonimmune chronic idiopathic neutropenia.*

Starkebaum G. Chronic neutropenia associated with autoimmune disease. *Semin Hematol.* 2002;39:121–127. *A nice review of neutropenia associated with autoimmune disorders.*

Neutropenia due to idiosyncratic drug reactions or chemotherapy

Aapro MS, Cameron DA, Pettengell R, et al. EORTC guidelines for the use of granulocyte-colony stimulating factor to reduce the incidence of chemotherapy-induced febrile neutropenia in adult patients with lymphomas and solid tumours. *Eur J Cancer.* 2006;42:2433–2453. *Guidelines for the use of myeloid growth factors for the prevention or treatment of neutropenia.*

Andersohn F, Konzen C, Garbe E. Systematic review: agranulocytosis induced by nonchemotherapy drugs. *Ann Intern Med.* 2007;146:657–665. *Systematic review of drug-induced neutropenia.*

Andres E, Maloisel F. Idiosyncratic drug-induced agranulocytosis or acute neutropenia. *Curr Opin Hematol.* 2008;15:15–21. *Systematic review of drug-induced neutropenia.*

Clark OA, Lyman GH, Castro AA, et al. Colony-stimulating factors for chemotherapy-induced febrile neutropenia: a meta-analysis of randomized controlled trials. *J Clin Oncol.* 2005;23:4198–4214. *Meta-analysis of myeloid growth factors to treat chemotherapy-induced febrile neutropenia showing shortened hospital stay, shortened neutrophil recovery, and a possible reduction in infection-related mortality.*

Crawford J, Althaus B, Armitage J, et al. Myeloid growth factors. Clinical practice guidelines in oncology. *J Natl Compr Canc Netw.* 2007;5:188–202.

Hughes WT, Armstrong D, Bodey GP, et al. 2002 Guidelines for the use of antimicrobial agents in neutropenic patients with cancer. *Clin Infect Dis.* 2002;34:730–751.

Smith TJ, Khatcheressian J, Lyman GH, et al. 2006 update of recommendations for the use of white blood cell growth factors: an evidence-based clinical practice guideline. *J Clin Oncol.* 2006;24:3187–3205. *Guidelines for the use of antibacterial, antifungal, and antiviral agents in patients with neutropenia and cancer.*

Disorders of neutrophil function

Boxer LA. Neutrophil abnormalities. *Pediatr Rev.* 2003;24:52–62. *Excellent review of congenital disorders of neutrophil function.*

Dinauer MC. Chronic granulomatous disease and other disorders of phagocyte function. *Hematology Am Soc Hematol Educ Program.* 2005;89–95. *Recent review of the molecular pathogenesis, clinical features, and treatment of chronic granulomatous disease.*

Drenth JPH, Van de Meer JWM. Hereditary periodic fever. *N Engl J Med.* 2001;345:1748–1757. *Review of autoinflammatory disorder.*

Engelhardt KR, McGhee S, Winkler S, et al. Large deletions and point mutations involving the dedicator of cytokinesis 8 (DOCK8) in the autosomal-recessive form of hyper-IgE syndrome. *J Allergy Clin Immunol.* 2009;124:1289–1302. *Original report of gene mutations in hyperimmunoglobulin IgE syndrome.*

Etzioni A. Leukocyte adhesion deficiencies: molecular basis, clinical findings, and therapeutic options. *Adv Exp Med Biol.* 2007;601:51–60. *Recent review of leukocyte adhesion deficiency.*

Holland SM, DeLeo FR, Elloumi HZ, et al. STAT3 mutations in the hyper-IgE syndrome. *N Engl J Med.* 2007;357:1608–1619. *Original report of gene mutations in hyperimmunoglobulin IgE syndrome.*

Minegishi Y, Saito M, Morio T, et al. Human tyrosine kinase 2 deficiency reveals its requisite roles in multiple cytokine signals involved in innate and acquired immunity. *Immunity.* 2006;25:745–755. *Original report of gene mutations in hyperimmunoglobulin IgE syndrome.*

Qasim W, Cavazzana-Calvo M, Davies EG, et al. Allogeneic hematopoietic stem-cell transplantation for leukocyte adhesion deficiency. *Pediatrics.* 2009;123:836–840. *Update on HSCT for leukocyte adhesion deficiencies.*

Seger RA. Modern management of chronic granulomatous disease. *Br J Haematol.* 2008;140:255–266. *Recent review of the molecular pathogenesis, clinical features, and treatment of chronic granulomatous disease.*

Yao Q, Furst DE. Autoinflammatory diseases: an update of clinical and genetic aspects. *Rheumatology (Oxford).* 2008;47:946–951. *Review of autoinflammatory disorder.*

Hemophagocytic lymphohistiocytosis

Arico M, Janka G, Fischer A, et al. Hemophagocytic lymphohistiocytosis. Report of 122 children from the International Registry FHL Study Group of the Histiocyte Society. *Leukemia.* 1996;10:197–203. *Registry study of FHL.*

Feldmann J, Callebaut I, Raposo G, et al. Munc13–4 is essential for cytolytic granules fusion and is mutated in a form of familial hemophagocytic lymphohistiocytosis (FHL3). *Cell.* 2003;115:461–473. *Initial report describing Munc13–4 mutations in FHL.*

Henter JI, Elinder G, Soder O, Hansson M, Andersson B, Andersson U. Hypercytokinemia in familial hemophagocytic lymphohistiocytosis. *Blood.* 1991;78:2918–2922. *Report describing the presence of elevated inflammatory cytokines in FHL.*

Henter JI, Horne A, Arico M, et al. HLH-2004: Diagnostic and therapeutic guidelines for hemophagocytic lymphohistiocytosis. *Pediatr Blood Cancer.* 2007;48:124–131. *Updated guidelines from the Histiocyte Society on the diagnosis and treatment of HLH.*

Henter JI, Samuelsson-Horne A, Arico M, et al. Treatment of hemophagocytic lymphohistiocytosis with HLH–94 immunochemotherapy and bone marrow transplantation. *Blood.* 2002;100:2367–2373. *Large series reporting the outcome of children treated with stem cell transplantation for HLH.*

Janka GE. Familial and acquired hemophagocytic lymphohistiocytosis. *Eur J Pediatr.* 2007;166:95–109. *Excellent recent review of HLH.*

Katano H, Cohen JI. Perforin and lymphohistiocytic proliferative disorders. *Br J Hematol.* 2005;128:739–750. *Excellent review describing spectrum of perforin mutations in HLH.*

Schneider EM, Lorenz I, Muller-Rosenberger M, Steinbach G, Kron M, Janka-Schaub GE. Hemophagocytic lymphohistiocytosis is associated with deficiencies of cellular cytolysis but normal expression of transcripts relevant to killer-cell-induced apoptosis. *Blood.* 2002;100:2891–2898. *Report describing NK cell defects found in HLH.*

Stepp SE, Dufourcq-Lagelouse R, Le Deist F, et al. Perforin gene defects in familial hemophagocytic lymphohistiocytosis. *Science.* 1999;286:1957–1959. *Classic paper describing identifying mutations in perforin as the cause for some cases of FHL.*

Langerhans cell histiocytosis

Arico M, Girschikofsky M, Genereau T, et al. Langerhans cell histiocytosis in adults. Report from the International Registry of the Histiocyte Society. *Eur J Cancer.* 2003;39:2341–2348. *Large registry study of 274 adults with LCH.*

Gadner H, Grois N, Arico M, et al. A randomized trial of treatment for multisystem Langerhans' cell histiocytosis. *J Pediatr.* 2001;138:728–734. *Study demonstrating similar outcomes with treatment with either vinblastine or etoposide for LCH.*

Grois N, Potschger U, Prosch H, et al. Risk factors for diabetes insipidus in Langerhans cell histiocytosis. *Pediatr Blood Cancer.* 2006;46:228–233. *Analysis of 1741 patients treated on clinical studies for LCH.*

Histiocyte Society. Langerhans Cell Histiocytosis Evaluation and Treatment Guidelines. http://www.histiocytesociety.org. Accessed May 7, 2010. *Clinical guidelines published by the Histiocyte Society.*

Titgemeyer C, Grois N, Minkov M, Flucher-Wolfram B, Gatterer-Menz I, Gadner H. Pattern and course of single-system disease in Langerhans cell histiocytosis data from the DAL-HX 83- and 90-study. *Med Pediatr Oncol.* 2001;37:108–114. *Describes the outcome of 170 patients with SS-LCH treated on German LCH studies.*

Valladeau J, Ravel O, Dezutter-Dambuyant C, et al. Langerin, a novel C-type lectin specific to Langerhans cells, is an endocytic receptor that induces the formation of Birbeck granules. *Immunity.* 2000;12:71–81. *Report describing Langerin as a novel receptor on Langerhans cells, which induces the formation of Birbeck granules.*

Vassallo R, Ryu JH, Schroeder DR, Decker PA, Limper AH. Clinical outcomes of pulmonary Langerhans'-cell histiocytosis in adults. *N Engl J Med.* 2002;346:484–490. *Retrospective review of pulmonary LCH outcomes.*

Weitzman S, Jaffe R. Uncommon histiocytic disorders: the non-Langerhans cell histiocytoses. *Pediatr Blood Cancer.* 2005;45:256–226. *Excellent review of non-LCH disorders.*

Willis B, Ablin A, Weinberg V, et al. Disease course and late sequelae of Langerhans' cell histiocytosis: 25-year experience at the University of California, San Francisco. *J Clin Oncol.* 1996;14:2073–2082. *Classic paper describine natural history of LCH.*

Willman CL, Busque L, Griffith BB, et al. Langerhans'-cell histiocytosis (histiocytosis X)—a clonal proliferative disease. *N Engl J Med.* 1994;331:154–160. *Classic paper describing the clonal nature of LCH.*

Lysosomal storage diseases

Barton NW, Brady RO, Dambrosia JM, et al. Replacement therapy for inherited enzyme deficiency–macrophage-targeted glucocerebrosidase for Gaucher's disease. *N Engl J Med.* 1991;324:1464–1470. *Classic paper describing effectiveness of enzyme replacement therapy in Gaucher disease.*

Cox T, Lachmann R, Hollak C, et al. Novel oral treatment of Gaucher's disease with N-butyldeoxynojirimycin (OGT 918) to decrease substrate biosynthesis. *Lancet.* 2000;355:1481–1485. *Report describing substrate reduction therapy with miglustat in Gaucher disease.*

Figueroa ML, Rosenbloom BE, Kay AC, et al. A less costly regimen of alglucerase to treat Gaucher's disease. *N Engl J Med.* 1992;327:1632–1636. *Report of alternative with more frequent low-dose regimen for enzyme replacement therapy in Gaucher disease.*

Hughes D, Cappellini MD, Berger M, et al. Recommendations for the management of the haematological and onco-haematological aspects of Gaucher disease. *Br J Haematol.* 2007;138:676–686. *Recent published guidelines on Gaucher disease.*

Schuchman EH. The pathogenesis and treatment of acid sphingomyelinase-deficient Niemann-Pick disease. *J Inherit Metab Dis.* 2007;30:654–663. *Recent review of Niemann-Pick disease.*

Weinreb NJ, Charrow J, Andersson HC, et al. Effectiveness of enzyme replacement therapy in 1028 patients with type 1 Gaucher disease after 2 to 5 years of treatment: a report from the Gaucher Registry. *Am J Med.* 2002;113:112–119. *Paper describing long-term results of ERT therapy in Gaucher disease.*

CHAPTER 14

Myeloproliferative neoplasms

Bruno C. Medeiros and Ross L. Levine

Epidemiology, 398
Chronic myelogenous leukemia,
  BCR-ABL1 positive, 398
Chronic neutrophilic leukemia, 406
Systemic mastocytosis, 407

Myeloid (and lymphoid) neoplasms
  associated with eosinophilia and abnormalities of PDGFRA, PDGFRB, or FGFR1, 410
Chronic eosinophilic leukemia, not
  otherwise specified, 413
Polycythemia vera, 414

Essential thrombocythemia, 425
Primary myelofibrosis, 431
Myeloproliferative neoplasm,
  unclassifiable, 437
Bibliography, 437

Myeloproliferative neoplasms (MPNs) are a phenotypically diverse group of stem cell–derived clonal disorders characterized by proliferation of 1 or more of the components of the myeloid lineage (ie, erythroid, granulocytic, megakaryocytic, or mast cell). In 1951, William Dameshek first used the term *myeloproliferative disorders* (MPDs) and grouped together these 4 similar and overlapping clinicopathologic entities (ie, chronic myelogenous leukemia [CML], primary myelofibrosis [PMF], polycythemia vera [PV], and essential thrombocythemia [ET]). In 2008, the World Health Organization (WHO) revised the classification of MPDs and renamed this group of disorders as MPNs to underscore their clonal nature (Table 14-1). The updated 2008 classification featured the following major modifications, aside from the nomenclature update: (i) mastocytosis has been included in the MPN category; (ii) diagnostic algorithms for ET, PV, and PMF have been updated; and (iii) a new category of myeloid or lymphoid neoplasms with eosinophilia and abnormalities of platelet-derived growth factor receptor α (PDGFRA), platelet-derived growth factor receptor β (PDGFRB), or fibroblast-growth factor receptor 1 (FGFR1) was created.

From a practical standpoint, classification of MPNs is currently in transition from traditional morphologic assessments toward a disease-defining and disease-associated molecular genetic defects classification. Genetic studies have identified clonal genetic abnormalities involving cytoplasmic or receptor tyrosine kinases (TKs) in the majority of MPN patients. These genetic abnormalities (translocations or point mutations) result in abnormal, constitutively active TK signaling that leads to pathologic proliferation of myeloid precursors. The 4 major or classic MPNs are *BCR-ABL*–positive CML, PV, ET, and PMF (formerly known as chronic idiopathic myelofibrosis or agnogenic myeloid metaplasia). At present, CML is the only one of the 4 major MPNs characterized by a disease-defining genetic abnormality—the t(9;22)(q34;q11) Philadelphia chromosome and its molecular equivalent, the aberrant *BCR-ABL* fusion TK. Although not specific for any MPN, activating point mutations of Janus kinase 2 (*JAK2*) TK (*JAK2* V617F) are observed in almost all patients with PV and in a significant proportion of patients with ET, PMF, and other myeloid disorders. More recent studies have identified somatic activating *JAK2* exon 12 mutations (*JAK2* V617F–negative PV) and myeloproliferative leukemia (*MPL*) mutations (in ET and PMF patients) in some *JAK2* V617F–negative MPN patients. In addition, systemic mastocytosis (SM) is frequently associated with somatic mutations in *c-KIT* (KIT D816V), and MPNs associated with eosinophilia (chronic eosinophilic leukemia [CEL] and other MPNs associated with eosinophilia) most commonly present with clonal rearrangements of *PDGFRA*, *PDGFRB*, or *FGFR1*. Unclassifiable MPN refers to clonal, TK-negative syndromes with features that may be shared by specific MPNs but have atypical findings and fail to meet specific diagnostic criteria for a specific MPNs or other related hematologic disorders. It is important to note, therefore, that the presence of a specific

Conflict-of-interest disclosure: *Dr. Medeiros*: consultancy: Millennium, Antisoma; research funding: Genentech; speakers' bureau: Celgene, Novartis. *Dr. Levine*: consultancy: Novartis, Cephalon, TargeGen (all on a one-time basis); honoraria: Novartis, Cephalon (paid talks).

Table 14-1 Current classification of myeloproliferative neoplasms.

Myeloproliferative neoplasms (MPNs)
    Chronic myelogenous leukemia, *BCR-ABL1* positive
    Chronic neutrophilic leukemia
    Polycythemia vera
    Primary myelofibrosis
    Essential thrombocythemia
    Chronic eosinophilic leukemia, not otherwise specified
    Systemic mastocytosis
    MPN, unclassifiable

Myeloid (and lymphoid) neoplasms associated with eosinophilia and abnormalities of *PDGFRA*, *PDGFRB*, or *FGFR1*
    Myeloid and lymphoid neoplasms associated with *PDGFRA* rearrangement
    Myeloid neoplasms associated with *PDGFRB* rearrangement
    Myeloid and lymphoid neoplasms associated with *FGFR1* abnormalities

MPN-associated mutation is of diagnostic significance, but the absence of *JAK2*, *MPL*, or other MPN-associated disease alleles does not exclude a diagnosis of a specific MPN.

The different MPNs share several clinical and laboratory features, including frequent organomegaly (hepatomegaly and/or splenomegaly) either caused by sequestration of excess blood cells or abnormal proliferation of hematopoietic cells; increased metabolic rate; hypercellularity of the bone marrow (due to clonal marrow hyperplasia) associated with increased numbers of granulocytes, red blood cells, and/or platelets; and absence of significant dysplasia. Despite insidious onset, each MPN has the potential to undergo a stepwise progression that terminates in marrow failure due to ineffective hematopoiesis caused by fibrosis or transformation to blast phase, which is clinically similar to acute leukemia. By definition, MPNs must have <20% undifferentiated blasts.

Epidemiology

Each of the specific MPNs is relatively uncommon. The incidence for each of the major MPNs varies from 0.4 to 2.8 cases per 100,000 persons per year. The National Cancer Institute's Surveillance, Epidemiology, and End Results (SEER) database began collecting data on chronic myeloproliferative disorders in 2001. The cumulative age-adjusted SEER incidence rate during this period varied between 2.1 and 2.4 per 100,000 persons per year. MPNs are primarily neoplasms of adults, with a peak in frequency between the fifth and seventh decades of life. In fact, it is assumed that only 5% of the patients with PV are younger than 40 years old at diagnosis. However, adult-type MPNs, especially *BCR-ABL*–positive CML and ET, can rarely occur in children.

Chronic myelogenous leukemia, *BCR-ABL1* positive

Clinical case

A 45-year-old man presents with a 3-month history of unintentional 20-pound weight loss, night sweats, and general malaise. He has diet-controlled hypercholesterolemia and takes no medications. He believes his weight loss is due to a shrinking stomach. Physical examination is unremarkable, except for painless splenomegaly (spleen tip palpable 8 cm below the left costal margin). The hemoglobin is 14.6 g/dL, hematocrit is 43%, white blood cell (WBC) count is 93,900/μL, and platelet count is 679,000/μL. Evaluation of the peripheral smear reveals neutrophilia with significant left shift, occasional eosinophils, and increased basophils. BCR-ABL fusion transcript is detected by molecular analysis.

CML is a clonal MPN originating from pluripotent hematopoietic stem cells characterized by the *BCR-ABL1* fusion gene, which is derived from a balanced translocation between the long arms of chromosomes 9 and 22, t(9;22)(q34;q11), also known as the Philadelphia (Ph) chromosome.

Epidemiology

CML accounts for 15% to 20% of leukemia cases in adults. The worldwide annual incidence of CML is 1 to 2 cases per 100,000 persons, with a slight male predominance (male-to-female ratio, 1.3:1). Although the disease may occur at any age, the median age at presentation is between 50 and 60 years. *BCR-ABL1*–positive CML accounts for 2% of childhood leukemia and is most common in the 10- to 14-year-old age group. A higher incidence of CML is noted among persons with heavy radiation exposure; however, there has been no evidence for a causal association between CML and organic solvents, industrial chemicals, or alkylating agents.

Pathobiology

The Ph chromosome [der(22q)] was initially identified in patients with CML in 1960. The t(9;22)(q34;q11) translocation in CML juxtaposes the 3′ segment of the *c-ABL* oncogene (normally encoding the Abelson TK) from the long arm of chromosome 9 to the 5′ part of the breakpoint cluster region (*BCR*) gene on the long arm of chromosome 22. The resultant hybrid oncogene is transcribed as a chimeric *BCR-ABL* mRNA, which, in turn, is translated into a functional abnormal protein. At diagnosis, characteristic t(9;22)(q34;q11) is present in approximately 95% of CML cases. The remaining cases have either variant translocations involving a third and, sometimes, fourth chromosome or cryptic translocations. In these cases, routine cytogenetic analysis is unable to detect the Ph chromosome, and the diagnosis relies on demonstration of the fusion transcript by either fluorescence in situ hybridization (FISH) or reverse transcriptase (RT) polymerase chain reaction (PCR).

Three separate breakpoint regions in the *BCR* gene are associated with distinct disease phenotypes. In typical CML, the *BCR* gene is interrupted at either its e13 or e14 loci (exons 12-16). Collectively, this region is referred to as the major breakpoint cluster region (M-BCR). In a rearrangement involving M-BCR, the 5′ *BCR* segments on chromosome 22 are joined with the sequences from *c-ABL* that are 3′ from the a2 breakpoint (a breakpoint near the 5′ end of *c-ABL*). This union gives rise to hybrid transcripts called e13a2 (b2a2) and e14a2 (b3a3). These transcripts are translated into 210-kd proteins, collectively known as p210BCR-ABL. Importantly, the rearranged *c-ABL* segment here includes sequences necessary for TK activity. As a result, the p210BCR-ABL oncoprotein functions as a constitutively active TK that can phosphorylate a number of cytoplasmic substrates with other activities of the chimeric protein, leading to alterations in cell proliferation, differentiation, adhesion, and survival.

Two alternative translocations involving *BCR* and *ABL* have also been implicated in the pathogenesis of hematologic malignancies (Figure 14-1). In one of these, a similar segment of *c-ABL* is transposed onto a locus of *BCR* that is downstream (3′) from the M-BCR locus, a region referred to as μ-BCR (exons 17-20). Translocations involving μ-BCR yield

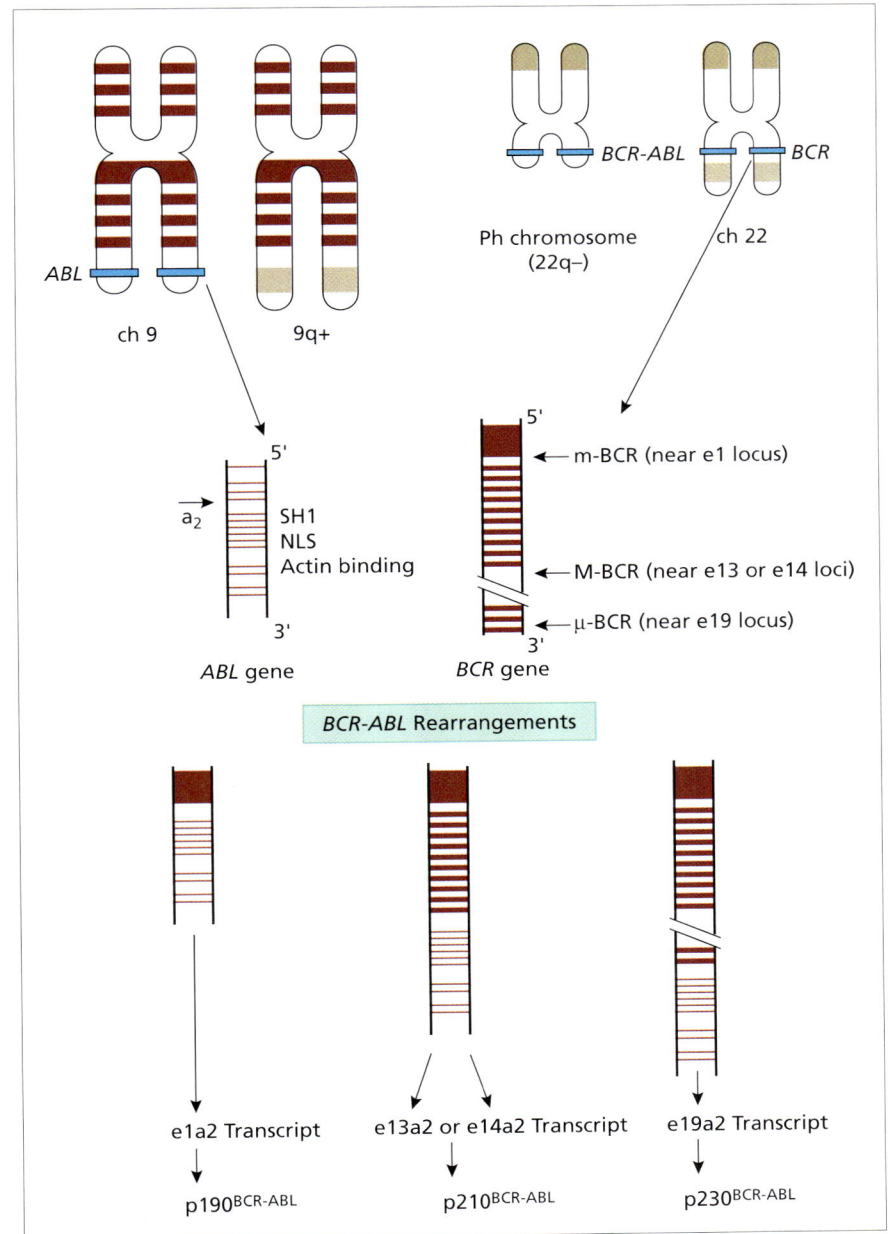

Figure 14-1 Schematic of molecular pathogenesis of t(9;22)(q34;q11) in chronic myelogenous leukemia (CML). The 3′ portion of the *ABL* gene on the telomeric region of the long arm of chromosome 9 is translocated to the *BCR* gene on chromosome 22 to form the characteristic 22q− abnormality referred to as the Philadelphia (Ph) chromosome. Breakpoints within the *ABL* gene occur within introns 1b or 2, both of which are 5′ (upstream) to the a2 exon. The a2 and downstream exons of *ABL* encode the Src homology (SH) domains of the *ABL* kinase, including the SH1/tyrosine kinase domain, DNA binding domain, nuclear localization signal (NLS), and actin binding site. The breakpoints on chromosome 22 occur at 1 of 3 different locations within *BCR*, yielding hybrid oncogenes of varying length consisting of 5′ BCR sequences and 3′ ABL sequences. Each hybrid oncogene gives rise to a chimeric transcript, which encodes a fusion protein with oncogenic activity. These include p190*BCR-ABL* (resulting from fusion at the minor breakpoint or m-*BCR* site), p210*BCR-ABL* gene product (resulting from fusion at the major breakpoint or M-*BCR* site), and p230*BCR-ABL* (resulting from fusion at the micro breakpoint or μ-*BCR* site).

a larger fusion gene than those involving M-BCR, and this larger fusion gives rise to a 230-kd p230BCR-ABL protein. The p230BCR-ABL product has been found in uncommon CML variant cases that are characterized by chronic neutrophilia with or without thrombocytosis and a more indolent disease course than CML associated with the p210BCR-ABL. Distinction between p230BCR-ABL CML and chronic neutrophilic leukemia can be challenging. The third type of *BCR-ABL* rearrangement juxtaposes the same *c-ABL* segment to the minor *BCR* breakpoint region (m-BCR), which is located upstream (5′) from the M-BCR (exons 1–2). The resultant smaller chimeric oncogene generated by this rearrangement gives rise to a 190-kd p190BCR-ABL protein product. The p190BCR-ABL transforming protein is most often found in a portion of de novo acute lymphoblastic leukemia (ALL) cases referred to as Ph-positive ALL. Rarely, the p190BCR-ABL product can be detected in CML, either coexpressed with p210BCR-ABL or detected alone in atypical cases that are associated with monocytosis. Coexpression of p190BCR-ABL and p210BCR-ABL is attributed to alternative splicing of the transcript arising from the M-BCR chimeric oncogene.

The leukemic clone in CML has a tendency to acquire additional oncogenic mutations over time. Clinically, the acquisition of additional cytogenetic or molecular abnormalities is associated with progression to accelerated and blast phases of disease or resistance to TK inhibitors. At the chromosomal level, additional mutations are identified in 50% to 80% of advanced-disease cases. These changes include monosomy 7, t(3;21), amplification of t(9;22), trisomy 8, trisomy 19, and abnormalities of chromosome 17. At the molecular level, mutations in the kinase domain of *BCR-ABL*, which are the most prevalent mechanism of imatinib resistance in patients with CML, have a reported annual resistance rate of <1% to 7% in newly diagnosed patients in chronic phase, with the incidence decreasing over time. To date, >50 different mutations have been associated with different degrees of clinical resistance to TK inhibitors.

Clinical features

Roughly 90% of patients with CML present in the chronic phase of disease, most commonly with an insidious onset. Nearly 20% to 40% of individuals are asymptomatic and are discovered incidentally. Common symptoms at presentation include fatigue, night sweats, and weight loss and are normally due to hypercatabolic symptoms, splenomegaly, anemia, and/or platelet dysfunction. Hyperleukocytosis alone does not routinely cause symptoms because of the relative maturity of the leukemic cells compared with those seen in acute leukemia; however, males with very high WBC counts rarely present with leukostasis-related priapism. Splenomegaly is detected in 50% to 90% of patients at diagnosis, and painless hepatomegaly may be present in up half of the patients. Thrombotic and hemorrhagic complications occur in <5% of patients, although purpura is a common complaint. Bleeding with CML becomes a major concern during the blast phase of disease.

Diagnostic criteria

The laboratory and marrow abnormalities in chronic phase, accelerated phase, and/or blast phase CML are summarized in Table 14-2. In the peripheral blood, neutrophilia and immature circulating myeloid cells are hallmark features of CML. More than 50% of patients present with a WBC count >100,000/μL, with blasts usually accounting for <2% of the WBCs. Absolute basophilia is invariably present, and eosinophilia is common. Anemia may be present in up to half of patients. Roughly 15% to 35% of patients present with platelet counts >700,000/μL, although extreme thrombocytosis (ie, >1,500,000/μL) is uncommon. Patients with very high platelet counts may be at greater risk of thrombotic or hemorrhagic complications. The high cell turnover and hypercatabolic state of CML are associated with elevated lactate dehydrogenase (LDH) and uric acid levels. The leukocyte alkaline phosphatase (LAP) score is almost always low or 0, in contrast to the high LAP scores observed in patients with other MPNs or with reactive neutrophilia. The marrow in chronic-phase CML typically shows myeloid hyperplasia and an elevated myeloid-to-erythroid ratio (often >10:1). Increased marrow blasts (>5%) are seen in approximately 5% of cases at diagnosis. Maturation of precursors is normal in CML, and dysplastic features are not routinely found. Marrow basophilia is noted in one fourth of cases. Increased reticulin fibrosis is found in 30% of the cases and may have negative prognostic impact on outcomes. Pseudo-Gaucher cells and sea-blue histiocytes, secondary to increased cell turnover, are frequently found.

The quickest and least expensive way to confirm a suspected case of CML is to assay the peripheral blood for either the *BCR-ABL* fusion gene or its chimeric transcripts. The most widely used techniques involve FISH and RT-PCR, and the sensitivity of peripheral blood is equal to that of bone marrow. FISH allows identification and quantitation of the chimeric oncogene among interphase nuclei on a peripheral blood smear; usually, 200 to 500 nuclei are screened. RT-PCR is carried out on peripheral blood–derived RNA and is an extremely sensitive technique; RT-PCR can detect the *BCR-ABL* transcript in <1 of 10^5 cells. Both methods can detect "masked" or cryptic chromosomal translocations that are missed by conventional cytogenetics in approximately 5% of cases. FISH has the advantage of identifying unusual variant rearrangements that are outside the regions amplified by the RT-PCR primers. The RT-PCR method, unlike FISH,

Table 14-2 Clinical features of chronic myeloid leukemia.

Symptoms	Laboratory abnormalities	WHO classification
Chronic phase		
Fatigue	Neutrophilic leukocytosis with immaturity	
Weight loss	Peripheral blasts <10%	
Nocturnal sweats	Thrombocytosis	
Left upper quadrant abdominal pain	Basophilia and/or eosinophilia	
Early satiety	Normocytic anemia	
Palpitations and/or dyspnea	BCR-ABL rearrangement (usually p210BCR-ABL)	
Bleeding/bruising	High LDH	
Priapism	Hyperuricemia	
	Marrow myeloid and megakaryocytic hyperplasia, mild/moderate fibrosis, <10% blasts, minimal dysplasia, t(9;22) ± other abnormalities	
Accelerated phase		
Progressive splenomegaly ± infarcts	Karyotypic evolution blasts	10%-19% of WBCs in peripheral blood and/or nucleated bone marrow cells
Progressive weight loss and sweats	Blood or marrow blasts ≥10%	Peripheral blood basophils = 20%
Unexplained fever or bone pain	Blasts and promyelocytes ≥20%	Persistent thrombocytopenia (<100 × 10^9/L) unrelated to therapy, or persistent thrombocytosis (>1000 × 10^9/L) unresponsive to therapy
Tissue chloromas	Basophils plus eosinophils ≥20%	Increasing spleen size and increasing WBC count unresponsive to therapy
	Platelet count <100,000/μL	Cytogenetic evidence of clonal evolution
	Increasing peripheral counts or cytopenias unresponsive to antileukemic therapy	Megakaryocytic proliferation?
	Increasing marrow fibrosis	
Blast phase		
Bleeding, bruising	Blood or marrow blasts ≥20%	Blasts ≥20% of peripheral blood white cells or of nucleated bone marrow cells
Infections	Myeloid blast phenotype	Extramedullary blast proliferation
Prominent constitutional symptoms	Lymphoid blast phenotype	Large foci or clusters of blasts in the bone marrow biopsy
Massive splenomegaly	Biphenotypic or undifferentiated blasts	
Tissue manifestations of extramedullary disease		

LDH = lactate dehydrogenase; WBC = white blood cell count; WHO = World Health Organization.

can differentiate between the fusion genes encoding the p210 BCR-ABL product and the p190BCR-ABL product. Because of the lower cost and ability to discriminate the breakpoints, RT-PCR is currently the preferred molecular assay for CML diagnosis. Quantitation of *BCR-ABL*, either by FISH or RT-PCR, is not particularly helpful at the time of diagnosis but becomes important for clinical decision making and monitoring of minimal residual disease in patients on therapy. With the use of TK inhibitors for chronic-phase CML, sensitive measures of treatment response have become critical in patient management decisions. Because the false-positive rate of FISH for *BCR-ABL* fusion gene is approximately 3%, quantitative real-time RT-PCR is the preferred technique for monitoring of disease response. Although a positive RT-PCR or FISH assay confirms the diagnosis of CML, a complete staging of the disease still requires a marrow evaluation to rule out advanced-stage CML (Table 14-2). The marrow sample is necessary to assess the percentage of undifferentiated blasts and to evaluate for the presence of additional cytogenetic abnormalities. Conventional cytogenetic studies identify a Ph chromosome in 90% to 95% of cases; more than half of the karyotypically negative cases will have a detectable *BCR-ABL* rearrangement by molecular assay. The clinical course of *BCR-ABL*–positive, Ph-negative patients is identical to that of patients with Ph-positive CML. Additional cytogenetic abnormalities are usually not found at diagnosis in patients with early-stage disease.

Treatment

The development of imatinib mesylate and second-generation TK inhibitors has completely changed standard therapeutic approaches for all phases of CML. However, other therapies can still serve an adjunctive role or, in the case of conventional allogeneic stem cell transplantation (SCT), can offer cure to a subset of patients. It is unknown whether TK therapy will offer a subset of patients the chance for life-long disease remission, although the majority of patients on TK therapy remain in clinical/cytogenetic remission for 5 to 7 years or longer.

Imatinib mesylate and other treatments aimed at achieving remission

The promise of targeted therapy for CML was realized with the approval of the first small-molecule TK inhibitor for cancer, imatinib mesylate, in May 2001. Imatinib binds the adenosine triphosphate (ATP) binding site in the catalytic domain of the BCR-ABL oncoprotein and inhibits the BCR-ABL TK activity. This interaction prevents the transfer of phosphate groups to tyrosine residues on substrate molecules involved in downstream signal transduction pathways. The drug also interferes with the TK activities of normal ABL and with the kinase activity of the ARG, PDGFRA, PDGFRB, and c-Kit TKs. These actions are useful for the treatment of other hematopoietic (eg, SM, CEL) and nonhematopoietic (eg, gastrointestinal stromal tumor) disorders, but can cause minor in vivo adverse effects (eg, anemia) in patients with CML when imatinib is used at the standard 400 mg/d dose. Higher doses of imatinib (eg, 600–800 mg/d) result in higher rates of cytogenetic and molecular remission; with these higher doses comes a modest increase in treatment adverse effects. In phase I clinical studies of chronic-phase CML patients who were either intolerant of or resistant to interferon alfa (IFNα), imatinib administered at doses >300 mg/d yielded a complete hematologic response (CHR) rate of 98%. The majority of the responses occurred by 4 to 6 weeks; 31% and 13% of patients achieved a major cytogenetic response (MCyR; ≤35% *BCR-ABL*–positive metaphases) or complete cytogenetic response (CCyR; negative *BCR-ABL* metaphases) at a median treatment time of 5 months. These responses were among patients who were, on average, 4 years from initial CML diagnosis. One third of patients in this pivotal study also had features of accelerated-phase disease (other than increased blast counts). With 2-year follow-up, the majority of patients maintained a durable response on imatinib therapy, and some achieved a delayed CCyR. The US Food and Drug Administration (FDA)-approved initial dose for chronic-phase disease, 400 mg/d, is very well tolerated. Infrequent adverse effects include nausea, muscle cramps, periorbital edema, diarrhea, and mild myelosuppression. In many patients who experience unacceptable adverse effects, transient dose reduction or treatment interruption allows for patients to resolve adverse effects and resume full-dose therapy.

In a phase II clinical trial, complete hematologic and cytogenetic responses were seen in 95% and 41% of patients, respectively. This led to the pivotal phase III study comparing imatinib to the combination of IFNα and cytarabine (the International Randomized Interferon and STI571 [IRIS] trial). The IRIS study demonstrated the superiority of imatinib compared with IFNα plus cytarabine, with higher rates of CHR, MCyR, CCyR, freedom from progression to accelerated-phase or blast crisis CML, and better tolerance of therapy. The majority of patients who were at high risk according to current prognostic models achieved MCyR at a rate of 69% to 78.9% in the imatinib arm. After a median follow-up time of 60 months, the cumulative best rate of CCyR among patients receiving imatinib was 87%. The estimated overall survival for these patients was 89%. An estimated 7% of patients progressed to accelerated-phase or blast crisis CML. Remarkably, patients who had a CCyR or MCyR had a significantly lower risk of disease progression than patients who did not achieve these outcomes. Adverse effects mirrored the initial experience with imatinib and diminished over time. Despite impressive results with imatinib, several attempts have been made to improve response rates and decrease resistance in newly diagnosed patients through the use of higher doses of imatinib (600–800 mg/d) or second-generation TK inhibitors (dasatinib and nilotinib). Phase II studies demonstrate that higher dose TK inhibition yields higher rates of CCyR and major molecular responses (MMRs) at earlier time points. However, the benefits of upfront higher dose TK inhibition versus reserving higher dose imatinib/second-generation TK inhibitor therapy for patients who do not achieve clinical milestones have not yet been reported, although phase III trials are currently being performed.

Second-generation TK inhibitors

Patients with CML who relapse while on imatinib therapy have been studied carefully to determine the molecular basis of imatinib resistance. In most patients, resistance is associated with reactivation of BCR-ABL TK activity and a number of possible mechanisms have been identified in tumor cell lines and patient samples, including amplification of the *BCR-ABL* gene and overexpression of the BCR-ABL protein. However, the acquisition of resistance in patients appears to be primarily due to point mutations that affect the TK domain (TKD) of ABL, the site of imatinib binding to BCR-ABL. Kinase domain mutations occur in 50% to 90% of reported imatinib-resistant cases, whereas gene amplification of *BCR-ABL* has been observed in <10% of cases.

To date, 50 different point mutations have been identified in patients with clinical resistance to imatinib. Moreover, the risk of acquisition of imatinib resistance mutations is associated with the phase of the disease. Acquired resistance to imatinib in early and late chronic-phase CML occurs in 15% and 25% of patients, respectively. In an analysis of 256 patients with various stages of CML, the overall incidence of TKD mutations was 26% in chronic phase, 44% in accelerated phase, 73% in myeloid blast crisis, and 81% in lymphoid blast crisis. Intriguingly, analysis of patients who have been prospectively followed during imatinib therapy demonstrates that *BCR-ABL* mutations were detectable in approximately 2% per year.

The FDA has recently approved 2 new ABL kinase inhibitors as second-generation TK inhibitors for CML. Both agents inhibit most, but not all, imatinib-resistant BCR-ABL TKDs; however, neither drug has activity against the "gatekeeper" T315I mutation. Dasatinib (Sprycel; Bristol-Myers Squibb, New York, NY), a TKI with no structural similarity to imatinib with activity against SRC family kinases in addition to ABL kinases, has been approved for the treatment of adults with chronic-phase, accelerated-phase, or myeloid or lymphoid blast-phase CML with resistance or intolerance to prior therapy. In contrast, nilotinib (Tasigna; Novartis Oncology, East Hanover, NJ), a structural derivative of imatinib that is a 30-fold more potent inhibitor of BCR-ABL activity, has been approved only for the treatment of chronic-phase and accelerated-phase Ph-positive CML in adult patients resistant or intolerant to prior therapy, including imatinib. Dasatinib does not rely on a conformational change of ABL for binding and thus appears to be less susceptible to the development of resistant TKD mutations that alter ABL conformation. A recent update of the START-C trial, where patients with chronic-phase CML with resistance or intolerance to imatinib were switched to dasatinib therapy (70 mg orally twice daily), demonstrated that a CHR was attained in approximately 90% of patients (median follow-up, 15 months), and MCyRs and CCyRs were noted in 59% and 49% of patients, respectively. Although no responses were seen in patients with the T315I mutation, disease control was noted across all other TK mutations. MMR rate at 12 months was 25%. Progression-free survival at 15 months was 90%, and overall survival was 96%. The average daily dose administered was approximately 100 mg. Toxicities include myelosuppression, diarrhea, fatigue, and pleural effusion. Similar response rates and decreased toxicity have been demonstrated with dasatinib 100 mg orally once daily. Similarly, nilotinib has demonstrated significant clinical activity and an acceptable safety and tolerability profile in patients with imatinib-resistant or -intolerant chronic-phase CML, except in those who carry the T315I mutation. Increasing the dose of imatinib has been demonstrated to work in the presence of some, but not all, point mutations that result in imatinib resistance or in moderate overexpression of the BCR-ABL protein. Many patients respond to dose escalation of imatinib, but the responses are not durable. Toxicities of imatinib therapy including cytopenias are more common at the higher dose. A recent study has compared the results of switching early to dasatinib therapy versus escalating to high-dose imatinib in chronic-phase CML resistant to imatinib at daily doses from 400 to 600 mg. With a minimum follow-up of 2 years, all end points of the study (CHR, MCyR, CCyR, MMR, and progression-free survival) favored the switch to dasatinib. Thus, imatinib dose escalation should only be considered in patients unable to obtain clinical milestones on imatinib therapy or who become intolerant to second-generation TK inhibitors. The T315I mutation results in resistance to imatinib as well as dasatinib and nilotinib because it causes a structural change that closes the ATP-binding pocket of BCR-ABL so that drugs cannot enter and inhibit the kinase domain. Patients who develop resistance to imatinib, nilotinib, or dasatinib in the setting of an acquired T315I mutation are considered resistant to all 3 TK inhibitors and should be considered for alternative therapies including allogeneic SCT or IFN therapy depending on the patient's age, comorbidity, and donor availability.

Stem cell transplantation
Allogeneic transplantation

Allogeneic SCT in CML is now generally reserved for adults who fail TK inhibitors, although transplantation is still a reasonable option as first-line therapy in children and younger adults (for whom the risk-to-benefit ratio is lower), given the lack of data on the long-term efficacy of imatinib. Children and younger adults with early chronic-phase CML who receive a matched sibling donor SCT have a 5-year disease-free survival rate of 60% to 85%. The relapse rate among these patients is 5% to 15%. Accelerated or blast phases of CML may also be treated with allogeneic SCT for curative intent; however, survival is significantly worse because of high relapse rates and other complications related to advanced disease. Across all ages, the incidences of acute graft-versus-host disease (GVHD) range from 8% to 63%, with severe and fatal GVHD affecting up to 20% and 13% of patients, respectively. Conditioning commonly involves use of cyclophosphamide and targeted-dose busulfan. In addition, the use of peripheral blood stem cells appears to offer an advantage for advanced-stage CML, with lower relapse rates and longer disease-free survival, compared with transplantation using marrow stem cells.

Graft-versus-leukemia effect and reduced-intensity conditioning regimens

CML cells are highly susceptible to the graft-versus-leukemia (GVL) effect of an allograft. The overall leukemia relapse rate after matched unrelated donor SCT is somewhat lower than after matched related transplantations, suggesting that minor antigen disparity enhances a GVL effect. In addition, relapse rates are higher after transplantation with T-cell–depleted stem cells compared with unmanipulated stem cells, implicating that donor graft immune function is important in clearing residual disease. The potency of the GVL effect is further illustrated by the success of donor lymphocyte infusion (DLI) for relapsed disease after SCT. DLI alone, without other therapy, induces remission in 54% to 93% of patients with early hematologic or cytogenetic relapse. A therapeutic approach that relies heavily on the GVL effect against CML is allogeneic SCT following reduced-intensity or nonmyeloablative conditioning. Initial results using nonmyeloablative regimens are intriguing and demonstrate durable responses with decreased transplantation-related toxicity. The use of imatinib after reduced-intensity allogeneic transplantation is also being explored. These approaches could prove useful for patients failing nontransplantation therapies or those who cannot tolerate a myeloablative transplantation due to age or comorbidity.

Therapy for advanced disease
Imatinib and cytoreductive therapies

The treatment approaches for advanced CML remain unsatisfactory. Accelerated-phase CML may respond to aggressive induction-type chemotherapy regimens (25%–30% response rates) or IFNα (~40% CHR rate). Unfortunately, these responses are usually transient and are followed by rapid progression to blast crisis. Imatinib appears superior to other modalities for treatment of accelerated-phase disease. In a published phase II study, overall hematologic responses occurred in approximately 80% of patients with accelerated-phase CML (CHR, MCyR, and CCyR occurred in 53%, 24%, and 17% of patients, respectively). Overall survival and disease progression rates at 12 months were also optimal among patients receiving 600 mg/d (78% and 44%, respectively). Toxicity was acceptable. Furthermore, imatinib therapy in accelerated-phase disease can serve as a bridge to SCT.

Imatinib can transiently control CML blast crisis in a proportion of patients. Both lymphoid and myeloid phenotypes respond, and optimal results are achieved with a dose of 600 mg/d, as for accelerated-phase disease. Imatinib induced overall hematologic responses in approximately 50% of study subjects; 8% to 21% achieved CHRs and approximately 30% achieved stable or sustained hematologic responses (lasting ~4 weeks). MCyRs occurred in 16% of patients, and CCyRs occurred in 7% of patients. The median overall survival for patients who achieved a sustained hematologic response was 19 months. Myelosuppression was common, and nonhematologic toxicities were mild to moderate and seldom required discontinuation of therapy. The remarkable and encouraging results for blast crisis with this well-tolerated single agent have led to ongoing studies combining imatinib with conventional acute leukemia chemotherapy regimens.

The second-generation TK inhibitors (dasatinib and nilotinib) have been evaluated in patients with accelerated-phase or blast crisis CML resistant or intolerant to imatinib. Recent studies demonstrate that second-generation TK inhibitors induce rapid and durable responses in patients with accelerated-phase CML who failed prior imatinib therapy due to intolerance or resistance, with a favorable toxicity profile. Dasatinib, at a dose of 70 mg orally twice daily, led to CHR, MCyR, and CCyR in 45%, 39%, and 32% of patients with accelerated-phase CML, respectively. Responses were achieved irrespective of imatinib status (resistant or intolerant). The 12-month progression-free survival and overall survival rates were 66% and 82%, respectively. Nilotinib, at a dose of 400 mg orally twice daily, led to CHR, MCyR, and CCyR in 30%, 32%, and 19% of patients, respectively. The 12-month overall survival rate was 82%. Dasatinib appears to have more activity in the management of myeloid and lymphoid blast crisis CML than nilotinib. However, the lack of long-term data with second-generation TK inhibitors in patients with myeloid and lymphoid blast crisis CML suggests that allogeneic transplantation should be considered in patients who achieve hematologic response after second-generation TK inhibitor therapy.

Allogeneic transplantation

Although myeloablative allogeneic SCT can cure up to 40% of adult patients with CML in accelerated phase, the salvage rate of patients who receive transplantation in the setting of blast crisis is dismal. If transplantation is delayed, patients are usually treated with induction therapy and/or TK inhibitors to help achieve a second chronic-phase CML that may help improve the success of an SCT. Transplantation in second chronic phase yields outcomes comparable to those for transplantation in accelerated phase (ie, 20%–40% long-term disease-free survival). With myeloid blast crisis, induction chemotherapy regimens used for acute myeloid leukemia (AML) can achieve a second chronic phase in 20% to 30%

of patients, whereas regimens for ALL are effective in 40% to 60% of cases with lymphoid blast crisis. Aggressive chemotherapy in these settings incurs all of the complications associated with treatment of de novo acute leukemia. Responses are unstable, and a second blast crisis develops within weeks to a few months without further therapy. Moreover, recent studies suggest that the combination of induction chemotherapy and TK inhibitor therapy might increase the likelihood of response in blast crisis; however, phase II and III data are not yet available.

Course and prognosis
Chronic phase

After diagnosis, the chronic phase of CML typically remains stable for an average of 3 to 5 years before patients progress to accelerated or blast crisis CML. The rate of transformation to blast phase is 5% to 10% per year during the first 2 years after diagnosis, but increases to 25% per year thereafter. Prior to the development of TK inhibitors, patients with CML who did not undergo SCT had a median survival of roughly 5 to 7 years, whereas 30% of patients survived beyond 10 years. Also prior to the development of TK inhibitors, multivariate prognostic models (eg, the 1984 Sokal score for patients treated with chemotherapy, the 1998 Gratwohl score for patients considering allogeneic SCT, and the 1998 Hasford [Euro] score for IFN-treated patients) were highly useful to help predict shorter survival and make decisions regarding earlier use of aggressive modalities such as SCT or experimental therapies. Recent studies suggest that these older prognostic models can still predict the probability of achieving a cytogenetic remission in patients treated with imatinib mesylate and second-generation TK inhibitors. In the current era of TK inhibitors, the most important prognostic indicator is the response to therapy. Currently, the CCyR rate to frontline TK inhibitors is 70% to 90%, with 5-year progression-free survival and overall survival rates between 80% and 95%. It is important to note that the likelihood of achieving good long-term outcomes is associated with patients achieving specific clinical milestones on imatinib therapy (Table 14-3), including:

- Achieving CHR at 3 months
- Achieving at least an MCyR at 12 months
- Achieving CCyR at 18 months

If patients do not achieve these responses, they should undergo full restaging, and if their clinical situation worsens, mutational testing and modification of therapy should be considered.

Accelerated phase

The accelerated phase of CML is accompanied by the acquisition of additional molecular lesions, genomic instability, and progressive impairment of myeloid cell differentiation. This latter feature leads to the accumulation of immature

Table 14-3 Expected milestones and definition of failure and suboptimal response for previously untreated patients in chronic-phase chronic myelogenous leukemia receiving first-line imatinib mesylate therapy at a dose of 400 mg daily.

Time	Failure	Suboptimal response
Diagnosis	NA	NA
3 months after diagnosis	No hematologic response (stable disease or disease progression)	Less than CHR
6 months after diagnosis	Less than CHR, no CyR (Ph$^+$ >95%)	Less than PCyR (Ph$^+$ >35%)
12 months after diagnosis	Less than PCyR (Ph$^+$ >35%)	Less than CCyR
18 months after diagnosis	Less than CCyR	Less than MMR
Anytime	Loss of CHR*, loss of CCyR[†], mutation	ACA in Ph$^+$ cells[‡], loss of MMR[§], mutation[‖]

Note: Failure implies that the patient should be moved to other treatments whenever available. Suboptimal response implies that the patient may still have a substantial benefit from continuing imatinib treatment but that the long-term outcome is not likely to be optimal so patients become eligible to other therapies.

* To be confirmed on 2 occasions unless associated with progression to accelerated phase/blast crisis.
[†] To be confirmed on 2 occasions, unless associated with CHR loss or progression to accelerated phase/blast crisis.
[‡] High level of insensitivity to imatinib.
[§] To be confirmed on 2 occasions, unless associated with CHR or CCyR loss.
[‖] Low level of insensitivity to imatinib.

Adapted from Baccarani M, Saglio G, Goldman J, et al. Evolving concepts in the management of chronic myeloid leukemia: recommendations from an expert panel on behalf of the European LeukemiaNet. *Blood*. 2006;108:1809–1820.

ACA = additional chromosome abnormalities; CCyR = complete cytogenetic response; CyR = cytogenetic response; CHR = complete hematologic response; MMR = major molecular responses; NA = not applicable; PCyR = partial cytogenetic response; Ph = Philadelphia chromosome.

precursors and undifferentiated blasts in the marrow, blood, and extramedullary tissue. The clinical symptoms associated with the accelerated phase (Table 14-2) may be minor, delayed, or completely absent. The median survival from the onset of accelerated phase, without an SCT or TK inhibitors, is only 12 to 18 months. Death occurs predominantly because of transformation to blast phase with the associated life-threatening complications of marked leukocytosis and complete failure of normal hematopoiesis. Various laboratory criteria have been proposed for defining entry into accelerated phase, some of which have been identified by multivariate analyses as prognostically useful. Patients with karyotypic evolution alone, except for the acquisition of chromosome 17 abnormalities, without accompanying clinical and other laboratory changes, may follow a more indolent course to blast transformation.

Blast phase (leukemic progression)

Progression of CML to acute leukemia, synonymous with "blast phase" and "blast crisis," evolves most commonly from a preceding accelerated phase and is reached when the proportion of blasts in the blood or marrow is ≥20% (Table 14-2). Blast crisis may develop suddenly, without an intervening accelerated phase, in up to one fourth of chronic-phase patients. By comparison, a sudden transformation from chronic phase to blast phase occurs in >5% of patients on IFNα therapy. Sudden transformation to blast phase in patients taking imatinib is observed with an annual rate of 1% to 2%. Myeloid lineage markers (eg, CD33, CD13, CD14, and/or CD15) are expressed by the blast cells in over half of the cases of blast-phase CML. Up to one third express B-cell–precursor lymphoid markers (eg, CD10, CD19, and/or CD20). Undifferentiated acute leukemia and cases displaying both myeloid and lymphoid cell surface markers account for the remainder. Most CML cases express the p210BCR-ABL gene product, and only rare cases are associated with p190BCR-ABL alone. Thus, a case of Ph-positive ALL that is subsequently found to be associated with p210BCR-ABL might actually represent CML presenting in lymphoid blast crisis. The clinical and laboratory features of blast-phase CML are summarized in Table 14-2. Cytogenetic abnormalities in addition to t(9;22) are found in 65% to 80% of cases. The overall median survival is 3 to 6 months for older patients and roughly 8 months for younger adults; patients with lymphoid blast crisis survive 4 to 5 months longer than those with myeloid blasts. In blast phase, the presence of >50% blast cells in the blood and cytogenetic progression have been identified as independent predictors of worse survival. Deaths are usually due to metabolic derangements, infection, bleeding, and end-organ extramedullary leukemic infiltration.

Chronic neutrophilic leukemia

Chronic neutrophilic leukemia (CNL) is a rare chronic MPN that has only recently been recognized as a distinct entity within the updated WHO classification. CNL is a diagnosis of exclusion because reactive neutrophilia and other MPNs need to be excluded.

Epidemiology

CNL is an extremely rare disorder with <200 cases described to date. It appears to occur more commonly in older patients, although cases in adolescents have been described. Males and females also appear to be equally affected.

Pathobiology

No known genetic lesions have been associated with CNL. Some patients may present with *JAK2* V617F mutations.

Clinical features

Splenomegaly is the most frequently found clinical feature in patients with CNL, often accompanied by hepatomegaly. Some patients have a history of bleeding from the gastrointestinal tract.

Diagnostic criteria

CNL is characterized by sustained, mature neutrophilic leukocytosis with few or no circulating immature granulocytes, monocytosis, or basophilia. The WBC count usually exceeds 25,000/μL. Granulocyte dysplasia is not detectable, but the granules may be coarse (toxic). Bone marrow biopsy demonstrates hypercellularity with a striking neutrophil proliferation with myeloid-to-erythroid ratio reaching up to 20:1. Blasts or promyelocytes are not increased in number in the beginning, and dysplasia and reticulin fibrosis are not evident. Cytogenetic studies are normal in approximately 90% of cases of CNL, but in the remaining cases, clonal karyotypic anomalies may include +8, +9, +21, del(20q), del(11q), and del(12p). No Ph chromosome or *BCR-ABL1* fusion gene is found. Furthermore, CNL should be differentiated from neutrophilic CML, which is a rare variant of *BCR-ABL* (e19/a2 junction)–driven Ph-positive CML. Occasionally, patients with a *JAK2* mutation have been described.

Treatment

Optimal treatment for patients with CNL remains to be defined. Splenectomy has resulted in worsening of neutrophilic leukocytosis and cannot be recommended. Treatment of CNL to date has consisted largely of cytoreductive agents such as hydroxyurea, where clinical responses are noted in 75% of cases. Median duration of responses is approximately 12 months. Similarly to other chronic MPNs, IFNα has been used successfully and may produce durable responses. Allogeneic sibling SCT is usually reserved for patients with accelerated or blastic transformation. However, given the potential for blastic transformation and progressive refractory neutrophilia, allogeneic SCT may be appropriate for younger patients.

Course and prognosis

The clinical course of CNL is heterogeneous. Disease acceleration often manifests with the development of progressive neutrophilia with resistance to previously effective therapy, progressive splenomegaly, or worsening thrombocytopenia, or with cytogenetic clonal evolution. Blastic transformation occurs in a significant proportion of patients at a median of 21 months from diagnosis. Progressive neutrophilia associated with anemia and a decrease in the platelet count have been reported, as has transformation to myelodysplasia and AML. Although, CNL is regarded as a relatively slowly progressive disease with survival ranging from 6 months to >20 years, one retrospective analysis of 40 patients with CNL reported a median survival time of 23.5 months. Most common causes of death included intracranial hemorrhage (n = 9), progressive disease (n = 5), blastic transformation (n = 4), infection (n = 1), and treatment-related complications (n = 1).

Systemic mastocytosis

> ### Clinical case
>
> A 50-year-old male patient was referred to a hematologist for the evaluation of lymphadenopathy, lymphocytosis, diarrhea, flushing, and headache. Medical history included urticaria pigmentosa–like skin lesions since early childhood. Physical examination showed cervical lymphadenopathy and maculopapular skin lesions. Laboratory examinations revealed leukocytosis (35,490/μL) and lymphocytosis (81%), an elevated LDH (302 U/L), increased β_2-microglobulin (2.94 mg/dL), and an elevated serum tryptase (163 ng/mL). The bone marrow histology demonstrated infiltration of sheets of mast cells. Staging investigations (ultrasound and computed tomography) revealed bilateral cervical and axillary nodes and abdominal lymphadenopathy but no hepatosplenomegaly. A skin biopsy confirmed cutaneous involvement by SM.

Mast cells are long-lived hematopoietic cells with unique biologic properties and a unique spectrum of mediators and cell surface antigens. Mature mast cells are best known for their involvement in allergic inflammation mediated by allergen-specific immunoglobulin E (IgE) and tend to reside in diverse organs, often in vicinity to smaller or larger blood vessels. Mastocytosis encompasses a heterogeneous spectrum of disorders characterized by clonal, neoplastic proliferation of mast cells accompanied by inappropriate tissue infiltration (Figure 14-2). Clinical manifestations of mastocytic disorders are caused by uncontrolled proliferation of tissue mast cells and the release of mast cell–derived mediators. Given that SM has a spectrum of clinical and pathobiologic features in common with MPNs, the revised 2008 WHO classification included SM under the broader umbrella of MPNs. Mastocytosis can be classified according to site and extent of involvement of mast cells as well as the biologic behavior of these cells (Table 14-4).

Epidemiology

The incidence of mastocytic disorders is poorly defined; SM is felt to be a very rare disease. Although mastocytosis can be diagnosed at any age, cutaneous mastocytosis (CM) is more common in children, whereas SM occurs predominantly in adults. These disorders appear to have a slight male predominance.

Pathobiology

Most cases of mastocytosis are associated with somatic activating point mutations of the *c-KIT*, the protein TK receptor for stem cell factor. The most common point mutations result from a Val for Asp substitution at codon 816 (D816V) and result in ligand-independent activation of KIT. Variants of Kit point mutations have been described more rarely. In addition, some patients present with mastocytosis and eosinophilia; in these cases, *PDGFRA* rearrangements, including the *FIP1L1-PDGFRA* fusion, are commonly observed.

Clinical features

Presenting clinical features for patients with mastocytosis depend on the extent of disease. Approximately 80% of patients with mastocytosis have evidence of cutaneous involvement. In SM, which represents 15% to 20% of mastocytosis cases, bone marrow involvement is necessary for the diagnosis, so bone marrow examinations should be performed in all patients with evidence of mast cell disease. Fifty percent of SM patients present with skin involvement. Other organs commonly involved include the liver, spleen, lymph nodes, and gastrointestinal mucosa.

Cutaneous manifestations of mastocytosis typically include a reddish-brown maculopapular eruption (urticaria pigmentosa) or, less often, a diffuse erythema, plaques, nodules, or the classic description of urticaria following stroking of the skin (Darier sign). Blistering can occur in pediatric patients and

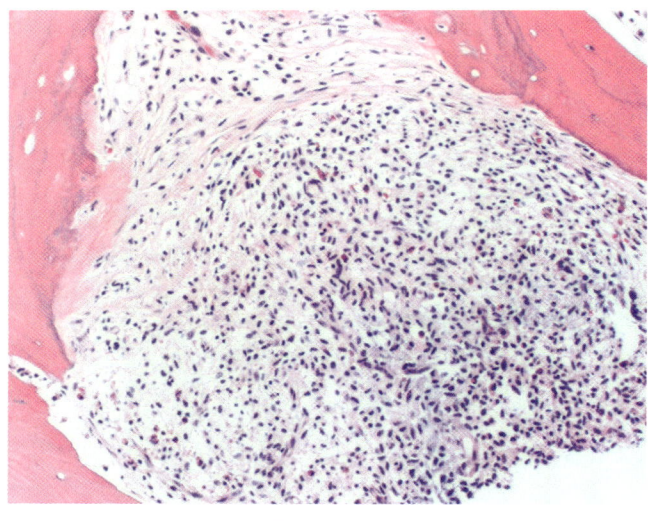
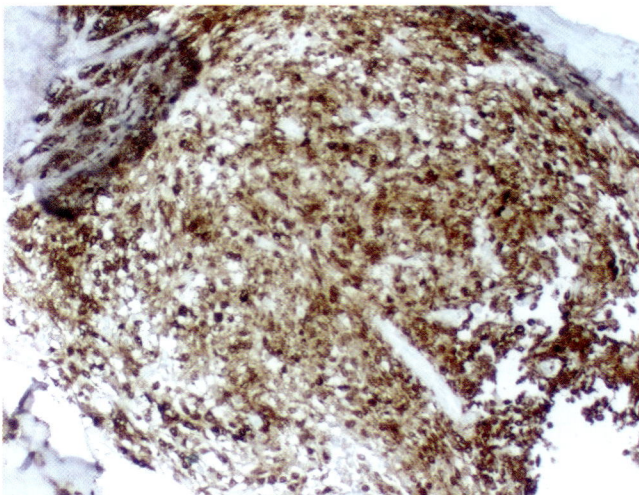
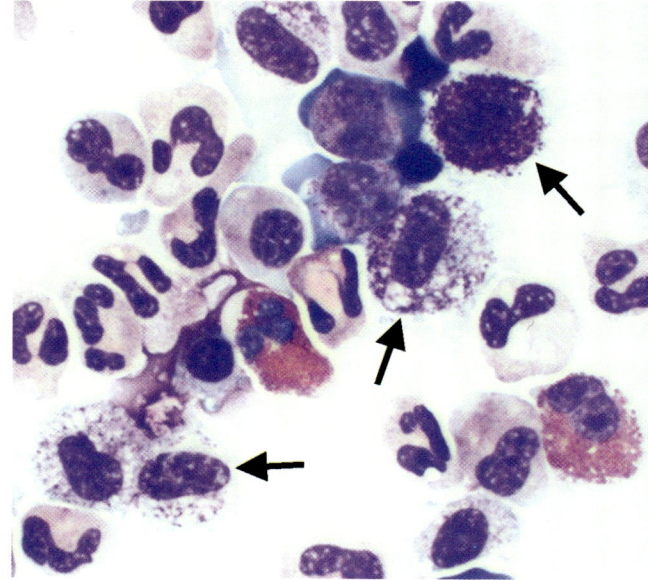

Figure 14-2 Bone marrow involvement with systemic mastocytosis. A, Marrow biopsy shows areas of scattered infiltration or complete replacement by elongated, spindle-shaped cells (hematoxylin-eosin stain; original magnification, 85×). B, Tryptase staining of the core marrow biopsy identifies the infiltrating cells as mast cells (magnification, 85×). C, Abnormal mast cells may also be identified in a marrow aspirate specimen (*arrows*); however, this is not a reliable assay for diagnosis (Wright-Giemsa stain; magnification, 425×). Photos courtesy of Steven J. Kussick, MD, PhD, University of Washington, Seattle, WA.

Table 14-4 The 2008 World Health Organization classification of mastocytosis.

1. Cutaneous mastocytosis
    Urticaria pigmentosa/maculopapular cutaneous mastocytosis
    Diffuse cutaneous mastocytosis
    Solitary mastocytoma of skin
2. Indolent systemic mastocytosis
    Bone marrow mastocytosis
    Smoldering systemic mastocytosis
3. Aggressive systemic mastocytosis
4. Systemic mastocytosis with associated clonal hematologic non–mast cell lineage disease (SM-AHNMD)
5. Mast cell leukemia
6. Mast cell sarcoma
7. Extracutaneous mastocytoma

Adapted from Horny H-P, Metcalfe DD, Bennett JM, et al. Mastocytosis. In: Swerdlow SH, Campo E, Harris NL, et al, eds. *World Health Organization Classification of Tumours of Haematopoietic and Lymphoid Tissues.* Lyon, France: IARC Press; 2008.

represents an aggressive form of urticaria pigmentosa. Clinical features of SM are grouped in 4 distinct groups: (i) constitutional symptoms (eg, fatigue, fever, weight loss); (ii) cutaneous manifestations; (iii) systemic mediator-related symptoms (eg, abdominal pain, flushing, headache, hypotension); and (iv) musculoskeletal complaints (eg, bone pain and myalgias, osteopenia, fractures). SM may present with indolent symptoms or very aggressive behavior. Serum tryptase levels are usually elevated in SM and represent a minor diagnostic criterion.

Diagnostic criteria

The diagnosis of CM is confirmed by the demonstration of pathologic mast cell infiltration of the skin. SM requires involvement of at least one extracutaneous tissue by clonal mast cells (bone marrow is the most commonly involved organ). Diagnostic criteria for CM, SM, and variant presentations of SM are summarized in Table 14-5.

Table 14-5 WHO criteria for diagnosis of cutaneous and systemic mastocytosis.

Cutaneous mastocytosis

Skin lesions demonstrating the typical clinical findings and typical infiltrates of mast cells in a multifocal or diffuse pattern in an adequate skin biopsy. Absence of features/criteria for the diagnosis of SM.

Systemic mastocytosis

The diagnosis of SM may be made if 1 major criterion and 1 minor criterion are present or if 3 minor criteria are fulfilled.

Major criterion

Multifocal, dense infiltrates of mast cells (≥15 mast cells in aggregates) detected in sections of bone marrow and/or other extracutaneous organ(s).

Minor criteria

    a. In biopsy sections of bone marrow or other extracutaneous organs, >25% of the mast cells in the infiltrate are spindle shaped or have atypical morphology or, of all mast cells in bone marrow aspirate smears, >25% are immature or atypical mast cells

    b. Detection of c-Kit point mutation at codon 816 in bone marrow, blood, or other extracutaneous organ(s)

    c. Mast cells in bone marrow, blood, or other extracutaneous organs that coexpress CD117 with CD2 and/or CD25

    d. Serum total tryptase persistently >20 ng/mL (unless there is an associated clonal myeloid disorder, in which case this parameter is not valid)

Indolent systemic mastocytosis

Meets criteria for SM

No evidence of an associated clonal hematologic non–mast cell lineage disease

No "C" findings

Mast cell burden is low, and skin lesions are almost invariably present

*Bone marrow mastocytosis: bone marrow involvement, but no skin lesions

*Smoldering systemic mastocytosis: with 2 or more "B" findings but no "C" findings

Aggressive systemic mastocytosis

Meets criteria for SM

One or more "C" findings

No evidence of mast cell leukemia

*Lymphadenopathic mastocytosis with eosinophilia (provisional subvariant): progressive lymphadenopathy with peripheral blood eosinophilia, often with extensive bony involvement and hepatosplenomegaly, but usually without skin lesions. Exclude cases with rearranged *PDGFRA*.

Systemic mastocytosis with associated clonal hematologic non–mast cell lineage disease

Meets criteria for SM *and*

Associated clonal hematologic non–mast cell lineage disorder (MDS, MPN, AML, lymphoma, or other hematologic neoplasm that meets the criteria for a distinct entity in the WHO classification)

Mast cell leukemia

Meets criteria for SM

Diffuse bone marrow infiltration by atypical immature mast cells. Bone marrow aspirate contains >20% mast cells. Usually >10% circulating mast cells on peripheral blood.

"B" findings

1. Bone marrow biopsy showing >30% infiltration by mast cells (focal, dense aggregates) and/or serum total tryptase level >200 ng/mL
2. Signs of dysplasia or myeloproliferation in non–mast cell lineage, but insufficient criteria for definitive diagnosis of hematopoietic neoplasm by WHO, with normal or only slightly abnormal blood counts
3. Hepatomegaly without impairment of liver function, and/or palpable splenomegaly without hypersplenism, and/or palpable or visceral lymphadenopathy

"C" findings

1. Bone marrow dysfunction manifested by one or more cytopenia (ANC $<1 \times 10^9$/L, hemoglobin <10 g/dL, or platelets $<100 \times 10^9$/L), but no frank non–mast cell hematopoietic malignancy
2. Palpable hepatomegaly with impairment of liver function, ascites, and/or portal hypertension
3. Skeletal involvement with large-sized osteolysis and/or pathologic fractures
4. Palpable splenomegaly with hypersplenism
5. Malabsorption with weight loss due to gastrointestinal mast cell infiltrates

Adapted from Horny H-P, Metcalfe DD, Bennett JM, et al. Mastocytosis. In: Swerdlow SH, Campo E, Harris NL, et al, eds. *World Health Organization Classification of Tumours of Haematopoietic and Lymphoid Tissues.* Lyon, France: IARC Press; 2008.

AML = acute myeloid leukemia; ANC = absolute neutrophil count; MDS = myelodysplastic syndrome; MPN = myeloproliferative neoplasm; SM = systemic mastocytosis; WHO = World Health Organization.

Treatment

Treatment of CM includes H1 and H2 antihistamines, cromolyn and other mast cell stabilizers, topical or intralesional glucocorticoids, and psoralen and ultraviolet A (PUVA) phototherapy. Adults with chronic CM may require long-term continuous or intermittent symptomatic treatment. For adult patients with indolent variants of SM, symptomatic treatment with combinations of H1 and H2 antihistamines, anticholinergic drugs, proton pump inhibitors, cromolyn and other mast cell stabilizers, or PUVA is sufficient to alleviate symptoms. Aspirin and nonsteroidal anti-inflammatory drugs have been helpful for some patients with flushing and syncope, but hypersensitivity to these drugs is relatively common and must be excluded. A major goal in the management of mastocytosis is the avoidance of known and possible inciting factors. Opioid analgesics, such as morphine and codeine, are known mast cell degranulators and may produce severe adverse reactions in sensitive individuals.

Symptomatic SM in the presence of a non–mast cell clonal hematologic disease should be treated as indicated both for the hematologic malignancy and for the SM complications. Generally, the underlying non-SM malignancy determines the overall clinical course. The aggressive variants of SM may progress to end-stage organ fibrosis or failure and may be complicated by pathologic fractures, severe cytopenias, or both. IFNα can be helpful for patients with painful skeletal lesions or mast cell tumors that threaten bony integrity. Corticosteroids are generally avoided in this case because of their potential adverse effects on bone density. Patients with evidence of end-organ damage without major bony complications should receive a combination of corticosteroids and IFNα. Roughly one half of patients will respond to this regimen, although most responses are only partial. Single-agent cladribine, given as 5-day treatment cycles every 4 to 6 weeks, induced clinical and laboratory responses (ie, decreased serum tryptase and urinary histamine metabolites) in 10 of 10 patients with symptomatic SM. Patients who fail to respond to these interventions and those who progress to mast cell leukemia should receive multiagent antileukemic chemotherapy. Allogeneic SCT should be considered for younger patients with aggressive SM who achieve a remission with chemotherapy.

The crucial role of *c-KIT* in normal mast cell development and the evidence that *c-KIT* mutations may be important in SM pathogenesis prompted treatment of mastocytosis patients with TK inhibitors. Imatinib mesylate, due to its inhibitory properties against KIT, was the first to enter the clinical arena. No clinical responses were seen among patients with the D816V mutation, and it was subsequently appreciated that the mutation, which affects the catalytic pocket of the c-Kit protein, prevents imatinib from binding and exerting its inhibitory activity. Nonetheless, a trial of imatinib should be considered in patients with aggressive SM who lack the D816V mutation. Other TK inhibitors also appear to have promising effects in patients with *KIT*-D816V–positive SM. PKC412 (midostaurin) is a novel TK inhibitor that has displayed potent activity (inhibitory concentration at 50% of 30–40 nM) against *KIT*-816 mutants. Based on these data, in one study, PKC412 100 mg twice a day was administered in continuous 28-day cycles until progression/intolerable toxicity for patients with aggressive SM. As of 2007, 15 patients were enrolled. Median age was 62 years (range, 24–76 years). Responses were observed in 11 (73%) of 15 patients, including major and partial responses in 5 and 6 patients, respectively. Among responders, the median duration of treatment was 10 cycles (range, 4–18+). Nilotinib, dasatinib, and MLN518 appear to have a similar preclinical cytotoxic profile against *KIT*-D816V–positive mast cells, although clinical experience is much more limited with these agents.

Course and prognosis

Life expectancy can be quite variable, ranging from only a few months in aggressive SM to normal life spans in more indolent disease. CM in children tends to have an indolent course and is often associated with spontaneous regression. Adults with CM may rarely evolve to SM. Presence of cutaneous involvement in SM appears to confer an indolent behavior, whereas lack of skin involvement is associated with aggressive behavior. Predictor factors of poor prognosis in SM include late onset of symptoms, absence of CM, low platelets, hepatosplenomegaly, anemia, and elevated LDH. Cytoreductive therapy should be considered for patients with aggressive variants of SM.

Myeloid (and lymphoid) neoplasms associated with eosinophilia and abnormalities of *PDGFRA*, *PDGFRB*, or *FGFR1*

> ### Clinical case
>
> A 29-year-old man of a medical history of bipolar disorder complains of abdominal discomfort, night sweats, progressive dyspnea on exertion, and general malaise. He has lost 25 pounds since the beginning of his symptoms. Physical examination shows a well-developed male and painless splenomegaly (spleen tip palpable 12 cm below the left costal margin). The hemoglobin is 8.2 g/dL, hematocrit is 23.9%, WBC count is 8600/μL, and platelet count is 126,000/μL. Normocytic and normochromic red blood cells and increased mature eosinophils are seen on the peripheral smear. No increase in blasts is noted. BCR-ABL testing is negative, and FISH analysis for *CHIC2* deletion confirms the diagnosis of *PDGFRA* rearrangement.

The revised 2008 WHO classification has recently recognized these 3 rare conditions as a new category of myeloid–lymphoid neoplasms associated with marked and persistent eosinophilia ($\geq 1.5 \times 10^9$/L) and chromosomal rearrangements, leading to constitutive activation of the *PDGFRA/PDGFRB* or *FGFR1* genes. These are separate entities from the previous subcategory of CEL/hypereosinophilic syndrome (HES), which remains a subcategory of MPNs and is now called *HES, CEL not otherwise specified* (CEL-NOS). Although the partner gene involved heavily influences the clinical features, separate consideration needs to be given to PDGFRA- and PDGFRB-rearranged eosinophilic disorders because they carry major therapeutic relevance due to the exquisite sensitivity to TK inhibitors. All 3 disorders can present with classic features of MPNs; however, it is still not clearly established whether *PDGFRB*-related rearrangements can manifest as lymphoid neoplasms.

Myeloid and lymphoid neoplasms associated with *PDGFRA* rearrangement

PDGFRA is a member of the family of class III receptor TKs, which also includes PDGFRB, c-KIT, and FLT3. The *PDGFRA* gene is located on the long arm of chromosome 4 (4q12) and has been implicated in the chronic eosinophilic syndromes as a result of a cryptic interstitial deletion at 4q12, leading to the juxtaposition and in-frame fusion of *FIP1L1* and *PDGFRA*. Although most cases of *PDGFRA*-related neoplasms present with clinical features of CEL with prominent involvement of mast cells, they may also present with features of AML or precursor T-cell lymphoblastic lymphoma. Furthermore, several other partner genes have been implicated in the pathogenesis of *PDGFRA*-related neoplasms, including *BCR*, *ETV6*, *KIF5B*, and *CDK5RAP2*.

Epidemiology

Although the true incidence of *PDGFRA*-related neoplasms is not really known, these are rare disorders. These neoplasms are considerably more common in men (male-to-female ratio, 9:1 to 17:1) and are usually diagnosed between the ages of 25 and 55 years (median age of onset is late 40s). *PDGFRA*-related neoplasms seem to represent approximately 50% of patients with HES.

Pathobiology

The classic *PDGFRA*-related chromosomal rearrangement, the *FIP1L1-PDGFRA* fusion gene, is generated by an 800-kilobase interstitial deletion on chromosome 4q12. This cryptic deletion, when using standard cytogenetic banding techniques, explains why most cases of CEL apparently have a normal karyotype. Expression of FIP1L1-PDGFR transformed a murine hematopoietic cell line and was constitutively active in these cells and led to increased STAT5 phosphorylation. Similar transforming properties were noted when *STRN-PDGFRA* or *ETV6-PDGFRA* fusion genes were transfected into murine hematopoietic cell lines.

Clinical features

PDGFRA-related neoplasms are multisystem disorders associated with bone marrow and peripheral blood eosinophilia. The most common presenting signs and symptoms are weakness, fatigue, cardiopulmonary symptoms, myalgias, angioedema, rash, and fever. Organ damage occurs as a result of release of cytokines or direct organ infiltration by eosinophils and possibly mast cells. The most serious complication of *PDGFRA*-related neoplasms is endomyocardial fibrosis with ensuing restrictive cardiomyopathy.

Diagnostic criteria

The revised 2008 WHO classification defines *PDGFRA*-related neoplasms as MPNs with prominent eosinophilia and the presence of the *FIP1L1-PDGFRA* fusion gene. Thus, the most prominent diagnostic feature of patients with *PDGFRA*-related neoplasms is the presence of peripheral blood mature eosinophilia. Anemia and thrombocytopenia are occasionally present. Bone marrow biopsy demonstrates marked hypercellularity with increased mature and precursor eosinophils and increased number of mast cells. Immunophenotyping is typical for activated eosinophils with expression of CD23, CD25, and CD69. Mast cells are usually double negative for CD2 and CD25. The gold standard for the diagnosis of these neoplasms is demonstration of the fusion gene. As previously mentioned, most cases of CEL present with normal karyotype; thus, FISH and RT-PCR are preferred methods. FISH testing relies on the probe for the *CHIC2* gene, which is uniformly deleted in patients with the *FIP1L1-PDGFRA* fusion gene. RT-PCR can be used both for diagnosis and monitoring of disease response and for minimal residual disease monitoring.

Treatment

As of 2009, the mainstay of therapy for patients with *PDGFRA*-related neoplasms is the use of TK inhibitors, such as imatinib mesylate. Since initially reported in 2001, several single- and multi-institution studies have looked at the efficacy of low to conventional doses of imatinib for the treatment of *PDGFRA*-related neoplasms. These studies report remarkably similar results, where patients found to have

PDGFRA gene rearrangements have rapid, deep, and durable responses to low to conventional doses of imatinib mesylate (100–400 mg/d). In 2 of these studies, the European LeukemiaNet reported the results of 11 patients treated for at least 12 months with imatinib. Overall, 11 of 11 evaluable patients achieved at least a 3-log reduction in *FIP1L1-PDGFRA* fusion transcripts, and 9 of 11 patients achieved a complete molecular remission. Similarly, an Italian multicenter study demonstrated high levels of durable (median, 25+ months) complete molecular remissions in 27 patients with *PDGFRA*-related neoplasms. Unfortunately, it appears that withdrawal of imatinib therapy is followed by a rapid increase in *FIP1L1-PDGFRA* transcript levels.

Course and prognosis

In the preimatinib era, the prognosis of patients with HES was poor; the median survival time was 9 months, and the 3-year survival was only 12%. Patients generally had advanced disease, with congestive heart failure accounting for 65% of the identified causes of death. More recently, an observed 5-year survival rate of 80%, decreasing to 42% at 15 years, was noted. Since the recognition that *PDGFRA*-related neoplasms are highly sensitive to TK inhibitors, most patients achieve and remain in complete hematologic and molecular remission within a few weeks of initiation of therapy.

Myeloid neoplasms associated with *PDGFRB* rearrangement

PDGFRB-related neoplasms are a distinct group of myeloid neoplasms associated with rearrangement of the *PDGFRB* gene, located on the long arm of chromosome 5 (5q31~33). Patients with *PDGFRB*-related neoplasms tend to present with features characteristic of chronic myelomonocytic leukemia with associated eosinophilia. In 1994, Golub et al (1994) were the first to characterize the t(5;12)(q31–q33;p13) translocation involving *ETV6*(12p13) and *PDGFRB* (5q33). Since then, >15 partner genes have been identified to collaborate in the development of *PDGFRB*-related neoplasms.

Epidemiology

Similarly to its counterpart, *PDGFRB*-related neoplasms are extremely uncommon disorders, and the true incidence of is not completely known. In fact, among >56,000 cytogenetically defined cases from the Mayo Clinic, only 0.04% exhibited the t(5;12) translocation. *PDGFRB*-related neoplasms are more common in men (male-to-female ratio, 2:1), with a median age of onset in late 40s.

Clinical features

PDGFRB-related neoplasms are also systemic disorders with extensive involvement of peripheral blood and bone marrow. Extramedullary manifestations, such as skin infiltration and splenomegaly, are common.

Diagnostic criteria

Confirmation of diagnosis for *PDGFRB*-related neoplasms requires demonstration of MPN with prominent eosinophilia and occasional neutrophilia or monocytosis and the presence of the *ETV6-PDGFRB* fusion gene or an alternative *PDGFRB* gene rearrangement. The classic t(5;12)(q31-q33;p13) can be easily detected by conventional metaphase analysis, so FISH or RT-PCR is usually used for the confirmation of diagnosis and determination of fusion gene. Peripheral blood usually presents with leukocytosis (neutrophilia or monocytosis) along with anemia and thrombocytopenia. Bone marrow is hypercellular, and mast cells can be increased in number.

Treatment

Imatinib mesylate is also the mainstay of therapy for patients with *PDGFRB*-related neoplasms. However, data to support this recommendation are scarcely available. A recent phase II study from a German group demonstrated that complete molecular remissions were achieved in 3 of 5 patients with *PDGFRB*-related neoplasms after 3 to 18 months of low to conventional doses of imatinib. Another multicenter study reports on the outcomes for 12 patients with *PDGFRB*-related neoplasms who received imatinib therapy for a median of 47 months. Eleven patients had prompt responses with normalization of peripheral blood cell counts and disappearance of eosinophilia; 10 had complete resolution of cytogenetic abnormalities and decrease or disappearance of fusion transcripts as measured by RT-PCR. Thus, it also appears that TK inhibitors impact positively on the outcome of patients with *PDGFRB*-related neoplasms.

Course and prognosis

Prognosis in the preimatinib era was also very poor for patients with *PDGFRB*-related neoplasms; the median survival time did not exceed 2 years. Although there are only small case series on the impact of imatinib on the survival of patients with *PDGFRB*-related neoplasms, these studies suggest a similar benefit to that seen in patients with *PDGFRA*-related neoplasms, with median survivals exceeding 5 years. Better recognition of these disorders and earlier initiation of therapy with TK inhibitors will undoubtedly continue to improve the outcome of these patients.

Myeloid and lymphoid neoplasms associated with *FGFR1* abnormalities

The revised 2008 WHO classification recognizes, for the first time, this extremely uncommon and heterogeneous group of neoplasms that arise from pluripotent hematopoietic stem cells and are associated with rearrangements in the *FGFR1* gene and eosinophilia. Formerly known as 8p11 myeloproliferative syndrome or 8p11 stem cell syndrome, *FGFR1*-related neoplasms can present as classic MPNs, precursor B- or T-cell lymphoblastic leukemia, or AML.

Epidemiology

FGFR1-related neoplasms have been reported across a wide age range (3–84 years), and the median age of diagnosis is 32 years. Females constitute approximately 40% of the cases.

Pathobiology

The molecular consequences of *FGFR1* rearrangements are remarkably well described for such an unusual disorder. In all *FGFR1*-related neoplasms, the N-terminal partner containing self-association motif is fused to the C-terminal TKD of *FGFR1*. These fusion genes (*ZNF198-FGFR1*), when expressed in primary murine hematopoietic cells, cause an MPN that recapitulates the human MPN phenotype. Furthermore, these constitutively active *FGFR1* fusion genes activate downstream effector molecules such as PLC-γ, STAT5, and PI3K/AKT.

Clinical features

Clinical manifestations include fever, weight loss, and night sweats. Lymphadenopathy is common in patients with lymphomatous presentation. Hypercatabolism and splenomegaly are common features of AML and MPN patients.

Diagnostic criteria

Diagnostic criteria established by the 2008 WHO classification include the presence of an MPN with prominent eosinophilia and occasional neutrophilia or monocytosis *or* the presence of AML or precursor B- or T-cell lymphoblastic leukemia *and* the presence of *FGFR1* rearrangement. The most common chromosomal translocation associated with *FGFR1*-related neoplasms is t(8;13)(p11;q12), which results in expression of the ZNF198-FGFR1 fusion TK. Nonetheless, several other translocation partners have been described over the last few years, including CEP110, FOP, and BCR.

Treatment

Early intensive therapy followed by allogeneic SCT remains the only potential curative therapy for patients with *FGFR1*-related neoplasms. Interestingly, PKC412 has demonstrated in vitro activity against one subtype of the *FGFR1* fusion gene.

Course and prognosis

The prognosis for patients with *FGFR1*-related neoplasms is currently very poor. The clinical aggressiveness and diminished awareness about the features of this entity and the lack of approved TK inhibitors make the management of these patients very challenging.

Chronic eosinophilic leukemia, not otherwise specified

CEL is a newly defined entity of MPNs characterized by an autonomous, clonal proliferation of eosinophil precursors resulting in persistent elevation of eosinophils in the peripheral blood, bone marrow, and peripheral tissues. By definition, in CEL-NOS, the absolute peripheral blood eosinophil count has to exceed $1.5 \times 10^9/L$, and patients must not have the Ph chromosome (*BCR-ABL1* fusion gene) or rearrangements of *PDGFRA/PDGFRB* or *FGFR1*. End-organ damage can be a manifestation of direct eosinophil leukemic infiltrate or secondary to the release of cytokines or other enzymes by release of their toxic granules. CEL-NOS requires demonstration of eosinophil clonality and must be differentiated from idiopathic HES. Idiopathic HES is defined as a persistent (>6 months) peripheral blood eosinophilia ($1.5 \times 10^9/L$), without clear underlying cause or associated end-organ damage or dysfunction and absence of eosinophil clonality.

Epidemiology

Although CEL-NOS is a rare MPN, the true incidence of these neoplasms is unknown. Complicating matters further, the revised 2008 WHO classification now separates previously classified patients with CEL into myeloid (and lymphoid) neoplasms associated with eosinophilia and abnormalities of *PDGFRA*, *PDGFRB*, or *FGFR1* or CEL-NOS depending on the presence or absence of rearrangements of *PDGFRA/PDGFRB* or *FGFR1*, respectively. Nonetheless, eosinophilic syndromes seem to occur much more often in men than in women, with a male-to-female ratio of approximately 9:1. The peak incidence is in the fourth decade, but CEL-NOS can occur at any age, including childhood. The true incidence of idiopathic HES will remain unclear until further defined.

Clinical features

Approximately 10% of cases of CEL-NOS are identified incidentally. More commonly, patients present with complaints of symptoms such as fever, fatigue, cough, pruritus, diarrhea, angioedema, and muscle pain. Most patients with idiopathic hypereosinophilia will develop signs of end-organ damage within 3 years of diagnosis. Clinically, CEL-NOS can manifest with a plethora of symptoms. The most serious clinical findings relate to endomyocardial fibrosis due to eosinophilic infiltration of the heart leading to constrictive pericarditis, fibroplastic endocarditis, myocarditis, or intramural thrombus formation (due to scarring of the mitral and/or tricuspid valves). Peripheral and central nervous system findings can include mononeuritis multiplex, peripheral neuropathy, and paraparesis, as well as cerebellar involvement, epilepsy, dementia, cerebral infarction, and eosinophilic meningitis. Pulmonary involvement includes idiopathic infiltrates, fibrosis, pulmonary effusions, and pulmonary emboli. Skin manifestations are common and can take many forms, including angioedema, urticaria, papulonodular lesions, and erythematous plaques. Gastrointestinal involvement by eosinophilia can result in ascites, diarrhea, gastritis, colitis, pancreatitis, cholangitis, or hepatitis.

Diagnostic criteria

The WHO criteria for diagnosis of CEL-NOS exclude patients with infectious, allergic, autoimmune, or collagen vascular disorders or pulmonary or neoplastic conditions (including clonal lymphoid disorders) that are known to be associated with secondary eosinophilia. The revised 2008 WHO criteria also require the presence of eosinophilia (1.5×10^9/L); presence of clonal cytogenetic or molecular abnormality or blasts cells >2% in the peripheral blood or >5% in the bone marrow; lack of *BCR-ABL1*, *PDGFRA/PDGFRB*, or *FGFR1* rearrangements; bone marrow blasts ≤20%; and absence of inv(16)(p13.1q22). Patients not fulfilling all of these diagnostic criteria should be classified as having secondary/reactive eosinophilia or idiopathic HES.

Treatment

Treatment is indicated for patients with evidence of end-organ damage. Therapy for CEL-NOS and idiopathic HES is primarily aimed at decreasing the eosinophil count, improving symptoms, and preventing end-organ damage or thromboembolic complications. Inadequate data exist to support initiation of therapy based on a specific eosinophil count in the absence of organ disease. In the past, corticosteroids (prednisone 1 mg/kg/d) have been the treatment of choice in HES to try to reduce eosinophil numbers and minimize the cytotoxic effects of the eosinophilic granules. Steroid-resistant patients have traditionally been treated with hydroxyurea. Lack of steroid responsiveness warrants consideration of cytotoxic chemotherapeutic agents, such as vincristine and etoposide; these agents have also been used in patients with HES resistant to other therapies and in patients with aggressive CEL. IFNα can elicit sustained hematologic and cytogenetic remissions in idiopathic HES and CEL-NOS patients refractory to other therapies including prednisone and hydroxyurea. Anti–interleukin (IL) 5 antibody approaches (eg, mepolizumab) have been undertaken in HES based on the cytokine's role as a differentiation, activation, and survival factor for eosinophils. Mepolizumab inhibits binding of IL-5 to the α chain of the IL-5 receptor expressed on eosinophils and has received orphan drug designation by the FDA for the treatment of CEL-NOS. Treatment with anti–IL-5 monoclonal antibodies could elicit rapid reductions in the peripheral blood eosinophil count (<48 hours) and/or decreases in serum levels of eosinophil mediators. The effective use of alemtuzumab (anti-CD52 monoclonal antibody) in refractory HES based on expression of the CD52 antigen on eosinophils has been reported in 2 separate case reports.

Course and prognosis

CEL-NOS and idiopathic HES have a variable course and overall survival, although both tend to be chronic disorders. Blast transformation can occur, usually many years after diagnosis. Poor prognostic features include marked splenomegaly, cytogenetic abnormalities, and dysplastic myeloid features in the bone marrow. In one series including patients with idiopathic HES and eosinophilic leukemia, 80% of patients were alive at 5 years from diagnosis, and 42% were alive at 15 years. Thus, close follow-up and judicious use of treatment interventions can lead to long survival.

Polycythemia vera

> ### Clinical case
>
> A 61-year-old man of Western European descent who smokes cigarettes regularly complains of headaches with exertion, vague epigastric discomfort, and general malaise. He has hypertension and takes 25 mg of hydrochlorothiazide and 1 adult aspirin tablet (325 mg) daily. He has lost 15 pounds in weight and has noted intermittent melena over the past year. Physical examination shows obesity, a ruddy complexion, painless splenomegaly (spleen tip palpable 4 cm below the left costal margin), and a stool specimen that is positive for occult blood. The hemoglobin is 17.6 g/dL, hematocrit is 54%, mean corpuscular volume is 75 fL, WBC count is 12,300/mL, and platelet count is 950,000/μL. Microcytic and hypochromic red blood cells, a few giant platelets, increased neutrophils, and occasional basophils are seen on the peripheral smear. JAK2 V617F mutation testing was positive.

PV is defined by an elevated red cell mass (RCM) in the absence of conditions that induce secondary erythrocytosis, such as hypoxia or inappropriate erythropoietin (EPO) production. Excessive red blood cell production by the bone marrow in PV is often associated with concomitant increases in circulating platelets and granulocytes because the acquired defect underlying PV involves a multipotential hematopoietic progenitor cell. PV is the most common MPN in the United States, with an annual incidence rate of roughly 1.1 cases per 100,000 persons per year. There is a slight male predominance. The median age at diagnosis is 60 to 65 years, with roughly 5% of cases occurring in those <40 years old. Radiation exposure, but not other environmental or toxic factors, has been linked to the disease.

Pathobiology
Clonality

PV was among the first hematopoietic disorders to be demonstrated to have a clonal origin; studies of blood cells from women with PV who were germline heterozygous for glucose-6-phosphate dehydrogenase (G6PD) isoenzyme types expressed either the normal G6PD type or the variant type, but not a balanced mix of normal- and variant-type cells, as would be expected in a polyclonal cell population. More recently, molecular analyses of other polymorphic X-linked genes have yielded similar findings. Moreover, circulating red blood cells, platelets, granulocytes, and sometimes B lymphocytes in patients with PV are all progeny of the malignant clone. By comparison, the majority of lymphocytes and natural killer cells are usually polyclonal and do not exhibit the karyotypic changes or other genetic abnormalities that characterize the abnormal clone. Despite this, clonal analysis using *JAK2* mutational analysis frequently identifies a subpopulation of *JAK2*-mutant hematopoietic cells in all hematopoiesis subtypes, including lymphocytes, demonstrating that PV and other *JAK2*-mutant MPNs arise in the pluripotent hematopoietic stem cell compartment.

JAK2 mutations

Recent genetic studies have shown that somatic activating mutations at codon 617 in the JAK2 TK are observed in 90% to 95% of patients with PV. JAK2 is an intracellular signaling molecule that is coupled to several cell surface hematopoietic growth factor receptors that lack intrinsic kinase domains, including the EPO receptor and the thrombopoietin (TPO) receptor. The specific *JAK2* point mutation most closely associated with MPN, V617F, causes constitutive activation of the JAK2 kinase domain, which results in erythropoiesis losing its dependence on EPO signaling and becoming virtually autonomous. *JAK2* V617F can be found in >90% of patients with PV, and diagnostic mutation assays are now available for routine clinical testing in numerous reference laboratories. This mutation is homozygous in at least one third of PV cases, a situation that arises by acquired uniparental disomy of the region including the mutated gene on chromosome 9p24. Analysis of *JAK2* V617F–negative PV patients led to the identification of acquired activating mutations in exon 12 of JAK2 in most, but not all, *JAK2* V617F–negative PV patients. Of note, unlike the more pleiotropic *JAK2* V617F allele, which is seen in a spectrum of myeloid malignancies, JAK2 exon 12 mutations are specific to *JAK2* V617F–negative PV and are most often identified in patients with erythrocytosis without associated thrombocytosis or leukocytosis.

Other biologic abnormalities

Prior to the discovery of *JAK2* V617F, a number of physiologic, growth, and survival abnormalities were identified in progenitor cells from PV patients. One such characteristic biologic feature, which has been used as a minor diagnostic criterion for PV by several groups, is the ability of erythroid progenitors to form colonies in serum-containing cultures in the absence of EPO, a phenomenon often called endogenous erythroid colony (EEC) growth. EEC growth is not specific for PV; it can also be observed in some cases of ET and PMF and in rare cases of congenital polycythemia. *JAK2* V617F provides a mechanistic explanation for this phenomenon in acquired MPNs. Additional phenotypic features of unclear pathogenic significance include decreased expression of c-Mpl (the TPO receptor) in PV megakaryocytes and platelets and overexpression of messenger RNA (mRNA) encoding polycythemia rubra vera 1 (PRV1) in mature granulocytes but not myeloid progenitors. Neither of these findings is specific for PV, although some groups use them as supportive evidence for a PV diagnosis in challenging cases. More recently, somatic loss-of-function mutations in the putative tumor suppressor genes *TET2* and *ASXL1* have been identified in a subset of PV, ET, and PMF patients. Although these mutations contribute to the pathogenesis of these MPNs, they are also frequently observed in myelodysplastic syndrome (MDS) and AML patients; thus, they are not useful from a diagnostic or clinicopathologic perspective other than as a marker of clonality.

Qualitative platelet defects and inappropriate granulocyte activation can occur in PV. Platelets may contain abnormally low levels of serotonin and adenine. In vitro aggregation responses to epinephrine and/or collagen may be incomplete or absent. Acquired type 2 von Willebrand disease (vWD) may occur with extreme thrombocytosis (usually >1,000,000/μL) and can contribute to clinical bleeding. The mechanism of acquired vWD in thrombocytosis appears to be related to platelet binding, cleavage, and ultimately clearance of large von Willebrand factor (vWF) multimers. Normal vWF activity is restored after the platelet count is normalized by cytoreductive drugs or plateletpheresis. Granulocyte activation may induce endothelial cell injury and plasma coagulation activation, contributing to thrombosis risk.

Clinical features

At presentation, approximately 80% of patients with PV are symptomatic; the rest are discovered incidentally as a result of a blood count performed for another reason. Up to one half of patients with PV complain of headache, pruritus (particularly after bathing in hot water), and fatigue. One third suffer from dyspnea, dizziness, visual changes, weight loss, epigastric pain, excessive sweating, or painful paresthesias of the hands and feet (erythromelalgia) (Table 14-6). These symptoms are believed to relate to hyperviscosity, hypercatabolism, elevated histamine release, and microvascular/vasomotor instability. Roughly 15% of patients diagnosed with PV will have suffered an arterial or, less commonly, a venous thrombotic event within the previous 2 years. One fifth of patients with PV present with a large-vessel thrombotic complication such as a transient ischemic attack, cerebrovascular accident, myocardial infarction, deep venous thrombosis, or hepatic vein thrombosis. It is important to consider the diagnosis of PV in people who develop an apparently unprovoked thromboembolic event, in particular at unusual sites (eg, dural sinuses or mesenteric veins). In particular, a substantial proportion of patients who present with Budd-Chiari syndrome are found to be *JAK2* V617F positive and have EEC formation and clinicopathologic features of PV not previously diagnosed. Epistaxis is reported by 15% to 20% of patients at diagnosis, and gastrointestinal bleeding is reported by approximately 5%. As illustrated by the clinical case, aspirin use may exacerbate bleeding from the upper gastrointestinal tract.

Clinical findings at PV diagnosis include splenomegaly (50%–80%), facial or conjunctival plethora (~60%), hypertension (~50%), hepatomegaly (~50%), and, less commonly, cutaneous ulcers or gouty features (Table 14-6). Pulmonary hypertension has been noted in some patients with PV, ET, or PMF. Myeloid progenitor cells can be seen in the lungs of these patients on bronchoscopic biopsy, and these cells elute vasoactive cytokines that may contribute to blood vessel damage and fibrosis. The median survival after developing pulmonary hypertension is only 18 months.

Differential diagnosis
Absolute polycythemia versus relative polycythemia

An elevated hematocrit may result from either an increase in the total RCM (absolute polycythemia) or a decrease in the total plasma volume (relative polycythemia). The latter condition is usually due to moderate to severe intravascular dehydration, such as that due to diarrhea or loss of fluid into third spaces (effusions or edema), sometimes exacerbated by diuretic use. It is important to remember that 2.5% of healthy people will have a hematocrit value above the normal laboratory reference range because laboratory normal ranges are based on statistical distributions. In contrast, in some cases, a normal hemoglobin and hematocrit can be a sign of disease; examination of old blood counts may demonstrate that the patient's hemoglobin has increased substantially from his or her personal baseline, although the level is still within the laboratory normal range. In addition, patients with fluid overload can present with a normal hematocrit in the setting of an elevated RCM; this is most common in patients with Budd-Chiari syndrome and resultant liver dysfunction, which masks erythrocytosis and can confound the diagnosis of PV.

Table 14-6 Classical features of polycythemia vera.

Symptoms*
Fatigue, headache, pruritus, weakness, dyspnea, dizziness, visual change, weight loss, epigastric pain, excessive sweating, paresthesias (erythromelalgia), symptoms related to large-vessel thrombosis (arterial or venous), epistaxis, gastrointestinal or other mucocutaneous bleeding

Clinical signs*
Systemic hypertension, splenomegaly, plethora, hepatomegaly, cutaneous ulcers, gouty features, pulmonary hypertension

Additional laboratory abnormalities
JAK2 V617F mutation, elevated LAP score, elevated B_{12} level, elevated LDH, elevated uric acid, EEC growth, *PRV1* granulocyte overexpression, decreased *c-Mpl* expression, marrow hypercellularity with megakaryocyte clustering

* More common → less common.
Updated and modified from Berlin NI. Polycythemia vera: diagnosis and treatment in 2002. *Expert Rev Anticancer Ther.* 2002;2:330–336.
EEC = endogenous erythroid colony; LAP = leukocyte alkaline phosphatase; LDH = lactate dehydrogenase.

Formerly, determination of RCM by isotope testing was routinely performed to evaluate an elevated hematocrit, with the goal of differentiating relative polycythemia from absolute polycythemia. In a nuclear medicine RCM assay, an aliquot of the patient's red blood cells is collected and labeled with a chromium-51 radiotracer and then reinfused into the patient. Radiolabeled albumin (iodine-125–albumin) is also injected to allow assessment of the plasma volume. Blood is then withdrawn after the radioisotopes have had time to dilute in the circulation, and photon emission from the radioisotopes is measured with a calibrated gamma counter. Absolute polycythemia is diagnosed when the total red blood cell volume is calculated to be >36 mL/kg in men or >32 mL/kg in women. The precise role of RCM testing in PV diagnosis has changed subsequent to the discovery of *JAK2* V617F; the revised WHO diagnostic criteria do not require demonstration of an elevated RCM in patients who present with an elevated hemoglobin (>18.5 g/dL in men or 16.5 g/dL in women) and are positive for *JAK2* V617F. Hemoglobin values >18.5 g/dL in men of European or Asian descent, >17.5 g/dL in African men, and >16.5 g/dL in women usually do not require formal RCM determination because these values almost always reflect a true elevation in RCM. Such levels of hemoglobin elevation generally cannot be achieved by conditions associated with plasma volume depletion alone, except in the most extreme circumstances, which should be clinically obvious. Diagnostic thresholds for hematocrit values have also been defined, with values >60% in men and >56% in women consistently correlating with absolute elevations in RCM. There are also some patients, who have an elevated platelet count or other MPN-associated features (eg, splenomegaly or unprovoked thrombosis in an unusual site) and a normal hemoglobin and hematocrit, in whom RCM testing will disclose an unsuspected elevated erythroid burden. Moreover, in patients in whom a *JAK2* mutation cannot be identified but in whom there is high clinical suspicion of PV, RCM can be used to support a diagnosis of PV. Finally, iron deficiency can result in a normal RCM in a patient with true PV, and microcytic indices in a nonthalassemic patient with MPN features should suggest this possibility. The revised WHO diagnostic criteria for PV are summarized in Table 14-7.

Primary erythrocytosis versus secondary erythrocytosis

In an adult with marked elevation of his or her hemoglobin and/or elevated RCM, additional studies are required to differentiate PV from secondary causes of erythrocytosis (Table 14-8). Rare patients may have both PV and a secondary cause of erythrocytosis. Most acquired secondary polycythemic states are associated with elevated or high-normal serum EPO levels, which may be appropriately elevated (eg, in the setting of chronic tissue hypoxemia) or inappropriately elevated (eg, due to exogenous administration of recombinant EPO or endogenous EPO overproduction by the kidney or liver or by a tumor). A smoking history (including exposure to secondhand smoke) should be obtained; arterial blood gas and carboxyhemoglobin determinations should be obtained in smokers or those with occupational exposure to hydrocarbon fumes. An oxygen saturation <92% suggests the possibility of EPO-driven polycythemia. Evidence for underlying lung or cardiac disease should be sought, and evaluation for sleep apnea through monitoring of nocturnal oxygen saturations should also be considered. An abdominal ultrasound is useful to assess for renal or hepatic cysts or tumors or for splenomegaly if it is not obvious from physical examination. In the absence of other causes of elevated EPO and with a normal oxygen saturation, an oxygen dissociation curve (partial pressure of oxygen at which hemoglobin is half saturated) should be determined to evaluate for a high oxygen-affinity hemoglobinopathy if there is sufficient

Table 14-7 Diagnostic criteria for polycythemia vera.

Disease	Polycythemia vera
Major	1. Hemoglobin >18.5 g/dL in men, >16.5 g/dL in women, *or* other evidence of increased red blood cell volume*
	2. Presence of *JAK2* V617F or other functionally similar mutation such as *JAK2* exon 12 mutation
Minor	1. Bone marrow biopsy showing hypercellularity for age with trilineage growth (panmyelosis) with prominent erythroid, granulocytic, and megakaryocytic proliferation
	2. Serum erythropoietin level below the reference range for normal
	3. Endogenous erythroid colony formation in vitro
Diagnosis	Requires the presence of both major criteria and 1 minor criterion *or* the presence of the first major criterion together with 2 minor criteria

* Hemoglobin or hematocrit >99th percentile of method-specific reference range for age, sex, altitude of residence *or* hemoglobin >17 g/dL in men, >15 g/dL in women if associated with a documented and sustained increase of at least 2 g/dL from an individual's baseline value that cannot be attributed to correction of iron deficiency, *or* elevated red bllod cell mass >25% above mean normal predicted value.
Adapted from Swerdlow SH, Campo E, Harris NL, et al, eds. *World Health Organization Classification of Tumours of Haematopoietic and Lymphoid Tissues*. Lyon, France: IARC Press; 2008.

Table 14-8 Causes of secondary polycythemia.

Neonatal
    Normal intrauterine environment (Hb F)
    Twin–twin transfusion syndrome or maternal–fetal bleeds
    Infants of diabetic mothers
    Intrauterine growth retardation
    Adrenal hyperplasia
    Thyrotoxicosis

Congenital
    Trisomies of 13, 18, or 21
    Mutant high oxygen-affinity hemoglobin
    Congenital low 2,3-bisphosphoglycerate
    Autonomous high EPO production (including Chuvash-type polycythemia associated with *VHL* mutations)
    Autosomal dominant polycythemia (including truncating EPO receptor mutations)
    Other congenital polycythemic states

Acquired
   Arterial hypoxemia
    High altitude
    Cyanotic congenital heart disease
    Chronic lung disease
    Sleep apnea and hypoventilation syndromes
   Other causes of impaired tissue oxygen delivery
    Smoking
    Carbon monoxide poisoning
   Renal lesions
    Renal tumors
    Renal cysts
    Diffuse parenchymal disease
    Hydronephrosis
    Wilms tumor
    Renal artery stenosis
    Renal transplantation
   Miscellaneous tumors
    Parotid tumors
    Cerebellar hemangiomas
    Lymphomas
    Uterine myomata
    Cutaneous leiomyomata
    Bronchial carcinoma
    Ovarian tumors
    Adrenal tumors
    Meningiomas
    Pheochromocytomas
   Drugs and chemicals
    Androgens
    Epoetin alfa or darbepoetin alfa
    Novel erythropoietic agents
    Nickel
    Cobalt
   Hepatic lesions
    Hepatomas
    Cirrhosis
    Hepatitis

Modified from Pearson TC, Messinezy M. Idiopathic erythrocytosis, diagnosis and clinical management. *Pathol Biol (Paris)*. 2001;49:170–177. EPO = erythropoietin; Hb = hemoglobin.

clinical suspicion. The family history is often suggestive in these cases. Alternative causes of secondary polycythemia must also be considered including EPO-producing renal or liver tumors; in addition, cerebellar hemangiomas, uterine myomas, ovarian tumors, parotid tumors, lymphomas, and adrenal tumors can be associated with pathologic EPO production. Budd-Chiari syndrome can be a presenting sign of PV; however, in the acute setting, hepatic necrosis can be associated with transiently elevated EPO levels, misleadingly suggesting a secondary, EPO-driven erythrocytosis. Therefore, it is important to assess patients after they recover from the acute complications of Budd-Chiari syndrome. Androgen replacement therapy or androgen abuse by aspiring athletes and bodybuilders may induce polycythemia. Absolute polycythemia may occur in up to 15% of patients after renal transplantation. This complication usually develops 8 to 24 months after transplantation and remits spontaneously in one fourth of patients; when treatment is required, therapy with angiotensin-converting enzyme inhibitors or angiotensin receptor blockers is often effective. It is important to recognize that *JAK2* V617F mutations have not been identified in patients with secondary polycythemia without a concurrent diagnosis of a MPN; therefore, the presence of the *JAK2* V617F allele supports a diagnosis of PV even in patients with concomitant secondary polycythemia.

Differentiation between PV and secondary polycythemia is important both for prognosis and treatment because secondary polycythemia does not carry a risk of leukemic or fibrotic transformation and has a lower risk of thrombosis. In either case, however, symptoms may result from increased viscosity of the blood. In secondary polycythemia, phlebotomy may occasionally be indicated to decrease blood viscosity and improve oxygenation when symptoms occur or prophylactically, especially when hematocrit values exceed 60%. With reduction in blood viscosity, symptoms such as headaches, plethora, and dizziness quickly abate. Caution must be exercised, however, when the cause of secondary polycythemia is physiologically appropriate, such as in cyanotic congenital heart disease, chronic hypoxia, or high-affinity hemoglobins. Tissue hypoxemia may be worsened by phlebotomy when the physiologically appropriate compensatory increase in hematocrit is reversed. If underlying severe cardiac disease exists, 0.9% normal saline should be given concurrently with phlebotomy to compensate for the blood volume that is removed.

Familial polycythemic states

Primary familial and congenital erythrocytosis is usually autosomal dominant and most commonly associated with low serum EPO levels. Approximately 10% of such cases have been linked to germline truncating mutations of the EPO receptor that abrogate an important inhibitory domain and lead to constitutive EPO receptor signaling. In contrast, normal or high EPO levels are found in patients with Chuvash-type congenital polycythemia due to abnormalities in cellular oxygen sensing. This autosomal recessive disorder was first recognized among the population of the Chuvash region in the center of the European part of Russia and is associated with a high risk of thrombotic and hemorrhagic complications. Sporadic cases of Chuvash-type polycythemia with homozygous or compound heterozygous inheritance patterns have subsequently been identified among other ethnic groups. These patients have mutations involving a region of the von Hippel-Lindau (*VHL*) gene that is distinct from the autosomal dominant *VHL* mutations associated with the von Hippel-Lindau syndrome. The Chuvash-type *VHL* mutations impair the function of the *VHL* gene product to facilitate degradation of hypoxia-inducible factor 1 (HIF1), an oxygen-responsive transcriptional factor that upregulates EPO expression. More recent studies of families with autosomal dominant heritable erythrocytosis have identified germline mutations in the *HIF2A* gene that lead to defective oxygen sensing and resultant polycythemia; of note, these mutations are heterozygous and result in dysregulation of the HIF transcriptional complex.

Diagnostic criteria and molecular testing

In the absence of causes for secondary polycythemia and a family history of erythrocytosis and in the presence of a low serum EPO level, PV is the most likely diagnosis. The Polycythemia Vera Study Group (PVSG) originally established criteria in the 1970s to standardize the diagnosis of PV to follow a uniform group of patients on treatment protocols. In light of the discovery of *JAK2* V617F and other MPN-associated molecular lesions, the WHO has published a set of diagnostic criteria that includes genetic testing for *JAK2* V617F as a major criterion (Table 14-7). *JAK2* V617F mutation testing by PCR-based assays is >90% sensitive for PV and appears to be 100% specific for clonal myeloproliferation. *JAK2* testing is useful as a first-intention diagnostic test for evaluation of an elevated hematocrit, before any other investigation, but it cannot distinguish inapparent PV from other clonal myeloid disorders. Therefore, it is important to note that *JAK2* V617F mutations are not specific for PV given their occurrence in ET, PMF, and other myeloid malignancies; however, the presence of the *JAK2* V617F allele and erythrocytosis does provide 2 major criteria for the diagnosis of PV using the new WHO criteria. For patients who are *JAK2* V617F negative, testing for *JAK2* exon 12 is of value; however, given the wide mutational spectra of *JAK2* exon 12 mutations in *JAK2* V617F–negative PV, the absence of a *JAK2* V617F or exon 12 mutation does not exclude a diagnosis of PV.

Ambiguous cases

Some patients present with an elevated RCM and a normal or near-normal serum EPO level in the absence of other diagnostic criteria for PV and without an apparent cause for secondary polycythemia. Typical features of PV will develop in 10% to 40% of such patients over time, but most cases will spontaneously resolve, or a cause of secondary polycythemia will ultimately become clear. *JAK2* testing is helpful to distinguish these groups. Some younger patients have been described with chronic "idiopathic erythrocytosis" that persists for many years without evolution to PV or development of thrombohemorrhagic complications. The etiology of this syndrome is unclear; however, a subset of patients with idiopathic erythrocytosis who do not meet the criteria for a diagnosis of PV are *JAK2* exon 12 mutation positive.

Laboratory and histopathologic features

A low or inappropriately normal serum EPO level is common with PV. Serum EPO levels within the normal range also occur in PV, especially when EPO levels are not measured until after the patient has undergone initial therapeutic phlebotomy. Normal EPO levels may also be seen in hypoxemia-induced secondary polycythemia after the elevated RCM has restored adequate renal oxygen delivery. Elevated EPO levels strongly suggest hypoxemia or another form of secondary erythrocytosis but may rarely be seen in PV if there is also a concomitant secondary polycythemic state. Assays for EEC growth, although not readily available to most clinicians, are minor criteria for the diagnosis of PV and are helpful in the evaluation of *JAK2* V617F–negative patients who present with polycythemia. Platelets show abnormal in vitro aggregation in up to 80% of cases. Additional laboratory abnormalities that are present in at least half of PV patients include an elevated LAP score, elevated LDH, and hyperuricemia (Table 14-6).

Bone marrow evaluation is not critical for the confirmation of suspected PV when other diagnostic criteria are present, including *JAK2* V617F, but is useful in supporting the diagnosis, in establishing prognosis, or in the diagnostic evaluation of *JAK2* V617F-negative patients. Common marrow findings with PV include erythroid and megakaryocytic hyperplasia, with abnormal megakaryocytes (typically large cells with hyperlobated nuclei) organized in clusters (Figure 14-3). Advanced reticulin fibrosis (ie, grades 3 or 4) is found in <5% of cases at diagnosis, but in at least 20% after 10 to 15 years and >50% after 20 years of disease. Karyotypic analysis may offer diagnostic utility in ambiguous

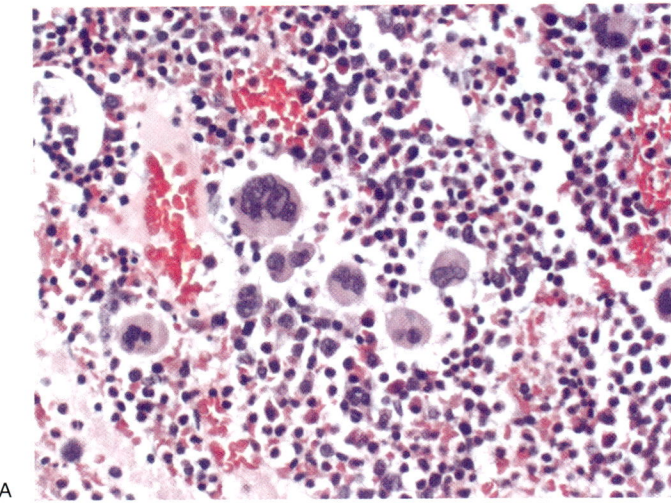

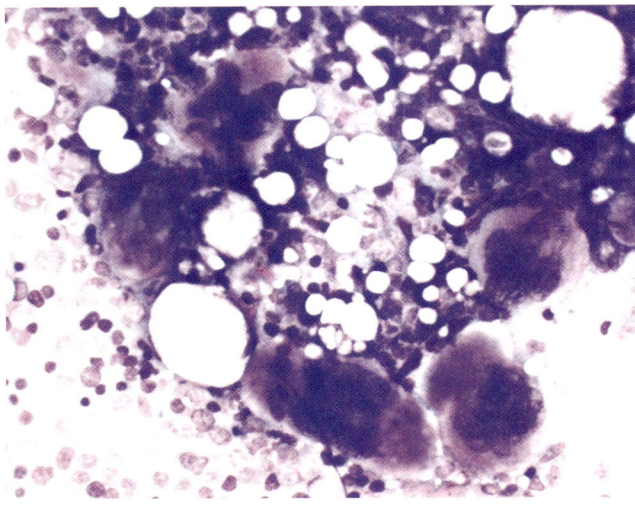

Figure 14-3 Megakaryocyte morphologic abnormalities observed in myeloproliferative disorders. A, Megakaryocyte hyperplasia, clustering, and nuclear hyperlobation in a bone marrow core biopsy sample from a patient with polycythemia vera (hematoxylin-eosin stain; original magnification, 170×) and B, a marrow aspirate from a patient with essential thrombocythemia (Wright-Giemsa stain; magnification, 170×). Photos courtesy of Steven J. Kussick, MD, PhD, University of Washington, Seattle, WA.

cases that are *JAK2* wild type. At diagnosis, approximately 15% of karyotypes from PV patients contain nonrandom chromosomal abnormalities, including trisomy 8, trisomy 9, del(13q), and del(20q). Monosomy 7, del(5q), and other abnormalities seen with AML and myelodysplasia are not common in PV. The frequency of a clonal karyotype in late-stage (>10 years) PV increases to 80%. Of note, there is no clear association between specific karyotypic abnormalities and progression to either AML or the preterminal stage of high-grade marrow fibrosis.

Course and prognosis

PV is a chronic disease that is incurable with current therapies other than SCT, which is reserved for high-risk, young patients in whom the risks of allogeneic SCT are acceptable. Although early studies suggested that untreated erythrocytosis and thrombocytosis lead to a median survival of only 18 months due to a high incidence of fatal thromboembolic events, more recent observational studies including younger individuals with PV and patients with chronic idiopathic erythrocytosis suggest that the clinical diagnosis of PV is often preceded by an asymptomatic prodrome of many years. Once the diagnosis is secure, treatment with phlebotomy, with aspirin, and with or without cytoreductive agents results in a near-normal life span for the average patient who is diagnosed at a median of 60 to 65 years of age. However, although it exceeds 10 years, the median survival of individuals diagnosed with PV before 40 years of age is considerably shorter than the life expectancy for a healthy person of similar age, even with active management.

Disease progression and leukemic transformation

Although PV patients commonly present with splenomegaly, marrow hyperplasia, erythrocytosis, and thrombocytosis, over time, a significant proportion of patients progress to develop progressive marrow fibrosis and compromised hematopoiesis, and then progress further to an end-stage condition often referred to as postpolycythemic myelofibrosis. Postpolycythemic myelofibrosis is characterized by progressive hepatosplenomegaly due to extramedullary hematopoiesis, advanced marrow fibrosis, and pancytopenia with leukoerythroblastosis. The median survival time in patients with postpolycythemic myelofibrosis is <3 years. At least 25% to 50% of patients with postpolycythemic myelofibrosis develop AML, although it is important to note that not all PV patients who transform to AML will progress through a postpolycythemic myelofibrosis phase. The presence or absence of splenomegaly and the degree of leukocytosis or thrombocytosis have not been useful predictors of the disease course. In addition, current studies do not clearly demonstrate that *JAK2* mutation status or allele burden predicts survival or transformation rate in a clinically meaningful manner, although the *JAK2* V617F allele burden does increase over time in most patients.

Transformation to AML occurs in roughly 1% to 3% of patients treated with phlebotomy alone. Phosphorus-32 (^{32}P) treatment, chlorambucil, busulfan, and alkylating agent combinations are associated with increased risk of transformation to AML (up to 15-fold increased risk in randomized PVSG trials). The European Collaboration on Low-dose Aspirin in Polycythemia Vera (ECLAP) study noted a higher rate of AML/MDS transformation with pipobroman use; this agent is no longer available in the United States but is still available for use in Europe and elsewhere. Leukemias that occur after chemotherapy or radiation may rarely be associated with abnormalities of chromosome 5 or 7. Although early observational studies suggested that AML transformation might be increased in patients receiving hydroxyurea, the largest prospective PV study to date, the ECLAP study, enrolled 1638 patients and noted no increase in AML in patients treated with hydroxyurea, with median a follow-up time of 8.4 years after PV diagnosis and 2.5 years after study enrollment. There is no evidence that IFNα or anagrelide are leukemogenic.

Thrombohemorrhagic risk

Thrombosis and bleeding are the major causes of morbidity and death with PV. Clinical risk factors for thrombosis and bleeding are listed in Table 14-9. Data from the ECLAP study revealed a thrombotic complication rate of 5.5 events per 100 patients per year at a median follow-up time of 2.7 years. Two thirds of those events were arterial, and one third were venous. The risk of a thrombotic complication in the ECLAP cohort was increased in PV patients >65 years old (hazard ratio [HR], 8.6), with a history of prior thrombosis (HR, 4.85), or >65 years old and with thrombosis (HR, 17.3); these represent the major factors used to assess thrombotic risk in PV patients. In addition, cardiovascular morbidity and mortality in PV were significantly linked to smoking, diabetes, and congestive heart failure. The etiology of hypercoagulability in PV is not well understood, but hyperviscosity due to uncontrolled erythrocytosis (at hematocrit >50%–55%), qualitative platelet dysfunction, and granulocyte activation likely contribute to the pathogenesis of thrombosis in PV.

Table 14-9 Risk factors for clinical complications of polycythemia vera.

Thrombosis
  Age >60 years old
  History of previous thrombosis (venous or arterial)
  High rate of phlebotomy
Hemorrhage
  Postoperative state with uncontrolled hematocrit or platelet count
  Platelet antiaggregating therapy (particularly in elderly)
  Thrombocytopenia during late-stage PPMM
Acute leukemia
  Previous therapy with chlorambucil, busulfan, or ^{32}P
  Evolution to late-stage PPMM
  Possibly hydroxyurea or pipobroman use

Multiple sources.
PPMM = postpolycythemic myeloid metaplasia.

Recent studies in patients treated with aspirin and hydroxyurea suggest that WBC count is an important predictor of thrombotic risk in patients with controlled erythrocytosis, suggesting that granulocyte activation contributes to thrombosis in patients treated with standard therapies. It is likely that patients with known genetic hypercoagulable states and concomitant PV are at higher risk of thrombosis, although this has not been confirmed in epidemiologic studies. The risk of postoperative thrombosis or bleeding is increased in patients with PV. Up to 80% of patients with PV who undergo surgery in the context of a hematocrit and/or platelet count markedly above the normal range will suffer a thrombohemorrhagic event. By contrast, only 5% to 10% of patients suffer these perioperative complications when their counts are normalized for at least several weeks preoperatively. Active treatment including phlebotomy, antiplatelet therapy, and cytoreductive agents decreases the risk of thrombosis and improves the disease course. The benefit of phlebotomy was clearly demonstrated by the PVSG trials. Randomized clinical trial data from the ECLAP study revealed that aspirin at a dose of 100 mg/d is safe and effective at reducing the rate of vascular events among PV patients without increasing the risk of bleeding, even in patients who are at low or unclear baseline risk for such events.

Therapy
Phlebotomy

The mainstay of treatment of PV remains phlebotomy to maintain the hematocrit closer to a normal physiologic range. Generally accepted goals include a hematocrit of <45% for men, <42% for women, and <37% for pregnant women late in gestation; however, there are no randomized trial data to support these specific guidelines. Additional cytoreductive or antithrombotic therapies are used as indicated for specific conditions and risk states (Table 14-10; Figure 14-4). In younger adults, weekly or even twice weekly phlebotomy may be required at the time of initial diagnosis to control presenting symptoms rapidly. Once the hematocrit is within the desired range, the interval between phlebotomies may be extended to 3 to 6 months. Aggressive initial phlebotomy without adjunctive myelosuppressive therapy may be associated with a higher risk of thrombosis, particularly in the elderly and those with a prior history of thrombosis; this has been hypothesized to be the result of new platelet formation in response to the thrombopoietic stimulus of rapid phlebotomy. Based on these clinical observations, myelosuppressive therapy is recommended as part of the initial treatment of patients >60 years of age and younger patients with thrombotic risk factors, particularly a history of thrombosis. Phlebotomy to the point of iron deficiency without concomitant

Table 14-10 Current treatment of polycythemia vera.

Risk categories	Treatment
Low	Low-dose aspirin + phlebotomy
Intermediate	Low-dose aspirin* + phlebotomy
High	Low-dose aspirin + phlebotomy + hydroxyurea

Risk stratification of PV according to thrombotic risk. High risk: age ≥60 years *or* previous thrombosis; intermediate risk: age <60 years *and* no previous thrombosis, *but* with either platelet count >1500 × 10^9/L *or* cardiovascular risk factors (tobacco use, diabetes mellitus, hypertension, hyperlipidemia); low risk: absence of any of the aforementioned risk factors.

* Clinically significant acquired von Willebrand disease should be excluded before the use of aspirin in patients with platelet count >1000 × 10^9/L. From Vanucchi AM, Guglielmelli P, Tefferi A. Advances in understanding and management of myeloproliferative neoplasms. *CA Cancer J Clin*. 2009;59:171–191.

cytoreductive therapy may be associated with reactive elevation in the platelet count, although the thrombohemorrhagic risk of reactive thrombocytosis in this clinical setting has not been delineated.

Thromboprophylaxis and symptomatic therapy

The ECLAP study, a double-blind randomized trial, compared low-dose aspirin with placebo among 518 patients who had no indication for anticoagulation and no preexisting clear indication or contraindication to aspirin therapy and demonstrated that low-dose aspirin (eg, 100 mg/d) reduces the rate of thrombosis and cardiovascular deaths in patients with PV receiving standard phlebotomy and supportive care. The aspirin-treated group suffered 60% fewer major thromboses and cardiovascular deaths (3.2% vs 7.9% absolute incidence) after roughly 3 years of follow-up. Low-dose aspirin can also effectively control erythromelalgia and other vasomotor symptoms in most patients. PVSG trials showed that higher doses of aspirin (ie, 500-900 mg/d) offer no added benefit but increase the risk of bleeding complications, especially when combined with dipyridamole. Elderly PV patients on high-dose aspirin are at highest risk of bleeding. However, the ECLAP trial observed only a modest increase in epistaxis and no increase in major bleeding on low-dose aspirin. The role of clopidogrel and other anticoagulants in thrombosis

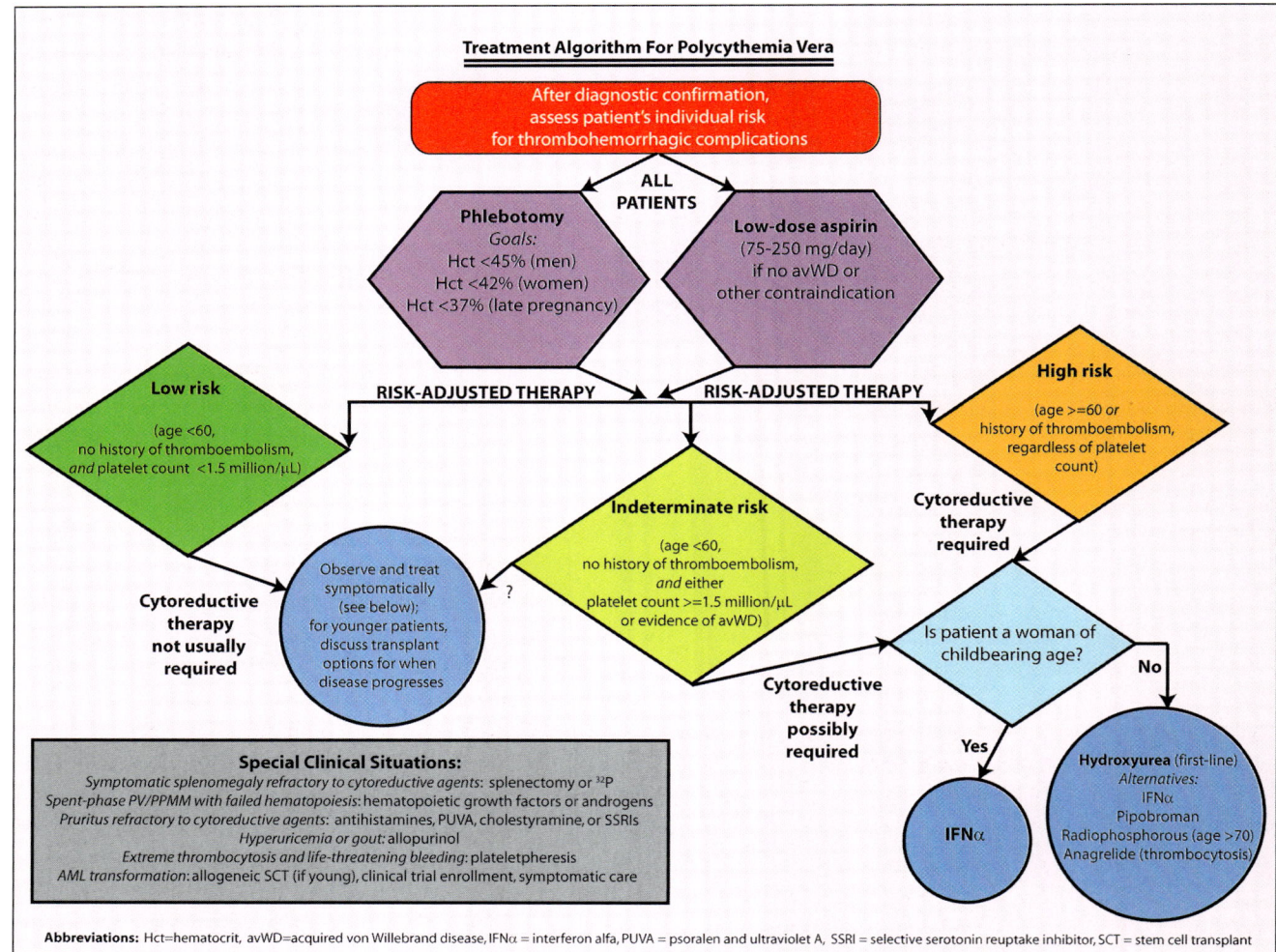

Figure 14-4 A suggested treatment algorithm for polycythemia vera. Assessment of the patient's thrombohemorrhagic risk is the key step.

prevention in PV is not well defined and is not considered standard of care.

Because of the observations from the PVSG regarding early thrombotic risk, hydroxyurea should be used in high-risk patients at the start of aggressive phlebotomy (Table 14-10). In general, patients with PV should also avoid practices that augment their hypercoagulability or risk of vascular complications, such as smoking and the use of oral contraceptives or estrogen hormone replacement therapy. For those requiring a surgical procedure, aggressive antithrombotic prophylaxis should be given postoperatively, in addition to ensuring that stable, normal hematocrit and platelet counts are maintained prior to surgery.

Pruritus may be a particularly disturbing symptom that is often unresponsive to phlebotomy or antiplatelet therapy. Antihistamines, PUVA, cholestyramine, or selective serotonin reuptake inhibitors (eg, paroxetine) may provide symptomatic relief. Cytoreductive therapy with hydroxyurea or IFNα may help in refractory cases. Painful splenomegaly and unacceptable hypercatabolic symptoms also usually require treatment with hydroxyurea or IFNα. Splenectomy or splenic irradiation may be necessary for palliation in selected patients who are intolerant of or unresponsive to cytoreductive agents.

Acute thrombosis management

Acute thrombotic events in patients with PV are managed with therapeutic systemic anticoagulation in a similar manner to other patients who present with acute thrombosis. It is also important to control the hematocrit and platelet count to minimize progression or recurrence; phlebotomy to normalize the hematocrit quickly should be initiated. The utility of plateletpheresis for thrombocythemic patients with acute thrombosis and the optimal target platelet count after depletion is unknown. Antiplatelet therapy in addition to warfarin may be useful in selected cases of PV-associated arterial thrombosis, but only after the acute event is stabilized with full anticoagulation and only if the potential additive risk of bleeding is considered acceptable.

Cytoreductive therapy

The choice of cytoreductive agent is based on the patient's age, the need to treat painful splenomegaly or troublesome hypercatabolic and constitutional symptoms, and whether or not concomitant thrombocytosis is present. Hydroxyurea, a ribonucleotide reductase inhibitor, reduces the thrombosis rate, can normalize the platelet count and spleen size, and frequently ameliorates hypercatabolic symptoms. It is the first choice for most patients with PV requiring cytoreductive therapy. The mutagenic and leukemogenic potential of hydroxyurea has been the subject of significant concern, but overall, the AML/MDS risk with chronic hydroxyurea therapy appears to be low based on data from the ECLAP (PV) and United Kingdom Medical Research Council Primary Thrombocythemia 1 (PT-1; ET) trials. Nevertheless, because of uncertainty regarding these concerns, hydroxyurea is often avoided in younger adults, and it should be used only after a thorough discussion of the potential risks and benefits. Additional adverse effects of hydroxyurea include cytopenias and, less commonly, chronic mucocutaneous ulcers.

Subcutaneous injections of IFNα, at initial doses of 3,000,000 to 5,000,000 IU 3 times per week (less in elderly patients), reliably control blood counts, splenomegaly, and constitutional symptoms in the majority of PV patients. IFNα therapy is safe during pregnancy, in contrast to hydroxyurea, which may be teratogenic (although experience from sickle cell anemia populations suggests that hydroxyurea is a low-risk agent, so abortion is not justified solely based on inadvertent fetal hydroxyurea exposure). Adjusted-dose IFNα can be useful for later-stage patients with progressive splenomegaly and poorly controlled peripheral blood leukoerythroblastosis. In general, the inconvenience, cost, and chronic adverse effects (including anorexia, depression, and fatigue) limit the practical use of IFNα to women who desire pregnancy and to those infrequent patients who do not tolerate or do not respond to other agents. Recent studies with pegylated IFNα have demonstrated significant clinical efficacy, including clinical/molecular remissions in a substantial proportion of patients with improved tolerability; current trials are aimed at assessing the efficacy and safety of pegylated IFNα in a larger cohort of PV patients.

Anagrelide, a prostaglandin synthetase inhibitor, selectively inhibits platelet production (although it can also cause mild anemia). It does not treat the hypercatabolic features of PV. The effect of anagrelide on thrombotic incidence has not yet been clearly established in patients with PV, and it should be considered a second-line agent. This is particularly true in light of data reported from the PT-1 trial comparing anagrelide and hydroxyurea in 809 patients with high-risk ET that suggested that anagrelide was associated with a higher risk of thrombosis compared with hydroxyurea (discussed later in this chapter), which has heightened concern. Studies of anagrelide in patients with ET have suggested that MPN-associated thrombotic complications are minimized if the platelet count is maintained below 400,000/μL; without good prospective data, this goal should be considered for PV patients with thrombocytosis who are being treated with cytoreductive agents. Anagrelide does not affect fertility, but it crosses the placenta and is of uncertain teratogenic potential; therefore, it is contraindicated during pregnancy. Anagrelide is a vasodilator, so it must be used cautiously in elderly patients and those with heart disease. Common adverse effects, including headache, palpitations, diarrhea, and fluid retention, may be avoided or minimized by starting at a lower dose and titrating up.

Conventional alkylating agents are generally avoided in patients with PV. Chlorambucil clearly increases the risk of AML/MDS, and busulfan probably does so as well. Occasional patients with disease manifestations that are refractory to other cytoreductive treatments, especially elderly patients with a limited life expectancy, may benefit from a limited schedule of busulfan (eg, intermittent 2-week courses). Similar to chlorambucil, ^{32}P has been demonstrated in randomized trials to increase the risk of hematologic and nonhematologic malignancies, particularly when combined with alkylating agents or hydroxyurea. However, it is well tolerated in the short term, and responses after a single treatment may last several months. Recent studies indicate that lower-dose ^{32}P may be equally effective as conventional doses, but with reduced and delayed risk of malignancy development. Therefore, low-dose ^{32}P is a reasonable palliative option for patients >70 years of age and may be especially useful in patients whose blood counts are difficult to control with hydroxyurea. Pipobroman is a neutral amide of piperazine, a metabolic competitor of pyrimidines that is chemically related to alkylating agents. Although unavailable in the United States since 1996, pipobroman appears to control PV disease manifestations as effectively as hydroxyurea. The ECLAP study, with shorter follow-up, revealed that pipobroman use was a significant risk factor for AML/MDS in PV, as had been previously shown for more conventional alkylating agents. None of the available cytoreductive therapies reliably modify established marrow fibrosis or prevent its progression in PV. Selective JAK2 TK inhibitors are currently entering clinical trials for PV and may supersede cytoreductive therapies.

Hematopoietic SCT

Allogeneic SCT offers the potential to restore normal hematopoiesis with donor cells, reverse marrow fibrosis, and eradicate the malignant PV clone. Data for SCT in PV are derived from small studies of patients younger than 65 years of age with rapidly progressive PV (ie, usually with clinicopathologic features indicating evolution to postpolycythemic myelofibrosis). Complete remissions and long-term survival are achievable after myeloablative allogeneic SCT from a histocompatible (human leukocyte antigen [HLA] matched) related or unrelated donor. However, reported overall survival and nonrelapse mortality rates vary widely among transplantation centers, likely reflecting differences in conditioning regimens, patient selection, and disease-related factors. Transplantation for untreated AML that has evolved from PV appears to be ineffective and cannot be recommended unless patients respond to induction/consolidation chemotherapy by returning to chronic-phase disease. There is little experience to date with outcomes of allogeneic transplantation after nonmyeloablative preparative regimens, although studies in PMF suggest that nonmyeloablative transplantation may offer significant efficacy with acceptable toxicity for patients with a related or unrelated donor. Currently, the high risks of morbidity and mortality with myeloablative allogeneic transplantation and the baseline favorable prognosis with PV restrict the use of SCT to younger patients with a poor prognosis.

Therapy for secondary AML in PV

Secondary AML arising from PV often, but not always, evolves during the postpolycythemic myelofibrosis stage of disease. AML in the setting of a previous diagnosis of PV is usually treated with conventional induction chemotherapy regimens. The response rate is low, and treatment-related morbidity and mortality are high, suggesting that these patients should be enrolled in clinical trials whenever possible. If remission is achieved, the duration is usually short lived. However, allogeneic myeloablative SCT can be considered during postinduction therapy remission in suitable younger patients with an acceptable donor. More generally, patients with MPNs who transform to AML do poorly for multiple reasons, including the preexisting marrow disorder and systemic complications associated with advanced disease, frequent leukemic cell chemotherapy resistance, and comorbidities of age and other medical conditions.

Pregnancy with PV

Because PV is uncommon in women of childbearing age, few pregnancy outcomes have been reported. One series of 18 pregnancies suggested poor outcomes unless the hematocrit was managed meticulously. Use of aspirin, phlebotomy, and, in some cases, low molecular weight heparin throughout pregnancy and for several weeks postpartum resulted in good maternal–fetal outcomes. The optimal regimen is undefined. Because severe iron deficiency may cause low birth weight and anemia in the neonate, some iron supplementation of phlebotomized women with PV may be indicated in selected cases during the first trimester of pregnancy. Because of the normal dilutional anemia of pregnancy, it is recommended that women with PV be phlebotomized to a hematocrit of <37% to minimize the risk of hyperviscosity, thrombotic, and hemorrhagic complications. Most of the myelosuppressive agents used for PV are contraindicated in pregnancy. If cytoreductive therapy is required, IFNα is the treatment of choice. It has been shown to be safe and effective in a small number of cases and is preferable to repeated apheresis procedures.

Key points

- PV is a stem cell disorder characterized by increased progenitor cell sensitivity to growth-promoting cytokines and is most commonly associated with activating somatic mutations in the JAK2 TK.
- PV (primary, absolute polycythemia) must be differentiated from relative and secondary polycythemias. Secondary polycythemias may be either physiologically appropriate (elevated EPO induced by tissue hypoxemia) or physiologically inappropriate (renal or ectopic overproduction of EPO or response to other erythropoietic stimuli). Familial polycythemic states are often associated with truncating EPO receptor mutations (low endogenous EPO level) or *VHL/HIF2A* mutations (high endogenous EPO level).
- Unless erythrocytosis is an incidental finding, at diagnosis, patients with PV have symptoms related to hyperviscosity, hypercatabolism, microvascular events, or thromboembolic complications.
- The median survival time of PV exceeds 10 years when patients are managed appropriately; thrombosis and bleeding are the major causes of morbidity and mortality. Transformation to AML is uncommon but is associated with use of radiophosphorous or alkylating agents.
- Major risk factors for thrombosis with PV include uncontrolled erythrocytosis and thrombocytosis, age >60 years, and a history of prior thromboembolic events. Smoking, established cardiovascular disease, and inherited or acquired thrombotic diatheses are likely also important risk factors.
- The hematocrit and platelet count should be normalized for several weeks prior to elective surgery to minimize the risk of perioperative thrombosis and bleeding in patients with PV. Postoperative thrombosis prophylaxis should be given whenever possible.
- All patients with PV should be phlebotomized to maintain the hematocrit closer to a physiologic range (ie, <45% for men, <42% for women, and <37% during late pregnancy). Aspirin at a dose of approximately 100 mg/d should be routinely used for thrombosis prophylaxis, unless a clear contraindication exists. Myelosuppressive agents, splenectomy, and hematopoietic SCT are indicated for specific patient populations.

Essential thrombocythemia

Clinical case

A 33-year-old woman is referred to the hematology clinic for evaluation of persistent thrombocytosis. Although her elevated platelet count was an incidental finding during an urgent care clinic visit for bronchitis 6 months ago, she now complains of episodic dizziness and headaches. Two months ago, she had a spontaneous abortion during the first trimester of her first pregnancy. At that time, her platelet count was 990,000/μL. Her past medical history, family history, and review of systems are otherwise unremarkable. A complete blood count from an insurance physical examination at age 25 years revealed a platelet count of 350,000/μL. The spleen tip is palpable on physical examination, but no other abnormalities are noted. The hemoglobin is 12.5 g/dL, hematocrit is 38%, mean corpuscular volume is 90 fL, WBC count is 12,000/μL, and platelet count is 1,500,000/μL. Giant platelets, increased neutrophils, and occasional basophils are seen on the peripheral smear. *JAK2* V617F mutation testing was positive.

ET is the second most common MPN in the United States, with an annual incidence rate of approximately 0.5 cases per 100,000 persons per year. The median age at diagnosis is approximately 60 years, although the diagnosis is increasingly made in younger adults. Women with ET outnumber men 1.5- to 2-fold, particularly among ETs diagnosed in the third to fifth decade of life. Morbidity and mortality from ET predominantly relate to thromboembolic, vasomotor, and, less commonly, hemorrhagic complications.

Pathobiology
Clonality

A clonal hematopoietic population can be demonstrated in most, but not all, women with ET when evaluating for G6PD isoenzyme expression or for inactivation patterns of polymorphic alleles of X-linked genes in myeloid populations (ie, granulocytes, platelets, and/or hematopoietic progenitors) and control somatic cell populations (usually T lymphocytes, skin fibroblasts, or buccal mucosal cells). Constitutive skewing is noted in 20% to 25% of normal women <50 years of age, and age-related skewing is present in >50% of women older than 75 years. Thus, these analyses of clonality are specific only for selected younger women. The inability to detect a clonal cell population in a portion of younger women with ET may relate to the infrequency of the affected clone as a proportion of total myeloid cells, restriction of clonal maturation to the megakaryocytic lineage, or alternative pathogenic mechanisms that lead to polyclonal platelet overproduction.

JAK2/MPL mutations

The *JAK2* V617F mutation is present in at least 40% to 50% of ET patients; using sensitive assays, it is possible to detect the mutant allele in different cell types (neutrophils, platelets) such that testing of peripheral blood neutrophils for the *JAK2*

V617F allele is appropriate as a diagnostic test. Patients with ET who have *JAK2* V617F have a higher median hemoglobin concentration and neutrophil count than those who lack the mutation, and they may have more thromboembolic events and require more cytoreductive therapy. Marrow karyotype is normal in 90% to 95% of cases. Recent studies have shown that 3% to 5% of ET patients have somatic activating mutations in the TPO receptor (MPL). By comparison, germline *TPO* or *MPL* mutations that lead to constitutive overexpression of the gene product have been identified in several kindreds with familial thrombocytosis. Familial thrombocytosis is rare.

Other biologic features

Biologic and functional abnormalities are frequently found in hematopoietic progenitor cells and platelets from ET patients. Myeloid progenitors demonstrate increased in vitro sensitivity to cytokines, with excessive colony growth in the majority of cases and endogenous megakaryocyte colony formation in a significant proportion of ET cases. A substantial proportion of ET patients demonstrate EEC growth, megakaryocytic progenitor sensitivity to TPO (the major megakaryocytic growth and differentiation factor), or both. Normal to elevated plasma levels of TPO are observed in most patients with ET, as well as many patients with PV. Some earlier studies attributed the higher TPO levels to decreased expression of the c-Mpl receptor on megakaryocytes and platelets, with decreased platelet-mediated clearance of bound ligand. More recent studies have not confirmed those earlier findings, suggesting that low c-Mpl expression levels and high plasma TPO levels are not specific or consistent abnormalities in ET. Increased mean platelet volume and qualitative platelet aggregation defects are also found in up to 90% of patients with ET; however, they are not useful clinical predictors of the risk of thrombosis or bleeding. Recent studies have identified somatic mutations in *TET2* and *ASXL1* in a small subset of ET patients; however, these mutations are not specific for ET (vs other myeloid neoplasms), and their pathogenetic role remains to be delineated.

Clinical features

At least one half of patients with ET are asymptomatic at diagnosis, but during the course of disease, vasomotor, thrombotic, or hemorrhagic manifestations will eventually occur in most individuals (Table 14-11). In contrast to PV, hypercatabolic signs and constitutional symptoms are uncommon in ET. Palpable splenomegaly is present in approximately 25% of ET patients at diagnosis, and ultrasound assessment reveals increased spleen length or volume

Table 14-11 Clinical features of essential thrombocythemia.

Vasomotor
  "Vascular" headaches, visual disturbances, dizziness, burning dysesthesia of the palms and soles (erythromelalgia), acrocyanosis, paresthesias, cutaneous ulcers, cognitive or psychiatric deficits, seizures

Thrombotic
  Arterial: cerebral (TIA, CVA), coronary, ophthalmic, distal/extremities
  Venous: deep extremities, pelvic, mesenteric, hepatic, portal

Hemorrhagic
  Gastrointestinal, mucosal, epistaxis, urogenital, deep hematoma, hemarthrosis

Obstetric
  First-trimester spontaneous abortion

Multiple sources.
CVA = cerebrovascular accident; TIA = transient ischemic attack.

in many patients with nonpalpable splenomegaly. Vasomotor manifestations, which appear to be due to platelet–endothelial interactions and inflammation in small arterioles, usually manifest as symptoms in the central nervous system or acral extremities (Table 14-11). In ET, thrombosis in the arterial system, including the cerebral, coronary, and peripheral arteries, is roughly 3 times more common than thromboembolic complications involving the veins. Approximately 10% to 25% of patients have a history of a thromboembolic event at the time they are diagnosed with ET. Hemorrhage is reported in only 6% of patients at diagnosis, most commonly as gastrointestinal or oral mucosal bleeding. Bleeding is more common in older individuals and in patients with platelet counts >1,500,000/μL. The bleeding risk with a platelet count >1,500,000/μL may be due, at least in some cases, to acquired vWD or to high-dose aspirin use.

ET is discovered as an incidental laboratory abnormality in 70% of patients who are diagnosed under the age of 40. However, upon careful questioning, less than one fourth of these individuals are truly completely asymptomatic, although the connection of nonspecific symptoms, such as headaches or episodic tinnitus, to ET is not always clear. Approximately 4% to 10% of younger patients with ET have suffered a thrombotic or bleeding complication prior to diagnosis. As illustrated by the previous clinical case, young women with ET have a significantly increased risk of first-trimester abortions (up to 36% of documented pregnancies) and may suffer recurrent fetal loss; studies have not identified clinical or laboratory risk factors for pregnancy-associated complications in ET with the exception of poorly managed platelet counts.

Table 14-12 Diagnostic criteria for essential thrombocythemia.

Disease	Essential thrombocytosis
Major	1. Sustained platelet count ≥450 × 10^9/L
	2. Bone marrow biopsy specimen showing proliferation mainly of the megakaryocytic lineage with increased numbers of enlarged, mature megakaryocytes; no significant increase or left-shift of neutrophil granulopoiesis or erythropoiesis
	3. Not meeting World Health Organization criteria for polycythemia vera, primary myelofibrosis, chronic myelogenous leukemia, myelodysplastic syndrome, or other myeloid neoplasm
	4. Demonstration of *JAK2* V617F or other clonal marker, *or* in the absence of a clonal marker, no evidence for reactive thrombocytosis
Diagnosis	Requires meeting all 4 major criteria

Adapted from Swerdlow SH, Campo E, Harris NL, et al, eds. *World Health Organization Classification of Tumours of Haematopoietic and Lymphoid Tissues.* Lyon, France: IARC Press; 2008.

Differential diagnosis and laboratory features
Distinction from reactive thrombocytosis or other myeloid disorders

The diagnosis of ET as the cause of persistent thrombocytosis (ie, >450,000/μL) relies on the exclusion of disorders associated with reactive thrombocytosis and the exclusion of other MPNs (especially PV and CML) and MDS [especially 5q– syndrome, chromosome 3(q21;q26) abnormalities, or refractory anemia with ringed sideroblasts associated with marked thrombocytosis (RARS-T)]. The revised WHO criteria lowered the threshold platelet count for ET to 450,000/μL (Table 14-12). A diagnosis of ET according to the revised WHO requires 4 features: thrombocytosis, bone marrow findings including megakaryocyte dysmorphology, absence of evidence of another clonal myeloid disorder, and the presence of a clonal marker (*JAK2* or *MPL* mutation or karyotypic abnormalities) or absence of reactive thrombocytosis. Iron deficiency, infection, inflammation, surgery, trauma, tissue injury or infarction, malignancy, and postsplenectomy state can all cause secondary or reactive thrombocytosis because platelets are an acute-phase reactant. Increased levels of inflammatory mediators, including IL-1β and IL-6 in addition to IL-11 (a direct thrombopoietic stimulator), have been associated with reactive thrombocytosis. An elevated C-reactive protein measurement is a surrogate marker for increased levels of IL-6, which can suggest an occult inflammatory process.

Laboratory features

The LAP score is typically elevated in ET, like PV but unlike CML. Moderate leukocytosis may be found in up to one half of ET patients. The peripheral blood smear is often notable for large or giant platelets (Figure 14-5) with occasional eosinophils, basophils, or circulating megakaryocyte fragments. Nucleated red blood cells or immature myeloid cells may be present in up to 25% of cases. Howell-Jolly bodies suggest hyposplenism; if the cause of this is not obvious (eg, prior splenectomy), then celiac disease, amyloidosis, or a hemoglobinopathy resulting in functional hyposplenism should be considered.

Because *JAK2* and *MPL* mutations are specific for clonal hematologic disease, their presence is valuable in excluding purely reactive thrombocytosis. However, given that as many as 30% to 40% of ET patients are negative for *JAK2/MPL* mutations, a negative *JAK2* result does not exclude a diagnosis of ET. The absolute value of the platelet count does not help distinguish reactive thrombocytosis from ET because platelet counts >2,000,000/μL can be seen with reactive conditions.

The significance of blood leukoerythroblastic features and their possible association with PMF rather than ET has been investigated. One study suggested that patients with more prominent circulating immature cells, teardrop erythrocytes, mild splenomegaly, and stainable marrow reticulin fibrosis more commonly progressed to overt myelofibrosis and had a significantly shorter survival, suggesting that their natural histories were more consistent with PMF and that they might have been classified as having "prefibrotic" or "early fibrotic" PMF rather than ET. This area is complex and requires an experienced morphologist and clinical correlation. Moreover, although patients with evidence of leukoerythroblastosis may be at higher risk for progression to post-ET

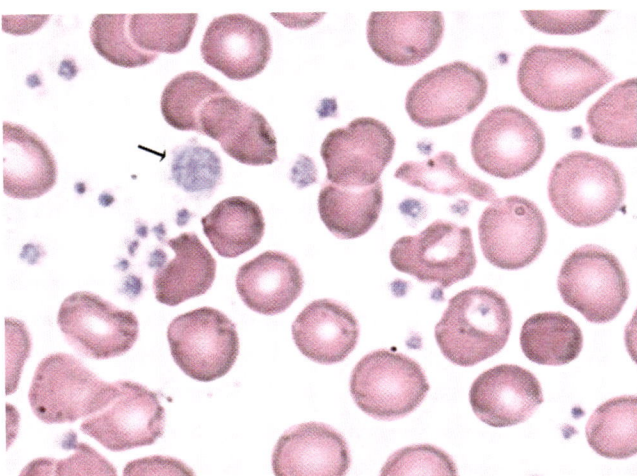

Figure 14-5 Increased numbers of platelets, including abnormally large platelets (*arrow*), are characteristic of essential thrombocythemia. Similar platelet abnormalities may also be seen in other myeloproliferative disorders. From American Society of Hematology Image Bank #100445.

myelofibrosis, the diagnostic and therapeutic strategy for patients with clonal thrombocytosis does not differ based on the likelihood for progression to overt myelofibrosis.

Bone marrow and cytogenetic findings

Marrow evaluation is important in suspected ET cases to assess for histopathologic features characteristic of ET to confirm the presence of adequate iron stores and to assess for fibrosis or other atypical features that might suggest an alternative diagnosis. Increased numbers and clusters of large megakaryocytes with hyperploid nuclei are seen in approximately 90% of marrow samples from patients with ET, and hypercellularity is seen in roughly three fourths of ET cases. Trilineage dysplasia and significant reticulin and collagen fibrosis are commonly minimal or absent. If >15% ringed sideroblasts are present, the rare provisional entity of RARS-T rather than ET must be considered, although the prognostic importance of this distinction is unclear. The presence of trilineage dysplastic morphologic features should raise the suspicion of MDS.

Alternative disorders to ET are particularly important to recognize in younger patients who might benefit from targeted therapy with imatinib (CML), treatment with lenalidomide [del(5q) MDS], or an early SCT if the diagnosis is revised. Cytogenetic studies are helpful in excluding CML or MDS (especially the 5q– syndrome), and specific assessment of *BCR-ABL* should be undertaken because CML can present with isolated thrombocytosis and a normal WBC count. Patients with isolated thrombocytosis in association with the t(9;22)(q34;q11) translocation detected on routine karyotyping or large proportions of cells positive for *BCR-ABL* detected by FISH follow a disease course similar to that of CML. Thus, such patients should be considered to have atypical CML and should be managed accordingly. However, the meaning of low-level *BCR-ABL* signals detected only by sensitive PCR assays in patients with suspected ET is less clear. *JAK2/MPL* mutational status or karyotypic abnormalities described in ET do not appear to have prognostic significance.

Course and prognosis
Disease progression

A single-institution observational study of 322 ET patients with a median follow-up time of 13.6 years showed that life expectancy is similar to age-matched controls in the first decade after diagnosis, but overall survival became significantly worse thereafter. Age at diagnosis of 60 years or older, leukocytosis, ongoing tobacco use, and diabetes mellitus were independent predictors of poor survival. Nevertheless, many patients can expect a normal or near-normal life span if major thrombotic or bleeding complications are avoided. Several studies have reported that transformation to AML is rare in the natural course of ET (<2%) in the first decade after diagnosis; however, the risk of leukemic progression or any myeloid disease transformation increases substantially in the second (8.1% and 28.3%, respectively) and third (24.0% and 58.5%, respectively) decades after diagnosis. It does not appear that hydroxyurea treatment by itself increases the risk of leukemic transformation; however, the AML transformation rate has been reported at 3.5% to 10% at 4 to 10 years when hydroxyurea is used in the setting of underlying cytogenetic abnormalities, marrow fibrosis, or concomitant use of additional chemotherapy agents.

Approximately 5% of patients with apparent ET with isolated thrombocytosis at diagnosis will later develop erythrocytosis consistent with transformation to PV; this most commonly occurs in patients with *JAK2* V617F because acquisition of *JAK2* V617F mutations after ET diagnosis does not commonly occur. Alternatively, 2% to 6% of patients progress to develop post-ET myelofibrosis, a disease that is clinically and pathologically indistinguishable from PMF. As noted previously, such patients may have had a prefibrotic or early fibrotic stage of PMF, rather than true ET. In general, these observations illustrate the overlapping clinical and pathophysiologic features of MPNs.

Thrombohemorrhagic risk

Between 10% and 50% of patients with ET will have a thrombotic episode during the first decade after diagnosis, and 4% will suffer a hemorrhagic complication. Older age and previous history of thrombohemorrhagic complications are the major risk factors in most studies. Complications of either type are uncommon in patients younger than age 40 years. One prospective observational study found no significant increase in the risk of thrombosis (1.91 cases per 100 patient-years, with 4.1 years of median follow-up) among untreated ET patients age <60 years with a negative prior thrombohemorrhagic event history and a platelet count <1,500,000/μL when compared with age-matched healthy controls. Older age and a platelet count >1,500,000/μL have been cited as predictors of bleeding risk in ET; however, the influence of comorbid factors must be taken into consideration (Table 14-13). Some ET patients with uncontrolled thrombocytosis and clinical bleeding are found to have vWD, as described previously for PV.

The overall risk of thrombotic complications in ET can be stratified based on age, history of prior thrombosis, and the presence of additional cardiovascular risk factors (Table 14-13). The relative importance of associated cardiovascular risk factors with arterial thromboembolism is not been

Table 14-13 Risk stratification for thrombotic and hemorrhagic complications of essential thrombocythemia.

Low risk (all of the following)
- Age <60 years old
- No history of thromboembolism
- Platelet count >1,500,000/μL (without bleeding history or acquired von Willebrand disease)
- No cardiovascular risk factors (smoking, hypercholesterolemia)

Indeterminate risk
- Neither low- nor high-risk disease

High risk (one or both)
- Age ≥60 years old
- History of thromboembolism

Adapted and modified from Tefferi A. Recent progress in the pathogenesis and management of essential thrombocythemia. *Leuk Res.* 2001;25:369–377.

Table 14-14 Current treatment of essential thrombocythemia.

Risk categories	Essential thrombocytosis
Low	Low-dose aspirin
Intermediate	Low-dose aspirin*
High	Low-dose aspirin + hydroxyurea

* Clinically significant acquired von Willebrand disease should be excluded before the use of aspirin in patients with platelet count >1000 × 10^9/L.

From Vanucchi AM, Guglielmelli P, Tefferi A. Advances in understanding and management of myeloproliferative neoplasms. *CA Cancer J Clin.* 2009;59:171–191.

clearly demonstrated; however, ET patients with a history of cigarette smoking, diabetes mellitus, and/or hypercholesterolemia are at higher risk of cerebral or cardiac thrombotic events. Although limited data exist, most experts consider oral contraceptive use, estrogen replacement therapy, and other acquired and congenital prothrombotic conditions to be modifiers of thrombotic risk with ET. Specifically, the presence of genetic thrombophilic states, including activated protein C resistance, prothrombin 20210A, or less common thrombophilic states (protein C/S deficiency, ATIII deficiency, or antiphospholipid antibodies), imparts a higher risk of thrombosis with ET. Although some studies have found an increased risk of bleeding in ET patients with a platelet count of 1,500,000/μL, there are no data to suggest that absolute platelet number is clearly predictive of thromboembolic complications in the absence of other clinical risk factors. Nevertheless, controlling the platelet count may be protective, and studies with hydroxyurea (targeted at maintaining the platelet count at <600,000/μL) and anagrelide (targeted at maintaining the platelet count at <400,000/μL) have shown that these drugs decrease the risk of primary or recurrent thrombotic events (from 24% to 3.6% during the 27-month observation period).

Therapy
General considerations

Treatment approaches for ET are based on the individualized risks for thrombosis or bleeding, the presence of vasomotor symptoms, and the risks and benefits of the available platelet-lowering agents (Table 14-14). The 3 platelet-lowering agents commonly used for ET in the United States are hydroxyurea, anagrelide, and IFNα. Alkylating agents are almost never used in ET because of their proven leukemogenicity in PV.

Cytoreductive therapy

Two important randomized trials of high-risk patients with ET inform current management principles. The first study from Italy, a randomized trial of 114 patients, convincingly showed a role for hydroxyurea in decreasing thromboembolic events in high-risk ET patients who either are older than age 60, have a previous history of thromboembolism, or both. A recent follow-up report of this study (median treatment time, 73 months) revealed a continued benefit for hydroxyurea; 45% of patients in the control group suffered a thrombotic event versus 9% of patients in the hydroxyurea group. Of note, 1.7% of control patients and 3.9% of the group receiving hydroxyurea developed secondary myeloid malignancies (AML/MDS), a difference that was not statistically significant. The second important randomized study in ET was the PT-1 trial. A total of 809 patients with ET at high risk of thrombosis were enrolled in the PT-1 study, received low-dose aspirin (75-100 mg daily), and were randomized to receive either hydroxyurea or anagrelide, with a goal platelet count of <400,000/μL. After a median follow-up of 39 months, patients in the anagrelide group were significantly more likely than those in the hydroxyurea group to have reached the adverse primary end point of thrombosis or serious hemorrhage. Specifically, compared with hydroxyurea plus aspirin, patients receiving anagrelide plus aspirin had increased rates of arterial thrombosis, serious hemorrhage, and development of marrow fibrosis but a decreased rate of venous thromboembolism. Patients receiving anagrelide were more likely to withdraw from their assigned treatment due to toxicity or treatment failure. Taken together, these 2 studies suggest that patients with ET at high risk of thrombosis should be treated with low-dose aspirin and hydroxyurea with a goal platelet count of <400,000 to 600,000/μL. Anagrelide should be reserved for patients with an insufficient response to hydroxyurea or with intolerable hydroxyurea-associated adverse effects. The use of hydroxyurea or anagrelide in patients at lower risk of thrombosis or the use of other cytoreductive agents in ET patients in general is not clear. Recent studies have reported excellent safety and efficacy of pegylated IFNα in ET, although this has not been assessed in randomized clinical trials.

Pregnancy

Based on case reports demonstrating safety and efficacy, IFNα remains the cytoreductive agent of choice for symptomatic or otherwise high-risk young women with ET (eg, those with thrombotic history) who desire pregnancy. Pegylated IFNα appears to have a more favorable safety and efficacy profile and should be considered as an alternative therapeutic regimen in pregnant women with ET. Although pregnancy is often successful in asymptomatic women with untreated ET, the increased risk of first-trimester abortions does not appear to be affected by the use of platelet-lowering agents or by prophylactic platelet depletion with apheresis. In addition, the outcome of a subsequent pregnancy is not predicted by the outcome of a first pregnancy. Aspirin is commonly recommended for women with ET and prior fetal loss; however, the benefit of this intervention has not been formally proven.

Prevention and management of thrombosis and hemorrhage

Low-dose aspirin as primary prophylaxis for ET patients is recommended in view of the beneficial results with aspirin in PV in the ECLAP study and the favorable outcomes of patients treated with aspirin and hydroxyurea in the PT-1 trial. In the setting of acute arterial or venous events, emergency plateletpheresis may occasionally be indicated to reduce the platelet count if it is very high. Standard heparin and warfarin therapy are indicated for venous thrombosis as for non-ET patients who present with thrombosis. Large-vessel arterial thrombotic events may require acute intervention with a heparin or thrombolysis. Lifelong warfarin is reserved for patients with recurrent events or if the primary event was catastrophic and unprovoked in a patient with a normal platelet count on cytoreductive therapy. In either circumstance, the patient should be monitored closely for bleeding while receiving anticoagulation. Platelet-lowering agents should be used to maintain the platelet count in a safe range, ideally <400,000/μL. Aspirin is indicated following an arterial thromboembolic event if the patient is not already taking it. As with PV, the risk of bleeding in ET appears to be elevated with high doses (>325 mg/d) of aspirin. Therefore, lower aspirin doses, in the range of 75 to 300 mg/d, are normally advised. As for PV, the role of clopidogrel or other antiplatelet agents in ET is unknown. The usefulness of aspirin after a venous thrombotic event is more questionable, and aspirin treatment should be deferred until warfarin therapy is discontinued. As in the case of PV, the platelet count in patients with ET should be normalized for several weeks prior to elective surgery to minimize the risk of perioperative thrombosis and bleeding.

SCT or transformation to acute leukemia

Despite the generally favorable prognosis with ET, occasional patients evolve to extensive myelofibrosis with myeloid metaplasia or AML. Allogeneic SCT is feasible and beneficial for selected high-risk younger patients who have developed myelofibrosis and have a suitable related or unrelated stem cell donor. Only small series have been reported. As with PV, the roles for nonmyeloablative SCT or autologous SCT remain undefined for high-risk ET. As in PV, patients with ET who transform to AML should be treated with standard induction and consolidation chemotherapy when clinically indicated, although the long-term prognosis of patients who transform to AML from ET is dismal.

> **Key points**
>
> - ET is a diagnosis of exclusion after evaluating patients for other myeloid disorders and for reactive thrombocytosis. Reactive or secondary thrombocytosis may be due to iron deficiency, infection, inflammation, tissue injury or trauma, malignancy, and postsplenectomy state or functional hyposplenism. The platelet count alone does not distinguish reactive thrombocytosis from ET.
> - *JAK2* and *MPL* mutations are present in 50% to 60% of ET patients; their presence proves the existence of a clonal myeloid disorder but is not specific for ET, and their absence does not exclude a diagnosis of ET.
> - The life expectancy of patients with ET is longer than for those with other MPNs, but patients are at risk for ET-related morbidity and mortality over time. Symptomatic bleeding, thromboembolic events (arterial > venous), and vasomotor complications affect most individuals eventually and are the major causes of morbidity and mortality.
> - Risk factors for bleeding and thrombosis should be identified and considered in a risk-based treatment approach for patients with ET.
> - Platelet-lowering agents and low-dose aspirin are indicated for high-risk patients with ET. Hydroxyurea should be the first choice because it is superior to anagrelide at preventing most thrombohemorrhagic events. Anagrelide can be a useful second-line agent. Low-dose aspirin alone should be used for low-risk patients and may effectively treat vasomotor symptoms.
> - ET is the most common MPN detected in young women and is associated with recurrent fetal loss. Aspirin and, if cytoreduction is required, IFNα can be used to strive for a favorable pregnancy outcome.

Primary myelofibrosis

> **Clinical case**
>
> A reclusive 78-year-old man comes to the clinic with complaints of abdominal pain, weight loss, and lower extremity swelling. He has not seen a doctor for several years. He has lost 50 pounds involuntarily over the last year. He suffers from fatigue, light-headedness, dyspnea on exertion, and nocturnal sweating. On physical examination, he is thin, with pale skin and conjunctivae. There is no lymphadenopathy. An early systolic crescendo–decrescendo murmur is heard over the entire precordium. The abdomen is markedly distended without a fluid wave or shifting dullness. The spleen extends to the pelvic brim and across the midline; it is firm and mildly tender. The liver edge is palpable 6 cm below the right costal margin on shallow inspiration. Gouty tophi are found on the pinnae and hands. The hemoglobin is 7.4 g/dL, hematocrit is 22%, WBC is 7400/μL, and platelet count is 68,000/μL. The peripheral blood smear is notable for moderate numbers of teardrop erythrocytes with occasional nucleated red blood cells, increased neutrophilic bands, metamyelocytes, basophils, and giant platelets. Serum uric acid level is 13 mg/dL, and the LDH is twice the upper limit of normal. *JAK2* and *MPL* mutational testing is negative.

PMF is the least common of the 4 major MPNs and carries the worst prognosis. The annual incidence is reported at 0.2 cases per 100,000 persons per year, with a predominance of men older than 50 years of age. The median survival time is 3.5 to 5.5 years, although the natural history of PMF is quite variable depending on the presence or absence of poor prognostic features. A subset of low-risk patients will live longer than 10 years and require minimal active management (see further details later in the chapter). The median age at diagnosis of PMF is approximately 65 years, with 70% of cases diagnosed after 60 years of age and approximately 10% of cases diagnosed at <45 years of age.

Pathobiology
Marrow microenvironment, CD34$^+$ cells, and clonality

The hallmarks of PMF are marrow fibrosis and extramedullary hematopoiesis; the latter most commonly affects the liver and spleen. These processes result from the proliferation and emigration of neoplastic hematopoietic cells and production of cytokines within the marrow microenvironment, leading to reactive proliferation of fibroblasts and other mesenchymal cells. Throughout all stages of disease, the circulating populations of red blood cells, granulocytes, and platelets are clonal. The number of circulating hematopoietic progenitors (CD34$^+$ cells) is significantly increased in PMF. This is also true for other MPNs, but the number of circulating CD34$^+$ cells in PMF patients can be 50-fold higher than in PV or ET. Higher levels of circulating CD34$^+$ cells in PMF are associated with more advanced bone marrow fibrosis and other disease characteristics. One study observed shorter survival and earlier transformation to AML among PMF patients with circulating CD34$^+$ cell counts <300/μL. A hostile marrow microenvironment alone does not appear to account for elevated CD34$^+$ counts because extensive myelofibrosis secondary to marrow involvement with carcinoma or lymphoid malignancies is associated with only mild increases in the numbers of circulating progenitor cells.

The marked reactive mesenchymal cell proliferation in PMF has been linked to inflammatory response cytokines and megakaryocyte- and monocyte-derived growth factors. Platelet-derived growth factor (PDGF) and basic fibroblast growth factor (bFGF) are constitutively overproduced by clonal megakaryocytes in PMF. Platelets and monocytes/macrophages in PMF marrow release increased amounts of transforming growth factor β (TGFβ), which also contributes to the stromal reaction. In PMF patients, elevated levels of IL-1 and tumor necrosis factor (TNF) are associated with augmented production or release of PDGF, bFGF, angiogenic factors such as vascular endothelial growth factor (VEGF), and osteogenic cytokines, in addition to direct or indirect effects of TGFβ. Neoangiogenesis is more significant in PMF compared with other MPNs, and high marrow microvascular density is associated with advanced splenomegaly and shorter survival.

Cytogenetic and molecular findings

JAK2 V617F is found in approximately 50% of patients with PMF. Several series have reported an association between *JAK2* V617F and elevated WBC count, older age, history of thrombosis, or pruritus. As in ET, approximately 5% to 10% of patients with PMF have somatic *MPL* mutations, which activate *JAK2* in a subset of *JAK2* V617F–negative PMF patients. However, 30% to 50% of PMF patients are negative for *JAK2/MPL* mutations, suggesting there are unidentified mutations that activate signaling and are responsible for clonal hematopoiesis in this subset of PMF. Mutations of the *p53* gene, the *RAS* family of proto-oncogenes, *p16*, or *c-Kit* have been described in a minority of PMF cases; whether these mutations represent disease-initiating events in PMF or are acquired during PMF disease progression are not known. Cytogenetic abnormalities are found in approximately one third to one half of patients with PMF at diagnosis and in approximately 90% at the time of disease progression to AML. The majority of patients with abnormal karyotypes have del(13q), del(20q), trisomy 8, trisomy 9, del(12p), or trisomy 1q. Pathobiologically relevant genes underlying these rearrangements are generally unknown.

Clinical features

Two thirds of patients with PMF are symptomatic at diagnosis, predominantly with constitutional complaints related to a cytokine-mediated hypercatabolic physiologic state (Table 14-15). As illustrated in the previous clinical case, fevers, night sweats, and weight loss are frequent hypercatabolic signs. Severe fatigue is the most common symptom in patients with PMF. Hyperuricemia is also common and results from increased myeloid cell turnover; gout or renal complications of hyperuricemia can develop. Splenomegaly is found in 85% to 100% of PMF patients at diagnosis. Ultimately, 35% of PMF patients will develop massive (ie, extending to the pelvic brim) splenomegaly. Extramedullary hematopoiesis in the spleen and, to a lesser degree, upstream effects of portal hypertension in the liver are responsible for the splenic enlargement. Extramedullary hematopoiesis can also cause hepatomegaly and lymphadenopathy. Rare patients with PMF develop nonhepatosplenic extramedullary hematopoiesis in locations such as the vertebral column (paraspinal or intraspinal lesions, which can lead to cord compression), lung, pleura, retroperitoneum, eye, kidney, bladder, mesentery, and skin. Lung extramedullary hematopoiesis is associated with pulmonary hypertension and marked reduction in overall survival and impaired quality of life.

Portal hypertension with ascites and varices develops in up to 7% of patients with PMF. This complication arises from thrombotic vasculopathy involving the portal circulation and extramedullary hematopoiesis. Portal hypertension and massive splenomegaly predispose to splenic infarction. Splenic infarction should be suspected in a patient with PMF who presents with acute or subacute left upper quadrant pain radiating to the shoulder, with or without associated nausea and fever. Splenic infarcts do not have clear prognostic value.

Anemia is the major hematologic complication of PMF. The cause of anemia in PMF is often multifactorial, including impaired erythropoiesis, hematopoietic failure, hemolysis, hemorrhage (usually gastrointestinal), and hypersplenism. Symptoms due to anemia are common among patients with PMF (Table 14-15). Approximately 50% to 70% of patients are anemic at presentation, and 25% of patients have hemoglobin levels <8 g/dL. Progressive thrombocytopenia, usually in the setting of hematopoietic failure and hypersplenism (ie, sequestration and destruction of circulating platelets in the spleen), significantly increases the risk of bleeding. Low-grade disseminated intravascular coagulopathy may also arise in some patients and can exacerbate the thrombotic and hemorrhagic risk. Secondary iron overload may develop because of inappropriate iron loading by the gut and red blood cell transfusion dependency. Autoimmune complications have been described with PMF, including hemolytic anemia and vasculitis.

Diagnosis

Diagnostic features have been published by the WHO (Table 14-16) that incorporate molecular, histopathologic, clinical, and laboratory features that distinguish PMF from other myeloid and nonmyeloid diseases. In most cases, the diagnosis of PMF is satisfied by finding increased bone marrow reticulin or collagen fibrosis, leukoerythroblastic peripheral blood findings, and splenomegaly, in the absence of a secondary cause for these findings or of features better fitting ET or PV. CML should always be ruled out by molecular studies for the *BCR-ABL* rearrangement. *JAK2* and *MPL* mutations demonstrate the presence of clonal hematopoiesis, but their presence is not specific for PMF, and their absence does not exclude a diagnosis of PMF. Acute myelofibrosis due to AML with megakaryocytic differentiation (ie, M7 AML by French-American-British [FAB] criteria and acute megakaryoblastic leukemia by WHO classification criteria) or other primary myeloid disorders may be confused with PMF. In most cases, acute megakaryoblastic leukemia is distinguished by a rapid disease onset, pancytopenia, mild splenomegaly, and a high frequency of marrow myeloblasts with a megakaryocytic immunophenotype (eg, positive for CD61). Many children

Table 14-15 Clinical features of primary myelofibrosis.

Mechanism	Symptoms
Hypercatabolic state (cytokine related)	Fatigue, weight loss, nocturnal sweating, pruritus
Splenomegaly	Pain, early satiety, diarrhea
Anemia	Dyspnea, palpitations, light-headedness
Portal hypertension/ascites	Abdominal pressure, peripheral edema
Splenic infarct	Acute left upper quadrant pain, fever, nausea, subscapular pain
Esophageal varices/hemorrhoids	GI bleeding (melena or hematochezia)
Hypertrophic osteoarthropathy, periostitis	Bone and musculoskeletal pain
Ectopic myeloid metaplasia	Tumor mass effect (lung, GI, GU, CNS, spine)
Thrombocytopenia/platelet dysfunction	Bleeding, bruising
Hyperuricemia	Monoarticular arthritis, nephrolithiasis (synovitis, hematuria)

Multiple sources.
CNS = central nervous system; GI = gastrointestinal; GU = genitourinary.

Table 14-16 Diagnostic criteria for primary myelofibrosis.

Disease	Criteria
Major	1. Presence of megakaryocyte proliferation and atypia, usually accompanied by either reticulin and/or collagen fibrosis, or, in the absence of significant reticulin fibrosis, the megakaryocyte changes must be accompanied by an increased bone marrow cellularity characterized by granulocytic proliferation and often decreased erythropoiesis (ie, prefibrotic cellular-phase disease). 2. Not meeting World Health Organization criteria for polycythemia vera, chronic myelogenous leukemia, myelodysplastic syndrome, or other myeloid neoplasm 3. Demonstration of *JAK2* V617F or other clonal marker (eg, *MPL* W515L/K), or, in the absence of a clonal marker, no evidence of bone marrow fibrosis due to underlying inflammatory or other neoplastic diseases
Minor	1. Leukoerythroblastosis 2. Increase in serum lactate dehydrogenase level 3. Anemia 4. Palpable splenomegaly
Diagnosis	Diagnosis requires meeting all 3 major criteria and 2 minor criteria.

Adapted from Swerdlow SH, Campo E, Harris NL, et al, eds. *World Health Organization Classification of Tumours of Haematopoietic and Lymphoid Tissues.* Lyon, France: IARC Press; 2008.

Table 14-17 Differential diagnosis of primary myelofibrosis.

Acute myelofibrosis (acute megakaryoblastic leukemia, AML-M7)
Myelodysplasia with fibrosis
Late-stage PV, ET, or CML with evolution to myelofibrosis
Malignant causes of secondary myelofibrosis
   Hairy cell leukemia
   Hodgkin lymphoma
   Non-Hodgkin lymphoma
   Plasma cell dyscrasias
   Acute lymphoblastic leukemia
   Metastatic carcinoma
   Multiple myeloma
   Chronic myelomonocytic leukemia
   Systemic mastocytosis
   Eosinophilic leukemia
Nonmalignant causes of secondary myelofibrosis
   Granulomatous infections (tuberculosis, histoplasmosis)
   Paget disease
Autoimmune disorders (eg, systemic lupus, Sjögren syndrome, psoriatic arthritis, primary autoimmune myelofibrosis)

CML = chronic myeloid leukemia; ET = essential thrombocythemia; PV = polycythemic vera.

who are diagnosed with PMF probably have acute megakaryoblastic leukemia. Other cases of acute myelofibrosis have a similar marrow histopathology and fulminant disease course to M7 AML but lack the 20% blast count required for the diagnosis of AML.

Patients with MDS may present with fibrosis in their bone marrow but usually lack the prominent splenomegaly and peripheral blood leukoerythroblastosis typical of PMF. The marrow in MDS with fibrosis should reveal trilineage dysplasia without osteosclerosis. Clonal abnormalities of chromosome 5 or 7 may be detected in either MDS or PMF and thus do not exclude a diagnosis of PMF. Late-stage PV or ET, where marrow fibrosis and myeloid metaplasia have developed, may be indistinguishable from PMF by morphologic and clinical criteria; it is important to note that the biology, prognosis, and treatment of PMF and postpolycythemic myelofibrosis/ET are identical. Other malignant and nonmalignant causes of marrow fibrosis are listed in Table 14-17. Of note, secondary marrow changes of increased reticulin fibrosis with megakaryocytic hyperplasia resembling PMF have been associated with systemic lupus erythematosus, Sjögren syndrome, psoriatic arthritis, and other chronic autoimmune diseases, most commonly in the absence of splenomegaly or significant leukoerythroblastic peripheral blood findings. These patients frequently have constitutional symptoms and anemia with positive antinuclear antibody and direct antiglobulin titers. Clinical, hematologic, and marrow fibrotic abnormalities in these conditions often respond to corticosteroids.

Laboratory features

In addition to a high frequency of anemia, patients with PMF present with leukocytosis, leukopenia, thrombocytosis, or thrombocytopenia in 50%, 7%, 28%, and 37% of cases, respectively. Egress of immature cells from the marrow into the blood is characteristic of this disorder. Erythroid precursors may account for up to 20% of the circulating nucleated cells, and circulating blast cells are found in up to 30% of cases at diagnosis (this does not necessarily indicate AML). In most cases, the peripheral blood smear reveals the typical leukoerythroblastic features of immature myeloid cells, nucleated red blood cells, teardrop erythrocytes, and large platelets. Although these findings are sensitive for the diagnosis of PMF, they are not highly specific. Secondary causes of marrow fibrosis (Table 14-17) may also give rise to a similar picture of peripheral blood leukoerythroblastosis. The LAP score in patients with PMF is usually elevated, although it may be normal or low in up to one fourth of patients. Because of the high marrow cell turnover, LDH, bilirubin, and uric acid levels are also commonly increased. Haptoglobin levels may be decreased, and there may be other clinical and laboratory indicators of low-grade idiopathic hemolysis.

Clinical, morphologic, and histopathologic features

Approximately 20% to 30% of patients with PMF are believed to present in the prefibrotic stage. The early prefibrotic stage of PMF, also referred to as the "cellular" or "proliferative" stage, may be associated with thrombocytosis and modest leukoerythroblastosis but may be difficult to distinguish from ET. This condition may cause diagnostic difficulties in the absence of clear evidence of megakaryocyte atypia on bone marrow biopsy. Splenomegaly may be present, and the marrow reveals hypercellularity, left-shifted myeloid maturation, and increased megakaryocyte numbers with clustering and nuclear dysplasia. The fibrotic stage of PMF is associated with reticulin or collagen fibrosis in addition to more characteristic clinical and peripheral blood changes and more prominent megakaryocyte atypia (Figure 14-6). With increasing degrees of fibrosis, a diagnostic marrow aspirate is often unobtainable, yielding a "dry tap." Progressive medullary fibrosis is characterized by accumulation of extracellular reticulin fibers (revealed by silver staining) and collagen (revealed by trichrome staining). In advanced stages of PMF, the hematopoietic space is completely replaced by fibroblasts and extracellular matrix material (Figure 14-6). Osteosclerosis may develop in some cases.

Course and prognosis

The outlook for PMF is more variable than for other MPNs. A number of studies have identified clinical and laboratory

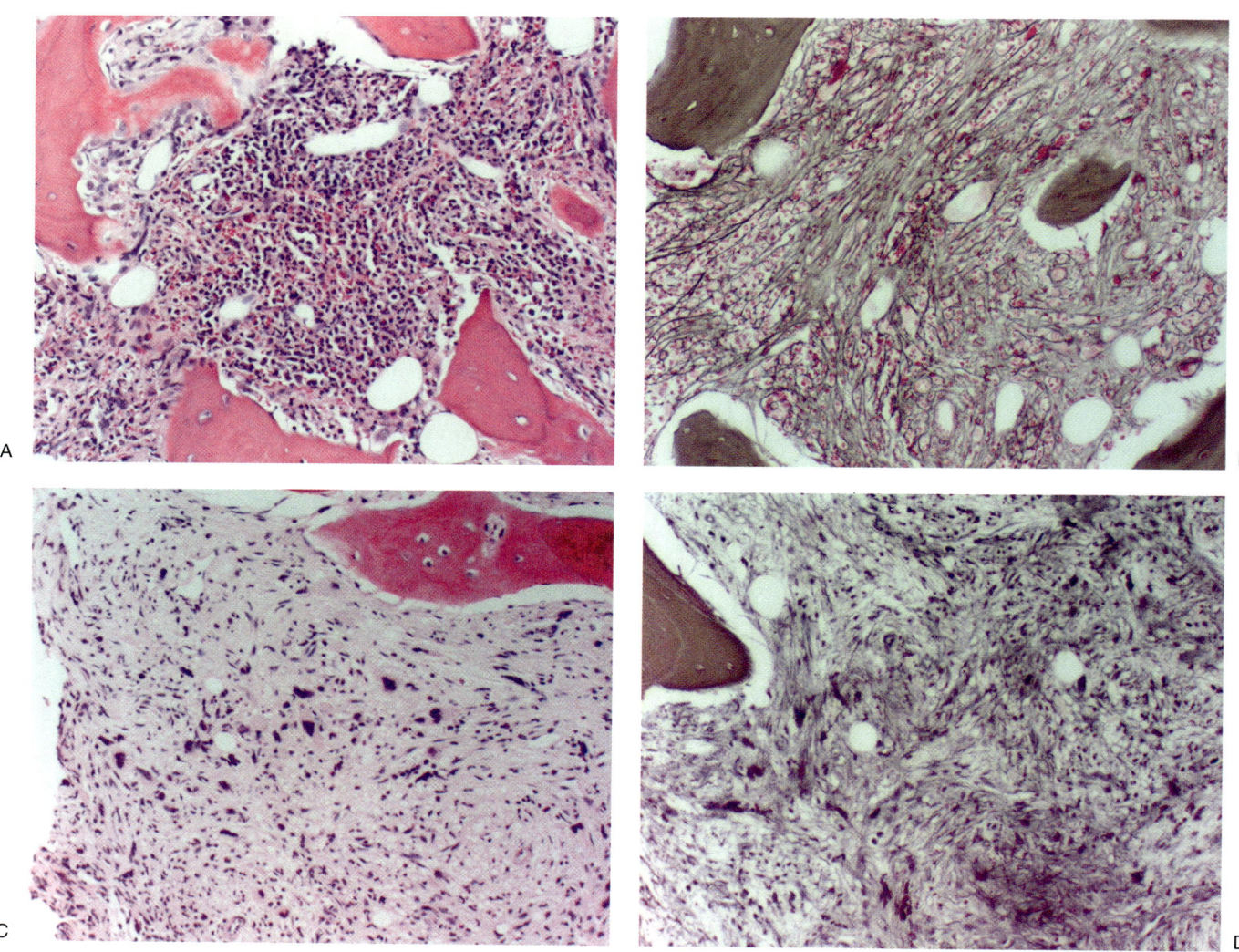

Figure 14-6 Bone marrow histopathologic findings in various stages of chronic idiopathic myelofibrosis. A, The early fibrotic, cellular stage is characterized by hypercellularity and myeloid hyperplasia (hematoxylin-eosin stain [H&E]; original magnification, 85×) with B, variable reticulin fibrosis (reticulin stain; magnification, 85×). C, The later fibrotic stage is associated with extensive collagen deposition and loss of hematopoietic precursors, except for occasional residual megakaryocytes (H&E stain; magnification, 85×), D, with more extensive reticulin fibrosis (reticulin stain; magnification, 85×). Photos courtesy of Steven J. Kussick, MD, PhD, University of Washington, Seattle, WA.

Table 14-18 Prognostic scoring system for primary myelofibrosis based on a study of the International Working Group for Myelofibrosis Research and Treatment.

Risk factor	Frequency in the series, %	Hazard ratio (95% CI)
Age [mt] 65 years	44.6	1.95 (1.61–2.36)
Constitutional symptoms	26.4	1.97 (1.62–2.40)
Hb <10 g/dL	35.2	2.89 (2.46–3.61)
WBC count >25 × 10^9/L	9.6	2.40 (1.83–3.14)
Blood blasts >1%	36.2	1.80 (1.50–2.17)

Risk group	No. of factors	Proportion of patients, %	Median survival, months (95% CI)
Low	0	22	135 (117–181)
Intermediate-1	1	29	95 (79–114)
Intermediate-2	2	28	48 (43–59)
High	>3	21	27 (23–31)

From Cervantes F, Dupriez B, Pereira A, et al. New prognostic scoring system for primary myelofibrosis based on a study of the International Working Group for Myelofibrosis Research and Treatment. *Blood.* 2009;113:2895–2901.
Hb = hemoglobin; WBC = white blood cell.

features that predict a more aggressive disease course and short survival with PMF (Table 14-18). In general, morbidity and mortality are related to hematopoietic failure, thrombosis, hypersplenism, advanced age, and evolution to AML. AML is the cause of death in 5% to 30% of patients. The risk of developing AML is increased among patients with severe anemia and a high number of circulating immature myeloid cells.

A hemoglobin <10 g/dL is the most consistent adverse prognostic indicator for patients with PMF. Age also appears to be important; patients <55 years of age at diagnosis have a median survival of 8 to 10 years, whereas the median survival of older patients (variously defined as >55, >60, or >65 years of age) is 3 to 5 years in most studies. Abnormal karyotype, constitutional symptoms, elevated WBC count, increased circulating immature precursors, and the presence of circulating blasts have also been identified as independent predictors of an adverse prognosis in multiple studies. Among 116 younger PMF patients, a hemoglobin <10 g/dL, the presence of constitutional symptoms, and circulating blasts >1% were independent adverse predictors and should be used in determining whether younger patients undergo evaluation for allogeneic SCT. In that cohort, patients with 0 or 1 adverse factor had a median survival of 176 months, whereas patients with 2 or 3 adverse factors had a median survival of only 33 months.

Therapy
General considerations

Conventional therapies for PMF are largely palliative and supportive; they do not alter the progression of marrow fibrosis and do not prolong survival. Asymptomatic PMF patients without adverse prognostic features, with no or mild splenomegaly, and with no or mild leukocytosis or thrombocytosis can be observed without treatment. If constitutional or hypercatabolic symptoms develop, spleen size increases, or progressive elevations occur in the WBC count or platelet count, hydroxyurea is the treatment of choice. Busulfan, 6-mercaptopurine, and 2-chlorodeoxyadenosine (cladribine) have also been used to try to ameliorate proliferative disease complications. IFNα can control blood counts and splenomegaly during the proliferative stage of disease in up to 50% of cases but is poorly tolerated by most patients given their preexisting constitutional symptoms. It is the drug of choice for the rare symptomatic young woman with PMF who requires treatment but is considering pregnancy. Anagrelide can be useful to control thrombocytosis after splenectomy or after a thromboembolic complication.

Anemia

Anemia may respond to high-dose recombinant EPO in up to 50% of cases; therapeutic success is most common in patients with endogenous EPO levels <120 U/L who have not yet progressed to transfusion dependence. One study noted an increased risk of leukemia associated with EPO therapy; this has not been evaluated or confirmed in larger epidemiologic studies. Anemia, thrombocytopenia, and, less commonly, splenomegaly improve in up to one half of patients who take low-dose thalidomide (ie, 50 mg/d), with or without a tapering-dose schedule of oral prednisone. Recent studies with pomalidomide therapy at 0.5 or 2 mg/d with an abbreviated course of prednisone resulted in improvement of anemia in 30% to 40% of patients, with a substantial proportion of responders becoming transfusion independent. A minority of patients respond to androgens, including oxymetholone, nandrolone, and testosterone enanthate. Occasionally, patients with PMF-associated hemolytic anemia respond to corticosteroids, danazol, or cyclophosphamide. Patients who survive for several years and are red blood cell transfusion dependent can develop complications of chronic tissue iron overload. Therefore, iron chelation therapy should be considered for transfusion-dependent PMF patients who have a prolonged life expectancy and ferritin >1000 μg/L.

Splenomegaly

Massive splenomegaly may cause portal hypertension and can be a major cause of morbidity in PMF due to pain, anemia, and thrombocytopenia. Splenectomy is indicated for palliation of portal hypertension, refractory anemia, and symptoms not controlled by cytotoxic agents. With the conventional laparotomy approach in experienced centers, postoperative mortality is approximately 10%, and the median survival is approximately 1 to 2 years, although patients without poor prognostic features of the underlying disease may have much longer survival. Patients with laboratory evidence of disseminated intravascular coagulopathy appear to be at highest risk of thrombohemorrhagic complications during and immediately after splenectomy. Laparoscopic splenectomy can be performed in selected cases by an experienced surgeon. Splenectomy significantly increases the hematocrit in 30% of anemic patients. By contrast, severe thrombocytopenia (ie, <20,000/μL) is unlikely to improve after splenectomy. Rebound thrombocytosis (ie, >600,000/μL) and massive hepatomegaly are potential complications of splenectomy in patients with PMF. The increased platelet count in this setting can lead to life-threatening thrombotic or hemorrhagic events. Patients at increased risk of thrombocytosis are those with preoperative platelet counts >50,000 to 100,000/μL; 18% to 50% of such patients will achieve postoperative levels >600,000/μL. In this setting, hydroxyurea or anagrelide should be started or the dose increased the moment the postoperative platelet count exceeds the normal range. Massive hepatomegaly resulting from accelerated extramedullary hematopoiesis develops in 16% to 24% of patients after splenectomy. This complication may be difficult to control but may respond to cladribine. Some recent studies, but not others, have suggested an increased incidence of transformation to AML among splenectomized patients with PMF. The interval from diagnosis to surgery, the duration of follow-up, and the median survival among splenectomized patients differed among these studies, and this may account for the discordant observations. On a practical level, splenectomy should not be withheld in cases with advanced disease because of a concern of subsequent AML transformation.

For patients with severe splenomegaly who are not surgical candidates due to comorbidities, low-dose splenic irradiation (ie, 1-5 Gy delivered over 5-10 fractions) can be administered. Benefits may last several months, but irradiation carries a substantial risk of severe, prolonged cytopenias, which cannot be predicted by baseline blood counts or by the dose of radiation. Therefore, the risks and benefits of splenic radiotherapy should be carefully considered and discussed for patients with known limited hematopoietic reserve. Nevertheless, irradiation can effectively palliate pain in >90% of patients, and treatment can be repeated if necessary. Local irradiation can be effective for palliation of painful or threatening focal areas of extramedullary hematopoiesis (eg, with spinal or retroperitoneal myeloid tumors).

Newer agents

A number of newer and experimental agents have been tested in PMF, with goals of controlling clinical manifestations and reversing myelofibrosis. In recent years, clinical trials with JAK2 inhibitors have been initiated for patients with PMF or post-PV/ET myelofibrosis. The early results from these trials suggest that JAK2 inhibitor therapy results in marked improvement in constitutional symptoms and splenomegaly but does not result in improvement in cytopenias or molecular remissions. Whether long-term JAK2 inhibitor therapy or the use of second-generation JAK2 inhibitors provides additional clinical benefit is not known, and the role of JAK2 inhibitors for patients who present with symptomatic, severe splenomegaly is also not yet known.

Stem cell transplantation

In younger individuals with PMF with poor prognostic features, allogeneic hematopoietic SCT should be considered because it represents the only potentially curative treatment. Studies using standard ablative conditioning regimens demonstrated that a subset of patients achieve long-term clinical and molecular remission after SCT. Results using unrelated donors were equivalent to those with HLA-matched sibling transplantations. An early multi-institutional experience, including patients <55 years old receiving marrow or peripheral blood stem cells predominantly from related donors, demonstrated a 47% 5-year probability of survival and a 40% rate of histologic and hematologic remission. Previously splenectomized patients engraft more rapidly after SCT; however, pretransplantation splenectomy is not recommended for this indication alone. Severe fibrosis may correlate with delayed engraftment and higher posttransplantation mortality in some patients but is not associated with graft failure. Responding patients had resolution of marrow fibrosis over months to years, and splenomegaly regressed to normal or minimally palpable in >90%. Inferior transplantation outcome was associated with higher pretransplantation disease risk features, high-grade marrow fibrosis, older age, and the presence of a marrow cytogenetic abnormality. Based on these recent data, a myeloablative allogeneic transplantation should be considered when poor prognostic features develop in children and adults with PMF up to 55 years of age who have an HLA-identical donor. The indications for transplantation at an earlier stage of disease, when the prognosis and survival are more favorable and less predictable, remain the subject of debate. Alternative transplantations approaches for PMF include allogeneic nonmyeloablative SCT, which may be the best transplantation option for patients 55 to 70 years of age. In a recent study of 21 patients (age 27–68 years), reduced-intensity conditioning resulted in long-term disease-free survival in the majority of patients with acceptable toxicities. Moreover, patients treated with reduced-intensity conditioning regimens can achieve stable donor chimerism, significant improvement in blood counts, and significant decrease in marrow fibrosis. Although SCT represents an important therapy for high-risk patients with a matched donor, acceptable comorbidities, and age <70, the majority of patients with PMF are not candidates for SCT; thus, new therapies are needed for the majority of patients with PMF.

> **Key points**
>
> - Over two-thirds of patients with PMF are diagnosed at age 60 years or older, and their median survival time is only 3.5 to 5.5 years.
> - PMF must be differentiated from advanced PV, ET, CML, acute megakaryoblastic leukemia, myelodysplasia with fibrosis, infiltrative malignant processes, and infectious or autoimmune diseases associated with reactive marrow fibrosis.
> - The majority of patients with PMF develop anemia, splenomegaly, and hypercatabolic symptoms during the course of their disease; anemia (hemoglobin <10 g/dL) and a high or low WBC count (>30 or <4 × 10^9/μL) predict a shorter survival.
> - Therapeutic approaches to PMF are guided by the presence of specific symptoms and disease-related complications.
> - Splenectomy should be considered for palliation of symptomatic massive splenomegaly; however, postsplenectomy complications include perioperative mortality, rebound thrombocytosis, and massive hepatomegaly.
> - Myeloablative allogeneic SCT should be considered for patients <55 years of age with poor prognostic features who have an HLA-compatible donor. Nonmyeloablative allogeneic SCT may benefit selected patients who are older or who are not candidates for conventional SCT.
> - New agents, including JAK2 inhibitors, are currently being investigated in PMF patients given the desperate need for novel therapies.

Myeloproliferative neoplasm, unclassifiable

The term MPN, unclassifiable (MPN-U) is a newly defined WHO entity, and it should be used only to describe patients who meet clinical, laboratory, and morphologic criteria of MPNs but fail to present features of any single MPN entity or patients who present with overlapping features of 2 or more MPN entities. The demonstration of pathognomonic molecular abnormalities, such a *BCR-ABL1* fusion or the *PDGFRA*, *PDGFRB*, or *FGFR1* rearrangements, excludes the diagnosis of MPN-U.

Epidemiology

The exact incidence, median age at onset, and sex distribution of MPN-U are not truly known.

Clinical features

The clinical features of patients with MPN-U can be quite variable. Patients can present with minimal to no organomegaly and well-preserved peripheral blood counts in the very early stages of the disease or massive organomegaly, extensive myelofibrosis, and severe cytopenias in advanced cases. Unexplained portal or splanchnic vein thrombosis may be the initial presenting feature in these patients.

Course and prognosis

The clinical course and prognosis for patients with MPN-U can also be extremely heterogeneous. Patients with early-stage disease can safely be followed every 6 months and generally will develop features of unique MPN entities. Patients in whom unique MPN entities are no longer recognizable tend to have aggressive clinical courses and very poor prognosis.

Bibliography

Introduction

Delhommeau F, Dupont S, Della Valle V, et al. Mutation in TET2 in myeloid cancers. *N Engl J Med*. 2009;360:2289–2301.

Johansson P. Epidemiology of the myeloproliferative disorders polycythemia vera and essential thrombocythemia. *Semin Thromb Hemost*. 2006;32:171–173.

Swerdlow SH, Campo E, Harris NL, et al, eds. *World Health Organization Classification of Tumors of Hematopoietic and Lymphoid Tissues*. Lyon, France: IARC Press; 2008.

Tefferi A. The history of myeloproliferative disorders: before and after Dameshek. *Leukemia*. 2008;22:3–13.

Chronic myelogenous leukemia, BCR-ABL1 positive

Apperley JF, Cortes JE, Kim DW, et al. Dasatinib in the treatment of chronic myeloid leukemia in accelerated phase after imatinib failure: the START A trial. *J Clin Oncol.* 2009;27:3472–3479.

Baccarani M, Gianantonio R, de Vivo A, et al. A randomized study of interferon-alpha versus interferon-alpha and low-dose arabinosyl cytosine in chronic myeloid leukemia. *Blood.* 2002;99:1527–1535.

Baccarani M, Rosti G, Saglio G, et al. Dasatinib time to and durability of major and complete cytogenetic response (MCyR and CCyR) in patients with chronic myeloid leukemia in chronic phase (CML-CP) [abstract]. *Blood.* 2008;112:450.

Bhatia R, Verfaillie CM, Miller JS, et al. Autologous transplantation therapy for chronic myelogenous leukemia. *Blood.* 1997;89:2623–2634.

Bonifazi F, de Vivo A, Rosti G, et al. Chronic myeloid leukemia and interferon-alpha: a study of complete cytogenetic responders. *Blood.* 2001;98:3074–3081.

Bose S, Deininger M, Gora-Tybor J, et al. The presence of typical and atypical BCR-ABL fusion genes in leukocytes of normal individuals: biologic significance and implications for the assessment of minimal residual disease. *Blood.* 1998;92:3362–3367.

Branford S, Rudzki Z, Parkinson I, et al. Real-time quantitative PCR analysis can be used as a primary screen to identify patients with CML treated with imatinib who have BCR-ABL kinase domain mutations. *Blood.* 2004;104:2926–2932.

Deininger MW, Druker BJ. Specific targeted therapy for chronic myelogenous leukemia with imatinib. *Pharmacol Rev.* 2003;55:401–423.

Druker BJ, Deininger M, Shah N, et al. Chronic myeloid leukemia. *Hematology Am Soc Hematol Educ Program.* 2005:174–194.

Druker BJ, Sawyers CL, Kantarjian H, et al. Activity of a specific inhibitor of the BCR-ABL TK in the blast crisis of chronic myeloid leukemia and acute lymphoblastic leukemia with the Philadelphia chromosome. *N Engl J Med.* 2001;344:1038–1042.

Druker BJ, Talpaz M, Resta DJ, et al. Efficacy and safety of a specific inhibitor of the BCR-ABL tyrosine kinase in chronic myeloid leukemia. *N Engl J Med.* 2001;344:1031–1037.

Garcia-Manero G, Faderl S, O'Brien S, et al. Chronic myelogenous leukemia: a review and update of therapeutic strategies. *Cancer.* 2003;98:437–457.

Goldman J, Melo J. Chronic myeloid leukemia—advances in biology and new treatment approaches to treatment. *N Engl J Med.* 2003;349:1451–1464.

Guilhot F, Chastang C, Michallet M, et al. Interferon-2b combined with cytarabine versus interferon alone in chronic myelogenous leukemia. French Chronic Myeloid Leukemia Study Group. *N Engl J Med.* 1997;337:223–229.

Hansen JA, Gooley TA, Martin PJ, et al. Bone marrow transplants from unrelated donors for patients with chronic myeloid leukemia. *N Engl J Med.* 1998;338:962–968.

Hughes TP, Kaeda J, Branford S, et al; International Randomized Study of Interferon Versus STI571 (IRIS) Study Group. Frequency of major molecular responses to imatinib or interferon alfa plus cytarabine in newly diagnosed chronic myeloid leukemia. *N Engl J Med.* 2003;349:1423–1432.

Kantarjian HM, Cortes J, O'Brien S, et al. Imatinib mesylate (STI571) therapy for Philadelphia chromosome-positive chronic myelogenous leukemia in blast phase. *Blood.* 2002;99:3547–3553.

Kantarjian HM, Keating MJ, Smith TL, et al. Proposal for a simple synthesis prognostic staging system in chronic myelogenous leukemia. *Am J Med.* 1990;88:1–8.

Kantarjian HM, O'Brien S, Smith TL, et al. Treatment of Philadelphia chromosome-positive early chronic phase chronic myelogenous leukemia with daily doses of interferon-alpha and low-dose cytarabine. *J Clin Oncol.* 1999;17:284–292.

Kantarjian H, Pasquini R, Lévy V, et al. Dasatinib or high-dose imatinib for chronic-phase chronic myeloid leukemia resistant to imatinib at a dose of 400 to 600 milligrams daily: two-year follow-up of a randomized phase 2 study (START-R). *Cancer.* 2009;115:4136–4147.

Kantarjian H, Sawyers C, Hochhaus A, et al. Hematologic and cytogenetic responses to imatinib mesylate in chronic myelogenous leukemia. *N Engl J Med.* 2002;346:645–652.

Kantarjian H, Talpaz M, O'Brien S, et al. High-dose imatinib mesylate therapy in newly diagnosed Philadelphia chromosome-positive chronic phase chronic myeloid leukemia. *Blood.* 2004;103:2873–2878.

Kurzrock R, Bueso-Ramos CE, Kantarjian H, et al. BCR rearrangement-negative chronic myelogenous leukemia revisited. *J Clin Oncol.* 2001;19:2915–2926.

Majlis A, Smith TL, Talpaz M, et al. Significance of cytogenetic clonal evolution in chronic myelogenous leukemia. *J Clin Oncol.* 1996;14:196–203.

McGlave PB, Shu XO, Wen W, et al. Unrelated donor marrow transplantation for chronic myelogenous leukemia: 9 years' experience of the national marrow donor program. *Blood.* 2000;95:2219–2225.

Michor F, Hughes TP, Iwasa Y, et al. Dynamics of chronic myeloid leukemia. *Nature.* 2005;435:1267–1270.

O'Brien SG, Guilhot F, Larson RA, et al. Imatinib compared with interferon and low-dose cytarabine for newly diagnosed chronic-phase chronic myeloid leukemia. IRIS Investigators. *N Engl J Med.* 2003;348:994–1004.

O'Dwyer ME, Mauro MJ, Blasdel C, et al. Clonal evolution and lack of cytogenetic response are adverse prognostic factors for hematologic relapse of chronic phase CML patients treated with imatinib mesylate. *Blood.* 2004;103:451–455.

Olavarria E, Ottmann OG, Deininger M, et al; Chronic Leukemia Working Party of the European Group of Bone and Marrow Transplantation (EBMT). Response to imatinib in patients who relapse after allogeneic stem cell transplantation for chronic myeloid leukemia. *Leukemia.* 2003;17:1707–1712.

Or R, Shapira MY, Resnick I, et al. Nonmyeloablative allogeneic stem cell transplantation for the treatment of chronic myeloid leukemia in first chronic phase. *Blood.* 2003;101:441–445.

Pane F, Frigeri F, Sindona M, et al. Neutrophilic-chronic myeloid leukemia: a distinct disease with a specific molecular marker (BCR/ABL with C3/A2 junction). *Blood*. 1996;88: 2410–2414.

Radich JP, Gooley T, Bryant E, et al. The significance of bcr-abl molecular detection in chronic myeloid leukemia patients "late," 18 months or more after transplantation. *Blood*. 2001;98: 1701–1707.

Sawyers CL, Hochhaus A, Feldman E, et al. Imatinib induces hematologic and cytogenetic responses in patients with chronic myelogenous leukemia in myeloid blast crisis: results of a phase II study. *Blood*. 2002;99:3530–3539.

Selleri C, Maciejewski JP. The role of FAS-mediated apoptosis in chronic myelogenous leukemia. *Leuk Lymphoma*. 2000;37: 283–297.

Shah NP, Tran C, Lee FY, et al. Overriding imatinib resistance with a novel ABL kinase inhibitor. *Science*. 2004;305:399–401.

Silver RT, Woolf SH, Hehlmann R, et al. An evidence-based analysis of the effect of busulfan, hydroxyurea, interferon, and allogeneic bone marrow transplantation in treating the chronic phase of chronic myeloid leukemia: developed for the American Society of Hematology. *Blood*. 1999;94:1517–1536.

Soverini S, Martinelli G, Rosti G, et al. ABL mutations in late chronic phase chronic myeloid leukemia patients with up-front cytogenetic resistance to imatinib are associated with a greater likelihood of progression to blast crisis and shorter survival: a study by the GIMEMA Working Party on Chronic Myeloid Leukemia. *J Clin Oncol*. 2005;23:4100–4109.

Talpaz M. Interferon-based treatment of chronic myeloid leukemia and implications of signal transduction inhibition. *Semin Hematol*. 2001;38:22–27.

Talpaz M, Silver RT, Druker BJ, et al. Imatinib induces hematologic and cytogenetic responses in patients with accelerated phase chronic myeloid leukemia: results of a phase 2 study. *Blood*. 2002;99:1928–1937.

von Bubnoff N, Peschel C, Duyster J. Resistance of Philadelphia chromosome positive leukemia towards the kinase inhibitor imatinib (STI571, Glivec): a targeted oncoprotein strikes back. *Leukemia*. 2003;17:829–838.

Wadhwa J, Szydlo RM, Apperley JF, et al. Factors affecting duration of survival after onset of blastic transformation of chronic myeloid leukemia. *Blood*. 2002;99:2304–2309.

Wang YL, Bagg A, Pear W, et al. Chronic myelogenous leukemia: laboratory diagnosis and monitoring. *Genes Chromosomes Cancer*. 2001;32:97–111.

Weisberg E, Manley PW, Breitenstein W, et al. Characterization of AMN107, a selective inhibitor of native and mutant Bcr-Abl. *Cancer Cell*. 2005;7:129–141.

Chronic neutrophilic leukemia

Elliott MA, Hanson CA, Dewald GW, Smoley SA, Lasho TL, Tefferi A. WHO-defined chronic neutrophilic leukemia: a long-term analysis of 12 cases and a critical review of the literature. *Leukemia*. 2005;19:313–317.

Thiele J. Philadelphia chromosome-negative chronic myeloproliferative disease. *Am J Clin Pathol*. 2009;132: 261–280.

Vannucchi AM, Guglielmelli P, Tefferi A. Advances in understanding and management of myeloproliferative neoplasms. *CA Cancer J Clin*. 2009;59:171–191.

Systemic mastocytosis

Butterfield JH. Systemic mastocytosis: clinical manifestations and differential diagnosis. *Immunol Allergy Clin North Am*. 2006;26:487–513.

Gotlib J. KIT mutations in mastocytosis and their potential as therapeutic targets. *Immunol Allergy Clin North Am*. 2006;26:575–592.

Gotlib J, George TI, Corless C, et al. The KIT tyrosine kinase inhibitor midostaurin (PKC412) exhibits a high response rate in aggressive systemic mastocytosis (ASM): interim results of a phase II trial [abstract]. *Blood*. 2007;110:3536.

Swerdlow SH, Campo E, Harris NL, et al, eds. *World Health Organization Classification of Tumors of Hematopoietic and Lymphoid Tissues*. Lyon, France: IARC Press; 2008.

Valent P. Diagnostic evaluation and classification of mastocytosis. *Immunol Allergy Clin North Am*. 2006;26:515–534.

Wilson TM, Metcalfe DD, Robyn J. Treatment of systemic mastocytosis. *Immunol Allergy Clin North Am*. 2006;26:549–573.

Myeloid (and lymphoid) neoplasms associated with eosinophilia and abnormalities of *PDGFRA*, *PDGFRB*, or *FGFR1*

Baccarani M, Cilloni D, Rondoni M, et al. The efficacy of imatinib mesylate in patients with FIP1L1-PDGFRalpha-positive hypereosinophilic syndrome. Results of a multicenter prospective study. *Haematologica*. 2007;92:1173–1179.

Chen J, Deangelo DJ, Kutok JL, et al. PKC412 inhibits the zinc finger 198-fibroblast growth factor receptor 1 fusion tyrosine kinase and is active in treatment of stem cell myeloproliferative disorder. *Proc Natl Acad Sci USA*. 2004;101:14479–14484.

Cools J, DeAngelo DJ, Gotlib J, et al. A tyrosine kinase created by fusion of the PDGFRA and FIP1L1 genes as a therapeutic target of imatinib in idiopathic hypereosinophilic syndrome. *N Engl J Med*. 2003;348:1201–1214.

David M, Cross NC, Burgstaller S, et al. Durable responses to imatinib in patients with PDGFRB fusion gene-positive and BCR-ABL-negative chronic myeloproliferative disorders. *Blood*. 2007;109:61–64.

Golub TR, Barker GF, Lovett M, et al. Fusion of PDGF receptor beta to a novel ets-like gene, tel, in chronic myelomonocytic leukemia with t(5;12) chromosomal translocation. *Cell*. 1994;77:307–316.

Gotlib J, Cools J, Malone JM 3rd, et al. The FIP1L1-PDGFRalpha fusion tyrosine kinase in hypereosinophilic syndrome and chronic eosinophilic leukemia: implications for diagnosis, classification, and management. *Blood*. 2004;103:2879–2891.

Gotlib J, Cross NC, Gilliland DG. Eosinophilic disorders: molecular pathogenesis, new classification, and modern therapy. *Best Pract Res Clin Haematol*. 2006;19:535–569.

Jovanovic JV, Score J, Waghorn K, et al. Low-dose imatinib mesylate leads to rapid induction of major molecular responses and achievement of complete molecular remission in FIP1L1-PDGFRA-positive chronic eosinophilic leukemia. *Blood*. 2007;109:4635–4640.

Metzgeroth G, Walz C, Erben P, et al. Safety and efficacy of imatinib in chronic eosinophilic leukaemia and hypereosinophilic syndrome: a phase-II study. *Br J Haematol*. 2008;143:707–715.

Stover EH, Chen J, Folens C, et al. Activation of FIP1L1-PDGFRalpha requires disruption of the juxtamembrane domain of PDGFRalpha and is FIP1L1-independent. *Proc Natl Acad Sci U S A*. 2006;103:8078–8083.

Swerdlow SH, Campo E, Harris NL, et al, eds. *World Health Organization Classification of Tumors of Hematopoietic and Lymphoid Tissues*. Lyon, France: IARC Press; 2008.

Chronic eosinophilic leukemia, not otherwise specified

Gotlib J, Cross NC, Gilliland DG. Eosinophilic disorders: molecular pathogenesis, new classification, and modern therapy. *Best Pract Res Clin Haematol*. 2006;19:535–569.

Hart TK, Cook RM, Zia-Amirhosseini P, et al. Preclinical efficacy and safety of mepolizumab (SB—240563), a humanized monoclonal antibody to IL-5, in cynomolgus monkeys. *J Allergy Clin Immunol*. 2001;108:250–257.

Pitini V, Teti D, Arrigo C, et al. Alemtuzumab therapy for refractory idiopathic hypereosinophilic syndrome. *Br J Haematol*. 2004;127:477.

Swerdlow SH, Campo E, Harris NL, et al, eds. *World Health Organization Classification of Tumors of Hematopoietic and Lymphoid Tissues*. Lyon, France: IARC Press; 2008.

Polycythemia vera, essential thrombocytosis, and primary myelofibrosis

Adamson JW, Fialkow PJ, Murphy S, Prchal JF, Steinman L. Polycythemia vera; stem cell and probable clonal origin of the disease. *N Engl J Med*. 1976;295:913–916.

Ang SO, Chen H, Hirota K, et al. Disruption of oxygen homeostasis underlies congenital Chuvash polycythemia. *Nat Genet*. 2002;32:614–621.

Arcasoy MO, Degar BA, Harris KW, Forget BG. Familial erythrocytosis associated with a short deletion in the erythropoietin receptor gene. *Blood*. 1997;89:4628–4635.

Argetsinger LS, Campbell GS, Yang X, et al. Identification of JAK2 as a growth hormone receptor-associated tyrosine kinase. *Cell*. 1993;74:237–244.

Baxter EJ, Scott LM, Campbell PJ, et al. Acquired mutation of the tyrosine kinase JAK2 in human myeloproliferative disorders. *Lancet*. 2005;365:1054–1061.

Beer P, Campbell P, Erber W, et al. Clinical significance of MPL mutations in essential thrombocythemia; analysis of the PT-1 cohort [abstract]. *Blood*. 2007;677:76.

Berk PD, Goldberg JD, Silverstein MN, et al. Increased incidence of acute leukemia in polycythemia vera associated with chlorambucil therapy. *N Engl J Med*. 1981;304:441–447.

Carbuccia N, Murati A, Trouplin V, et al. Mutations of ASXL1 gene in myeloproliferative neoplasms. Mutations of ASXL1 gene in myeloproliferative neoplasms. *Leukemia*. 2009;23: 2183–2186.

Cervantes F, Dupriez B, Pereira A, et al. New prognostic scoring system for primary myelofibrosis based on a study of the International Working Group for Myelofibrosis Research and Treatment. *Blood*. 2009;113:2895–2901.

Cortelazzo S, Finazzi G, Ruggeri M, et al. Hydroxyurea for patients with essential thrombocythemia and a high risk of thrombosis. *N Engl J Med*. 1995;332:1132–1136.

Dameshek W. Some speculations on the myeloproliferative syndromes. *Blood*. 1951;6:372–375.

Delhommeau F, Dupont S, Della Valle V, et al. Mutation in TET2 in myeloid cancers. *N Engl J Med*. 2009;360:2289–2301.

Ding J, Komatsu H, Wakita A, et al. Familial essential thrombocythemia associated with a dominant-positive activating mutation of the c-MPL gene, which encodes for the receptor for thrombopoietin. *Blood*. 2004;103:4198–4200.

El Kassar N, Hetet G, Li Y, Briere J, Grandchamp B. Clonal analysis of haemopoietic cells in essential thrombocythaemia. *Br J Haematol*. 1995;90:131–137.

Epstein E, Goedel A. Hemorrhagic thrombocythemia with a vascular, sclerotic spleen. *Virchows Arch A Pathol Anat Histopathol*. 1934;293:233–48.

Fruchtman SM, Mack K, Kaplan ME, Peterson P, Berk PD, Wasserman LR. From efficacy to safety: a Polycythemia Vera Study group report on hydroxyurea in patients with polycythemia vera. *Semin Hematol*. 1997;34:17–23.

Gilliland DG, Blanchard KL, Levy J, Perrin S, Bunn HF. Clonality in myeloproliferative disorders: analysis by means of the polymerase chain reaction. *Proc Natl Acad Sci U S A*. 1991;88:6848–6852.

Harrison CN, Campbell PJ, Buck G, et al. Hydroxyurea compared with anagrelide in high-risk essential thrombocythemia. *N Engl J Med*. 2005;353:33–45.

Heuck G. Two cases of leukemia with peculiar blood and bone marrow findings, respectively. *Arch Pathol Anat*. 1879;78: 475–496.

James C, Ugo V, Le Couedic JP, et al. A unique clonal JAK2 mutation leading to constitutive signalling causes polycythaemia vera. *Nature*. 2005;434:1144–1148.

Kiladjian JJ, Cassinat B, Turlure P, et al. High molecular response rate of polycythemia vera patients treated with pegylated interferon alpha-2a. *Blood*. 2006;108:2037–2040.

Kralovics R, Passamonti F, Buser AS, et al. A gain-of-function mutation of JAK2 in myeloproliferative disorders. *N Engl J Med*. 2005;352:1779–1790.

Landolfi R, Marchioli R, Kutti J, et al. Efficacy and safety of low-dose aspirin in polycythemia vera. *N Engl J Med*. 2004;350: 114–124.

Levine RL, Wadleigh M, Cools J, et al. Activating mutation in the tyrosine kinase JAK2 in polycythemia vera, essential thrombocythemia, and myeloid metaplasia with myelofibrosis. *Cancer Cell*. 2005;7:387–397.

Migliaccio AR, Martelli F, Verrucci M, et al. Altered SDF-1/CXCR4 axis in patients with primary myelofibrosis and in the Gata1 low mouse model of the disease. *Exp Hematol*. 2008;36:158–171.

Osler W. Chronic cyanosis with polycythaemis and enlarged spleen: a new entity. *Am J Med Sci*. 1903;126:187–192.

Pardanani AD, Levine RL, Lasho T, et al. MPL515 mutations in myeloproliferative and other myeloid disorders: a study of 1182 patients. *Blood*. 2006;108:3472–3476.

Percy MJ, Furlow PW, Lucas GS, et al. A gain-of-function mutation in the HIF2A gene in familial erythrocytosis. *N Engl J Med*. 2008;358:162–168.

Pikman Y, Lee BH, Mercher T, et al. MPLW515L is a novel somatic activating mutation in myelofibrosis with myeloid metaplasia. *PLoS Med*. 2006;3:e270.

Prchal JF, Axelrad AA. Letter: bone-marrow responses in polycythemia vera. *N Engl J Med*. 1974;290:1382.

Rondelli D, Barosi G, Bacigalupo A, et al; Myeloproliferative Diseases-Research Consortium. Allogeneic hematopoietic stem-cell transplantation with reduced-intensity conditioning in intermediate- or high-risk patients with myelofibrosis with myeloid metaplasia. *Blood*. 2005;105:4115–4119.

Rosti V, Massa M, Vannucchi AM, et al. The expression of CXCR4 is down-regulated on the CD34+ cells of patients with myelofibrosis with myeloid metaplasia. *Blood Cells Mol Dis*. 2007;38:280–286.

Scott LM, Tong W, Levine RL, et al. JAK2 exon 12 mutations in polycythemia vera and idiopathic erythrocytosis. *N Engl J Med*. 2007;356:459–468.

Tefferi A, Verstovsek S, Barosi G, et al. Pomalidomide is active in the treatment of anemia associated with myelofibrosis. *J Clin Oncol*. 2009;27:4563–4569.

Vaquez H. On a special form of cyanosis accompanied by excessive and persistent erythrocytosis. *Comp Rend Soc Biol*. 1892;12:384–388.

Verstovek S, Kantarjian H, Pardanani A, et al. INCB018424, an oral, selective JAK2 inhibitor shows significant clinical activity in a phase I/II study in patients with primary myelofibrosis (PMF) and post-polycythemia vera/essential thrombocythemia myelofibrosis (post-PV/ET MF) [abstract]. *Blood*. 2007:558.

Wernig G, Kharas MG, Okabe R, et al. Efficacy of TG101348, a selective JAK2 inhibitor, in treatment of a murine model of JAK2V617F-induced polycythemia vera. *Cancer Cell*. 2008;13:311–320.

Myeloproliferative neoplasm, unclassifiable

Swerdlow SH, Campo E, Harris NL, et al, eds. *World Health Organization Classification of Tumors of Hematopoietic and Lymphoid Tissues*. Lyon, France: IARC Press; 2008.

Thiele J, Kvasnicka HM, Orazi A. Bone marrow histopathology in myeloproliferative disorders–current diagnostic approach. *Semin Hematol*. 2005;42:184–195.

Thiele J, Kvasnicka HM, Vardiman J. Bone marrow histopathology in the diagnosis of chronic myeloproliferative disorders: a forgotten pearl. *Best Pract Res Clin Haematol*. 2006;19:413–437.

CHAPTER 15

Marrow failure syndromes

Jaroslaw P. Maciejewski and David P. Steensma

Congenital bone marrow failure syndromes, 443 | Acquired bone marrow failure conditions, 450 | Bibliography, 472

Bone marrow failure refers to the inability of hematopoiesis to meet physiologic demands for production of healthy blood cells. Pancytopenia may result from marrow failure, or cytopenias involving a single myeloid lineage may dominate; usually lymphopoiesis is relatively preserved.

The causes of marrow failure are diverse and may either be extrinsic to the marrow, as in the disordered immune response that characterizes aplastic anemia, or intrinsic, as in the hematopoietic progenitor or stem cell defects that underlie the myelodysplastic syndromes. Bone marrow failure syndromes can be acquired or, more rarely, congenital.

The range of molecular mechanisms responsible for congenital marrow failure states is broad, including abnormal DNA damage response (Fanconi anemia), defective ribogenesis (Diamond-Blackfan anemia), abnormal telomere dynamics (dyskeratosis congenita), and altered hematopoietic growth factor receptor/kinase signaling (congenital amegakaryocytic thrombocytopenia). In some congenital marrow failure syndromes, the mechanism of hematopoietic failure is currently unclear (eg, the congenital dyserythropoietic anemias).

This chapter reviews common acquired marrow failure syndromes, as well as several congenital marrow failure syndromes in which the chief cytopenia is anemia or thrombocytopenia. For a discussion of marrow failure syndromes in which neutropenia dominates the clinical picture (eg, severe congenital neutropenia, cyclic neutropenia, Shwachman-Diamond syndrome, WHIM syndrome, Chédiak-Higashi syndrome), please refer to Chapter 13.

Conflict-of-interest disclosure: *Dr. Maciejewski* declares no competing financial interest. *Dr. Steensma*: research funding: Amgen, Johnson & Johnson, Novartis.
Off-label drug use: *Dr. Maciejewski* cyclosporine A, prednisone, danazol.

Congenital bone marrow failure syndromes

Fanconi anemia

> **Clinical case**
>
> A 12-year-old boy presents to his primary care physician with pallor and bruising. His past medical history is remarkable only for an orchiopexy during the first year of life to correct an undescended testis. Pancytopenia is now noted. The patient and his parents do not report any medication or toxin exposures. There are no siblings. On initial examination, the boy appears to be a normal prepubescent male. On closer examination, however, his thumbs appear underdeveloped, and patches of cutaneous hyperpigmentation are noted on his trunk. Bone marrow aspiration and biopsy are performed. The marrow cellularity is only 10%; the marrow aspirate shows hypocellular spicules and rare megakaryocytes, most of which are abnormal uninucleate forms. Cytogenetic studies are normal. Exposure of peripheral blood mononuclear cells to diepoxybutane (DEB) results in numerous chromosomal breakages, confirming a diagnosis of Fanconi anemia.

Epidemiology

Although the inherited bone marrow failure syndromes are rare disorders, collectively affecting just a few dozen new patients in the United States each year, a diagnosis with one of these syndromes has profound implications for medical management and treatment. Fanconi anemia (FA) is the most common and the best defined of these rare congenital conditions (common is a relative term here, as the incidence of FA in the United States has been estimated at approximately 1 in 360,000 live births).

Several inherited marrow failure syndromes are compared in Table 15-1. Bone marrow failure is usually not the only

Table 15-1 Comparison of congenital marrow failure syndromes.

Syndrome	Male:female ratio	Median age at diagnosis (years)	% diagnosed after age 15	Potential nonhematologic characteristics*	Hematology/oncology	Screening test	Genetics (genes)
Fanconi anemia (FA)	1.2:1	6.6	9	Skin hyperpigmentation and café-au-lait spots, short stature, triangular face, abnormal thumbs/radii, microcephaly, abnormal kidneys, decreased fertility	Pancytopenia; hypocellular marrow; MDS, leukemia, solid tumors (head and neck, gynecologic, liver, CNS)	Chromosome breakage in cells cultured with DNA cross-linkers (diepoxybutane or mitomycin C)	Autosomal/X-linked recessive (~13 FANC genes)
Dyskeratosis congenita (DC)	4:1	15	46	Dyskeratotic nails, lacey reticular rash, oral leukoplakia; hypogonadism, urethral stricture, lacrimal duct stenosis, exudative retinopathy, pulmonary fibrosis, liver fibrosis, esophageal strictures, early gray hair, osteoporosis, cerebellar hypoplasia	Pancytopenia; hypocellular marrow; MDS, leukemia, solid tumors (head and neck)	Telomere length assay	X-linked (DKC1), autosomal dominant (TERC), autosomal recessive (?)
Diamond-Blackfan anemia (DBA)	1.1:1	0.25	1	Short stature, abnormal thumbs; hypertelorism, cardiac septal defect, cleft lip or palate, short neck	Macrocytic anemia; erythroid hypoplasia in marrow; MDS, leukemia, solid tumors (osteosarcoma)	Elevated red blood cell adenosine deaminase (ADA)	Autosomal dominant (RPS19 in 25%; other ribosomal genes in some cases)
Shwachman-Diamond syndrome (SDS)†	1.5:1	1	5	Short stature, exocrine pancreatic insufficiency with malabsorption	Neutropenia; anemia, thrombocytopenia, aplastic anemia; MDS, leukemia	Decreased serum trypsinogen and pancreatic isoamylase	Autosomal recessive (SBDS)
Severe congenital neutropenia (SCN)†	1.2:1	3	13	None	Neutropenia; MDS or leukemia risk	Bone marrow exam for promyelocyte arrest	Autosomal dominant or recessive (ELA2)
Congenital amegakaryocytic thrombocytopenia (CAMT)	0.8:1	0.1	0	None	Thrombocytopenia; decreased megakaryocytes in marrow early in disease course, later aplastic anemia; MDS, leukemia	Bone marrow exam for megakaryocytes	Autosomal recessive (MPL)
Thrombocytopenia-absent radius syndrome (TAR)†	0.7:1	<0.6	0	Absent radii, abnormal ulnae or humerii (phocomelia), thumbs present, occasional cryptorchidism, hypertelorism, strabismus, horseshoe kidney, hemangiomas, micrognathia, cows' milk allergy, cardiac anomalies	Thrombocytopenia; MDS or leukemia	Bone marrow exam for megakaryocytes	Autosomal recessive? (200-kilobase chromosome 1q21.1 microdeletion is necessary but not sufficient to cause disease)

*Some patients with these syndromes have no family history and either none of the physical features or none of the hematologic figures. A high index of suspicion is required.
†These syndromes are not discussed in this chapter.

Modified from Alter BP. Diagnosis, genetics, and management of inherited bone marrow failure syndromes. *Hematology Am Soc Hematol Educ Program.* 2007:29–39. Reproduced with permission.

CNS = central nervous system; MDS = myelodysplastic syndrome.

feature of the congenital marrow failure disorders, and marrow failure may even be absent in some patients. Alternatively, isolated marrow failure or development of a malignancy may be the first clinical manifestation of FA in the absence of other clinical stigmata, and occasionally, patients with FA may first come to clinical attention as young adults.

Pathobiology

A hallmark of cells from patients with FA is hypersensitivity to genetic damage induced by DNA-damaging and cross-linking agents such as DEB, mitomycin C (MMC), and ionizing radiation. The underlying molecular defects resulting in the FA phenotype involve components of a critical pathway that regulates cellular DNA damage recognition and response.

FA is a heterogeneous disease at the molecular level, with at least 13 distinct complementation groups (ie, distinct genes; *complementation* in molecular biology means that 2 different gene loci encode proteins of distinct function that can each provide something the other lacks, facilitating identification in vitro) identified to date. More than 75% of patients fall into complementation groups A or C. Molecular cloning of the genes corresponding to each of these complementation groups led to the identification of a complex DNA repair pathway comprised of distinct FA proteins (Figure 15-1). Each of these genes, when biallelically mutated, can cause FA.

DNA damage activates an 8-protein core complex consisting of Fanconi A, B, C, E, F, G, L, and M proteins, which results in monoubiquitylation of the Fanconi I protein and the Fanconi D2 (FANCD2) protein, probably by a ubiquitin ligase domain of FANCL. (Confusingly, there is no Fanconi H protein; it turned out to be the same complementation group as Fanconi A. There is also no Fanconi K protein.) The modified FANCD2 protein then translocates to chromatin nuclear foci and localizes to sites of DNA repair, where it interacts with the breast cancer susceptibility protein BRCA1,

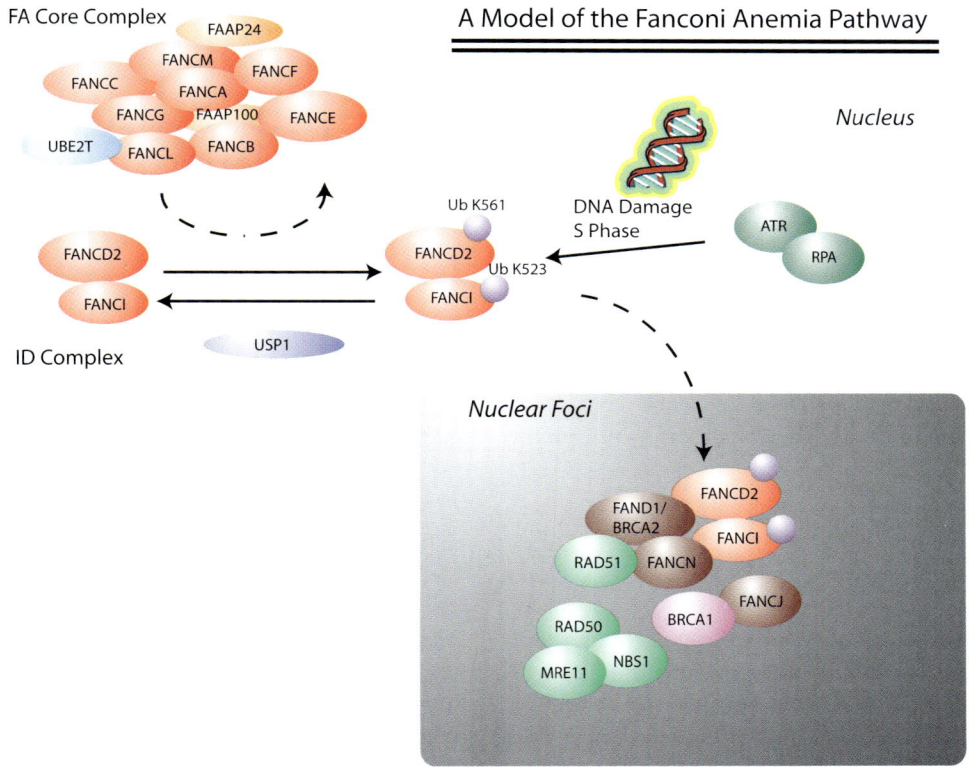

Figure 15-1 Current model of the Fanconi anemia (FA) pathway. The FA core complex consists of 8 proteins (FANCA, -B, -C, -E, -F, -G, -L, and -M) plus a FANCM-interacting protein called FAAP24 and another factor, FAAP100. This core complex has E3 ubiquitin ligase activity; FANCL is the catalytic subunit, interacting with the E2 ubiquitin conjugating enzyme UBE2T. In response to exogenous DNA damage or during normal S phase progression, the FANCD2 protein is monoubiquitylated on lysine 561 (K561) and the FANCI protein is monoubiquitylated on lysine 523 (K523) in an FA core complex– and UBE2T-dependent manner. DNA damage–induced monoubiquitylation of FANCD2 also requires ATR and RPA, linking the FA pathway with ATM/ATR/Chk1. USP1 negatively regulates the Fanconi anemia pathway by deubiquitylating FANCD2. Monoubiquitylation of FANCD2 and FANCI targets these proteins into nuclear foci, where they colocalize with BRCA1, FANCJ (which itself interacts with BRCA1), FANCD1/BRCA2, FANCN, RAD51, and other proteins including RAD50/MRE11/NBS1. Normal resistance to DNA cross-linking agents requires all of these agents. Adapted with modifications from Jacquemont C, Taniguchi T. The Fanconi anemia pathway and ubiquitin. *BMC Biochemistry*. 2007;8(Suppl 1):S10.

as well as with effector proteins FANCJ (a structure-specific helicase that binds to BRCA1) and FANCN. FANCD2 is also phosphorylated by the ataxia-telangiectasia mutated (ATM) protein kinase in response to ionizing radiation, linking the Fanconi pathway to the ATM/ATR/Chk1 DNA damage–sensing and checkpoint response pathway.

Biallelic mutations in the *BRCA2* gene, encoding a DNA repair enzyme for which heterozygous mutations had been linked to breast, ovarian, and prostate cancer susceptibility, were shown to be the underlying abnormality in FA patients who were previously assigned to complementation group D1; thus, BRCA2 and FANCD1 turned out to be identical. FANCD1/BRCA2 is essential for recruiting the homologous recombination-promoting protein RAD51 into DNA damage–inducible nuclear foci. These data clearly establish a defect in the ability to repair certain types of DNA damage appropriately as the underlying abnormality in FA, although the precise molecular mechanisms are still being elucidated.

Despite progress in identifying the genetic and biochemical defects in FA, it is not known why affected individuals develop bone marrow failure or are at risk for development of clonal hematopoietic neoplasms, including myelodysplastic syndromes (MDS) and acute myeloid leukemia (AML). The cause of the progressive aplastic anemia (AA) in FA has been thought to be due to the loss of hematopoietic stem cells (HSCs) due to cumulative DNA damage. However, it is unknown whether children with FA have a developmental defect that leads to a reduction in the size of the stem cell pool, whether there is rapid attrition of stem cells during the first years of life, or whether both mechanisms are operative.

Cells from patients with FA also have been shown to have increased sensitivity to apoptosis, and elevated levels of apoptosis may contribute to the hematopoietic failure phenotype. Additionally, FA hematopoietic progenitor cells are hypersensitive to interferon-γ, a known inhibitor of hematopoiesis.

Clinical features and diagnosis of FA

FA is an autosomal recessive or X-linked disorder that is generally characterized by pancytopenia and congenital defects in the cutaneous, musculoskeletal, and urogenital systems. Patients with FA were recognized historically by characteristic physical findings including short stature, microcephaly, intense patchy brown pigmentation of the skin, gonadal abnormalities, and malformations of the thumb and kidney. Hemoglobin F levels are increased in FA, and 80% of patients develop signs of bone marrow failure by age 20 years. It is now clear that many patients with FA lack any abnormal physical findings, and some may not demonstrate overt marrow failure, so a high index of suspicion is required. Chromosome breakage testing now secures the diagnosis in most patients.

Contemporary diagnosis of FA is based on the analysis for chromosome breaks in phytohemagglutinin-stimulated peripheral blood lymphocytes cultured with and without clastogenic agents (DEB or MMC). Results are usually reported as percentage of cells with chromosome aberrations; the percentage of such cells inducible in samples from healthy individuals depends on the specific laboratory protocol but is dramatically increased in FA. Alternatively, the finding of an increased percentage of cells arrested at the G2/M phase (4 N DNA) of the cell cycle, ascertained by flow cytometry, is also consistent with a diagnosis of FA. Bone marrow cells should not be used for chromosome breakage studies because false-negative results are more likely. These in vitro diagnostic tests have revealed that approximately 30% of patients with FA lack typical physical findings, and approximately 10% of patients first present at age >16 years.

Diagnosis may be complicated by the development of somatic mosaicism in the lymphocytes. Somatic mosaicism results from a genetic reversion to normal (non-FA), such that a subset of lymphocytes is no longer susceptible to chromosomal breakage in response to DEB or MMC. Because reversion to wild type confers a growth advantage over the nonreverted FA cells, the diagnosis of FA may be missed. In patients for whom there is a strong suspicion for FA, the diagnosis may be made by testing for chromosomal breakage in response to DEB or MMC using cultured skin fibroblasts obtained from a punch biopsy.

Although spontaneous chromosomal alterations can be observed in Bloom syndrome and ataxia telangiectasia, DEB-induced chromosomal alterations are not seen in those disorders. Patients with Nijmegen breakage syndrome (NBS) may exhibit increased chromosomal breakage with MMC, and this condition must be distinguished from FA; immunologic abnormalities are characteristic of NBS but not FA, and in doubtful cases, testing of the *NBS1* gene can help diagnostically.

Complications of marrow failure are the most common causes of death in FA, but FA is also characterized by an increased incidence of malignancies. Approximately 10% to 15% of FA patients develop MDS or AML, often in the context of a hypoplastic marrow and monosomy 7. Patients with FA are also at increased risk for liver tumors, and squamous cell carcinomas (particularly esophageal, oral, and vulvar/vaginal tumors) are also much more common in patients with FA than in the general population. In addition to hepatocellular carcinoma, peliosis hepatis and hepatic adenomas also occur with increased frequency, especially in patients treated with androgens. The risk of AML is 700-fold in patients with FA compared with the general population but plateaus after the second decade of life, whereas the risk of solid tumors increases with age; 30% of patients with FA will develop a solid tumor by age 45 years.

The clinical significance of an abnormal marrow cytogenetic clone (eg, monosomy 7) in the absence of morphologic dysplasia is not always clear because these clones may be stable or even regress with time. The exquisite sensitivity of FA patients to the DNA-damaging effects of chemotherapy and radiation poses a formidable obstacle to the treatment of malignancies in these patients. The most successful treatment of solid tumors in FA results from early detection and complete surgical excision. For this reason, regular tumor surveillance is an important aspect of medical management beginning in the late teenage years.

Treatment

The only potentially curative option for marrow failure in FA patients is allogeneic HSC transplantation (HSCT). However, because of the increased sensitivity of FA cells to DNA damage–inducing agents, it is necessary to use modified transplantation conditioning regimens, such as attenuated alkylating agent and radiation doses, or alternative non–DNA-damaging agents such as fludarabine or antithymocyte globulin (ATG). For this reason, it is critical to identify patients with FA as having the condition prior to proceeding to stem cell transplantation. Patients with FA who present with MDS or AML without an observed bone marrow failure phase may go unrecognized until the use of standard transplantation conditioning results in a disaster.

Stem cell transplantation in FA is associated with an increased risk of subsequent solid tumors, particularly in the setting of chronic graft-versus-host disease (GVHD). Stem cell transplantation corrects only the hematopoietic defect, and the patient remains at risk for FA-related complications in other tissues, such as solid tumors. Despite these limitations, stem cell transplantation from a matched (unaffected) sibling may be considered as the initial treatment of choice for patients with FA who present with marrow failure. Unrelated donor stem cell transplantation is complicated in these patients because the intensive conditioning regimens required for engraftment can exacerbate cellular damage and increase the risk for GVHD. Transplantation outcomes are better if transplantation occurs prior to the development of leukemia, so regular surveillance of the peripheral blood counts and bone marrow is recommended.

Androgens (eg, oxymetholone with a starting dose of 2 mg/kg/d) may elevate the blood counts in a subset of patients. Although the response to androgen therapy is typically most pronounced in the red blood cell lineage, improvements in platelet and neutrophil counts have also been seen. Responses may be delayed, particularly for platelets, where first responses have been reported as far as 6 months out from initiation of treatment. The neutrophil count may also respond to granulocyte colony-stimulating factor (G-CSF) or granulocyte-macrophage colony-stimulating factor (GM-CSF). Some patients who initially responded to androgens may become refractory over time. Supportive therapy with transfusions can be considered, but in the patient who is a candidate for allogeneic stem cell transplantation, the use of transfusions should be minimized to prevent alloimmunization, and transfusions should never be from family members. Iron overload may develop in patients receiving chronic red blood cell transfusions.

Because of the risk of neoplasia, patients with FA should undergo regular screening for cancer. Although there is no consensus on optimal frequency of such screening evaluations, annual gynecologic examination for female patients is recommended after menarche, and regular dental care is also important, with careful examination for head and neck cancer. Surveillance with liver ultrasound at least once yearly is recommended for patients undergoing treatment with androgens.

> **Key points**
>
> - FA is an autosomal or X-linked recessive cause of bone marrow failure that is due to a defect in DNA repair.
> - Approximately 80% of patients develop signs of marrow failure, but the absence of marrow failure does not rule out FA if typical physical stigmata are present.
> - The diagnostic test for FA is a DEB or MMC chromosome breakage study.
> - FA can present in adulthood and without classic features other than bone marrow failure. These patients remain at risk for marrow failure, leukemia, and solid tumors.
> - Chemotherapeutic agents and radiation are poorly tolerated; attenuated conditioning regimens are necessary for stem cell transplantation.
> - Stem cell transplantation is the only curative option for FA-associated hematologic manifestations.
> - Careful monitoring for malignancies allows early institution of treatment, with attention to minimizing exposure to chemotherapy and radiation.

Diamond-Blackfan anemia
Clinical features

Diamond-Blackfan anemia (DBA) classically presents within the first year of life with a hypoproliferative, macrocytic anemia. Bone marrow examination typically reveals a paucity of erythroid precursors. Approximately one half of patients have associated nonhematologic physical findings, which may include radial ray anomalies, midline craniofacial defects or cleft palate, urogenital abnormalities, or cardiac defects. Red blood cell adenosine deaminase levels and fetal hemoglobin levels are usually elevated, and this can help in diagnosis. An increased risk of AML has been reported in DBA patients, but the risk is less than in patients with FA.

Pathobiology

Heterozygous germline mutations in the *RPS19* gene, which encodes a ribosomal protein, have been reported in 25% of patients with DBA. The clinical manifestations among family members with identical *RPS19* gene mutations are highly variable, and anemia may be absent. It is not clear how a defect in 1 allele of a gene encoding a ribosomal protein leads to red blood cell hypoplasia and not other dramatic phenotypic manifestations, because ribosomes are essential for cellular protein synthesis broadly. However, intact ribosomes appear to be particularly important for normal erythropoiesis; in patients with MDS associated with deletion of chromosome 5q, acquired haploinsufficiency of *RPS14*, a gene at 5q31 that encodes another ribosomal component, contributes to disease-associated anemia.

Germline mutations in 6 other genes encoding ribosome-associated proteins (*RPS24*, *RPS17*, *RPL35A*, *RPL5*, *RPL11*, and *RPS7*) have now been described in families with DBA who have wild-type *RPS19*, and an additional unknown gene has been mapped to chromosome 8p23. Although the overall inheritance pattern is autosomal dominant, many cases of DBA appear to be sporadic, presumably resulting from new germline mutations.

Treatment

For unclear reasons, in the majority of patients with DBA (~80%), the hemoglobin level improves with corticosteroid treatment. It is vital to use the minimal dose of steroids required to support erythropoiesis to minimize adverse effects of chronic steroid use. Patients who fail to respond to steroids, become refractory to steroids, or require high steroid doses may be supported with red blood cell transfusions instead. Careful attention to iron overload and timely initiation of iron chelation therapy are important for patients undergoing chronic transfusions.

Currently, the only curative treatment of marrow failure is stem cell transplantation, but the risks of transplantation must be weighed against the benefits for each patient. Some patients with DBA will undergo spontaneous remission and maintain adequate hemoglobin levels independent of steroids. In a few patients, a diet supplemented with leucine and isoleucine has resulted in improved erythropoiesis and growth; this approach needs to be investigated further.

> **Key points**
>
> - DBA typically presents with macrocytic anemia and red blood cell hypoplasia in infancy.
> - Approximately one half of patients with DBA have physical signs including radial ray and craniofacial abnormalities.
> - Autosomal dominant mutations in *RPS19* are seen in 25% of patients with DBA. At least 6 other ribosomal proteins have also been described as mutated in other DBA pedigrees.
> - Treatment options for DBA include corticosteroids, red blood cell transfusion support, and stem cell transplantation.
> - Spontaneous remissions may occur in a subset of patients.

Congenital dyserythropoietic anemias
General clinical features

The congenital dyserythropoietic anemias (CDAs) are a heterogeneous group of conditions characterized by ineffective erythropoiesis and anemia, multinucleated erythroid precursors in the marrow (Figure 15-2), and excess iron even in the absence of blood transfusions. Beyond these commonalities, the subtypes of CDA have differing clinical features and modes of inheritance. Two types of CDA—CDA I and the more common CDA II—are fairly well defined, but CDA III is poorly understood, and the other forms of CDA are very rare and poorly characterized. The differential diagnosis of dyserythropoiesis includes other conditions, such as hemoglobinopathies, hereditary sideroblastic anemias, *GATA1* mutations, and MDS, and these should be ruled out.

CDA type I

CDA I is a rare autosomal recessive disorder (eg, ~80 pedigrees are listed in the pan-European registry) that usually

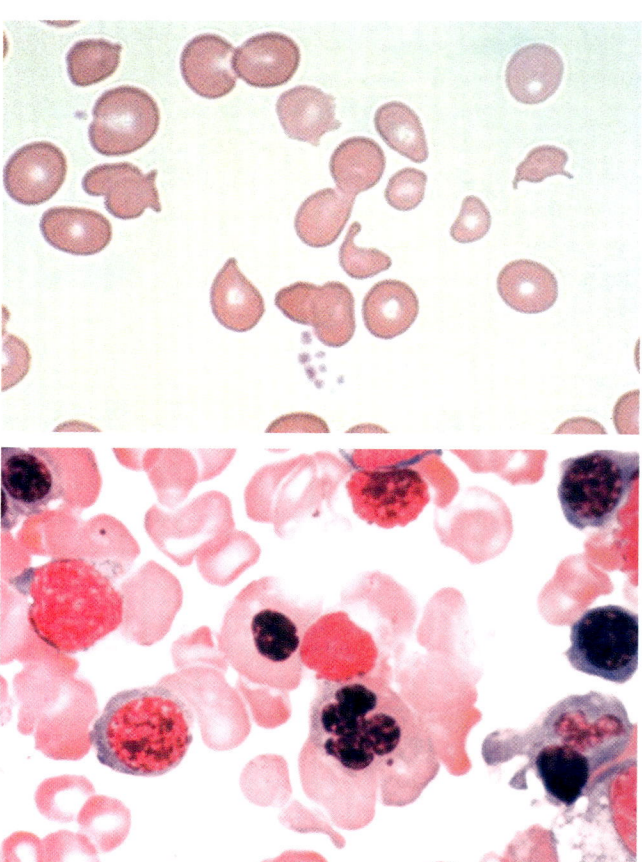

Figure 15-2 Peripheral blood smear and marrow aspirate from a patient with congenital dyserythropoietic anemia type II (CDA II, HEMPAS). Key features include anisopoikilocytosis and multinucleated erythroid precursors. Images from ASH slide bank #953, #1532.

presents in childhood or adolescence. CDA I is characterized by hemolytic anemia (usually moderate, with hemoglobin in the range of 9-10 g/dL), anisopoikilocytosis with reduced levels of erythrocyte membrane protein 4.1R, normal or elevated reticulocyte count, macrocytosis, and high serum iron levels. Serum bilirubin levels are often elevated, and some patients develop pigment gallstones or jaundice. Splenomegaly is a frequent feature. Some patients have dysmorphologic features, including syndactyly, absent or hypoplastic distal phalanges or nails, skin pigmentation abnormalities, hypoplastic right third rib, and sensorineural deafness. Bone marrow examination shows erythroid hyperplasia, binucleated erythroblasts, and a distinctive pattern of internuclear chromatin bridging.

CDA I has been linked to defects in the gene codanin 1 (*CDAN1*) at chromosome 15q15, a gene encoding a protein of unknown function and without well-defined domains. At least 1 kindred with CDA I lacked *CDAN1* mutations, and linkage analysis failed to link the condition in this pedigree to chromosome 15q, so another gene may also be responsible in some cases.

For unclear reasons, the anemia in type I CDA typically responds to recombinant interferon-α_{2a}, interferon-α_{2b}, or peginterferon-α_{2b}. Folate supplementation is helpful, given the chronic hemolysis. Most patients with type I CDA do not typically require transfusions, and transfusions can exacerbate the tendency to iron overload.

CDA type II

CDA II is more common than CDA I (>340 patients have been collected in European registries) and usually presents during childhood with anemia of variable severity. Transfusion dependence is uncommon. The reticulocyte count is low, and the bone marrow typically shows multinucleated erythroid precursors, karyorrhexis, and pseudo-Gaucher cells. The red blood cell membrane in patients with this disorder demonstrates abnormal glycosylation, apparently due to a defect in Golgi processing in erythroblasts. Abnormal migration of band 3 and band 4.5 on sodium dodecyl sulfate (SDS) gels may be useful diagnostically. Although some cases have been linked to chromosome 20q11, the precise gene defect in CDA II is yet unknown.

CDA II was formerly known as HEMPAS (hereditary erythroblastic multinuclearity with a positive acidified serum test). A characteristic feature of HEMPAS is the ability of some group-compatible sera to lyse the patient's erythrocytes, resulting in a positive acid hemolysis test (Ham test, described below in the section on paroxysmal nocturnal hemoglobinuria [PNH]). However, the sucrose hemolysis test is negative, and the cells are not lysed by autologous serum, unlike the situation in PNH. The cell lysis is secondary to increased immunoglobulin M (IgM) binding to erythrocytes and not to increased sensitivity to complement.

Like other patients with congenital dyserythropoiesis, patients with CDA II can have problems with iron overload. Phlebotomy and chelation have been used to treat iron overload in these patients. Because the osmotic fragility test is usually abnormal in CDA II, some patients are misdiagnosed as having hereditary spherocytosis and undergo splenectomy. Splenectomy may be useful in treating anemia in some patients, but results are variable.

Other CDA types

CDA III is a rare autosomal dominant disorder characterized by the presence of multinucleated erythroid precursors in the marrow (gigantoblasts) in addition to mild anemia and low reticulocyte counts. The causative gene is unknown, but in 1 kindred, the disorder was linked to chromosome 15q21. The peripheral smear shows marked anisopoikilocytosis and basophilic stippling of the red blood cells, a picture similar to severe β thalassemia. Additional exceptionally rare types of CDA (eg, CDA IV, V, VI, and VII) have also been proposed.

> **Key points**
>
> - CDA I is characterized by moderate hemolytic anemia, internuclear chromatin bridging, iron overload, germline mutations in *CDAN1*, and responsiveness to interferon-α therapy.
> - CDA II is the most common form of CDA and can be misdiagnosed as hereditary spherocytosis. Patients typically have a positive acid hemolysis (Ham) test, multinucleated giant cells, and a low reticulocyte count. The genetic cause is unknown.
> - There are several rare forms of CDA that have not yet been genetically characterized.

Dyskeratosis congenita
Clinical features

Dyskeratosis congenita (DC) is an inherited marrow failure syndrome classically characterized by the clinical triad of abnormal nails, reticulated skin rash, and oral leukoplakia. Additional features may include sparse hair, dry eyes and mouth, scleroderma-like skin changes, osteopenia, hyperhidrosis, and genitourinary abnormalities. The diagnosis is easily missed in young patients in whom the marrow failure may precede the typical skin and nail findings, because the skin and nail findings typically do not develop until the second decade of life. The clinical features of DC may be difficult to differentiate from chronic GVHD in patients who undergo transplantation at an early age for AA. A careful family history and special laboratory testing (discussed later in this section) may distinguish between these 2 diagnoses.

Patients with DC are at risk for restrictive pulmonary disease. Vascular inflammatory disease and immune deficiencies have also been described in these patients. Patients with DC are also at increased risk for developing MDS, AML, and squamous cell carcinomas.

Pathobiology

Three inheritance patterns have been described for DC: X-linked, autosomal dominant, and autosomal recessive. Mutations in the *DKC1* gene, which encodes the dyskerin protein, are responsible for the X-linked form of DC. Dyskerin is involved in telomere maintenance as well as ribosomal RNA/small nuclear RNA pseudouridylation. The autosomal dominant form of DC is associated with mutations in the *TERC* gene, which encodes the RNA component of telomerase. Additional genes may also be involved in the autosomal dominant form of DC. The gene(s) involved in the autosomal recessive form of DC have yet to be identified.

Consistent with these genetic data, patients with DC exhibit extremely short telomeres. Telomeres are required to stabilize the ends of chromosomes and prevent chromosomal rearrangements. Telomeres undergo progressive shortening with successive rounds of chromosomal duplication during cell division. Progressive accelerated telomere shortening has been described in successive generations in DC families.

Treatment

DC patients with marrow failure may respond to androgens. Responses to G-CSF and recombinant erythropoietin have also been reported. Allogeneic stem cell transplantation offers potentially curative therapy for marrow failure in DC patients, but patients may be at increased risk of adverse events from the conditioning regimen of chemotherapy and radiation. The role of nonmyeloablative regimens is currently under investigation, and the ongoing risk of leukemia in the setting of chimerism posttransplantation remains a potential concern.

> **Key points**
>
> - DC is a marrow failure syndrome characterized by the clinical triad of dystrophic nails, reticulated skin rash, and oral leukoplakia.
> - Nonhematologic clinical features develop later in life and may be absent in young children.
> - Nonhematologic features of DC may be mistaken for chronic GVHD in patients who received marrow transplantations for AA.
> - DC is associated with an increased risk for MDS, AML, and squamous cell carcinomas.
> - DC is associated with genetic defects in telomere maintenance. Very short telomere lengths are typically seen in these patients.
> - Patients with DC may have mutations in the *DKC1* or *TERC* genes, but absence of these mutations does not rule out DC.

Congenital amegakaryocytic thrombocytopenia

Clinical features

Congenital amegakaryocytic thrombocytopenia (CAMT) is a very rare autosomal recessive disorder characterized by hypoproductive thrombocytopenia. Megakaryocytes are absent or greatly diminished in the bone marrow. Patients typically present shortly after birth with petechiae, bruising or bleeding, and a very low platelet count. Patients with CAMT are at risk for developing pancytopenia and a picture similar to AA. There are also case reports of patients with CAMT developing MDS and leukemia.

Pathobiology

CAMT is caused by biallelic mutations in the *MPL* gene, which encodes the thrombopoietin (TPO) receptor. Development of AA in CAMT patients is consistent with findings that TPO signaling plays an important role in the maintenance and expansion of HSCs and multipotent progenitors. TPO levels are typically high in CAMT.

Treatment

Supportive care consists largely of platelet transfusions. Antifibrinolytic agents may be useful to help treat bleeding. Marrow failure may be cured with an HSCT. The platelet count is not responsive to TPO.

> **Key points**
>
> - CAMT is caused by autosomal recessively inherited defects in the *MPL* gene encoding the TPO receptor.
> - CAMT presents in the neonatal period with bruising or bleeding and severe thrombocytopenia; pancytopenia may evolve in later childhood.
> - CAMT may be treated with HSCT.

Acquired bone marrow failure conditions

Aplastic anemia

Definition

AA is an HSC disease associated with bone marrow with markedly reduced cellularity and deficient blood cell production. Classification and clinical prognosis are related to the severity in the depression of blood counts. *Severe AA* is defined by severe depression of blood counts of at least 2 hematopoietic lineages (absolute reticulocyte count <60 × 10^9/L, absolute neutrophil count <0.5 × 10^9/L, or platelet

Clinical case

A 19-year-old male college student presents to the emergency room complaining of excessive bruising. He takes occasional acetaminophen but no other medications. On physical examination, he is noted to be pale without icterus. He has scattered ecchymoses of varying ages on his upper extremities and torso, and petechiae are noted over his lower extremities. He has no palpable lymphadenopathy or splenomegaly. He is of normal height and weight and does not have any dysmorphic features or musculoskeletal abnormalities. Family history is negative for hematologic problems. A complete blood count shows a hemoglobin of 4.2 g/dL, an absolute reticulocyte count of 35×10^9/L, a platelet count of 4×10^9/L, a total white blood cell count of 1.5×10^9/L and an absolute neutrophil count of 0.4×10^9/L. His vitamin B_{12} and serum folate levels are within the normal range. A bone marrow biopsy shows 10% cellularity. Aspirated marrow spicules are markedly hypocellular, with mostly lymphoid and plasma cell elements. A few early erythroid progenitors are seen, some with megaloblastic changes. No megakaryocytes are noted. There is no obvious dysplasia of the few myeloid elements. Cytogenetic studies reveal a normal karyotype. Severe AA is diagnosed.

Epidemiology, etiology, and pathogenesis

AA is rare in Western Europe and the United States (3-6 cases per million population per year), but the incidence in China, Southeast Asia, and Mexico is 3 to 4 times higher. AA is primarily a disease of children and younger adults, with another peak in patients >60 years old; in the latter group, some of the cases may reflect diagnostic overlap with hypocellular MDS.

AA can arise during pregnancy or in association with hepatitis. Hepatitis-associated AA accounts for 2% to 5% of cases of AA in Europe and 4% to 10% of cases in East Asia. AA has been reported to occur in 28% to 33% of patients requiring orthotopic liver transplantation for fulminant non-A, non-B, non-C hepatitis. Seronegative hepatitis in patients with posthepatitic AA does not appear to be caused by any of the known hepatitis viruses and is often referred to as to *hepatitis/AA syndrome*. AA evolves with a typical delay of several months after the episode of hepatitis, usually after improvement of liver tests.

AA can be acquired or constitutional. Acquired idiopathic AA, presumably the result of a T-cell–mediated autoimmune process, is more common than AA associated with medication exposure and accounts for most cases in North America. The association of AA with chloramphenicol is well documented and serves as a model for drug-induced AA, but this condition is rarely observed in the United States because chloramphenicol is rarely used. Many other drugs have been associated with AA; the link with some drugs has been doubtful, whereas with others, the evidence is more convincing. Indomethacin, diclofenac, butazones such as phenylbutazone, clopidogrel, antithyroid medications such as propylthiouracil, and gold salts are the medications most clearly associated with development of AA.

Irrespective of the etiology, hematopoiesis is markedly reduced in all patients with AA, as reflected by marrow histology, low numbers of circulating or marrow $CD34^+$ cells, diminished numbers of long-term culture-initiating cells (a surrogate measure of HSCs), and poor hematopoietic colony formation by aplastic marrow. The inhibition of hematopoiesis involves all stages of hematopoiesis, including immature and more committed progenitor cells.

count $<20 \times 10^9$/L) and bone marrow hypocellularity (<30%). *Very severe AA* has an absolute neutrophil count of $<0.2 \times 10^9$/L, whereas *moderate AA* is characterized by depression of blood counts not fulfilling the definition of severe disease (Table 15-2). AA is associated with normal cytogenetics; an abnormal karyotype is more consistent with a diagnosis of MDS, although some investigators believe that certain chromosomal abnormalities such as trisomy 8 can still be compatible with the diagnosis of AA.

AA may be acquired and idiopathic, or it can arise in the context of an inherited marrow failure syndrome such as those described earlier (Tables 15-3 and 15-4). This distinction carries profound implications for management and treatment. Diagnosis of AA requires exclusion of systemic causes for marrow failure and nutritional deficiency. The diagnosis of AA is usually reserved for naturally occurring conditions and excludes those patients with a recent history of cytotoxic chemotherapy or exposure to toxins such as ionizing radiation.

Table 15-2 Classification of aplastic anemia by severity.

Severe aplastic anemia*	Moderate aplastic anemia
Bone marrow cellularity <30%	Decreased bone marrow cellularity
Depression of at least 2 of the following 3 hematopoietic lineages: Absolute neutrophil count $<0.5 \times 10^9$/L Transfusion dependence, with absolute reticulocyte count $<60 \times 10^9$/L Platelet count $<20 \times 10^9$/L	Depression of at least 2 of 3 hematopoietic lineages not fulfilling the severity criteria as specified in the left column

*Some investigators also define a "very severe" aplastic anemia category: severe aplastic anemia with an absolute neutrophil count $<0.2 \times 10^9$/L.
From Young NS, Maciejewski J. The pathophysiology of acquired aplastic anemia. *N Engl J Med*. 1997;336:1365–1372.

Table 15-3 Classification of aplastic anemia by etiology.

Acquired aplastic anemia	Inherited disorders that present with or can evolve to aplastic anemia
Primary	Fanconi anemia
Idiopathic aplastic anemia	Dyskeratosis congenita
Pregnancy-associated aplastic anemia	Reticular dysgenesis (severe combined immunodeficiency with leukopenia)
Aplastic anemia/paroxysmal nocturnal hemoglobinuria syndrome	Shwachman-Diamond syndrome
	Genetic primary nonhematologic syndromes
Secondary	
Drug associated	
Iatrogenic/cytotoxic	
Idiosyncratic	
Radiation associated	
Iatrogenic	
Accidental	
Viruses	
Epstein-Barr virus	
Cytomegalovirus	
Hepatitis/aplastic anemia syndrome (presumed viral)	
Pancytopenia of autoimmune diseases	

Obligatory involvement of all blood lineages points toward HSCs as main target of the pathophysiologic mechanism involved in AA (Figure 15-3).

Clinical response to immunosuppressive therapy targeting T cells (eg, antithymocyte globulin) supports an immune-mediated pathogenesis of AA. Activated cytotoxic T cells produce interferon-α and tumor necrosis factor α (TNFα), which suppress hematopoiesis. Fas ligand (CD95) expression by hematopoietic progenitor and stem cells is increased in patients with AA and is likely induced by interferon-α and TNFα. Ligand binding to the Fas death receptor on the surface of hematopoietic progenitors could contribute to marrow aplasia by triggering apoptosis. Inhibitory cytokines also exert a direct inhibitory effect on hematopoietic progenitors. Although the T-cell–mediated process is intrinsically polyclonal, oligoclonal expansion of CD8$^+$ T cells has been observed in some AA patients, raising the possibility that these might represent immunodominant autoreactive clones. Human leukocyte antigen (HLA)-DR15 (a split of HLA-DR2) is overrepresented in AA (40%–50%, compared with an antigen frequency of approximately 20% in the general population), which also suggests an immune pathogenesis of idiopathic AA. Although diverse triggers such as viruses or chemical haptens may serve as inciting

Table 15-4 Differential diagnosis of idiopathic aplastic anemia and pancytopenia.

Pancytopenia	
Hypocellular bone marrow	**Hypercellular bone marrow**
Primary marrow disorders	*Direct marrow involvement*
Acquired aplastic anemia	Myelodysplastic syndrome
Fanconi anemia	Paroxysmal nocturnal hemoglobinuria
Aleukemic acute myeloid leukemia	Primary myelofibrosis
Hairy cell leukemia	Lymphoma
Rarely:	Metastatic carcinomas and sarcomas
Lymphoma	
Myeloma	
Primary myelofibrosis	
Systemic illnesses	*Systemic disorders*
Hypothyroidism	Systemic lupus erythematosus
Anorexia nervosa	Hypersplenism
Infections	Sepsis
Tuberculosis	Alcohol
Q fever	Brucellosis
	Ehrlichiosis

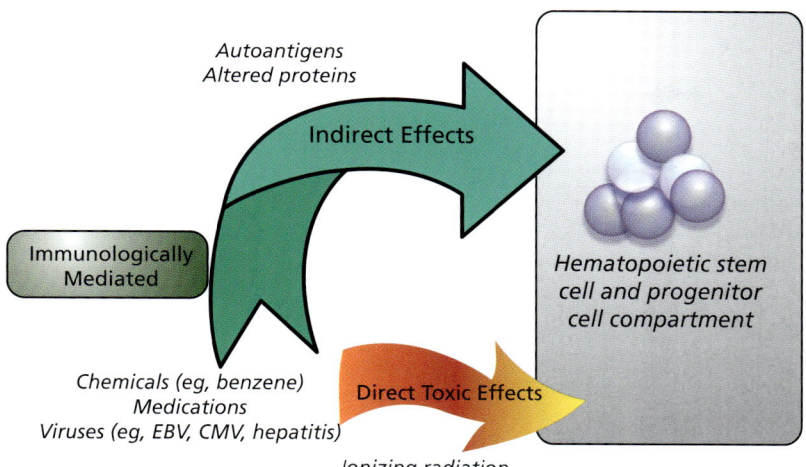

Figure 15-3 Types of stem cell injury in aplastic anemia. Aplastic anemia can result both from direct toxic effects on hematopoietic stem cells and progenitors and from an aberrant T-cell–driven immune response. CMV = cytomegalovirus; EBV = Epstein-Barr virus.

events in individual cases, the final autoimmune pathway appears to be uniform.

Recent data also implicate intrinsic HSC defects in some AA cases. Mutations in 2 of the 3 genes encoding telomerase components, *TERC* and *TERT*, have been described in patients who lack the overt clinical stigmata of DC, a condition associated with germline *TERC* and *TERT* mutations (and, most commonly, mutations in *DKC1* [dyskerin]). Telomeres consist of short TTAGGG nucleotide repeats associated with telomeric proteins and protect the ends of chromosomes. Telomeres progressively shorten over successive cell divisions. When a critically short telomere length is reached, cell death ensues. Telomerase is a ribonucleoprotein that is important for telomere length maintenance. The RNA component of telomerase is encoded by the *TERC* gene, and the reverse transcriptase activity is encoded by the *TERT* gene. Although telomerase expression is generally low in most somatic cells, telomerase dysfunction is associated with accelerated telomere shortening and may result in premature death of rapidly proliferating cells. Hematopoiesis requires sustained rapid cell proliferation and division. So it is likely that shorter telomeres, due to defects of the telomerase complex, contribute to premature HSC attrition and a lower compensatory capacity of hematopoiesis, thereby predisposing to development of bone marrow failure.

Clinical presentation

Symptoms of AA are a consequence of lack of production of blood cell elements. Patients present with pallor and fatigue due to anemia, with increased bruising or hemorrhage due to thrombocytopenia, or with infection due to neutropenia. AA usually arises in a previously healthy patient who has no history of malignancy and no exposure to cytotoxic drugs or history of radiation exposure. A family history of marrow failure or dysmorphology may help identify inherited causes of pancytopenia such as FA. Drug associations have to be explored, and all potentially offending agents need to be discontinued.

Splenomegaly and hepatomegaly are not typical features of AA and should raise the question of another underlying disease. Short stature, musculoskeletal abnormalities (particularly radial ray anomalies), dysplastic nails, skin rashes, oral leukoplakia, exocrine pancreatic insufficiency, or other congenital anomalies may suggest an inherited bone marrow failure state (see "Differential Diagnosis," below). The absence of characteristic physical findings or a suggestive family history does not rule out an inherited marrow failure syndrome, however. Patients with inherited marrow failure syndromes may first present in adulthood with marrow failure or a malignancy (eg, MDS). The peripheral blood smear is remarkable for erythrocyte normocytosis or macrocytosis, thrombocytopenia, and a decrease in all granulocytic cells and monocytes.

Malignant or markedly dysplastic cells are not seen in the marrow or peripheral blood, although mild dysplastic features are sometimes noted in the marrow, which can cause diagnostic confusion with hypocellular MDS. In the marrow, all hematopoietic cell lines are diminished, whereas macrophages, mast cells, and fibroblasts are present. The marrow is characterized by hypocellularity, an expansion of the fatty marrow, and no increase in reticulin.

Marrow biopsy is the gold standard for assessing marrow cellularity. Because residual marrow cellularity in AA may be patchy and variable, results should be interpreted within the clinical context of the patient. Cytogenetic results are typically normal in AA, but in some instances, profound depletion of stem cells may lead to occurrence of transient clonal abnormalities seen in a proportion of metaphases examined. Such clonal defects may be transient and usually disappear with hematopoietic improvement.

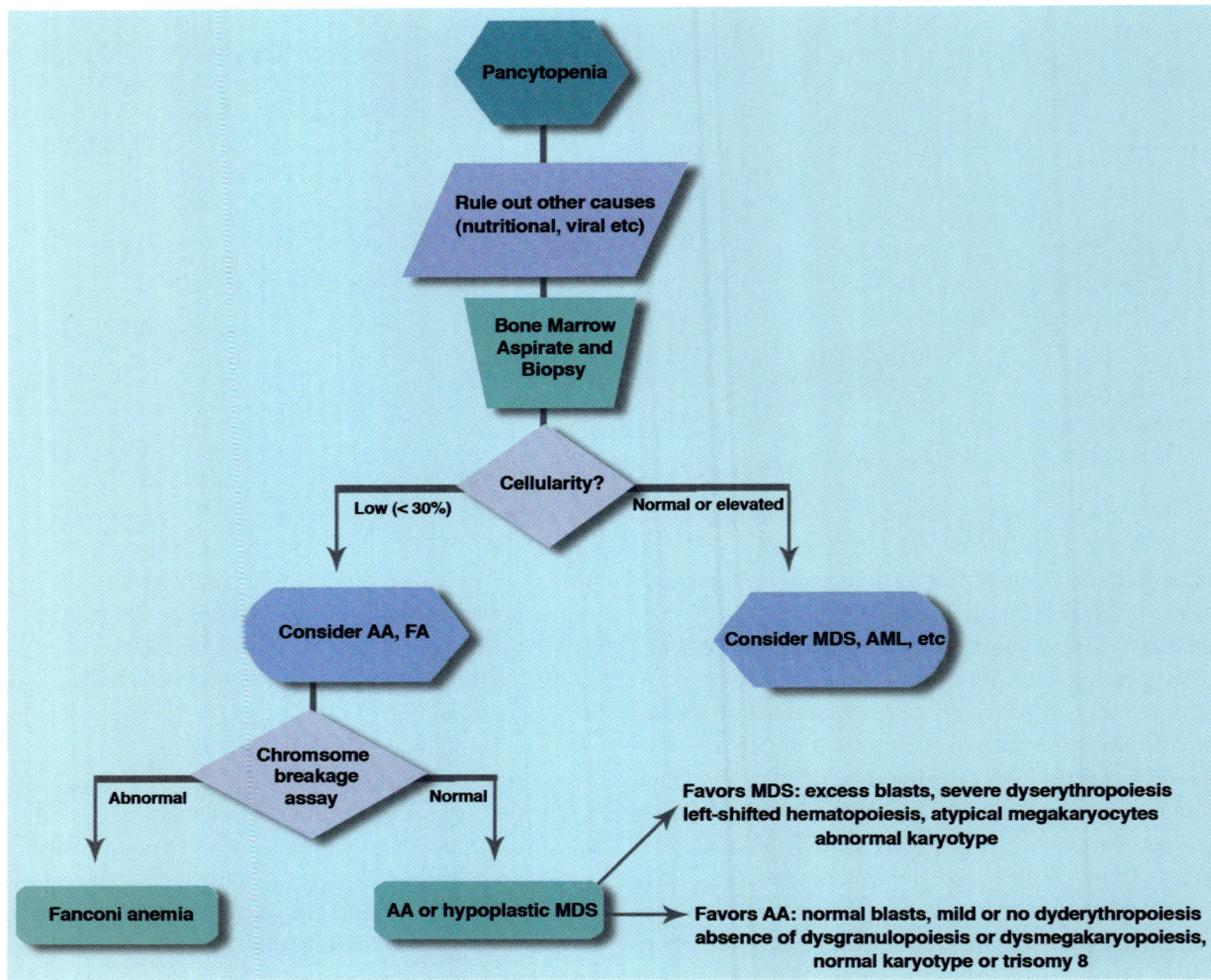

Figure 15-4 Diagnostic algorithm for evaluation of suspected aplastic anemia (AA). AML = acute myeloid leukemia; FA = Fanconi anemia; MDS = myelodysplastic syndrome.

Differential diagnosis

When evaluating a patient with pancytopenia and a hypocellular marrow, the physician must exclude a number of other diagnoses before a diagnosis of AA can be made (Figure 15-4). The most common disorders include MDS, aleukemic leukemia, PNH, myelofibrosis, hairy cell leukemia, tuberculosis, nutritional deficiency (eg, anorexia nervosa), T-cell large granular lymphocyte (T-LGL) disease (T-LGL can coexist with AA), and human immunodeficiency virus (HIV) infection.

The presence of immature hematopoietic cells or blast cells should lead to a diagnosis of hypocellular acute leukemia or a hypocellular MDS. Similarly, marrow cytogenetic analysis may detect a cytogenetic abnormality diagnostic of lymphoid or myeloid leukemic disorders. Hairy cell leukemia frequently presents as pancytopenia with difficulty in aspirating the marrow, or a "dry tap." Pancytopenia can arise in the setting of anorexia nervosa as an epiphenomenon of the eating disorder. Pancytopenia in that setting is associated with a hypocellular marrow and replacement of the marrow with eosinophilic material. Vitamin B_{12} and folate levels should be determined in all patients, although the marrow in B_{12} or folate deficiency is typically hypercellular and megaloblastic. HIV infection or acquired immunodeficiency syndrome (AIDS) is associated with cytopenia, morphologic dysplasia, and marrow hypocellularity in approximately 10% of cases. A careful inquiry into HIV risk factors and an HIV test are prudent because this diagnosis would entail different medical management.

T-LGL disease is a rare condition characterized by more circulating T cells bearing the CD57 activation marker of effector/cytotoxic T cells. T-LGL disease, like PNH, can coexist with AA or MDS. T-LGL disease should be considered if increased large granular lymphocytes are noted on the peripheral blood smear or if the patient has rheumatoid arthritis, which is known to be associated with T-LGL disease. Testing for a clonal T-cell receptor gene rearrangement is appropriate when T-LGL is suspected.

A possible underlying cause of AA is FA, which can present with AA, even in adult patients without other classic features of this disease. Therefore, DEB or MMC testing to exclude chromosome fragility should be considered in patients even in the absence of musculoskeletal abnormalities. These studies are indicated in the 19-year-old patient described in the earlier clinical case.

The distinction between AA and hypoplastic MDS may be difficult, and there is increasing evidence to suggest that immune-mediated mechanisms similar to those postulated to cause AA may contribute to the cytopenias associated with hypocellular MDS and some cases of normocellular or hypercellular MDS (even in the absence of a preceding diagnosis of AA). Such evidence includes the identification of clonal activated cytotoxic T-cell populations in both AA and MDS, the coexistence of PNH and T-LGL clones in both AA and MDS, and improved blood counts in a subset of MDS patients treated with ATG or cyclosporine immunosuppression (see next section). Hypolobated neutrophils, dysplastic megakaryocytes, or abnormally localized immature precursors favor a diagnosis of hypoplastic MDS rather than AA. Sometimes the only way to make the distinction between AA and MDS is by detection of an abnormal cytogenetic clonal population, but even this may not be diagnostic of MDS because sometimes cytogenetically abnormal clones are transiently seen in AA.

In typical AA, PNH clones can be detected by flow cytometry in 30% of cases. Detection of a PNH clone at diagnosis provides support for the diagnosis of idiopathic AA. PNH can also appear in the later course of disease. PNH clones can remain stable over time or expand and lead to evolution of frank hemolytic PNH. Indicators of the presence of PNH include elevated lactate dehydrogenase (LDH), absent haptoglobin, increased reticulocytes, and erythroid predominance in the marrow.

Therapy

Without treatment, patients with severe or very severe AA will eventually succumb to infection or to hemorrhagic complications. Therefore, such patients require urgent therapy. The standard of care for moderate AA, in contrast, is not established. Except for cases where there is transfusion dependence, therapy is optional because survival is not affected by treatment. Rarely, patients with AA can spontaneously recover normal hematopoiesis. Spontaneous remission can be seen with drug-induced AA and usually occurs within 2 months of discontinuing the offending drug.

Therapy of severe AA consists of allogeneic HSCT or various types of immunosuppressive therapies. At the time of diagnosis, all potential transplantation candidates should

> **Key points**
>
> - Differential diagnosis for pancytopenia with hypocellular marrow includes the following:
>   - Idiopathic AA
>   - Constitutional forms of bone marrow failure
>   - Hypocellular MDS
>   - Aleukemic leukemia
>   - PNH
>   - Myelofibrosis
>   - Rheumatologic disorders (eg, systemic lupus erythematosus)
>   - Hairy cell leukemia
>   - Tuberculosis, histoplasmosis, HIV, Epstein-Barr virus, hepatitis
>   - Anorexia nervosa
>   - T-LGL disease
>   - Folate or vitamin B_{12} deficiency (marrow typically hypercellular)
>   - Drugs or toxins
> - Diagnostic approach to the patient with pancytopenia includes the following:
>   - History including medications, previous chemotherapy/radiation, occupational toxic exposures, HIV risk factors, family history
>   - Physical examination, paying particular attention to presence of organomegaly, lymphadenopathy, or congenital abnormalities
>   - Complete blood count, including reticulocyte count and peripheral smear examination
>   - Liver function tests
>   - Vitamin B_{12} and folate levels
>   - LDH, haptoglobin, and flow cytometry for PNH
>   - Bone marrow aspirate and biopsy
>   - Cytogenetic studies
>   - Consider chromosome fragility tests, in particular in children and younger adults

be HLA typed to identify a sibling donor or a potential unrelated donor. Because registries of unrelated donors frequently take several months to identify a donor, this process should be initiated immediately if a sibling donor cannot be identified.

Supportive care, transfusions, and hematopoietic growth factors

Supportive care is instituted to sustain a pancytopenic patient and alleviate symptoms of pancytopenia. Potential marrow toxins should be withdrawn. Supportive therapy consists of transfusion of irradiated, leukocyte-depleted blood products because patients are at risk for posttransfusion GVHD. If the patient is cytomegalovirus (CMV) negative, it is best to use CMV-negative blood products or leukocyte-depleted products. Transfusions should not be withheld from symptomatic patients, but in patients who are candidates for allogeneic stem cell transplantation, the use of transfusions should be limited to decrease the risk of alloimmunization, and transfusions should never be given from family members. Transfusions should be limited to prevent sensitization to transplantation antigens. Target platelet counts, which should be maintained to limit the risk of bleeding, are not well established. The role of preventive antibiotics in neutropenic patients is also not clear.

Most patients with AA have an elevated serum erythropoietin level and do not respond to recombinant erythropoietin. Although typical AA will also not respond to G-CSF or GM-CSF, some patients do respond, and these growth factors may have a role in decreasing infectious morbidity (either for primary or secondary prevention of infection) while awaiting definitive treatment with immunosuppression or stem cell transplantation. No significant improvement in survival has been seen in patients receiving G-CSF compared with those who did not receive G-CSF. The role of newer thrombopoietic agents in AA is not clear.

> **Key points**
> - In candidates for stem cell transplantation:
>   - Limit transfusions when possible.
>   - Use irradiated, leukocyte-depleted blood products.
>   - Transfusions should not be from family members.
> - Growth factors may have a role in decreasing infectious morbidity pending definitive treatment with immunosuppression or stem cell transplantation for severe AA.
> - Typical AA does not respond to G-CSF or erythropoietin.

Bone marrow transplantation

In AA, the pretransplantation conditioning regimen is primarily administered to provide immunosuppression, which enables the donor stem cells to engraft and also eliminates activated immune cells that may be causing the marrow aplasia. Bone marrow has been a traditional source for the stem cell graft, but the use of peripheral blood stem cells is growing. The standard conditioning regimen in matched sibling transplantation includes high-dose cyclophosphamide and ATG conditioning, which results in a 92% long-term survival rate and is superior to conditioning regimens involving total lymphoid irradiation and cyclophosphamide. The latter conditioning regimen has been shown to result in a much higher incidence of secondary malignancies, infertility, and, in children, retardation of growth and development.

GVHD and infection remain limiting factors to the success of transplantation for patients with severe AA. GVHD increases in frequency and severity in recipients older than 20 years of age. Cyclosporine prophylaxis appears to have reduced the incidence of both acute and chronic GVHD. The increased risk of GVHD contributes to the poor survival in older patients. Standard therapy of GVHD includes cyclosporine and methotrexate.

Patients with AA exhibit higher rates of engraftment problems than patients receive transplantation for other indications.

Marrow transplantation using unrelated donors carries higher morbidity and mortality than transplantations using matched sibling donors in AA and has been generally reserved for patients who lack a matched sibling donor and fail to respond to 1 or more rounds of ATG/cyclosporine therapy. Transplantation results are typically best in young patients (ie, <21 years of age) who have not had significant infections or heavy transfusion loads. For older patients (>55 years old), reduced-intensity transplantation conditioning regimens using lower doses of total-body irradiation or fludarabine have shown early promise, although patient numbers are still few and follow-up is limited.

> **Key points**
> - Outcomes with stem cell transplantation are better in younger patients (especially patients ≤20 years old); in patients >40 years old, transplantation-related mortality and morbidity markedly increase.
> - Matched unrelated donor transplantation should currently be reserved for patients who have failed immunosuppression.

Immunosuppressive therapy

Initial investigations using ATG or cyclosporine alone in AA were succeeded by studies of ATG and cyclosporine in combination, with improved response rates. The addition of mycophenolate mofetil did not improve results. The median time to response is approximately 12 weeks. In most studies, responses are defined as achieving blood counts that no longer fulfill criteria for severe disease, as well as transfusion independence. Total restoration of blood counts will occur in a minority of patients, and recovery can be very protracted. The overall response rate at 3 months in patients receiving ATG and cyclosporine is between 60% and 80%. Although most patients who will respond to immunosuppressive therapy will do so by 6 months, in a small minority of patients, time to recovery may be longer.

Hepatitis-associated AA and drug-related AA appear to be equally responsive to immunosuppressive therapy; 7 of 10 patients in one study experienced hematologic improvement after cyclosporine/ATG therapy. Repeated cycles of ATG/cyclosporine may be given to refractory patients, which results in additional responses in approximately 35% of refractory patients. However, the survival of refractory patients is poor. Positive predictors of response include HLA-DR15 and the presence of PNH clones, whereas low lymphocyte counts at presentation are associated with poor outcomes from immunosuppressive therapy. The addition of G-CSF did not improve the response rate or decrease early morbidity of treatment with ATG/cyclosporine in a recently completed controlled trial.

In responders to ATG/cyclosporine, relapse has been reported in 35% of patients by 5 years. Relapses are often temporally related to the discontinuation of cyclosporine or reduction of cyclosporine dose. Consequently, cyclosporine should be continued for at least 6 months, followed by a protracted tapering of the dose. In patients without restoration of counts to nearly normal levels, cyclosporine therapy may be continued for prolonged periods of time because relapse is almost certain with discontinuation. Relapsed patients may respond to an increase of cyclosporine dose or a second course of ATG, which results in responses in most of the patients. Approximately 25% of patients remain cyclosporine dependent to maintain their blood counts.

As alternative therapy to ATG/cyclosporine, high-dose cyclophosphamide has been used, with high response rates. However, the recovery of blood counts is slow. In a small randomized trial of ATG/cyclosporine versus cyclophosphamide/cyclosporine immunosuppressive therapy in 19 patients with severe AA who lacked a marrow donor, responses were comparable, but adverse events were more common in the cyclophosphamide-treated group.

Immunosuppression versus bone marrow transplantation

Although the response rate of severe AA to ATG/cyclosporine combination is incomplete and patients may suffer from relapse and have a risk of evolution of clonal diseases, the morbidity and mortality of patients who receive bone marrow transplantation is substantial. Transplantation outcomes are age dependent. Therefore, matched sibling allogeneic marrow transplantation is the treatment of choice for children and adolescents and may be considered as a first treatment option in adults up to the age of 40 years with severe AA, for whom transplantation-related morbidity and mortality are relatively low and potential remaining life span is relatively long. For the older population, immunosuppressive therapy is the treatment of choice. In immunosuppression-refractory adult patients, matched-related bone marrow transplantation may constitute a second-line therapy. Stem cell transplantation is associated with several long-term complications, including increased frequency of solid tumors.

Despite significant progress with matched unrelated donor marrow transplantation, survival rates remain poor compared with matched related donor transplantation. Patients who do not have a sibling donor should receive ATG/cyclosporine as a first-line therapy, regardless of age. Children who received 1 cycle of ATG/cyclosporine followed by unrelated matched donor transplantation showed superior survival compared with patients who received transplantation after several cycles of ATG/cyclosporine, but this has not been formally established for adults.

Late clonal complications

Although a significant proportion of patients with AA will have PNH clones at presentation, the frequency of evolution of frank PNH has been reported to be as high as 20% in 10 years after initial diagnosis. However, PNH that occurs after treatment is frequently subclinical and rarely associated with overt hemolysis or thrombosis. MDS, most frequently associated with either del7/7q– or trisomy 8, can evolve in up to 20% of patients in the first 20 years after diagnosis, an event usually associated with decrease in blood counts or refractoriness to immunosuppression. The prognosis of patients with MDS with chromosome 7 abnormalities is poor, whereas those with trisomy 8 can respond to cyclosporine therapy.

> **Key points**
>
> - Allogeneic stem cell transplantation from a matched sibling donor is the treatment of choice for patients with severe AA who are <20 years old.
> - For older patients, those without sibling donors, and those who refuse transplantation, immunosuppression with ATG/cyclosporine combination should be initiated as soon as possible once the diagnostic workup is completed.
> - In patients without matched sibling donors, regardless of age, ATG/cyclosporine may constitute the initial treatment.
> - Matched unrelated donor transplantation may be considered for refractory patients, but survival is poorer than for sibling donor transplantation.
> - The combination of ATG and cyclosporine is more effective than single-agent immunosuppression in severe AA.
> - Relapses are common, especially after cyclosporine is discontinued, but often respond well to reinstitution of immunosuppressive therapy.
> - Repeated courses of ATG/cyclosporine may be given to refractory patients, resulting in a salvage rate of approximately 35%.
> - There is an increased incidence of late clonal disorders (eg, PNH, MDS, AML) in AA patients treated with immunosuppression.

> **Clinical case (continued)**
>
> Based on the existing data, the recommended treatment of the 19-year-old student with AA presented in the earlier clinical case is transplantation from an HLA-matched sibling, provided chromosome fragility testing is normal. Transplantation would still be indicated if the patient proved to have FA; however, it is important to use a modified conditioning regimen in such individuals. In the absence of a matched sibling donor, immunosuppression with the combination of ATG and cyclosporine is the treatment of choice, followed by transplantation from a matched unrelated donor if the patient fails to respond to immunosuppression.

Paroxysmal nocturnal hemoglobinuria

Clinical case

A previously healthy 37-year-old woman is admitted to the hospital for evaluation of severe midabdominal pain. Evaluation reveals an acute mesenteric vein thrombosis. The patient is treated with thrombolytic therapy and heparin, leading to clinical improvement. She has no prior or family history of thrombosis. She is currently taking an oral contraceptive. Her examination is significant for mild scleral icterus and jaundice. There is no abdominal tenderness. Mild splenomegaly is noted. Laboratory studies are significant for a hematocrit of 32% with a corrected reticulocyte count of 8%. The absolute neutrophil count and platelet count are slightly depressed. Indirect bilirubin is elevated at 4 mg/dL, but aspartate aminotransferase (AST), alanine aminotransferase (ALT), and alkaline phosphatase are normal. LDH is also increased at 1024 U/L. Blood bank evaluation confirms a Coombs-negative hemolytic anemia. Testing for inherited prothrombotic diatheses such as factor V Leiden and the prothrombin 20210 A>G mutation is unrevealing, homocysteine level is normal, and antiphospholipid antibodies are not detected.

Definition

PNH is a clonal bone marrow failure disorder due to a somatic mutation in the *PIGA* gene in HSCs, which results in failure to synthesize the glycophosphatidylinositol (GPI) anchor. The consequence of failure to synthesize this anchor is deficiency of all GPI-anchored proteins on the surface of progeny cells of all hematopoietic lineages derived from the affected stem cell (Figure 15-5).

Clinically, PNH is characterized by a triad:
- Intravascular hemolysis
- Thrombophilia
- Bone marrow failure

Pathophysiology

There are 2 classes of cell membrane–associated proteins: transmembrane proteins and GPI-anchored proteins. In PNH, due to the defect of the enzyme encoded by the mutant *PIGA* gene, the first step in biosynthesis of the GPI anchor cannot be completed, and all GPI-anchored proteins are absent in the membrane of affected cells. Abnormalities in the

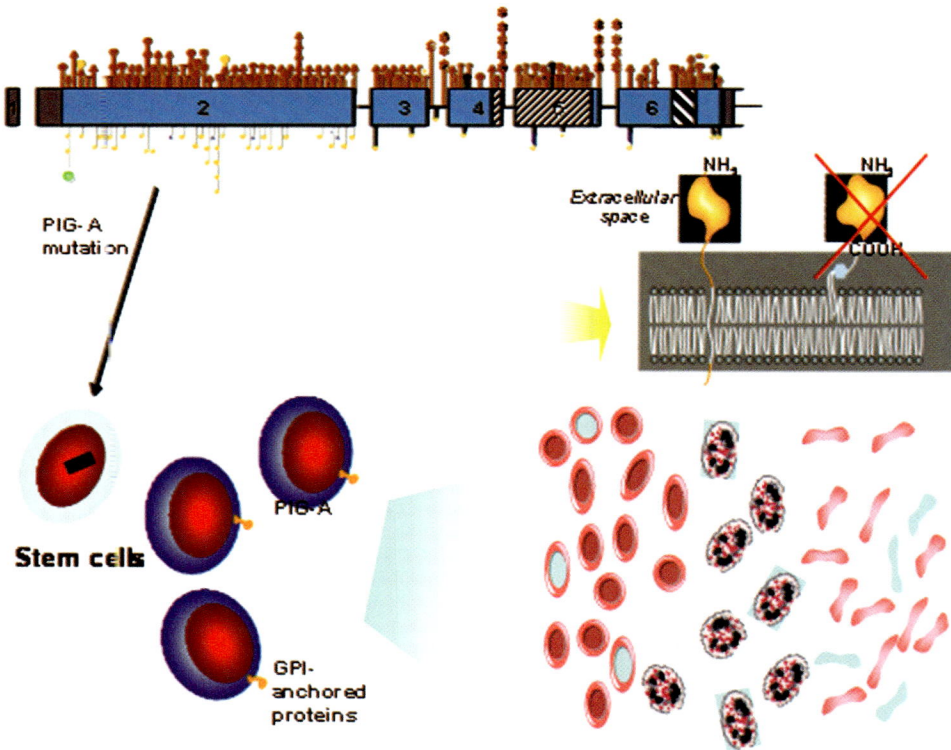

Figure 15-5 Pathogenesis of paroxysmal nocturnal hemoglobinuria (PNH). In hematopoietic stem cells, acquired somatic mutations of the *PIGA* gene may occur. Mutations occur across the gene and without a specific hot spot. Such mutations can decrease the function or totally inactivate the enzyme encoded by *PIGA*, which controls the key step in the biosynthesis of glycophosphatidylinositol (GPI) in the lip anchor of the GPI-linked class of membrane proteins. As a consequence, all proteins using this type of anchor are deficient from the membrane of affected progeny derived from the mutant stem cells. With the expansion of PNH clone, presumably because the clone can evade an aberrant immune response, the contribution of normal stem cells to blood cell production decreases.

PIGA gene identified in patients with PNH include deletions; insertions; and missense, nonsense, and splice site mutations. *PIGA* mutations have been found in asymptomatic individuals, and patients with PNH may harbor multiple clones with distinct *PIGA* mutations. The relative size of the PNH clone measured by the flow cytometry correlates generally with the severity of disease. Although there are many GPI-anchored proteins with diverse functions, it is hypothesized that symptoms of PNH are related to the deficiency of specific GPI-linked proteins, such as those that protect cells from complement-mediated lysis (Figure 15-6).

Hemolysis

Intravascular hemolysis in PNH is due to the lack of decay-accelerating factor (DAF; CD55) and membrane inhibitor of reactive lysis (MIRL; CD59), proteins that attenuate complement activation on the surface of erythrocytes. Depending on the type of mutation in the *PIGA* gene, various degrees of CD59 and CD55 deficiency can occur. Patients with PNH may have in their circulation an admixture of normal complement-resistant red blood cells (so-called PNH I cells), as well as mildly (PNH II) or markedly (PNH III) abnormal complement-sensitive cells. The difference in the proportion of these red blood cell populations contributes to the variability in intravascular hemolysis between patients and in an individual patient over time. The enhanced hemolysis observed during infections can be accounted for by increased complement activation on the red bllod cell surface.

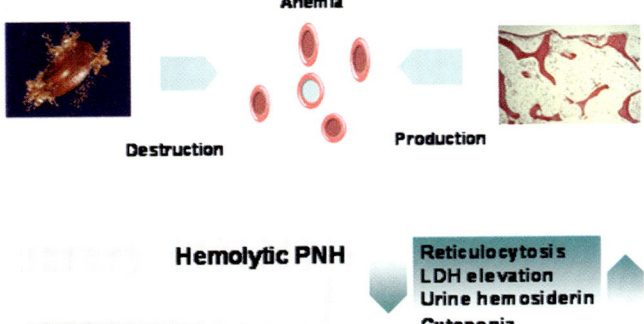

Figure 15-6 Pathogenesis of paroxysmal nocturnal hemoglobinuria (PNH)–associated anemia. Anemia in PNH can be a result of increased red blood cell (RBC) destruction due to intravascular hemolysis of glycophosphatidylinositol (GPI)-deficient RBCs, decreased production of RBCs due to immune-mediated bone marrow failure, or a combination of these 2 mechanisms. Hemolysis can be compensated for by increased production (patients with increased reticulocytes), or compensation may be inadequate (patients with low reticulocyte counts). Hemolytic PNH can develop from aplastic anemia (AA) or myelodysplastic syndrome (eg, AA/PNH syndrome), or it can be a primary disease.
LDH = lactate dehydrogenase

Thrombosis

Several theories have been postulated to account for the hypercoagulability observed in PNH patients, but the mechanism has not been clearly defined. It is believed that thrombophilia is related to the degree of hemolysis and thereby indirectly to the size of PNH clone. Possible prothrombotic pathways include platelet activation by complement components, procoaguable microparticles derived from GPI-deficient erythrocytes, lack of GPI-anchored urokinase plasminogen activator receptor, slowing of the microcirculation due to vasoconstriction induced by products of hemolysis, and deficiency of proteinase 3 that is normally displayed on neutrophils via GPI-anchored CD177. It has also been suggested that intravascular hemolysis exposes red blood cell phospholipids that may serve to initiate coagulation.

Bone marrow failure and evolution of PNH

PNH clones evolve only in the context of immune-mediated bone marrow failure, explaining the close association between AA and PNH. According to the most predominant hypothesis, PNH stem cells, which can be found in very low frequencies in healthy individuals, have a selective advantage in certain circumstances of immune dysregulation. Under conditions of T-cell–mediated immune attack on HSCs, GPI-deficient stem cells appear to enjoy selective survival advantage compared with healthy stem cells, which facilitates their expansion. The molecular nature of this growth advantage has not been clarified but is likely related to a deficiency of certain immunomodulatory GPI-anchored proteins from the surface of PNH stem cells. This close association between immune-mediated depletion of normal stem and progenitor cells explains the coexistence of hematopoietic failure and frequent cytopenias related to impaired blood cell production.

> **Key points**
> - PNH is an acquired clonal HSC disorder characterized by deficiency of GPI-linked proteins in blood and bone marrow cells due to a somatic mutation in the *PIGA* gene.
> - Patients may experience chronic hemolytic anemia, cytopenias, or a thrombotic tendency.
> - Flow cytometric techniques to identify cell populations lacking GPI-linked proteins have replaced the Ham and sucrose lysis tests and can be used to estimate the size of PNH clone.
> - Bone marrow failure often precedes or follows clinical PNH, and AA is frequently associated with the presence of PNH clones.

Laboratory findings and diagnosis

In patients with frank hemolytic PNH, macrocytic anemia is typically present, but some patients with iron deficiency due to urinary iron losses may have microcytic red blood cell indices. In the absence of hematopoietic suppression, patients will show high reticulocyte counts, contributing to the macrocytosis. Elevated LDH and absent haptoglobin together with urine hemosiderin indicate the presence of intravascular hemolysis. Patients with PNH who do not receive transfusions develop various degrees of iron deficiency anemia over time. Various degrees of thrombocytopenia and neutropenia may be present in patients with AA overlap syndromes. The bone marrow shows relative expansion of erythroid series and is most often hypercellular.

The laboratory diagnosis of PNH formerly relied on the demonstration of abnormally complement-sensitive erythrocyte populations. Thomas Hale Ham first described the acidified serum lysis test in 1938. In that test, acidification of the serum activates the alternative pathway of complement, and increased amounts of C3 are fixed to red blood cells lacking complement regulatory proteins. Complement sensitivity of PNH red blood cells can also be demonstrated in high-concentration sucrose solutions, which is the basis for the "sugar water" or sucrose lysis test. These 2 tests are primarily of historical interest because they lack sensitivity; in the presence of significant hemolysis, PNH clones can be missed.

Currently, the diagnosis of PNH is secured by flow cytometry, in which the percentage of circulating granulocytes deficient in GPI-anchored proteins is assayed. PNH granulocytes are defined by the absence of 2 otherwise constitutive GPI-anchored proteins, such as CD55, CD59, CD66b, or CD16. Flow cytometric methods are very sensitive and can detect even small PNH clones that are of unclear clinical significance. Recently, an exceptionally sensitive flow cytometric assay that makes use of fluorescent-labeled aerolysin (a toxin with high affinity for the GPI anchor) has been developed (FLAER assay).

Clinical manifestations

Chronic hemolytic anemia of various degrees is the most common manifestation of PNH. Despite the name of the disease, hemoglobinuria with dark-stained urine is reported by only a minority of patients; this symptom correlates with the size of the PNH clone. Symptoms related to episodes of hemolysis include back and abdominal pain, headache, esophageal spasm, and fever. Exacerbations of hemolysis can occur with infections, surgery, or transfusions and manifest as acute worsening of anemia. If severe, hemolysis can result in acute renal failure. Icterus is often present intermittently and typically worsens during hemolytic exacerbations. Reported fatigue is worse than expected from the degree of anemia and has been hypothesized to be related to impaired microcirculation due to microthrombi or vasoconstriction associated with hemolysis. In the presence of coexistent bone marrow failure, reticulocytosis may be absent, and patients may display various degrees of pancytopenia.

Some patients may initially present with thrombotic complications, including mesenteric, hepatic, or splenic vein clots, or cerebral sinus thrombosis. In some patients, anemia may be mild and well compensated, and a diagnosis of PNH requires a high index of suspicion. PNH can be associated with Budd-Chiari syndrome, and a diagnosis of PNH is often missed in this setting. For unclear reasons, thrombotic complications are less common in PNH patients of Asian descent. The thrombotic propensity is particularly enhanced during pregnancy.

Conceptually, PNH can be classified as follows:
- Primary hemolytic PNH
- Secondary hemolytic PNH (history of antecedent AA)
- AA/PNH syndrome (ie, coexistence of a sizable PNH clone and bone marrow failure)
- Small PNH clones detected in the context of otherwise typical AA or MDS, which are of uncertain significance but should be monitored because they can expand and come to dominate the clinical picture

Treatment

Except for allogeneic stem cell transplantation, there are no curative treatments for PNH, but long-term remissions are possible. The variability in the clinical manifestations of PNH makes it necessary to individualize the treatment plan.

Anemia is often the dominant issue to be addressed. Anemia due to hemolysis should be distinguished from bone marrow failure–related anemia. Chronic hemolysis should be treated with supportive measures such as supplementation of folate and iron and, in the context of renal failure, recombinant erythropoietin administration. Some patient may benefit from low-dose or alternating doses of prednisone or androgenic steroids.

Acute hemolytic attacks may require hydration, increased doses of corticosteroids, and transfusions. Recently, a humanized monoclonal antibody to the C5 terminal complement component, eculizumab, has shown efficacy in decreasing intravascular hemolysis, decreasing the need for transfusion, and improving the quality of life in patients with PNH. Eculizumab effectively stops hemolysis and alleviates the need for transfusions in >50% of patients. Treatment with eculizumab is associated with remarkably few complications, but because the terminal components of complement are important in protection from *Neisseria meningitis*, vaccination is important prior to initiation of eculizumab therapy. The decision about when to start eculizumab needs to take into consideration the degree of chronic hemolysis, frequency of acute hemolytic attacks, severity of constitutional symptoms, and frequency of transfusions—parameters that should be balanced against the need for chronic biweekly infusions and the high cost of the drug.

The clinician should have a high index of suspicion for thrombosis in patients with PNH who develop new symptoms potentially consistent with a clotting event. Conversely, patients who present with thrombotic complications in unusual sites should be investigated for the presence of PNH, especially if anemia is present. Thrombosis is a major source of morbidity and mortality in patients with PNH.

Once the diagnosis of a thrombosis is made, aggressive treatment is warranted. Thrombolytic therapy is effective in the management of hepatic vein thrombosis and should also be considered as an initial option for other major venous thrombotic events. The administration of heparin followed by chronic warfarin using standard approaches is recommended. Unless the patient undergoes therapy resulting in elimination of the PNH clone (as discussed later in this section), indefinite anticoagulant therapy should be considered for patients who have had a thrombotic event.

For the patient without thrombosis, prophylactic therapy is indicated for provocative clinical settings (eg, surgery and prolonged immobilization), as for other hypercoagulable conditions. A prospective study has also suggested that patients with a large PNH clone (PNH granulocytes >50%) and no contraindication to anticoagulation benefit with a substantial reduction of spontaneous thrombosis when given prophylactic warfarin. However, preventive anticoagulation of all PNH patients remains controversial; thrombotic complications occur in only approximately 30% of patients over a lifetime. In some patients, anticoagulation may not be possible due to the presence of thrombocytopenia.

Recently, eculizumab has been shown to decrease the rate of thrombosis, suggesting a close pathophysiologic link between hemolysis and thrombosis. However, it remains unclear whether patients receiving eculizumab may discontinue chronic anticoagulation that had been instituted after a thrombotic event.

The approach to bone marrow failure associated with PNH should be similar to that taken for severe AA. Immunosuppressive therapy with ATG/cyclosporine or cyclosporine alone can be effective in improving blood counts and allowing better compensation for hemolysis. However, immunosuppressive drugs other than corticosteroids are mostly ineffective in patients with purely hemolytic forms of PNH who have adequate marrow reserve.

Bone marrow transplantation appears to be the only curative therapy modality for PNH. Although only small series of PNH patients who have received transplantation have been published, the outcomes appear to be less favorable than in AA. Application of minimal-intensity transplantation may change this situation. Undisputed indications for bone marrow transplantation include the presence of severe bone marrow failure and intractable thrombotic events despite adequate anticoagulation.

Prognosis

The median survival time for patients with PNH is 10 to 15 years. Thrombotic events, progression to pancytopenia, and age >55 years at diagnosis are poor prognostic factors. The development of an MDS or acute leukemia markedly shortens survival. Patients without leukopenia, thrombocytopenia, or other complications can anticipate long-term survival.

Key points

- Steroid therapy and supportive measures can ameliorate the hemolytic anemia.
- Eculizumab, a monoclonal antibody against the C5 terminal complement component, effectively blocks hemolysis in patients with symptomatic PNH and alleviates the need for transfusions.
- Prompt evaluation of PNH patients is indicated when symptoms are suggestive of thrombosis because the risk of clotting is high.
- PNH can be a cryptic cause of unusual thrombotic events.
- Thrombotic complications of PNH require indefinite anticoagulation, which has been shown to decrease the rate of recurrent thrombosis.
- Treatment of bone marrow aplasia with immunosuppressive therapy will not eliminate the PNH clone and is generally ineffective in primary hemolytic PNH. However, immunosuppression may be helpful in patients with AA/PNH syndrome.
- Allogeneic hematopoietic cell transplantation has curative potential but is currently indicated only in patients with severe cytopenias and severe thrombotic complications.

Clinical case (continued)

The 37-year-old female patient described in the earlier clinical case likely has PNH, possibly related to an underlying bone marrow failure syndrome. The diagnosis can be confirmed by flow cytometry performed on peripheral blood red blood cells or, preferably, leukocytes, revealing a population of cells with absence of GPI-linked antigens. PNH may be diagnosed in association with other causes of bone marrow failure, such as AA or MDS. Treatment is aimed at the major clinical presentation; hemolysis may be controlled with corticosteroids or eculizumab. Thrombosis is treated with chronic anticoagulation. If pancytopenia is marked, immunosuppressive therapy, such as with ATG/cyclosporine, has been used with varying success. Stem cell transplantation has been performed in selected cases.

Myelodysplastic syndromes

> ### Clinical case
>
> A 78-year-old retired man with an unremarkable past medical history develops fatigue and shortness of breath with exertion. Physical examination demonstrates generalized pallor; splenomegaly and lymphadenopathy are absent. A complete blood count reveals a hemoglobin of 8.1 g/dL, white blood cell count of 2.9×10^9/L with 33% neutrophils, and a platelet count of 88×10^9/L. Vitamin B_{12} and folate levels are normal; the ferritin level is 348 ng/mL. Peripheral smear shows hypogranular, hypolobated neutrophils. The patient undergoes marrow aspiration and biopsy, which reveals a hypercellular marrow for age (80% cellularity) with erythroid hyperplasia, megaloblastoid erythroid maturation, reduced granulocyte progenitors, and abnormal dysplastic megakaryocytes. There are 8% undifferentiated blasts in the bone marrow, and the karyotype is 47, XY, +8, del(20)(q11q13).

Introduction and classification

MDS include a heterogeneous group of clonal, acquired disorders of ineffective hematopoiesis, characterized by peripheral blood cytopenias and a variable risk of progression to AML. Cases of MDS may arise de novo or may be secondary to exposure to DNA-damaging agents, such as alkylating drugs, ionizing radiation, or topoisomerase II inhibitors. Among the potential peripheral blood cytopenias, anemia (often macrocytic) is the most common. So-called *dysplastic* cell morphology (Figure 15-7; discussed further later) is diagnostically important, reflects failure of cells to differentiate and mature normally, and is often accompanied by cellular dysfunction that exacerbates the signs and symptoms of cytopenias (eg, hypogranular neutrophils with impaired bactericidal activity compound the infection risk associated with neutropenia). The bone marrow in MDS is usually hypercellular for age, but approximately 10% of cases are accompanied by a hypocellular marrow, and such cases may be difficult to distinguish from AA, as described earlier.

The current prevailing classification of MDS is the fourth edition of the World Health Organization (WHO) *Classification of Tumors of Hematopoietic and Lymphoid Tissues*, published in 2008 (Table 15-5). The 2008 WHO MDS classification is a minor modification of the third edition WHO classification formally published in 2001, which in turn was built on the 1982 MDS classification by the French-American-British (FAB) Cooperative Group. Important classification factors in the current WHO MDS schema include the specific cell lineages in which dysplasia is present, the marrow blast proportion, the presence of ring sideroblasts, and, to a limited extent, the presence of cytogenetic abnormalities, such as an interstitial deletion of the long arm of chromosome 5. By definition, MDS are associated with <20% marrow blasts. Treatment-related MDS (t-MDS) are grouped together with treatment-related AML (t-AML) by the WHO because the outcome in such patients is poor regardless of the blast count.

The natural history of MDS includes progression to treatment-refractory AML, but most patients with MDS do not develop AML. Instead, most patients who die from MDS suffer complications of cytopenias (eg, infection due to neutropenia and neutrophil dysfunction or bleeding due to thrombocytopenia and intrinsic platelet defects). Because MDS are primarily diseases of older persons, some patients succumb to unrelated conditions that are common in the elderly and die with MDS rather than from MDS.

Epidemiology and etiology

Aging is the most important risk factor for MDS; the median age at diagnosis is approximately 70 years. Overall, there is a slight male predominance that is possibly related to occupational exposures, but 1 specific MDS subtype, MDS associated with isolated deletion of the long arm of chromosome 5 and a specific marrow morphology including hypolobated megakaryocytes (*5q– syndrome*), is more common in women than in men.

MDS are rare in the pediatric age group and represent approximately 5% of hematologic malignancies in patients under age 18. When MDS do arise in children, they are frequently associated with Down syndrome or with congenital marrow failure syndromes and defects of DNA repair, such as those described at the beginning of this chapter. Children with Shwachman-Diamond syndrome, congenital neutropenia, or FA are all at markedly increased risk of developing MDS. In all of these inherited conditions, MDS arise in the context of hematopoietic deficits and typically present in late childhood or in adolescence. Children who develop MDS without excess blasts but who appear to lack a predisposing congenital syndrome are provisionally classified by the WHO as having *refractory cytopenia of childhood*.

Refractory anemia with excess blasts is also relatively common in children, and the bone marrow is often hypocellular rather than the hypercellular marrow characteristic of adults; there is also a high incidence of unfavorable biologic features such as monosomy 7. Refractory anemia with ring sideroblasts and 5q– syndrome are rare in children, although there are a number of forms of congenital sideroblastic anemia, such as those due to mutations of *ALAS2* or *ABCB7*, which do not carry a risk of progression to AML. MDS or AML with monosomy 7 has been reported in at least 10 families in

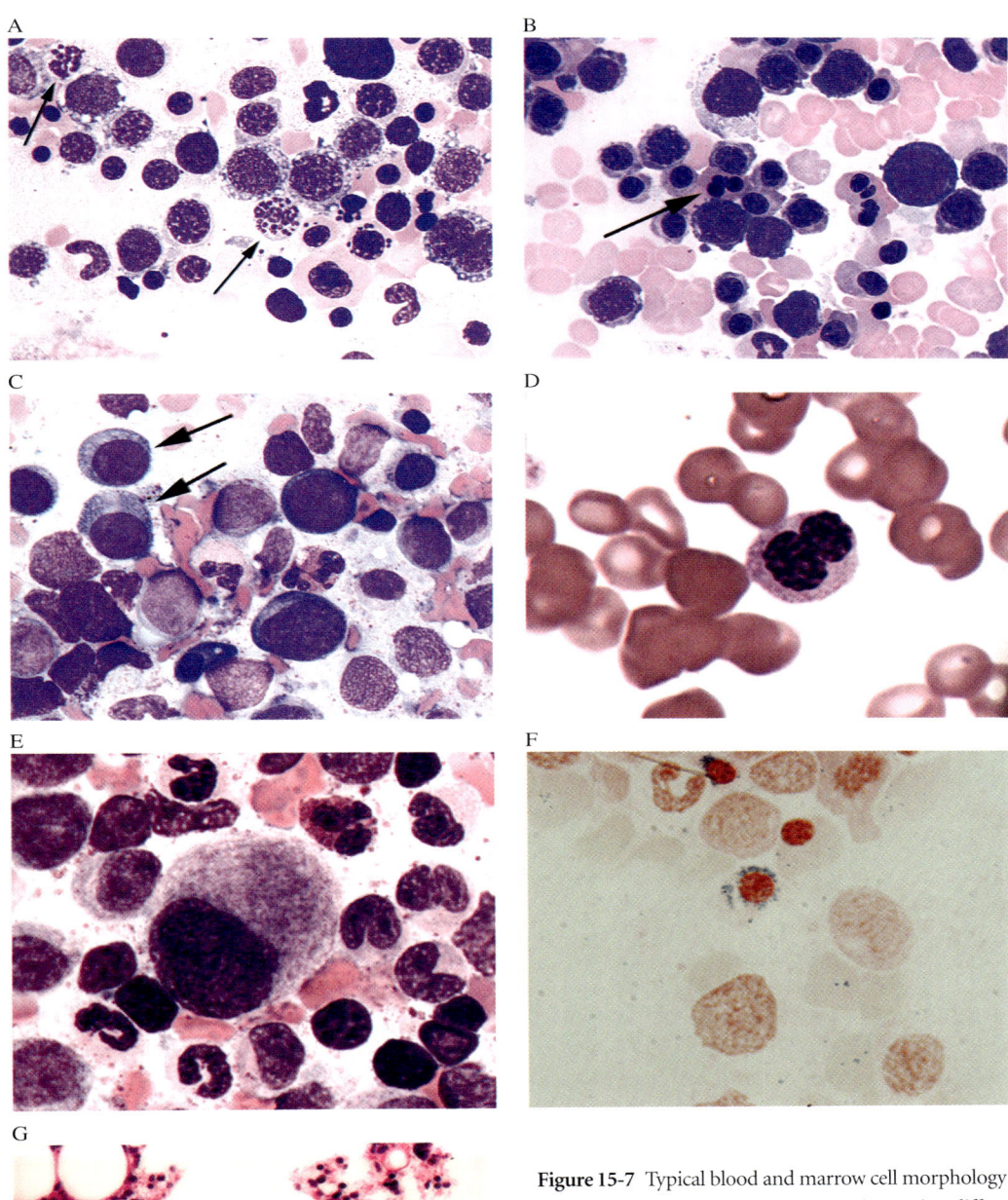

Figure 15-7 Typical blood and marrow cell morphology in patients with MDS. A and B, Multinuclear red blood cell precursors (*arrows*) at different stages of maturation. These cells are characteristic of MDS. Figure 15-7A source: ASH Image Bank (2006); doi: 10.1182/ashimagebank-2006-6-00038, Figure 1. Figure 15-7B source: ASH Image Bank (2006); doi: 10.1182/ashimagebank-2006-6-00037, Figure 7. C, Asynchronous maturation of erythroid cells (*arrows*). The chromatin pattern of these cells is fine, suggesting relative immaturity, whereas the lightening of the cytoplasm indicative of hemoglobinization is an event associated with later stages of maturation. Source: ASH Image Bank (2006); doi: 10.1182/ashimagebank-2006-6-00038, Figure 6. D, Hypolobated neutrophil (pseudo–Pelger-Huët cell) found in the peripheral blood of a patient with refractory anemia. Source: ASH Image Bank (2004); doi: 10.1182/ashimagebank-2004-101151. E, Micromegakaryocytes may have an eccentric, hypolobulated or round nucleus. Source: ASH Image Bank (2004); doi: 10.1182/ashimagebank-2004-101142. F, Ring sideroblast (a Prussian blue reaction on a marrow aspirate, seen at low power). Source: ASH Image Bank (2006); doi: 10.1182/ashimagebank-2006-6-00022. G, The bone marrow biopsy in this middle-aged woman with isolated del(5q) reveals a marrow that is normocellular with increased numbers of megakaryocytes that have hypolobulated nuclei (hematoxylin and eosin stain). Source: ASH Image Bank (2004); doi: 10.1182/ashimagebank-2004-101163.

Table 15-5 2008 World Health Organization (WHO) classification of myelodysplastic syndromes/neoplasms.

Name	Abbreviation	Peripheral blood: key features	Bone marrow: key features	WHO-estimated % of patients with MDS
Refractory cytopenias with unilineage dysplasia (RCUD)				
Refractory anemia	RA	Anemia; <1% blasts	Unilineage erythroid dysplasia (in ≥10% of cells); <5% blasts	10%–20%
Refractory neutropenia	RN	Neutropenia; <1% blasts	Unilineage granulocytic dysplasia; <5% blasts	<1%
Refractory thrombocytopenia	RT	Thrombocytopenia; <1% blasts	Unilineage megakaryocytic dysplasia; <5% blasts	<1%
Refractory anemia with ring sideroblasts	RARS	Anemia; no blasts	Unilineage erythroid dysplasia; ≥15% of erythroid precursors are ring sideroblasts; <5% blasts	3%–11%
Refractory cytopenias with multilineage dysplasia	RCMD	Cytopenia(s); <1% blasts; no Auer rods	Multilineage dysplasia ± ring sideroblasts; <5% blasts; no Auer rods	30%
Refractory anemia with excess blasts, type 1	RAEB-1	Cytopenia(s); <5% blasts; no Auer rods	Unilineage or multilineage dysplasia; 5%-9% blasts; no Auer rods	40%*
Refractory anemia with excess blasts, type 2	RAEB-2	Cytopenia(s); 5%–19% blasts; ± Auer rods	Unilineage or multilineage dysplasia; 10%-19% blasts; ± Auer rods	
Myelodysplastic syndrome (MDS) associated with isolated del(5q)	Del(5q)	Anemia; normal or high platelet count; <1% blasts	Isolated 5q31 chromosome deletion; anemia, hypolobated megakaryocytes	<5%
Childhood MDS, including refractory cytopenia of childhood (provisional)	RCC	Pancytopenia	<5% marrow blasts for RCC; marrow usually hypocellular	<1%
MDS, unclassifiable	MDS-U	Cytopenias; ≤1% blasts	Does not fit other categories; dysplasia; <5% blasts; if no dysplasia, MDS-associated karyotype	?

Note: If peripheral blood blasts are 2% to 4%, the diagnosis is RAEB-1 even if marrow blasts are <5%. If Auer rods are present, the WHO considers the diagnosis RAEB-2 if the blast proportion is <20% (even if <10%) or acute myeloid leukemia (AML) if ≥20% blasts. For all subtypes, peripheral blood monocytes are <1 × 10^9/L. Bicytopenia may be observed in RCUD subtypes, but pancytopenia with unilineage marrow dysplasia should be classified as MDS-U. Therapy-related MDS (t-MDS), whether due to alkylating agents, topoisomerase II inhibitors, or radiation, is classified together with therapy-related AML (t-MDS/t-AML) in the WHO classification of AML and precursor lesions. The listing in this table excludes MDS/myeloproliferative neoplasm overlap categories, such as chronic myelomonocytic leukemia, juvenile myelomonocytic leukemia, and the provisional entity RARS with thrombocytosis.
*This 40% figure represents the proportion of patients with RAEB-1 or RAEB-2, collectively.
From Swerdlow SH, Campo E, Harris NL, et al, eds. *WHO Classification of Tumours of Haematopoietic and Lymphoid Tissues.* 4th ed. Lyon, France: IARC Press; 2008:87–107.

the absence of either phenotypic abnormalities or any history of hematologic disorders. These kindreds typically include 2 or more affected children. Occasionally, bone marrow monosomy 7 is detected in an asymptomatic sibling with a normal physical examination and normal blood counts who is being evaluated as a possible donor for transplantation.

In most adult patients with MDS, the etiology is unknown, and there is no specific predisposing factor other than advanced age. Occupational exposure to organic solvents such as benzene is associated with the development of MDS, but such exposures rarely occur in the developed world. MDS can occur after treatment for another malignancy. The observation that alkylating agents and radiation predispose patients to both MDS and AML and the existence of shared cytogenetic abnormalities, such as deletions or gains in all or parts of chromosomes 5, 7, 8, or 20, imply a biologic continuum between MDS and AML. However, whereas loss or gain of chromosomal material is common in MDS, chromosomal translocations are less common. The good-risk AML-associated translocations, t(8;21), t(15;17), and inv(16), are extremely rare in patients with dysplasia, and the WHO classifies patients with these abnormalities as having AML regardless of the blast count.

> **Key points**
>
> - MDS are characterized by ineffective hematopoiesis, leading to peripheral blood cytopenias. The marrow is often hypercellular for age.
> - Aging and exposure to alkylating agents, topoisomerase II inhibitors, and ionizing radiation are risk factors for developing MDS.
> - MDS are rare in children, and when they occur, are often associated with congenital marrow failure syndromes.
> - The 2008 WHO classification of MDS is the current standard.

Diagnosis

After a thorough history and physical examination, diagnosis of MDS is readily established in most patients by a complete blood count, careful review of the peripheral blood smear, bone marrow examination, and basic laboratory tests to rule out other disorders. Vitamin B_{12} and folate deficiency, HIV infection, copper deficiency, alcohol abuse, and medication effects (eg, antimetabolites such as methotrexate) need to be excluded. The diagnosis of MDS is based primarily on morphologic criteria demonstrating dysplastic features in the peripheral blood and >10% of bone marrow precursors in 1 or more lineages (Figure 15-7).

In one large study, the median hemoglobin of patients diagnosed with MDS was 9.5 g/dL, and 75% of patients had a level <11 g/dL. Only 20% of patients had both a platelet count $>100 \times 10^9$/L and an absolute neutrophil count $>1.0 \times 10^9$/L, indicating that a presentation with anemia alone is relatively uncommon. Although patients with MDS often seek medical attention because of symptoms related to cytopenias, many are asymptomatic at diagnosis and are discovered because of a complete blood count performed to evaluate another condition.

Oval macrocytic red blood cells, hypogranular and hypolobulated granulocytes, and giant platelets can be identified in the peripheral blood of many patients with MDS. Peripheral blood smears may be highly suggestive of the diagnosis, but they are never conclusive by themselves. A bone marrow aspirate is mandatory to establish definitively a diagnosis of MDS, and the bone marrow core biopsy provides complementary information on cellularity and architecture, megakaryocyte morphology, and the presence of fibrosis—information that is important to complete the evaluation and informs therapeutic decisions.

The bone marrow biopsy usually demonstrates hypercellularity, which, in the setting of cytopenias in the peripheral blood, indicates ineffective hematopoiesis. On the marrow aspirate, megaloblastoid red blood cell precursors with asynchronous maturation of the nucleus and the cytoplasm are usually evident, and multinucleated erythroid precursors are common (Figure 15-7). Ring sideroblasts—erythroid precursors with iron-stuffed mitochondria surrounding at least one third of the nucleus—may be identified, and often there is predominance of immature myeloid cells and dysplastic granulocytic precursors. Megakaryocytes may be smaller than normal and may be hypolobated. Dysplastic features in all lineages can include nuclear and cytoplasmic blebs and misshapen nuclei.

Cytogenetic studies can further support a diagnosis of MDS, and specific aberrations correlate with prognosis and response to treatment (see Table 15-8). In a small percentage of cases, fluorescence in situ hybridization (FISH) analysis reveals specific chromosomal translocations and losses or gains of DNA segments that were not detected with standard cytogenetic methods. The clinical relevance of small clones detectable only by FISH is uncertain.

Flow cytometric analysis of the bone marrow, which is now a standard procedure for diagnosing and subclassifying patients with acute leukemia, is being used increasingly to evaluate patients suspected of having MDS. A number of investigative groups have described abnormal cell populations and inappropriate antigen expression detected by flow cytometry, but the diagnostic specificity of many of these findings remains uncertain. Because accurate classification according to WHO criteria is based, at least in part, on bone marrow morphology, flow cytometry should be viewed as a complementary test that is best interpreted in the context of the appearance of the marrow morphology. Specifically, flow cytometric enumeration of marrow blasts should not replace a manual differential from the marrow aspirate. The diagnosis of MDS is evolving toward the approach used in AML, in which morphologic, cytogenetic, and flow cytometric data are assessed together to make an accurate diagnosis and determine the optimal treatment. This strategy will become increasingly important as biologically distinct subsets of MDS patients who respond to specific therapies are defined.

> **Key points**
>
> - Complete blood counts, peripheral blood morphology, bone marrow aspirate and core biopsy, and cytogenetic testing are the keys to establishing a diagnosis of MDS.
> - Flow cytometry may provide complementary information but cannot be used to establish a diagnosis of MDS in the absence of marrow morphology.
> - Vitamin B_{12} and folate deficiency, HIV infection, copper deficiency, alcohol abuse, and medication effects (eg, antimetabolites such as methotrexate) can cause dysplastic changes in blood cells and need to be excluded.
> - Anemia is the most common cytopenia in patients with MDS.
> - Functional defects of neutrophils and platelets exacerbate the clinical problems associated with neutropenia and thrombocytopenia.

Table 15-6 The 1997 International Prognostic Scoring System (IPSS) for myelodysplastic syndromes.

Prognostic factor	Category Score (sum all 3 for overall IPSS score)				
	0 (best)	0.5	1	1.5	2 (worst)
Marrow blasts (%)	<5	5–10	–	11–20	21–30*
Karyotype	Good: normal, isolated –Y, isolated del(5q), or isolated del(20q)	Intermediate: all karyotypes not defined as good or poor	Poor: abnormal chromosome 7 or a complex karyotype (≥3 anomalies)	–	–
Peripheral blood cytopenias†	0 or 1	2 or 3	–	–	–

*No longer considered myelodysplastic syndrome (redefined as acute myeloid leukemia by World Health Organization in 2001).
†IPSS definition of peripheral blood cytopenias: hemoglobin <10 g/dL; absolute neutrophil count <1800/μL; and platelet count <100,000/μL.
From Greenberg P, Cox C, LeBeau MM, et al. International scoring system for evaluating prognosis in myelodysplastic syndromes. *Blood*. 1997;89:2079–2088.

Prognosis

The 1997 International Prognostic Scoring System (IPSS) (Tables 15-6 and 15-7) was developed to help stratify patients with MDS by their risk of disease progression to acute leukemia and death. The overall IPSS score is based on the sum of 3 subscores—subscores for the karyotype, percentage of bone marrow blasts, and number of cytopenias. Patients over age 60 with a low IPSS score have a median survival of 4.8 years, whereas patients with a high IPSS score have a median survival of only 4 months. Younger patients have better outcomes than older patients.

The IPSS differs from the WHO classification system in that it assigns patients with 21% to 30% blasts to the MDS category, whereas the WHO system defines 20% or more blasts as acute leukemia. A major limitation of the IPSS is that it does not distinguish between patients with severe and modest degrees of cytopenias, which may influence outcome. For example, a platelet count of $<10 \times 10^9/L$ is not weighted any differently by the IPSS than a count of $90 \times 10^9/L$, although several studies have shown that severe thrombocytopenia is an important risk factor for disease progression and death. The IPSS has also only been validated for patients with de novo disease treated with supportive care alone, and includes only a limited number of MDS-associated karyotypes. Despite these shortcomings, the IPSS has greater prognostic value than the WHO classification system for individual patients and remains widely used for clinical trial enrollment purposes.

Several newer MDS prognostic systems have been introduced since 2007, such as the WHO-based Prognostic Scoring System (WPSS), which integrates the WHO classification with karyotyping data and transfusion requirements; a modified form of the WPSS that includes the presence or absence of marrow fibrosis; and a general risk model proposed by investigators at the M.D. Anderson Cancer Center, which is valid across a broad spectrum of MDS patients, including those with exposure-related MDS and those who have been previously treated (eg, with a hypomethylating agent). These systems have some advantages over the IPSS but are not used universally. The IPSS is currently under revision and will likely incorporate features of these systems, as well as a broader range of cytogenetic abnormalities than the small subset included in the 1997 IPSS version.

Cytogenetics and molecular biology

Chromosome analysis provides strong evidence that MDS are clonal disorders. Approximately one half of patients with de novo MDS and most patients with secondary MDS have

Table 15-7 Risk stratification of International Prognostic Scoring System (IPSS).

Risk category	Total score	Median survival (years)	Median survival (years) for patients ≤60 years old (n = 205)	Median survival (years) for patients >60 years old (n = 611)	Time until 25% of surviving patients in category developed leukemia (years)
Low risk	0	5.7	11.8	4.8	9.4
Intermediate-1 (INT-1)	0.5 to 1.0	3.5	5.2	2.7	3.3
Intermediate-2 (INT-2)	1.5 to 2.0	1.2	1.8	1.1	1.1
High	≥2.5	0.4	0.3	0.5	0.2

Scoring system: A point value from 0 to 2.0 is determined for each of the 3 prognostic factors in Table 15-6, and the 3 values are summed to obtain the total IPSS score.
From Greenberg P, Cox C, LeBeau MM, et al. International scoring system for evaluating prognosis in myelodysplastic syndromes. *Blood*. 1997;89:2079–2088.

Table 15-8 Combined-database cytogenetic risk stratification system.

Risk group	Karyotypes (22 groups)	Median survival (months)	Time until 25% of patients developed AML (months)
Favorable	5q−, 12p−, 20q−, +21, −Y, 11q−, t(11(q23)), normal, any 2 abnormalities including 5q−	51	71.9
Intermediate-1	+1q, 3q21/q26 abnormalities, +8, t(7q), +19, −21, any other single abnormality, any double abnormality not including abnormalities of chromosomes 5q or 7	29	16
Intermediate-2	−X, −7 or 7q−, any double abnormality with −7 or 7q−, complex with 3 abnormalities	15.6	6
Unfavorable	Complex with >3 abnormalities	5.9	2.8

Derived by Haase D, et al, based on combined German-Austrian, Spanish Myelodysplastic Syndrome Registry, and International Myelodysplasia Risk Analysis Workshop cohorts. Univariate analysis. Data presented at the 10th International Myelodysplastic Syndrome Symposium, Patras, Greece, May 2009.
AML = acute myeloid leukemia.

cytogenetic abnormalities detectable on routine G-banded karyotyping. Cytogenetic results have independent prognostic significance (Table 15-8). New clonal cytogenetic aberrations emerge in 20% to 35% of patients with MDS during the course of their disease, which suggests genomic instability of some form, although microsatellite instability is not common.

One particular clonal abnormality involving interstitial or terminal deletion of part of the long arm of chromosome 5 (5q−) has received a great deal of attention in recent years because patients with deletions of chromosome 5q preferentially respond to lenalidomide therapy (see section on treatment). There is also new evidence that haploinsufficiency of a 5q-encoded ribosomal factor, RPS14, contributes to defective erythropoiesis, just as mutations of ribosomal components contribute to DBA (see earlier section on DBA). As originally described, the 5q− syndrome is associated with a refractory macrocytic anemia, normal or increased platelet count, giant thrombocytes, dyserythropoiesis, hypolobulated megakaryocytes, female predominance, prolonged survival, and a low rate of leukemic transformation. It is important to differentiate the 5q− syndrome from other myeloid disorders where the same deletion is found. Patients with the 5q− abnormality without the characteristic clinical and morphologic features of 5q− syndrome may have a more aggressive clinical course and shorter survival, although they may still respond to lenalidomide treatment.

The clinical and genetic heterogeneity found in MDS and the typical advanced age at disease onset support the idea that multiple cooperating genetic lesions contribute to leukemogenesis. However, it has been difficult to uncover the mutations that initiate MDS or to identify processes in addition to defective apoptosis (see "Cell Biology," below) that contribute to disease evolution. Unlike AML and myeloproliferative neoplasms (MPNs), which frequently demonstrate chromosomal translocations, gains and losses of entire chromosomes (eg, monosomy 5 and 7 or trisomy 8) or of large DNA segments (eg, many mega base pairs of chromosomes 5q, 7q, 13q, or 20q) are more common in MDS, which has made pinpointing individual genes that contribute to the development or progression of MDS a formidable challenge.

Activating mutations in proto-oncogenes such as NRAS, FLT3, and JAK2 are detected in many cases of AML or MPN but are uncommon in MDS. Although RAS mutations are common in the MDS-MPN overlap syndromes of chronic myelomonocytic leukemia and juvenile myelomonocytic leukemia (discussed in Chapter 14), these mutations are rare in MDS without MPN features and are usually found only after progression to acute leukemia. These data suggest that aberrant activation of signal transduction pathways may not be a major mechanism of aberrant cell growth in MDS, which distinguishes these diseases from other myeloid malignancies.

By contrast, the TP53 tumor suppressor gene, which regulates cell cycle progression, DNA repair, and apoptosis, is mutated in 5% to 10% of MDS cases, especially t-MDS. RUNX1 point mutations are also relatively common in patients with secondary t-MDS. Recently, TET2 mutations were described in approximately 25% of patients with MDS.

Patients who develop MDS secondary to exposure to mutagenic or carcinogenic agents have similar findings in terms of the types and significance of the chromosomal abnormalities. t-MDS is usually associated with previous treatment with alkylating agents or exposure to ionizing radiation, and these cases frequently demonstrate losses involving chromosomes 5 or 7. The latency period for t-MDS arising after alkylating agent therapy is typically 3 to 7 years. Patients treated with epipodophyllotoxins (eg, etoposide) can develop specific translocations involving the breakpoint at 11q23; the latency period is typically 1 to 3 years. These 11q23 translocations lead to transcription of a fusion protein involving the mixed lineage leukemia (*MLL*) gene. Translocations and inversions of 3q21/3q26 can also arise after etoposide treatment and involve rearrangement of the *MDS1-EVI1* genes. Such patients usually have a normal or elevated platelet count.

In patients with MDS who have a normal karyotype, more sensitive analytical techniques such as single nucleotide polymorphism arrays and array-based comparative genomic hybridization frequently detect areas of loss of heterozygosity and uniparental disomy, which are often clonally restricted (ie, not present in germline tissue). Such techniques have highlighted the diversity of MDS and may help better define the molecular biology of MDS in the years to come.

> **Key points**
>
> - One half of patients with de novo MDS and most patients with secondary, t-MDS have a clonal cytogenetic abnormality.
> - 5q– syndrome has a relatively benign prognosis, but not all patients with del(5q) have 5q– syndrome.
> - Patients with t-MDS who have been exposed to alkylating agents or ionizing radiation usually have abnormalities of chromosomes 5 and 7, whereas those who have been exposed to epipodophyllotoxins usually have abnormalities of chromosome 11q23.
> - Despite the frequency of chromosomal abnormalities, little is known about the molecular biology of MDS.

Cell biology

A major challenge in unraveling the complex pathogenesis of MDS is distinguishing primary events from secondary effects of specific initiating mutations within HSCs/progenitor cells or the marrow microenvironment. As noted previously, this is particularly challenging because the critical genetic lesions that initiate MDS are largely unknown except in rare familial syndromes.

MDS arises from clonal expansion of multipotent or pluripotent HSCs/progenitor cells. Most studies of adults with MDS have shown that ineffective hematopoiesis, as opposed to a lack of hematopoietic activity as in AA, is the major factor contributing to pancytopenia in MDS. Abnormal responses to cytokine growth factors, impaired cell survival, and defects in the bone marrow microenvironment are all implicated in the pathogenesis of MDS.

Analysis of X-linked polymorphisms and other molecular techniques indicate that the malignant clone in MDS includes $CD34^+$ cells and differentiated myeloid, erythroid, and megakaryocytic cells. The B-cell lineage may also be involved, which may partially explain the immunologic disorders identified in some patients. Cell culture studies have shown reduced growth of multilineage colony-forming unit (CFU)–granulocyte-erythroid-monocyte-megakaryocyte progenitors and of lineage-restricted burst-forming unit–erythroid, CFU–erythroid, CFU–granulocyte-macrophage, and CFU–megakaryocyte progenitors. These abnormalities in the progenitor compartment likely contribute to the development of peripheral blood cytopenias and might underlie the responses of some patients to pharmacologic doses of hematopoietic growth factors.

Experimental evidence implicates inhibitory cytokines and increased apoptosis as contributors to ineffective hematopoiesis in early MDS. Death receptor ligand binding may contribute to excessive apoptosis of hematopoietic precursors, resulting in ineffective hematopoiesis. For example, in several studies, bone marrow cells from patients with MDS demonstrated increased expression of Fas and Fas ligand or of TNFα and its receptors. In marrow cultures, strategies that block TNFα-mediated signals, such as the use of anti-TNFα antibodies, significantly increase the numbers of hematopoietic colonies compared with untreated cells. Increased apoptosis has been identified in both mature cells and immature $CD34^+$ cells from patients with lower risk MDS, compared with healthy controls and patients with higher risk MDS or de novo AML. In patients with higher-risk MDS or AML, cell survival signals dominate.

Several studies have suggested that the bone marrow microenvironment is abnormal in MDS. The growth of stromal progenitors is defective with reduced colony growth and failure of cultures to grow to confluence. Furthermore, stromal support of the growth and maturation of normal hematopoietic progenitors is also impaired, consistent with a functional defect. Stromal cells may also play an important role in the development and maintenance of abnormal signaling networks mediated by TNFα, Fas, and other soluble factors.

> **Key points**
>
> - MDS is clonal disorder that arises in HSCs/progenitor cells and affects the entire myeloid compartment. The heterogeneous nature of MDS and the advanced age at disease onset infer the existence of multiple cooperating genetic lesions.
> - Both the "soil" (microenvironment) and the "seed" (hematopoietic progenitor cells) may be abnormal in MDS, contributing to failed hematopoiesis.
> - Abnormal responses to cytokine growth factors, impaired cell survival/excessive apoptosis, and defects in the bone marrow microenvironment are all implicated in the pathogenesis of MDS.

Hypocellular MDS

Some patients with MDS have a hypocellular marrow resembling AA. Factors used to differentiate MDS from AA include morphologic evidence of dysplasia and an abnormal karyotype, both of which would be more consistent with MDS than AA (Figure 15-4). Given the subjectivity of the histologic criteria and the presence of transient chromosomal abnormalities in some patients with AA, however, differentiating these 2 disorders can be difficult. Although clinical characteristics and prognosis of hypocellular MDS do not appear significantly different than the more typical hypercellular MDS, recent evidence has shown that a subgroup of these hypocellular MDS patients may respond to immunosuppressive therapy, as described later.

Idiopathic cytopenias of undetermined significance

Some patients present with cytopenias and nondiagnostic bone marrow findings (ie, minimal or no dysplastic changes and no increase in marrow myeloblasts) and without any cytogenetic abnormalities—a situation where MDS is a diagnostic possibility and an alternative diagnosis is often not apparent, yet WHO-defined diagnostic criteria for MDS are not met. Such patients have been termed as having *idiopathic cytopenias of undetermined significance* (ICUS). Close observation is recommended. Some patients with ICUS will develop overt MDS over time, whereas others will be stable for a prolonged period, with or without complications from the cytopenias.

A related situation is when patients have cytopenias and a nondiagnostic bone marrow, yet a clonal cytogenetic abnormality typical for MDS [eg, del(5q)] is present. The clinical behavior of such patients is typical for MDS, with a risk of death from cytopenias and progression to AML. In the 2008 version of the WHO classification of MDS, such patients with unremarkable morphology but an abnormal karyotype can now be considered as having MDS, unclassifiable subtype. However, certain MDS-associated karyotypes [eg, trisomy 8, del(20q), and loss of the Y chromosome] are not specific enough for MDS to define a case as MDS in the absence of dysplastic morphology.

Treatment of MDS

With the exception of allogeneic HSCT, no therapeutic options in MDS have demonstrated curative potential. However, 3 medications now have specific US Food and Drug Administration (FDA) approval for MDS-related indications (azacitidine, decitabine, and lenalidomide) and offer benefit to a subset of patients. Advanced age, the presence of comorbidities, and a lack of a suitable donor limit the availability of allogeneic HSCT, but use of reduced-intensity conditioning approaches and alternative stem cell sources (eg, umbilical cord blood) are expanding the roster of potentially eligible patients. Therefore, patients with MDS who are potentially candidates for transplantation should be evaluated early in the disease course by a physician with expertise in stem cell transplantation.

Goals of MDS therapy depend in part on the stage of disease and include symptom control, reduction of transfusion needs, delay of disease progression, and extension of survival. The IPSS classification and newer prognostic systems allow clinicians to incorporate risk factors, median survival, and the risk of progression into therapeutic decisions.

Supportive care: transfusions and iron chelation

Despite the availability of several active treatments for MDS, transfusion support remains a mainstay of therapy for many patients. Patients receiving red blood cell transfusions at least once every 8 weeks have a poorer survival than those who do not require regular transfusions, probably because a need for transfusions is a marker of more advanced hematopoietic failure and higher risk disease. In one study, lower risk patients with MDS who had a ferritin >1000 ng/mL had a poorer survival than lower risk MDS patients with a ferritin <1000 ng/mL, suggesting that transfusion-related iron overload might also be a contributing factor to poorer outcomes in transfusion-dependent patients.

Because the correlation between ferritin and iron burden is relatively poor and patients receiving transfusions develop iron overload at different rates, newer techniques for noninvasively measuring hepatic iron concentration, such as quantitative (R2*) magnetic resonance imaging may be useful in determining which patients are candidates for iron chelation. Consideration should be given to initiation of iron chelation therapy with parenteral deferoxamine or oral deferasirox in patients who have a reasonable life expectancy, are red blood cell transfusion dependent, and have evidence of tissue iron overload. However, no controlled prospective data support a survival benefit from iron chelation in MDS, and such therapy is costly and can have adverse effects. Platelet transfusions may also be necessary in some patients with MDS, but development of alloimmunization is problematic.

Growth factors

Hematopoietic growth factors have become an integral part of the treatment of MDS, despite the lack of a specific FDA-approved indication (which has implications for reimbursement). Growth factors may reduce the risk of infectious complications or transfusion requirements by improving peripheral blood counts, and these agents are generally well tolerated.

Studies with recombinant erythropoiesis-stimulating agents (ESAs; epoetin and darbepoetin) demonstrated erythroid response rates in the range of 10% to 40%. The combination of ESA and G-CSF may be more effective than treatment with ESA alone. No prospective studies have shown an alteration in survival with ESAs in MDS, although retrospective studies suggest that ESAs may improve survival in MDS.

A 2- to 3-month trial of an ESA is appropriate for anemic patients with serum erythropoietin levels <500 U/L; patients with serum erythropoietin levels >500 U/L only rarely respond, and patients who have heavy transfusion needs are less likely to respond than those who do not require transfusions.

Both G-CSF (filgrastim) and GM-CSF (sargramostim) have been evaluated in patients with MDS and increase the neutrophil count in up to 80% to 90% of patients, which may help in patients who have recurrent infections. Concerns regarding use of G-CSF and risk of leukemic transformation were addressed in a randomized controlled trial of 102 patients with high-risk MDS who were treated with either G-CSF or supportive care. No differences in frequency or time to progression to AML were seen between the 2 groups, but survival was shorter in patients with 5% to 19% blasts who received G-CSF. Pegfilgrastim has been associated with splenic rupture and leukemoid reactions in MDS and, if used, should be administered only with caution and started at low doses (eg, 1-2 mg, rather than the standard 6-mg vial).

The newer TPO receptor agonists romiplostim and eltrombopag are undergoing evaluation in patients with MDS-associated thrombocytopenia. In an early clinical trial of romiplostim in MDS, the platelet count improved in many patients, but a small number of patients developed circulating blast cells that disappeared after discontinuation of the study drug. This is a concern because some myeloblasts have functional TPO receptors; another concern is the possibility of development of marrow fibrosis with long-term use, because mice engineered to overexpress TPO develop a myelofibrosis-like picture. When romiplostim was used in pilot studies in combination with azacitidine, decitabine, or lenalidomide, development of circulating blasts was not observed. Thrombocytopenic patients who have bleeding from mucosal surfaces (eg, urinary bladder or gut) may benefit from careful use of the antifibrinolytic agent ε-aminocaproic acid.

Key points

- Transfusion support with leukocyte-depleted blood products is an integral part of supportive care for most patients with MDS; iron chelation may become necessary in carefully selected low-risk patients
- There are insufficient data to determine whether treating MDS patients with hematopoietic growth factors alters disease progression or survival.
- ESAs lead to a red blood cell response in approximately 20% to 30% of patients; adding G-CSF to ESAs can lead to red blood cell response in approximately 40% of patients.
- ESAs are less effective in patients with high serum erythropoietin levels (>500 U/L).
- TPO receptor agonists can raise the platelet count in some patients with MDS, but whether such agents increase the risk of AML progression is still being evaluated.

Hypomethylating agents

The cytidine residues in mammalian DNA can be methylated; DNA methylation is a dynamic process that affects transcription rates. Methylated cytidine residues cluster in so-called *cytosine-phosphate-guanine (CpG) islands*, which are located near the promoter regions of many genes. When these regions are hypermethylated, they are associated with gene silencing and represent a mechanism for regulating gene expression. DNA methyltransferase 1 (DNMT1) is the enzyme responsible for maintenance of cytidine methylation patterns, and the cytosine analogs azacitidine and decitabine can inhibit DNMT1, resulting in generalized hypomethylation of DNA and reversal of gene silencing. Although these so-called *epigenetic* changes occur in vitro in cells exposed to DNMT1 inhibitors, it is not clear whether these epigenetic effects are responsible for the clinical activity of azacitidine or decitabine in MDS or whether other biologic effects (eg DNA damage) also play a role.

Azacitidine is the first and, as of this writing, only medication that has been shown to improve survival in higher risk MDS patients. In a multicenter trial (AZA-001), 358 patients with IPSS intermediate-2 or high-risk MDS were randomized to receive either azacitidine 75 mg/m^2 subcutaneously for 7 consecutive days every 28 days or conventional care (ie, best supportive care, low-dose cytarabine, or AML-like chemotherapy with 7+3). The median survival time was 24 months in patients receiving azacitidine versus 15 months in patients receiving conventional care. Although the complete response rate in the azacitidine treated group was a modest 17%, subsequent analysis demonstrated that a complete response was not necessary for patients to achieve a survival benefit. Azacitidine is approved for intravenous administration and subcutaneous dosing. Intravenous administration avoids injection-site reactions, but the AZA-001 survival study used the subcutaneous regimen, and it is not clear whether the benefit is identical with intravenous dosing.

Decitabine is also active in MDS, but a European multicenter study designed to show a survival benefit was negative, possibly because a median of only 3 cycles of decitabine were administered, compared with 9 treatment cycles in the AZA-001 azacitidine survival study. Clinical response to hypomethylating agents may be delayed, and an adequate therapeutic trial of either agent requires at least 4 to 6 treatment cycles. Although the initial FDA approval of decitabine was for a regimen of 15 mg/m^2 administered every 8 hours for 9 doses intravenously (in a hospital-based setting), the most commonly used regimen in clinical practice is 20 mg/m^2 intravenously once daily for 5 consecutive days every 4 to 6 weeks. In a multicenter study of this 5-day decitabine regimen, 17% of patients achieved a complete response, 15%

achieved a marrow response, and 18% experienced hematologic improvement (similar to the response rates observed with azacitidine therapy).

The most common adverse events for both hypomethylating agents are neutropenia and thrombocytopenia, which often improve over time with continued treatment. The optimal maintenance dosing once patients achieve a response is unknown, but some maintenance therapy appears to be required to maintain responses. Thus far, no therapy has been demonstrated to improve survival for patients with lower risk MDS.

Histone deacetylase inhibitors

Histone deacetylase (HDAC) inhibitors are another therapeutic strategy for MDS that is also based on the principle of epigenetic modification. HDAC inhibitors are agents that maintain chromatin in a transcriptionally active state by inhibiting deacetylation of histone tails on chromatin. These agents lead to reversal of transcription repression and gene silencing in vitro. In vitro, HDAC inhibitors are synergistic in reactivating silenced genes when combined with hypomethylating agents. Several HDAC inhibitors are currently under clinical investigation in MDS and AML. These compounds appear to have limited activity as single agents in MDS but are being studied in combination with hypomethylating agents.

Immunomodulatory drugs

Thalidomide has multiple mechanisms of action, including alteration of immune cell subsets, inhibition of TNFα, and angiogenesis. When thalidomide was used in MDS, responses were seen in approximately 20% of patients, but the drug was difficult to tolerate (especially for elderly patients) due to sedation, constipation, peripheral neuropathy, and other adverse events.

Lenalidomide was generated by chemical modification of thalidomide and has an improved toxicity profile without the neurologic toxicity seen with thalidomide. Lenalidomide has more potent immunomodulatory, anti-TNFα, and anti–vascular endothelial growth factor effects than the parent compound. Lenalidomide was tested in a phase II trial in patients with IPSS low-risk or intermediate-1–risk disease who were red blood cell transfusion dependent and had a deletion of chromosome 5q31, either alone or in association with other chromosomal abnormalities. Of 148 patients enrolled, 67% achieved transfusion independence, with a median time to response of 4.6 weeks. The median increase in hemoglobin was 5.4 g/dL, and the median duration of response was >2 years. A major cytogenetic response (elimination of the clonal abnormality) occurred in 44% of patients. The major adverse effect was myelosuppression, with grade 3 to 4 neutropenia and thrombocytopenia seen in up to 55% of patients. These results led to the approval of lenalidomide by the FDA in 2005 for patients with del(5q) with IPSS low-risk or intermediate-1–risk disease who are red blood cell transfusion dependent. A second phase II trial was conducted in patients with the same eligibility who did not have del(5q). In this patient population, responses were less frequent and of shorter duration compared with those in patients with del(5q); 26% of patients became red blood cell transfusion independent, with a median response duration of 41 weeks.

Immunotherapy

Investigators have hypothesized that a T-cell–mediated process may contribute to the pancytopenia in some patients with MDS; therefore, immunosuppressive therapy, analogous to immunosuppressive treatment of AA, may be beneficial to some patients with MDS. ATG and cyclosporine have shown benefit in some patients with lower risk disease, especially those who are younger, lack transfusion dependence, and have either a normal karyotype or trisomy 8. Selection of patients most likely to respond to ATG/cyclosporine therapy remains challenging, because marrow hypocellularity and HLA-DRB15 positivity have predicted response to immunosuppressive therapy in some studies but not others.

> **Key points**
>
> - Azacitidine has been demonstrated to improve survival by a median of 9 months in patients with higher risk MDS. Decitabine, another hypomethylating cytosine analog, also produces responses in MDS. Both drugs are approved by the FDA for the treatment of MDS.
> - Azacitidine and decitabine induce DNA hypomethylation through the inhibition of DNMT1, but it is not clear whether this mechanism is responsible for the clinical effects.
> - Lenalidomide led to transfusion independence in 67% of patients with deletions of chromosome 5q, and some patients also achieved a cytogenetic remission.
> - Some patients with MDS respond to ATG or cyclosporine immunotherapy, but selecting the most appropriate patients for this therapy remains challenging. Younger patients and those with lower risk disease (ie, those who are not yet transfusion dependent or have required transfusions for only a short time) seem most likely to benefit.

Allogeneic HSCT

Allogeneic HSCT is the only routinely curative therapy in MDS, but <10% of patients are eligible for myeloablative HSCT due to age and comorbidities. Younger patients

(<40 years) with low disease burden may have a disease-free survival rate as high as 75% after an HLA-matched HSCT. However, patients with high IPSS scores or chemotherapy-resistant disease have survival rates as low as 30% after HSCT.

Allogeneic HSCT should be seriously considered for patients with higher risk MDS who have a matched sibling donor and a good performance status. Allogeneic transplantations performed from matched unrelated donors or umbilical cord blood are also a consideration in patients without a sibling donor. The use of reduced-intensity conditioning regimens may permit allogeneic HSCT in older individuals. This procedure remains investigational because long-term follow-up is not available.

Given the risks of allogeneic HSCT, defining the optimal time to refer patients for transplantation is an important consideration. One analysis indicated that performing transplantation in patients with lower risk disease (IPSS low and intermediate-1 risk) only at the time of progression of disease resulted in greater life expectancy than when HSCT was performed earlier in the course. In contrast, patients with higher risk disease (IPSS intermediate-2 and high risk) benefited from HSCT shortly after diagnosis. Unfortunately, disease relapse occurs in the majority of high-risk patients after HSCT and thus represents a continuing challenge. Strategies to reduce relapse rates are being studied and include pre- and posttransplantation interventions with novel therapies. No clear benefit has been shown for the administration of 1 or more courses of cytotoxic chemotherapy or hypomethylating agent therapy before HSCT, although pretransplantation therapy may be useful to reduce the burden of marrow blasts to <5% prior to the HSCT.

HSCT is the treatment of choice for children with MDS. It is imperative to perform a DEB test to exclude FA before performing a transplantation in a child with MDS because patients with FA suffer severe toxicity with conventional conditioning regimens. As mentioned earlier, although most children with FA have dysmorphic features, many do not. It is also important to exclude FA carefully in potential sibling donors. A bone marrow examination and cytogenetic testing should be performed on any related donor when the recipient is a child with bone marrow monosomy 7 because there are a number of instances in which an unsuspected clonal disorder has been detected in the prospective donor. Particular care must be exercised in determining the proper conditioning regimen and best time to perform HSCT in infants and young children due to the toxic effects of radiation on the developing central nervous system and because of differences in drug metabolism compared with older children and adults.

Key points

- Allogeneic HSCT remains the only routinely curative approach in MDS and is an important consideration if the patient is young, is otherwise healthy, and has an HLA-identical sibling or a matched unrelated donor.
- Reduced-intensity conditioning regimens are associated with a lower transplantation-related mortality but higher relapse rate in MDS; overall survival is similar with reduced-intensity and conventional myeloablative conditioning. Reduced-intensity conditioning regimens may permit HSCT to be performed in older and sicker patients.
- Transplantation at the time of progression for patients with lower risk disease and at the time of diagnosis for patients with higher risk disease yields the greatest life expectancy.
- HSCT is the treatment of choice for pediatric MDS; however, donors and recipients must be screened carefully to exclude familial disorders such as FA that would alter the management.

Clinical case (continued)

The patient's IPSS score is 1.5: 0.5 point for being pancytopenic, 0.5 point for an intermediate-risk karyotype, and 0.5 point for having a blast count between 5% and 10%. This places him in the IPSS intermediate-2 risk group, with an expected median survival of just over 1 year. The AZA-001 randomized trial demonstrated that IPSS intermediate-2– and high-risk patients gain a median survival benefit of 9 months from azacitidine, which would be an appropriate therapy in this situation. Unfortunately, the patient is too old to consider allogeneic HSCT using currently available approaches.

Bibliography

Inherited bone marrow syndromes

Alter BP. Diagnosis, genetics, and management of inherited bone marrow failure syndromes. *Hematology Am Soc Hematol Educ Program*. 2007:29–39. *An excellent general review of congenital marrow failure states.*

Bagby GC, Meyers G. Myelodysplasia and acute leukemia as late complications of marrow failure: future prospects for leukemia prevention. *Hematol Oncol Clin North Am*. 2009;23:361–376. *MDS and AML represent feared late complications of several inherited marrow failure states. This review summarizes what is currently known about clonal evolution of marrow failure.*

Dokal I, Vulliamy T. Inherited aplastic anaemias/bone marrow failure syndromes. *Blood Rev*. 2008;22:141–153. *Another excellent summary of the inherited marrow failure syndromes.*

Teo JT, Klaassen R, Fernandez CV, et al. Clinical and genetic analysis of unclassifiable inherited bone marrow failure syndromes. *Pediatrics*. 2008;122:e139–e148. *Some congenital marrow failure syndromes are difficult to fit into the framework presented in this chapter. This article discusses analysis of such cases.*

Fanconi anemia

Ameziane N, Errami A, Leveille F, et al. Genetic subtyping of Fanconi anemia by comprehensive mutation screening. *Hum Mutat.* 2008;29:159–166. *Now that FA has been linked to 13 different genes, the subtyping has become quite complex. This article nicely summarizes typing of FA.*

Rosenberg PS, Alter BP, Ebell W. Cancer risks in Fanconi anemia: findings from the German Fanconi Anemia Registry. *Haematologica.* 2008;93:511–517. *Patients with FA are at risk not only for MDS and AML but also for a number of solid tumors. This registry study summarizes the risk of cancer in FA.*

Diamond-Blackfan anemia

Ganapathi KA, Shimamura A. Ribosomal dysfunction and inherited marrow failure. *Br J Haematol.* 2008;141:376–387. *DBA appears to be due primarily to defective ribogenesis. This article discusses the contribution of ribosomal failure to DBA and potential role in other syndromes.*

Congenital dyserythropoietic anemia

Iolascon A, Delaunay J. Close to unraveling the secrets of congenital dyserythropoietic anemia types I and II. *Haematologica.* 2009;94:599–602. *An editorial that crisply summarizes contemporary understanding of the molecular biology of CDA types I and II.*

Renella R, Wood WG. The congenital dyserythropoietic anemias. *Hematol Oncol Clin North Am.* 2009;23:283–306. *A comprehensive and highly readable review of the current state of knowledge about CDA.*

Dyskeratosis congenita

Alter BP, Giri N, Savage SA, Rosenberg PS. Cancer in dyskeratosis congenita. *Blood.* 2009;113:6549–6557. *A detailed review of the risk of cancer development in DC.*

Savage SA, Alter BP. Dyskeratosis congenita. *Hematol Oncol Clin North Am.* 2009;23:215–231. *Thorough and very readable review of the various molecular and clinical aspects of DC.*

Congenital amegakaryocytic thrombocytopenia

Ballmaier M, Germeshausen M. Advances in the understanding of congenital amegakaryocytic thrombocytopenia. *Br J Haematol.* 2009;146:3–13. *A nice summary of the current state of knowledge in CAMT.*

Aplastic anemia

Brodsky RA, Jones RJ. Aplastic anaemia. *Lancet.* 2005;365:1647–1656. *An excellent recent general review of AA.*

Brown KE, Tisdale J, Barrett AJ, et al. Hepatitis associated aplastic anemia. *N Engl J Med.* 1997;336:1059–1064. *Description of the clinical presentations, course, and response to treatment of hepatitis-associated AA.*

Calado RT, Young NS. Telomere maintenance and human bone marrow failure. *Blood.* 2008;111:4446–4455. *Review of the pathogenic role of telomerase complex mutations in AA.*

Gluckman E, Rokicka-Milewska R, Hann I, et al. Results and follow-up of a phase III randomized study of recombinant human-granulocyte stimulating factor as support for immunosuppressive therapy in patients with severe aplastic anaemia. European Group for Blood and Marrow Transplantation Working Party for Severe Aplastic Anemia. *Br J Haematol.* 2002;119:1075–1082. *A phase III study defining the role of the hematopoietic growth factor therapy in AA.*

Locasciulli A, Oneto R, Bacigalupo A, et al. Outcome of patients with acquired aplastic anemia given first line bone marrow transplantation or immunosuppressive treatment in the last decade: a report from the European Group for Blood and Marrow Transplantation (EBMT); Severe Aplastic Anemia Working Party of the European Blood and Marrow Transplant Group. *Haematologica.* 2007;92:11–18. *Describes current results of allogeneic bone marrow transplantation for AA contrasted with immunosuppressive therapy.*

Maciejewski JP, Risitano A, Sloand EM, Nunez O, Young NS. Distinct clinical outcomes for cytogenetic abnormalities evolving from aplastic anemia. *Blood.* 2002;99:3129–3135. *A study of the frequency and outcomes of MDS evolution in AA.*

Margolis DA, Casper JT. Alternative-donor hematopoietic stem-cell transplantation for severe aplastic anemia. *Semin Hematol.* 2000;37:43–55. *Review of unrelated donor transplantations for AA.*

Rosenfeld S, Follman D, Nunez O, et al. Antithymocyte globulin and cyclosporine for severe aplastic anemia. *JAMA.* 2003;289:1130–1135. *An update on the long-term outcome of a series of patients with AA treated with ATG and cyclosporine.*

Yamaguchi H, Calado RT, Ly H, et al. Mutations in TERT, the gene for telomerase reverse transcriptase, in aplastic anemia. *N Engl J Med.* 2005;352:1413–1424. *A study describing TERT mutations in patients with AA unresponsive to immunosuppressive therapy.*

Young NS, Calado RT, Scheinberg P. Current concepts in the pathophysiology and treatment of aplastic anemia. *Blood.* 2006;108:2509–2519. *A thoughtful review of immunosuppression versus HSCT.*

Paroxysmal nocturnal hemoglobinuria

Hill A, Richards SJ, Hillmen P. Recent developments in the understanding and management of paroxysmal nocturnal haemoglobinuria. *Br J Haematol.* 2007;137:181–192. *Review of current therapies for PNH.*

Parker C. Eculizumab for paroxysmal nocturnal haemoglobinuria. *Lancet.* 2009;373:759–767. *Current overview of the role of eculizumab in the therapy of PNH*

Parker C, Omine M, Richards S, et al; International PNH Interest Group. Diagnosis and management of paroxysmal nocturnal hemoglobinuria. *Blood.* 2005;106:3699–3709. *Comprehensive description of diagnostic and clinical aspects of PNH*

Young NS, Maciejewski JP. Genetic and environmental effects in paroxysmal nocturnal hemoglobinuria: this little PIG-A goes "Why? Why? Why?" *Clin Invest.* 2000;106:637–641. *Overview of the pathogenesis of PNH and its association with AA.*

Myelodysplastic syndromes
Classification, prognosis, and biology

Greenberg P, Cox C, LeBeau MM, et al. International scoring system for evaluating prognosis in myelodysplastic syndromes. *Blood.* 1997;89:2079–2088. *The original IPSS description, which is still the most commonly used prognostic system in MDS.*

Kantarjian H, O'Brien S, Ravandi F, et al. Proposal for a new risk model in myelodysplastic syndrome that accounts for events not considered in the original International Prognostic Scoring System. *Cancer.* 2008;113:1351–1361. *Description of the M.D. Anderson Cancer Center risk model for MDS, which, unlike the IPSS, is also valid for patients with secondary, t-MDS and patients with prior therapy for MDS. However, it is more complex than the IPSS.*

Malcovati L, Germing U, Kuendgen A, et al. Time-dependent prognostic scoring system for predicting survival and leukemic evolution in myelodysplastic syndromes. *J Clin Oncol.* 2007;25:3503–3510. *Description of the WPSS, which has some advantages over the IPSS.*

Mufti GJ. Pathobiology, classification, and diagnosis of myelodysplastic syndrome. *Best Pract Res Clin Haematol.* 2004;17:543–557. *A detailed review of the tantalizing clues to the still mysterious pathobiology of MDS.*

Niemeyer CM, Kratz CP. Paediatric myelodysplastic syndromes and juvenile myelomonocytic leukaemia: molecular classification and treatment options. *Br J Haematol.* 2008;140:610–624. *Pediatric MDS is distinct from adult MDS in a number of respects; this readable review summarizes current thinking on pediatric MDS and a related MDS-MPN overlap syndrome, juvenile myelomonocytic leukemia.*

Vardiman JW, Thiele J, Arber DA, et al. The 2008 revision of the WHO classification of myeloid neoplasms and acute leukemia: rationale and important changes. *Blood.* 2009;114:937–951. *Discussion of the specific changes and reasoning behind the latest WHO revision of MDS classification.*

Treatment

de Witte T, Oosterveld M, Muus P. Autologous and allogeneic stem cell transplantation for myelodysplastic syndrome. *Blood Rev.* 2007;21:49–59. *A contemporary review of transplantation outcomes in MDS.*

Fenaux P, Mufti GJ, Hellstrom-Lindberg E, et al. Efficacy of azacitidine compared with that of conventional care regimens in the treatment of higher-risk myelodysplastic syndromes: a randomised, open-label, phase III study. *Lancet Oncol.* 2009;10:223–232. *Azacitidine was the first agent shown to improve survival in patients with higher risk MDS. This report describes the AZA-001 clinical trial comparing azacitidine to conventional care.*

List A, Dewald G, Bennett J, et al. Lenalidomide in the myelodysplastic syndrome with chromosome 5q deletion. *N Engl J Med.* 2006;355:1456–1465. *Lenalidomide is very effective in patients with lower risk MDS and deletions of chromosome 5q31. This paper describes a 148-patient clinical trial of lenalidomide in 5q deletion MDS in which 67% of patients responded and no longer required transfusions.*

Moyo V, Lefebvre P, Duh MS, et al. Erythropoiesis-stimulating agents in the treatment of anemia in myelodysplastic syndromes: a meta-analysis. *Ann Hematol.* 2008;87:527–536. *A meta-analysis of trials of ESAs in MDS.*

Schiffer CA. Myelodysplasia: the good, the fair and the ugly. *Best Pract Res Clin Haematol.* 2007;20:49–55. *A pithy and refreshingly honest review of the current state of MDS therapy.*

Steensma DP. Myelodysplasia paranoia: iron as the new radon. *Leuk Res.* 2009;33:1158–1163. *A review of some of the controversy regarding the role of iron chelation in MDS.*

Steensma DP, Baer MR, Slack JL, et al. Multicenter study of decitabine administered daily for 5 days every 4 weeks to adults with myelodysplastic syndromes: the Alternative Dosing for Outpatient Treatment (ADOPT) Trial. *J Clin Oncol.* 2009;27:3842–3848. *This paper describes a multicenter trial of 1 of the 3 FDA-approved drugs for MDS, decitabine, using the 5-day outpatient regimen currently used by most hematologists using decitabine.*

CHAPTER 16

Acute myeloid leukemia

Gail J. Roboz and Lillian Sung

Definition and epidemiology, 475
Clinical manifestations, 475
Subtype classification, 476
Prognostic factors, 477
Treatment, 479
Monitoring residual disease, 480
AML relapse, 480
Older patients with AML, 481
Acute promyelocytic leukemia, 481
Pediatric AML, including Down syndrome, 483
Bibliography, 483

Definition and epidemiology

Acute myeloid leukemia (AML) is a heterogeneous clonal stem cell malignancy in which immature hematopoietic cells proliferate and accumulate in bone marrow, peripheral blood, and other tissues. This results in inhibition of normal hematopoiesis, characterized by neutropenia, anemia, thrombocytopenia, and the clinical features of bone marrow failure. AML comprises 90% of all acute leukemias in adults, with approximately 13,000 new cases and 9000 deaths in the United States in 2009. The annual incidence is approximately 3.5 per 100,000 and increases with age, with approximately a 10-fold increased risk between ages 30 (1 case per 100,000) and 65 years (1 case per 10,000). The median age at diagnosis is 67 years, with approximately 6% of patients <20 years old and 34% of patients ≥75 years old at diagnosis. Overall survival in adults remains poor, with <50% 5-year survival in patients under age 45 years and <5% in patients over age 65 years at diagnosis. In children, overall survival has improved to approximately 50% to 60%.

Most cases of AML have no apparent cause. Risk factors associated with increased incidence include exposure to chemotherapy (especially topoisomerase II inhibitors and alkylating agents), benzene, and ionizing radiation; inherited bone marrow failure syndromes (eg, Fanconi anemia, Shwachman-Diamond syndrome, severe congenital neutropenia); and genetic disorders (eg, Down syndrome). Therapy-related AML (t-AML) accounts for approximately 10% to 20% of all AML cases. Those that arise after exposure to alkylating agents or radiation therapy have increased incidence with age, typically have a 5- to 10-year latency period, and are frequently associated with an antecedent therapy-related myelodysplastic syndrome (MDS) and unbalanced loss of genetic material involving chromosomes 5 and/or 7. t-AML associated with exposure to topoisomerase II inhibitors encompasses 20% to 30% of patients, has a shorter latency period of 1 to 5 years, is less often preceded by a myelodysplastic phase, and may be associated with balanced recurrent chromosomal translocations involving 11q23 (*MLL*) or 21q22 (*RUNX1*). Patients with MDS and myeloproliferative disorders are also at increased risk for developing AML and have poor treatment outcomes.

Clinical manifestations

Patients with AML generally present with nonspecific signs and symptoms related to infiltration of the bone marrow with leukemic blasts, including pallor, anemia, fatigue, bone pain, hepatosplenomegaly, shortness of breath, fever, infection, bruising, and bleeding. Tissue infiltration of the skin, gingiva, and central nervous system is more common with monocytic subtypes. Patients with leukocytosis and leukemic blasts >50,000/mL are at increased risk of pulmonary and central nervous system complications from leukostasis caused by leukemic cell upregulation of surface adhesion molecules and inflammatory cytokines. Pathologically, this process shows a combination of microinfarction and hemorrhage. AML may be associated with a variety of laboratory derangements in addition to abnormal blood counts. Coagulation abnormalities are particularly common and severe in patients with acute promyelocytic leukemia (APL), but may be seen in all subtypes. Metabolic abnormalities related to tumor lysis syndrome may also be present, including hyperuricemia, hyperkalemia, hyperphosphatemia, and hypocalcemia.

Conflict-of-interest disclosure: *Dr. Roboz*: honoraria: Celgene, Eisai, Genzyme, Novartis, Cephalon. *Dr. Sung* declares no competing financial interest.

Subtype classification

In the 1970s, AML was subclassified according to the French-American-British (FAB) classification using morphologic and cytochemical criteria to define 8 major AML subtypes (M0-M7) on the basis of ≥30% blasts, lineage commitment, and the degree of blast cell differentiation (Table 16-1). The FAB system has been largely replaced by the World Health Organization (WHO) classification, which was developed to incorporate epidemiology, clinical features, biology, immunophenotype, and genetics into the diagnostic criteria. The WHO has identified 7 subgroups of AML (Table 16-2). AML is now defined as ≥20% myeloblasts and/or monoblasts/promonocytes and/or megakaryoblasts in the peripheral blood or bone marrow, except in patients with the following cytogenetic abnormalities, who are classified as having AML irrespective of blast count: t(8;21)(q22;q22), inv(16)(p13q22), t(16;16)(p13;q22), and t(15;17)(q22;q12). Immunophenotypic characterization using surface antigens remains important in AML and may include progenitor-associated antigens (eg, HLA-DR [except in APL], CD34, CD117) and myeloid antigens (eg, CD13, CD33), but complex composite immunophenotypes, including nonlineage-restricted lymphoid markers, may also be seen.

Key points

- The FAB classification for AML has been largely replaced by the WHO classification.
- AML is defined by the presence of ≥20% myeloblasts and/or monoblasts/promonocytes and/or megakaryoblasts in the peripheral blood or bone marrow.
- Certain cytogenetic abnormalities are classified as AML regardless of the blast count.

Table 16-1 French-American-British (FAB) classification of acute myeloid leukemia (AML).

FAB subtype	Name	% of adult AML patients	Features
M0	Undifferentiated acute myeloblastic leukemia	5%–10%	MPO <3%
M1	Acute myeloblastic leukemia without maturation	15%–20%	MPO ≥3%, <10% maturation beyond blast stage
M2	Acute myeloblastic leukemia with maturation	25%–30%	MPO ≥3%, >10% maturation beyond blast stage
M3	Acute promyelocytic leukemia (APL)	10%–15%	≥30 blasts + hypergranular promyelocytes, strongly MPO or Sudan black B positive; microgranular variant (M3v) has inconspicuous granules, 15% of APL
M4	Acute myelomonocytic leukemia	10%–20%	>20% monocytes, NSE positive
M4 eos	Acute myelomonocytic leukemia with eosinophilia	5%	Abnormal marrow eosinophils, associated with inv(16) or t(16;16)
M5	Acute monocytic leukemia	10%–20%	M5a (poorly differentiated, monoblastic) M5b (differentiated, promonocytes, monocytes); strongly NSE positive
M6	Acute erythroid leukemia (erythroleukemia)	5%	Erythroblasts ≥50%, dyserythropoiesis, glycophorin A(+)
M7	Acute megakaryoblastic leukemia	5%	Associated with marrow fibrosis, CD41 or CD61 often positive

MPO = myeloperoxidase; NSE = nonspecific esterase.

Table 16-2 World Health Organization 2008 classification of acute myeloid leukemia (AML) and related myeloid neoplasms.

1. AML with recurrent genetic abnormalities
    a. AML with balanced translocations/inversions
        i. AML with t(8;21)(q22;q22); *RUNX1-RUNX1T1*
        ii. AML with inv(16)(p13.1q22) or t(16;16)(p13.1;q22); *CBFB-MYH11*
        iii. Acute promyelocytic leukemia with t(15;17)(q22;q12); *PML-RARα*
        iv. AML with t(9;11)(p22;q23); *MLLT3-MLL*
        v. AML with t(6;9)(p23;q34); *DEK-NUP214*
        vi. AML with inv(3)(q21q26.2) or t(3;3)(q21;q26.2); *RPN1-EVI1*
        vii. AML (megakaryoblastic) with t(1;22)(p13;q13); *RBM15-MLK1*
    b. AML with gene mutations
        i. Provisional entity: AML with mutated *NPM1* (nucleophosmin)
        ii. Provisional entity: AML with mutated *CEBPA* (CCAAT/enhancer binding protein α)
2. AML with myelodysplasia-related changes
3. Therapy-related myeloid neoplasms
4. AML, not otherwise specified
    a. AML with minimal differentiation
    b. AML without maturation
    c. AML with maturation
    d. Acute myelomonocytic leukemia
    e. Acute monoblastic/monocytic leukemia
    f. Acute erythroid leukemia
        i. Pure erythroid
        ii. Erythroleukemia, erythroid/myeloid
    g. Acute megakaryoblastic leukemia
    h. Acute basophilic leukemia
    i. Acute panmyelosis with myelofibrosis
5. Myeloid sarcoma
6. Myeloid proliferations related to Down syndrome
    a. Transient abnormal myelopoiesis
    b. Myeloid leukemia associated with Down syndrome
7. Blastic plasmacytoid dendritic cell neoplasm

Prognostic factors

AML is a clinically and biologically heterogeneous disease. Adverse clinical prognostic features include advanced age, extramedullary disease, and the presence of an antecedent hematologic disorder (MDS or myeloproliferative disorders). Patients older than 60 years, and especially those older than 75 years, have poor long-term survival due to both disease- and host-related factors, including increased expression of multidrug resistance genes, medical comorbidities, and poor performance status. White blood cell count >50,000/μL at diagnosis is associated with increased risk of early death from hemorrhage and/or leukostasis.

Cytogenetics and molecular genetics are of critical prognostic importance in newly diagnosed AML patients and must be included as part of the initial diagnostic workup. Acquired, nonrandom, clonal chromosomal abnormalities including balanced translocations, inversions, deletions, monosomies, and trisomies are found in >50% of patients with AML. The abnormal karyotype is complex (generally defined as ≥3 abnormalities) in 10% to 20% of patients. Cytogenetic abnormalities are often classified into favorable, intermediate, and unfavorable risk groups, but it should be noted that clinical study groups in AML assign certain abnormalities differently (Table 16-3). However, it is universally agreed that patients with the t(15;17)(q22;q12-21) found in APL have excellent outcomes. Balanced abnormalities of t(8;21)(q22;q22), inv(16)(p13.1 q22), and t(16;16)(p13.1;q22) involve the heterodimeric components of core binding factor (CBF) and are associated with a relatively favorable prognosis. Complex karyotype involving ≥3 abnormalities, inv(3)(q21q26)/t(3;3)(q21;q26), and monosomal karyotype (at least 2 autosomal monosomies or 1 single autosomal monosomy combined with at least 1 structural abnormality) are associated with particularly poor outcomes.

AML is a genetically heterogeneous disease that has been associated with numerous acquired somatic genetic alterations in hematopoietic cells (Figure 16-1). The presence or absence of specific gene mutations and/or changes in gene expression have been shown to be of prognostic significance in AML. Currently, this is particularly important for patients with cytogenetically normal AML, who comprise the largest cytogenetic subset of AML and are generally assigned to an intermediate-risk group. These patients have variable outcomes with conventional treatment strategies, which may be explained by the striking molecular heterogeneity associated with their disease. For example, 20% to 30% of patients with AML have activating mutations of the receptor tyrosine kinase fms-like tyrosine kinase 3 (*FLT3*), and internal tandem duplications (*FLT3*-ITD) within the juxtamembrane domain are consistently associated with inferior outcome in patients with cytogenetically normal AML. In addition, heterozygous mutations in exon 12 of the nucleophosmin member 1 (*NPM1*) gene have been found in 40% to 60% of AML patients with a normal karyotype, and mutated *NPM1*, in conjunction with wild-type *FLT3*, is associated with a favorable prognosis. Finally, mutations of CCAAT/enhancer binding protein α (*CEBPA*), a gene encoding a myeloid transcription factor important for normal granulopoiesis, also appear to be associated with favorable clinical outcomes. The field of molecular diagnostics in AML is evolving rapidly, and several additional mutations and abnormalities of gene expression have already been identified. These are expected to provide additional prognostic information and

Table 16-3 Variation in cytogenetic risk group classification across clinical trial groups.

	Original MRC	SWOG/ECOG	CALGB	GIMEMA/AML10	German AMLCG	HOVON/SAKK	Refined MRC
Favorable	t(15;17)	t(15;17)	t(15;17)	t(15;17)	t(15;17)	t(15;17)	t(15;17)
	t(8;21)	t(8;21) [lacking del(9q), complex, re, ≥3 unrel abn]	t(8;21)	t(8;21)	t(8;21)	t(8;21) alone inv/del(16) and lacking unfav abn	t(8;21)
	inv(16)/t(16;16)	inv(16)/t(16;16)/del(16q)	inv(16)/t(16;16)	inv(16)/t(16;16)	inv(16)/t(16;16)		inv(16)/t(16;16)
Intermediate	Normal	Normal	Normal	Normal	Normal	Normal	Normal
	Other non-complex	+6, +8, −Y, del(12p)	Other non-complex	−Y	Other non-complex	Other non-complex	Other non-complex
				Other			
Adverse	abn(3q)	abn(3q),(9q),(11q),(21q)	inv(3)/t(3;3)		inv(3)/t(3;3)	abn(3q)	abn(3q) [excluding t(3;5)]
	−5/del(5q)	abn(17p)	−7		−5/del(5q)	−5/del(5q)	inv(3)/t(3;3)
	−7	−5/del(5q)	t(6;9)		−7/del(7q)	−7/del(7q)	add(5q)/del(5q)/−5, −7/add(7q)
	complex [≥ 5 unrel abn]	−7/del(7q)	t(6;11)		abn(11q23)	abn(11q23)	t(6;11)
		t(6;9)	t(11;19)		del(12p)	t(6;9)	t(10;11)
		t(9;22)	+8		abn(17p)	t(9;22)	t(9;22)
		complex [≥3 unrel abn]	complex (≥ 3 unrel abn)		complex (≥ 3 unrel abn)	complex (≥ 3 unrel abn)	−17
							abn(17p) with other changes
							Complex (> 3 unrel abn)
	Excluding those with favorable changes		Excluding those with favorable changes				Excluding those with favorable changes

Unrel abn = unrelated abnormality; abn = abnormal.

References for the various classification systems can be found in Grimwade D. Impact of cytogenetics on clinical outcome in AML. In: Karp JE, ed. *Acute Myelogenous Leukemia*. Totowa, New Jersey: Humana Press; 2007:177–192.

The HOVON/SAKK cytogenetic classification was derived from the study by Cornelissen JJ, van Putten WL, Verdonck LF, et al. Results of a HOVON/SAKK donor versus no-donor analysis of myeloablative HLA-identical sibling stem cell transplantation in first remission acute myeloid leukemia in young and middle-aged adults: benefits for whom? *Blood*. 2007;109:3658–3666.

The revised MRC classification system was based on an analysis of 5635 patients aged 16 to 59 years enrolled in the MRC AML10, AML12 and AML15 trials. (Grimwade D, Hills RK, Moorman AV, et al. Refinement of cytogenetic classification in AML: determination of prognostic significance of rare recurring chromosomal abnormalities amongst 5635 younger adults treated in the UK MRC trials. *Haematologica/Haematology J*. 2009;94:217).

Table adapted from Grimwade D, Hills RK. Independent prognostic factors for AML outcome. *Hematology Am Soc Hematol Educ Program*. 2009:385–95, p. 387. With permission.

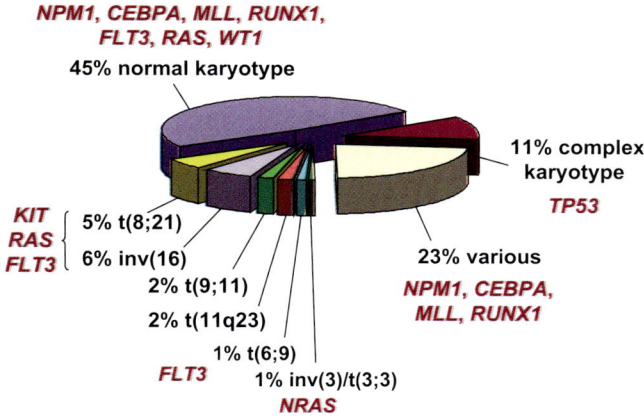

Figure 16-1 Major cytogenetic subgroups of acute myeloid leukemia (AML) (excluding acute promyelocytic leukemia) and associated gene mutations.

therapeutic targets. Gene expression profiling has also been shown to identify prognostically distinct AML subgroups and is rapidly becoming more feasible and readily available. Recently, highly parallel DNA sequencing techniques have been used to analyze the entire genome of 2 cases of AML, and recurrent cooperative (driver) mutations have been identified.

> **Key points**
> - The most important prognostic indicators in AML are age, cytogenetics, and molecular genetics.
> - Complex cytogenetic abnormalities and monosomal karyotypes are associated with poor clinical outcomes.
> - t(15;17), t(8;21), and inv(16) are cytogenetic abnormalities associated with favorable outcomes.
> - Patients with cytogenetically normal AML and *FLT3*-ITD mutations have an unfavorable prognosis, whereas those with wild-type *FLT3* and mutations of *NMP1* or *CEBPA* have a more favorable prognosis.

Treatment

Treatment for AML is generally divided into remission induction and postremission therapy. Standard remission induction regimens in the United States for all AML subtypes, excluding APL (see later section on APL), almost always include 7 days of infusional cytarabine and 3 days of an anthracycline, commonly known as "7+3." This strategy (with or without a second induction course with identical or different drugs, depending on the treatment protocol) results in complete remission (CR) in 70% to 80% of adults under age 60 and 30% to 50% of selected adults over age 60 with a good performance status. The Cancer and Leukemia Group B (CALGB) established that 3 days of daunorubicin and 7 days of cytarabine were more effective than 2 and 5 days, respectively, and that 10 days of cytarabine was not better than 7 days. Also, 100 mg/m^2 of cytarabine for 7 days was as effective as 200 mg/m^2 for the same duration. Daunorubicin at a dose of 30 mg/m^2 was inferior to 45 mg/m^2, and recently, daunorubicin 90 mg/m^2 has been shown, in large cooperative group trials, to be superior to 45 mg/m^2 even in selected patients over age 60 years. Many modifications to the standard "7+3" backbone have been attempted. Remission rates were similar or slightly improved when idarubicin or mitoxantrone was substituted for daunorubicin, but there was no convincing improvement in overall survival when equivalent doses were used. Randomized prospective trials also failed to demonstrate that induction with high-dose cytarabine (HiDAC) improved survival compared with standard induction. Similarly, addition of 6-thioguanine, etoposide, or dexamethasone to the anthracycline/cytarabine backbone did not improve overall survival. Finally, despite compelling scientific rationale, neither the addition of multidrug resistance modulators nor the addition of cytokines to chemotherapy has improved outcomes in AML to date. Trials combining targeted antibodies and *FLT3* inhibitors with chemotherapy are ongoing.

Once remission has been achieved, further therapy is required to prevent relapse. Options include repeated courses of consolidation chemotherapy or hematopoietic stem cell transplantation (HSCT). Autologous HSCT was developed to permit escalation to myeloablative doses of chemotherapy, and allogeneic HSCT allows combination of the myelotoxic effects of chemotherapy with a hoped graft-versus-leukemia effect from the donor cells. Several studies have prospectively evaluated the role of intensive consolidation with HiDAC. The CALGB randomized patients in first remission to 4 courses of cytarabine using either a continuous infusion of 100 mg/m^2 for 5 days or a 3-hour infusion of 400 mg/m^2 or 3 g/m^2 twice daily on days 1, 3, and 5. Significant central nervous system toxicity was observed in patients >60 years old randomized to the high-dose arm, and thus, this regimen is not recommended for older patients. In patients <60 years old, there was a significant improvement in disease-free survival associated with the high-dose regimen, and this was most pronounced in patients with favorable cytogenetics, including t(8;21) and inv(16). Although it has become standard to offer 3 to 4 cycles of HiDAC at 3 g/m^2 on days 1, 3, and 5 to younger patients with AML, it should be noted that there are no clear data defining the optimal number or intensity of HiDAC cycles. Also, the original CALGB protocol that defined this regimen included 4 additional maintenance cycles of cytarabine and daunorubicin administered after HiDAC, which have not been adopted as part of common practice.

Although it is clear that patients with CBF leukemias specifically benefit from HiDAC, some of these patients also have mutations in *KIT*, which are associated with an inferior outcome; clinical trials of chemotherapy combined with tyrosine kinase inhibitors are ongoing in these patients. Consolidation chemotherapy, in general, has not been proven to be of benefit for patients >60 years old, but older patients able to tolerate additional treatment are often offered 1 or 2 cycles of 5 days of cytarabine combined with 2 days of an anthracycline after induction.

Several studies of postremission therapy in AML have compared intensive chemotherapy consolidation to HSCT by assigning younger patients with a human leukocyte antigen (HLA)-matched sibling donor to allogeneic HSCT and randomizing other patients to chemotherapy or autologous HSCT. Meta-analyses have shown that autologous HSCT decreases relapse risk but increases treatment-related mortality compared with chemotherapy consolidation, thus resulting in similar overall survival rates of approximately 40% to 45% at 3 to 5 years. Although autologous HSCT remains a reasonable postremission therapy for AML, there is no specific indication, to date, for its use in any prognostic subgroup.

Allogeneic HSCT is probably the most effective antileukemic therapy currently available and offers a combination of the therapeutic efficacy of the conditioning regimen and the graft-versus-leukemia effect from the donor cells. However, it is associated with significant morbidity and mortality. A recent comprehensive meta-analysis by Koreth et al (2009) of prospective clinical trials of allogeneic HSCT in AML patients in first CR evaluated 24 trials and >6000 patients. In this analysis, allogeneic HSCT resulted in significantly improved 5-year overall survival, from 45% to 52% for patients with intermediate-risk cytogenetics and from 20% to 31% in patients with poor-risk cytogenetics. There was no benefit for allogeneic HSCT for patients with good-risk cytogenetics. Retrospective analyses of uniformly treated patients have shown that allogeneic HSCT was also beneficial for cytogenetically normal AML patients with *FLT3*-ITD$^+$, *FLT3*-ITD$^-$/*NPM1*$^-$, and *FLT3*-ITD$^-$/*CEBPA*$^-$, and prospective trials using molecular and cytogenetic risk stratification are underway.

There is tremendous momentum in the field of allogeneic transplantation in AML, with many more questions than answers. Important areas of investigation include:

- Optimal conditioning strategies: myeloablative versus nonmyeloablative and reduced-intensity
- Unrelated donor and umbilical cord transplantations
- Strategies for stem cell expansion
- The need for consolidation chemotherapy prior to transplantation
- Strategies for prevention and treatment of graft-versus-host disease, including optimization of T-cell depletion techniques
- Optimization of supportive care
- Refinement of risk stratification systems to incorporate molecular diagnostics and medical comorbidities

Key points

- Treatment of AML generally involves remission induction followed by postremission therapy.
- Three days of an anthracycline combined with 7 days of cytarabine remains the standard of care for induction for all AML subtypes in adults, excluding APL (FAB-M3).
- Consolidation chemotherapy with 3 to 4 cycles of HiDAC is of particular benefit for patients <60 years old with favorable prognosis cytogenetics involving CBF [t(8;21) and inv(16)]; it is not routinely recommended for patients >60 years old.
- Allogeneic stem cell transplantation appears to be of benefit for AML patients in first remission who have intermediate- or poor-risk cytogenetics.
- Retrospective data suggest that allogeneic transplantation may also be of benefit for patients with *FLT3*-ITD.

Monitoring residual disease

Although morphologic methods remain the gold standard for determining the status of disease in AML, more sensitive immunologic and molecular methods for detecting the presence of minimal residual disease (MRD) are available. Although not a standard practice, so-called leukemia-associated immunophenotypes can be identified as "signatures" for some patients with AML, and the presence of MRD as measured by immunophenotype has been shown to predict for disease relapse in some studies. The genetic abnormalities associated with a significant proportion of AML cases provide unique markers that can be also used to monitor MRD. Polymerase chain reaction (PCR) offers a qualitative detection of abnormal gene rearrangements or fusion genes, whereas real-time PCR offers both the advantage of higher sensitivity and the possibility of quantification. The optimal sensitivity for detection methods remains to be determined, and prospective clinical trials are required to assess whether additional postremission treatment with chemotherapy, allogeneic transplantation, or other agents will improve outcomes for patients with persistent MRD.

AML relapse

The majority of adult patients with AML experience relapse, despite initially attaining CR. The prognosis of relapsed disease is poor, and these patients should be considered for investigational trials. Most AML relapses occur within 2 years of diagnosis. The duration of first remission is of critical prognostic importance, and patients with an initial CR of <6 months are unlikely to respond to standard chemotherapeutic agents. Patients whose initial CR duration was >12 months may have up to a 50% chance of responding to an HiDAC-containing regimen, even if they had previous exposure to this agent. Gemtuzumab ozogamicin, an immunoconjugate of an anti-CD33 monoclonal antibody linked to calicheamicin, a potent cytotoxic, is approved by the US Food and Drug Administration for patients ≥60 years old with AML in first relapse and produces remission in approximately 25% of patients. Patients who achieve second remission should be considered for standard or reduced-intensity allogeneic transplantation if possible because the duration of second remission with chemotherapy alone is generally short. The prognosis for patients who relapse after allogeneic transplantation is dismal.

There are many categories of novel agents under investigation for AML, including chemotherapeutics (eg, topoisomerase II inhibitors, purine nucleoside analogs), FLT3 inhibitors, DNA methyltransferase inhibitors, and farnesyltransferase inhibitors. In general, so-called "targeted" agents have had limited single-agent activity in relapsed AML and may be more effective in combination with chemotherapy.

Older patients with AML

> **Clinical case**
>
> An 82-year-old woman with a history of myocardial infarction, diabetes, and peripheral vascular disease presents with shortness of breath and is found to be pancytopenic. Bone marrow biopsy shows 40% myeloblasts with monosomy 7.

Most patients with AML are >60 years old, and their prognosis is dismal, with median survival times of only 8 to 12 months among the most "fit" patients. Older patients have a high frequency of poor prognostic features, including antecedent hematologic disorders, unfavorable cytogenetics, and multidrug resistance (*MDR1*) phenotypes. Also, older patients are often less able to tolerate intensive chemotherapy because of medical comorbidities, polypharmacy, poor performance status, and limited social supports. There is no universally accepted standard of care for treatment of older patients, but they are generally offered either conventional "7+3" induction, repeated cycles of low-dose subcutaneous cytarabine, supportive care with antibiotics and transfusions, hospice care, or an investigational trial. Although remission can be attained in approximately 50% of selected older patients with a good performance status using 7+3, relapse is almost certain, and <10% of patients are long-term survivors. Major cooperative group trials, which generally favor patients <75 years old with de novo AML and a good performance status, show 3- to 5-year overall survival rates of only 10% to 20%. Many older patients are not offered any treatment for AML, despite randomized data clearly demonstrating a survival benefit favoring treatment with chemotherapy over supportive care in this population. Clinical experience suggests that quality of life is better for those who achieve CR, but data are sparse. Although there are clearly frail and debilitated older patients who cannot tolerate any treatment, emerging data suggest that age alone should not be used as the major determinant of treatment because several intensive options, including intensified doses of daunorubicin and reduced-intensity stem cell transplantations, are both feasible and effective in selected patients >60 years old. It is notable that many, if not most, older patients with AML fail to benefit from therapy because of lack of therapeutic efficacy, not intolerable toxicity. Novel therapies are clearly needed for this population, and there are many ongoing clinical trials with cytotoxics, antibodies, farnesyltransferase inhibitors, hypomethylating agents, and nonmyeloablative transplantations. Older AML patients should be encouraged to participate in clinical trials whenever possible.

Acute promyelocytic leukemia (APL)

> **Clinical case**
>
> A 23-year-old Hispanic female presents with 2 weeks of dyspnea, bruising, and menorrhagia. Laboratory evaluation shows pancytopenia with elevated prothrombin and partial thromboplastin times and markedly decreased fibrinogen. Bone marrow aspiration shows intensely myeloperoxidase-positive promyelocytes and t(15;17).

APL (FAB-M3) is a clinically, cytogenetically, and prognostically distinct subtype of AML that accounts for approximately 5% to 15% of all adult AML cases, with a higher incidence among Hispanics. It is the most curable form of AML in adults. Almost all leukemic cells from patients with APL have a balanced reciprocal translocation between chromosomes 15 and 17, which results in the fusion of the promyelocytic leukemia (*PML*) and retinoic acid receptor α (*RARα*) genes, a *PML-RARα* fusion gene product, and disruption of normal differentiation. APL blasts contain granules with proteolytic enzymes, the release of which induces severe coagulopathy and fibrinolysis, which predispose patients to both hemorrhage and thrombosis.

APL exists in hypergranular ("typical") and microgranular forms. In hypergranular APL, the promyelocytes are

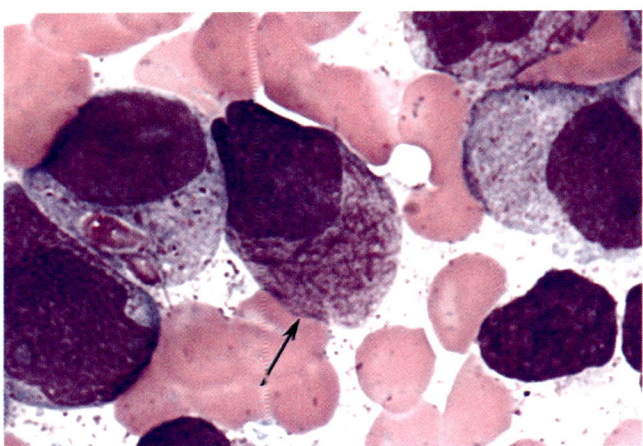

Figure 16-2 Faggot cell. From Maslak P. American Society of Hematology Image Bank, April 2008, 7-00039.

strongly myeloperoxidase positive and have bilobed or kidney-shaped nuclei. The cytoplasm has densely packed, large granules, and characteristic cells containing bundles of Auer rods ("faggot cells") may be found in most cases (Figure 16-2). Cases of microgranular APL have predominantly bilobed nuclei, are also strongly myeloperoxidase positive, and often have a very high leukocyte count and doubling time. APL is characterized by low expression or absence of HLA-DR, CD34, CD117, and CD11b. The diagnosis is confirmed with cytogenetics, reverse transcriptase PCR (RT-PCR) for the *PML-RAR* fusion transcript, fluorescence in situ hybridization with probes for *PML* and *RARα*, and/or anti-*PML* antibodies.

APL promyelocytes have the unique ability to undergo differentiation with exposure to all-*trans* retinoic acid (ATRA). Detection of t(15;17) or the underlying *PML-RARα* rearrangement is predictive of response to ATRA in virtually 100% of cases. Some infrequent APL variants, such as t(11;17)(q23;q21) with *ZBTB16-RARα* and cases with *STAT5B-RARα* fusions, are resistant to ATRA. It is crucial that ATRA is started as soon as the diagnosis of APL is suspected, prior to pathologic confirmation. Combination regimens with ATRA and an anthracycline with or without cytarabine induce remission in >90% of patients, and long-term cures are achieved in >70% to 80% of patients in many series. Primary resistance to chemotherapy is virtually nonexistent, and bone marrow aspiration and biopsy should be deferred until the time of peripheral count recovery, not on day 14 of induction, as is often done in other AML subtypes. There have been 2 prospective trials comparing ATRA, with or without chemotherapy, with chemotherapy alone in APL induction, all of which show benefits in event-free survival, disease-free survival, and overall survival with the addition of ATRA. Thus, standard treatment generally includes anthracycline-based chemotherapy plus ATRA. There is some controversy regarding the best chemotherapy to include with ATRA during induction, but an anthracycline alone appears to be sufficient, and either daunorubicin 60 mg/m^2 for 3 days or idarubicin 12 mg/m^2 on days 2, 4, 6, and 8 can be used. Consolidation protocols differ between the United States and European cooperative groups but generally include several cycles of anthracycline-based chemotherapy. The role of infusional cytarabine during induction is not clear, but patients presenting with white blood cell count ≥10,000/μL may benefit from intermediate-dose cytarabine or HiDAC during either induction or consolidation. Some protocols for high-risk patients have also incorporated prophylactic intrathecal chemotherapy. The role of maintenance therapy is also controversial in APL, but ATRA with or without 6-mercaptopurine is frequently offered to patients in CR. The optimal combination and duration of maintenance have not been defined.

Despite the success of ATRA-based regimens, there is still an early mortality of approximately 10% in APL patients, primarily due to hemorrhagic complications. Predictors of early death due to hemorrhage include WBC count at presentation, abnormal creatinine, peripheral blast count, presence of coagulopathy, and age. Also, patients must be closely monitored for the development of APL differentiation syndrome, a potentially fatal constellation of findings, including interstitial pulmonary infiltrates, hypoxemia, respiratory distress, fluid retention, weight gain, pleural or pericardial effusions, and sometimes renal failure. Rapid administration of dexamethasone 10 mg twice daily for at least 3 days at the earliest manifestations of the syndrome is lifesaving.

The persistence or reappearance of *PML-RARα* fusion gene transcripts in patients with APL is highly predictive of clinical relapse, and frequent monitoring, approximately every 3 months by RT-PCR, is considered standard of care. Relapsed disease can be treated effectively with arsenic trioxide, which causes differentiation and apoptosis of APL cells, alone or in combination with ATRA. Autologous stem cell transplantation can be considered for patients in second remission if the stem cells are negative for *PML-RARα*. Allogeneic stem cell transplantation is generally not recommended for patients with APL but may be considered for relapsed patients.

Arsenic trioxide may be the single most active agent in APL and appears to offer a survival benefit when given as consolidation for newly diagnosed patients. It also produces high rates of durable CR when combined with ATRA in newly diagnosed patients. Treatment with the combination of arsenic and ATRA has allowed reduction or elimination of chemotherapy for selected newly diagnosed patients with APL and is frequently offered to older patients who cannot tolerate conventional chemotherapy.

> **Key points**
>
> - APL is a unique subtype of AML that is exquisitely sensitive to ATRA, anthracyclines, and arsenic trioxide.
> - ATRA should be started immediately if the diagnosis of APL is suspected.
> - Cure rates are high in APL.
> - APL may be complicated by a life-threatening coagulopathy and/or differentiation syndrome.
> - APL differentiation syndrome should be treated promptly with dexamethasone 10 mg twice daily for at least 3 days.

Pediatric AML, including Down syndrome

> **Clinical case**
>
> A 6-year-old boy presents with a 4-week history of fatigue and fever and a 1-week history of bruising and pallor. Laboratory evaluation shows pancytopenia. Bone marrow aspiration shows myeloblasts with granules and an occasional Auer rod. Cytogenetic studies reveal t(8;21).

Pediatric AML has unique clinical features, risk stratification, and therapeutic approaches. Cutaneous involvement is more common in children, particularly in infants diagnosed at <1 year of age. Poor-prognosis cytogenetics are less frequent in children, and within the pediatric spectrum, age is not a critical prognostic indicator, except for children with Down syndrome. Also, children may tolerate intensive chemotherapy better than adults, and this may impact on the optimal therapeutic approach. Standard induction chemotherapy in pediatrics typically includes cytarabine and an anthracycline with the addition of a third agent such as etoposide. Most current pediatric AML protocols use at least 4 to 5 cycles of chemotherapy with HiDAC-based consolidation. The current phase III trial being conducted by the Children's Oncology Group is designed to determine whether the addition of gemtuzumab ozogamicin to standard chemotherapy improves outcomes. Autologous HSCT has been abandoned by most pediatric groups, whereas the role of allogeneic HSCT is variable. In North America, most children with favorable features are treated with chemotherapy alone, whereas most children with poor-risk features are offered allogeneic HSCT from either a related or unrelated donor. Those with intermediate-risk AML are typically treated with allogeneic HSCT if a matched family donor is available. Children with favorable cytogenetics have an overall survival rate of approximately 70% irrespective of response to the first cycle of induction, whereas children with adverse cytogenetics or poor response to the first cycle of induction therapy with >15% residual blasts have an overall survival rate of only 15%.

Children with Down syndrome have a 46- to 83-fold increased risk of AML and are generally younger than other pediatric AML patients. AML associated with Down syndrome tends to be classified as FAB-M7 (acute megakaryoblastic leukemia [AMKL]), and *GATA1* mutations have been described in the leukemic blasts. AMKL in Down syndrome may be preceded by transient myeloproliferative disorder (TMD), a condition unique to children with Down syndrome. TMD is a clonal disorder characterized by circulating blasts and dysplastic features and is usually diagnosed in the first few weeks after birth. Although TMD typically resolves spontaneously within the first 3 months, intensive supportive care may be required, and early death has been reported in as many as 15% to 20% of cases. For those who survive, approximately 20% to 30% will later develop AMKL. Children with Down syndrome and AML who are younger than 2 to 4 years of age have better prognosis compared with both non–Down syndrome AML and Down syndrome AML patients >4 years of age at diagnosis. This superior prognosis may be related to enhanced sensitivity of the leukemic blast to cytarabine. Children with Down syndrome have greater toxicities with treatment and are not offered HSCT in first remission.

Bibliography

Advani R, Saba HI, Tallman MS, et al. Treatment of refractory and relapsed acute myelogenous leukemia with combination chemotherapy plus the multidrug resistance modulator PSC 833 (Valspodar). *Blood.* 1999;93:787–795. *Explores the benefits of the multidrug resistance modulator, PSC 833, in patients with relapsed and refractory AML.*

Anderson JE, Gooley TA, Schoch G, et al. Stem cell transplantation for secondary acute myeloid leukemia: evaluation of transplantation as initial therapy or following induction chemotherapy. *Blood.* 1997;89:2578–2585. *Prompt transplantation can be considered following diagnosis of secondary AML or high-risk myelodysplasia, especially in patients with low peripheral blood blast counts. Outcome was not statistically different from that achieved with transplantation following induction chemotherapy in second remission or first untreated relapse.*

Appelbaum FR, Clift RA, Buckner CD, et al. Allogeneic marrow transplantation for acute nonlymphoblastic leukemia after first relapse. *Blood.* 1983;61:949–953. *Shows that for patients not undergoing allogeneic transplantation in first remission, such a strategy can be considered as soon as possible after first relapse.*

Aversa F, Tabilio A, Velardi A, et al. Treatment of high-risk acute leukemia with T-cell-depleted stem cells from related donors with one fully mismatched HLA haplotype. *N Engl J Med.* 1998;339:1186–1193. *Reports results with full-haplotype mismatched donors in patients with high-risk leukemia with a transplantation-related mortality rate of 40%.*

Berman E, Heller G, Santorsa J, et al. Results of a randomized trial comparing idarubicin and cytosine arabinoside with daunorubicin and cytosine arabinoside in adult patients with newly diagnosed acute myelogenous leukemia. *Blood.* 1991;77:1666–1674. *Shows that idarubicin plus cytarabine is as effective as daunorubicin plus cytarabine in younger adults with newly diagnosed AML.*

Bishop JF, Matthews JP, Young GA, Bradstock K, Lowenthal RM. Intensified induction chemotherapy with high-dose cytarabine and etoposide for acute myeloid leukemia: a review and updated results of the Australian Leukemia Study Group. *Leuk Lymphoma.* 1998;28:315–327. *Intensifying induction with etoposide or HiDAC improves relapse-free survival but has less impact on overall survival. Such benefits appear confined to younger patients.*

Bishop JF, Matthews JP, Young GA, et al. A randomized study of high-dose cytarabine in induction in acute myeloid leukemia. *Blood.* 1996;87:1710–1717. *This study shows that the addition of HiDAC to a standard dose of daunorubicin plus cytarabine in induction may prolong disease-free survival and remission duration.*

Bloomfield CD, Lawrence D, Byrd JC, et al. Frequency of prolonged remission duration after high-dose cytarabine intensification in acute myeloid leukemia varies by cytogenetic subtype. *Cancer Res.* 1998;58:4173–4179. *The outcome of patients with CBF leukemia is superior to that of patients with normal karyotypes and other karyotype abnormalities when treated with HiDAC.*

Buchner T, Hiddemann W, Wormann B, et al. Double induction strategy for acute myeloid leukemia: the effect of high-dose cytarabine with mitoxantrone instead of standard-dose cytarabine with daunorubicin and 6-thioguanine: a randomized trial by the German AML Cooperative Group. *Blood.* 1999;93:4116–4124. *The incorporation of HiDAC with mitoxantrone induction may be beneficial for patients with low-risk AML.*

Burnett AK, Goldstone AH, Stevens RMF, et al. Randomized comparison of addition of autologous bone-marrow transplantation to intensive chemotherapy for acute myeloid leukaemia in first remission: results of MRC AML 10 trial. *Lancet.* 1998;351:700–708. *The addition of autologous transplantation to four courses of intensive chemotherapy reduces the relapse risk with an improvement in overall survival.*

Byrd JC, Dodge RK, Carroll A, et al. Patients with t(8;21)(q22;q22) and acute myeloid leukemia have superior failure-free and overall survival when repetitive cycles of high-dose cytarabine are administered. *J Clin Oncol.* 1999;17:3767–775. *Shows that failure-free survival and overall survival are improved in patients with t(8;21) AML with repetitive cycles of HiDAC.*

Cassileth PA, Harrington DP, Appelbaum FR, et al. Chemotherapy compared with autologous or allogeneic bone marrow transplantation in the management of acute myeloid leukemia in first remission. *N Engl J Med.* 1998;339:1649–1656. *One of only a handful of randomized trials in postremission therapy for AML.*

Dastugue N, Payen C, Lafage-Pochitaloff M, et al. Prognostic significance of karyotype in de novo adult acute myeloid leukemia. The BGMT Group. *Leukemia.* 1995;9:1491–1498. *Prognostic importance of cytogenetics in outcome is described. Complex karyotypes found were predictive of shorter continuous CR in older adults.*

De Lima M, Strom SS, Keating M, et al. Implications of potential cure in acute myelogenous leukemia: development of subsequent cancer and return to work. *Blood.* 1997;90:4719–4724. *Provides impact of cure in AML on development of second malignancies and ability to resume employment.*

Döhner K, Döhner H. Molecular characterization of acute myeloid leukemia. *Haematologica.* 2008;93:976–982.

Döhner H, Estey EH, Amadori S, et al; and European LeukemiaNet. Diagnosis and management of acute myeloid leukemia in adults: recommendations from an international expert panel, on behalf of the European LeukemiaNet. *Blood.* 2010;115(3):453–474.

Elonen E, Almqvist A, Hanninen A, et al. Comparison between four and eight cycles of intensive chemotherapy in adult acute myeloid leukemia: a randomized trial of the Finnish Leukemia Group. *Leukemia.* 1998;12:1041–1048. *Once in remission after two cycles of induction, six additional cycles were not better than two cycles, with no difference in either relapse-free survival or overall survival.*

Estey E. Treatment of refractory AML. *Leukemia.* 1996;10:932–936. *Shows that an important prognostic variable in refractory AML is the duration of first remission.*

Estey E, Thall P, Beran M, Kantarjian H, Pierce S, Keating M. Effect of diagnosis (refractory anemia with excess blasts, refractory anemia with excess blasts in transformation, or acute myeloid leukemia [AML]) on outcome of AML-type chemotherapy. *Blood.* 1997;90:2969–2977. *After accounting for karyotype, age, and other factors, results of AML-type chemotherapy are the same in AML, refractory anemia with excess blasts, or refractory anemia with excess blasts in transformation.*

Estey E, Thall PF, Pierce S, Kantarjian H, Keating M. Treatment of newly diagnosed acute promyelocytic leukemia without cytarabine. *J Clin Oncol.* 1997;15:483–490.

Fenaux P, Chastang C, Chevret S, et al. A randomized comparison of all trans-retinoic acid (ATRA) followed by chemotherapy and ATRA plus chemotherapy and the role of maintenance therapy in newly diagnosed acute promyelocytic leukemia. The European APL Group. *Blood.* 1999;94:1192–1200. *Randomized study showing that concurrent ATRA plus chemotherapy is associated with lower relapse rate and better overall survival than sequential ATRA until remission followed by chemotherapy. Also shows benefit of maintenance in APL.*

Fernandez HF, Sun Z, Yao X, et al. Anthracycline dose intensification in acute myeloid leukemia. *N Engl J Med.* 2009;361:1249–1259.

Gale RP, Horowitz MM, Weiner RS, et al. Impact of cytogenetic abnormalities on outcome of bone marrow transplants in acute myelogenous leukemia in first remission. *Bone Marrow Transplant.* 1995;16:203–208.

Demonstrates that cytogenetics influence outcome after allogeneic transplantation.

Giralt S, Estey E, Albitar M, et al. Engraftment of allogeneic hematopoietic progenitor cells with purine analog-containing chemotherapy: harnessing graft-versus-leukemia without myeloablative therapy. *Blood.* 1997;89:4531–4536. *Shows that purine analog-containing nonmyeloablative chemotherapy followed by allogeneic hematopoietic progenitor cell infusion is feasible in patients with advanced leukemia who might not otherwise be candidates for transplantation.*

Goldstone AH, Burnett AK, Wheatley K, Smith AG, Hutchinson RM, Clark RE. Attempts to improve treatment outcomes in acute myeloid leukemia (AML) in older patients: the results of the United Kingdom Medical Research Council AML11 trial. *Blood.* 2001;98:1302–1311. *Reports outcome for older adults given one of three induction regimens and shows improved remission rate with daunorubicin, cytarabine, and 6-thioguanine (vs cytarabine, daunorubicin, and etoposide or mitoxantrone and cytarabine) but no difference in overall survival. In addition, no benefit was seen with the addition of granulocyte colony-stimulating factor when given from day 8 onward as supportive care.*

Gorin NC, Labopin M, Rocha V, et al. Marrow versus peripheral blood for geno-identical allogeneic stem cell transplantation in acute myelocytic leukemia: influence of dose and stem cell source shows better outcome with rich marrow. *Blood.* 2003;102:3043–3051. *This report suggests that increasing the dose of stem cells collected from patient's bone marrow is actually associated with lower transplantation-related mortality compared with patients who receive peripheral blood.*

Greenberg P, Cox C, LeBeau MM, et al. International scoring system for evaluating prognosis in myelodysplastic syndromes. *Blood.* 1997;89:2079–2088. *Describes prognostic scoring system for patients with myelodysplasia, which is based on percentage of marrow blasts, cytogenetics, and number of cytopenias.*

Grimwade D, Hills RK. Independent prognostic factors for AML outcome. *Hematol Am Soc Educ Program.* 2009;385–395.

Grimwade D, Walker H, Oliver F, et al. The importance of diagnostic cytogenetics on outcome in AML: analysis of 1612 patients entered into the MRC AML 10 trial. The Medical Research Council Adult and Children's Leukaemia Working Parties. *Blood.* 1998;92:2322–2333. *Provides large data set correlating cytogenetics with outcome in patients with AML. Provides evidence that cytogenetically defined prognostic groups have predictive value in secondary AML and in patients undergoing transplantation.*

Hann IM, Stevens RF, Goldstone AH, et al. Randomized comparison of DAT versus ADE as induction chemotherapy in children and younger adults with acute myeloid leukemia. Results of the Medical Research Council's 10th AML trial (MRC AML10). Adult and Childhood Leukaemia Working Parties of the Medical Research Council. *Blood.* 1997;89:2311–2318. *Shows that the addition of etoposide to a standard induction regimen of daunorubicin and cytarabine did not confer a benefit in disease-free survival or overall survival.*

Harousseau JL, Cahn JY, Pignon B, et al. Comparison of autologous bone marrow transplantation and intensive chemotherapy as postremission therapy in adult acute myeloid leukemia. Groupe Ouest Est Leucemies Aigues Myeloblastiques (GOELAM). *Blood.* 1997;90:2978–2986. *Prospective trial of autologous transplantation, allogeneic transplantation, and consolidation chemotherapy showing no difference in outcome among the three strategies.*

Karanes C, Kopecky KJ, Head DR, et al. A phase III comparison of high-dose ARA-C (HIDAC) versus HIDAC plus mitoxantrone in the treatment of first relapsed or refractory acute myeloid leukemia. *Leuk Res.* 1999;23:787–94. *Randomized trial of HiDAC versus HiDAC plus mitoxantrone in relapsed and refractory AML showing a trend toward higher CR rate with the combination but less advantage in overall survival.*

Koreth J, Schlenk R, Kopecky KJ, et al. Allogeneic stem cell transplantation for acute myeloid leukemia in first complete remission. *JAMA.* 2009;301:2349–361.

Kottaridis PD, Gale RE, Frew ME, et al. The presence of a FLT3 internal tandem duplication in patients with acute myeloid leukemia (AML) adds important prognostic information to cytogenetic risk group and response to the first cycle of chemotherapy: analysis of 854 patients from the United Kingdom Medical Research Council AML 10 and 12 trials. *Blood.* 2001;98:1752–1759. *Describes important prognostic value of FLT3-ITD in AML.*

Laughlin MJ, Barker J, Bambach B, et al. Hematopoietic engraftment and survival in adult recipients of umbilical-cord blood from unrelated donors. *N Engl J Med.* 2001;344:1815–1822. *Umbilical cord blood stem cells from unrelated donors can restore hematopoiesis with acceptable rates of severe acute and chronic graft-versus-host disease.*

Leith CP, Kopecky KJ, Chen IM, et al. Frequency and clinical significance of the expression of the multidrug resistance proteins MDR1/P-glycoprotein, MRP1, and LRP in acute myeloid leukemia: a Southwest Oncology Group Study. *Blood.* 1999;94:1086–1099.

Leith CP, Kopecky KJ, Godwin J, et al. Acute myeloid leukemia in the elderly: assessment of multidrug resistance (MDR1) and cytogenetics distinguishes biologic subgroups with remarkably distinct responses to standard chemotherapy. A Southwest Oncology Group study. *Blood.* 1997;89:3323–3329.

Levi I, Grotto I, Yerushalmi R, et al. Meta-analysis of autologous bone marrow transplantation versus chemotherapy in adult patients with acute myeloid leukemia in first remission. *Leuk Res.* 2004;28:605–612.

Ley TJ, Mardis ER, Ding L, et al. DNA sequencing of a cytogenetically normal acute myeloid leukaemia genome. *Nature.* 2008;456:66–72.

Lowenberg B, van Puttten W, Theobald M, et al. Effect of priming with granulocyte colony-stimulating factor on the outcome of chemotherapy for acute myeloid leukemia. *N Engl J Med.* 2003; 349:743–752. *Randomized study showing no increase in CR rate but better disease-free survival for patients who received granulocyte colony-stimulating factor (G-CSF) with both cycles of induction chemotherapy. Standard-risk patients had better event-free survival, disease-free survival, and overall survival if they received G-CSF.*

Lowenberg B, Ossenkoppele GJ, van Putten W, et al. High-dose daunorubicin in older patients with acute myeloid leukemia. *N Engl J Med.* 2009;361:1235–1248.

Mardis ER, Ding L, Dooling DJ, et al. Recurring mutations found by sequencing an acute myeloid leukemia genome. *N Engl J Med.* 2009;361:1058–1066.

Mayer RJ, Davis RB, Schiffer CA, et al. Intensive post-remission chemotherapy in adults with acute myeloid leukemia. *N Engl J Med.* 1994;331:896–903. *Randomized study of three different cytarabine regimens in postremission therapy of AML. Benefit of HiDAC is limited to younger patients. HiDAC is suggested to be harmful to older patients.*

Ravindranath Y, Yeager AM, Chang MN, et al. 'Autologous' bone marrow transplantation versus intensive consolidated chemotherapy for acute myeloid leukemia in childhood. Pediatric Oncology Group. *N Engl J Med.* 1996;334:1428–1434. *Discusses role of autologous transplantation in childhood AML.*

Roboz GJ. Treatment of acute myeloid leukemia in older patients. *Expert Rev Anticancer Ther.* 2007;7:285–295. *Review of strategies for treatment of older patients with AML.*

Rowe JM, Andersen JW, Mazza JJ, et al. A randomized placebo-controlled phase III study of granulocyte-macrophage colony-stimulating factor in adult patients (>55 to 70 years of age) with acute myelogenous leukemia: a study of the Eastern Cooperative Oncology Group (E1490). *Blood.* 1995;86:457–462.

San Miguel JF, Vidriales MB, Lopez-Berges C, et al, et al. Early immunophenotypical evaluation of minimal residual disease in acute myeloid leukemia identifies different patient risk groups and may contribute to postinduction treatment stratification. *Blood.* 2001;98:1746–1751. *Concludes that immunophenotypical evaluations to detect MRD in the CR marrow after induction have important prognostic value.*

Sanz MA, Grimwade D, Tallman MS, et al. Management of acute promyelocytic leukemia: recommendations from an expert panel on behalf of the European LeukemiaNet. *Blood.* 2009;113:1975–1991.

Sanz MA, Martin G, Rayon C, et al. A modified AIDA protocol with anthracycline-based consolidation results in high antileukemic efficacy and reduced toxicity in newly diagnosed PML/RARalpha-positive acute promyelocytic leukemia. PETHEMA group. *Blood.* 1999;94:3015–3021.

Schiffer CA. Hematopoietic growth factors as adjuncts to the treatment of acute myeloid leukemia. *Blood.* 1996;88:3675–3685. *Presents perspective on use of hematopoietic growth factors in AML.*

Schlenk RF, Dohner K. Impact of new prognostic markers in treatment decisions in acute myeloid leukemia. *Curr Opin Hematol.* 2009;16:98–104.

Schlenk RF, Dohner K, Krauter J. et al. Mutations and treatment outcome in cytogenetically normal acute myeloid leukemia. *N Engl J Med.* 2008;358:1909–1918.

Sierra J, Granena A, Garcia J, et al. Autologous bone marrow transplantation for acute leukemia: results and prognostic factors in 90 consecutive patients. *Bone Marrow Transplant.* 1993;12:517–523. *Describes prognostic variables predictive of success after autologous transplantation and reports that disease stage at transplantation, FAB subtype, leukocytosis, splenomegaly, and time to first CR influence outcome.*

Slovak ML, Kopecky KJ, Cassileth PA, et al. Karyotypic analysis predicts outcome of preremission and postremission therapy in adult acute myeloid leukemia: a Southwest Oncology Group/Eastern Cooperative Oncology Group Study. *Blood.* 2000;96:4075–4083. *Reports the association of cytogenetics with complete remission rate, DFS, and overall survival in patients treated with allogeneic autologous or consolidation chemotherapy. Patients with favorable-risk cytogenetics did better with allogeneic transplantation.*

Stone RM, Berg DT, George SL, et al. Granulocyte macrophage colony-stimulating factor after initial chemotherapy for elderly patients with primary acute myelogenous leukemia. Cancer and Leukemia Group B. *N Engl J Med.* 1995;332:1671–1677. *Shows lack of benefit in outcome for granulocyte-macrophage colony-stimulating factor in older adults with AML.*

Suciu S, Mandelli F, De Witte T, et al. Allogeneic compared with autologous stem cell transplantation in the treatment of patients younger than 46 years with acute myeloid leukemia (AML) in first complete remission (CR1): an intention-to-treat analysis of the EORTC/GIMEMA AML-10 trial. *Blood.* 2003;102:1232–1240. *A large retrospective analysis of 1198 patients younger than 46 years of age who either received allogeneic transplantation, intensive consolidation with chemotherapy, or autologous transplantation after achieving CR. Patients' outcome was stratified based on their karyotype. Patients with poor cytogenetics had better disease-free survival and overall survival with consolidation with allogeneic transplantation after achieving their first CR as compared with other postremission modalities.*

Swerdlow SH, Campo E, Harris NL et al, eds. *World Health Organization Classification of Tumours of Haematopoietic and Lymphoid Tissues.* Lyon, France: IARC; 2008.

Tallman MS, Andersen JW, Schiffer CA, et al. All-trans-retinoic acid in acute promyelocytic leukemia. *N Engl J Med.* 1997;337:1021–1028. *The US Intergroup trial in newly diagnosed APL indicates that ATRA either during induction or postremission therapy is essential in treating this disease.*

Tallman MS, Rowlings PA, Milone G, et al. Effect of post-remission chemotherapy before human leukocyte antigen-identical sibling transplantation for acute myelogenous leukemia in first complete remission. *Blood.* 2000;96:1254–1258. *Shows that there appears to be no benefit to consolidation chemotherapy prior to HLA-matched allogeneic transplantation for patients with AML in first CR.*

Tallman UG, Andersen JW, Schiffer CA, et al. All-trans retinoic acid in acute promyelocytic leukemia: long term outcomes and prognostic factor analysis from the North American Intergroup protocol. *Blood.* 2002;100:4298–4302. *Shows excellent long-term outcome for ATRA plus chemotherapy.*

Tsukimoto I, Tawa A, Horibe K, et al. Risk-stratified therapy and the intensive use of cytarabine improves the outcome in childhood acute myeloid leukemia: the AML99 trial from the

Japanese Childhood AML Cooperative Study Group. *J Clin Oncol.* 2009;27:4007–1013.

Weick JK, Kopecky KJ, Appelbaum FR, et al, et al. A randomized investigation of high-dose versus standard-dose cytosine arabinoside with daunorubicin in patients with previously untreated acute myeloid leukemia: a Southwest Oncology Group study. *Blood.* 1996;88:2841-2851. *Reports outcome of high-dose cytarabine in induction, which proved to be too toxic for older adults.*

Wiernik PH, Banks PL, Case DC Jr, et al. Cytarabine plus idarubicin or daunorubicin as induction and consolidation therapy for previously untreated adult patients with acute myeloid leukemia. *Blood.* 1992;79:313–319. *Prospective randomized trial of cytarabine plus idarubicin versus cytarabine plus daunorubicin reports superiority of the idarubicin-containing regimen with respect to CR rate and percentage of resistant disease in patients with hyperleukocytosis.*

Woods WG, Kobrinsky N, Buckley JD, et al. Timed-sequential induction therapy improves post-remission outcome in acute myeloid leukemia: a report from the Children's Cancer Group. *Blood.* 1996;87:4979–4989.

Woods WG, Neudorf S, Gold S, et al. A comparison of allogeneic bone marrow transplantation, autologous bone marrow transplantation, and aggressive chemotherapy in children with acute myeloid leukemia in remission: a report from the Children's Cancer Group. *Blood.* 2001;97:56–62. *Matched sibling bone marrow transplantation improves disease-free survival. There was no benefit for autologous bone marrow transplantation.*

Zittoun RA, Mandelli F, Willernze R, et al. Autologous or allogeneic bone marrow transplantation compared with intensive chemotherapy in acute myelogenous leukemia. European Organization for Research and Treatment of Cancer (EORTC) and the Gruppo Italiano Malattie Ematologiche Maligne dell'Adulto (GIMEMA) Leukemia Cooperative Groups. N Engl J Med. 1995;332:217–223. *Extends observations of Mayer et al (1994) to induction therapy with HiDAC.*

CHAPTER 17

Acute lymphoblastic leukemia and lymphoblastic lymphoma

Wendy Stock and Ching-Hon Pui

Classification and diagnosis of ALL, 489	Molecular genetics, 491	Lymphoblastic lymphoma, 503
Immunophenotyping, 489	Prognostic factors, 492	Late complications of therapy, 504
Cytogenetics, 490	Treatment of ALL, 493	Bibliography, 504

Acute lymphoblastic leukemia (ALL) is the most common leukemia in children (representing 23% of cancer diagnoses among children younger than 15 years of age) but accounts for only 20% of adult acute leukemia. The prognosis for both adult and especially childhood ALL has improved substantially in recent years with the use of risk-directed induction-consolidation-continuation (maintenance) regimens that include central nervous system (CNS) prophylaxis. In children, treatment now results in complete remission (CR) rates of 97% to 99% and in 5-year event-free survival rates of 75% to 86% (Pui et al, 2008, 2009). The use of similar treatment regimens in adults with ALL has also improved the prognosis, with CR rates of 65% to 90% and 5-year survival rates of 25% to 50% (Gökbuget and Hoezler, 2009). The less favorable prognosis for adults with ALL is related to several factors, including a much higher frequency of poor-risk prognostic factors based on disease biology, comorbidities associated with older age that impair the ability to tolerate intensive multiagent chemotherapeutic regimens that have been used successfully in children, subtle differences in the treatment regimens used by medical oncologists treating adults, and treatment compliance.

Classification and diagnosis of ALL

The French-American-British (FAB) morphologic classification of ALL was based largely on morphology and contained little prognostic or therapeutic information that might help to guide treatment choice. The World Health Organization (WHO) classification was revised in 2008 and has changed the classification to reflect increased understanding of the biology and molecular pathogenesis of the diseases (Swerdlow et al, 2008). In addition to discarding the FAB terms, the WHO classification divides these heterogeneous lymphoid diseases into 2 major categories: precursor lymphoid neoplasms and mature lymphoid neoplasms. The precursor lymphoid diseases include both B lymphoblastic leukemia/lymphoma and T lymphoblastic leukemia/lymphoma. The new classification further subdivides the precursor B-cell ALL cases by recurring molecular-cytogenetic abnormalities to provide prognostic and therapeutic information and to facilitate the implementation of specific molecularly targeted therapies (Swerdlow et al, 2008). Burkitt lymphoma/leukemia is the one subset of ALL that is classified as a mature B lymphoid neoplasm.

Examination of a bone marrow aspirate is preferable to blood for diagnosis of ALL because as many as 10% of patients lack circulating blasts at the time of diagnosis and because bone marrow cells are better than blood cells for genetic studies. Fibrosis or tightly packed marrow can occasionally lead to difficulties with marrow aspiration that necessitate a biopsy to make the diagnosis. In patients with marrow necrosis, multiple marrow aspirations are sometimes needed to obtain diagnostic tissue.

Immunophenotyping

Because leukemic lymphoblasts lack specific morphologic and cytochemical features, immunophenotyping by flow cytometry and genetic analyses are essential for diagnosis. Most leukocyte antigens lack lineage specificity; hence, a panel of antibodies is needed to establish the diagnosis and to distinguish among the different immunologic subclasses

Conflict-of-interest disclosure: *Dr. Stock*: consultancy: Hana Biosciences; research funding: Enzon; honoraria: Enzon; *Dr. Pui*: honoraria: EUSA Pharma, Sanofi-Aventis.

of leukemic cells. In general, the panel includes antibodies to at least one very sensitive marker for each hematopoietic and lymphoid lineage (CD19 for B-lineage cells, CD7 for T-lineage cells, and CD13 or CD33 for myeloid cells) and antibodies to a relatively specific marker (cytoplasmic CD79a and CD22 for B-lineage cells, cytoplasmic CD3 for T-lineage cells, and CD20 and surface immunoglobulin for mature B cells) (Pui and Evans, 2006).

The distribution of the immunophenotypic subsets in adult and pediatric ALL is similar, with precursor B-cell ALL accounting for the majority (70%–85%) of all cases, precursor T-cell ALL accounting for approximately 15% to 25% of cases; Burkitt ALL accounting for approximately 2% to 5% of cases. The main distinctions of therapeutic importance are those between precursor B-cell ALL, precursor T-cell ALL, and Burkitt ALL. Typically, precursor B-cell ALL cases are terminal deoxynucleotidyl transferase (TdT) positive, human leukocyte antigen (HLA)-DR positive, and almost always positive for CD19 and CD79a. CD10 and CD22 are positive in most cases. The lymphoblasts in precursor T-cell ALL are TdT positive and most often express CD7 and cytoplasmic CD3; CD4 and CD8 are frequently coexpressed on the blasts. Recently, a distinct subset of precursor T-cell ALL has been identified in adults and children, termed early thymic precursor (or early precursor T) ALL. It has the same gene expression profile of normal early thymic precursor cells, a population of recent immigrants from bone marrow to the thymus that retain multilineage differentiation potential (Coustan-Smith, Mullighan, et al, 2009). These cases are associated with a dismal treatment outcome with chemotherapy. The mature B-cell ALL, Burkitt ALL, has a unique immunophenotype with expression of surface immunoglobulin and strong expression of CD20 with distinctive morphologic and cytogenetic features. These ALLs are associated with chromosome translocations involving the c-MYC proto-oncogene on chromosome 8.

Myeloid-associated antigens may be expressed on otherwise typical lymphoblasts. The pattern of myeloid-associated antigen expression is correlated with certain genetic features of blast cells. CD15, CD33, and CD65 are expressed in ALL patients with a rearranged *MLL* gene, and CD13 and CD33 are expressed in patients with the *ETV6-RUNX1* (also known as *TEL-AML1*) fusion. A subset of patients coexpress both lymphoid and myeloid markers but do not cluster with precursor T-cell, precursor B-cell, or acute myeloid leukemia in gene expression profiling. These patients may not respond to myeloid-directed therapy but may attain remission with ALL-directed induction treatment (Rubnitz et al, 2009). The presence of myeloid-associated antigens lacks prognostic significance but can be useful in immunologic monitoring of patients for minimal residual leukemia (Campana, 2009).

A summary of CD markers and specific immunophenotypic techniques and findings in ALL is found in Chapter 10.

Cytogenetics

ALL arises from a lymphoid progenitor cell that has sustained multiple specific genetic damages that lead to malignant transformation and proliferation. Thus, genetic classification of blast cells is expected to yield more relevant biologic information than that obtained by other means. More than 75% of adult and childhood cases can be readily classified into prognostically or therapeutically relevant subgroups based on the modal chromosome number (or DNA content estimated by flow cytometry), specific chromosomal rearrangements, and molecular genetic changes (Pui et al, 2004, 2008; Moorman et al, 2007; Pullarkat et al, 2008; Meijerink et al, 2009). Table 17-1 lists selected cytogenetic and molecular genetic abnormalities with prognostic and therapeutic relevance. Increasingly, as described in later sections on therapy, treatment strategies are being specifically "tailored" to the different molecular genetic subsets of ALL.

According to the modal chromosomal number, ALL can be classified into several ploidy subgroups. Hyperdiploidy >50 chromosomes, which is seen in approximately 25% of childhood cases and 6% to 7% of adult cases, is associated with a favorable prognosis in childhood ALL and in some studies of adult ALL, and may reflect an increased cellular accumulation of methotrexate and its polyglutamates, an increased sensitivity to antimetabolites, and a marked propensity of these cells to undergo apoptosis (Pui and Evans, 2006; Moorman et al, 2007). It should be noted that the outcome of hyperdiploid cases in adults is not comparable to the excellent outcome of childhood cases and that hyperdiploidy lacked favorable prognosis in some adult studies (Mancini et al, 2005). By contrast, hypodiploidy <44 chromosomes, especially near-haploidy, is consistently associated with an adverse prognosis in both children and adults with ALL (Nachman et al, 2007; Moorman et al, 2007; Pullarkat et al, 2008). Flow cytometric determination of cellular DNA content is a useful adjunct to cytogenetic analysis because it is automated, rapid, and inexpensive, and its measurements are not affected by the mitotic index of the cell population; results can be obtained in almost all cases. Flow cytometric studies can sometimes identify a small but drug-resistant subpopulation of near-haploid cells that may have been missed by standard cytogenetic analysis.

Specific reciprocal translocations have important biologic and clinical significance. Some translocations can mobilize the promoter/enhancer element of the immunoglobulin heavy or light chain gene or the T-cell antigen receptor β/γ or α/δ gene to sites adjacent to a variety of transcription factor genes and result in the overexpression

Table 17-1 Clinical and biologic characteristics of selected genetic subtypes of ALL.

Genetic abnormality	Frequency (%)		Estimated event-free survival (%)		Therapeutics
	Adult	Pediatric	Adult	Pediatric	
B cell					
t(8;14); t(2;8); t(8;22); *c-MYC* overexpression	5	2	50–80 at 3 years	75–85 at 3 years	Short-term intensive multiagent chemotherapy with rituximab
t(12;21)(p13;q22)/*ETV6-RUNX1* fusion	0–3	20–25	Unknown	85–95 at 5 years	Intensive asparaginase
Hyperdiploidy >50 chromosomes	6–7	23–29	30–50 at 5 years	80–90 at 5 years	Antimetabolites
t(1;19)(q23;p13.3)/*TCF3-PBX1* fusion	2–3	4–5	40–70 at 3 years	85–90 at 5 years	High-dose methotrexate
t(9;22)(q34;q11)/ *BCR-ABL1* fusion	25–30	2–3	40–60 at 2 years	80–90 at 3 years	Tyrosine kinase inhibitors (imatinib/dasatinib)
t(4;11)(q21;q23)/*MLL-AF4* fusion	3–7	2	10–20 at 3 years	30–40 at 5 years	*FLT3* inhibitors (PKC412/CEP-701)
BCR-ABL1–like/*IKZF1* alterations	Unknown	15–20	Unknown	40–50 at 5 years	–
Hypodiploid <44 chromosomes	2	1	10–20 at 3 years	30–40 at 3 years	–
iAMP21	Unknown	2	Unknown	~30 at 5 years	–
T cell					
NOTCH1 mutations	60–70	>50	~50 at 4 years	90 at 5 years	? γ-secretase inhibitors
HOX11 overexpression	30	7	70–80 at 3 years	90 at 5 years	–
HOX11L2	13	20	~20 at 2 years	~45 at 5 years	–
t(9;9)(q34;q34)/*NUP214-ABL1* fusion	5	4	Unknown	? unfavorable	ABL kinase inhibitors (imatinib/dasatinib)

ALL, acute lymphoblastic leukemia; iAMP21, intrachromosomal amplification of chromosome 21.

of the transcription factor. An example of this type of translocation occurs in Burkitt ALL, where the transcription factor *c-MYC* is translocated to the promoter/enhancer element of the immunoglobulin heavy or light chain and, consequently, is aberrantly expressed. More often, the genetic rearrangements result from the fusion of 2 genes encoding different transcription factors. These chimeric transcription factors may regulate genes involved in the differentiation, self-renewal, proliferation, and drug resistance of hematopoietic stem cells (Pui et al, 2004). Included in this group of translocations are those involving the *MLL* gene on chromosome 11q23, the most common of which is t(4;11), which results in the creation of the *MLL-AF4* fusion gene. Other fusion genes result in the aberrant activation of tyrosine kinases that play a critical role in pathogenesis of these diseases. An important example of this type of translocation is the Philadelphia chromosome, where t(9;22) results in the *BCR-ABL1* fusion gene and causes constitutive activation of the ABL tyrosine kinase, which is directly linked to disease pathogenesis.

Molecular genetics

In addition to cytogenetic analysis, there are compelling reasons to perform molecular genetic studies. First, molecular analyses can identify several important submicroscopic genetic alterations not visible by standard karyotyping procedures, such as the *ETV6-RUNX1* (also known as *TEL-AML1*) fusion, intrachromosomal amplification of chromosome 21, deletions of tumor suppressor genes, and mutations of proto-oncogenes. Second, cases with clinically important genetic rearrangements can be missed because of technical errors (eg, karyotyping residual normal metaphase cells rather than leukemic metaphase cells). Hence, fluorescence in situ hybridization (FISH) and reverse transcriptase polymerase chain reaction (RT-PCR) assays are used frequently.

More recently, the application of microarray-based genome-wide analysis of gene expression and DNA copy number, complemented by transcriptional profiling, resequencing, and epigenetic approaches, has identified specific genetic alterations with biologic and therapeutic implications. For example, genetic expression profiling studies have classified precursor T-cell ALL cases into several distinct genetic subgroups that correspond to specific T-cell development stages: *HOX11L2*, *LYL1* plus *LMO2*, *TAL1* plus *LMO1* or *LMO2*, *HOX11*, and *MLL-ENL*. Whereas *HOX11L2* generally confers a poor outcome, *HOX11* and *MLL-ENL* are associated with a favorable outcome (Baak et al, 2008; Ballerini et al, 2008; Meijerink et al, 2009). Among many other mutations in precursor T-cell ALL, *NOTCH1* or *FBXW7* mutations are associated with a favorable prognosis in childhood ALL, and the *NUP214-ABL1* fusion is responsive to tyrosine kinase inhibition (Breit et al, 2006; Asnafi et al, 2009;

Meijerink et al, 2009). In a recent adult study with small number of patients, NOTCH1 and FBXW7 mutations failed to correlate with treatment outcome (Mansour et al, 2009).

In precursor B-cell ALL with BCR-ABL1 fusion, IKZF1 is deleted in both pediatric and adult cases (75%-85%) (Mullighan et al, 2008; Iacobucci et al, 2009). Of interest, there is a subgroup of B-cell precursor ALL with IKZF1 deletion that has a genetic profile similar to that of cases with BCR-ABL1 fusion and also has poor prognosis with conventional treatment (den Boer et al, 2009; Mullighan, Su, et al, 2009). Recent genome-wide studies have identified another high-risk subgroup characterized by JAK mutation (Mullighan, Zhang, et al, 2009).

Prognostic factors

Of the many variables that influence prognosis, genetic subsets, initial white blood cell (WBC) count, age at diagnosis, and early treatment response are the most important (Pui et al, 2008). Although improved treatment has abolished the prognostic strength of many prognostic indicators in pediatric ALL, it should be stressed that even so-called low-risk patients need a certain degree of treatment intensification to avoid unacceptable rates of relapse. Table 17-2 lists the prognostic factors in adults and children that may be used for risk stratification in current clinical trials.

Clinical prognostic factors

Children age 1 to 9 years have a better outcome than either infants or adolescents, who, in turn, fare significantly better than adults with ALL. Among adults, the outcome of therapy worsens with increasing age. Leukocyte count is a continuous variable, with increasing counts conferring a poorer outcome. In childhood ALL, there is a general agreement of using a presenting age between 1 and 9 years and a leukocyte count of $<50 \times 10^9$/L as minimal criteria for low-risk precursor B-cell ALL; age and leukocyte count have little prognostic value in precursor T-cell ALL. In adult ALL, age <35 years and leukocyte count $<30 \times 10^9$/L are considered favorable prognostic indicators, and leukocyte count $>100 \times 10^9$/L is considered a poor prognostic feature for precursor T-cell ALL in some studies (Hoelzer and Gökbuget, 2009).

Cytogenetic and molecular genetic prognostic factors

The prognostic impact of age and, to a lesser extent, leukocyte count can be explained by their association with specific genetic abnormalities. For example, there is a preponderance of cases with favorable genetic abnormalities of hyperdiploidy >50 chromosomes or ETV6-RUNX1 in patients age 1 to 9 years (Pui et al, 2008). ETV6-RUNX1 mutations are rare in adults. Adverse genetic abnormalities such as MLL rearrangements occur in 70% to 80% of infant cases. The Philadelphia chromosome (Ph^+) occurs in 25% to 30% of adult patients, and the incidence of Ph^+ ALL increases with increasing age. Approximately 50% of cases of precursor B-cell ALL in patients over the age of 60 years are Ph^+.

Although many genetic abnormalities are associated with clinical outcome, only a few are routinely used for treatment stratification (Table 17-1). The Children's Oncology Group also uses trisomy of chromosomes 4, 10, and 17 (triple trisomy) as a favorable prognostic factor in its clinical trials (Schultz et al, 2007). There is clinical heterogeneity within each specific genetic subtype. For example, among patients with Ph^+ ALL, patients age 1 to 9 years fare significantly better than older patients (Aricó et al, 2000). In adults, Ph^+ ALL is associated not only with a high initial leukocyte count but also a dismal prognosis with standard chemotherapeutic regimens (Gökbuget and Hoelzer, 2009). Treatment intensification with allogeneic stem cell transplantation (allo-SCT)

Table 17-2 Prognostic factors used for risk stratification.

Prognostic factors	Favorable	Adverse
Adult		
Age (years)	<35	>60
Leukocyte count ($\times 10^9$/L)	<30	>100
Immunophenotype	Thymic T-ALL	Early T cell
Genotype	–	BCR-ABL1; MLL-AF4
Minimal residual disease after induction	<0.01%	>0.01%
Pediatric		
Age (years)	1 to 9	<1 or ≥10
Leukocyte count ($\times 10^9$/L)	<50	>50
Immunophenotype	Precursor B cell	Early thymic precursor
Genotype	Hyperdiploidy >50; ETV6-RUNX1	Hypodiploidy <44; BCR-ABL1; MLL-AF4
Minimal residual disease after induction	<0.01%	≥1%

in first remission remains a standard curative approach for these adults. In patients with *MLL-AF4* fusion, infants and adults have a worse prognosis than children (Pui et al, 2002; Mancini et al, 2005; Gleissner et al, 2005). The basis of these differences may be related to some combination of secondary genetic events, the developmental stage of the target cell undergoing malignant transformation, and the pharmacogenetic or pharmacokinetic features of the patient. In addition to t(4;11), the *MLL* gene is involved in a number of other translocations in ALL [eg, t(11;19), t(9;11)] (Pui et al, 2002). Due to their poor prognosis, allogeneic transplantation in first CR (CR1) is recommended for adult patients with translocations involving the *MLL* gene.

The clinical significance of many prognostic factors changes with improvements in treatment. For example, the outcome for patients with Ph$^+$ ALL has improved substantially with the addition of tyrosine kinase inhibitors to treatment, which is described in detail later. In fact, children with this genotype who are treated with chemotherapy and imatinib (without allo-SCT) have a 3-year event-free survival rate of >80% (Schultz et al, 2009). If the favorable outcome is confirmed with longer follow-up, Ph chromosome may join a long list of other factors such as male sex and African American ethnicity that have lost adverse prognostic impact with improved treatment in childhood ALL (Silverman et al, 2001; Möricke et al, 2008; Pui, Sandlund, et al, 2003; Pui et al, 2009). The recent finding of adverse prognosis of CD20 expression in adult ALL (Thomas et al, 2009), albeit not childhood ALL (Jeha et al, 2006), may have therapeutic implications as a result of the availability of the anti-CD20 monoclonal antibody rituximab.

Minimal residual disease detection

A useful adjunct in risk assessment is the response to early treatment, which is measured by the rate of clearance of leukemic cells from the blood or bone marrow. This measure accounts for the drug sensitivity or resistance of leukemic cells and the pharmacodynamics of the drugs, which are affected by the pharmacogenetics of the host. Flow cytometric profiling of aberrant immunophenotypes and PCR amplification of fusion transcripts or antigen-receptor genes, which are at least 100-fold more sensitive than conventional morphologic determinations, have allowed minimal residual disease (MRD) to be detected at very low levels (<0.01%), providing a useful means to identify patients at very low or high risk of relapse. Patients with 1% or more leukemic cells after remission induction fare almost as poorly as those who fail to achieve clinical remission by the conventional morphologic standard (≥5% leukemic cells), whereas those who achieve molecular or immunologic remission (<0.01%) have an excellent outcome (Borowitz et al, 2008; Campana, 2009; Pui et al, 2009). MRD can be measured by the current techniques in nearly all patients and has become a crucial factor for risk stratification in childhood ALL (Pui et al, 2009). MRD detection after achievement of morphologic remission in adults with ALL has also been associated with a significantly worse prognosis (for review, see Abutalib, Wetzler, and Stock, 2007). Monitoring of MRD can also be used for early detection of impending relapse and hence for early treatment intervention (Raff et al, 2007). Finally, MRD level is also a strong predictor of treatment outcome at the time of second remission and before allo-SCT for relapsed leukemia in both pediatric and adult ALL (Coustan-Smith et al, 2004; Paganin et al, 2008; Bader et al, 2009).

MRD measurement is now used to improve risk stratification and to allocate patients to allo-SCT in many pediatric trials and in at least 1 adult clinical trial (Pui et al, 2009; Bassan et al, 2009). MRD detection before and after allo-SCT in adults with Ph$^+$ ALL has also been associated with poor disease-free survival (DFS). Based on these insights, some investigators are examining the efficacy of posttransplantation therapy with imatinib or other targeted tyrosine kinase inhibitors to eradicate MRD and improve posttransplantation progression-free survival (Wassmann et al, 2005; Carpenter et al, 2007)

Treatment of ALL
Supportive care

Optimal management of patients with ALL requires careful attention to supportive care. Hyperuricemia and hyperphosphatemia with secondary hypocalcemia are frequently encountered at diagnosis, even before chemotherapy is initiated, especially in patients with high leukemic cell burden and those with precursor T-cell or mature B-cell ALL. Patients should be given intravenous fluids; allopurinol or rasburicase (recombinant urate oxidase) should be given to patients at high risk of tumor lysis syndrome to treat or prevent hyperuricemia (Coiffier et al, 2008); and a phosphate binder, such as aluminum hydroxide, calcium acetate or carbonate (if the serum calcium concentration is low), lanthanum carbonate, or sevelamer, should be given to treat hyperphosphatemia. Infections are common in febrile patients with newly diagnosed ALL. Therefore, any patient presenting with fever, especially patients with neutropenia, should be given broad-spectrum antibiotics until infection is excluded. Usually, all patients with ALL are given trimethoprim-sulfamethoxazole, 2 to 3 days per week, as prophylactic therapy for *Pneumocystis carinii* (*Pneumocystis jiroveci*) pneumonia. Many adult trials also recommend some form of antiviral and antifungal prophylaxis during the active phases of treatment. The use of hematopoietic growth factors for adults with ALL has been found to be safe and reduces the number of induction deaths. These studies are reviewed later in the treatment section of adult ALL. All blood products should be irradiated to prevent graft-versus-host disease. Other important supportive care measures include the use of indwelling catheters, amelioration of nausea and vomiting, pain control, and continuous psychosocial support for the patient and family.

Treatment of Burkitt lymphoma/leukemia in children and adults

The outcome for both children and adults with Burkitt lymphoma/leukemia has improved dramatically during the last decade. The improved outcomes have resulted from the use of fractionated high doses of alkylating agents such as cyclophosphamide or ifosfamide with high-dose methotrexate. These agents are combined with vincristine, an anthracycline (doxorubicin or daunorubicin), and high-dose cytarabine and administered in rapid succession over 4 to 6 months. To reduce the large tumor bulk often present at diagnosis and limit the severity of tumor lysis syndrome, a "reduction" phase consisting of a week of glucocorticoid treatment and a dose of vincristine and cyclophosphamide before intensive chemotherapy has often been incorporated into treatment regimens. Because of a predisposition to central nervous system (CNS) involvement in ALL, aggressive CNS-directed therapy is given with high doses of systemically administered cytarabine and methotrexate and intrathecal administration with these agents in combination with hydrocortisone (triple therapy). CNS irradiation is typically omitted and reserved for adult patients with overt CNS disease. Recurrence after the first year rarely, if ever, occurs; therefore, maintenance therapy has not been shown to be beneficial and is not recommended. Using this aggressive approach, the survival for these patients has ranged from 50% to 60% in many adult series to well over 80% in pediatric series. Because the lymphoblasts in mature B-cell ALL exhibit strong expression of CD20, ongoing studies have incorporated the anti-CD20 monoclonal antibody rituximab into frontline regimens in an attempt to further improve outcome. The data from the first of these trials appear very promising, with survival rates of >80% reported in 2 recent adult series (Thomas et al, 2006; Gökbuget and Hoelzer, 2009). The addition of rituximab to frontline therapies for Burkitt lymphoma/leukemia is also being tested in children.

Treatment of precursor B-cell and precursor T-cell ALL in children

Although risk-directed therapy is a standard therapeutic strategy for childhood ALL, there is no consensus on the risk criteria and the terminology for defining prognostic subgroups. Usually, childhood ALL cases are divided into low- (standard-) risk, high- (intermediate- or average-) risk, and very high–risk groups, although the US Children's Oncology Group advocates 4 categories, including a very low–risk group. Often infants are treated with a separate regimen. Treatment typically consists of a remission induction phase, an intensification (consolidation) phase, and prolonged continuation therapy to eradicate residual disease. CNS-directed therapy is started early and is given for different lengths of time, depending on the patient's risk of relapse and the intensity of the primary systemic treatment.

Remission induction

Rates of CR range from 97% to 99% with contemporary chemotherapy (Pui and Evans, 2006). The induction regimen typically includes a glucocorticoid (prednisone, prednisolone, or dexamethasone), vincristine, and asparaginase. Children with high- or very high–risk ALL receive 1 or more additional drugs including an anthracycline and cyclophosphamide. Intensive induction can lead to increased early morbidity and mortality. In a recent study, the use of high-dose dexamethasone (10 mg/m^2/d) instead of prednisone (60 mg/m^2/d) during remission induction resulted in a high induction death rate, especially in adolescent patients, but significantly improved treatment outcome for patients with precursor T-cell ALL (Schrappe et al, 2008). However, intensification of induction is not necessary for children with standard-risk ALL, particularly if they receive postinduction intensification therapy (Gaynon et al, 2000; Harms and Janka-Schaub, 2000).

Although dexamethasone provided better control of systemic and CNS disease than did prednisone in 2 randomized studies (Bostrom et al, 2003; Mitchell et al, 2005), a small study showed that an augmented dose of prednisolone produced results comparable to those achieved with dexamethasone (Igarashi et al, 2005). Similarly, the pharmacodynamics of asparaginase differ by formulation, and in terms of leukemic control, the dose-intensity and duration of asparaginase treatment (ie, the amount of asparagine depletion) are far more important than the type of asparaginase used. Because of the lower immunogenicity, less frequent dosing, and feasibility in intravenous administration of PEG-asparaginase (a polyethylene glycol form of the *Escherichia coli* asparaginase), compared with the native product (Silverman et al, 2001; Hak et al, 2004), PEG-asparaginase has replaced the asparaginase as the first-line treatment for children in the United States and is also increasingly used in other clinical trials around the world. Because antibodies to *E coli* asparaginase cross-react with PEG-asparaginase (Hak et al, 2004), patients with allergic reactions to either form of the asparaginase should be treated with the product derived from

Erwinia chrysanthemi. It should also be noted that antibodies can develop against polyethylene glycol and adversely affect the efficacy of the drug (Armstrong et al, 2007). Of the various anthracyclines given to patients with ALL, none has proved superior to any other; however, daunorubicin is used most commonly.

Intensification (consolidation) therapy

When normal hematopoiesis is restored, patients in remission become candidates for intensification therapy. Although there is no dispute on the importance of this treatment, there is no consensus on the best regimen and duration of treatment. More commonly used regimens include high-dose methotrexate with or without mercaptopurine, high-dose asparaginase given for an extended period, or a combination of dexamethasone, vincristine, asparaginase, and doxorubicin, followed by thioguanine, cytarabine, and cyclophosphamide (Pui and Evans, 2006). This phase of therapy has improved outcome, even for patients with low-risk ALL. Patients with *ETV6-RUNX1* have an especially good outcome in clinical trials featuring intensive postremission treatment with glucocorticoids, vincristine, and asparaginase (Loh et al, 2006; Pui et al, 2009). High-dose methotrexate (5 g/m^2) is associated with improved outcome in T-cell ALL (Schrappe et al, 2000; Pui et al, 2009), whereas lower doses appear to be sufficient for low-risk precursor B-cell ALL (Evans et al, 1998).

Delayed intensification (or reinduction), first introduced by investigators of the Berlin-Frankfurt-Münster consortium, is a widely used approach consisting of a repetition of the first remission induction therapy 3 months after the end of remission induction. Investigators at the Children's Cancer Group reported that double delayed intensification improved patient outcome in patients with intermediate-risk ALL (Lange et al, 2002). Although extended and stronger intensification therapy with asparaginase, methotrexate, and vincristine was shown to significantly improve outcome for children and adolescents with high-risk ALL and slow response to initial induction therapy (Nachman et al, 1998), recent studies demonstrated that early intensive (rather than extended) postinduction treatment benefits the patients (Nachman et al, 2009; Pui et al, 2009). Double or prolonged intensification probably is not necessary for patients with low-risk ALL.

Maintenance (continuation) therapy

A combination of methotrexate administered weekly and mercaptopurine administered daily constitutes the usual continuation regimen for ALL. In the past, boys were treated with a longer duration of continuation therapy than girls because male sex was associated with a poorer prognosis. With improved outcome, both boys and girls are now treated with the same duration of 2 to 2.5 years of continuation therapy in most clinical trials. Accumulation of higher intracellular concentrations of the active metabolites of methotrexate and mercaptopurine and administration of this combination to the limits of tolerance (as indicated by low leukocyte counts) have been associated with improved clinical outcome (Schmiegelow et al, 1995). Many investigators advocate that the drug dosage be adjusted to maintain leukocyte counts below 3×10^9/L and neutrophil counts between 0.5 and 1.5×10^9/L to ensure adequate dose-intensity during the continuation treatment in childhood ALL. In 1 study, the dose intensity of mercaptopurine was the most important pharmacologic factor influencing treatment outcome (Relling et al, 1999). However, overzealous use of mercaptopurine is counterproductive, resulting in interruption of chemotherapy due to neutropenia and reduction of overall dose intensity. Mercaptopurine should be taken in the evening. Although methotrexate is used orally in most clinical trials, parenteral administration could circumvent problems of decreased bioavailability and poor compliance, especially in adolescents. Antimetabolite treatment should not be withheld because of isolated increases of liver enzymes; such liver function abnormalities are tolerable and reversible.

A few patients (1 in 300) have an inherited homozygous deficiency of thiopurine *S*-methyltransferase, the enzyme that catalyzes the *S*-methylation (inactivation) of mercaptopurine. Mercaptopurine should be markedly reduced (eg, 10-fold reduction) in these patients to avoid potentially fatal hematologic toxicity. Approximately 10% of patients are heterozygous for the enzyme deficiency and have intermediate levels of thiopurine methyltransferase. This subgroup can be treated safely with only moderate reductions in mercaptopurine dosage and appears to have better clinical outcomes than patients with the homozygous wild-type phenotype (Relling et al, 1999). Importantly, patients with this enzyme deficiency are at risk for therapy-related leukemia (Pui and Relling, 2000; Schmiegelow et al, 2009). Whether dose reduction of mercaptopurine can reduce the risk of therapy-related leukemia in these patients is unknown. Although thioguanine is more potent than mercaptopurine, leads to higher concentrations of thioguanine nucleotides in cells and cytotoxic concentrations in cerebrospinal fluid, and produces superior antileukemic response, its prolonged use at a dose >40 mg/m^2 has been associated with profound thrombocytopenia, an increased risk of death, and an unacceptable rate of hepatic veno-occlusive disease (Vora et al, 2006). Therefore, mercaptopurine remains the drug of choice for ALL.

Intermittent pulses of vincristine and a glucocorticoid have improved the efficacy of antimetabolite-based continuation regimens (Childhood ALL Collaborative Group, 1996) and have been widely adopted in the treatment of childhood ALL. However, in a randomized trial featuring intensive reinduction, the addition of 6 pulses of vincristine and dexamethasone during early continuation treatment failed to improve outcome of children with intermediate-risk ALL (Conter et al, 2007). Thus, whether this pulse therapy is necessary in contemporary regimens featuring early intensification of therapy remains to be determined.

CNS-directed treatment

Prophylactic cranial irradiation, once a standard treatment, is being replaced by intrathecal and systemic chemotherapy to reduce radiation-associated late complications. Two early clinical trials tested the feasibility of complete omission of prophylactic cranial irradiation from treatment (Vilmer et al, 2000; Manera et al, 2000); although the cumulative risks of an isolated CNS relapse were relatively low (4% and 3%), the event-free survival rates were only 68.4% and 60.7%. In another study, prophylactic cranial irradiation appeared to improve outcome in T-cell ALL with leukocyte count $>100 \times 10^9$/L (Conter et al, 1997). Thus, virtually all childhood study groups continue to rely on prophylactic cranial irradiation for up to 20% of patients (Pui and Howard, 2008). A radiation dose of 12 Gy appeared to provide adequate protection against CNS relapse, even in high-risk patients (eg, those with T-cell ALL and leukocyte counts $>100 \times 10^9$/L) (Schrappe et al, 2000). However, 2 recent studies tested the feasibility of total omission of prophylactic cranial irradiation, even in patients with T-cell ALL, hyperleukocytosis, or overt CNS leukemia at diagnosis (Pui et al, 2009; Veerman et al, 2009). In these 2 studies, the 5-year survival rates were 85.6% and 81%, and the cumulative risks of an isolated CNS relapse were only 2.7% and 2.6%, respectively. Importantly, all 11 patients with isolated CNS relapse in the first study remained in second remission for 0.4 to 5.5 years (Pui et al, 2009). These promising results suggest that prophylactic cranial irradiation can be safely omitted in all patients in the context of the effective intrathecal and systemic chemotherapy.

Systemic treatment, including high-dose methotrexate, intensive asparaginase, and dexamethasone, and optimal intrathecal therapy are important to control CNS leukemia (Pui and Howard, 2008). Triple intrathecal therapy with methotrexate, cytarabine, and hydrocortisone is more effective than intrathecal methotrexate alone in preventing CNS relapse (Matloub et al, 2006). Because the presence of ALL blasts in the cerebrospinal fluid, even from traumatic lumbar puncture, has been associated with an increased risk of CNS relapse and poor event-free survival (Gajjar et al, 2000; Bürger et al, 2003), special precaution should be taken to decrease the rate of traumatic lumbar puncture (eg, transfusion to increase platelet count to $>100 \times 10^9$/L for initial intrathecal treatment, having the most experienced clinician perform the procedure with the patient under deep sedation or general anesthesia), and intrathecal therapy should be intensified in patients with this feature (Pui and Howard, 2008). Patients should remain in a prone position for at least 30 minutes after the procedure.

Stem cell transplantation

The indications for hematopoietic stem cell transplantation (SCT) during first remission should be continuously reviewed as treatment improves and new agents become available. At this time, poor early response to remission induction treatment (eg, $\geq$1% blasts after remission induction) is the most frequent indication for transplantation. Except in some small studies, transplantation failed to improve outcome of infant patients with *MLL* rearrangement (Pui et al, 2002). Hypodiploid cases also did not appear to benefit from transplantation, but the number of patients treated with this modality was very small (Nachman et al, 2007). The use of imatinib has dramatically improved early treatment results in children with *BCR-ABL1*–positive ALL, including those with poor early response (Schultz and Alayton, 2009), raising the question of whether transplantation should be performed in first remission even in children with this subtype of ALL. In fact, because of this remarkable early result, many pediatric oncologists are not recommending transplantation for children with *BCR-ABL1*–positive ALL while awaiting the long-term results of the study. Whether transplantation would benefit patients with early thymic precursor ALL remains to be determined.

Treatment for relapse in children

Marrow relapse, with or without extramedullary involvement, remains the most common type of relapse and portends a poor outcome for most patients. Factors indicating an especially poor prognosis include relapse while on therapy or after a short initial remission, T-cell immunophenotype, the presence of the Philadelphia chromosome, and an isolated hematologic relapse (Rivera et al, 2005; Nguyen et al, 2008). Prolonged second remissions ($>$3 years) can be achieved with chemotherapy in as many as half of patients with late relapses (ie, $>$6 months after cessation of therapy) but in only approximately 10% of patients with early relapse. The presence of MRD after reinduction treatment also portends a very poor prognosis (Coustan-Smith et al, 2004; Paganin et al, 2008). In patients who experience hematologic relapse while on therapy or shortly thereafter and in patients with high levels of MRD after remission induction for relapse, allogeneic hematopoietic SCT is the treatment of choice. For patients without histocompatible related donors, transplantation of stem cells from cord blood or marrow from matched unrelated donors has yielded encouraging results (Borgmann et al, 2003). Outcome may be further improved by a new strategy using a reduced-intensity conditioning regimen and selection of donor-derived alloreactive natural killer cells for haploidentical transplantation (Leung et al, 2004; Triplett et al, 2006). Among various chemotherapeutic regimens tested in relapsed ALL, the combination of clofarabine, etoposide, and cyclophosphamide appears to be particularly promising and warrants additional studies (Hijya et al, 2009).

Although extramedullary relapse is frequently an isolated clinical finding, many occurrences are associated with MRD in the marrow. CNS relapses are associated with a higher level of MRD in the bone marrow than testicular relapses (Hagedorn et al, 2007). Importantly, submicroscopic bone marrow involvement at a level of 10^{-4} or higher at the time of overt extramedullary relapse confers a very poor outcome. Hence, patients with extramedullary relapse and MRD in bone marrow require intensive treatment to prevent subsequent hematologic relapse. The efficacy of retrieval therapy in children with an isolated CNS relapse depends partly on duration of CR1 and partly on whether CNS irradiation was previously performed. The strategy of delaying cranial or craniospinal irradiation for 6 to 12 months to allow initial intensification of systemic chemotherapy has yielded long-term second event-free survival rates of 70% to 80% in children with isolated CNS relapse (Ribeiro et al, 1995; Ritchey et al, 1999). In 1 study, 12 months of intensive systemic chemotherapy and reduced-dose cranial irradiation (18 Gy) resulted in an excellent 4-year event-free survival rate among children with precursor B-cell ALL who had not received cranial irradiation during initial treatment and had an initial remission duration of ≥18 months (Barredo et al, 2006). One-third of patients with early testicular relapse and two-thirds of patients with late testicular recurrence became long-term survivors after salvage chemotherapy and testicular irradiation (Nguyen et al, 2008). For patients with bilateral testicular relapse, local irradiation (22-26 Gy) is usually recommended, but the optimal dose of irradiation is unclear. In patients with unilateral testicular relapse, some leukemia therapists advocate unilateral orchiectomy with reduced irradiation (15 Gy) to the "uninvolved testicle," but others would rely on intensive chemotherapy alone to spare the testicular function. Indeed, successful treatment in some patients with testicular relapse has been achieved without the use of any testicular irradiation (van den Berg et al, 1997).

Targeted therapies

The best example of targeted therapy is the use of the tyrosine kinase inhibitor imatinib in *BCR-ABL1*–positive ALL. Second-generation tyrosine kinase inhibitors (eg, dasatinib, nilotinib) that are more potent have been developed to partly address the problem of resistance to imatinib. Other novel agents include inhibitors of FLT3, farnesyltransferase, proteasome, DNA methylation, and histone deacetylase (Pui and Jeha, 2007). Immunotherapeutic options are progressively emerging. Rituximab (anti-CD20), gemtuzumab ozogamicin (anti-CD33), alemtuzumab (anti-CD52), and epratuzumab (anti-CD22) have already been incorporated into some clinical trials (Pui and Jeha, 2007). Recombinant immunotoxins and bispecific antibodies (blinatumomab) are being tested (Reichert and Valge-Archer, 2007; Bargou et al, 2008). Other promising investigational drugs include nelarabine and forodesine for T-cell ALL (Pui and Jeha, 2007).

Special subgroups of ALL in children

Patients with Down syndrome have a 10- to 20-fold higher relative risk for leukemia, and they constitute approximately 2% of pediatric ALL. They have the same age range as the general pediatric population with the exception of a lack of cases in the infant age group. ALL patients with Down syndrome lack T-cell and mature B-cell ALL and have a low frequency of other specific genetic subtypes of precursor B-cell ALL (Forestier et al, 2008) but have a high frequency of activating somatic *JAK2* mutations, affecting approximately 20% of the cases (Bercovich et al, 2008). A recent study showed that 55% of Down syndrome cases have *CRLF2* overexpression, frequently in association with activating *JAK* mutations (Mullighan et al, 2009). Although the outcome has improved with modern treatment, these patients still fared significantly worse than other children with ALL, due to poor tolerance to chemotherapy, such as dexamethasone and methotrexate, and excessive treatment-related deaths (Aricó et al, 2008; Rabin and Whitlock, 2009).

Infant ALL accounts for 2% to 3% of childhood ALL and is characterized by a high frequency of 11q23 chromosomal abnormalities and rearrangements of the *MLL* gene (70%-80%), a CD10-negative pro-B immunophenotype, hyperleukocytosis, and an inferior outcome. A recent clinical trial featuring intensive lymphoid- and myeloid-directed therapy resulted in improved outcome of infants with ALL, with a 4-year event-free survival rate of 47% (Pieters et al, 2007).

Several studies have shown that adolescents and young adults treated on pediatric trials fared significantly better than the same age groups treated on adult protocols (Boissel et al, 2003; de Bont et al, 2004; Hallböök et al, 2006; Ramanujachar et al, 2007; Barry et al, 2007; Nachman et al, 2009). The superior outcome with pediatric regimens has been attributed to more effective treatment and to the better compliance by patients, parents, and clinicians. Several combined adult and pediatric consortia are using common regimens to treat children and young adults to understand the basis for this difference

Treatment of precursor B-cell and T-cell ALL in adults

Tailoring treatment to assessed risk has resulted in improved outcomes in pediatric ALL. In adults with ALL, although risk stratification has been used with success in the treatment of Burkitt ALL and, more recently, Ph$^+$ ALL (described later), over the last 2 decades, the majority of patients with precursor B- and T-cell ALL have been treated without specific consideration of biologic risk. Treatment for these adults has, in general, followed the same basic strategy of induction, consolidation-intensification, CNS prophylaxis, and maintenance therapy that has been used so successfully in pediatric ALL. The relative contribution of each of these phases toward improved prognosis and disease curability has not been rigorously determined in adult ALL. Nevertheless, the use of regimens patterned after those used in childhood ALL has resulted in the achievement of remission in the majority (75%-90%) of adults with ALL, although cure rates are only approximately 30% to 40% overall. The general treatment strategy for adults with ALL is described in the following sections. Due to the lower survival rates in adults with ALL treated with aggressive combination chemotherapy approaches, the use of allo-SCT in CR1 has been explored, and results of these studies are also reviewed briefly in this chapter. Current clinical research efforts are focused on better risk stratification with implementation of biologically directed therapies tailored to disease subset, as described in the following sections, for adolescents and young adults with ALL and those with Ph$^+$ ALL.

Induction phase

Over the last 20 years, intensification of the induction regimen for adults with ALL has resulted in significant improvement in CR rates, with >80% of patients achieving remission in many current multicenter studies. Building on a backbone of vincristine, a glucocorticoid (prednisone or dexamethasone), and often asparaginase, the addition of an anthracycline (daunorubicin or doxorubicin) has resulted in improved CR rates ranging from 72% to 92% (Hoelzer et al, 1992; Larson et al, 1995). Given the high CR rate observed with these 4-drug induction regimens, it has been difficult to demonstrate further improvements in overall CR rates with the addition of other drugs such as cyclophosphamide or cytarabine during induction (Annino et al, 2002). The Italian Gruppo Italiano Malattie Ematologiche Maligne dell'Adulto (GIMEMA) reported that, similar to childhood ALL, a good response to 1 week of pretreatment prednisone prior to chemotherapy, defined as a decrease in circulating blasts to ≤1000/μL, was predictive of a longer CR duration and survival. An alternative treatment regimen known as Hyper-CVAD was developed at the M.D. Anderson Cancer Center and uses hyperfractionated cyclophosphamide (similar to the approach used for Burkitt lymphoma/leukemia), dexamethasone, vincristine, and doxorubicin without asparaginase during induction and high-dose cytarabine and methotrexate during consolidation (Kantarjian et al, 2000). In their trial of 204 patients, 91% achieved CR with 3- and 5-year DFS rates of 50% and 38%, respectively. Pioneered in the treatment of pediatric ALL, the contribution of asparaginase to response rates and duration of response in adults is not clear. The toxicities of asparaginase in adults include pancreatitis, hepatotoxicity, and coagulopathy. An analysis of the Cancer and Leukemia Group B (CALGB) 8811 study showed a marginal benefit in DFS at 3 years for patients who received all prescribed doses of asparaginase (55% vs 48%, with overlapping 95% confidence intervals) (Larson et al, 1998). Eighty-five percent of the 197 patients in that trial achieved CR after induction (Larson et al, 1995). Ongoing trials by the German Multicenter ALL (GMALL) group of the long-acting asparaginase, PEG-asparaginase, suggest a potential survival benefit in older adults with ALL when the drug is administered at slightly lower doses than have been used by the pediatricians (Gökbuget et al, 2008).

The goal of using granulocyte colony-stimulating factor (G-CSF) is to shorten the period of neutropenia to prevent possibly fatal infections, and previous studies demonstrate the utility of this drug with induction regimens for ALL (Ottmann et al, 1995; Geissler et al, 1997; Larson et al, 1998; Thomas X et al, 2004). In the Leucémie Aigüe Lymphoblastique de l'Adulte (LALA)-94 trial, patients were randomized to receive G-CSF, granulocyte-macrophage colony-stimulating factor (GM-CSF), or no colony-stimulating factor (CSF) (Thomas X et al, 2004). When given on day 4 of induction until return of absolute neutrophil count >1000/μL, patients receiving G-CSF had significantly shorter hospital stays, less time to neutrophil recovery, and fewer severe infections compared with patients who did not receive CSF. The previously discussed CALGB 9111 trial highlighted the benefit of using this drug in patients prone to difficulty with hematologic recovery, specifically older patients (Larson et al, 1998). The study observed a trend toward increased CR rates in patients 60 years of age or older in the G-CSF arm compared with the placebo arm. Although G-CSF does not affect DFS or overall survival (OS), it appears to be safe and assists patients to proceed with postremission therapy.

Consolidation therapy

Traditionally, agents similar to the 4 or 5 drugs used during remission induction, with the addition of antimetabolites such as methotrexate, mercaptopurine, or thioguanine, are used for postremission treatment. The postremission treatment modules in adult series have typically been modeled after the pediatric regimens. Cyclophosphamide, high-dose cytarabine, and etoposide have also been incorporated into many postremission strategies, although it has been difficult to analyze critically the contribution of each drug or schedule to outcome in adult ALL series.

Although induction chemotherapy leads to CR rates that are >90% in many series, the relapse rate in adult ALL patients is 50% to 75%, leading to many variations of postremission consolidation treatment in an attempt to eradicate MRD and improve DFS. Adult consolidation regimens have evolved from pediatric schedules that have been shown to be successful (Nachman et al, 1998). Postremission therapy in ALL can include a wide range of drugs, including cytarabine, etoposide, teniposide, methotrexate, mercaptopurine, and thioguanine. In addition, the use of autologous SCT (auto-SCT) and allo-SCT has been incorporated into ALL treatment, as will be discussed in a separate section.

The CALGB compared a more intensive consolidation regimen that included both early and late intensification using 8 drugs with previous CALGB trials in a phase II study (Larson et al, 1998). The results showed that median remission duration improved to 29 months, whereas median survival extended to 36 months. Likewise, the M.D. Anderson group used extended consolidation within its Hyper-CVAD regimen by alternating cyclophosphamide, doxorubicin, vincristine, and dexamethasone (cycles 1, 3, 5, and 7) with high doses of methotrexate and cytarabine (cycles 2, 4, 6, and 8) in a single-arm trial (Kantarjian et al, 2000). In this study of 204 patients treated between 1992 and 1998, median survival time was 35 months, and the 5-year survival rate was 39%. The Italian GIMEMA group conducted a study that included randomization of 388 patients to postremission intensification followed by maintenance chemotherapy versus early maintenance therapy without intensification (Annino et al, 2002). The results showed no significant difference between the 2 groups at 8 years, with 36% DFS in patients treated with consolidation versus 37% in patients who went directly to maintenance therapy. However, only 35% of patients who were randomized to the consolidation/maintenance arm completed treatment as prescribed due to compliance problems and treatment-related toxicity.

The French LALA-94 trial investigated the use of intensive versus less intense consolidation treatment in patients with standard-risk ALL (Thomas X et al, 2004). In this trial, patients were considered to be at standard risk if they had (1) precursor B-cell ALL without CNS involvement; (2) absence of the Ph chromosome, t(4;11), t(1;19), or other abnormalities involving 11q23 rearrangements; (3) WBC count $<30 \times 10^9$/L; (4) an immunophenotype characterized by $CD10^+/CD19^+$ or $CD20^+/CD19^+$; (5) absence of myeloid markers; and (6) achievement of CR after 1 course of chemotherapy. Intensive consolidation included the use of high-dose cytarabine and mitoxantrone, whereas standard consolidation included cyclophosphamide, lower dose cytarabine, and mercaptopurine. Of 307 patients who had standard-risk disease in this trial, there was no significant difference in OS between the more intense versus less intense consolidation arms (45% vs 43%, respectively; $P = .73$).

In summary, all of these regimens result in similar DFS rates of approximately 30% to 40% in adult patients with ALL who are entered into cooperative group trials. However, outcomes vary considerably. Younger patients with favorable-risk cytogenetics can have DFS rates of >60%; in contrast, older adults >60 years old still have a dismal prognosis, with fewer than 10% to 15% achieving long-term survival. Ongoing clinical trials are testing the incorporation of novel agents, including targeted monoclonal antibodies, such as rituximab for $CD20^+$ lymphoblasts and alemtuzumab for $CD52^+$ cases, and targeted tyrosine kinase inhibitors, into standard regimens in an attempt to eradicate MRD and improve DFS.

CNS prophylaxis

Although <10% of adults with ALL present with CNS involvement (Cortes et al, 1995; Reman et al, 2008), CNS relapse will occur in 35% to 75% of patients at 1 year if prophylactic CNS-directed therapy is not incorporated into treatment (Omura et al, 1980). A lumbar puncture at the time of ALL diagnosis is essential. CNS disease is present when more than 5 leukocytes per microliter of cerebrospinal fluid are seen along with the presence of lymphoblasts in the cerebrospinal fluid. Symptoms may include headache, meningismus, fever, or cranial nerve palsies. However, some patients have no symptoms. Risk factors for CNS involvement in adults include mature B-cell ALL, high serum lactate dehydrogenase levels (>600 U/L), and the presence of a high proliferative index at diagnosis (>14% of lymphoblasts in the S and G_2/M phase of the cell cycle) (Kantarjian et al, 1988). If symptomatic CNS disease is present at diagnosis, concurrent radiation therapy and chemotherapy are used.

Initially, CNS-directed therapy included the use of intrathecal methotrexate and 24 Gy of cranial radiation in the pediatric population. This strategy was incorporated into an early adult trial that compared CNS prophylaxis with no CNS treatment, resulting in an improved CNS relapse rate of 19% versus 42% at 24 months (Omura et al, 1980). Although in children it is known that combination treatment can result in toxicities that include seizures, early dementia, cognitive dysfunction, and slow growth, the long-term effects on adults are less clear. It is known that combined radiation and intrathecal chemotherapy in adults can cause substantial acute toxicities that may delay postremission consolidation treatment. An alternative strategy that combines intrathecal chemotherapy without radiation has been investigated. This treatment regimen includes so-called *triple therapy* that uses intrathecal methotrexate, cytarabine, and corticosteroids without radiation (Pullen et al, 1993).

CNS relapse rates as low as 5% have been achieved without radiation by using combination intrathecal treatment in conjunction with high-dose systemic treatment that can penetrate the cerebrospinal fluid (Kantarjian et al, 2000; Annino et al, 2002). However, the German GMALL investigators have reported higher CNS relapse rates of 9% versus 5% when CNS-directed radiation was postponed (Gökbuget, 2000).

Therefore, although CNS-directed therapy is required in ALL treatment, there is no single modality or combination that has been proven to be superior. Of note, the pediatric groups generally still recommend cranial irradiation as part of CNS prophylaxis for high-risk precursor T-cell ALL, as do the German study groups

Maintenance therapy

The rationale behind the use of maintenance treatment is the elimination of slowly growing subclones that persist after induction and consolidation treatments by exposing them to antimetabolite drugs over long periods of time, ranging from 18 months up to 3 years after initial diagnosis. Commonly used components of maintenance therapy include daily mercaptopurine and oral weekly methotrexate, supplemented by monthly pulses of vincristine, corticosteroids, and periodic intrathecal methotrexate.

Despite the lack of randomized trials investigating the importance of maintenance treatment in adults with ALL, 2 older trials showed inferior results compared with historical controls when maintenance therapy is not included (Cuttner et al, 1991; Dekker et al, 1997). Thus, based on these data and the clear success of prolonged maintenance therapy in pediatric studies, maintenance regimens mimicking those used in pediatric protocols are routinely incorporated into the treatment regimens of adult pre–B- and T-cell ALL.

Risk-directed treatment of adult ALL

The focus of current treatment studies for adults with ALL is to begin to adapt treatment according to biologic risk. Similar to the progress that has been made in Burkitt lymphoma/leukemia when a specific therapeutic approach is applied based on the underlying biology of the disease, targeted treatment of Ph^+ ALL that incorporates the tyrosine kinase inhibitor imatinib into frontline therapy and application of a pediatric-inspired regimen for older adolescents and young adults may be changing the treatment paradigm for adults with ALL and resulting in improvements in survival. The role of allo-SCT in first remission based on risk group is also reviewed.

Ph^+ ALL

Treatment and outcome of patients with Ph^+ ALL has changed dramatically during the last decade with the addition of imatinib, a targeted ABL tyrosine kinase inhibitor, to frontline therapy. Previously, the standard approach for adult patients in whom the presence of the Ph chromosome portended a very poor prognosis with standard therapy alone (median survival of <1 year) was to recommend, whenever possible, allo-SCT in first remission. Allo-SCT in first remission resulted in improved DFS rates ranging from 30% to 65% in the pre-imatinib era, and this approach still remains the treatment of choice for eligible patients. However, recent studies have demonstrated that the addition of imatinib to frontline chemotherapy is feasible, does not add to systemic toxicities, and significantly increases remission rates. Several studies have recently reported CR rates $>90\%$ for these high-risk patients (Thomas DA et al, 2004; de Larbarthe et al, 2007). Results from these studies also suggest that the addition of imatinib to standard therapy can rapidly reduce MRD. Because it has been demonstrated that patients with Ph^+ ALL have improved DFS when allo-SCT is performed without evidence of MRD, the addition of imatinib before and/or after allogeneic transplantation appears to be improving OS in this high-risk group (Lee et al, 2005; Yanada, Matsuo, et al, 2006). When imatinib is added to frontline therapy, followed by allo-SCT (and sometimes followed by posttransplantation imatinib), DFS rates of 60% to 75% have been reported in these studies. For patients >60 years old with precursor B-cell ALL where the incidence of the Ph^+ disease approaches 50%, the addition of imatinib to standard regimens appears to be improving remission duration, even without the addition of allo-SCT (Vignetti et al, 2007; Ottmann et al, 2007). However, longer follow-up will be needed to confirm these promising results. Concern about CNS relapses and emergence of imatinib resistance remain potential obstacles to long-term survival. Thus, a new generation of trials is under way that incorporate the second-generation tyrosine kinase inhibitor dasatinib, which has the following several potential advantages over imatinib: it is a more potent tyrosine kinase, it can penetrate the CNS, and it maintains activity in cases with a variety of ABL kinase domain mutations that result in imatinib resistance (Ravandi et al, 2009). Thus, the addition of molecularly targeted therapy in ALL has created a new paradigm for improving outcome for these high-risk patients. At the present time, incorporation of a targeted tyrosine kinase inhibitor into frontline therapy followed by allo-SCT in first remission for eligible patients appears to be the standard of care. For patients who are not suitable candidates for transplantation, current studies are evaluating the benefit of prolonged tyrosine kinase inhibitor therapy in combination with more traditional CNS prophylaxis and maintenance chemotherapy.

Adolescents and young adults

Increasing age is one of the most important poor prognostic factors of outcome in newly diagnosed patients with ALL. The 5-year DFS is approximately 80% for children and 40% for adults with ALL. These divergent outcome results can be explained, in part, by the much higher incidence of poor-risk cytogenetics (eg, Ph$^+$) and the lower incidence of favorable-risk molecular genetics (eg, *RUNX-ETV1*) in older adults with ALL. In addition, older patients with ALL have a higher incidence of associated comorbid conditions with poorer baseline performance status that frequently preclude the use of intensive chemotherapy regimens and enrollment onto clinical trials. Recent retrospective data suggest that younger patients between the ages of 16 and 21 years fare better when treated according to current intensive pediatric regimens rather than with conventional adult ALL treatment regimens. Despite slight differences in treatment approaches across the different cooperative groups, all of the retrospective studies have demonstrated significantly better outcome for the patients when treated on pediatric studies, where survival has been reported to be in the range of 60% to 65%. In contrast, when the same age group is treated on adult cooperative group ALL treatment trials, survival has been only 30% to 40% (Stock et al, 2008; Boissel et al, 2003; de Bont et al, 2004; Ramanujachar et al, 2007).

From these retrospective studies, it appears that the major differences in treatment between the adult and pediatric regimens are the more intensive use of the nonmyelosuppressive agents (glucocorticoids, asparaginase, and vincristine), earlier and more intensive CNS-directed therapy, and more prolonged maintenance therapy used in the pediatric regimens. In addition to the obvious treatment differences between adult and pediatric trials, there has been much debate about potential differences in adherence to protocol therapy among pediatric and adult medical hematologists and the patients that they treat.

Several new prospective European and American studies that apply the pediatric approach to younger adults have recently been published and confirm promising outcomes for patients age 16 to 30 years old, with reported DFS rates of 60% to 65% (Ribera et al, 2008; Huguet et al, 2009; Nachman et al, 2009). The Dana-Farber consortium has also presented preliminary results applying this pediatric approach to adults up to the age of 50 years with an event-free survival rate of 63% with short follow-up (DeAngelo et al, 2007). The US Intergroup is currently performing a large phase II trial (C-10403) for younger adults up to age 40 years that is testing the successful approach used by the Children's Oncology Group for treatment of high-risk adolescents with ALL. However, older adults over the age of 50 years may not benefit from this approach due, in part, to their inability to tolerate the intensive asparaginase, glucocorticoid, and vincristine dosing upon which these regimens are based (Huguet et al, 2009).

Allo-SCT in adult ALL in CR1

The efficacy of allo-SCT in ALL was first reported in 1973 (Storb et al, 1973), and the graft-versus-leukemia effect was described as early as 1979 (Weiden et al, 1979). The role of allo-SCT has been established in patients with well-known risk factors such as t(9;22) and t(4;11) cytogenetics and may represent the optimal approach to curing these patients. Determining whether other patients may also benefit from allo-SCT in CR1 has been an area of intense study. Results from recent trials suggest that specific disease subsets may benefit from an allo-SCT in CR1.

In an earlier Dutch trial, 54 patients (age 15-51 years) with ALL and 15 patients with lymphoblastic lymphoma were treated with induction and consolidation chemotherapy. Thirty patients had an HLA-matched sibling, and 22 of those patients were scheduled to undergo allo-SCT (De Witte et al, 1994). The DFS of these patients was 58% ($\pm$11%) at 5 years, a result not significantly different from the outcomes of the other patients in the study who did not receive transplantation as part of their regimens.

The French LALA-87 trial was designed to evaluate the best postremission strategy in ALL, comparing consolidation chemotherapy versus auto-SCT versus allo-SCT (Thiebaut et al, 2000). The results of this trial analyzing 572 patients with 10 years of follow-up data showed that survival was 46% for patients who received an allo-SCT versus 31% for patients who received chemotherapy ($P = .04$). When broken into high-risk and standard-risk groups (with high risk including Ph$^+$ status, age >35 years, WBC >30 × 10^6/μL, and time to CR >4 weeks), OS at 10 years was 44% in the allo-SCT group versus 11% for the chemotherapy group ($P = .009$). In the standard-risk group, survival rates in the allo-SCT group (49%) and the chemotherapy group (39%) were similar ($P = .6$). Thus, this study demonstrated a survival benefit for allo-SCT in high-risk patients.

Similarly, the LALA-94 trial reevaluated the benefit of allogeneic transplantation in high-risk patients (Thomas X et al, 2004). In this study, 922 adult patients were divided into the following 4 risk groups: (1) standard-risk ALL, (2) high-risk ALL, (3) Ph$^+$ ALL, and (4) ALL with CNS involvement (Thomas X et al, 2004). Patients in all but the standard-risk group were assigned to receive allo-SCT if they had an HLA-matched sibling. Patients in groups 3 and 4 were assigned to auto-SCT if no family donor was available, whereas patients in group 2 were randomized to either auto-SCT or further chemotherapy. The results of this intent-to-treat analysis showed that patients with high-risk ALL and patients with CNS involvement had a better outcome if a donor was available for transplantation. Among high-risk patients, those allocated to the allo-SCT arm had a better median DFS of 20.8 months compared with a median DFS of 15.2 months in the auto-SCT arm and a median DFS of only 11 months in the chemotherapy arm ($P = .007$). These results confirm the findings of the LALA-87 trial showing benefit of allo-SCT in high-risk patients if a sibling donor is available.

The Medical Research Council United Kingdom ALL (MRC UKALL) 12/Eastern Cooperative Oncology Group (ECOG) 2993 study is the largest prospective, randomized trial comparing allo-SCT with chemotherapy as a postremission treatment strategy (Goldstone et al, 2008). In this study, 1913 patients age 15 to 59 years were enrolled between 1993 and 2006, with the upper age limit extended to 64 years in 2003. The study schema allocated all patients younger than 50 years (later amended to 55 years) having an HLA-matched sibling to receive a transplantation. All Ph$^+$ patients were assigned to transplantation, using a matched unrelated donor if necessary. Younger patients without a family member donor and patients older than age 50 years (or >55 years old later in the study) were randomized to either auto-SCT or further chemotherapy for consolidation treatment. High-risk patients throughout the study period were defined by the following factors: (1) age >35 years; (2) WBC count >30,000/μL in B-lineage disease or >100,000/μL in T-lineage disease; and (3) Ph$^+$ status. The median follow-up time was 4 years, 11 months (range, 1 month to 13 years, 11 months). Ph$^-$ patients with a donor had a 5-year OS rate of 53% versus 45% for patients without a donor ($P = .01$). Standard-risk patients had the most benefit from transplantation, with 5-year OS rates of 62% versus 52% ($P = .02$) in patients who had a donor versus those who did not, respectively. The benefit from transplantation in high-risk patients was not statistically significant ($P = .2$), with OS rates of 41% and 35% in the donor group and no-donor group, respectively. The trial also showed that in all groups, auto-SCT offered no more benefit than chemotherapy alone. In contrast to the LALA trials, the joint MRC UKALL/ECOG trial showed that transplantation was most beneficial to standard-risk patients, as defined, rather than high-risk patients. Thus, allo-SCT in CR1 was not significantly better for patients >35 years old (high risk) due to unacceptably high transplantation-related mortality.

Auto-SCT has been studied as a treatment option for patients who do not have an HLA-matched sibling donor. In a review of the French LALA-85, -87, and -94 trials, investigators studied 175 patients who received auto-SCT and 174 patients who were treated with chemotherapy. Their results showed that receiving auto-SCT was associated with a lower incidence of relapse compared with treatment with chemotherapy (66% vs 78% at 10 years, respectively; $P = .05$). However, DFS and OS were not significantly different between the groups (Dhedin et al, 2006). Similarly, Yanada, Matsuo, et al (2006) performed a meta-analysis of 7 trials conducted by Japanese and European cooperative groups that included 1274 patients. No benefit was seen when auto-SCT was compared with chemotherapy in patients who lacked an HLA-matched sibling donor.

Relapsed disease

Although the majority of adult ALL patients reach CR, most will eventually relapse and subsequently be much less responsive to salvage therapy. First relapse typically occurs within the first 2 years after induction, and remissions lasting longer than 18 months are associated with improved response to salvage regimens (Thomas et al, 1999; Fielding et al, 2007). CR rates for salvage regimens range from 31% to 78%, and survival for these patients remains poor (Thomas et al, 1999; Weiss et al, 2002; Tavernier et al, 2007). The more effective salvage regimens are multidrug regimens and usually contain intermediate- to high-dose cytarabine. For patients with relapsed or refractory precursor T-cell ALL, nelarabine, a deoxyguanosine analog prodrug, is approved as single-agent therapy with proven favorable results. The CALGB used nelarabine to treat relapsed and refractory patients and demonstrated a CR rate of 41% and OS rate of 28% at 1 year (DeAngelo et al, 2007). These results are especially impressive given that many of the patients had failed 2 or more inductions or had not achieved CR with their last induction regimen. Despite this difficult patient population, nelarabine allowed patients to proceed to transplantation and achieve increased survival.

Allo-SCT beyond CR1

To evaluate the role of SCT in relapsed disease, the large MRC UKALL 12/ECOG 2993 trial evaluated the outcome of

609 relapsed patients treated with chemotherapy, auto-SCT, or allo-SCT (Fielding et al, 2007). The 5-year OS rates for the chemotherapy, auto-SCT, matched unrelated donor SCT, and sibling SCT arms were 4%, 15%, 16%, and 23%, respectively, with a significant survival difference between the chemotherapy and transplantation groups. The LALA-94 trial observed similar results in relapsed patients with active disease or in second CR (CR2), with SCT producing improved DFS and OS with a 5-year OS rate of 25%. In these trials, initial postremission therapy and risk stratification group did not affect relapse rates; however, achieving CR2 prior to SCT did improve outcomes. These studies, as well as previous studies, show that allo-SCT is the only potentially curative therapy in relapsed or refractory ALL. Available data from the Center for International Blood and Marrow Transplant Research (CIBMTR) show that patients receiving transplantation with an HLA-identical sibling donor for ALL in CR2 have approximately a 35% to 40% chance of long-term DFS, whereas patients receiving transplantation with disease not in remission have a DFS of only 10% to 20%.

Novel therapies

Several new agents are currently in clinical trials for patients with relapsed disease, some of which are now being incorporated into frontline therapies (for review, see Abutalib et al, 2009). These range from newer formulations of active drugs, including a liposomal form of vincristine, to more biologically targeted therapies, including monoclonal antibodies such as rituximab, alemtuzumab, and novel antibodies directed against CD19; drugs that target aberrant *NOTCH1* expression resulting from activating mutations in *NOTCH1*, which have been reported in up to 60% of both adults and children with T-cell ALL; and the newer generation of ABL (or multitargeted) tyrosine kinase inhibitors, including nilotinib and dasatinib. Recently, 2 novel purine nucleosides have received US Food and Drug Administration approval. Nelarabine has been approved for treatment of relapsed T-cell ALL, and clofarabine has been approved for relapsed ALL in children. Based on their significant activity in relapsed disease, several studies have begun that incorporate nelarabine into frontline therapies to further improve outcome of T-cell ALL. Exploration of allo-SCT using reduced-intensity conditioning regimens is another novel approach to treatment of these high-risk patients that might result in a potent antileukemia effect while minimizing the unacceptably high treatment-related mortality (Forman, 2009). Of note, adults >60 years old with ALL, in whom survival remains dismal at <10%, are excellent candidates for trials that incorporate some of these novel approaches into frontline treatment.

Key points

- The prognosis for adolescent and adult ALL has improved, but cure rates remain inferior compared with children with ALL. The majority of adults (75%-90%) will achieve remission, but OS at 5 years remains at 30% to 40%.
- Cytogenetic abnormalities provide important prognostic information that is beginning to result in risk-adapted therapies. MRD detection using sensitive methods identifies patients at high risk of relapse.
- Therapy for precursor B- and T-cell ALL consists of multiagent induction, consolidation-intensification, CNS prophylaxis, and maintenance phases. These regimens are typically modeled after the successful regimens used by pediatricians; however, alternative regimens have been used with equivalent results.
- Treatment outcomes for older adolescents and young adults appear to be improving with the use of pediatric regimens that focus on dose-intensive glucocorticoids, vincristine, and asparaginase.
- Allo-SCT in CR1 has been demonstrated to improve survival of specific subsets of patients in several studies; however, the optimal selection of patients for this approach remains controversial. Allo-SCT is recommended as the only potentially curable strategy for eligible patients in CR2.
- The prognosis for patients over the age of 60 remains poor, with a DFS rate of <10%. Older adults with ALL are excellent candidates for novel therapeutic approaches.
- Therapy for Burkitt ALL in adults is modeled after successful pediatric regimens using intensive short-course cyclic therapy and has resulted in significant improvements in outcome for adults, with OS rates of 50% of 60%. Recent studies incorporating rituximab, a monoclonal antibody directed against CD20, have resulted in even more promising survival rates of >70%.
- Treatment of Ph$^+$ ALL now includes the addition of a targeted tyrosine kinase inhibitors to frontline therapy, which has improved remission rates and prolonged DFS. Currently, eligible patients are still recommended to receive an allo-SCT in CR1. Studies are under way to determine the utility of posttransplantation tyrosine kinase inhibitor therapy and to evaluate the effect of prolonged tyrosine kinase inhibitor therapy in combination with lower dose chemotherapy for older adults with Ph$^+$ ALL who are not transplantation candidates.

Lymphoblastic lymphoma

Lymphoblastic lymphoma represents approximately 2% and 30% of adult and pediatric non-Hodgkin lymphomas, respectively. The peak incidence is in the second decade of life, with a smaller peak in adults >40 years of age. Males are affected twice as often as females. The vast majority of patients have advanced-stage disease with a precursor T-cell immunophenotype. The immunophenotype of T-cell lymphoblastic lymphoma overlaps with that of T-cell ALL. The clinical distinction between the 2 entities is arbitrarily determined by the degree of bone marrow involvement. Patients with ≥25% bone marrow replacement by lymphoblasts are considered to have T-cell ALL, whereas patients with a lesser degree of replacement or no detectable abnormal lymphoblasts in the marrow are classified as having T-cell lymphoma. In fact, lymphoma cells can be detected in the bone marrow in <20% of patients with T-cell lymphoma using conventional morphologic examination of bilateral bone marrow aspirates and biopsies. Distinguishing lymphoma cells from normal activated lymphocytes and lymphoid progenitors (hematogones) by morphology alone can be difficult, and hence, the true extent of disease dissemination at diagnosis in T-cell lymphoma was uncertain in the past. Using a flow cytometric method that allows the detection of 1 lymphoma cell among 10,000 normal cells, it has recently been reported that marrow involvement was present in bone marrow samples of 71 (72%) of 99 children with newly diagnosed T-cell lymphoblastic lymphoma, a proportion that is much higher than that previously established by morphologic examination. The levels of involvement ranged from 0.01% to 31.6%. Interestingly, lymphoma cells were as prevalent in peripheral blood as they were in bone marrow, suggesting that examination of blood samples can be used for disease staging and monitoring in these patients. Moreover, high levels of disease dissemination (≥1%) were significantly associated with a poorer event-free survival.

The treatment strategy for lymphoblastic lymphoma is similar to that used for T-cell ALL (Patte et al, 1992; Anderson et al, 1993; Reiter et al, 2000; Burkhardt et al, 2006; Abromowitch et al, 2008). Intensive multiagent systemic chemotherapy regimens incorporating CNS-directed therapy have resulted in event-free survival rates of 75% to 90% in children and 40% to 80% in adults (Hoelzer and Gökbuget, 2009). The Berlin-Frankfurt-Münster 95 trial showed that prophylactic cranial irradiation could be omitted from treatment in patients with stage III or IV disease and without CNS involvement at diagnosis (Burkhardt et al, 2006). In a recent single-institution pilot study, a 5-year event-free survival rate of 83% and 5-year OS rate of 90% were achieved without the use of cranial irradiation in all patients, regardless of the CNS status at diagnosis (Sandlund et al, 2009), a result similar to that for childhood ALL (Pui et al, 2009).

Late complications of therapy

Emphasis on the intensive use of methotrexate and glucocorticoids has led to an increased frequency of neurotoxicity (Waber et al, 2000; Laningham et al, 2007) and osteonecrosis (Kadan-Lottick et al, 2008), underscoring the need for judicious use of even seemingly benign agents. Many long-term survivors of childhood ALL, especially those who received high cumulative doses of glucocorticoid, methotrexate, or cranial irradiation, have developed severe osteoporosis (Rai et al, 2008; Thomas et al, 2008). Such development highlights the need for early identification of bone lesions and therapeutic intervention to prevent fractures. Treatment with anthracyclines can produce severe cardiomyopathy, especially when they are given in high cumulative and peak doses to young girls. Cardiac abnormalities are persistent and progressive years after anthracycline therapy (Lipshultz et al, 2005). In one study, dexrazoxane prevented or reduced anthracycline-induced cardiotoxicity without interfering with antileukemic activity (Lipshultz et al, 2004). In current clinical trials, only limited doses of anthracyclines are used, even for high-risk cases, to decrease the risk of subsequent cardiomyopathy.

Cranial irradiation has been implicated as the cause of numerous late sequelae in children, including second cancer, neurocognitive deficits, and endocrine abnormalities that can lead to obesity, short stature, precocious puberty, and osteoporosis (Oeffinger et al, 2006; Pui et al, 2003; Hijiya et al, 2007; Geenen et al, 2007). In general, these complications are seen in girls more often than in boys and in young children more often than in older children. A long-term follow-up study of survivors of childhood ALL revealed a >10% cumulative risk of second neoplasms at 30 years and a higher than average mortality rate among patients who had received cranial irradiation (Pui et al, 2003; Hijiya et al, 2007). The most devastating complication is the development of malignant brain tumors. The median time to the diagnosis of secondary high-grade brain tumor is 9 years, and the median time to diagnosis of meningioma is 20 years (Pui et al, 2003).

Knowledge of potential treatment sequelae to modify treatment strategy and of appropriate screening measures to permit early detection of complications should greatly improve the quality of life of survivors of ALL.

Bibliography

Abromowitch M, Sposto R, Perkins S, et al. Shortened intensified multi-agent chemotherapy and non-cross resistant maintenance therapy for advanced lymphoblastic lymphoma in children and adolescents: report from the Children's Oncology Group. *Br J Haematol*. 2008;143:261–267.

Abutalib SA, Wetzler M, Stock W. Looking towards the future: novel strategies based on molecular pathogenesis of acute lymphoblastic leukemia. *Hematol Oncol Clin North Am*. 2009;23:1099–1119.

Anderson JR, Jenkin RD, Wilson JF, et al. Long-term follow-up of patients treated with COMP or LSA2L2 therapy for childhood non-Hodgkin's lymphoma: a report of CCG-551 from the Children's Cancer Group. *J Clin Oncol*. 1993;11:1024–1032.

Annino L, Vegna ML, Camera A, et al. Treatment of adult acute lymphoblastic leukemia (ALL): long-term follow-up of the GIMEMA ALL 0288 randomized study. *Blood*. 2002;99:863–871.

Aricó M, Valsecchi MG, Camitta B, et al. Outcome of treatment in children with Philadelphia chromosome-positive acute lymphoblastic leukemia. *N Engl J Med*. 2000;342:998–1006.

Aricó M, Ziino O, Valsecchi MG, et al. Acute lymphoblastic leukemia and Down syndrome: presenting features and treatment outcome in the experience of the Italian Association of Pediatric Hematology and Oncology (AIEOP). *Cancer*. 2008;113:515–521.

Armstrong JK, Hempel G, Koling S, et al. Antibody against poly(ethylene glycol) adversely affects PEG-asparaginase therapy in acute lymphoblastic leukemia patients. *Cancer*. 2007;110:103–111.

Asnafi V, Buzyn A, Le NS, et al. NOTCH1/FBXW7 mutation identifies a large subgroup with favorable outcome in adult T-cell acute lymphoblastic leukemia (T-ALL): a Group for Research on Adult Acute Lymphoblastic Leukemia (GRAALL) study. *Blood*. 2009;113:3918–3924.

Baak U, Gökbuget N, Orawa H, et al. Thymic adult T-cell acute lymphoblastic leukemia stratified in standard- and high-risk group by aberrant HOX11L2 expression: experience of the German multicenter ALL study group. *Leukemia*. 2008;22:1154–1160.

Bachanova V, Verneris MR, DeFor T, et al. Prolonged survival in adults with acute lymphoblastic leukemia after reduced-intensity conditioning with cord blood or sibling donor transplantation. *Blood*. 2009;113:2902–2905.

Bader P, Kreyenberg H, Henze GH, et al. Prognostic value of minimal residual disease quantification before allogeneic stem-cell transplantation in relapsed childhood acute lymphoblastic leukemia: the ALL-REZ BFM Study Group. *J Clin Oncol*. 2009;27:377–384.

Ballerini P, Landman-Parker J, Cayuela JM, et al. Impact of genotype on survival of children with T-cell acute lymphoblastic leukemia treated according to the French protocol FRALLE-93: the effect of TLX3/HOX11L2 gene expression on outcome. *Haematologica*. 2008;93:1658–1665.

Bargou R, Leo E, Zugmaier G, et al. Tumor regression in cancer patients by very low doses of a T cell-engaging antibody. *Science*. 2008;321:974–977.

Barredo JC, Devidas M, Lauer SJ, et al. Isolated CNS relapse of acute lymphoblastic leukemia treated with intensive systemic chemotherapy and delayed CNS radiation: a Pediatric Oncology Group study. *J Clin Oncol*. 2006;24:3142–3149.

Barry E, DeAngelo DJ, Neuberg D, et al. Favorable outcome for adolescents with acute lymphoblastic leukemia treated on Dana-Farber Cancer Institute Acute Lymphoblastic Leukemia Consortium Protocols. *J Clin Oncol*. 2007;25:813–819.

Bassan R, Spinelli O, Oldani E, et al. Improved risk classification for risk-specific therapy based on the molecular study of minimal residual disease (MRD) in adult acute lymphoblastic leukemia (ALL). *Blood*. 2009;113:4153–4162.

Bercovich D, Ganmore I, Scott LM, et al. Mutations of JAK2 in acute lymphoblastic leukaemias associated with Down's syndrome. *Lancet*. 2008;372:1484–1492.

Boissel N, Auclerc MF, Lhéritier V, et al. Should adolescents with acute lymphoblastic leukemia be treated as old children or young adults? Comparison of the French FRALLE-93 and LALA-94 trials. *J Clin Oncol*. 2003;21:774–780.

Borgmann A, von Stackelberg A, Hartmann R, et al. Unrelated donor stem cell transplantation compared with chemotherapy for children with acute lymphoblastic leukemia in a second remission: a matched-pair analysis. *Blood*. 2003;101:3835–3839.

Borowitz MJ, Devidas M, Hunger SP, et al. Clinical significance of minimal residual disease in childhood acute lymphoblastic leukemia and its relationship to other prognostic factors: a Children's Oncology Group study. *Blood*. 2008;111:5477–5485.

Bostrom BC, Sensel MR, Sather HN, et al. Dexamethasone versus prednisone and daily oral versus weekly intravenous mercaptopurine for patients with standard-risk acute lymphoblastic leukemia: a report from the Children's Cancer Group. *Blood*. 2003;101:3809–3817.

Breit S, Stanulla M, Flohr T, et al. Activating NOTCH1 mutations predict favorable early treatment response and long-term outcome in childhood precursor T-cell lymphoblastic leukemia. *Blood*. 2006;108:1151–1157.

Bürger B, Zimmermann M, Mann G, et al. Diagnostic cerebrospinal fluid examination in children with acute lymphoblastic leukemia: significance of low leukocyte counts with blasts or traumatic lumbar puncture. *J Clin Oncol*. 2003;21:184–188.

Burkhardt B, Woessmann W, Zimmermann M, et al. Impact of cranial radiotherapy on central nervous system prophylaxis in children and adolescents with central nervous system-negative stage III or IV lymphoblastic lymphoma. *J Clin Oncol*. 2006;24:491–499.

Cairo MS, Gerrard M, Sposto R, et al. Results of a randomized international study of high-risk central nervous system B non-Hodgkin lymphoma and B acute lymphoblastic leukemia in children and adolescents. *Blood*. 2007;109:2736–2743.

Campana D. Minimal residual disease in acute lymphoblastic leukemia. *Semin Hematol*. 2009;46:100–106.

Carpenter PA, Snyder DS, Flowers ME, et al. Prophylactic administration of imatinib after hematopoietic cell transplantation for high-risk Philadelphia chromosome-positive leukemia. *Blood*. 2007;109:2791–2793.

Childhood ALL Collaborative Group. Duration and intensity of maintenance chemotherapy in acute lymphoblastic leukaemia: overview of 42 trials involving 12,000 randomized children. *Lancet*. 1996;347:1783–1788.

Coiffier B, Altman A, Pui CH, et al. Guidelines for the management of pediatric and adult tumor lysis syndrome: an evidence-based review. *J Clin Oncol*. 2008;26:2767–2778.

Conter V, Schrappe M, Aricó M, et al. Role of cranial radiotherapy for childhood T-cell acute lymphoblastic leukemia with high WBC count and good response to prednisone. Associazione Italiana Ematologia Oncologia Pediatrica and the Berlin-Frankfurt-Munster groups. *J Clin Oncol*. 1997;15:2786–2791.

Conter V, Valsecchi MG, Silvestri D, et al. Pulses of vincristine and dexamethasone in addition to intensive chemotherapy for children with intermediate-risk acute lymphoblastic leukaemia: a multicentre randomized trial. *Lancet*. 2007;369:123–131.

Cortes J, O'Brien SM, Pierce S, et al. The value of high-dose systemic chemotherapy and intrathecal therapy for central nervous system prophylaxis in different risk groups of adult acute lymphoblastic leukemia. *Blood.* 1995;86:2091–2097.

Coustan-Smith E, Gajjar A Hijiya N, et al. Clinical significance of minimal residual disease in childhood acute lymphoblastic leukemia after first relapse. *Leukemia.* 2004;18:499–504.

Coustan-Smith E, Mullighan CG, Onciu M, et al. Early T-cell precursor leukaemia: a subtype of very high-risk acute lymphoblastic leukaemia. *Lancet Oncol.* 2009;10:147–156.

Coustan-Smith E, Sandlund JT, Perkins SL, et al. Minimal disseminated disease in childhood T-cell lymphoblastic lymphoma: a report from the Children's Oncology Group. *J Clin Oncol.* 2009;27:3533–3539.

Cuttner J, Mick R, Budman DR, et al. Phase III trial of brief intensive treatment of adult acute lymphocytic leukemia comparing daunorubicin and mitoxantrone: a CALGB study. *Leukemia.* 1991;5:425–431.

DeAngelo DJ, Yu D, Johnson JL, et al. Nelarabine induces complete remissions in adults with relapsed or refractory T-lineage acute lymphoblastic leukemia or lymphoblastic lymphoma: Cancer and Leukemia Group B study 19801. *Blood.* 2007;109:5136–5142.

de Bont JM, Holt B, Dekker AW, et al. Significant difference in outcome for adolescents with acute lymphoblastic leukemia treated on pediatric vs adult protocols in the Netherlands. *Leukemia.* 2004;18:2032–2035.

Dekker AW, van't Veer MB, Sizoo W, et al. Intensive postremission chemotherapy without maintenance therapy in adults with acute lymphoblastic leukemia. Dutch Hemato-Oncology Research Group. *J Clin Oncol.* 1997;15:476–482.

de Labarthe A, Rousselot P, Huguet-Rigal F, et al. Imatinib combined with induction or consolidation chemotherapy in patients with de novo Philadelphia chromosome-positive acute lymphoblastic leukemia: results of the GRAAPH-2003 study. *Blood.* 2007;109:1408–1413.

den Boer ML, van SM, De Menezes RX, et al. A subtype of childhood acute lymphoblastic leukaemia with poor treatment outcome: a genome-wide classification study. *Lancet Oncol.* 2009;10:125–134.

De Witte T, Awwad B, Boezeman J, et al. Role of allogeneic bone marrow transplantation in adolescent or adult patients with acute lymphoblastic leukaemia or lymphoblastic lymphoma in first remission. *Bone Marrow Transplant.* 1994;14:767–774.

Dhedin N, Dombret H, Thomas X, et al. Autologous stem cell transplantation in adults with acute lymphoblastic leukemia in first complete remission: analysis of the LALA-85, -87 and -94 trials. *Leukemia.* 2006;20:336–344.

Evans WE, Relling MV, Rodman JH, et al. Conventional compared with individualized chemotherapy for childhood acute lymphoblastic leukemia. *N Engl J Med.* 1998;338:499–505.

Fielding AK, Richards SM, Chopra R, et al. Outcome of 609 adults after relapse of acute lymphoblastic leukemia (ALL); an MRC UKALL12/ECOG 2993 study. *Blood.* 2007;109:944–950.

Forestier E, Izraeli S, Beverloo B, et al. Cytogenetic features of acute lymphoblastic and myeloid leukemias in pediatric patients with Down syndrome: an iBFM-SG study. *Blood.* 2008;111:1575–1583.

Forman SJ. The role of reduced intensity transplantation in the treatment of acute lymphoblastic leukemia: if and when? *Best Pract Res Clin Haematol.* 2009;22:557–566.

Gajjar A, Harrison PL, Sandlund JT, et al. Traumatic lumbar puncture at diagnosis adversely affects outcome in childhood acute lymphoblastic leukemia. *Blood.* 2000;96:3381–3384.

Gaynon PS, Trigg ME, Heerema NA, et al. Children's Cancer Group trials in childhood acute lymphoblastic leukemia: 1983–1995. *Leukemia.* 2000;14:2223–2233.

Geenen MM, Cardous-Ubbink MC, Kremer LC, et al. Medical assessment of adverse health outcomes in long-term survivors of childhood cancer. *JAMA.* 2007;297:2705–2715.

Geissler K, Koller E, Hubmann E, et al. Granulocyte colony-stimulating factor as an adjunct to induction chemotherapy for adult acute lymphoblastic leukemia: a randomized phase-III study. *Blood.* 1997;90:590–596.

Gleissner B, Gökbuget N, Rieder H, et al. CD10- pre-B acute lymphoblastic leukemia (ALL) is a distinct high-risk subgroup of adult ALL associated with a high frequency of MLL aberrations: results of the German Multicenter Trials for Adult ALL (GMALL). *Blood.* 2005;106:4054–4056.

Gökbuget N, Baumann A, Beck J, et al. PET-asparaginase in adult acute lymphoblastic leukemia: efficacy and feasibility analysis with increasing dose levels. *Blood.* 2008;122(Suppl):Abstact 302.

Gökbuget N, Hoelzer D. Treatment of adult acute lymphoblastic leukemia. *Semin Hematol.* 2009;46:64–75.

Gökbuget N, Hoelzer D, Arnold R, et al. Treatment of adult ALL according to protocols of the German Multicenter Study Group for Adult ALL (GMALL). *Hematol Oncol Clin North Am.* 2000;14:1307–25.

Goldberg JM, Silverman LB, Levy DE, et al. Childhood T-cell acute lymphoblastic leukemia: the Dana-Farber Cancer Institute acute lymphoblastic leukemia consortium experience. *J Clin Oncol.* 2003;21:3616–3622.

Goldstone AH, Richards SM, Lazarus HM, et al. In adults with standard-risk acute lymphoblastic leukemia, the greatest benefit is achieved from a matched sibling allogeneic transplantation in first complete remission, and an autologous transplantation is less effective than conventional consolidation/maintenance chemotherapy in all patients: final results of the International ALL Trial (MRC UKALL XII/ECOG E2993). *Blood.* 2008;111:1827–1833.

Hagedorn N, Acquaviva C, Fronkova E, et al. Submicroscopic bone marrow involvement in isolated extramedullary relapses in childhood acute lymphoblastic leukemia: a more precise definition of "isolated" and its possible clinical implications, a collaborative study of the Resistant Disease Committee of the International BFM Study Group. *Blood.* 2007;110:4022–4029.

Hak LJ, Relling MV, Cheng C, et al. Asparaginase pharmacodynamics differ by formulation among children with newly diagnosed acute lymphoblastic leukemia. *Leukemia.* 2004;18:1072–1077.

Hallböök H, Gustafsson G, Smedmyr B, et al. Treatment outcome in young adults and children >10 years of age with acute lymphoblastic leukemia in Sweden: a comparison between a pediatric protocol and an adult protocol. *Cancer.* 2006;107:1551–1561.

Harms DO, Janka-Schaub GE. Co-operative study group for childhood acute lymphoblastic leukemia (COALL): long-term follow-up of trials 82, 85, 89 and 92. *Leukemia*. 2000;14:2234–2239.

Hijiya N, Gaynon P, Barry E, et al. A multi-center phase I study of clofarabine, etoposide and cyclophosphamide in combination in pediatric patients with refractory or relapsed acute leukemia. *Leukemia*. 2009;23:2259–2264.

Hijiya N, Hudson MM, Lensing S, et al. Cumulative incidence of secondary neoplasms as a first event after childhood acute lymphoblastic leukemia. *JAMA*. 2007;297:1207–1215.

Hoelzer D, Gökbuget N. T-cell lymphoblastic lymphoma and T-cell acute lymphoblastic leukemia: a separate entity? *Clin Lymphoma Myeloma*. 2009;9(Suppl 3):S214–S221.

Hoelzer D, Thiel E, Ludwig WD, et al. The German multicentre trials for treatment of acute lymphoblastic leukemia in adults. The German Adult ALL Study Group. *Leukemia*. 1992;6(Suppl 2):175–177.

Huguet F, Leguay T, Raffoux E, et al. Pediatric-inspired therapy in adults with Philadelphia chromosome-negative ALL: the GRAALL 2003 study. *J Clin Oncol*. 2009;20:911–918.

Iacobucci I, Storlazzi CT, Cilloni D, et al. Identification and molecular characterization of recurrent genomic deletions on 7p12 in the IKZF1 gene in a large cohort of BCR-ABL1-positive acute lymphoblastic leukemia patients: on behalf of Gruppo Italiano Malattie Ematologiche dell'Adulto Acute Leukemia Working Party (GIMEMA AL WP). *Blood*. 2009;114:2159–2167.

Igarashi S, Manabe A, Ohara A, et al. No advantage of dexamethasone over prednisolone for the outcome of standard- and intermediate-risk childhood acute lymphoblastic leukemia in the Tokyo Children's Cancer Study Group L95–14 protocol 24. *J Clin Oncol*. 2005;23:6489–6498.

Jeha S, Behm F, Pei D, et al. Prognostic significance of CD20 expression in childhood B-cell precursor acute lymphoblastic leukemia. *Blood*. 2006;108:3302–3304.

Kadan-Lottick NS, Dinu I, Wasilewski-Masker K, et al. Osteonecrosis in adult survivors of childhood cancer: a report from the childhood cancer survivor study. *J Clin Oncol*. 2008;26:3038–3045.

Kantarjian HM, O'Brien S, Smith TL, et al. Results of treatment with hyper-CVAD, a dose-intensive regimen, in adult acute lymphocytic leukemia. *J Clin Oncol*. 2000;18:547–561.

Kantarjian HM, Walters RS, Keating MJ, et al. Identification of risk groups for development of central nervous system leukemia in adults with acyte lymphocytic leukemia. *Blood*. 1988;72:1784–1789.

Lange BJ, Bostrom BC, Cherlow JM, et al. Double-delayed intensification improves event-free survival for children with intermediate-risk acute lymphoblastic leukemia: a report from the Children's Cancer Group. *Blood*. 2002;99:825–833.

Laningham FH, Kun LE, Reddick WE, et al. Childhood central nervous system leukemia: historical perspectives, current therapy, and acute neurological sequelae. *Neuroradiology*. 2007;49:873–888.

Larson RA, Dodge RK, Burns CP, et al. A five-drug remission induction regimen with intensive consolidation for adults with acute lymphoblastic leukemia: Cancer and Leukemia Group B study 8811. *Blood*. 1995;85:2025–2037.

Larson RA, Fretzin MH, Dodge RK, et al. Hypersensitivity reactions to L-asparaginase do not impact on the remission duration of adults with acute lymphoblastic leukemia. *Leukemia*. 1998;12:660–665.

Lee S, Kim YJ, Min CK, et al. The effect of first-line imatinib interim therapy on the outcome of allogeneic stem cell transplantation in adults with newly diagnosed Philadelphia chromosome-positive acute lymphoblastic leukemia. *Blood*. 2005;105:3449–3457.

Leung W, Iyengar R, Turner V, et al. Determinants of antileukemia effects of allogeneic NK cells. *J Immunol*. 2004;172:644–650.

Lipshultz SE, Lipsitz SR, Sallan SE, et al. Chronic progressive cardiac dysfunction years after doxorubicin therapy for childhood acute lymphoblastic leukemia. *J Clin Oncol*. 2005;23:2629–2636.

Lipshultz SE, Rifai N, Dalton VM, et al. The effect of dexrazoxane on myocardial injury in doxorubicin-treated children with acute lymphoblastic leukemia. *N Engl J Med*. 2004;351:145-153.

Loh ML, Goldwasser MA, Silverman LB, et al. Prospective analysis of TEL/AML1-positive patients treated on Dana-Farber Cancer Institute Consortium Protocol 95–01. *Blood*. 2006;107:4508–4513.

Mancini M, Scappaticci D, Cimino G, et al. A comprehensive genetic classification of adult acute lymphoblastic leukemia (ALL): analysis of the GIMEMA 0496 protocol. *Blood*. 2005;105:3434–3441.

Manera R, Ramirez I, Mullins J, et al. Pilot studies of species-specific chemotherapy of childhood acute lymphoblastic leukemia using genotype and immunophenotype 123. *Leukemia*. 2000;14:1354–1361.

Mansour MR, Sulis ML, Duke V, et al. Prognostic implications of NOTCH1 and FBXW7 mutations in adults with T-cell acute lymphoblastic leukemia treated on the MRC UKALLXII/ECOG E2993 protocol. *J Clin Oncol*. 2009;27:4352–4356.

Matloub Y, Lindemulder S, Gaynon PS, et al. Intrathecal triple therapy decreases central nervous system relapse but fails to improve event-free survival when compared with intrathecal methotrexate: results of the Children's Cancer Group (CCG) 1952 study for standard-risk acute lymphoblastic leukemia, reported by the Children's Oncology Group. *Blood*. 2006;108:1165–1173.

Meijerink JP, den Boer ML, Pieters R. New genetic abnormalities and treatment response in acute lymphoblastic leukemia. *Semin Hematol*. 2009;46:16–23.

Mitchell CD, Richards SM, Kinsey SE, et al. Benefit of dexamethasone compared with prednisolone for childhood acute lymphoblastic leukaemia: results of the UK Medical Research Council ALL97 randomized trial. *Br J Haematol*. 2005;129:734–745.

Moorman AV, Harrison CJ, Buck GA, et al. Karyotype is an independent prognostic factor in adult acute lymphoblastic leukemia (ALL): analysis of cytogenetic data from patients treated on the Medical Research Council (MRC) UKALLXII/Eastern Cooperative Oncology Group (ECOG) 2993 trial. *Blood*. 2007;109:3189–3197.

Möricke A, Reiter A, Zimmermann M, et al. Risk-adjusted therapy of acute lymphoblastic leukemia can decrease treatment burden and improve survival: treatment results of 2169 unselected pediatric and adolescent patients enrolled in the trial ALL-BFM 95. *Blood.* 2008;111:4477–4489.

Mullighan CG, Collins-Underwood JR, Phillips LA, et al. Rearrangement of CRLF2 in B-progenitor- and Down syndrome-associated acute lymphoblastic leukemia. *Nat Genet.* 2009;41:1243–1246.

Mullighan CG, Miller CB, Radtke I, et al. BCR-ABL1 lymphoblastic leukaemia is characterized by the deletion of Ikaros. *Nature.* 2008;453:110–114.

Mullighan CG, Su X, Zhang J, et al. Deletion of IKZF1 and prognosis in acute lymphoblastic leukemia. *N Engl J Med.* 2009;360:470–480.

Mullighan CG, Zhang J, Harvey RC, et al. JAK mutations in high-risk childhood acute lymphoblastic leukemia. *Proc Natl Acad Sci U S A.* 2009;106:9414–9418.

Nachman JB, Heerema NA, Sather H, et al. Outcome of treatment in children with hypodiploid acute lymphoblastic leukemia. *Blood.* 2007;110:1112–1115.

Nachman JB, La MK, Hunger SP, et al. Young adults with acute lymphoblastic leukemia have an excellent outcome with chemotherapy alone and benefit from intensive postinduction treatment: a report from the Children's Oncology Group. *J Clin Oncol.* 2009;27:5189–5194.

Nachman JB, Sather HN, Sensel MG, et al. Augmented post-induction therapy for children with high-risk acute lymphoblastic leukemia and a slow response to initial therapy. *N Engl J Med.* 1998;338:1663–1671.

Nguyen K, Devidas M, Cheng SC, et al. Factors influencing survival after relapse from acute lymphoblastic leukemia: a Children's Oncology Group study. *Leukemia.* 2008;22:2142–2150.

Oeffinger KC, Mertens AC, Sklar CA, et al. Chronic health conditions in adult survivors of childhood cancer. *N Engl J Med.* 2006;355:1572–1582.

Omura GA, Moffitt S, Vogler WR, et al. Combination chemotherapy of adult acute lymphoblastic leukemia with randomized central nervous system prophylaxis. *Blood.* 1980;55:199–204.

Oriol A, Ribera JM, Bergua J, et al. High-dose chemotherapy and immunotherapy in adult Burkitt lymphoma: comparison of results in human immunodeficiency virus-infected and noninfected patients. *Cancer.* 2008;113:117–125.

Ottmann OG, Hoelzer D, Gracien E, et al. Concomitant granulocyte colony-stimulating factor and induction chemoradiotherapy in adult acute lymphoblastic leukemia: a randomized phase III trial. *Blood.* 1995;86:444–450.

Ottmann OG, Wassmann B, Pfeifer H, et al. Imatinib compared with chemotherapy as front-line treatment of elderly patients with Philadelphia chromosome-positive acute lymphoblastic leukemia (Ph+ALL). *Cancer.* 2007;109:2068–2076.

Paganin M, Zecca M, Fabbri G, et al. Minimal residual disease is an important predictive factor of outcome in children with relapsed 'high-risk' acute lymphoblastic leukaemia. *Leukemia.* 2008;22:2193–2200.

Patte C, Auperin A, Michon J, et al. The Société Francaise d'Oncologie Pédiatrique LMB89 protocol: highly effective multiagent chemotherapy tailored to the tumor burden and initial response in 561 unselected children with B-cell lymphomas and L3 leukemia. *Blood.* 2001;97:3370–3379.

Patte C, Kalifa C, Flamant F, et al. Results of the LMT81 protocol, a modified LSA2L2 protocol with high dose methotrexate, on 84 children with non-B-cell (lymphoblastic) lymphoma. *Med Pediatr Oncol.* 1992;20:105–113.

Patte C, Philip T, Rodary C, et al. High survival rate in advanced-stage B-cell lymphomas and leukemias without CNS involvement with a short intensive polychemotherapy: results from the French Pediatric Oncology Society of a randomized trial of 216 children. *J Clin Oncol.* 1991;9:123–132.

Pieters R, Schrappe M, De LP, et al. A treatment protocol for infants younger than 1 year with acute lymphoblastic leukaemia (Interfant-99): an observational study and a multicentre randomised trial. *Lancet.* 2007;370:240–250.

Pui CH, Cheng C, Leung W, et al. Extended follow-up of long-term survivors of childhood acute lymphoblastic leukemia. *N Engl J Med.* 2003;349:640–649.

Pui CH, Campana D, Pei D, et al. Treating childhood acute lymphoblastic leukemia without prophylactic cranial irradiation. *N Engl J Med.* 2009;360:2730–2741.

Pui CH, Evans WE. Treatment of acute lymphoblastic leukemia. *N Engl J Med.* 2006;354:166–178.

Pui CH, Gaynon PS, Boyett JM, et al. Outcome of treatment in childhood acute lymphoblastic leukaemia with rearrangements of the 11q23 chromosomal region. *Lancet.* 2002;359:1909–1915.

Pui CH, Howard SC. Current management and challenges of malignant disease in the CNS in paediatric leukaemia. *Lancet Oncol.* 2008;9:257–268.

Pui CH, Jeha S. New therapeutic strategies for the treatment of acute lymphoblastic leukaemia. *Nat Rev Drug Discov.* 2007;6:149–165.

Pui CH, Relling MV. Topoisomerase II inhibitor-related acute myeloid leukaemia. *Br J Haematol.* 2000;109:13–23.

Pui CH, Relling MV, Downing JR. Acute lymphoblastic leukemia. *N Engl J Med.* 2004;350:1535–1548.

Pui CH, Robison LL, Look AT. Acute lymphoblastic leukaemia. *Lancet.* 2008;371:1030–1043.

Pui CH, Sandlund JT, Pei D, et al. Results of therapy for acute lymphoblastic leukemia in black and white children. *JAMA.* 2003;290:2001–2007.

Pullarkat V, Slovak ML, Kopecky KJ, et al. Impact of cytogenetics on the outcome of adult acute lymphoblastic leukemia: results of Southwest Oncology Group 9400 study. *Blood.* 2008;111:2563–2572.

Pullen J, Boyett J, Shuster J, et al. Extended triple intrathecal chemotherapy trial for prevention of CNS relapse in good-risk and poor-risk patients with B-progenitor acute lymphoblastic leukemia: a Pediatric Oncology Group study. *J Clin Oncol.* 1993;11:839–849.

Rabin KR, Whitlock JA. Malignancy in children with trisomy 21. *Oncologist.* 2009;14:164–173.

Raff T, Gökbuget N, Luschen S, et al. Molecular relapse in adult standard-risk ALL patients detected by prospective MRD monitoring during and after maintenance treatment: data from the GMALL 06/99 and 07/03 trials. *Blood.* 2007;109:910–915.

Rai SN, Hudson MM, McCammon E, et al. Implementing an intervention to improve bone mineral density in survivors of childhood acute lymphoblastic leukemia: BONEII, a prospective placebo-controlled double-blind randomized interventional longitudinal study design. *Contemp Clin Trials*. 2008;29:711–719.

Ramanujachar R, Richards S, Hann I, et al. Adolescents with acute lymphoblastic leukaemia: outcome on UK national paediatric (ALL97) and adult (UKALLXII/E2993) trials. *Pediatr Blood Cancer*. 2007;48:254–261.

Ravandi F, Kantarjian HM, Thomas DA, et al. Phase II study of combination of the HyperCVAD regimen with dasatinib in the front line therapy of patients with Philadelphia chromosome (Ph) positive acute lymphoblastic leukemia. *Blood*. 2009;114:Abstract 837.

Reichert JM, Valge-Archer VE. Development trends for monoclonal antibody cancer therapeutics. *Nat Rev Drug Discov*. 2007;6:349–356.

Reiter A, Schrappe M, Ludwig WD, et al. Intensive ALL-type therapy without local radiotherapy provides a 90% event-free survival for children with T-cell lymphoblastic lymphoma: a BFM group report. *Blood*. 2000;95:416–421.

Relling MV, Hancock ML, Boyett JM, et al. Prognostic importance of 6-mercaptopurine dose intensity in acute lymphoblastic leukemia. *Blood*. 1999;93:2817–2823.

Relling MV, Hancock ML, Rivera GK, et al. Mercaptopurine therapy intolerance and heterozygosity at the thiopurine S-methyltransferase gene locus. *J Natl Cancer Inst*. 1999;91:2001–2008.

Reman O, Pigneux A, Huguet F, et al. Central nervous system involvement in adult acute lymphoblastic leukemia at diagnosis and/or at first relapse: Results from the GET-LALA group. *Leuk Res*. 2008;32:1741–1750.

Ribeiro RC, Rivera GK, Hudson M, et al. An intensive re-treatment protocol for children with an isolated CNS relapse of acute lymphoblastic leukemia. *J Clin Oncol*. 1995;13:333–338.

Ribera JM, Oriol A, Sanz MA, et al. Comparison of the results of the treatment of adolescents and young adults with standard-risk acute lymphoblastic leukemia with the Programa Espanol de Tratamiento en Hematologia pediatric-based protocol ALL-96. *J Clin Oncol*. 2008;26:1843–1849.

Ritchey AK, Pollock BH, Lauer SJ, et al. Improved survival of children with isolated CNS relapse of acute lymphoblastic leukemia: a Pediatric Oncology Group study. *J Clin Oncol*. 1999;17:3745–3752.

Rivera GK, Zhou Y, Hancock ML, et al. Bone marrow recurrence after initial intensive treatment for childhood acute lymphoblastic leukemia. *Cancer*. 2005;103:368–376.

Rubnitz JE, Onciu M, Pounds S, et al. Acute mixed lineage leukemia in children: the experience of St Jude Children's Research Hospital. *Blood*. 2009;113:5083–5089.

Sandlund JT, Pui CH, Zhou Y, et al. Effective treatment of advanced-stage childhood lymphoblastic lymphoma without prophylactic cranial irradiation: results of St. Jude NHL13 study. *Leukemia*. 2009;23:1127–1130.

Schmiegelow K, Al-Modhwahi I, Andersen MK, et al. Methotrexate/6-mercaptopurine maintenance therapy influences the risk of a second malignant neoplasm after childhood acute lymphoblastic leukemia: results from the NOPHO ALL-92 study. *Blood*. 2009;113:6077–6084.

Schmiegelow K, Schroder H, Gustafsson G, et al. Risk of relapse in childhood acute lymphoblastic leukemia is related to RBC methotrexate and mercaptopurine metabolites during maintenance chemotherapy. Nordic Society for Pediatric Hematology and Oncology. *J Clin Oncol*. 1995;13:345–351.

Schrappe M, Reiter A, Ludwig WD, et al. Improved outcome in childhood acute lymphoblastic leukemia despite reduced use of anthracyclines and cranial radiotherapy: results of trial ALL-BFM 90. German-Austrian-Swiss ALL-BFM Study Group. *Blood*. 2000;95:3310–3122.

Schrappe M, Zimmermann M, Möricke A, et al. Dexamethasone in induction can eliminate one third of all relapses in childhood acute lymphoblastic leukemia (ALL): results of an international randomized trial in 3655 patients (Trial AIEOP-BFM ALL 2000). *Blood*. 2008;112:9.

Schultz KR, Alayton W. Improved early event free survival with imatinib in Philadelphia chromosome-positive acute lymphoblastic leukemia: a Children's Oncology Group study. *J Clin Oncol*. 2009;27:5175–5181.

Schultz KR, Pullen DJ, Sather HN, et al. Risk- and response-based classification of childhood B-precursor acute lymphoblastic leukemia: a combined analysis of prognostic markers from the Pediatric Oncology Group (POG) and Children's Cancer Group (CCG). *Blood*. 2007;109:926–935.

Silverman LB, Gelber RD, Dalton VK, et al. Improved outcome for children with acute lymphoblastic leukemia: results of Dana-Farber Consortium Protocol 91–01. *Blood*. 2001;97:1211–1218.

Stock W, La M, Sanford B, et al. Adolescents and young adults with acute lymphoblastic leukemia (ALL) have improved outcomes when treated on pediatric oncology cooperative group treatment regimens: A comparison of Children's Cancer Group (CCG) and Cancer and Leukemia Group B (CALGB) studies. *Blood*. 2008;112:1646–1654.

Storb R, Bryant JI, Buckner CD, et al. Allogeneic marrow grafting for acute lymphoblastic leukemia: leukemic relapse. *Transplant Proc*. 1973;5:923–926.

Swerdlow SH, Campo E, Harris NL, et al, eds. *WHO Classification of Tumours of Haematopoietic and Lymphoid Tissues*. 4th ed. Geneva, Switzerland: World Health Organization Press; 2008:168–178.

Tavernier E, Boiron JM, Huguet F, et al. Outcome of treatment after first relapse in adults with acute lymphoblastic leukemia initially treated by the LALA-94 trial. *Leukemia*. 2007;21:1907–1914.

Thiebaut A, Vernant JP, Degos L, et al. Adult acute lymphocytic leukemia study testing chemotherapy and autologous and allogeneic transplantation. A follow-up report of the French protocol LALA 87. *Hematol Oncol Clin North Am*. 2000;14:1353–1366.

Thomas DA, Faderl S, Cortes J, et al. Treatment of Philadelphia chromosome-positive acute lymphocytic leukemia with hyper-CVAD and imatinib mesylate. *Blood*. 2004;103:4396–4407.

Thomas DA, Faderl S, O'Brien S, et al. Chemoimmunotherapy with hyper-CVAD plus rituximab for the treatment of adult Burkitt and Burkitt-type lymphoma or acute lymphoblastic leukemia. *Cancer*. 2006;106:1569–1580.

Thomas DA, Kantarjian H, Smith TL, et al. Primary refractory and relapsed adult acute lymphoblastic leukemia: characteristics, treatment results, and prognosis with salvage therapy. *Cancer.* 1999;86:1216–1230.

Thomas DA, O'Brien S, Jorgensen JL et al. Prognostic significance of CD20 expression in adults with de novo precursor B-lineage acute lymphoblastic leukemia. *Blood.* 2009;113:6330–6337.

Thomas IH, Donohue JE, Ness KK, et al. Bone mineral density in young adult survivors of acute lymphoblastic leukemia. *Cancer.* 2008;113:3248–3256.

Thomas X, Boiron JM, Huguet F, et al. Outcome of treatment in adults with acute lymphoblastic leukemia: analysis of the LALA-94 trial. *J Clin Oncol.* 2004;22:4075–4086.

Triplett B, Handgretinger R, Pui CH, et al. KIR-incompatible hematopoietic-cell transplantation for poor prognosis infant acute lymphoblastic leukemia. *Blood.* 2006;107:1238–1239.

van den Berg H, Langeveld NE, Veenhof CH, Behrendt H. Treatment of isolated testicular recurrence of acute lymphoblastic leukemia without radiotherapy. Report from the Dutch Late Effects Study Group. *Cancer.* 1997;79:2257–2262.

Veerman AJ, Kamps WA, van den Berg H, et al. Dexamethasone-based therapy for childhood acute lymphoblastic leukaemia: results of the prospective Dutch Childhood Oncology Group (DCOG) protocol ALL-9 (1997–2004). *Lancet Oncol.* 2009;10:957–966.

Vignetti M, Fazi P, Cimino G, et al. Imatinib plus steroids induces complete remissions and prolonged survival in elderly Philadelphia chromosome-positive patients with acute lymphoblastic leukemia without additional chemotherapy: results of the Gruppo Italiano Malattie Ematologiche dell'Adulto (GIMEMA) LAL0201-B protocol. *Blood.* 2007;109:3676-3678.

Vilmer E, Suciu S, Ferster A, et al. Long-term results of three randomized trials (58831, 58832, 58881) in childhood acute lymphoblastic leukemia: a CLCG-EORTC report. Children Leukemia Cooperative Group. *Leukemia.* 2000;14:2257–2266.

Vora A, Mitchell CD, Lennard L, et al. Toxicity and efficacy of 6-thioguanine versus 6-mercaptopurine in childhood lymphoblastic leukaemia: a randomised trial. *Lancet.* 2006;368:1339–1348.

Waber DP, Carpentieri SC, Klar N, et al. Cognitive sequelae in children treated for acute lymphoblastic leukemia with dexamethasone or prednisone. *J Pediatr Hematol Oncol.* 2000;22:206–213.

Wassmann B, Pfeifer H, Stadler M, et al. Early molecular response to posttransplantation imatinib determines outcome in MRD$^+$ Philadelphia-positive acute lymphoblastic leukemia (Ph$^+$ ALL). *Blood.* 2005;106:458–463.

Weiden PL, Flournoy N, Thomas ED, et al. Antileukemic effect of graft-versus-host disease in human recipients of allogeneic-marrow grafts. *N Engl J Med.* 1979;300:1068–1073.

Weiss MA, Aliff TB, Tallman MS, et al. A single, high dose of idarubicin combined with cytarabine as induction therapy for adult patients with recurrent or refractory acute lymphoblastic leukemia. *Cancer.* 2002;95:581–587.

Woessmann W, Seidemann K, Mann G, et al. The impact of the methotrexate administration schedule and dose in the treatment of children and adolescents with B-cell neoplasms: a report of the BFM Group Study NHL-BFM95. *Blood.* 2005;105:948–958.

Yanada M, Takeuchi J, Sugiura I, et al. High complete remission rate and promising outcome by combination of imatinib and chemotherapy for newly diagnosed BCR-ABL-positive acute lymphoblastic leukemia: a phase II study by the Japan Adult Leukemia Study Group. *J Clin Oncol.* 2006;24:460–466.

Yanada M, Matsuo K, Suzuki T, et al. Allogeneic hematopoietic stem cell transplantation as part of postremission therapy improves survival for adult patients with high-risk acute lymphoblastic leukemia: a metaanalysis. *Cancer.* 2006;106:2657–2663.

CHAPTER 18

Lymphomas

Kerry J. Savage and Stephanie A. Gregory

Overview of lymphocyte development, 511
Non-Hodgkin lymphomas, 516
Immunodeficiency-associated lymphoproliferative disorders, 539
Hodgkin lymphoma, 541
Acknowledgment, 547
Bibliography, 548

Overview of lymphocyte development

Lymphocytes develop from a common lymphoid progenitor cell. B cells mature primarily in the bone marrow, whereas T cells mature in the thymus. Although the process and signals of maturation differ between the 2 cell types, they rely on similar genetic events to generate specific antibodies or cell surface receptors. These gene rearrangements are critical for the development of a broad immune repertoire and also provide molecular markers of clonality that can be used to diagnose lymphoid malignancies.

B-cell development

B-cell maturation consists of early (antigen-independent) and late (antigen-dependent) stages. Early development is initiated by the rearrangement of genes for the heavy and light chains of antibodies, a process referred to as V/(D)/J recombination. The earliest B-precursor cell shows rearrangement of the immunoglobulin heavy chain, which is then followed by light chain rearrangement. The κ light chain genes rearrange first; if neither κ locus is productively rearranged, then the λ gene loci undergo rearrangement. Once a successful light chain rearrangement occurs, the cell will express the complete immunoglobulin molecule on its surface, which identifies it as a mature B cell. Mature B cells will typically express either immunoglobulin M (IgM) or immunoglobulin D (IgD) on their surface, and this surface expression is critical to cell survival. Further, the combination of the *VDJ* gene sequences is unique for each immunoglobulin molecule variable region and, hence, each B cell and is referred to as the idiotype.

Cell surface markers are also used to define the early stages of B-cell development. CD10 (CALLA, the common acute lymphoblastic leukemia antigen) and CD19 are expressed on immature B cells (pro-B and B precursor) that have begun heavy chain rearrangement. Terminal deoxynucleotidyl transferase (TdT), a DNA polymerase important for nucleotide chain elongation during gene rearrangement, is also expressed at this stage. CD20 is then expressed as cells rearrange light chains and express surface immunoglobulin, and the expression of CD10 and TdT is lost. The mature but antigen-naive B cell leaves the bone marrow to circulate and populate lymphoid organs such as lymph nodes, spleen, and mucosa-associated lymphoid tissue (MALT).

The late, or antigen-dependent, stages of B-lymphocyte development begin when a naive B cell recognizes an antigen with its membrane-bound antibody. These B cells collect in germinal centers of the various lymphoid organs and begin to divide and undergo several types of genetic modification. Somatic hypermutation is a process by which cells introduce mutations into the variable region (V) genes. These mutations result in antibodies that may have a higher or lower affinity for the antigen. Those that produce a higher affinity antibody will persist and become either plasma cells or memory B cells, whereas those that fail to produce functional antibody at this stage will undergo apoptosis. Class switching involves changing the heavy chain that is expressed to produce other antibody classes: immunoglobulin G (IgG), immunoglobulin A (IgA), or immunoglobulin E (IgE).

Conflict-of-interest disclosure: *Dr. Savage:* honoraria: Roche, Eli Lilly. *Dr. Gregory:* consultancy: Amgen, Genentech; research funding: Amgen, Boehringer Ingelheim, Celgene, CTI, Genentech, GenMab, GlaxoSmithKline, Gloucester Pharmaceuticals, Millennium, NCIC CTG, Rigel Pharmaceuticals; speakers' bureau: Genentech, GlaxoSmithKline, Millennium.

Off-label drug use: *Dr. Savage and Dr. Gregory:* rituximab maintenance after rituximab chemotherapy in lymphoma; radioimmunotherapy for consolidation therapy after chemotherapy for initial treatment of lymphoma; bortezomib and combinations in Waldenström macroglobulinemia, rituximab in hairy cell leukemia, R-CHOP in localized DLBCL, thalidomide in mantle cell lymphoma.

Although this switch does not alter antibody affinity, the change in class of antibody will alter its effector function and thereby affect the immune response.

T-cell development

T-cell maturation occurs in the thymus, where T-cell precursor–thymic stroma interactions guide the maturation and selection of mature T cells. The differentiation steps of the T lymphocyte are in many ways parallel to those of B lymphocytes. The 4 T-cell receptor (TCR) genes, α, β, γ, and δ, undergo rearrangement analogous to that seen in the immunoglobulin gene locus. These proteins form heterodimeric receptors in mature lymphocytes, and any given T cell expresses either an α-β or a γ-δ TCR on its surface, but not both. Once a TCR is expressed on the surface of the developing thymocyte, the cell undergoes both positive and negative selection. Positive selection requires the TCR to recognize a self-peptide major histocompatibility complex (MHC) molecule, and negative selection then ensures that the TCR–MHC binding affinity is not high, which could indicate an autoreactive clone. Cells that survive positive and negative selection then exit the thymus as mature T cells.

In addition to the TCR, other surface molecules expressed on mature T cells include the CD3, CD4, and CD8 proteins. The TCR is expressed in association with the CD3 antigen, expression of which is considered to be the definitive marker of T-cell identity. Coreceptors with the TCR–CD3 complex are CD4 and CD8, which identify helper and cytotoxic/suppressor subtypes, respectively. Most mature T cells will express either CD4 or CD8, although there are occasional cells that express both. In addition, virtually all T cells express the pan-T-cell marker CD5; this same marker is expressed on a subset of normal and malignant B cells such as chronic lymphocytic leukemia (CLL) and mantle cell lymphoma (MCL) (see the Non-Hodgkin lymphomas section). Absence of CD5 expression on circulating lymphocytes with some characteristics of T cells is a marker of natural killer (NK) cells; however, it can also be an important marker for lymphoproliferation because many neoplasms of phenotypically mature T cells lack CD5 expression.

Biology of lymphomas

The transforming events in lymphoproliferative disorders are best understood for B-cell processes. Analysis of V genes from a variety of B-cell neoplasms reveals evidence of somatic mutation, which indicates that they arise from germinal center or post–germinal center B cells. This suggests that the germinal center is a site of initiation of the transforming event, as cells undergo a number of DNA-modifying events including class switching and somatic hypermutation. Failure of these processes may result in inappropriate translocations

Table 18-1 Risk factors in the development of non-Hodgkin lymphoma.

Viral	EBV, HTLV-1, HHV-8, hepatitis C
Bacterial	*Helicobacter pylori*
Impaired/altered immunity	Ataxia-telangiectasia
Congenital	Wiskott-Aldrich syndrome
Acquired	Severe combined immunodeficiency
	AIDS (HIV infection)
	Organ or stem cell transplantation
	Aging
	Autoimmune disease
Environmental or occupational	Herbicides
	Pesticides

AIDS = acquired immunodeficiency syndrome; EBV = Epstein-Barr virus; HHV-8 = human herpesvirus 8; HIV = human immunodeficiency virus; HTLV-1 = human T-cell lymphotropic virus 1.

(oncogene to immunoglobulin switch region) or point mutations in oncogenes, resulting in unregulated oncogene activation. Similar errors in DNA rearrangement can occur during V/(D)/J recombination, resulting in precursor B- or T-cell malignancies. Several viral infections are also associated with the development of lymphoproliferative disorders, including Epstein-Barr virus (EBV) and human herpesvirus 8 (HHV-8) (Table 18-1).

Diagnostic testing in lymphoproliferative disorders

In general, there are no surface markers that are diagnostic of malignancy in lymphocytes. Several methods are used to document a lymphoid malignancy including morphology (lymph node, peripheral blood, or bone marrow), immunophenotyping, molecular genetics, and cytogenetics.

Morphology

Many lymphoproliferative malignancies are diagnosed by characteristic morphology of a lymph node or other biopsy. Examination of patterns of growth, degree of cytologic atypia, degree and type of differentiation, and the presence of reactive components are important for diagnosis. Fine needle aspiration can be used to identify an abnormal population of cells but furnishes none of the structural information provided by a core or excisional biopsy. For that reason, an excisional biopsy is recommended for the initial diagnosis of a suspected lymphoproliferative disorder.

Immunophenotyping

Diagnosis by immunophenotyping is based on finding increased expression of a certain marker (or markers) that is usually present only on a small percentage of normal cells. For B-cell malignancies, clonality can be identified by light

Table 18-2 Phenotypic markers and chromosomal translocations in non-Hodgkin lymphomas.

NHL	sIg	CD5	CD10	CD20	Other	Cyclin D1	Cytogenetics	Oncogene	Function
CLL/SLL	Weak	+	−	Weak	CD23$^+$, FMC$^-$	−	No diagnostic abnormalities*	−	−
Follicular	++	−	+	+		−	t(14;18)	BCL2	Antiapoptosis
Mantle cell	++	+	−	+	CD23$^-$, FMC$^+$	+	t(11;14)	Cyclin D1	Cell cycle regulator
Marginal zone/ extranodal marginal zone lymphoma	+	−	−	+		−	t(11;18)	AP12-MALT	Resistance to *Helicobacter pylori* treatment
Lymphoplasmacytic lymphoma	++	−	−	+	CD25$^{+/-}$, CD38$^{+/-}$	−	t(9;14)	−	−
Hairy cell leukemia	++	−	−	+	CD11c$^+$, CD25$^+$, CD103$^+$	Weak	−	−	−
DLBCL	+	Rare	+/−	+		−	t(14;18), t(3;14), t(3;v) t(8;14), t(2;8), t(2;22) Rare	BCL2 BCL6 CMYC	Antiapoptosis Transcription factor Transcription factor
Burkitt lymphoma	+	−	+	+	TdT$^-$	−	t(8;14), t(2;8), t(2;22)	CMYC	Transcription factor
ALCL, ALK-positive	−	−	−	−	CD2$^+$, CD3$^{-/+}$, EMA$^+$	−	t(2;5)	ALK	Tyrosine kinase

*See chapter on CLL/SLL (Chapter 19) for prognostic cytogenetic abnormalities.
ALCL = anaplastic large-cell lymphoma; CLL = chronic lymphocytic leukemia; DLBCL = diffuse large B-cell lymphoma; MALT = mucosa-associated lymphoid tissue; sIg = surface immunoglobulin; SLL = small lymphocytic lymphoma; TdT = terminal deoxynucleotidyl transferase.

chain restriction of the surface immunoglobulin. B cells normally express κ and λ light chains in a ratio of 2:1. A clonal expansion can be identified by a marked predominance of either κ- or λ-expressing B cells. This would not be expected in a reactive process. Some pan-B-cell surface markers are frequently coexpressed, such as CD19, CD20, and CD22. Others, including CD5, CD10, and CD23, are helpful in the differential diagnosis of B-cell neoplasms, such as differentiating CLL/small lymphocytic lymphoma (SLL) (CD5$^+$, CD19$^+$, CD23$^+$) from follicular lymphoma (CD5$^-$, CD10$^+$, CD19$^+$) or MCL (CD5$^+$, CD19$^+$, CD23$^-$) (Table 18-2).

The immunophenotyping of T-cell neoplasms is less conclusive than for B-cell disorders because T cells lack the equivalent of light chain restriction. Several findings can be suggestive of neoplasia, including expression of CD4 or CD8 on the majority of the T cells, lack of expression of CD4/CD8 or a pan-T-cell marker on the majority of T cells, or coexpression of CD4 and CD8 on the majority of T cells. Often, however, molecular techniques to look at TCR gene rearrangements are necessary to differentiate reactive from clonal T-cell processes.

Molecular genetics/cytogenetics

Molecular genetic techniques can be helpful in assessing clonality when morphology and immunophenotyping are inconclusive. These involve isolating the DNA from a sample and subjecting it to Southern blot analysis or polymerase chain reaction (PCR) to detect rearrangements of immunoglobulin or TCR genes. The demonstration of a dominant rearrangement of the immunoglobulin or TCR genes is indicative of a clonal process. PCR testing has several advantages over Southern analysis, including increased sensitivity, smaller amounts of clinical sample with which to run the assay, and decreased time to perform the test.

Chromosomal translocations are common in lymphoproliferative disorders and can therefore provide useful markers of malignancy. Many oncogene translocations may contribute to the transformation process or cellular proliferation. The finding of particular translocations can help confirm a diagnosis [eg, the t(11;14) in MCL] and can be used for monitoring of disease status following treatment (Table 18-2).

The use of microarray technology has also been used to define the gene expression profile of various lymphoid malignancies and to compare them to normal lymphoid populations. This has been successfully applied to a number of B-cell lymphomas, including diffuse large B-cell lymphoma, follicular lymphoma, CLL, and MCL to identify expression patterns that correlate with patient outcome. It has also identified novel genes that may be important for malignant transformation, which could increase our understanding of lymphomagenesis and potentially elucidate novel therapeutic targets.

Classification of lymphomas

The classification of lymphoproliferative disorders has evolved as a result of an increased understanding of the biology of these diseases. The current classification system used is the *WHO Classification of Tumors of Hematopoietic and Lymphoid Tissues*, which was updated in 2008 (Tables 18-3 and 18-4). This classification recognizes B-cell and T-cell/NK-cell neoplasms and Hodgkin lymphoma (HL). The B- and T-cell neoplasms are separated into precursor (lymphoblastic) neoplasms and mature B- or T-cell neoplasms. The precursor neoplasms are reviewed in Chapter 17, and B-cell and T-cell prolymphocytic leukemia are discussed in Chapter 19. There have been a number of updates and disease refinements in both the B-cell lymphoma and T-cell lymphoma sections of the World Health Organization (WHO) classification. Changes to the classification of mature B- and T-cell lymphomas, including molecular subclassification, will be briefly reviewed here and further highlighted in later sections.

In the updated WHO classification, there are a number of new designations in the category of diffuse large B-cell lymphoma (DLBCL), with morphologic, molecular, and immunophenotypical subgroups as well as distinct disease entities recognized. DLBCL–not otherwise specified (DLBCL-NOS) comprises all DLBCL cases that do not belong to specific subtypes or disease entities. It includes morphologic (eg, centroblastic and immunoblastic), molecular (ie, germinal center B-cell like [GCB] and activated B-cell like [ABC]), and immunohistochemical (eg, GCB vs non-GCB) subgroupings (Table 18-4). Specific DLBCL disease subtypes include the new designations primary central nervous system (CNS) DLBCL and EBV-positive DLBCL of the elderly, and in addition, there are a number of recognized lymphomas of large B cells (eg, primary mediastinal large B-cell lymphoma [PMBCL], intravascular lymphoma, lymphomatoid granulomatosis) (Table 18-4). Of note, borderline cases are also distinguished, including an overlapping category between DLBCL and Burkitt lymphoma and an overlapping category between DLBCL and classical Hodgkin lymphoma (CHL) (Table 18-4).

Few changes have been introduced to the indolent B-cell lymphoma classification. There are a variety of entities that are considered small B-cell clonal lymphoproliferations but that do not fall into the established categories of small B-cell lymphomas, including splenic B-cell lymphoma/leukemia, unclassifiable. In addition, a new category called primary cutaneous follicle center lymphoma has been introduced, where patients typically present with solitary lesions on the head and trunk tumors are composed of neoplastic follicle center cells including centrocytes and a variable number of centroblasts. It should be distinguished from primary cutaneous DLBCL, leg type, which is comprised of a diffuse monotonous pattern of centroblasts or immunoblasts, irrespective of site, and is considered aggressive (Table 18-4).

For the peripheral T/NK-cell neoplasms, the previously established categories of predominantly leukemia, predominantly nodal, and predominantly extranodal have been eliminated given that the subdivisions were often overlapping. The classification system has been further refined with a number important modifications, including recognition of several new distinct and provisional disease categories (Table 18-4). Anaplastic lymphoma kinase (ALK)-positive anaplastic large-cell lymphoma (ALCL) is now recognized as a distinct entity and ALK-negative ALCL is a provisional entity (see section on ALCL). The rare peripheral T-cell lymphoma, subcutaneous panniculitis-like T-cell lymphoma (SCPTCL), is confined to cases with an α-β phenotype. Several new primary cutaneous PTCL categories have been created due to differences in clinical behavior, including primary cutaneous γ-δ T-cell lymphoma, which also includes the γ-δ subtype of SCPTCL due to a similar aggressive course. Of note, one entity has been removed from this section of the WHO classification, blastic NK-cell lymphoma, and is listed in a new category called acute leukemias of ambiguous lineage.

Table 18-3 Subtypes of Hodgkin lymphoma.

Classical Hodgkin lymphoma
    Nodular sclerosis
    Mixed cellularity
    Lymphocyte-rich
    Lymphocyte-depleted
Nodular lymphocyte-predominant Hodgkin lymphoma

Key points

- B and T cells undergo maturation in the bone marrow and thymus, respectively.
- Both B and T cells rearrange antigen receptor genes and acquire cell surface markers as they differentiate.
- B cells may undergo neoplastic transformation during immunoglobulin gene rearrangement, class switch, or somatic hypermutation as a result of errant chromosomal translocation and dysregulation of oncogene expression.
- Specific patterns of surface marker expression and chromosomal translocation characterize many lymphoproliferative diseases.
- The WHO classification represents an important advance in characterizing clinical and biologic subtypes of hematologic malignancies
- Excisional biopsy is critical for accurate diagnosis and hematopathology review for lymphoma classification and management.

Table 18-4 World Health Organization classification of B-cell and T-cell neoplasms.

B-cell neoplasms	T-cell neoplasms
Precursor B-cell neoplasms*	**Precursor T-cell neoplasms***
B lymphoblastic leukemia/lymphoma NOS	T lymphoblastic leukemia/lymphoma
B lymphoblastic leukemia/lymphoma with recurrent genetic abnormalities	
Mature B-cell neoplasms	**Mature T-cell neoplasms**
Aggressive lymphomas	*Aggressive lymphomas*
Diffuse large B-cell lymphoma: variants, subgroups and subtypes/entities	T-cell prolymphocytic leukemia
Diffuse large B-cell lymphoma, NOS	Aggressive NK-cell leukemia
Common morphologic variants: centroblastic, immunoblastic, anaplastic	Peripheral T-cell lymphoma, NOS
Rare morphologic variants	Angioimmunoblastic T-cell lymphoma
Molecular subgroups: germinal center B-cell like (GCB) and activated B-cell like (ABC)	Anaplastic large-cell lymphoma, ALK positive
Immunohistochemical subgroups: $CD5^+$ DLBCL, GCB, and non-GCB	Anaplastic large-cell lymphoma, ALK negative
Diffuse large B-cell lymphoma subtypes	Extranodal NK/T-cell lymphoma, nasal type
T-cell/histiocyte-rich large B-cell lymphoma	Enteropathy-type T-cell lymphoma
Primary DLBCL of the CNS	Hepatosplenic T-cell lymphoma
Primary cutaneous DLBCL, leg type	Subcutaneous panniculitis-like T-cell lymphoma
EBV-positive DLBCL of the elderly	Adult T-cell leukemia/lymphoma
Other lymphomas of large B cells	Primary cutaneous γ-δ T-cell lymphoma
Primary mediastinal large B-cell lymphoma	Primary cutaneous $CD8^+$ aggressive epidermotropic T-cell lymphoma
Intravascular large B-cell lymphoma	
DLBCL associated with chronic inflammation	
Lymphomatoid granulomatosis	
ALK-positive large B-cell lymphoma	
Plasmablastic lymphoma	
Large B-cell lymphoma arising in HHV-8–associated multicentric Castleman disease	
Primary effusion lymphoma	
Borderline cases	
B-cell lymphoma, unclassifiable, with features intermediate between DLBCL and Burkitt lymphoma	
B-cell lymphoma, unclassifiable, with features intermediate between DLBCL and classical Hodgkin lymphoma	
Burkitt lymphoma	
Mantle cell lymphoma	
Indolent lymphomas	*Indolent lymphomas*
Follicular lymphoma	T-cell large granular lymphocytic leukemia[†]
Primary cutaneous follicle center lymphoma	Chronic lymphoproliferative disorders of NK cells
Extranodal marginal zone lymphoma of mucosa-associated lymphoid tissue (MALT)	Mycosis fungoides
Nodal marginal zone lymphoma	Sézary syndrome
Splenic marginal zone lymphoma	Primary cutaneous $CD30^+$ T-cell lymphoproliferative disorder
Splenic B-cell lymphoma/leukemia, unclassifiable	Primary cutaneous $CD4^+$ small/medium T-cell lymphoma
Lymphoplasmacytic lymphoma	
Heavy chain disease	
Plasma cell neoplasms	
CLL/SLL	
B-cell prolymphocytic leukemia	
Hairy cell leukemia	

*All precursor neoplasms are considered aggressive.
[†]Course is usually indolent but in some cases is aggressive.
CLL = chronic lymphocytic leukemia; CNS = central nervous system; DLBCL = diffuse large B-cell lymphoma; HHV-8 = human herpesvirus 8; NK = natural killer; NOS = not otherwise specified; SLL = small lymphocytic lymphoma.

Non-Hodgkin lymphomas

The non-Hodgkin lymphomas (NHLs) are a biologically and clinically heterogeneous group of lymphoproliferative diseases that reflect the diverse cell types comprising our immune system. These neoplasms are characterized by the clonal expansion of malignant cells of B-cell, T-cell, NK-cell, or, rarely, histiocytic/dendritic-cell origin. The natural history, prognosis, and therapeutic approach for an individual with NHL depend on the specific subtype of lymphoma and the clinical stage; thus, accurate diagnosis and staging are essential to optimal management.

Classification

The WHO classification of the tumors of hematopoietic and lymphoid tissues, based on the earlier Revised European-American Lymphoma (REAL) classification, represents an important advance in defining hematologic malignancies and was the first lymphoma classification to integrate morphologic, immunophenotypic, molecular genetic, and clinical features to define individual entities. The third edition of the WHO classification served to update the REAL and add several new entities, and the recently published fourth edition of the WHO classification has refined the classification further as our understanding of lymphoid neoplasms has expanded over the last decade (Swerdlow et al, 2008).

As described above, NHLs are divided into precursor and mature B- or T/NK-cell categories (Table 18-4). Overall, approximately 90% of all NHLs in Western countries are of mature B-cell origin, with DLBCL and follicular lymphoma being the most common subtypes. In children, HL is more predominant, and the aggressive NHLs of lymphoblastic lymphoma, Burkitt lymphoma, and DLBCL are much more commonly encountered than indolent neoplasms. The incidence of NHL is lower among Asian populations, in whom T-cell neoplasms are more frequent.

For clinical purposes, the NHLs can be broadly separated into indolent or aggressive categories (Table 18-4). *Indolent lymphomas* are generally incurable with most standard therapeutic approaches and are typified by a chronic course with repeated relapses and progression with standard therapy. However, some of these patients survive many years with remarkably stable disease even in the absence of specific therapy. Median survival is usually 8 to 10 years but not uncommonly may exceed 15 to 20 years. Most, but not all, *aggressive lymphomas* are potentially curable with combination chemotherapy. Aggressive subtypes usually have a more acute presentation often with B-symptoms and a more rapid progression than the indolent entities. In the event of failure to achieve complete remission following treatment or with relapse after an initial therapeutic response, survival is usually measured in months rather than years. Some of these patients, however, are cured by second-line chemotherapy and stem cell transplantation approaches, as described later in this chapter.

Epidemiology, pathogenesis, and molecular characterization

Data from cancer registries show that the incidence of NHL has been steadily increasing in North America, Europe, and Australia at a rate of approximately 2% to 3% per year for the past 30 years. Over 65,000 new cases of NHL were diagnosed in the United States in 2009, compared with approximately 8000 cases of HL, making NHL the sixth most common cancer in adult men and fifth in adult women. The reasons for this increasing incidence are unknown but are the subject of ongoing epidemiologic investigations. Associations have been made with occupational exposure to certain pesticides and herbicides (Table 18-1). Agricultural workers with cutaneous exposure to these agents have an approximately 2- to 6-fold increased incidence of NHL, possibly contributing to the relatively greater frequency of lymphoma in rural versus urban populations. In children, NHL accounts for approximately 8% of all childhood cancers.

Immunosuppression associated with human immunodeficiency virus (HIV) infection or iatrogenically induced immune suppression in the organ transplantation setting is associated with an increased incidence of aggressive B-cell lymphomas, likely due to dysregulated B-cell proliferation and susceptibility to viruses such as EBV (Table 18-1). In some cases, these neoplasms are polyclonal and may respond to reduced immunosuppression when feasible after transplantation. More subtle, chronic immunoregulatory disorders such as rheumatoid arthritis, Sjögren syndrome, and Hashimoto thyroiditis also carry an increased risk of NHL. In children, the incidence of NHL is increased in several disorders that have in common immunodeficiency from primary immune disorders, including ataxia-telangiectasia, Wiskott-Aldrich syndrome, common variable or severe combined immunodeficiency, and X-linked lymphoproliferative disorder.

In general, there is no particular predilection for lymphoma among specific ethnic groups, although NHL is more frequent in Western than in Asian populations. Familial predisposition to NHL is rare; however, kindreds with high frequencies of NHL have been reported. In particular, CLL and Waldenström macroglobulinemia are seen more frequently in first-degree relatives.

Infection with the bacterium *Helicobacter pylori* is strongly associated with gastric MALT lymphoma. Interestingly, patients with MALT limited to the stomach often achieve complete remission following successful therapy to eradicate

H pylori, indicating that the lymphoma remains dependent in part on continued antigenic drive. Recently, associations have been made between orbital infection by *Chlamydia psittaci* and orbital adnexal MALT lymphoma, infection with *Campylobacter jejuni* and immunoproliferative small intestinal disease, and *Borrelia burgdorferi* and cutaneous MALT lymphoma. These intriguing associations need to be firmly established by additional investigation, including assessment of lymphoma regression following eradication of the infectious agent.

Certain viral infections have been linked with specific subtypes of NHL. EBV has a clear pathogenic role in endemic as well as some cases of sporadic Burkitt lymphoma and in many cases of HIV-related aggressive B-cell lymphoma. EBV is also strongly associated with extranodal NK/T-cell lymphoma, nasal type most commonly seen in Asia and in Central and South America. It is also detected in 70% to 80% of cases of angioimmunoblastic T-cell lymphoma (AITL); however, its role, if any, in disease pathogenesis is unknown. A new entity in the 2008 WHO classification classifies a DLBCL of the elderly that is EBV-associated. Evidence of EBV is also seen at a moderate frequency in HL, particularly the mixed cellularity subtype; however, a direct causal link has not yet been proven. The γ-herpesvirus HHV-8 (Kaposi sarcoma–associated herpesvirus [KSHV]) was first described in Kaposi sarcoma but also has been associated with an unusual primary body cavity lymphoma (primary effusion lymphoma) most commonly seen in patients with acquired immunodeficiency syndrome (AIDS). HHV-8 has also been described in association with multicentric Castleman disease. The retrovirus human T-cell lymphotropic virus 1 (HTLV-1) is associated with adult T-cell leukemia/lymphoma endemic to Japan, central Africa, and the Caribbean. Chronic hepatitis C virus infection has been linked to the development of lymphoplasmacytic lymphoma. Studies using highly sensitive PCR techniques have reported that approximately 40% of NHL, primarily diffuse large B-cell and follicular histologies, have detectable simian virus 40 (SV40) sequences. SV40 was found to be a contaminant of polio vaccines administered in the late 1950s and early 1960s, and it has been suggested that this exposure may be a contributing factor to the increasing occurrence of NHL. However, these SV40 findings need to be verified in additional studies before causation is established.

Specific chromosomal translocations are strongly associated with individual subtypes of B-cell NHL (Table 18-2). The majority of these arise early in B-cell differentiation during the process of immunoglobulin gene rearrangement, when errant fusion of immunoglobulin promoter and enhancer elements with other genes leads to dysregulated oncogene expression. Careful study of such translocations has provided important insights into pathogenetic mechanisms in lymphoma. The most frequent of these translocations are (i) t(14;18), with resultant overexpression of the antiapoptotic gene *BCL2*, which is present in >85% of follicular lymphomas; (ii) t(11;14) with cyclin D1 overexpression, which is present in virtually all MCLs; and (iii) t(8;14), t(2;8), and t(8;22) of Burkitt lymphoma, which fuse an immunoglobulin heavy or light chain gene promoter to the *CMYC* transcription factor. *BCL6*, a chromosome 3 transcription factor gene capable of promiscuous rearrangement with multiple translocation partners, is most commonly identified in DLBCL. It has been reported that lymphomas that overexpress *BCL6* mRNA or protein, either as a result of chromosomal translocation or another mechanism, may have a better prognosis for survival compared with those that are *BCL6* negative.

The t(2;5)(p23;q35) fuses the *ALK* gene with nucleophosmin, the nucleophosmin promoter, and is associated with Ki-1 (CD30)-positive ALCL. Several other translocation partners for *ALK* also have been described in this disease. This translocation and *ALK* expression are associated with a more favorable prognosis in ALCL (see also section on peripheral T-cell lymphomas).

Gene signatures in lymphoma

The diagnostic accuracy of lymphomas is now significantly improved; however, within any given lymphoma subtype, there is a diverse spectrum of clinical behavior that reflects the underlying molecular genetic alterations inherent within tumor cells. For example, even those disease entities defined by specific genetic abnormalities that are important in disease initiation [eg, t(14;18) in follicular lymphoma] have additional aberrant pathways composed of multiple genes that contribute to the malignant phenotype. The recent sequencing of the human genome facilitates more genome-wide approaches using large-scale gene expression analyses that have been applied to simultaneously monitor the expression of thousands of genes from human tumor samples. Such studies have the potential to further refine the classification of heterogeneous disease sets, define molecular signatures of prognosis, and elucidate novel therapeutic targets.

Multiple techniques have been developed to analyze the expression of a large number of genes, but microarrays have emerged as the most commonly used method. Oligonucleotide arrays are commonly used today, and the most widely used is the Affymetrix chip (Affymetrix, Santa Clara, CA), which is composed of 25-mers that overcome the difficulty of cross-hybridization by having multiple probes representing each transcript and inclusion of a second oligonucleotide probe that contains a single variant in the center of the probe (Ramaswamy et al, 2002). With the availability of the full human genome sequence, current-generation chips are representative of all known genes. Furthermore, investigators wishing more "customized" arrays can have them individually built.

There are 2 main approaches to gene expression data analysis: unsupervised and supervised learning. In unsupervised learning, samples are aggregated into groups based on the overall similarity of their gene expression profiles without any a priori knowledge of the sample labels, thus facilitating class discovery. In contrast, in supervised learning, tumors are grouped based on known differences, and a model can then be trained to distinguish between 2 classes. Incorporation of both of these techniques and various array platforms described has been instrumental to our current understanding of lymphoid biology. Furthermore, multivariate models can also be used if clinical data are available to correlate specific gene signatures and prognosis.

This technology has provided new insights into biologically and clinically relevant subsets of lymphoma, as well as being a tool for gene discovery and identification of novel therapeutic targets. These insights are discussed with the relevant NHL entities later in the chapter.

Staging and prognostic factors

Staging procedures define the anatomic extent of the disease and generally include careful physical examination for lymphadenopathy and organomegaly; computed tomography (CT) scans of the neck, chest, abdomen, and pelvis; and bone marrow biopsy. CT or magnetic resonance imaging (MRI) of the brain and evaluation of the cerebrospinal fluid are indicated in patients with Burkitt or lymphoblastic lymphomas and should also be considered in patients with aggressive histology lymphoma involving the bone marrow, paraspinal region, sinonasal region, or testis. The Ann Arbor staging system, identifying patients as having stage I (localized) to stage IV (extensive) disease, was originally devised for use in HL but was later adopted for use in NHL. Patients are further stratified as to the absence (A) or presence (B) of symptoms, namely, fevers, drenching night sweats, or weight loss of 10% or more within 6 months of diagnosis (Table 18-5). Several limitations become apparent when the Ann Arbor classification is applied to NHL. Unlike HL, which has a contiguous pattern of lymphatic involvement, NHLs have a tendency to spread hematogenously and involve noncontiguous lymph node sites. In addition, the Ann Arbor staging system does not reflect the unique natural history of specific NHL subtypes or the consequences of lymphomatous involvement of certain extranodal disease sites (eg, sinus, CNS, testicular). In addition, important factors reflecting tumor burden (eg, lactate dehydrogenase [LDH], number of nodal or extranodal sites involved, tumor bulk, β_2-microglobulin, B-symptoms) and physiologic reserve of the patient (eg, age, performance status) are not included in this conventional staging system.

To more fully incorporate additional relevant prognostic features, more broadly relevant models have been developed in the most common NHLs, DLBCL and follicular lymphoma.

The most widely used clinical prognostic model to stratify patients with aggressive NHLs is the International Prognostic Index (IPI) (Shipp et al, 1993). Institutions from all over the world provided clinical and laboratory information on patients with aggressive large-cell lymphoma diagnosed by the Working Formulation, Kiel, and Rappaport classifications, and thus, immunophenotyping information was not available or incorporated into the model. Based on disease frequency, the most common subtype submitted for the development of the IPI would have been DLBCL. The purpose was to identify pretreatment variables that predict relapse-free and overall survival (OS) with doxorubicin-containing combination chemotherapy. The following 5 risk factors were independently associated with clinical outcome

Table 18-5 Ann Arbor staging system.*

Stage	Definition[†]
I	Involvement of a single lymph node or of a single extranodal organ or site (IE)
II	Involvement of 2 or more lymph node regions on the same side of the diaphragm, or localized involvement of an extranodal site or organ (IIE) and 1 or more lymph node regions on the same side of the diaphragm
III	Involvement of lymph node regions on both sides of the diaphragm, which may also be accompanied by localized involvement of an extranodal organ or site (IIIE) or spleen (IIIS) or both (IIISE)
IV	Diffuse or disseminated involvement of 1 or more distant extranodal organs with or without associated lymph node involvement

*Fever >38°C, night sweats, and/or weight loss >10% of body weight in the 6 months preceding admission are defined as systemic symptoms.
[†]The spleen is considered nodal.

Table 18-6 International Prognostic Index (IPI) and age-adjusted index for aggressive lymphoma patients treated with doxorubicin-containing combination chemotherapy.

Risk group	Risk factors (no.)	Distribution of cases (%)	CR rate (%)	5-year OS (%)
All ages*				
Low (L)	0, 1	35	87	73
Low-intermediate (LI)	2	27	67	51
High-intermediate (HI)	3	22	55	43
High (H)	4, 5	16	44	26
Age-adjusted index (≤60)†				
Low (L)	0	22	92	83
Low-intermediate (LI)	1	32	78	69
High-intermediate (HI)	2	32	57	46
High (H)	3	14	46	32

*IPI risk factors are age >60 years, LDH > normal, PS ≥2, stage III or IV, and >1 extranodal sites.
†Age-adjusted IPI risk factors are age >60, LDH > normal, PS ≥ 2, and stage III or IV.
Shipp MA, Harrington DP, Anderson JR, et al. A predictive model for aggressive non-Hodgkin's lymphoma. The International Non-Hodgkin's Lymphoma Prognostic Factors Project. *N Engl J Med*. 1993;329:987-994.
CR = complete remission; LDH = lactate dehydrogenase; OS = overall survival; PS = performance status.

and are often referred to as *APLES*: (i) age ≥60; (ii) performance status ≥2; (iii) elevated serum LDH; (iv) number of extranodal sites of disease >1; and (v) stage III or IV. The IPI score is derived as a simple additive score from 0 to 5 and has been widely adopted to estimate prognosis in patients with NHL (Table 18-6). Four prognostic risk categories were identified that had the following 5-year OS rates: low risk, 0 to 1 factor = 73%; low-intermediate risk, 2 factors = 51%; high-intermediate risk, 3 factors = 43%; and high risk, 4 to 5 factors = 26%. Of note, these survival estimates are prior to the use of rituximab.

An age-adjusted score has been developed for patients ≤60 years of age, where stage, performance status, and elevated LDH, but not extranodal disease, correlate with outcome (Table 18-6). It is recognized that these clinical IPI factors likely represent surrogate markers of the underlying biology of the lymphoma. Other serum and tumor markers, plus recent cDNA microarray analyses, hold promise to provide additional insights into pathogenesis and prognosis that in the future may have clinical utility to develop the treatment approach for individual patients. The IPI score is also predictive of survival in indolent lymphomas, namely follicular lymphoma, although using the IPI, the majority of these patients fall into the low- or low-intermediate–risk categories (Table 18-7). As such, a new index was developed specifically for follicular lymphoma called the *Follicular Lymphoma International Prognostic Index* (FLIPI) in hopes of better stratifying patients by risk. This index is often remembered by "No-LASH." The 5 clinical factors that are the strongest predictors of outcome in multivariate analysis are age > 5 nodal sites of disease, elevated LDH, age > 60 years, stage III or IV disease, and hemoglobin < 10 g/L. Compared with the IPI, the FLIPI provides a better distribution of patients across the risk categories of good risk (0 to 1 factor), intermediate risk (2 factors), or poor risk (≥3 factors) (Table 18-7). The 5- and 10-year OS rates were 90% and 70%, respectively, for good-risk patients but decreased to 53% and 36%, respectively, for poor-risk patients (Table 18-7).

Although the IPI scoring system provides useful prognostic information, there is no definitive evidence that outcome is altered by using intensive regimens in high-risk patients. Numerous studies have been reported, and others are still in progress, assessing the utility of the IPI and "risk-adjusted" or "risk-adapted" therapeutic strategies. These include trials

Table 18-7 Comparison of the Follicular Lymphoma International Prognostic Index (FLIPI) and the International Prognostic Index (IPI) in follicular lymphoma.

Risk model and group	No. of factors	Distribution of cases (%)	5-year OS (%)	10-year OS (%)
FLIPI				
Low	0–1	36	91	71
Intermediate	2	37	78	51
High	≥3	27	53	36
IPI				
Low	0–1	49	88	67
Low-intermediate	2	31	71	50
High-intermediate	3	15	57	28
High	4–5	5	44	36

OS = overall survival.

Histology	Pretreatment	Mid-treatment	Response assessment	Posttreatment surveillance
Routinely FDG avid				
DLBCL	Yes*	Clinical trial	Yes	No
HL	Yes*	Clinical trial	Yes	No
Follicular NHL	No†	Clinical trial	No†	No
MCL	No†	Clinical trial	No†	No
Variably FDG avid				
Other aggressive NHLs	No†	Clinical trial	No†‡	No
Other indolent NHLs	No†	Clinical trial	No†‡	No

Table 18-8 Recommended timing of PET/CT scans in lymphoma clinical trials.

*Recommended but not required before treatment.
†Recommended only if ORR/CR is a primary study end point.
‡Recommended only if PET is positive before treatment.
CR = complete remission; CT = computed tomography; DLBCL = diffuse large B-cell lymphoma; FDG = fluorodeoxyglucose; HL = Hodgkin lymphoma; MCL = mantle cell lymphoma; NHL = non-Hodgkin lymphoma; ORR = overall response rate; PET = positron emission tomography.

of high-dose therapy (HDT) and autologous stem cell transplantation (ASCT) for aggressive lymphoma patients with high IPI scores; however, such strategies are not currently established as standard approaches and remain experimental. The IPI is useful in comparing studies and also in the investigation of new prognostic factors to determine the independent effect on outcome.

The use of positron emission tomography (PET) scanning is proving increasingly useful both for staging and assessing response to lymphoma therapy. The International Harmonization Project in lymphoma has recently outlined recommendations on the role of PET scans in staging and response assessment (Juweid et al, 2007). PET scanning in the curative lymphomas, DLBCL and HL, is recommended because it will facilitate assessment of disease extent and also provide a pretreatment comparison for response assessment (Table 18-8). However, given that PET is not widely available, it is not absolutely required. Residual abnormalities on CT scans frequently lead to a "partial remission" assessment, although it is recognized that many of these patients may in fact be in a complete remission (CR) (PET negative) and that the abnormal tissue visualized may represent fibrosis rather than residual lymphoma (Cheson et al, 2007). PET scanning in such cases may provide evidence for a "functional CR." Several recent reports have suggested that the achievement of early PET negativity, for example, after only 2 to 4 cycles of treatment, may be highly predictive of very low relapse rates in aggressive lymphoma (Spaepen et al, 2002). In one comprehensive analysis where treatment was not modified based on the PET results, the 2-year event-free survival (EFS) rate was 0% to 35% if the mid-treatment PET was positive compared with 72% to 93% if the mid-treatment PET was negative (Kasamon and Wahl, 2008). Overall, relapse or progression occurs in 71% to 100% of patients with a positive mid-treatment PET. However, whether PET scanning can be used to alter therapy is the subject of ongoing clinical trials, and thus the use of mid-therapy PET scans should be restricted to use in clinical trials. Furthermore, the specificity of a PET scan is not 100% because uptake can occur in the setting of inflammation, including granulomatous disease and infection, and a biopsy should be performed in a PET-positive patient in a remission by CT scan if HDT and SCT are under consideration.

Patient follow-up

Patient surveillance following treatment of lymphoma should address both long-term complications of therapy and disease recurrence. Long-term effects of therapy depend on the type of treatment and whether radiotherapy was also administered. Radiotherapy to the head and neck region leads to decreased salivation with dental caries; thus, close dental follow-up should be performed. Additionally, if the thyroid was included in the radiation field, a large proportion of patients may eventually become hypothyroid and the thyroid-stimulating hormone level should monitored with each follow-up visit. Women who have had mantle radiation should receive a mammogram 10 years after radiation or at age 40. Long-term survivors are also at risk of second malignancies. Once primary therapy has been completed and remission documented, patients are typically followed every 3 months for the first 2 years, then every 6 months until 5 years, and then annually thereafter. Most recurrences of aggressive lymphoma occur in the first 2 years after treatment, although late relapses beyond 5 years do occur in a small minority of patients. Patients with indolent lymphoma have a lifelong risk of relapse and are typically seen every 3 months for the first 2 years and then every 3 to 6 months indefinitely. There is no evidence that routine CT imaging impacts outcome in the surveillance of patients (Weeks et al, 1991), because most relapses are detected by patients or their physicians based on the development of new symptoms or signs. However, it can be considered in high-risk young patients with curable lymphomas. Currently, there are insufficient data to support the use of routine fluorodeoxyglucose PET in the follow-up of patients with lymphoma.

> **Key points**
>
> - NHLs are biologically and clinically heterogeneous; accurate diagnosis using the WHO classification is essential to optimal management.
> - The majority of NHLs are of B-cell origin and are broadly categorized as indolent versus aggressive subtypes.
> - The incidence of NHL is increasing 2% to 3% per year in Western countries.
> - Specific chromosomal translocations are associated with specific subtypes of lymphoma and are pathogenetically involved in malignant transformation and progression.
> - The IPI score provides important prognostic information for outcome and survival in both aggressive and indolent lymphomas. The FLIPI has been developed specifically for follicular lymphoma.

Indolent B-cell NHL

The indolent B-cell lymphomas include the cell types shown in Table 18-4, and the most commonly encountered subtype is follicular lymphoma, which accounts for 20% of all lymphomas. Other subtypes include marginal zone lymphomas, including extranodal marginal zone lymphomas, or what was previously referred to as MALT lymphomas, and lymphoplasmacytic lymphoma. This category also includes CLL/SLL, discussed separately in Chapter 19.

Follicular lymphoma

Follicular lymphomas are derived from germinal center B cells and are graded based on the number of centroblasts per high-power field: grade 1 (0-5); grade 2 (6-15); and grade 3 (>15). The tumor cells are $CD20^+$, $CD10^+$, $BCL6^+$, $BCL2^+$, and $CD5^-$. Up to 90% of follicular lymphomas have a t(14;18) with a higher frequency observed in grade 1 or 2 follicular lymphomas. Many clinicians distinguish between follicular grade 1 or 2 and grade 3 and treat the latter with anthracycline-based chemotherapy, but data are discrepant as to whether a clear plateau can be seen in the survival curve. This suggests that cure is possible in patients with grade 3 follicular lymphoma or follicular large-cell lymphoma, the latter term referring to the designation in earlier classifications. Furthermore, in the third edition of the WHO classification, grade 3A (centrocytes present) was distinguished from grade 3B (solid sheets of centroblasts), and there may be important clinical and biologic differences within this category. Abnormalities of 3q27 and/or BCL6 rearrangement are more commonly found in grade 3B cases. Follicular grade 3B may behave more like DLBCL; however, as a result of only relatively recent recognition in the WHO classification, clinical studies of the natural history and outcome differences compared with the other grades of follicular lymphoma are limited.

In the updated WHO classification, there are a number of identified variants of follicular lymphoma. Primary intestinal follicular lymphoma, which primarily occurs as localized disease in the small intestine, particularly the duodenum, is one such variant. Other extranodal follicular lymphomas and pediatric follicular lymphoma are also considered variants. Of note, primary cutaneous follicular center lymphoma, a provisional entity in the updated WHO classification, should be distinguished from follicular lymphoma. It is derived from follicle center cells including centrocytes and a variable number of centroblasts and can have a follicular, follicular and diffuse, or diffuse growth pattern. It typically occurs as solitary or localized skin lesions on the scalp, forehead, or trunk, and only 15% present with multifocal lesions.

Gene expression profiling has been explored in follicular lymphoma to determine whether molecular subgroupings could be identified that have prognostic significance. In the largest study, whole tumor biopsies of 191 untreated patients with follicular lymphoma were used, and RNA was hybridized to the U133A and U133B microarrays. Using a supervised method to determine signature patterns associated with survival, a molecular signature was constructed that could divide patients into 4 quartiles with widely disparate median survival times (3.9, 10.8, 11.1, and 13.6 years; Dave et al, 2004). Interestingly, the signatures largely consisted of nonmalignant cells from the microenvironment. One signature was termed *immune response-1* and was associated with a more favorable prognosis and had high expression of genes expressed in T cells. In contrast, *immune response-2* had high expression of genes expressed in monocytes and/or dendritic cells. Whether these signatures can be used to develop new targeted therapies or are still relevant in rituximab-treated patients is unknown.

Management of patients with localized follicular lymphoma

The standard management of stage I and some stage II patients with typically nonbulky, follicular lymphoma consists of radiotherapy alone, using involved-field or extended-field irradiation. There are no randomized or comparative studies of these 2 radiotherapy approaches, but there is no clear evidence that OS is improved by more extensive radiation fields. In addition, late-onset radiation-induced second primary cancers remain a concern and are increased in patients with more extensive fields. MacManus and Hoppe

(1996) found that approximately 40% of limited-stage patients with follicular lymphoma remained disease free at 10 years after radiation treatment; late relapses beyond 10 years were unusual. Other studies also reported a 10-year disease-free survival rate of approximately 40% to 50%, suggesting that cure is possible in a proportion of patients with this approach (Wilder et al, 2001; Campbell et al, 2009). Recent data also support that radiation fields can be reduced without impacting outcome (Campbell et al, 2009). An alternative approach is the use of combined-modality therapy with chemotherapy plus involved-field radiation (IFRT), although no randomized studies demonstrate that there is an added benefit of chemotherapy in early-stage indolent NHL. A recent Stanford report of stage I and II patients with follicular lymphoma who received no initial therapy showed that over half of the 43 patients did not require therapy at a median of 6 or more years of follow-up, emphasizing the indolent course for many patients with this presentation.

> ### Clinical case
>
> A 78-year-old man with a history of angina and insulin-dependent diabetes is referred for evaluation of bilateral cervical adenopathy. He has been more fatigued in recent weeks and has noted several episodes of angina responsive to nitroglycerin. He denies fevers, night sweats, and weight loss. Eastern Cooperative Oncology Group (ECOG) performance status is 2. Examination confirms 2- to 3-cm bilateral cervical adenopathy as well as bilateral axillary and inguinal adenopathy that is causing some mild discomfort. The spleen is palpable 3 cm below the costal margin. Laboratory studies show a normal LDH and normal renal and hepatic function. The hemoglobin is 11.5 g with a normal white blood cell count and platelet count. Excisional biopsy of a cervical node shows replacement by grade 1 follicular lymphoma positive for CD20, CD10, and κ light chains. Bone marrow biopsy is positive for lymphoma. FLIPI score is 3 (age, stage, and number of nodal sites >4).

Patients with indolent lymphoma are generally of older age and usually present with advanced-stage disease that is very responsive to chemotherapy but not curable with standard therapeutic approaches. In the few randomized controlled studies that are available, it has not been shown that early treatment of asymptomatic advanced-stage patients improves survival, so a common approach in such patients who also have nonthreatening, typically nonbulky disease is watchful waiting and treatment when symptoms or disease progression become apparent. However, it is important that patients be evaluated at regular intervals and are educated as to the signs and symptoms of progressive disease. The patient presented in the clinical case has symptomatic stage IV follicular lymphoma with fatigue, anemia, high-risk FLIPI score, and significant comorbid disease. Treatment with palliative intent is indicated for this individual but must take into account his age and generally poor health. It is important that the primary care physician also be involved in the patient's care to optimize his cardiac status and discuss the best timing of initiating therapy with his competing comorbidities.

An increasing array of therapeutic options are available for advanced-stage follicular lymphoma, ranging from single-agent chemotherapy, which today is uncommonly used, to a variety of combination chemotherapy regimens to newer approaches with monoclonal antibody therapy alone or in combination with cytotoxic drugs. Additional options include HDT with stem cell rescue for selected patients and targeted radioimmunotherapy. This discussion will focus on some of the benefits and limitations of traditional versus newer approaches, but the reader should recognize that this is a dynamic and rapidly evolving field of clinical investigation with considerable promise for favorably altering the natural history of follicular and other indolent lymphomas.

Primary therapy of advanced-stage follicular lymphoma

The majority of patients enrolled into clinical trials for indolent lymphomas have follicular lymphoma. There are no randomized clinical trials specifically in the more uncommon indolent lymphomas, and results are often extrapolated to these other groups. For the purposes of this review, the data will focus on follicular lymphoma, but the principles and therapy approaches can be applied, for the most part, to the other subtypes. The median survival for patients with follicular lymphoma is approximately 9 years; however, this number can vary depending on the FLIPI score. As described, prior studies have found no clear survival benefit to initiating chemotherapy in asymptomatic patients with nonthreatening disease; thus, the watch-and-wait approach is still an appropriate approach to these patients (Ardeshna et al, 2003). When patients require systemic therapy, there are a number of existing options. The standard first-line therapy for advanced-stage indolent lymphoma is alkylator-based chemotherapy. Single-agent therapy with oral chlorambucil or cyclophosphamide delivered in varying schedules, with or without prednisone, will palliate symptoms in most patients, although few achieve CR. Such regimens are useful for elderly patients and those with significant comorbidities, as in the earlier clinical case. Thus, oral chlorambucil or cyclophosphamide would be a reasonable approach for the patient in the clinical case; prednisone should be withheld in view of his diabetes unless close monitoring is assured.

Combination chemotherapy with cyclophosphamide, vincristine, and prednisone (CVP); cyclophosphamide, doxorubicin, vincristine, and prednisone (CHOP); fludarabine in combination with cyclophosphamide or cyclophosphamide

Table 18-9 Chemotherapy combinations used in the treatment of non-Hodgkin lymphomas in the primary and relapsed setting.

Newly diagnosed patients	Relapsed and refractory patients
CVP	ICE
Cyclophosphamide	Ifosfamide
Vincristine	Carboplatin
Prednisone	Etoposide
CHOP	DHAP
Cyclophosphamide	Dexamethasone
Doxorubicin	High-dose cytarabine
Vincristine	Cisplatin
Prednisone	
R-CHOP	GDP
CHOP + rituximab	Dexamethasone
	Gemcitabine
	Cisplatin
MACOP-B	ESHAP
Methotrexate/leucovorin	Etoposide
Doxorubicin	Methylprednisolone
Cyclophosphamide	High-dose cytarabine
Vincristine	Cisplatin
Prednisone	
Bleomycin	
M-BACOD	EPOCH
Methotrexate/leucovorin	Etoposide
Bleomycin	Vincristine
Doxorubicin	Doxorubicin
Cyclophosphamide	Cyclophosphamide
Vincristine	Prednisone
Dexamethasone	
ProMACE-CytaBOM	
Prednisone	
Doxorubicin	
Cyclophosphamide	
Etoposide	
Cytarabine	
Vincristine	
Prednisone	
Bleomycin	

and mitoxantrone (FC or FCM) (Table 18-9); and numerous other regimens have been shown to increase response rates compared with single agents but have not been established in randomized controlled trials to improve OS. These combination chemotherapy approaches are often used in younger patients in whom the goal is to achieve a more durable remission. They are also useful in the setting of bulky, rapidly progressing, or highly symptomatic disease where a quick response is desirable. Local radiation therapy can be useful for control of locally bulky or obstructing disease that fails to respond adequately to chemotherapy. Furthermore, there are no published randomized controlled trials demonstrating an OS benefit of one combination over another in the primary therapy of follicular lymphoma; thus, practices vary around the world.

Rituximab, an anti-CD20 chimeric monoclonal antibody, is a targeted monoclonal antibody that has improved outcomes in virtually all B-cell lymphomas, both indolent and aggressive subtypes. Targeted monoclonal antibodies have several mechanisms of activity, including activation of complement and antibody-dependent cellular cytotoxicity and induction of apoptosis. Rituximab was initially approved in relapsed follicular lymphoma based on an overall response rate (ORR) of approximately 60% with a median response duration of approximately 1 year (McLaughlin et al, 1998). Rituximab's nonoverlapping toxicities, differing mechanisms of action, and in vitro synergy with chemotherapy have led to numerous trials evaluating chemotherapy/rituximab combinations. Virtually all of the randomized trials have demonstrated improved responses for concurrent rituximab/chemotherapy combinations compared with chemotherapy alone or sequential chemotherapy and rituximab.

One of the first published studies evaluating a rituximab/chemotherapy combination in advanced-stage follicular lymphoma compared CVP to rituximab plus CVP (R-CVP) for a total of 8 cycles and showed that all end points including ORR, time to treatment failure, and progression-free survival (PFS) were improved in the R-CVP arm (Marcus et al, 2005). Longer follow-up confirmed an improvement in 4-year OS in the R-CVP arm (83% vs 77%, $P = .029$; Marcus et al, 2008). The ECOG evaluated the benefit of maintenance rituximab in advanced-stage indolent lymphomas, the majority of which were follicular lymphomas. All patients received induction therapy with CVP followed by randomization for patients achieving a CR or partial remission (PR) to scheduled rituximab retreatment 4 times weekly every 6 months for 2 years versus observation (Hochster et al, 2009). A significant benefit was identified in the maintenance rituximab arm with regard to PFS (3-year PFS, 68% maintenance rituximab vs 33% observation; $P = 4.4 \times 10^{-10}$) and OS (3-year OS, 92% maintenance rituximab vs 86% observation; one-sided $P = .05$). Similar results have been seen comparing CHOP with rituximab plus CHOP (R-CHOP) (Hiddemann et al, 2005) and rituximab plus mitoxantrone, chlorambucil, and prednisolone with mitoxantrone, chlorambucil, and prednisolone (Herold et al, 2007). Thus, in symptomatic and fit patients, rituximab combinations have become routine in the primary treatment of indolent lymphomas.

A study by the Southwest Oncology Group (SWOG) evaluating the impact of rituximab on the natural history of advanced-stage follicular lymphoma showed an improvement in survival in more recent studies incorporating rituximab or radioimmunotherapy compared with chemotherapy alone as first-line therapy (Fisher et al, 2005). This observational analysis suggests that rituximab is prolonging survival and changing the natural history of follicular lymphoma; however, it is unknown whether earlier treatment in lower risk, asymptomatic patients will impact outcome. This question is currently the subject of clinical trials.

First-line therapy with rituximab alone and the use of rituximab as maintenance therapy are also being investigated. Two phase II studies of rituximab as first-line therapy, one by Hainsworth et al (2002) incorporating maintenance rituximab therapy every 6 months for 2 years and another by Ghielmini et al (2004, 2009) using an abbreviated maintenance regimen, have shown high response rates and delayed disease progression. In the latter trial, patients who were either treatment naive or relapsed received 1 dose every week for 4 weeks of rituximab; those demonstrating at least stable disease were randomized to either 4 additional doses of rituximab given at 2-month intervals or no further treatment. The results were recently updated with a median follow-up time of 8.9 years, and the EFS in the consolidation arm was 26% at 5 years compared with 10% in the observation arm (Hainsworth et al, 2002; Ghielmini et al, 2000, 2009).

Radioimmunotherapy has recently been evaluated in the primary therapy setting of follicular lymphoma in the First-Line Indolent Trial (FIT), and the first report was presented at the American Society of Hematology (ASH) 2008 meeting. Patients could receive any alkylator-based induction chemotherapy, and patients who had achieved a response were randomized to observation versus treatment with yttrium-90 (^{90}Y)-ibritumomab tiuxetan (Zevalin) which is targeted against CD20 (Morschhauser et al, 2008). The first analysis demonstrated an improvement in PFS in the treatment arm. However, few patients were treated with rituximab, and with the established benefit of rituximab in this setting, it is unknown whether additional radioimmunotherapy will improve outcome in patients who have received rituximab with their upfront therapy.

Therapy for relapsed and refractory follicular lymphoma

Multiple options exist for the treatment of patients who have failed first-line therapy, and the decision of what chemotherapy to use depends on a number of factors including the duration of prior response, patient age, and comorbid illnesses. If a durable remission was achieved with alkylator therapy (>2 years), it may be used again. Of note, if CHOP was used as first-line therapy, a ceiling dose for the anthracyclines may have been reached. For shorter remission durations, fludarabine can be used. However, it must be used with caution in heavily pretreated or elderly patients due to immunosuppression. Patients are at increased risk of *Pneumocystis carinii* and reactivation of herpes zoster. Prophylaxis with trimethoprim/sulfamethoxazole and acyclovir should be considered. Furthermore, if ASCT is considered as a future treatment option, the number of cycles with fludarabine should be minimized to avoid stem cell toxicity.

Rituximab combinations have also been tested in the relapsed setting, although the current published data only include patients who did not receive rituximab with initial study. A recent study enrolling patients with relapsed follicular lymphoma compared CHOP with R-CHOP, with a second randomization to maintenance rituximab (375 mg/m^2 every 3 months for 8 doses) versus no therapy in patients achieving a response (van Oers et al, 2006). Similar to studies in the primary setting, R-CHOP was superior to CHOP with regard to PFS and OS. Furthermore, patients who received maintenance rituximab, regardless of whether rituximab was received with CHOP therapy, had an improvement in PFS (median, 51.5 months vs 14.9 months; $P < .001$) and OS. This study has established the benefit of rituximab maintenance in the relapsed setting. The Primary Rituximab and Maintenance (PRIMA) study is currently evaluating whether the benefit of maintenance rituximab can be extrapolated to the primary therapy setting.

Radioimmunotherapy targeted to CD20 is also a viable option for patients with indolent B-cell NHL if the bone marrow is minimally involved and disease is not bulky. The 2 approved radioimmunotherapy treatments for relapsed follicular lymphomas are both murine monoclonal antibodies incorporating either radioimmunotherapy with iodine-131 (^{131}I) (tositumomab) or ^{90}Y (ibritumomab tiuxetan). These agents are the most active single agents in the relapsed disease setting, although their use is limited to patients with adequate leukocyte and platelet counts and <25% marrow involvement by lymphoma. Response duration is, on average, 11 to 15 months, and radioimmunotherapy can also be effective in transformed lymphoma.

Single-agent rituximab can also be used in relapsed lymphoma, although now that most patients have received it with their primary therapy and maybe on maintenance, few receive for relapsed lymphoma today. The exception is an elderly patient who has failed an alkylator-based regimen. In this situation, it remains a viable treatment option, given its virtual lack of myelosuppression and relatively low adverse effect profile compared with standard second- and third-line chemotherapy regimens. Single-agent rituximab remains an important treatment option for select patients with relapsed indolent NHL.

Bendamustine has recently emerged as a highly active agent in indolent lymphomas. It is described as a bifunctional agent that is an alkylator with purine analog characteristics. The mechanism of action of the alkylator component is through activation of a base excision DNA repair pathway rather than an alkyltransferase DNA repair mechanism. It is now approved in the United States for use in patients with rituximab-refractory indolent B-cell lymphomas and CLL. A 77% ORR was seen in heavily pretreated patients with a response duration of >6 months. Similar results were seen in a pivotal trial of 100 patients. A phase III trial comparing bendamustine plus rituximab to R-CHOP as first-line treatment of patients with follicular lymphoma, other indolent lymphoma, and MCL was presented at the ASH meeting in 2007, and the second interim analysis was reported last year. With a median follow-up time of 28 months, there was no difference in response rate or EFS, and the toxicity profile favored the bendamustine plus rituximab regimen.

High-dose chemotherapy and ASCT

The use of high-dose chemotherapy with autologous bone marrow or peripheral blood stem cell rescue is being investigated as a therapeutic option in the treatment of indolent lymphomas, especially for higher risk disease in first or second relapse. van Besien et al (2003) reviewed 904 patients in the International Bone Marrow Transplant Registry who underwent autologous or allogeneic transplantation for follicular lymphoma. Durable remissions could be induced with either technique. Allogeneic transplantation remains the only known curative option; however, a lower 5-year recurrence rate with allogeneic transplantations is offset by a higher treatment-related mortality compared with autologous transplantation, leading to similar 5-year survival rates of 51% to 62%. There is a suggestion of benefit for purged versus unpurged autologous transplantations. The randomized CUP (chemotherapy, unpurged high dose therapy [U] or purged high dose therapy [P]) study, in which patients received an ASCT following remission with CHOP-type chemotherapy, suggested an improvement in PFS ($P = .0037$) but not OS (comparing chemotherapy alone with unpurged ASCT and purged ASCT) for ASCT (Schouten et al, 2003). However, these studies were performed prior to the use of rituximab. Further studies, including on the use of monoclonal antibody therapy as an in vivo purge or for consolidation treatment, and improvement in patient stratification are needed to establish the role of these aggressive therapeutic approaches in indolent NHL.

Tumor vaccine approaches

As described earlier, each B cell expresses a unique immunoglobulin molecule, and the variable region contains a unique recombination gene sequence referred to as an idiotype (Id). B-cell lymphomas represent clonal proliferation of lymphocytes, and thus, the immunoglobulin they express is unique for each patient. This observation led to studies exploring active immunization of patients against their own tumor idiotype. In early studies, the tumor-specific idiotype was isolated from the B-cell lymphoma and fused to a myeloma cell line, resulting in hybrid cells that secreted the tumor-derived immunoglobulins that were then purified to generate a vaccine. Recombinant DNA technology has more recently been used to clone the immunoglobulin variable region from the tumor, which can then be transfected to produce large amounts of idiotype protein in a more efficient and timely manner than the hybridoma methodology. Immune adjuvants such as granulocyte-macrophage colony-stimulating factor (GM-CSF) are given to enhance the immune response. Early testing of this approach in follicular lymphoma suggested that the development of an anti-idiotype response correlated with outcome (freedom from progression, 7.9 years in responders vs 1.3 years in nonresponders; Kwak et al, 1992). Encouraging results from this and other studies led to the development of 3 randomized controlled studies to determine the efficacy of idiotype vaccination (Biovest, Genitope, Favrille; Houot and Levy, 2009). These trials have been reported in abstracts, but the full publications are not yet available. In 2 of the trials (Genitope and Biovest), vaccination occurred following alkylator-type chemotherapy and at least a PR was necessary to proceed to randomization to either vaccine or placebo. These trials initially did not include the addition of rituximab; however, as data emerged regarding the efficacy of rituximab with combination chemotherapy, the Biovest trial was amended in July 2006 to include R-CHOP as an alternative to the cisplatin, doxorubicin, cyclophosphamide, and etoposide chemotherapy. In the third trial (Favrille), patients were first treated with rituximab, and if stable disease or better was achieved, they proceeded to the vaccine portion. Of note, rituximab has been shown to delay humoral responses, and thus in the latter trial, the vaccine was continued until disease progression. Unfortunately, the results have been somewhat mixed. The Genitope trial failed to meet its primary end point with no difference in PFS between the vaccine arm (idiotype–keyhole limpet hemocyanin plus GM-GSF) and the control arm (KLM [keyhole limpet hemocyanin] plus GM-CSF). However, in subgroup analysis, superior PFS was observed in patients who did mount an immune response, consistent with prior observations (Levy et al, 2008). The Favrille trial was reported at the ASH 2008 meeting and no improvement in time to progression was observed in the vaccine arm (Freedman et al, 2008). In contrast, the Biovest trial was stopped early due to an apparent benefit observed in disease-free survival in patients who received the idiotype vaccination and who had achieved a CR (33.8 months vs 21.2 months; $P = .047$). The details of this study are also not yet available for review. Thus, the role of vaccination remains unclear, particularly now that rituximab is routinely incorporated into primary therapy regimens.

The array of therapeutic options in follicular and indolent lymphomas is thus increasingly complex and ranges from watchful waiting to aggressive chemotherapy/immunotherapy or stem cell transplantation. The management of individual patients therefore requires a thorough understanding of the natural history of these diseases, an assessment of potential risk and benefit for a particular therapy, the pathologic subtype of lymphoma, and the clinical features of disease (eg, stage, bulk) and comorbid disease. It is important that the therapeutic goals and treatment algorithm be thoroughly considered and discussed with the patient at diagnosis so that the sequencing of treatment options can be logically applied.

Marginal zone lymphomas

The WHO classification separates the marginal zone B-cell lymphomas (MZL) into extranodal MZL of MALT, nodal MZL, and splenic MZL. The morphology of these disorders is characterized by an infiltrate of centrocyte-like small cleaved cells, monocytoid B cells, or small lymphocytes and may exhibit an expanded marginal zone surrounding lymphoid follicles. The immunophenotype is characterized by expression of CD20 but lack of CD5 or CD10 expression (Table 18-2); this marker profile is useful in distinguishing MZL from SLL, MCL, and follicular lymphoma.

MALT lymphomas

MALT lymphomas constitute 50% to 70% of all MZLs. They occur in mucosal sites, predominantly gastric or intestinal, and some nonmucosal extranodal sites, including the lung, salivary gland, periorbital or soft tissue, skin, and thyroid. Often these sites are affected by chronic infection or inflammation, such as Sjögren syndrome involving the parotid gland or Hashimoto thyroiditis. The typical presentation of MALT lymphoma is an isolated mass in any of these extranodal sites or an ulcerative lesion in the stomach. Clinically, they behave as indolent disorders. At a molecular level, MALT lymphomas are characterized by the t(11;18)(q21;q21) translocation in approximately 40% of cases and, less commonly, the t(1;14)(p22;q32) translocation. Interestingly, these distinct translocations appear to mimic one another in activating the nuclear factor (NF)-κB pathway, potentially leading to antigen-independent growth and clonal progression. Trisomy 3 and 3q27 amplification have also been reported as frequent anomalies.

The stomach is the most common site of MALT lymphoma. The majority of cases of gastric MALT lymphoma are associated with *H pylori* infection. Gastric MALT lymphoma is thought to arise as a result of chronic stimulation of the B and T cells in the stomach by *H pylori*. These T lymphocytes release cytokines that stimulate the B cells in the marginal zone of the acquired lymphoid follicles, which eventually leads to the emergence of a clonal B-cell neoplasm that, at least in its early stages, is antigen driven by *H pylori*. Most commonly, these tumors present with a gastric ulcer and occasionally with a gastric mass. At clinical presentation, they are usually confined to the stomach but may involve draining lymph nodes. A remarkable observation has been that up to 70% of gastric MALT lymphomas regress and are cured following effective antibiotic therapy to eradicate *H pylori*, with a 5- and 10-year OS of approximately 90% and 80%, respectively (Stathis et al, 2009). The most widely used antibiotic regimen is a combination of amoxicillin, omeprazole, and clarithromycin. Metronidazole is an effective alternative antibiotic in patients with a penicillin allergy. Responses can be slow, taking up to 6 months to 1 year. Repeat assessment of *H pylori* either by histologic examination or a urea breath test is necessary to ensure that the bacteria have been eradicated. Patients failing to remit may have previously unrecognized large-cell transformation or may carry the t(11;18) translocation, which has been associated with resistance to eradication with *H pylori* therapy. These tumors are usually antigen independent and thus fail to respond to *H pylori* eradication. In patients who do not respond to antibiotics, IFRT has been highly effective in localized MALT lymphomas with disease-free survival or PFS rates of >80% at 5 and 10 years (Tomita et al, 2009; Tsai et al, 2007). Similar regimens as those used in follicular lymphoma, including rituximab-based combinations, can be used in patients with advanced-stage disease.

Nongastric MALT lymphomas usually have an indolent course, including most of the 20% to 25% of patients who present with stage IV disease. Treatment approaches depend on both stage and site of primary involvement and may include surgery, radiation therapy, or chemotherapy. Patients with resected stage IE lesions, as in the lung, may be followed expectantly without systemic or other therapy until evidence of progression. Other localized MALT lymphomas are often treated with radiotherapy with excellent results (Isobe et al, 2007).

Nodal MZL

Nodal MZL, previously known as monocytoid B-cell lymphoma, also arises from marginal zone B cells. Whenever nodal MZL is diagnosed, a careful history and physical examination should be pursued for a possible coexisting extranodal MALT lymphoma component, which may be identified in up to one third of cases. It more commonly presents with advanced stage than MALT-type MZL, with peripheral and intra-abdominal lymphadenopathy and bone marrow involvement present in 28% to 45% of cases (Arcaini et al, 2009). Evaluation should include endoscopy or other procedures as clinically indicated. The t(11;18) and t(1;14) karyotypic changes identified in MALT are absent in nodal MZL, and no specific or recurring karyotypic anomaly has been described. IgM monoclonal gammopathy can occur in approximately 10% of cases. HCV infection is reported in up to 25% of patients. Across reported series, the 5-year OS is 60% to 70%; however, the EFS is only 30%, which likely reflects more commonly encountered advanced-stage disease.

In the recent updated WHO classification, a new category was introduced—pediatric nodal MZL, which has distinctive clinical and morphologic characteristics. There is a male predominance (20:1), and patients usually present with localized asymptomatic adenopathy in the head and neck region. Morphologically, the infiltrate is similar to that seen in adults, except that progressively transformed germinal centers are often seen.

Splenic MZL

Splenic MZLs are rare and occur in older individuals approximately 70 years of age. Patients present with splenomegaly in the absence of peripheral node involvement. Splenic MZL may have associated mesenteric or hepatic involvement, and the bone marrow and blood are typically involved. Some cases have been associated with hepatitis C infection, and responses have been reported with clearance of the virus with pegylated interferon and ribavirin (Hermine et al, 2002); similar results have been seen in other indolent B-cell lymphomas with associated HCV infection (Vallisa et al, 2005). Diagnosis is usually based on spleen histology following splenectomy, bone marrow involvement, or the presence of circulating villous lymphocytes. The disease is very indolent, with median survival times exceeding 10 years. Splenectomy is considered the optimal first-line therapy in symptomatic patients or in the case of cytopenias not felt to be related to bone marrow infiltration.

Lymphoplasmacytic lymphoma and Waldenström macroglobulinemia

Lymphoplasmacytic lymphoma (LPL) is defined in the WHO classification as an indolent neoplasm of small B lymphocytes, plasmacytoid lymphocytes, and plasma cells. The lymphoma cells may express B-cell markers CD19 and CD20 and are CD5 and CD10 negative, much like the MZLs (Table 18-2). They may also express CD25 and CD38, but it is not a consistent finding. Waldenström macroglobulinemia (WM) is found in a significant subset of patients with lymphoplasmacytic lymphoma and is defined as lymphoplasmacytic lymphoma with bone marrow involvement and an IgM monoclonal gammopathy. The disease affects predominantly older patients; however, a familial predisposition can occur in up to 20% of patients who present at a younger age. Symptoms may be due to tumor infiltration (marrow, spleen, liver, and lymph nodes), circulating IgM macroglobulin (hyperviscosity, cryoglobulinemia, or cold agglutinin hemolytic anemia), and tissue deposition of IgM or other proteins (neuropathy, glomerular disease, and/or amyloid) can occur. Coagulopathies result from IgM binding to clotting factors, platelets, and fibrin.

When serum viscosity is significantly elevated due to the IgM paraprotein, patients may experience visual disturbances, headaches, dizziness, decreased level of consciousness, cardiopulmonary symptoms, or a bleeding diathesis, which constitute the hyperviscosity syndrome. Symptomatic patients with hyperviscosity should be treated promptly with plasmapheresis to lower the circulating monoclonal protein, followed by prompt institution of chemotherapy to control the malignant proliferation and further paraprotein production.

The treatment approach to lymphoplasmacytic lymphoma is more like that of indolent lymphoma or CLL than for a plasma cell dyscrasia. Patients without symptoms are best managed by close monitoring without treatment. Prognostic factors at the time of initial treatment associated with decreased survival include age >65 and anemia. The use of these 2 factors can identify those patients at high (2 factors), intermediate (1 factor), and low risk (0 factors). The median survival times in a study of 122 patients for the high-, intermediate-, and low-risk groups were 46, 107, and 172 months, respectively.

Recently, treatment guidelines have been put forth from the International Workshop on Waldenström macroglobulinemia (Dimopoulos et al, 2009). Given disease rarity, there are no randomized controlled studies to support one first-line regimen over another. Either alkylator-based chemotherapy or nucleoside analogs represent reasonable first-line options. Vincristine is often omitted due to underlying neuropathy. Response rates of 75% have been observed using the nucleoside analogs fludarabine and cladribine in newly diagnosed patients compared with approximately 50% using alkylator-based regimens; however, these regimens have not been compared with alkylators in a randomized clinical trial. Several studies have demonstrated that the anti-CD20 monoclonal antibody rituximab has significant activity both as initial therapy and in relapsed patients. Rituximab has been combined with other agents including cyclophosphamide and dexamethasone (ORR, 83%), CHOP (PR, 91%), and fludarabine/cyclophosphamide (PR, 79% in primarily relapsed disease). Abrupt increases in IgM can occur following rituximab therapy, particularly if the pretreatment IgM level is >5000 mg/dL with worsening symptoms of hyperviscosity (Treon et al, 2004). Recent reports suggest that there may be an increased incidence of transformation and development of myelodysplastic syndrome (MDS)/acute myeloid leukemia (AML) in WM patients treated with nucleoside containing therapy (Treon et al, 2009). More recently, thalidomide and lenalidomide have been tested in WM and are highly active agents. The proteasome inhibitor bortezomib is also active in WM with an ORR of 78% to 85%; however, peripheral neuropathy can be problematic. The combination of bortezomib, dexamethasone, and rituximab was evaluated in untreated patients with WM with an ORR of 96%. Autologous or allogeneic transplantation are considered in patients with aggressive high-risk disease.

Hairy cell leukemia

The typical presentation of hairy cell leukemia is that of a middle-aged man (median age, 50-55 years) with pancytopenia, splenomegaly, cytopenic complications (eg, infections, bleeding), and an inaspirable bone marrow (dry tap). The male-to-female ratio is 3:1 to 5:1. Hairy cell leukemia may be misdiagnosed as myelofibrosis, aplastic anemia, or MDS. Hairy cell leukemia is rare, and making the proper diagnosis is crucial because of its generally favorable prognosis, with a 10-year OS exceeding 90%, and the excellent treatment responses to nucleoside analogs. Long-term survivors have been reported to have an increased risk of second cancers, with a cumulative incidence of 30% by 25 years after the diagnosis.

The disease is diagnosed by its typical peripheral blood morphology with cytoplasmic "hairy" projections on the cell surface, a positive tartrate-resistant acid phosphatase stain, and an immunophenotype positive for surface immunoglobulin, CD19, CD20, CD22, CD11c, CD25, and CD103 (Table 18-2). Marrow biopsy demonstrates a mononuclear cell infiltrate with a "fried egg" appearance of a halo around the nuclei and increased reticulin and collagen fibrosis.

Hairy cell leukemia has a unique sensitivity to purine analogs. The nucleoside analogs cladribine or pentostatin are the treatments of choice in hairy cell leukemia in view of the high response rates and durable remissions achieved. Cladribine may be superior because of the short duration of therapy required (the majority of patients remit after a single course of cladribine) and a more favorable toxicity profile. In one large series of 233 patients with long-term follow-up, the response rate with either of these agents was 80%, and median recurrence-free survival was 16 years (Else et al, 2009). Hairy cell leukemia has high-density CD20 expression and thus has been responsive to anti-CD20 monoclonal antibody therapy with rituximab. Rituximab has been used as a single agent in relapsed patients with an ORR of 80% and has also been explored in combination with purine analogs. Splenectomy and interferon alfa were the treatments of choice in years past but have been largely supplanted by these newer approaches.

Transformation to aggressive lymphoma in indolent lymphomas

Transformation is the development of aggressive NHL in patients with underlying indolent lymphomas. It most commonly occurs in follicular lymphoma but can occur in any of the indolent lymphomas. The British Columbia Cancer Agency recently reported on the incidence and outcome of 600 patients with follicular lymphoma who subsequently developed transformed lymphoma (Al-Tourah et al, 2008). Diagnoses were either made clinically (sudden increase in LDH >2× the upper limit of normal, discordant nodal growth, or unusual extranodal sites of involvement) (37%) or pathologically (63%). In this series, the annual risk of transformation was 3% per year, with a 10- and 15-year risk of 30% and 45%, respectively. Overall, the median posttransformation survival time was 1.7 years, with superior outcomes observed in limited-stage patients. Similar results were observed in a series from St. Bartholomew's, where histologic transformation was observed in 28% of patients with follicular lymphoma by 10 years (Montoto et al, 2007).

> **Key points**
>
> - Advanced stage indolent NHL is treatable but not curable with standard chemotherapy.
> - Follicular NHL is the most common indolent NHL.
> - IFRT for stage I and II indolent lymphoma will lead to long-term remission and potentially cure in a subset of patients.
> - Patients with asymptomatic, advanced-stage indolent NHL may be followed without specific therapy to assess the pace of disease; a variety of chemotherapeutic and targeted monoclonal antibody therapies may be used for symptomatic or progressive disease.
> - Newer approaches, including monoclonal antibody plus cytotoxic chemotherapy combinations and stem cell transplantation, hold promise for improved survival in selected patients.

Aggressive B-cell lymphomas

The most prevalent of the aggressive lymphomas is DLBCL. Other histologies in this category include MCL, Burkitt lymphoma, lymphoblastic lymphoma, and most of the T- and NK-cell lymphomas (Table 18-4). These neoplasms are characterized by a more acute presentation and, although often curable (except for MCL), are associated with relatively short survival in the absence of therapy-induced remission. This chapter focuses on the mature B- and T/NK-cell neoplasms. For further discussion on B- and T-cell lymphoblastic lymphoma, please see Chapter 17.

Diffuse large B-cell lymphoma

DLBCL is composed of large B cells with a diffuse growth pattern. There are number of subtypes that fall under the

> **Clinical case**
>
> A 68-year-old woman is diagnosed with stage IIIA DLBCL, with the largest nodal mass measuring 4 cm in the left internal iliac chain. There is no splenomegaly by examination or CT scan, and bone marrow biopsy is negative. Laboratory studies show a normal complete blood cell count and chemistries except for an LDH elevated 1.5× normal. Her ECOG performance status is 1. Immunophenotypic stains of the lymphoma cells reveal them to express CD19, CD20, κ light chains, and BCL2 but to be negative for CD10 and BCL6 expression.

category of DLBCL but have distinct features that distinguish them as a separate disease category. The new WHO classification recognizes several disease categories of DLBCL including molecular subtypes (GBC and ABC; see later sections), distinct subtypes including T-cell–rich B-cell lymphoma or primary CNS lymphoma, and disease entities including PMBCL. Other than primary CNS lymphoma, treatment approaches are similar for the DLBCL subtypes.

DLBCL constitutes 25% to 30% of all NHLs and can present with nodal or extranodal disease. Bone marrow involvement occurs in approximately 11% to 27% of cases, but a proportion of these cases are discordant with the presence of a low-grade B-cell lymphoma in the bone marrow. In addition to the B-cell markers CD20 and CD19, the neoplastic cells may also express CD10 (30%-60%), BCL6 (60%-90%), and IRF4/MUM1 (35%-65%). Rare cases may express CD5 (10%) and must be distinguished from the blastoid variant of MCL, which is cyclin D1 positive. Subsets of DLBCL with markedly differing biology and prognoses have been identified using microarray technology, which is capable of analyzing genome-wide expression of thousands of genes. These analyses have identified 2 molecularly distinct subtypes of DLBCL that are recognized as molecular subtypes of DLBCL-NOS: GCB, which has a gene expression profile similar to germinal center B cells; and ABC, which has a profile similar to activated peripheral B cells. Initially a "type 3" subtype was identified in an expanded series; however, now it is not felt to represent a distinct subgroup but includes cases that cannot be classified into the GCB and ABC subtypes (Rosenwald et al, 2002). Recurrent chromosomal aberrations have been found to be associated with these subtypes. Gains of 3p, 18q21-22, and losses of 6q21-22 are seen in the ABC subtype, and gains in 12q12 are observed frequently in the GCB subtype. The latter also can also be found to be associated with t(14;18). Importantly, the GCB subtype has an improved survival versus the non-GCB types, and this information may prove useful in developing risk-adapted treatment strategies. The prognostic value of the subtype appears independent of but complementary to the IPI score (see below). However, this molecular technique is currently impractical and not yet widely available for routine clinical use. Hans et al (2004) have recently reported the ability to distinguish GCB versus non-GCB using a small set of immunophenotypic markers: CD10, BCL6, and IRF4/MUM1. Using the cDNA microarray as the gold standard, the sensitivity of the tissue microarray was 71% for the GCB group and 88% for the non-GCB group. However, the results have been inconsistent as to whether this immunophenotypic distinction can be applied to rituximab-treated patients. Currently, cell-of-origin information, whether by molecular profiling or immunohistochemistry, is not used to direct treatment decisions outside of clinical trials.

Treatment of advanced-stage DLBCL

The backbone of treatment of all subtypes of DLBCL is anthracycline-based treatment with CHOP chemotherapy. With this approach, approximately 40% of patients are cured. Dose-intensive second- and third-generation regimens were explored in the 1990s, and although more complex regimens (eg, low-dose methotrexate with leucovorin rescue, bleomycin, doxorubicin, cyclophosphamide, vincristine, and dexamethasone [m-BACOD]; prednisone, doxorubicin, cyclophosphamide, and etoposide, followed by cytarabine, bleomycin, vincristine, and methotrexate with leucovorin rescue [ProMACE-CytaBOM]; and methotrexate with leucovorin rescue, doxorubicin, cyclophosphamide, vincristine, prednisone, and bleomycin [MACOP-B]) showed promise for improved CR rates and survival in phase II studies, a large cooperative group study revealed that CHOP therapy was equivalent but less toxic than the other regimens, and thus, it remains the standard of care (Fisher et al, 1993). Furthermore, no higher risk subset of patients could be identified who benefited from a regimen other than CHOP. Consequently, the use of these earlier regimens has been largely abandoned, and 6 to 8 cycles of CHOP has become generally accepted as standard therapy.

Rituximab has several mechanisms of action, including the ability to sensitize otherwise resistant lymphoma cells to chemotherapy agents in vitro, perhaps in part via downregulation of the Bcl-2 protein. In 2002, Coiffier et al (2002) from the GELA group presented preliminary results at the ASH annual meeting plenary session of a phase III clinical trial in which 399 patients 60 to 80 years of age with previously untreated advanced-stage CD20$^+$ DLBCL were randomized to receive 8 cycles of standard CHOP chemotherapy or R-CHOP given on day 1 of each 3-week cycle. An improvement in all end points including CR rate, EFS, and OS favoring R-CHOP over CHOP was demonstrated. With longer follow-up, the results held, and R-CHOP quickly became the standard of care for advanced-stage DLBCL around the world (Coiffier et al, 2002). In a follow-up analysis of outcome based on Bcl-2 protein expression, the benefit of R-CHOP appeared largely restricted to the Bcl-2–positive subset. A similar study carried out by the US ECOG intergroup study comparing 6 to 8 cycles of CHOP versus R-CHOP in aggressive lymphoma was presented at the ASH 2003 annual meeting plenary session. This study enrolled 632 previously untreated patients >60 years of age, and complete responders underwent a second randomization to no maintenance therapy versus rituximab maintenance therapy every 6 months for 2 years (Habermann et al, 2006). Results from this trial, unlike the Groupe d'Etude des Lymphomes de l'Adulte (GELA) study, showed no difference in response rates or OS for the CHOP versus R-CHOP arms, although there was a benefit in time to treatment failure for the R-CHOP arm at 2.7 years of median follow-up. The analysis was confounded to some extent by the secondary randomization to maintenance versus no-maintenance rituximab. Maintenance therapy was beneficial for the time to treatment failure only in the CHOP-induction subset. As such, interpretation of these results supports the use of R-CHOP induction without subsequent maintenance rituximab therapy.

Two other randomized controlled studies have been published supporting the benefit of the addition of rituximab to anthracycline-based chemotherapy in DLBCL. The MabThera International Study Group (MINT) study included young (≤60 years) low-risk (IPI 0 or 1) patients with DLBCL who received either the investigators' choice of anthracycline-based regimen versus the same regimen with rituximab. Most of the patients on this trial received standard CHOP (48%) or CHOP with etoposide (44%). The rituximab-containing regimens demonstrated an improvement in EFS and OS. Of interest, in a prior study by the German High-Grade NHL Study Group (DSHNHL), CHOP plus etoposide appeared to show an improvement in EFS in young patients with DLBCL compared with CHOP in a prior study (Pfreundschuh et al, 2004); however, with the addition of rituximab, this benefit disappears, and as a result, rituximab has been referred to as the great equalizer (Pfreundschuh et al, 2006). The Rituximab With CHOP Over Age 60 Years (RICOVER) trial by the same group evaluated a CHOP-14 regimen (biweekly) with or without rituximab in elderly patients (>60 years) and also demonstrated an improvement in all end points with the rituximab combination (Pfreundschuh et al, 2008). Of note, the latter study had a second randomization comparing 6 cycles to 8 cycles of chemotherapy and demonstrated that although patients receiving 6 or 8 cycles of R-CHOP-14 had an improvement in EFS and PFS, only patients who had received 6 cycles had an improvement in OS, suggesting that this may be the optimal number of cycles.

The interval reduction from 3 weeks (CHOP-21) to 2 weeks (CHOP-14) has been shown to improve the outcome of DLBCL in elderly patients without increasing toxicity (Pfreundschuh et al, 2004). In the largest randomized trial of DLBCL performed to date, the projected survival of elderly patients with DLBCL after 6 cycles of R-CHOP-14 was 74% at 2.5 years, which compares favorably with 64% in the GELA study. Trials are currently ongoing to determine whether reducing the cycle length of R-CHOP to 2 weeks results in improved outcomes compared with the standard 21-day cycle. A population-based retrospective analysis has also been reported from the British Columbia Cancer Agency (BCCA) comparing the outcomes of CHOP versus R-CHOP in patients with DLBCL (Sehn et al, 2005). Based on the results from the GELA study, R-CHOP was adopted as the standard of care in British Columbia in newly diagnosed patients >16 years of age with DLBCL in March 2001. The outcomes for patients treated in the 18-month period prior to (n = 142) and after (n = 152) the routine addition of rituximab to CHOP demonstrated highly statistically significant differences in favor of R-CHOP for 2-year PFS (52% vs 71%; $P = .002$) and OS (53% vs 77%; $P < .001$). Importantly, both younger and older patients benefited from the addition of rituximab. As described earlier, the IPI was initially developed in approximately 4000 patients with large-cell lymphoma with diagnoses based on the Working Formulation. Thus, the majority of cases would be considered DLBCL by today's diagnostic criteria. A study of similar magnitude has not yet been performed in the post–rituximab treatment era. However, limited studies suggest that the IPI is still prognostic of survival in DLBCL patients who have been treated with rituximab-containing regimens. The BCCA evaluated the IPI in R-CHOP–treated patients and demonstrated that 3 groups could be defined: very good risk (0 risk factors; 5-year PFS of 90%), good risk (2 risk factors; 5-year PFS of 70%), and poor risk (≥3 risk factors; 5-year PFS of 50%) (Sehn et al, 2007). The patient described earlier in the clinical case has an IPI score of 3 (age, stage, and LDH), placing her in a high-intermediate–risk group with an expected 5-year probability of survival of approximately 40% after therapy with CHOP or an equivalent regimen. However, with R-CHOP, the expectation is that the projected 5-year OS is approximately 55%.

It has been proposed that patients in IPI poor-risk groups might benefit from a more aggressive treatment approach, such as high-dose chemotherapy and ASCT or allogeneic stem cell transplantation. A recent European randomized trial in aggressive NHL patients tested 8 cycles of CHOP versus 2 cycles of cyclophosphamide, epirubicin, vindesine, and prednisone followed by high-dose chemotherapy and ASCT and found higher 5-year EFS for patients in the transplantation arm. There was an OS benefit for transplantation in the high-intermediate IPI risk subgroup. Whether these results would hold using R-CHOP as the standard chemotherapy arm versus HDT and stem cell transplantation is under study in a US intergroup trial of IPI high-intermediate- and high-risk patients (age-adjusted IPI score of 2 or 3) with aggressive NHL.

Patients with bone marrow involvement by large-cell lymphoma and patients with sinonasal, paraspinal, or testicular involvement are at increased risk for CNS dissemination or relapse. However, there has been no definitive study that proves that there is a benefit of CNS prophylaxis for such patients. The exception may be patients with sinus involvement, in whom intrathecal prophylaxis appears to have reduced the frequency of CNS disease. Despite this, intrathecal prophylaxis is often administered given the potential devastating consequence of secondary CNS disease, which is rarely curable. It appears that rituximab is reducing but not eliminating the risk of CNS relapse in DLBCL patients; thus, this complication still remains problematic in the post–rituximab treatment era (Boehme et al, 2007; Villa et al, 2009).

Treatment of localized DLBCL

Localized or limited-stage DLBCL usually includes patients with stage I and nonbulky (<10 cm) stage II disease. Some groups or studies will also include patients with bulky stage I disease and exclude patients with B-symptoms. A large randomized trial established that 3 cycles of CHOP followed by IFRT is superior to 8 cycles of CHOP alone for the treatment of localized intermediate- and high-grade NHL (Miller et al, 1998). In this SWOG study, the 5-year OS for CHOP followed by radiotherapy was superior to that of CHOP alone (82% vs 72%), but a recent update with longer follow-up showed that the treatment advantage for the combined-modality therapy was not sustained due to an excess of late relapses in the combined-modality arm, which was offset by increased toxicity in the chemotherapy alone arm. A stage-adjusted IPI has been proposed for limited-staged disease that includes nonbulky stage II disease, advanced age (>60 years), poor performance status (>1), and elevated LDH as poor-risk factors. The 5-year OS rates reported in the updated follow-up for patients with 0, 1 or 2, and 3 risk factors were 94%, 71%, and 50%, respectively (Miller et al, 2003).

The recently published GELA study did not reveal any added benefit of consolidative radiotherapy after 4 cycles or CHOP chemotherapy for elderly patients with low-risk localized aggressive lymphoma (Bonnet et al, 2007). The benefit of rituximab has not been specifically analyzed in a randomized controlled trial in localized DLBCL. The MINT study did include some patients with localized disease by nature of the inclusion criteria, but a large proportion also received radiotherapy to sites of bulky disease (>5 cm). The SWOG recently published a phase II study evaluating 3 cycles of R-CHOP followed by IFRT (40-46 Gy if CR and 50-55 Gy if PR) in patients with localized (stage I, IE, nonbulky [<10 cm] II or IIE) aggressive B-cell lymphoma, the majority of whom had DLBCL with at least 1 risk factor by the stage-modified IPI (Persky et al, 2008). The study population was similar to the prior SWOG study described earlier, and thus, a study to compare outcomes could be performed to determine the impact of the addition of rituximab to the combined-modality therapy. The 2-year PFS was superior in the R-CHOP patients (95% vs 83%). Although there has not been a randomized controlled trial, 3 cycles of R-CHOP followed by IFRT is considered the standard therapy for localized DLBCL.

Assessment of therapeutic response in DLBCL

Assessment of response to therapy has varied among clinical studies and practitioners. A CT scan is usually performed after 4 cycles to assess response; patients will receive 2 additional cycles if in a CR, and patients with residual abnormalities after 4 cycles will often receive a total of 6 to 8 treatments, although the RICOVER study would suggest that 6 cycles is optimal. One of the difficulties in assessing response is the inability to determine, even with repeat biopsy in some cases, whether residual lesions on CT scans represent fibrosis or lymphoma. PET scanning has been shown to be more sensitive than CT scan or gallium scan for both initial staging and assessment of response. As outlined earlier, several studies have suggested that the achievement of early PET negativity, after only 2 to 4 cycles of chemotherapy, strongly correlates with durable remission, whereas patients who remain PET positive have high rates of relapse or progression. Although PET scans are not mandatory in staging and assessment of response, given more widespread use in addition to use in clinical trials, the revised response criteria now include PET scan in the assessment of response to treatment (Cheson et al, 2007). If a PET scan is negative, a patient is considered to be in CR, even if a residual mass is present. In the past, such patients were considered as having either unconfirmed CR or PR depending on the degree of tumor shrinkage. PET scans are strongly recommended in DLBCL patients before treatment but not absolutely required given limited availability. A pretreatment PET scan facilitates interpretation of the mid- or posttreatment response assessment. However, it is unknown whether patients with DLBCL who have a positive PET scan mid-treatment benefit from a change of therapy, and this question is currently being tested in clinical trials. Given the possibility of false-positive PET scans, a biopsy should be performed if a change of therapy or high-dose chemotherapy or stem cell transplantation are under consideration.

Relapsed and refractory DLBCL

Patients with DLBCL that has relapsed after initial response should receive a second-line chemotherapy regimen such as ESHAP, ICE, DHAP, GDP, or EPOCH (see Table 18-9 for regimens) followed by HDT with autologous stem cell rescue if chemotherapy-sensitive disease is demonstrated. There are no randomized controlled trials confirming the efficacy of the addition of rituximab to any of these regimens, but it is often added given the strong data in the primary setting. Further phase II studies support that higher response rates are observed using rituximab in combination with chemotherapy. The use of HDT and ASCT in relapsed DLBCL is based on the PARMA study in which patients with relapsed aggressive lymphoma–the majority of whom had DLBCL–received 2 cycles of DHAP salvage chemotherapy; if a PR or a CR was attained, they were randomized to receive either further chemotherapy with DHAP or HDT (with carmustine, etoposide, cytarabine, and cyclophosphamide) and ASCT. The latter resulted in an improvement in the 5-year EFS (46% vs 12%; $P = .038$; Philip et al, 1995). The optimal second-line therapy combination is unknown. The ongoing Collaborative Trial in Relapsed Aggressive Lymphoma (CORAL) study is designed to compare rituximab plus DHAP with rituximab plus ICE as well as to study the role of maintenance rituximab in relapsed and refractory DLBCL (Gisselbrecht et al, 2007). An early report from this study at the ASH 2007 meeting suggests that patients who relapse following prior treatment with rituximab may have lower response rates and an inferior outcome compared with rituximab-naive patients.

Patients with primary refractory lymphoma and those with chemotherapy-resistant disease have a very poor prognosis and should be considered for investigational regimens. The roles of allogeneic transplantation, ^{131}I-tositumomab or ^{90}Y-ibritumomab tiuxetan radiolabeled monoclonal antibodies, and novel biologic agents are currently under study in these settings.

Primary mediastinal (thymic) large B-cell lymphoma

PMBCL is a specific subtype of DLBCL that was distinguished based on unique clinicopathologic characteristics. Patients are typically females with a median age of 35 years who present with a bulky anterior mediastinal disease that can be locally invasive into the lung and chest wall occasionally with symptoms of superior vena cava syndrome. Distant spread, including bone marrow involvement, is uncommon at diagnosis. Clinically, there are many similarities in presentation to CHL, in particular the nodular sclerosis subtype including predominant mediastinal disease. At relapse, involvement of unusual extranodal sites can occur in PMBCL, including the kidneys, adrenals, ovaries, liver, spleen, and CNS.

Histologically, sclerosis is typically present, and phenotypically, the cells may lack surface immunoglobulin expression but express B-cell markers such as CD19 and CD20. CD30 is present in >30% of cases; however, it is usually weak and heterogeneous. Interestingly, recent gene expression analysis has shown that PMBCL is molecularly distinct from typical DLBCL and shares many components of the molecular signature with Hodgkin Reed-Sternberg cell lines (Savage et al, 2003; Rosenwald et al, 2003). There is also evidence of NF-κB activation in PMBCL, similar to findings in CHL (Feuerhake et al, 2005).

Treatment of PMBCL is similar to DLBCL, with R-CHOP chemotherapy considered to be the standard therapy, and some centers in Europe use MACOP-B in addition to rituximab, but a direct comparison in a randomized trial has not been performed. IFRT is often administered to the mediastinum followed by chemotherapy, but it is unknown whether this reduces relapse rate in a patient otherwise in CR. The outcome of patients with PMBCL is excellent even in the pre–rituximab treatment era (5-year OS, 70%; Savage et al, 2006), and retrospective studies suggest that a similar magnitude of benefit of rituximab that is seen in DLBCL is also achieved in PMBCL. The role of PET scanning to identify patients with residual disease at the bulky site (as opposed to fibrosis only) and who thus may be at increased risk for relapse and candidates for other therapeutic intervention, including radiotherapy, is currently under study.

Burkitt lymphoma

Burkitt lymphoma is among the most aggressive of all human malignancies, with a rapid doubling time, acute onset, and progression of symptoms. Originally described in its endemic form in African children presenting with jaw or facial masses, it also occurs in sporadic form in the Western world, predominantly in children and young adults. It is also seen in HIV-infected patients. Most endemic and some sporadic cases show evidence of EBV infection and presence of the EBV genome.

Clinically, most patients with Burkitt lymphoma present with a bulky abdominal mass, B-symptoms, and frequent extranodal and bone marrow involvement (up to 70%; Perkins et al, 2008). CNS dissemination, usually in the form of leptomeningeal involvement, may be present at diagnosis in up to 40% of patients; as a result, high-dose methotrexate and intrathecal chemoprophylaxis are integrated into the therapy for all Burkitt lymphoma patients.

Histologically, Burkitt lymphoma has a diffuse growth pattern of medium-sized cells and a high mitotic rate, as depicted by nearly 100% of cells showing positivity for Ki-67 due to deregulated high-level expression of c-MYC arising from reciprocal translocation with immunoglobulin heavy (t8;14) or light chain gene loci (t8;2 or t8;22). There is also a high rate of cell death or apoptosis, and the dead cells are phagocytosed by histiocytes, which gives a "starry sky" appearance at low power. The B cells are positive for CD19, CD20, and CD10. BCL2 is usually negative, but in the updated WHO classification, weakly positive cases (~20%) can be included. Lack of TdT is critical to rule out acute lymphoblastic leukemia/lymphoma. Recent gene expression profiling studies show that Burkitt lymphoma has a distinct molecular signature distinguishing it from DLBCL (Hummel et al, 2006; Dave et al, 2006).

Therapy for Burkitt lymphoma must be instituted quickly due to the rapid clinical progression of the disease. Admission to hospital and tumor lysis precautions are essential and include vigorous alkalinization, hydration, allopurinol, and close monitoring of laboratory studies including electrolytes and renal function. Early dialysis is indicated at the first signs of decreasing renal function, hyperkalemia, and/or hyperphosphatemia. Recently, recombinant uric acid oxidase (rasburicase) has been shown to be very effective in preventing uric acid nephropathy and its secondary metabolic complications. CHOP chemotherapy is inadequate for the treatment of Burkitt lymphoma. Multiagent combination chemotherapy that includes high doses of alkylating agents and CNS prophylaxis have improved the outcome for adults and children with the disease. The most commonly used approaches today include intensive short-duration chemotherapy, acute lymphoblastic leukemia–type chemotherapy, and intensive chemotherapy followed by high-dose chemotherapy and ASCT. Given disease rarity, there are no randomized controlled treatment trials in adults comparing these approaches. Magrath et al (1996) at the National Cancer Institute demonstrated a risk-adapted strategy that is useful for treatment stratification in both adults and children. Low-risk patients were those with a single extra-abdominal mass or completely resected abdominal disease and a normal LDH, and all other patients were considered high risk. Low-risk patients received 3 cycles of cyclophosphamide, vincristine, doxorubicin, and methotrexate (CODOX-M) only, and high-risk patients received CODOX-M alternating with ifosfamide, etoposide, and cytarabine (IVAC) for a total of 4 cycles (ie, 2 cycles each of CODOX-M and IVAC). All patients received intrathecal chemoprophylaxis with each cycle, and those with CNS disease at presentation received additional intrathecal therapy during the first 2 cycles. Approximately half of the patients were adults, and the 2-year EFS for all patients was 92%. Of note, some of the patients in this study had what has been previously referred to as *Burkitt-like lymphoma*, and the median age of adult patients was still only 24 years. Two other phase II studies have used the Magrath regimen with minor modifications. In a United Kingdom study, adult (age range, 16-60 years; median, 26.5 years), non-HIV patients were treated with dose-modified CODOX-M (3 g/m2) for 3 cycles if determined to be low risk (ie, normal LDH, performance status of 0 or 1, Ann Arbor stage I or II, and no tumor mass >10 cm), and all other patients were considered high risk and treated with alternating dose-modified CODOX-M/IVAC. The 2-year PFS for the patients with Burkitt lymphoma was 64%. At the Dana-Farber Cancer Institute, an older population (median age, 47 years) of patients was studied (n = 14), and the reported 2-year EFS was 71% with a modified Magrath regimen (Lacasce et al, 2004). Other therapeutic approaches have included the hyperfractionated cyclophosphamide, vincristine, doxorubicin, and dexamethasone (HyperCVAD)/methotrexate-cytarabine regimen and acute lymphoblastic leukemia–type regimens. Of note, in the modern treatment era, there is no role for radiotherapy in the treatment of Burkitt lymphoma, even for localized disease. The role of consolidative ASCT in Burkitt lymphoma is unknown.

Given the limited data in older patients, the results from 12 large treatment series (10 prospective and 2 retrospective) were combined to better determine outcome in patients with Burkitt lymphoma in patients >40 years of age (Friedberg et al, 2005). In total, 470 patients were identified, 183 of whom were >40 years. The median OS at 2 years with intensive short-duration chemotherapy was inferior compared with patients ≤40 years (39% vs 71%). Patients in the older age group who underwent ASCT appeared to have a more favorable prognosis (median OS at 2 years, 62%), but this was a small group, and selection bias may have been introduced.

Mantle cell lymphoma

In many ways, MCL falls between the indolent and aggressive lymphomas, unfortunately combining the poorer attributes of each, namely the lack of curability with standard therapy typical of the indolent subtypes and a relatively aggressive clinical course with median survival historically of 3 to 4 years. However, in recent years with more dose-intensive regimens including stem cell support, the median survival may be shifting to 5 years or more (Geisler et al, 2007).

The clinical features of MCL include median age of 60, a striking male predominance, advanced stage at presentation frequently with bone marrow and peripheral blood involvement, and splenomegaly. Extranodal involvement is present in the majority of cases, with a peculiar tendency to invade the gastrointestinal (GI) tract, which may present as a distinctive syndrome of multiple lymphomatous polyposis of the large bowel. Even patients without overt colonic polyposis frequently have subclinical GI epithelial invasion by biopsy. Other extranodal sites may include the Waldeyer ring, lungs, kidneys, prostate, or CNS. Hypogammaglobulinemia is not uncommon, and IgM monoclonal gammopathy may occur in approximately 25% of the patients.

Cytologically, the majority of MCLs consist of small lymphocytes with notched nuclei. The architectural pattern of the lymph node is usually diffuse but may show a vaguely nodular or mantle zone growth pattern. A spectrum of morphologic variants has been recognized, including small cell, mimicking SLL/CLL, and marginal zone, which has been associated with a more indolent course. The aggressive variants are blastoid, which has a high mitotic rate, and pleomorphic. The immunophenotype of MCL is that of a B-cell lymphoma, and in addition, they are typically $CD5^+$, FMC^+, and $CD43^+$ but $CD10^-$ (Table 18-2). Some of the salient features that distinguish MCL from SLL or CLL are the expression in MCL of cyclin D1 and FMC-7 and the lack of CD23 expression (Table 18-2). Furthermore, MCL has a more intense or bright surface IgM and/or IgD and CD20 expression than SLL and CLL. Virtually all MCLs carry the t(11;14)(q13;q32) on karyotypic analysis or by fluorescence in situ hybridization technique. This reciprocal translocation juxtaposes the immunoglobulin heavy chain locus and the cyclin D1 (*CCND1*) gene. cDNA microarray analysis has demonstrated that genes associated with cellular proliferation show striking variability among MCL cases, ranging from low to very high expression. Patients in the lowest quartile of expression have median survival times of 6 to 8 years, whereas patients in the highest expression quartile have survivals of <1 year (Rosenwald et al, 2003).

MCL is chemotherapy sensitive, but response duration is typically short with standard chemotherapy such as chlorambucil, CVP or CHOP, or nucleoside analogs. There is no evidence of superiority of anthracycline-based chemotherapy in the treatment of MCL; however, given a higher ORR, CHOP or other more intensive regimens are often used as the backbone of therapy. The benefit of rituximab is less established in MCL compared with DLBCL. The German Low Grade Lymphoma Study Group (GLSG) compared CHOP with R-CHOP in untreated advanced-stage MCL, with a second randomization in responding patients to ASCT or interferon alfa maintenance therapy. R-CHOP had superior ORR (94% vs 75%), CR rate (34% vs 7%), and time to treatment failure; however, the PFS and OS were equivalent in the 2 arms. In the relapsed setting, rituximab plus FCM (R-FCM) was compared with FCM in patients with follicular lymphoma and MCL, with a second randomization to observation versus rituximab maintenance. In the first randomization, the trial was stopped because R-FCM was shown to be superior to FCM at reducing the risk of relapse, and all subsequent patients received R-FCM. Response duration was prolonged in MCL patients receiving maintenance rituximab ($P = .049$); however, the median duration of response was similar, and the estimated 3-year OS was not statistically significant (77% vs 57%; $P = .11$) (Forstpointner et al, 2006). Rituximab has also been evaluated at a single institution with HyperCVAD alternating with rituximab plus high-dose methotrexate and cytarabine with reported high ORR and encouraging PFS at 2 years of 60% (Romaguera et al, 2005); however, these results have not been replicated in a subsequent multicenter trial.

Given the poor results with standard chemotherapy, autologous transplantation has been explored in the hope of prolonging response duration and possible cure. A matched-pair analysis comparing standard chemotherapy with up-front ASCT plus rituximab in vivo purging showed a superior PFS at 3 years (89% vs 29%; $P < .00001$) and a trend toward improved OS in patients receiving the high-dose approach (Mangel et al, 2004). The Nordic group evaluated intensive induction immunochemotherapy with alternating cycles of "maxi" R-CHOP and rituximab plus cytarabine followed by in vivo purge (with rituximab) and ASCT in a phase II trial. The ORR was 96%, and the 6-year EFS and OS were 56% and 70%, respectively, with no relapses observed after 5 years; however, follow-up is still short, and it is too early to determine whether this represents a curative approach (Geisler et al, 2007).

Allogeneic stem cell transplantation still remains the only known curative therapeutic option in MCL but is not applicable to the majority of MCL patients, who are generally of older age. Other investigational approaches include nonmyeloablative stem cell transplantation, reported by Khouri et al (2003) to have a high and durable response rate with acceptable toxicity in 18 patients, most with chemotherapy-sensitive disease.

Bendamustine in combination with rituximab has been tested in relapsed MCL and is highly active, with an ORR of approximately 90% and a median duration of response of 19 to 24 months. As described earlier, first-line therapy with bendamustine plus rituximab is being compared with R-CHOP in indolent lymphomas and MCL and appears to be equivalent. Bortezomib has moderate activity in MCL, with an ORR of 45% in MCL patients, but the time to progression is only 6 months. Thalidomide in combination with rituximab had a high ORR (81%) in a small phase II trial, and lenalidomide is also highly active in relapsed MCL. Cyclin D1–inhibitory agents such as flavopiridol and temsirolimus are under evaluation in MCL.

Radioimmunotherapy has been evaluated in MCL, with an ORR of 30% to 40%, but remission duration is disappointingly short. Overall, young patients should be treated aggressively with R-CHOP or similar induction followed by

ASCT or with up-front dose-intensification rituximab plus HyperCVAD. Older patients can be treated with a variety of regimens depending on additional comorbidities including R-CHOP, R-CVP, or fludarabine-containing regimens.

Peripheral T-cell lymphomas

Peripheral T-cell lymphomas (PTCLs) represent 12% of all NHLs in Western populations and are a heterogenous group of mature T-cell neoplasms arising from postthymic T cells at various stages of differentiation. NK-cell lymphomas are included in this group because of the close relationship between these 2 cell types. The importance of the T-cell phenotype and impact on prognosis is now well established but is a relatively recent advance. Progress in elucidating the pathobiology and appropriate therapy of these neoplasms has been slow, primarily due to their rarity but also because until the early 1990s, they were generally grouped together and combined with B-cell lymphomas. It is now understood that the majority of PTCLs are highly aggressive, respond poorly to standard chemotherapy, and thus have a significantly poorer prognosis than their B-cell counterparts. A recent large retrospective study, the International Peripheral T-Cell Lymphoma Project (ITLP), collected 1153 cases of PTCLs from 22 centers from around the world and highlighted the geographic, clinicopathologic, and prognostic differences of this diverse group of diseases (Vose et al, 2008). The most common subtypes encountered in North America are PTCL–not otherwise specified (PTCL-NOS), AITL, and ALCL.

Given disease rarity, there are no randomized controlled trials establishing that an alternate regimen is superior to CHOP, and thus CHOP remains the standard therapy of PTCLs. However, there is a range of disease in this category (Table 18-4), and a minority have a more favorable prognosis or a more indolent course.

Indolent PTCLs
Mycosis fungoides and Sézary syndrome

Mycosis fungoides (MF) is an epidermotropic, primary cutaneous T-cell lymphoma and represents the most common of all primary cutaneous lymphomas (50%). Most cases occur in adults, and there is a male predominance. The disease is limited to the skin in its early phases and appears as plaques or patches, but with time, it evolves to diffuse erythroderma or cutaneous nodules or tumors, usually with associated adenopathy. Extracutaneous disease can occur in advanced stages and may indicate histologic transformation. MF has an indolent clinical course with slow progression from patches to plaques and tumors over years and remains incurable. The overall 5-year disease-specific survival is approximately 90% (Willemze et al, 2005). The histology varies with stage of the disease, but typical epidermotropism is seen with typical plaques and intradermal collections of so-called Pautrier microabscesses. Immunophenotypic analysis reveals T-cell markers, typically with a $CD4^+/CD8^-$ (T-helper) phenotype. Progression to nodal disease, organ infiltration, and circulating clonal T cells (Sézary syndrome) represents the advanced stage of disease. Often early-stage disease is misdiagnosed as psoriasis or another chronic skin condition, at times for several years, prior to biopsy and recognition of its true nature. A unique clinical staging system has been proposed by the International Society for Cutaneous Lymphomas (ISCL) and the Cutaneous Lymphoma Task Force of the European Organization of Research and Treatment of Cancer (EORTC) for MF and Sézary syndrome (Olsen et al, 2007). The extent of cutaneous and extracutaneous disease is the most important prognostic factor in MF, with a 10-year disease-specific survival ranging from 97% to 98% for patients with limited patch/plaque disease (<10% of skin surface; stage I) to 20% for patients for patients with lymph node involvement.

Sézary syndrome is a distinct disorder characterized by erythroderma, generalized lymphadenopathy, and the presence of Sézary cells in the skin, lymph nodes, and peripheral blood. One of the following is also required: Sézary cell count >1000/μL; CD4/CD8 ratio of >10 resulting from an expanded CD4 population; or loss of ≥1 T-cell antigen (CD2, CD3, CD4, or CD5) (Swerdlow et al, 2008). Sézary syndrome is much rarer than MF, and patients often have intense pruritus, alopecia, and hyperkeratosis on the palmar and plantar surfaces. It also is associated with a more aggressive course, with a 5-year OS rate of 20% to 30%. The prognosis is more favorable with Sézary cell counts of <1000 Sézary cells/L (7.6 years) versus 10,000 Sézary cells/L (2.4 years).

For MF, control of the cutaneous phase may be accomplished by topical nitrogen mustard, electron-beam radiotherapy, or cutaneous photochemotherapy with oral psoralen plus ultraviolet A (PUVA). Patients with progressive disease and those with systemic dissemination may be palliated with methotrexate and/or corticosteroids, although responses are usually poor and transient. Combination chemotherapy regimens are not particularly effective and provide only transient responses (Prince et al, 2009). Interferon alfa, bexarotene, vorinostat, and denileukin diftitox all have efficacy in advanced-stage MF and Sézary syndrome. Denileukin diftitox is a recombinant fusion protein that combines interleukin 2 (IL-2) with the cytotoxic A chain of diphtheria toxin with an ORR of 49%. It has recently been approved by the US Food and Drug Administration (FDA) for patients with relapsed cutaneous T-cell lymphoma whose tumors express the IL-2 receptor subunit (CD25). The FDA has also recently approved suberoylanilide hydroxamic acid (SAHA; vorinostat) for the treatment of cutaneous T-cell lymphoma, which is an orally available hydroxamic acid with an ORR of 24%. A number of chemotherapy agents have activity in MF and Sézary syndrome. Single-agent treatment is preferred, particularly with slowly progressive disease, due to a high risk of myelosuppression and infection and only modest response durations seen with combination chemotherapy. Gemcitabine, pentostatin, and liposomal doxorubicin have good single-agent activity. Alemtuzumab, the humanized monoclonal antibody targeting CD52, has also been used in MF and Sézary syndrome with some success; however, patients are at high risk of opportunistic infections.

Primary cutaneous ALCL

Primary cutaneous ALCL (C-ALCL) is part of a spectrum of diseases in the category of primary cutaneous $CD30^+$ T-cell lymphoproliferative disorders that also includes the lymphomatoid papulosis and "borderline" cases that have overlapping features of both disorders. C-ALCL must be distinguished from systemic ALCL with secondary cutaneous involvement through staging procedures. Patients with C-ALCL typically present with a solitary nodule and have a favorable outcome, with a 10-year disease-specific survival of 90%. For localized disease, surgery with or without radiation is the preferred therapy, and the impact of chemotherapy is unknown. Progression to systemic involvement can occur in a minority of cases.

Primary cutaneous $CD4^+$ small/medium T-cell lymphoma

This is a new provisional entity in the updated WHO classification and is characterized by the presence of localized plaques or nodular lesions that most commonly occur on the face, neck, or upper trunk. Epidermotropism is uncommon and, if present, is focal. The malignant cells are $CD3^+$, $CD4^+$, and $CD8^-$ and may be accompanied by a loss of pan-T-cell markers. The prognosis is excellent, with a 5-year OS of 80%. Localized lesions are typically treated with surgery with or without radiotherapy.

T-cell large granular lymphocytic leukemia

T-cell large granular lymphocytic leukemia is defined by a persistent (>6 months) increase in the number of peripheral blood large granular lymphocyte cells without an identifiable cause. Concurrent rheumatoid arthritis can also occur. Most cases have an indolent clinical course, with a median survival time of approximately 13 years, but rare cases with an aggressive course have also been described. Of note, T-cell large granular lymphocytic leukemia should be distinguished from NK-cell leukemia, which does have a fulminant aggressive course (see following Aggressive NK-cell leukemia section). In T-cell large granular lymphocytic leukemia, moderate splenomegaly is the most common clinical finding, and lymphadenopathy is rare. Severe neutropenia with or without anemia is common, but thrombocytopenia is rare. Red blood cell aplasia may also occur. The immunophenotype is $CD3^+$ and $CD8^+$, with clonality demonstrated by TCR gene rearrangement studies. CD57 and CD16 are expressed in $>80\%$ of cases. If treatment is required for cytopenias, cyclosporine A, chlorambucil, cyclophosphamide, or corticosteroids can be effective. Splenectomy may also be useful in cases with an accompanying splenomegaly and or cytopenias (Mohan and Maciejewski, 2009). The anti-CD52 monoclonal antibody alemtuzumab has been reported to be effective (Rosenblum et al, 2004).

Aggressive PTCLs
Adult T-cell leukemia/lymphoma

Adult T-cell lymphoma/leukemia is caused by infection with HTLV-1 and occurs in endemic areas of infection (eg, Caribbean basin and southwestern Japan). HTLV-1 alone is not sufficient to result in neoplastic transformation, and the cumulative incidence of adult T-cell lymphoma/leukemia among HTLV-1 carriers is 2.5% in Japan. The virus can be transmitted in breast milk and through exposure to blood products. Pathologically, the malignant cells have a distinct cloverleaf appearance and lack CD7, and the majority are $CD4^+$/$CD8^-$. The following clinical variants have been recognized: acute type with a rapidly progressive clinical course, bone marrow and peripheral blood involvement, hypercalcemia with or without lytic bone lesions, skin rash, generalized lymphadenopathy, hepatosplenomegaly, and pulmonary infiltrates; lymphoma type with prominent adenopathy but lacking peripheral blood involvement but also associated with an aggressive course; chronic type with lymphocytosis and occasionally associated with lymphadenopathy, hepatosplenomegaly, and cutaneous lesions but having an indolent course; and smoldering type with $<5\%$ circulating neoplastic cells, skin involvement, and prolonged survival.

Survival time in the acute and lymphomatous variants ranges from 2 weeks to >1 year. The chronic and smoldering subtypes have a longer survival but can transform into the more acute forms. Underlying immunodeficiency associated with adult T-cell lymphoma/leukemia leads to a high rate of infections throughout the disease course.

Aggressive NK-cell leukemia

This is a rare form of leukemia that is almost always associated with EBV infection and an aggressive course, with a median survival of 3 months. It is seen more often in Asians, and the median age of onset is 42 years. Typically, the bone marrow and peripheral blood are involved in addition to the liver and spleen. Patients often have fever and constitutional symptoms and multiorgan failure with coagulopathy and hemophagocytic syndrome. It is unclear whether aggressive NK-cell leukemia represents the leukemic phase of extranodal NK/T-cell lymphoma. There is no known curative therapy, and responses to chemotherapy are usually brief. Some encouraging results have been seen with L-asparaginase–based treatment in this disease and extranodal NK/T-cell lymphoma but require further study.

PTCL–not otherwise specified

PTCL-NOS is the most common subgroup of PTCLs, accounting for up to 30% of cases worldwide. This is the default PTCL category for any mature T-cell neoplasm that does not fit into any of the "specified" categories in the WHO classification. Patients typically present with advanced-stage disease, and the 5-year survival is 20% to 30% in most series. Recognizing that the division of PTCLs into leukemic, nodal, and extranodal is somewhat artificial, these categories have been eliminated in the updated WHO classification (Table 18-4). The morphologic spectrum of PTCL-NOS is wide, including the histiocyte-rich lymphoepithelioid or Lennert lymphoma. Typically, the neoplastic cells are T-helper ($CD4^+$/$CD8^-$) phenotype; CD5 and CD7 are frequently downregulated, and approximately 30% are $CD30^+$. CHOP chemotherapy is considered the standard of care in PTCL-NOS, but it is largely ineffective. Consolidative therapy with HDT and ASCT is being explored with conflicting results in phase II studies and is still considered experimental.

Gene expression profiling has been explored in heterogeneous PTCL-NOS to determine whether there are reproducible, molecular subsets and to better define prognostic markers within PTCL-NOS. However, in comparison to B-cell lymphomas, large-scale studies are lacking. A recent study evaluating 35 cases of nodal PTCL-NOS found that high expression of proliferation-associated genes was associated with a worse prognosis (Cuadros et al, 2007). Another study by the same Spanish group found that expression of NF-κB pathway genes was associated with a more favorable prognosis in PTCL-NOS (Martinez-Delgado et al, 2005).

Angioimmunoblastic T-cell lymphoma

AITL is a well-defined, distinct PTCL subtype, with unique pathobiologic features. Similar to PTCL-NOS, patients are typically older and have advanced-stage disease, often with B-symptoms and hepatosplenomegaly. It was originally believed to be a form of immune dysregulation, with polyclonal gammopathy being a common finding. Survival is similar to PTCL-NOS; however, a small proportion may have a more indolent course.

Key morphologic findings of AITL include an expanded $CD21^+$ follicular dendritic cell network and prominent arborizing high endothelial venules. The neoplastic cells in AITL are mature $CD4^+$/$CD8^-$ T cells, expressing most pan-T-cell antigens. In recent years, a number of studies support that the follicular helper T cell is the normal physiologic cell counterpart of AITL. Consistent with this, the tumor cells are CD10, BCL6, and CXCL13 positive. A follicular helper T-cell derivation is also supported by recent gene expression profiling (de Leval et al, 2007). EBV is identified in most cases in the surrounding B cells.

Anaplastic large-cell lymphoma

ALCL was originally described as a lymphoma composed of large anaplastic lymphoid cells, uniformly strongly positive for CD30 and with a predilection for a sinusoidal and cohesive growth pattern (Stein et al, 1985). Since then, there has been significant progress made in further classifying this subgroup of PTCLs. It includes cases that have T-cell or null-cell lineage, the latter implying loss of T-cell antigens but monoclonality demonstrable. B-cell cases are considered a subtype of DLBCL. In the WHO classification, primary systemic ALCL is separated from primary cutaneous ALCL, and more recently, ALK-positive ALCL has been defined a distinct entity in the updated classification (Table 18-4). Cases of ALK-positive ALCL are associated with a characteristic chromosomal translocation, t(2;5)(p23;q35), resulting in a fusion gene, *NPM-ALK*, encoding a chimeric protein. With the availability of antibodies to the ALK protein, ALK expression can be demonstrated in 60% to 85% of all systemic ALCL, with higher frequencies seen in the pediatric and young adult age groups. In contrast, although ALK-negative ALCL lacks any defining features, there is accumulating evidence that it should be separated from other PTCLs; as a result, it is considered a provisional entity in the updated WHO classification.

ALK-positive ALCL

Morphologically, ALK-positive ALCL has a spectrum of appearances, and all subtypes have a variable proportion of the pathognomonic "hallmark cells" recognized by their eccentric, horseshoe, or kidney-shaped nuclei. In addition to strong expression of CD30, ALK-positive ALCL is usually positive for epithelial membrane antigen (EMA) and cytotoxic markers (TIA1, granzyme B, and perforin). Several studies have now firmly established that patients with ALK-positive ALCL have a much more favorable prognosis with anthracycline-based chemotherapy than patients who have ALK-negative ALCL and other PTCLs, as well as DLBCL, at least in the pre–rituximab treatment era (Gascoyne et al, 1999). The improved outcome may in part be related to the young age at presentation. As indicated earlier, ALK-positive ALCL has a characteristic genetic rearrangement forming a fusion gene that encodes for the 80-kd NPM-ALK chimeric protein, which possesses significant oncogenic potential resulting from constitutive activation of the tyrosine kinase ALK.

ALK-negative ALCL

In the fourth edition of the WHO classification, ALK-negative ALCL is considered a provisional entity, distinct from both ALK-positive ALCL and PTCL-NOS. Patients with ALK-negative ALCL tend to be older at presentation; otherwise, the clinical presentation is similar to ALK-positive cases, although sites of extranodal disease may vary. ALK-negative ALCL has been difficult to define, in part due to a lack of uniformly applied diagnostic criteria across studies. Moreover, a specific oncogenic abnormality comparable to the *ALK* gene rearrangement has not been identified. Like ALK-positive ALCL, ALK-negative ALCL is composed of large lymphoid cells that are strongly positive for CD30 with abundant cytoplasm. It is not reproducibly distinguished from ALK-positive ALCL other than lacking the ALK protein. The prognosis of ALK-negative ALCL is poor, but there is some recent evidence that it may be more favorable than PTCL-NOS (Savage et al, 2008).

Extranodal NK/T-cell lymphoma, nasal-type

Extranodal NK/T-cell lymphomas, nasal-type, display great variation in racial and geographic distribution, with the majority of cases occurring in the East Asia. The designation NK/T is used to reflect the fact that, although most are NK-cell derived [$CD2^+$, $CD56^+$, $CD3\varepsilon(cytoplasmic)^+$, EBV^+], rare cases with identical clinical and cytologic features exhibit an EBV^+/$CD56^-$ cytotoxic T-cell phenotype. The qualifier *nasal-type* is used because although most cases present in the nasal region and associated structures, identical tumors can also occur at extranasal sites, such as the skin, soft tissue, GI tract, and testis. From the International T-Cell Lymphoma Project and other studies, it appears that cases that occur in extranasal regions may have a more aggressive course (Au et al, 2009). Accumulating evidence supports that radiotherapy is the most important treatment modality for localized disease. Alternate chemotherapy combinations in extranodal NK/T-cell lymphomas, nasal-type, including asparaginase and methotrexate, have shown encouraging results but await further study (Jaccard et al, 2009).

Rare PTCL subtypes
Subcutaneous panniculitis-like T-cell lymphoma

Subcutaneous panniculitis-like T-cell lymphoma (SCPTCL) is an extremely uncommon PTCL subtype that preferentially infiltrates the subcutaneous tissue. Recently, it has been determined that tumors with γ-δ phenotype have a far inferior prognosis to those with α-β phenotype (5-year OS, 11% for γ-δ vs 82% for α-β). The more common α-β SCPTCL typically has a $CD4^-$, $CD8^+$, and $CD5^-$ phenotype and is rarely associated with hemophagocytic syndrome, which is associated with a worse prognosis. The updated WHO specifies that SCPTCL should be restricted to cases with the α-β phenotype. The γ-δ subtype has been combined in the new WHO classification with a new, rare PTCL entity, termed *primary cutaneous γ-δ T-cell lymphoma* (see later section) due to similar aggressive behavior (Table 18-4). Durable responses have been observed with both CHOP and immunosuppressive agents.

Hepatosplenic T-cell lymphoma

Hepatosplenic T-cell lymphoma is a recently recognized and uncommon PTCL subtype. The majority of patients are young men (median age, 34 years) presenting with hepatosplenomegaly and bone marrow involvement. Up to 20% of hepatosplenic T-cell lymphomas occur in the setting of immunosuppression, most commonly following solid organ transplantation (WHO). It has also been observed in patients treated with azathioprine and infliximab for Crohn disease. The splenic red pulp is diffusely involved, and the liver will show a sinusoidal pattern. Most tumor cells are $CD3^+$, $CD4^-$, and $CD8^-$, and most are associated with isochrome 7q. The majority of cases are of the γ-δ TCR type; however, rare cases that are of the α-β TCR type have been reported. The prognosis is extremely poor with rare long-term survivors. The optimal therapy is unknown; however, some long-term survivors have been reported with high-dose chemotherapy and ASCT or allogeneic stem cell transplantation.

Enteropathy-associated T-cell lymphoma

Enteropathy-associated T-cell lymphoma is a rare, aggressive intestinal tumor with a male predominance and occurs in the setting of celiac disease. It most commonly involves the jejunum or ileum. Patients often present with abdominal pain, and intestinal perforation can occur. The prognosis is extremely poor due to chemotherapy resistance and difficult treatment delivery related to abdominal complications that can arise in the setting of malabsorption. In some cases, there is a childhood history of celiac disease, but more commonly, the disease occurs in adulthood. Alternatively, there is a prodrome of refractory disease, or a concomitant diagnosis of celiac disease is found at the time the lymphoma is discovered. In the updated WHO classification, a sporadic, monomorphic variant, type II enteropathy-associated T-cell lymphoma, is more clearly defined that occurs in 10% to 20% of cases and has a broader geographic distribution that includes Asia. An association with celiac disease has not been definitively proven in this subtype; thus, this may represent a distinct disease entity. In the common subtype, the neoplastic cells are $CD3^+$, $CD7^+$, $CD4^-$, $CD8^{-/+}$, and $CD56^-$ and contain cytotoxic proteins.

Primary cutaneous PTCL, rare aggressive subtypes
Primary cutaneous γ-δ T-cell lymphoma

In the updated WHO classification, primary cutaneous γ-δ T-cell lymphoma is now considered a distinct entity, which also includes cases previously known as SCPTCL with a γ-δ phenotype, as described earlier. Clinically, the extremities are commonly affected, and the presentation can be variable, with patch/plaque disease or subcutaneous and deep dermal tumors that may exhibit necrosis and ulceration. The clonal T cells have an activated γ-δ cytotoxic phenotype, with most cases being negative for both CD4 and CD8 and positive for TCR-δ. Prognosis is poor in this disease, particularly with subcutaneous fat involvement, with a fulminant clinical course and primary resistance to combination chemotherapy.

Primary cutaneous aggressive epidermotropic CD8$^+$ T-cell lymphoma

This provisional entity typically presents with generalized cutaneous lesions appearing as eruptive papules, nodules, and tumors with central ulceration and necrosis. Histologically, there is marked epidermotropism, and invasion into the dermis and adnexal structures is common. The tumor cells are CD3$^+$, CD4$^-$, CD8$^+$, and cytotoxic marker positive, and the clinical course is aggressive.

Immunodeficiency-associated lymphoproliferative disorders

Congenital or acquired immunodeficiency states are associated with an increased incidence of lymphoproliferative disorders. The WHO classification identifies 4 such categories: (i) primary immunodeficiency disorders including Wiskott-Aldrich syndrome, ataxia-telangiectasia, common variable or severe combined immunodeficiency, X-linked lymphoproliferative disorder, Nijmegen breakage syndrome, hyper-IgM syndrome, and autoimmune lymphoproliferative syndrome; (ii) HIV infection; (iii) post solid organ or marrow transplantation with iatrogenic immunosuppression; and (iv) methotrexate- or other iatrogenic-related immunosuppression for autoimmune disease. The lymphomas seen in these settings are heterogeneous and may include HL or, more commonly, aggressive NHL. Chédiak-Higashi syndrome has also been associated with an increased incidence of pseudolymphoma and true NHL.

Lymphoproliferative disorders associated with primary immune deficiencies (PIDs) are most commonly seen in pediatric patients and are frequently associated with EBV infection. Extranodal disease including the CNS is common. Lymphomas occurring in patients with PID do not differ morphologically compared with immunocompetent hosts. DLBCL is the most frequent histologic type, although T-cell lymphomas are more common in ataxia-telangiectasia. EBV-related lymphomatoid granulomatosis is associated with Wiskott-Aldrich syndrome. These malignancies respond poorly to standard therapy. Therapy depends on both the underlying disorder and the specific lymphoma subtype; allogeneic transplantation has been used successfully in some patients. Novel immunotherapeutic or pharmacologic strategies targeting EBV are being explored (Heslop, 2005).

HIV-associated lymphomas are typically monoclonal B-cell aggressive subtypes, usually DLBCL or Burkitt lymphoma. Approximately two thirds of cases are EBV associated, and many carry *c-MYC* oncogene translocations. CNS involvement is frequent. The entity of primary effusion lymphoma (body cavity lymphoma) usually presents in HIV-positive patients as ascites or a pleural effusion but may involve soft tissue or visceral masses. It is pathogenetically associated with HHV-8 (KSHV) and generally carries a poor prognosis. HL also occurs in the HIV setting but with much lower incidence and is usually the mixed cellularity of lymphocyte-depleted subtypes. Therapy for HIV-associated lymphomas has used both full-dose and dose-modified combination chemotherapy regimens, usually with cytokine support with granulocyte colony-stimulating factor (G-CSF) or GM-CSF and erythropoietin, and can lead to durable remissions. Appropriate HIV management such as highly active antiretroviral therapy (HAART) is essential and should be given concurrently with chemotherapy and in communication with the HIV specialist to avoid antiretrovirals that can exacerbate chemotherapy toxicity. Several registries have reported a significant decline in the incidence of HIV-associated lymphoma since the introduction of HAART. The role of rituximab with anthracycline combinations in HIV-associated DLBCL is unknown, with one small randomized study showing no improvement in outcome relating to an increase in treatment-related infectious deaths. The toxicity was higher in patients with a CD4 count <50 (Kaplan et al, 2005). This is in contrast to a phase II French study of R-CHOP in aggressive lymphomas that demonstrated a 2-year OS of 75% without an increase in life-threatening infections, which likely reflects the exclusion of poor-prognosis patients with a CD4 cell count of <100 or a performance status >2 (Boue et al, 2006). Thus, R-CHOP can be considered in HIV patients if the CD4 count is >50; however, it should be given in conjunction with G-CSF given the high rate of infection in this population.

Posttransplantation lymphoproliferative disorders (PTLDs) occur as a consequence of immunosuppression in recipients of solid organ, bone marrow, or stem cell allograft. PTLDs are comprised of a spectrum of disorders ranging from EBV-positive infectious mononucleosis (early lesions) to polymorphic PTLD to full blown monomorphic PTLD that can be either EBV positive (common) or EBV negative and are indistinguishable from B-cell lymphomas (common) and T-cell lymphomas (rare) that occur in immunocompetent hosts. HL-type PTLDs can also occur; however, indolent B-cell lymphomas arising in transplantation recipients are not among the PTLDs. Aggressive lymphomas occur in approximately 2% to 5% of patients after solid organ or marrow and stem cell transplantation. The risk of lymphoma is directly correlated with the degree of immunosuppression. These PTLDs may arise within the first 6 months of transplantation or have a later onset beyond 1 to 2 years; the former is more commonly associated with EBV. More than 90% of PTCLs in solid organ recipients are of host origin; however, in contrast, most PTLDs in bone marrow allograft recipients are of donor origin. Although a minority of patients will respond to a reduction in intensity of immunosuppression, particularly in polymorphic PTCL, most require additional systemic therapy. The prognosis for such patients has been poor due to both inadequate response and poor tolerance of chemotherapy. Single-agent rituximab in PTLD has demonstrated an ORR of approximately 40% to 75% and is extremely well tolerated (Svoboda et al, 2006); however, remission duration may be short in many patients. In one large phase II prospective study of 60 patients treated with single-agent rituximab, the median PFS was only 6 months; however, the 1- and 2-year OS rates were 72.5% and 51.8%, respectively, suggesting that these patients could be salvaged with either chemotherapy or re-treatment with rituximab (Choquet et al, 2006). Another approach is the infusion of graded doses of EBV-specific cytotoxic lymphocytes. Durable CR rates of up to 80% have been reported with this therapy.

Primary CNS lymphoma

Primary CNS lymphoma (PCNSL) is distinguished in the updated WHO classification as DLBCL subtype. Most intraparenchymal lymphomas show a diffuse growth pattern typically in the perivascular space. In addition to B-cell markers, CD10 expression is observed in 10% to 20%, and BCL6 expression is common (60% to 80%). PCNSLs are rare and may occur in immunocompetent patients or in association with immunosuppression related to HIV infection or organ or marrow transplantation. With the introduction of HAART, the incidence of PCNSL has decreased in HIV-infected persons. Of note, most cases of PCNSL are DLBCLs, but rare cases of PTCL, low-grade lymphoma, and Burkitt lymphoma have also been reported (Batchelor and Loeffler, 2006). PCNSL may be multifocal in 20% to 49% of cases, with or without meningeal involvement (5%). A contrast-enhanced MRI should be performed, along with lumbar puncture with cerebrospinal fluid analysis. A slit-lamp examination is important in the staging evaluation to rule out concurrent ocular involvement, which can occur in up to 20% of patients at the time of diagnosis. Patients typically present with neurologic symptoms, and systemic symptoms are uncommon. A prognostic scoring system has been developed in PCNSL given the limitations of the Ann Arbor staging system and the IPI in this disease. The following factors are associated with a poor prognosis: age >60; performance status >1; elevated LDH; high cerebrospinal fluid protein concentration; and tumor location within the deep regions of the brain. Patients with 0, 1 to 4, or 5 of these factors had 2-year OS rates of 80%, 48%, or 15%, respectively (Ferreri et al, 2003).

Surgery in PCNSL is typically used to obtain a diagnostic biopsy, and full surgical resection confers no survival benefit over biopsy alone. The median survival after surgery alone is approximately 1 to 4 months. Whole-brain radiation is associated with a high response rate of 90%, but the median survival is only 12 months. Although there have been no randomized controlled studies to establish the best therapy, in retrospective analyses, outcomes are superior when high-dose methotrexate (2-8 g/m^2) is incorporated into first-line regimens. With this approach, the median survival is approximately 55 to 60 months, and 5-year survival is approximately 30%, suggesting that cure is possible in a proportion of patients. Rituximab has poor penetration across the blood–brain barrier but is currently being tested in clinical trials given synergy with chemotherapy. In younger patients, the combination of whole-brain radiation and methotrexate is often used, but it has not been directly compared with methotrexate alone. Furthermore, in patients >60, the risk of neurotoxicity is high and manifests as dementia, ataxia, and incontinence, with a median time to onset of approximately 1 year. HDT and ASCT have been used in the salvage setting with a median survival from the time of relapse of 24 months. Temozolomide either alone or in combination with rituximab has shown an ORR of 26% and 53%, respectively, in relapsed and refractory patients.

NHLs in children

NHLs comprise 8% of cancers in children. There are striking variations of incidence by sex (male-to-female ratio of 2-3:1) and race (white-to-black ratio of 2:1, rare in Asian populations). There is an increased incidence in patients with congenital (ataxia-telangiectasia, Wiskott-Aldrich syndrome, and others) or acquired (posttransplantation) immunodeficiency states. Prior EBV infection has been implicated in the pathogenesis of endemic (African) Burkitt lymphoma but is less common in sporadic American and European cases.

The histologic subtypes of childhood NHL are significantly different from those in adults. Burkitt lymphomas (mature B-cell) account for one third of cases, lymphoblastic lymphomas (primarily T cell) account for 30%, and large-cell lymphomas of multiple lineages account for 25% to 30%.

Follicular lymphomas are rare in children. However, chromosomal translocations and molecular features are similar to those in adults with the same lymphoma subtype.

Childhood NHLs are staged using the Murphy staging system. Therapy depends on the stage. Ninety percent of patients with stage I or II Burkitt or large-cell lymphoma can be cured with 9 weeks of CHOP-like chemotherapy. Using the same regimen, only 70% of patients with stage I or II lymphoblastic lymphoma are cured; adding a 1- to 2-year continuation phase of treatment with methotrexate, mercaptopurine, vincristine, and prednisone may decrease the relapse rate, although this has not been definitively established. CNS prophylaxis may be limited to patients with lower stage NHL who have head and neck primary sites.

Stage III and IV (initial involvement of the CNS and/or bone marrow) lymphomas require more intensive chemotherapy. Burkitt and large B-cell lymphomas can be cured in 80% to 85% of cases with 3 to 8 months of chemotherapy that includes cyclophosphamide, doxorubicin, dexamethasone, vincristine, high-dose methotrexate, and high-dose cytarabine. A similar protocol that also includes ifosfamide and etoposide has cured almost 80% of children with advanced-stage ALCLs. Lymphoblastic lymphomas are cured in a similar fraction of cases with 2 to 3 years of treatment with protocols similar to those for higher risk acute lymphocytic leukemia in children (see Chapter 17). CNS chemoprophylaxis with intrathecal medications is an important component of treatment of all subtypes in children with advanced-stage NHLs. Some protocols still use low-dose (12-18 Gy) cranial irradiation as part of CNS prophylaxis for patients with advanced lymphoblastic lymphomas.

Key points

- DLBCL is the most common subtype of aggressive NHL in Western populations; T- and NK-cell subtypes are more common in Asian populations.
- The IPI score and the cell of origin phenotype provide useful prognostic information in DLBCL.
- R-CHOP chemotherapy results in cure in >50% of patients with DLBCL. The IPI and cell of origin phenotype remain prognostic in the rituximab treatment era.
- Relapsed aggressive lymphoma patients who have chemotherapy-sensitive disease to a second-line regimen (at least a PR) should be referred for HDT with ASCT.
- PTCLs have an inferior outcome to DLBCL. The exception is ALK-positive ALCL, which has a high cure rate with CHOP chemotherapy.
- Most children with NHL have aggressive subtypes; however, high cure rates are seen with multidrug chemotherapy regimens.
- Patients with congenital or acquired immunodeficiency have an increased risk of lymphoma and often respond poorly to therapy.

Hodgkin lymphoma

HL is a relatively uncommon malignant lymphoma, with an average incidence of approximately 8000 cases per year in the United States; HL accounts for approximately 30% of all lymphomas. HL is most commonly diagnosed in younger patients, with an average age at diagnosis of 30 years. Patients with HL often present with an asymptomatic mass, typically in the cervical region, but constitutional symptoms including fever, night sweats, and weight loss can also occur. With high cure rates, a reduction in the long-term treatment-related morbidity and mortality is now a major goal of newer therapeutic approaches.

Pathology

The classic histologic finding associated with HL is the Hodgkin Reed-Sternberg (HRS) cell, a large cell that may be bi- or multinucleate and that contains large acidophilic nucleoli. The origin of these cells has long been debated but now has been demonstrated to be of B-cell origin in most cases. The use of micromanipulation and PCR analysis of single cells reveals that these cells usually comprise a monoclonal population of B cells, likely derived from germinal centers. Because the origin of the HRS cell is now firmly established to be a lymphoid cell, the term *Hodgkin lymphoma* is preferred over Hodgkin disease.

It is now known that HL is composed of 2 disease types due to differences in pathology and also clinical behavior (Table 18-3): CHL and nodular lymphocyte-predominant Hodgkin lymphoma (NLPHL). CHL has 4 subtypes: nodular sclerosis, mixed cellularity, lymphocyte-rich, and lymphocyte-depleted, which all differ in their sites of presentation, clinical features, and histologic appearance.

Classical Hodgkin lymphoma

CHL accounts for 95% of all HLs, with the majority of patients presenting at age 15 to 35 years. A recent population-based study has demonstrated an increased risk of HL in patients with a diagnosis of infectious mononucleosis in the previous 2 years, suggesting an association of the disease with recent primary EBV infection. EBV is postulated to play a role in the development of CHL, but it is only found in a proportion of cases, predominantly in the mixed cellularity and lymphocyte-depleted subtypes. EBV-positive CHL is also more commonly encountered in the setting of HIV infection, and the incidence has not declined in the era of HAART. EBV-infected HRS cells express the EBV protein LMP-1, which is postulated to have transforming and anti-apoptotic properties. CHL is characterized by a variable number of HRS cells admixed with a rich inflammatory background, the composite of which varies according to the CHL subtype. The classic HRS cells are large with at least 2 nuclear lobes of nuclei giving the appearance of "owl's eyes." The HRS cells represent a minority of the cellular infiltrate ranging in frequency from 1% to 10%. The classic phenotype of the HRS cell is $CD15^+$, $CD30^+$, and $CD45^-$.

Nodular sclerosis CHL

Nodular sclerosis CHL accounts for 70% of CHL in Western populations. There is an equal prevalence in males and females, and the average age of presentation is 15 to 35 years. Typically patients present with mediastinal adenopathy, often with bulky disease, and B-symptoms are common (40%). The second most common site of involvement is the cervical region. Splenic and/or lung involvement is seen in approximately 10%, and bone marrow involvement is rare (3%). Morphologically, a nodular growth pattern is seen, with nodules separated by characteristic fibrotic bands. LMP-1 EBV protein is found in approximately 10% to 40% of cases.

Mixed cellularity CHL

Mixed cellularity CHL accounts for 20% to 25% of CHL and is more frequently encountered in patients with HIV infection and in developing countries. The median age of presentation is 38 years, and 70% of patients are male. B-symptoms are more common than in nodular sclerosis CHL. Peripheral adenopathy is common, but mediastinal involvement is rare. Bone marrow disease is found in 10% of patients, and splenic involvement occurs in 30%. Scattered HRS cells are seen in a diffuse or occasionally vaguely nodular mixed inflammatory background without the bands of fibrosis encountered in nodular sclerosis CHL. The prognosis of patients with mixed cellularity CHL was less favorable compared with nodular sclerosis CHL when radiotherapy was used as a single modality. However, with combination chemotherapy, outcomes approximate those seen in nodular sclerosis CHL.

Lymphocyte-rich CHL

Lymphocyte-rich CHL comprises 5% of all CHLs, and patients most frequently present with peripheral adenopathy and stage I or II disease. Mediastinal involvement and B-symptoms are rare. Morphologically, lymphocyte-rich CHL can be difficult to distinguish from NLPHL most commonly occurring with a nodular growth pattern (see later section on NLPHL), but they can be distinguished by immunophenotyping. The atypical cells of lymphocyte-rich CHL have the same immunophenotype as the HRS cells of other subtypes of CHL. The prognosis is excellent in part because of predominantly early-stage disease.

Lymphocyte-depleted CHL

Lymphocyte-depleted CHL is a rare subtype of CHL comprising <1% of cases in Western populations. Most patients are male, the median age of onset is 30 to 37 years, and like mixed cellularity CHL, it is more commonly encountered in HIV patients and in developing countries. There is a predilection for intra-abdominal lymphadenopathy and extranodal involvement, including the bone marrow. Lymphocyte-depleted CHL is more likely to occur as advanced-stage disease with B-symptoms. The morphology is variable; however, there is a predominance of HRS cells compared with the background lymphocytes. Coexpression of CD30 and Pax5 can be helpful in differentiating lymphocyte-depleted CHL from ALK-ALCL. With combination chemotherapy, the prognosis is similar to other stage-matched CHL subtypes.

Nodular lymphocyte-predominant HL

NLPHL is differentiated from CHL based on distinct pathologic and clinical features. The neoplastic cells in NLPHL are known as lymphocyte-predominant cells or the so-called "popcorn cells" based on their characteristic appearance. They differ immunophenotypically by expression of B-cell markers such as CD20, CD79a, BCL6, and CD45 but lack CD15 and CD30. Morphologically, a nodular pattern is typically seen predominantly composed of nonneoplastic cells including small lymphocytes intermixed with lymphocyte-predominant cells. At the molecular level, clonally rearranged immunoglobulin genes are found. Differentiating NLPHL from T-cell–rich B-cell lymphoma (TCRBCL) can be challenging; however, the presence of small B cells and $CD4^+$/$CD57^+$ T cells favors NLPHL, whereas the absence of small B cells and the presence of $CD8^+$ cells and $TIA1^+$ cells favors primary TCRBCL. As outlined earlier, immunophenotyping can differentiate NLPHL from the morphologically similar lymphocyte-rich CHL.

Clinically, patients are typically male, ranging in age from 30 to 50 years and presenting with localized peripheral adenopathy with stage I or II disease. Mediastinal and splenic involvement is rare. Late relapses are more common in NLPHL compared with CHL. There is also an increased risk of secondary NHL, most commonly DLBCL, including TCRBCL, compared with patients with CHL. A recent study evaluated the frequency of transformation to aggressive lymphoma in a cohort of patients with NLPHL with mature follow-up and found that the 10-, 15-, 20-, and 25-year risks were 7%, 15%, 31%, and 36%, respectively, with no apparent plateau (Al-Mansour et al, 2010). Because this development can occur decades after the primary diagnosis, patients need to have ongoing surveillance, and biopsy is imperative at the time of disease recurrence. It has been speculated that given the B-cell

Table 18-10 Prognostic factors for advanced-stage Hodgkin lymphoma.

Male sex
Stage IV disease
Age >45
Serum albumin <4 g/dL
Hemoglobin <10.5 g/dL
White blood cell count >15,000/μL
Lymphocyte count <600/μL or <8% of total white blood cell count

From Hasenclever D, Diehl V. A prognostic score for advanced Hodgkin disease. *N Engl J Med*. 1998;339:1506–1514.

Table 18-11 Rates of freedom from progression and overall survival at 5 years according to grouped prognostic scores.

Prognostic score	Frequency (%)	5-year freedom from progression (%)	5-year overall survival (%)
0–3	81	70	83
≥4	19	47	59

From Hasenclever D, Diehl V. A prognostic score for advanced Hodgkin disease. *N Engl J Med*. 1998;339:1506–1514.

phenotype and observation of late relapses that NLPHL maybe more related to indolent B-cell lymphoma. However, recent gene expression profiling studies demonstrated a high degree of similarity to CHL as well as the tumor cells of TCR-BCL; in contrast, the signature had a low degree of relatedness to follicular lymphoma (Brune et al, 2008).

Staging and prognostic factors

The Ann Arbor staging system for HL has been used for >25 years (Table 18-5). The same staging procedures as described earlier for NHL are also performed in HL, including CT scans of the neck, chest, abdomen, and pelvis; bone scans are indicated in the presence of bone pain or other localizing symptom. Bone marrow aspiration and biopsy are indicated in the presence of advanced-stage disease, B-symptoms, or cytopenias, but they have a small yield of positive findings in asymptomatic clinically early-stage patients. PET scanning has excellent sensitivity, and several studies have demonstrated improved sensitivity and specificity over CT alone for detecting residual disease. In the recently revised response criteria, PET is recommended before treatment but not required due to current limitations of cost and availability. PET is recommended after treatment and may be particularly helpful if there is a residual mass on CT imaging (Table 18-8). As indicated earlier, in the revised response criteria, a CR is assigned if the PET scan is negative even if a residual mass is present on CT imaging. Staging laparotomy and splenectomy and bipedal lymphangiograms are no longer required in HL management.

A prognostic scoring system has been developed for advanced-stage HL after analyzing outcome data for >5000 patients who were primarily treated with doxorubicin, bleomycin, vinblastine, and dacarbazine (ABVD) or mechlorethamine, vincristine, procarbazine, and prednisone (MOPP)/ABVD. Regression analysis identified 7 factors, consisting of 3 clinical risk factors and 4 laboratory risk factors, that were predictive of outcome; these factors are shown in Table 18-10 (Hasenclever and Diehl, 1998). Each factor has approximately equal weight in reducing the freedom from progressive disease, so a simple additive score is possible. A score of 0 to 3 results in a 5-year freedom from progression of 70% compared with 47% for a score of ≥4 (Table 18-11).

> **Key points**
> - HL is most common in adolescents and young adults.
> - There are 2 subtypes of HL: CHL and NLPHL.
> - Most HLs are derived from B cells; nodular sclerosis is the most common subtype in Western populations.
> - Accurate staging is the most important factor in determining the therapeutic approach.

Treatment of HL

In North America, patients are typically divided into those with limited- or early-stage disease (stage I or II disease, nonbulky [<10 cm], and no B-symptoms) and advanced-stage disease (stage III or IV disease, bulky stage II, or B-symptoms) for treatment stratification (Table 18-12). Of note, stage I patients rarely present with B-symptoms, but if they do, they are typically treated with limited-stage protocols. In Europe, other staging categories have also been developed. European HL study groups have further stratified early-stage patients into those with favorable versus unfavorable risk factors (large mediastinal mass, elevated erythrocyte sedimentation rate, >3–4 involved nodal groups, age >50 years, and extranodal disease).

Treatment of early-stage HL

The prognosis of patients with early-stage HL is excellent, with a 5-year OS rate of 95% (Meyer et al, 2005). Thus, the current challenge is to maintain high cure rates and minimize long-term toxicities of therapy, particularly given the young

Table 18-12 Staging of patients with Hodgkin lymphoma in North America for treatment stratification.

Early (limited) stage
  Stage I or II, no bulky disease, no B-symptoms

Advanced stage
  Stage III or IV, bulky stage II, or B-symptoms

age of presentation of most patients. Options for these patients include radiation therapy alone, a combination of chemotherapy and radiation therapy, or chemotherapy alone.

Irradiation has been historically used in the treatment of early-stage HL largely because it predated chemotherapy. Radiation therapy alone was used for early-stage disease for patients staged by laparotomy and confirmed to have pathologic stage IA or IIA disease. With a negative laparotomy, extended-field radiation (eg, mantle with or without periaortic fields) induces CRs in >95%. Long-term disease-free survival is achieved in approximately 80% of patients, and because they generally remain chemotherapy sensitive at relapse, >90% are alive >10 years from diagnosis. However, approximately 20% of patients are upstaged at the time of laparotomy and require an extended course of chemotherapy. Because laparotomy is no longer used, there are significant advantages to incorporating chemotherapy into the treatment of early-stage HL. A current approach for early-stage patients is the combination of brief chemotherapy with radiation therapy. The inclusion of chemotherapy plus irradiation eliminates the need for surgical staging with laparotomy because the systemic therapy will eliminate microscopic disease, and reducing the number of cycles may decrease the short- and long-term toxicities of the chemotherapy. From studies in advanced-stage HL (see next section on treatment of advanced-stage HL), ABVD emerged as the obvious choice for patients with early-stage HL, balancing high efficacy with low toxicity. Several studies have demonstrated that brief chemotherapy with ABVD (2–4 cycles) followed by irradiation is very effective for treating early-stage HL. However, there is also great interest in reducing the dose and field of radiation to minimize long-term toxicities such as secondary malignancies and cardiac disease (Aleman, van den Belt-Dusebout, et al, 2003), while maintaining high cure rates. Mature follow-up from a small randomized controlled study from the Milan group that compared ABVD plus subtotal nodal radiotherapy with ABVD plus IFRT demonstrated 12-year freedom from progression and OS rates of 94%, with no difference in outcome between the radiation groups (Bonadonna et al, 2004). More recently, studies of involved nodal radiation, which reduces radiation field size even further, support that margins can be limited to ≤5 cm without compromising relapse rates (Campbell et al, 2008).

The German Hodgkin Study Group has recently evaluated the optimal number of cycles of ABVD with IFRT in patients with early-stage HL. More than 1000 patients were randomized to receive either 2 or 4 cycles of ABVD followed by a second randomization of 30 or 20 Gy of IFRT. At a median follow-up of just over 2 years, there was no difference in the freedom from treatment failure or OS between any of the treatment groups (Engert et al, 2005); however, follow-up remains short.

Recognizing that there are long-term complications of RT, chemotherapy alone has been explored in the treatment of early-stage HL. Many of the early trials, however, lack relevance today because they relied on staging laparotomy, included patients who would be considered advanced stage, and used chemotherapy less effective than ABVD. A recently published randomized study in early-stage HL conducted by the National Cancer Institute of Canada and the ECOG compared ABVD alone versus either extended-field radiation for patients with favorable risk factors or ABVD for 2 cycles followed by extended-field radiation in patients with unfavorable risk factors (age ≥ 40 years, erythrocyte sedimentation rate ≥50 mm/h, mixed cellularity and lymphocyte-depleted histology, and ≥4 disease sites). There was a modest but statistically significant difference in PFS favoring the radiation-containing therapy (93% in ABVD alone vs 87% in RT-containing therapies; $P = .006$); however, OS was similar (96% in ABVD alone vs 94% in RT-containing therapies; $P = .06$), suggesting that the advantage in PFS is offset due to deaths related to other causes. Interestingly, in a subgroup analysis, for patients who achieved a CR by CT imaging after 2 cycles of ABVD, a similar PFS was observed comparing the chemotherapy alone and RT-containing arms. Most centers still consider brief chemotherapy with ABVD and IFRT to be the standard approach in patients with early-stage disease, and trials are planned to study chemotherapy alone integrating a PET-adapted approach in the hope of avoiding radiotherapy in patients who are otherwise cured with chemotherapy alone.

Several studies in children have investigated the use of chemotherapy alone for early-stage HL. Results in limited numbers of patients suggest that CR and EFS rates are similar to those seen with irradiation alone. Further studies with larger numbers of patients are necessary to evaluate the relative efficacy and toxicities of these approaches (see discussion later in this section).

Treatment of advanced-stage HL

Patients with B-symptoms, bulky disease, or stage III or IV disease require an extended course of chemotherapy. Multiagent chemotherapy with MOPP was first developed in the 1960s and achieved high response rates and long-term survival in approximately 50% to 60% of patients (Table 18-13). ABVD was developed by the Milan group in 1973 and has partial non–cross-resistance with MOPP and can cure approximately 20% of patients who are not cured with MOPP. Hybrid and alternating regimens were tested in the 1980s and were shown to be superior to MOPP alone. However, in a large randomized Cancer and Leukemia Group B trial comparing ABVD versus MOPP/ABVD versus MOPP, both ABVD-containing regimens had a superior 5-year

Table 18-13 Chemotherapy regimens for Hodgkin lymphoma.

ABVD
  Doxorubicin
  Bleomycin
  Vinblastine
  Dacarbazine

MOPP
  Mechlorethamine
  Vincristine
  Procarbazine
  Prednisone

MOPP/ABVD
  MOPP and ABVD alternated every 28 days

MOPP/ABV hybrid
  MOPP and ABV alternating within each treatment cycle

Stanford V (12-week regimen)
  Meclorethamine
  Doxorubicin
  Vinblastine
  Vincristine
  Bleomycin
  Etoposide
  Prednisone
  Plus irradiation 36 Gy to initial sites of disease ≥ 5 cm

BEACOPP
  Bleomycin
  Etoposide
  Doxorubicin
  Cyclophosphamide
  Vincristine
  Procarbazine
  Prednisone
  Plus irradiation to initial sites of disease

failure-free survival ($P = .04$); however, ABVD alone emerged as being the optimal choice because it had equivalent efficacy to the alternating regimen but did not cause sterility or premature menopause and was less leukemogenic. For this reason, ABVD is the current standard regimen for advanced HL in adults. Of note, there was no statistically significant difference in OS across the arms, which reflects the high salvage rate with secondary treatment. Treatment is generally given for 6 to 8 cycles. There is no role for additional radiotherapy in patients with stage III or IV disease who achieve a CR using conventional imaging. A recent study by Aleman, Raemaekers, et al (2003) evaluated the role of IFRT for patients with advanced disease in CR after chemotherapy with MOPP/doxorubicin, bleomycin, vinblastine (ABV). No improvement was seen for those receiving radiation versus observation after chemotherapy, and there was a trend toward decreased 5-year survival in the group that received radiation. Patients in PR all received IFRT and had an outcome that was similar to those who achieved a CR. However, given the high frequency of residual disease in this population, a substantial proportion of these patients may have actually been in a CR and would not have required the additional radiotherapy. With the availability of PET scanning, studies are ongoing evaluating whether radiotherapy can be withheld in patients in PR by CT imaging but in CR by PET criteria (ie, PET negative).

Patients with a bulky mediastinal mass (>10 cm or more than one third of the maximum diameter of the chest) may benefit from adjuvant radiation therapy to the residual mass after chemotherapy because of a higher rate of local relapse. Whether PET scanning will be useful in identifying patients with active residual disease versus fibrosis, and thus the need for local irradiation, remains to be determined.

Two newer regimens have also been used in advanced-stage HL. The Stanford V regimen (ie, mechlorethamine, doxorubicin hydrochloride, vinblastine, vincristine, bleomycin, etoposide, and prednisone) involves weekly chemotherapy for 12 weeks, with myelosuppressive agents alternating with nonmyelosuppressive agents. Patients also receive 36 Gy of irradiation to sites of original tumor bulk (defined as ≥5 cm) following completion of chemotherapy. The initial single-arm study of 142 patients reported by Horning et al (2002) included 96 patients with stage III or IV disease and 46 patients with stage I or II disease plus a mediastinal mass greater than one third of the maximum chest diameter. The disease-free survival was 89% with a median follow-up of 5.4 years. One quarter of the patients required hospitalization during therapy due to acute toxicities, usually related to myelosuppression; there were no treatment-related deaths. Late toxicity at 5 to 6 years appeared minimal, although longer follow-up will be required to assess any late effects or second malignancies related to the combined chemotherapy plus irradiation. The results of an ongoing intergroup study comparing the Stanford V regimen with ABVD are awaited to determine its role in first-line therapy. The German Hodgkin Study Group studied a dose-escalated and accelerated regimen—bleomycin, etoposide, doxorubicin, cyclophosphamide, vincristine, procarbazine, and prednisone (BEACOPP)—in >1200 patients with advanced HL (Table 18-13). When compared with cyclophosphamide, vincristine, procarbazine, and prednisone (COPP)/ABVD, BEACOPP and an increased-dose version of BEACOPP (escalated) had improved freedom from treatment failure at 5 years, and escalated BEACOPP had a superior 5-year OS compared with COPP/ABVD ($P = .002$). Of note, a large proportion of patients in this study received radiotherapy to sites of bulky disease (≥5 cm) or residual tumor. This analysis was updated at the ASH meeting in 2007 with a median follow-up of 112 months. At 10 years, the freedom from treatment failure rates were 64%, 70%, and 82% and OS rates were 75%, 80%, and 86% for COPP/ABVD (arm A), BEACOPP baseline (arm B), and BEACOPP escalated (arm C), respectively ($P < .0001$). Benefits were seen across the prognostic subgroups; however, they were most profound in the group with ≥ 4 factors. Escalated BEACOPP was superior to standard BEACOPP, but there was also a higher rate of secondary AML after escalated BEACOPP. Furthermore, there is a high rate of infertility in men and women (Sieniawski et al, 2008; Behringer et al, 2005). Because of the toxicity of therapy with BEACOPP, there is interest in targeting the patient population who would benefit the most (ie, those with high-risk disease). A trial is currently ongoing comparing ABVD with BEACOPP in patients with ≥ 3 Hasenclever prognostic risk factors.

Recent interest has also turned to the use of PET scan to guide the use of more dose-intensive therapy. The prognostic value of a PET scan after 2 cycles of ABVD in patients with advanced-stage HL (stages IIB-IVB) was recently reported whereby therapy was not changed based on the results of the PET. The 2-year PFS for patients with a PET-positive scan after 2 cycles of ABVD was 12.8% compared with 95% for patients with a PET-negative result ($P < .0001$) (Gallamini et al, 2007). The results of the interim PET overshadowed the prognostic value of the IPS, and even patients with a score of 3 to 7 who achieved a PET-negative status had an excellent outcome. Studies are under way in the United Kingdom and the United States evaluating the role of escalation of therapy from ABVD to BEACOPP in patients who have a PET-positive result after 2 cycles of ABVD.

Studies have also evaluated the benefit of HDT with ASCT in first remission for patients with high-risk disease. A recent European intergroup trial randomized 163 patients with unfavorable advanced disease with a CR or PR to 4 cycles of standard induction therapy to receive 4 more cycles of standard therapy versus HDT with autologous stem cell rescue. Although there was a slightly lower risk of relapse in the high-dose arm, there was no difference in OS, indicating that standard-dose chemotherapy is appropriate for high-risk patients.

Treatment of relapsed/refractory disease

The approach to patients with relapsed HL depends on the primary therapy and duration of initial remission. Those treated with irradiation alone for early-stage disease are generally chemotherapy sensitive at relapse, and 50% to 80% achieve long-term disease-free survival with standard chemotherapy. However, the majority of patients who relapse will have received chemotherapy as a component of their primary therapy. Patients who relapse late (>12 months) after a CR may be treated with combination chemotherapy; 50% to 60% remain disease free at 5 years. Patients who relapse within 12 months are much less likely to achieve remission and long-term disease-free survival with chemotherapy alone. Other poor prognostic signs in patients at relapse include advanced stage, relapse in extranodal sites, relapse in previously irradiated sites, and the presence of B-symptoms. Patients who have high-risk factors or relapse <12 months after completion of primary chemotherapy should be considered for HDT and ASCT. Patients who relapse >12 months after completion of chemotherapy or in previously unirradiated sites can potentially be treated with chemotherapy with or without radiotherapy; however, given the excellent results with HDT and ASCT, some groups also consider this approach in this subgroup of patients.

Hematopoietic stem cell transplantation

For patients whose disease is refractory to primary therapy or relapses shortly after an initial response, standard-dose chemotherapy is unlikely to be beneficial. High-dose chemotherapy with autologous stem cell support has been demonstrated to provide long-term disease-free survival to some patients in this circumstance. Additional irradiation to areas of bulky disease may also be helpful. The 5-year PFS is approximately 30% in patients with refractory HL who undergo HDT and ASCT. The most commonly used HDT regimens are carmustine, etoposide, cytarabine, and melphalan (BEAM) or cyclophosphamide, carmustine, and etoposide (CBV). Prior to transplantation, a salvage regimen is often given if the patient is symptomatic or to arrange for the logistics of the transplantation. Unlike in aggressive lymphoma, the purpose of this chemotherapy is not to test chemosensitivity because even disease that does not respond to standard-dose chemotherapy can be cured with HDT/ASCT.

HL in children

HL represents 5% of childhood cancers. The disease is uncommon before age 10. Males are affected more frequently than females, especially in patients younger than 10 years. The incidence of EBV-associated disease varies widely by age, histologic subtype, and racial group (Asian 93%, white 46%, African American 17%). The incidence of histologic subtypes also differs from adults, with lymphocyte predominant in 1% to 15%, mixed cellularity in 30%, and nodular sclerosis in 40% to 70%. Lymphocyte-depleted HL is rare, except in HIV-infected patients.

Treatment of HL in children must take into account 2 important differences from adults: ongoing growth and development and a longer expected life span after cure. Thus, there is increasing concern regarding late complications for treatment in children, including second cancers (AML, breast cancer, and NHL), cardiomyopathy, sterility, and others. To address this problem, several studies have investigated the use of chemotherapy alone for treatment. In one trial for lower stage (IA, IIA, or IIIA) HL, disease-free survival was 87% for 83 patients treated with chemotherapy (MOPP × 3, ABVD × 3) alone and 91% for 85 patients treated with chemotherapy plus irradiation (25.5 Gy IFRT). In a similar trial for patients with higher stage (IIB, IIIA2, IIIB, or IV) disease, EFS was 79% for 81 patients treated with MOPP × 4 plus ABVD × 4 alone and 80% for 80 patients treated with chemotherapy plus irradiation (21 Gy). OS in the latter study was 96% after chemotherapy alone and 87% after combined-modality treatment. In a third trial, 501 patients (all stages) who achieved a CR after 2 or 3 courses of COPP/ABV were randomized to receive irradiation (21 Gy IFRT) or no further therapy. EFS at 3 years favored the irradiated cohort (93% vs 85%), but OS was 98% in both groups. Thus, chemotherapy alone may cure 80% to 90% of children with HL. Patients who relapse will often respond to subsequent treatments including chemotherapy, irradiation, and stem cell transplantation. Current studies are directed at development of less toxic chemotherapy regimens and prediction of chemotherapy failure by assessment of the rapidity of response to initial chemotherapy.

Long-term complications of HL therapy

An important issue in the current management of patients with HL concerns the long-term morbidity of the various approaches. As increased numbers of patients were cured of their diseases in the 1970s and 1980s, long-term follow-up has demonstrated a high rate of late toxicity. In large cohorts of patients followed at Stanford from 1960 to 1995 and at the Dana-Farber Cancer Institute and Massachusetts General Hospital from 1969 to 1997, the risk of death from other causes surpasses that from HL at approximately 15 years. The causes of these late deaths are predominantly second malignancies and cardiovascular events, many of which can be attributed to radiation or chemotherapy. Thus, long-term follow-up of HL patients is an important component of management, as is appropriate patient education regarding health maintenance and comorbid risk factors such as tobacco use.

Second solid tumors are attributed to prior radiation, the majority of which occur within or on the border of the prior radiation field. The malignancies commonly identified are breast, lung, GI, or thyroid carcinomas and sarcomas of soft tissue and bone. There is typically a latent period of at least 5 to 10 years, and the risk of secondary cancers continues for >30 years from initial treatment. The best-studied secondary tumor is breast cancer, which has its highest incidence in adolescent girls treated with radiation as well as women treated before 30 years of age. Breast cancers begin to appear at the end of the first decade following treatment and continue to increase with time, with an estimated incidence of >30% by 40 years of age in these patients. For this reason, mammographic and self-examination surveillance is recommended to start within 10 years of irradiation and to continue indefinitely.

Cardiovascular complications also occur following radiation therapy. These include myocardial infarction from damage to the coronary arteries, pericardial disease, and diffuse myocardial disease. Males and older patients are at highest risk, but all patients are at risk for vascular damage within their radiation ports. Another common adverse effect of radiation therapy is hypothyroidism, which occurs in approximately 50% of patients treated with radiation to the thyroid bed.

The long-term toxicities of chemotherapy depend on the regimen. MOPP is associated with sterility, an increased risk of MDS, and secondary AML. ABVD has not been associated with sterility or MDS/leukemia but does have the risks of pulmonary and cardiac toxicity from bleomycin and doxorubicin, respectively. The risks of high-dose chemotherapy and combined chemotherapy and radiation therapy have become more of a concern as more patients receive this therapy. An increased incidence of MDS/AML has been documented within 5 to 7 years of HDT, which is in addition to the acute toxicity of transplantation. This likely reflects the cumulative marrow toxicity of alkylating agents, etoposide, and radiation therapy. Patients with a history of HL also have an increased incidence of NHL, but the contributions of radiation, chemotherapy, or the immune suppression of HL itself are unclear.

Key points

- ABVD is the standard therapy for advanced-stage HL.
- Limited-stage HL shows high rates of durable remission following 2 to 4 cycles of chemotherapy and IFRT or extended-field radiation therapy.
- Patients with primary refractory disease or those relapsing after initial chemotherapy-induced remission should be evaluated for HDT and autologous stem cell rescue.
- Late radiation-induced complications include solid tumors within the radiation field and cardiovascular disease; the risk persists >20 years after treatment.
- Late chemotherapy-induced complications include cardiac dysfunction, lung disease, development of MDS or AML, and sterility.

Acknowledgment

The authors thank Dr. Bruce M. Camitta for providing the discussion regarding NHL and HL in children.

Bibliography

Overview of lymphocyte development

Jennings CD, Foon KA. Recent advances in flow cytometry. *Blood.* 1997;90:2863–2892. *A thorough review of the technical aspects of flow cytometry and its use in the diagnosis and follow-up of hematologic malignancies.*

Kuppers R, Klein U, Hansmann M-L, Rajewsky K. Cellular origin of human B-cell lymphomas. *N Engl J Med.* 1999;341:1520–1529. *An overview of the biology of lymphocyte development and its relation to lymphomagenesis.*

Staudt LM. Molecular diagnosis of the hematologic cancers. *N Engl J Med.* 2003;348:1777–17785.

Swerdlow SH, Campo E, Harris NL, et al. *WHO Classification of Tumors of Hematopoietic and Lymphoid Tissues.* 4th ed. Lyon, France: IARC Press; 2008. *The current state-of-the-art classification integrating morphologic, phenotypic, and biologic features for all hematologic neoplasms.*

Thorley-Lawson DA, Gross A. Persistence of the Epstein-Barr virus and the origins of associated lymphomas. *N Engl J Med.* 2004;350:1328–1337.

Non-Hodgkin lymphoma

Advani R, Rosenberg SA, Horning SJ. Stage I and II follicular non-Hodgkin lymphoma: long-term follow-up of no initial therapy. *J Clin Oncol.* 2004;22:1454–1459. *Over half of patients with early stage follicular lymphoma who received no initial therapy remained untreated at a median of ≥6 years.*

Alizadeh AA, Eisen MB, Davis RE, et al. Distinct types of diffuse large B-cell lymphoma identified by gene expression profiling. *Nature.* 2000;403:503–511. *A seminal paper demonstrating the utility of molecular profiling based on gene expression patterns within histologically and immunophenotypically defined DLBCL; a germinal center subtype had significantly better outcome and survival than an ABC subtype.*

Al-Mansour MM, Connors JM, Gascoyne RD, Skinnider B, Savage KJ. Transformation to aggressive lymphoma in nodular lymphocyte predominant Hodgkin lymphoma. *J Clin Oncol.* In press.

Al-Tourah AJ, Gill KK, Chhanabhai M, et al. Transformed indolent non-Hodgkin lymphoma, a population-based analysis of incidence and outcome. *J Clin Oncol.* 2008;26:5165–5169.

Arcaini L, Lucioni M, Boveri E, Paulli M. Nodal marginal zone lymphoma: current knowledge and future directions of an heterogeneous disease. *Eur J Haematol.* 2009;83(3):165–174.

Ardeshna KM, Smith P, Norton A, et al. Long-term effect of a watch and wait policy versus immediate systemic treatment for asymptomatic advanced-stage non-Hodgkin lymphoma: a randomised controlled trial. *Lancet.* 2003;362:516–522.

Au WY, Weisenburger DD, Intragumtornchai T, et al. Clinical differences between nasal and extranasal natural killer/T-cell lymphoma: a study of 136 cases from the International Peripheral T-Cell Lymphoma Project. *Blood.* 2009;113:3931–3937.

Batchelor T, Loeffler JS. Primary CNS lymphoma. *J Clin Oncol.* 2006;24:1281–1288.

Boehme V, Zeynalova S, Kloess M, et al. Incidence and risk factors of central nervous system recurrence in aggressive lymphoma: a survey of 1693 patients treated in protocols of the German High-Grade Non-Hodgkin's Lymphoma Study Group (DSHNHL). *Ann Oncol.* 2007;18:149–157.

Bonnet C, Fillet G, Mounier N, et al. CHOP alone compared with CHOP plus radiotherapy for localized aggressive lymphoma in elderly patients: a study by the Groupe d'Etude des Lymphomes de l'Adulte. *J Clin Oncol.* 2007;25:787–792.

Bosga-Bouwer AG, van Imhoff GW, Boonstra R, et al. Follicular lymphoma grade 3B includes 3 cytogenetically defined subgroups with primary t(14;18), 3q27, or other translocations: t(14;18) and 3q27 are mutually exclusive. *Blood.* 2003;101:1149–1154.

Campbell BA, Woods R, Gascoyne RD, et al. Long-term outcomes for patients with limited stage, follicular lymphoma: involved regional radiotherapy versus involved nodal radiotherapy. *Eur J Cancer.* 2009;7(Suppl):560.

Cheson BD, Pfistner B, Juweid ME, et al. Revised response criteria for malignant lymphoma. *J Clin Oncol.* 2007;25:579–586.

Coiffier B, Lepage E, Briere J, et al. CHOP chemotherapy plus rituximab compared with CHOP alone in elderly patients with diffuse large B-cell lymphoma. *N Engl J Med.* 2002;346:235–242. *The report of a prospective randomized trial of CHOP versus R-CHOP in patients 60 to 80 years of age with newly diagnosed large B-cell lymphoma, demonstrating an EFS and OS advantage for the R-CHOP arm at 2 years.*

Cuadros M, Dave SS, Jaffe ES, et al. Identification of a proliferation signature related to survival in nodal peripheral T-cell lymphomas. *J Clin Oncol.* 2007;25:3321–3329.

Dave SS, Fu K, Wright GW, et al. Molecular diagnosis of Burkitt's lymphoma. *N Engl J Med.* 2006;354:2431–2442.

Dave SS, Wright G, Tan B, et al. Prediction of survival in follicular lymphoma based on molecular features of tumor-infiltrating immune cells. *N Engl J Med.* 2004;351:2159–2169.

de Leval L, Rickman DS, Thielen C, et al. The gene expression profile of nodal peripheral T-cell lymphoma demonstrates a molecular link between angioimmunoblastic T-cell lymphoma (AITL) and follicular helper T (TFH) cells. *Blood.* 2007;109:4952–4963.

Dimopoulos MA, Gertz MA, Kastritis E, et al. Update on treatment recommendations from the Fourth International Workshop on Waldenstrom's Macroglobulinemia. *J Clin Oncol.* 2009;27(1):120–126.

Else M, Dearden CE, Matutes E, et al. Long-term follow-up of 233 patients with hairy cell leukaemia, treated initially with pentostatin or cladribine, at a median of 16 years from diagnosis. *Br J Haematol.* 2009;145:733–740.

Elstrom R, Guan L, Baker G, et al. Utility of FDG-PET scanning in lymphoma by WHO classification. *Blood.* 2003;101:3875–3876.

Feuerhake F, Kutok JL, Monti S, et al. NFkappaB activity, function, and target-gene signatures in primary mediastinal large B-cell lymphoma and diffuse large B-cell lymphoma subtypes. *Blood.* 2005;106(4):1392–1399.

Fillet G, Bonnet C, Mounier N, et al. No role for chemoradiotherapy when compared with chemotherapy alone in elderly patients with localized low risk aggressive lymphomas. Final results of the LNH93–4 GELA study [abstract]. *Blood*. 2005;106:15.

Fisher RI, Gaynor ER, Dahlberg S, et al. Comparison of a standard regimen (CHOP) with three intensive chemotherapy regimens for advanced non-Hodgkin's lymphoma. *N Engl J Med*. 1993;328:1002–1006. *The randomized, 4-arm intergroup study demonstrating the equivalency of CHOP chemotherapy with m-BACOD, ProMACE-CytaBOM, and MACOP-B for 3-year survival in advanced-stage aggressive NHL. Subsequent reports with longer follow-up have not demonstrated an advantage for any of the regimens.*

Fisher RI, LeBlanc M, Press OW, Maloney DG, Unger JM, Miller TP. New treatment options have changed the survival of patients with follicular lymphoma. *J Clin Oncol*. 2005;23:8447–8452.

Forstpointner R, Unterhalt M, Dreyling M, et al. Maintenance therapy with rituximab leads to a significant prolongation of response duration after salvage therapy with a combination of rituximab, fludarabine, cyclophosphamide, and mitoxantrone (R-FCM) in patients with recurring and refractory follicular and mantle cell lymphomas: results of a prospective randomized study of the German Low Grade Lymphoma Study Group (GLSG). *Blood*. 2006;108:4003–4008.

Freedman A, Neuberg D, Gribben J, et al. High-dose chemoradiotherapy and anti-B-cell monoclonal antibody-purged autologous bone marrow transplantation in mantle-cell lymphoma: No evidence for long-term remission. *J Clin Oncol*. 1998;16:13–18.

Friedberg JW, Ciminello L, Kelly J, et al. Outcome of patients > age 40 with Burkitt lymphoma (BL) treated with aggressive chemotherapeutic regimens: results from the International Burkitt Lymphoma Collaborative Group [abstract]. *Blood*. 2005;106:928.

Friedberg JW, Cohen P, Chen L, et al. Bendamustine in patients with rituximab-refractory indolent and transformed non-Hodgkin's lymphoma: results from a phase II multicenter, single-agent study. *J Clin Oncol*. 2008;26:204–210.

Gascoyne R, Aoun P, Wu D, et. al. Prognostic significance of anaplastic lymphoma kinase (ALK) protein expression in adults with anaplastic large cell lymphoma. *Blood*. 1999;93:3913.

Geisler CH, Elonen E, Kolstad A, et al. Mantle cell lymphoma can be cured by intensive immunochemotherapy with in-vivo purged stem-cell support; final report of the Nordic Lymphoma Group MCL2 Study [abstract]. *Blood*. 2007;110:LB1.

Ghielmini M, Schmitz S, Burki K, et al. The effect of Rituximab on patients with follicular and mantle-cell lymphoma. Swiss Group for Clinical Cancer Research (SAKK). *Ann Oncol*. 2000;11:123–126.

Ghielmini M, Schmitz SF, Cogliatti SB, et al. Prolonged treatment with rituximab in patients with follicular lymphoma significantly increases event-free survival and response duration compared with the standard weekly × 4 schedule. *Blood*. 2004;103(12):4416–4423.

Ghielmini M, Schmitz S, Martinelli G, et al. Long-term follow-up of patients with follicular lymphoma (FL) receiving single agent rituximab at two different schedules in study SAKK 35/98. *J Clin Oncol*. 2009;27(15s):8512a.

Gisselbrecht C, Schmitz N, Mounier N, et al. R-ICE versus R-DHAP in relapsed patients with CD20 diffuse large B-cell lymphoma (DLBCL) followed by stem cell transplantation and maintenance treatment with rituximab or not: first interim analysis on 200 patients. CORAL Study [abstract]. *Blood*. 2007;110:517.

Habermann TM, Weller EA, Morrison VA, et al. Phase III trial of rituximab-CHOP versus CHOP with a second randomization to maintenance rituximab or observation in patients 60 years of age and older with diffuse large B-cell lymphoma [abstract]. *Blood*. 2003;102:6a.

Hainsworth JD, Litchy S, Burris H, et al. Rituximab as first-line and maintenance therapy for patients with indolent non-Hodgkin lymphoma. *J Clin Oncol*. 2002;20:4261–4267.

Hans CP, Weisenburger DD, Greiner TC, et al. Confirmation of the molecular classification of diffuse large B-cell lymphoma by immunohistochemistry using a tissue microarray. *Blood*. 2004;103:275–282.

Hermine O, Lefrere F, Bronowicki JP, et al. Regression of splenic lymphoma with villous lymphocytes after treatment of hepatitis C virus infection. *N Engl J Med*. 2002;347:89–94.

Herold M, Haas A, Srock S, et al. Rituximab added to first-line mitoxantrone, chlorambucil, and prednisolone chemotherapy followed by interferon maintenance prolongs survival in patients with advanced follicular lymphoma: an East German Study Group Hematology and Oncology Study. *J Clin Oncol*. 2007;25:1986–1992.

Hiddemann W, Kneba M, Dreyling M, et al. Frontline therapy with rituximab added to the combination of cyclophosphamide, doxorubicin, vincristine, and prednisone (CHOP) significantly improves the outcome for patients with advanced-stage follicular lymphoma compared with therapy with CHOP alone: results of a prospective randomized study of the German Low-Grade Lymphoma Study Group. *Blood*. 2005;106:3725–3732.

Hochster H, Weller E, Gascoyne RD, et al. Maintenance rituximab after cyclophosphamide, vincristine, and prednisone prolongs progression-free survival in advanced indolent lymphoma: results of the randomized phase III ECOG1496 study. *J Clin Oncol*. 2009;27:1607–1614.

Houot R, Levy R. Vaccines for lymphomas: idiotype vaccines and beyond. *Blood Rev*. 2009;23:137–142.

Hummel M, Bentink S, Berger H, et al. A biologic definition of Burkitt's lymphoma from transcriptional and genomic profiling. *N Engl J Med*. 2006;354:2419–2430.

International T-Cell Lymphoma Project. International peripheral T-cell and natural killer/T-cell lymphoma study: pathology findings and clinical outcomes. *J Clin Oncol*. 2008;26:4124–4130.

Isobe K, Kagami Y, Higuchi K, et al. A multicenter phase II study of local radiation therapy for stage IEA mucosa-associated lymphoid tissue lymphomas: a preliminary report from the Japan Radiation Oncology Group (JAROG). *Int J Radiat Oncol Biol Phys*. 2007;69(4):1181–1186.

Jaccard A, Petit B, Girault S, et al. L-asparaginase-based treatment of 15 western patients with extranodal NK/T-cell lymphoma and leukemia and a review of the literature. *Ann Oncol*. 2009;20(1):110–116.

Juweid ME, Stroobants S, Hoekstra OS, et al. Use of positron emission tomography for response assessment of lymphoma:

consensus of the Imaging Subcommittee of International Harmonization Project in Lymphoma. *J Clin Oncol.* 2007;25:571–578.

Kaminski MS, et al. Pivotal study of iodine I[131] tositumomab for chemotherapy-refractory low-grade or transformed low-grade B-cell non-Hodgkin lymphomas. *J Clin Oncol.* 2001;19:3918–3928.

Kasamon YL, Wahl RL. FDG PET and risk-adapted therapy in Hodgkin's and non-Hodgkin's lymphoma. *Curr Opin Oncol.* 2008;20:206–219.

Khouri IF, Lee MS, Saliba RM, et al. Nonablative allogeneic stem-cell transplantation for advanced/recurrent mantle cell lymphoma. *J Clin Oncol.* 2003;23:4407–4412.

Kwak L, Campbell M, Czerwinski D, Hart S, Miller R, Levy R. Induction of immune responses in patients with B-cell lymphoma against the surface-immunoglobulin idiotype expressed by their tumors. *N Engl J Med.* 1992;327:1209–1215.

Lacasce A, Howard O, Lib S, et al. Modified Magrath regimens for adults with Burkitt and Burkitt-like lymphomas: preserved efficacy with decreased toxicity. *Leuk Lymphoma.* 2004;45:761–767.

Lenz G, Dreyling M, Hoster E, et al. Immunochemotherapy with rituximab and cyclophosphamide, doxorubicin, vincristine, and prednisone significantly improves response and time to treatment failure, but not long-term outcome in patients with previously untreated mantle cell lymphoma: results of a prospective randomized trial of the German Low Grade Lymphoma Study Group (GLSG). *J Clin Oncol.* 2005;23:1984–1992.

Levy R, Robertson MJ, Ganjoo K, Vose J, Denney D. Results of a phase 3 trial evaluating safety and efficacy of specific immunotherapy, recombinant idiotype (Id) conjugated to KLH (Id-KLH) with GM-CSF in patients with follicular non-Hodgkin's lymphoma (fNHL) [abstract]. *Proc Am Assoc Cancer Res.* 2008:LB-204.

Link MP, Shuster JJ, Donaldson SS, Berard CW, Murphy SB. Treatment of children and young adults with early stage non-Hodgkin's lymphoma. *N Engl J Med.* 1997;337:1259–1266. *A summary of clinical trials comparing an abbreviated, 9-week chemotherapy regimen without radiation therapy with more protracted chemotherapy protocols for early-stage NHL in patients <21 years of age. Five-year survival rates were >85% with both abbreviated and more protracted regimens; only lymphoblastic lymphoma patients appeared to benefit from the more protracted therapy.*

MacManus MP, Hoppe RT. Is radiotherapy curative for stage I and II low-grade follicular lymphoma? Results of a long-term follow-up study of patients treated at Stanford University. *J Clin Oncol.* 1996;14:1282–1290.

Magrath I, Adde M, Shad A, et al. Adults and children with small noncleaved-cell lymphoma have a similar excellent outcome when treated with the same chemotherapy regimen. *J Clin Oncol.* 1996;14:925–934. *A strategy incorporating treatment stratification of patients into low-versus high-risk groups based on presenting clinical stage and LDH levels. Treatment consisted of CODOX-M alone for low-risk patients and alternating cycles of CODOX-M and IVAC for high-risk patients.*

Mangel J, Buckstein R, Imrie K, et al. Immunotherapy with rituximab following high-dose therapy and autologous stem-cell transplantation for mantle cell lymphoma. *Semin Oncol.* 2002;29(1 Suppl 2):56–69.

Marcus R, Imrie K, Belch A, et al. CVP chemotherapy plus rituximab compared with CVP as first-line treatment for advanced follicular lymphoma. *Blood.* 2005;105:1417–1423.

Marcus R, Imrie K, Solal-Celigny P, et al. Phase III study of R-CVP compared with cyclophosphamide, vincristine, and prednisone alone in patients with previously untreated advanced follicular lymphoma. *J Clin Oncol.* 2008;26:4579–4586.

Martinez-Delgado B, Cuadros M, Honrado E, et al. Differential expression of NF-kappaB pathway genes among peripheral T-cell lymphomas. *Leukemia.* 2005;19:2254–2263.

McLaughlin P, Grillo-Lopez AJ, Link BK, et al. Rituximab chimeric anti-CD20 monoclonal antibody therapy for relapsed indolent lymphoma: half of patients respond to a four-dose treatment program. *J Clin Oncol.* 1998;16(8):2825–2833.

Mead GM, Sydes MR, Walewski J, et al. An international evaluation of CODOX-M and CODOX-M alternating with IVAC in adult Burkitt's lymphoma: results of United Kingdom Lymphoma Group LY06 study. *Ann Oncol.* 2002;13:1264–1274. *An analysis of 72 adult patients confirming the high response rates and favorable outcomes reported by Magrath et al (1996).*

Miller TP, Dahlberg S, Cassady R, et al. Chemotherapy alone compared with chemotherapy plus radiotherapy for localized intermediate and high-grade non-Hodgkin lymphoma. *N Engl J Med.* 1998;339:21–26.

Miller TP, LeBlanc-Straceski J, Spiers A, Chase E, Fisher RI. CHOP alone compared to CHOP plus radiotherapy for early stage aggressive non-Hodgkin's lymphomas: update of the Southwest Oncology Group (SWOG) [abstract]. *Blood.* 2003:3024a.

Milpied N, Deconinck E, Gaillard F, et al. Initial treatment of aggressive lymphoma with high-dose chemotherapy and autologous stem-cell support. *N Engl J Med.* 2004;350:1287–1295. *A randomized study of CHOP chemotherapy versus induction chemotherapy followed by HDT and transplantation for aggressive NHL patients with low, intermediate, or high-intermediate IPI scores, demonstrating EFS benefit for transplantation and OS benefit for patients in the high-intermediate subgroup.*

Mohan SR, Maciejewski JP. Diagnosis and therapy of neutropenia in large granular lymphocyte leukemia. *Curr Opin Hematol.* 2009;16:27–34.

Montoto S, Davies AJ, Matthews J, et al. Risk and clinical implications of transformation of follicular lymphoma to diffuse large B-cell lymphoma. *J Clin Oncol.* 2007;25:2426–2433.

Morschhauser F, Bischof-Delaloye A, Rohatiner AZS, et al. Extended follow-up of the international randomized phase 3 First-Line Indolent Trial (FIT) shows durable benefit of 90 y-ibritumomab tiuxetan (Zevalin) consolidation of first remission in advanced stage follicular non-Hodgkin's lymphoma [abstract]. *Blood.* 2008;112:2002.

Olsen E, Vonderheid E, Pimpinelli N, et al. Revisions to the staging and classification of mycosis fungoides and Sézary syndrome: a proposal of the International Society for Cutaneous Lymphomas (ISCL) and the Cutaneous Lymphoma Task Force of the European Organization of Research and Treatment of Cancer (EORTC). *Blood.* 2007;110:1713–1722.

Perkins AS, Friedberg JW. Burkitt lymphoma in adults. *Hematology.* 2008;2008(1):341–348

Persky DO, Unger JM, Spier CM, et al. Phase II study of rituximab plus three cycles of CHOP and involved-field radiotherapy for patients with limited-stage aggressive B-cell lymphoma: Southwest Oncology Group study 0014. *J Clin Oncol.* 2008;26:2258–2263.

Peterson BA, Petroni GR, Frizzera G, et al. Prolonged single-agent versus combination chemotherapy in indolent follicular lymphomas: a study of the Cancer and Leukemia Group B. *J Clin Oncol.* 2003;12:5–15.

Pfreundschuh M, Schubert J, Ziepert M, et al. Six versus eight cycles of bi-weekly CHOP-14 with or without rituximab in elderly patients with aggressive CD20$^+$ B-cell lymphomas: a randomised controlled trial (RICOVER-60). *Lancet Oncol.* 2008;9:105–116.

Pfreundschuh M, Trumper L, Kloess M, et al. Two-weekly or 3-weekly CHOP chemotherapy with or without etoposide for the treatment of young patients with good-prognosis (normal LDH) aggressive lymphomas: results of the NHL-B1 trial of the DSHNHL. *Blood.* 2004;104:626–633.

Pfreundschuh M, Trumper L, Kloess M, et al. Two-weekly or 3-weekly CHOP chemotherapy with or without etoposide for the treatment of elderly patients with aggressive lymphomas: results of the NHL-B2 trial of the DSHNHL. *Blood.* 2004;104:634–641.

Pfreundschuh M, Trumper L, Osterborg A, et al. CHOP-like chemotherapy plus rituximab versus CHOP-like chemotherapy alone in young patients with good-prognosis diffuse large-B-cell lymphoma: a randomised controlled trial by the MabThera International Trial (MInT) Group. *Lancet Oncol.* 2006;7:379–391.

Philip T, Guglielmi C, Hagenbeek A, et al. Autologous bone marrow transplantation as compared with salvage chemotherapy in relapses of chemotherapy-sensitive non-Hodgkin's lymphoma. *N Engl J Med.* 1995;333:1540–1545.

Press OM, Unger J, Maloney D, et al. An update of a phase II trial of CHOP followed by tositumomab (Bexxar) for front-line treatment of advanced stage follicular lymphoma: Southwest Oncology Group Protocol 9911 [abstract]. *Blood.* 2005;106:352.

Prince HM, Whittaker S, Hoppe RT. How I treat mycosis fungoides and Sézary syndrome. *Blood.* 2009;114:4337–4353.

Romaguera JE, Fayad L, Rodriguez MA, et al. High rate of durable remissions after treatment of newly diagnosed aggressive mantle-cell lymphoma with rituximab plus hyper-CVAD alternating with rituximab plus high-dose methotrexate and cytarabine. *J Clin Oncol.* 2005;23:7013–7023.

Romaguera JE, Khouri IF, Kantarjian HM, et al. Untreated aggressive mantle cell lymphoma: results with intensive chemotherapy without stem cell transplant in elderly patients. *Leuk Lymphoma.* 2000;39:77–85. *A report of the HyperCVAD regimen given in alternating cycles with high-dose methotrexate-cytarabine for 25 newly diagnosed MCL patients age 65 or older. The CR rate was 68%, and median failure-free survival was 15 months. More recent studies are testing the inclusion of rituximab with the regimen as an effort to increase responses and survival in this non–transplantation-eligible group.*

Rosenblum MD, LaBelle JL, Chang C-C, et al. Efficacy of alemtuzumab treatment of refractory T-cell large granular lymphocytic leukemia. *Blood.* 2004;103:1969–1971.

Rosenwald A, Wright G, Chan WC, et al. The use of molecular profiling to predict survival after chemotherapy for diffuse large-B-cell lymphoma. *N Engl J Med.* 2002;346:1937–1947.

Rosenwald A, Wright G, Wiestner A, et al. The proliferation gene expression signature is a quantitative integrator of oncogenic events that predicts survival in mantle cell lymphoma. *Cancer Cell.* 2003;3:185–197.

Rummel MJ, Al-Batran SE, Kim SZ, et al. Bendamustine plus rituximab is effective and has a favorable toxicity profile in the treatment of mantle cell and low-grade non-Hodgkin's lymphoma. *J Clin Oncol.* 2005;23:3383–3389.

Rummel MJ, von Gruenhagen U, Niederle N, et al. Bendamustine plus rituximab versus CHOP plus rituximab in the first-line treatment of patients with follicular, indolent and mantle cell lymphomas: results of a randomized phase III study of the Study Group Indolent Lymphomas (StiL) [abstract]. *Blood.* 2008;112:2596a.

Savage KJ, Al-Rajhi N, Voss N, et al. Favorable outcome of primary mediastinal large B-cell lymphoma in a single institution: the British Columbia experience. *Ann Oncol.* 2006;17:123–130.

Savage KJ, Harris NL, Vose JM, et al. ALK- anaplastic large-cell lymphoma is clinically and immunophenotypically different from both ALK$^+$ ALCL and peripheral T-cell lymphoma, not otherwise specified: report from the International Peripheral T-Cell Lymphoma Project. *Blood.* 2008;111:5496–5504.

Savage KJ, Monti S, Kutok LJ, et al. The molecular signature of mediastinal large B-cell lymphoma differs from that of other diffuse large B-cell lymphomas and shares features with classic Hodgkin lymphoma. *Blood.* 2003;102:3871–3879.

Saven A, Burian C, Koziol JA, Piro LD. Long-term follow-up of patients with hairy cell leukemia after cladribine treatment. *Blood.* 1998;92:1918–1926. *A summary of 349 evaluable patients treated with cladribine, including duration of response and survival data, second treatment responses, and complication rates.*

Schouten HC, Qian W, Kvaloy S, et al. High-dose therapy improves progression-free survival and survival in relapsed follicular non-Hodgkin's lymphoma: results from the randomized European CUP trial. *J Clin Oncol.* 2003;21:3918–3927. *An analysis of 89 patients who received CHOP chemotherapy only versus an unpurged or purged ASCT, indicating a PFS and OS advantage for transplantation.*

Sehn LH, Berry B, Chhanabhai M, et al. The revised International Prognostic Index (R-IPI) is a better predictor of outcome than the standard IPI for patients with diffuse large B-cell lymphoma treated with R-CHOP. *Blood.* 2007;109:1857–1861.

Sehn LH, Donaldson J, Chhanabhai M, et al. Introduction of combined CHOP plus rituximab therapy dramatically improved outcome of diffuse large B-cell lymphoma in British Columbia. *J Clin Oncol.* 2005;23:5027–5033.

Shipp MA, Harrington DP, Anderson JR, et al. A predictive model for aggressive non-Hodgkin's lymphoma. The International

Non-Hodgkin's Lymphoma Prognostic Factors Project. *N Engl J Med*. 1993;329:987–994.

Shipp MA, Ross KN, Tamayo P, et al. Diffuse large B-cell lymphoma outcome prediction by gene-expression profiling and supervised machine learning. *Nat Med*. 2002;8:68–74. *A report of microarray analysis of pretreatment biopsy samples from 77 patients with large B-cell lymphoma treated with CHOP chemotherapy, identifying prognostic markers and patient categories with strikingly different clinical outcomes.*

Spaepen K, Stroobants S, Dupont P, et al. Early restaging positron emission tomography with (18)F-fluorodeoxyglucose predicts outcome in patients with aggressive non-Hodgkin's lymphoma. *Ann Oncol*. 2002;13:1356–1363.

Stathis A, Chini C, Bertoni F, et al. Long-term outcome following *Helicobacter pylori* eradication in a retrospective study of 105 patients with localized gastric marginal zone B-cell lymphoma of MALT type. *Ann Oncol*. 2009;20:1086–1093.

Stein H, Mason D, Gerdes J, et al. The expression of Hodgkin's disease associated antigen Ki-1 in reactive and neoplastic lymphoid tissue: evidence that the Reed Sternberg cells and histiocytic malignancies are derived from activated lymphoid cells. *Blood*. 1985;66:848–85.

Swerdlow SH, Campo E, Harris NL, et al. *WHO Classification of Tumors of Hematopoietic and Lymphoid Tissues*. 4th ed. Lyon, France: IARC Press; 2008.

Swerdlow SH, Williams ME. From centrocytic to mantle cell lymphoma: a clinicopathologic and molecular review of 3 decades. *Hum Pathol*. 2002;33:7–20. *A review of the clinicopathologic characteristics of MCL and its molecular pathogenesis.*

Todeschini G, Secchi S, Morra E, et al. Primary mediastinal large B-cell lymphoma: long-term results from a retrospective multicenter Italian experience in 138 patients treated with CHOP or MACOP-B/VACOP-B. *Br J Cancer*. 2006;90:372–376. *A retrospective analysis suggesting improved EFS and OS in PMLBCL with MACOP-B or VACOP-B versus CHOP. Involved-field radiation therapy improved the outcomes for each of the chemotherapy regimens.*

Tomita N, Kodaira T, Tachibana H, Nakamura T, Mizoguchi N, Takada A. Favorable outcomes of radiotherapy for early-stage mucosa-associated lymphoid tissue lymphoma. *Radiother Oncol*. 2009;90:231–235.

Treon SP, Branagan AR, Hunter Z, Santos D, Tournhilac O, Anderson KC. Paradoxical increases in serum IgM and viscosity levels following rituximab in Waldenström's macroglobulinemia. *Ann Oncol*. 2004;15:1481–1483.

Treon SP, Branagan AR, Ioakimidis L, et al. Long-term outcomes to fludarabine and rituximab in Waldenstrom macroglobulinemia. *Blood*. 2009;113(16):3673–3678.

Tsai HK, Li S, Ng AK, Silver B, Stevenson MA, Mauch PM. Role of radiation therapy in the treatment of stage I/II mucosa-associated lymphoid tissue lymphoma. *Ann Oncol*. 2007;18(4):672–678.

Vallisa D, Bernuzzi P, Arcaini L, et al. Role of anti-hepatitis C virus (HCV) treatment in HCV-related, low-grade, B-cell, non-Hodgkin's lymphoma: a multicenter Italian experience. *J Clin Oncol*. 2005;23(3):468–473.

van Besien K, Loberiza FR, Bajorunaite R, et al. Comparison of autologous and allogeneic hematopoietic stem cell transplantation for follicular lymphoma. *Blood*. 2003;102:3521–3529.

van Oers MH, Klasa R, Marcus RE, et al. Rituximab maintenance improves clinical outcome of relapsed/resistant follicular non-Hodgkin lymphoma in patients both with and without rituximab during induction: results of a prospective randomized phase 3 intergroup trial. *Blood*. 2006;108:3295–3301.

Villa D, Connors JM, Shenkier TN, Gascoyne RD, Sehn LH, Savage KJ. Incidence and risk factors for central nervous system relapse in patients with diffuse large B-cell lymphoma: the impact of the addition of rituximab to CHOP chemotherapy. *Ann Oncol*. 2009;21(5):1046–1052.

Weeks J, Yeop B, Canellos G, Shipp M. Value of follow-up procedures in patients with large-cell lymphoma who achieve a complete remission. *J Clin Onc*. 1991;9:1196–1203.

Wilder RB, Jones D, Tucker SL, et al. Long-term results with radiotherapy for Stage I-II follicular lymphomas. *Int J Radiat Oncol Biol Phys*. 2001;51(5):1219–1227.

Willemze R, Jaffe ES, Burg G, et al. WHO-EORTC classification for cutaneous lymphomas. *Blood*. 2005;105:3768–3785.

Willemze R, Jansen PM, Cerroni L, et al. Subcutaneous panniculitis-like T-cell lymphoma: definition, classification, and prognostic factors: an EORTC Cutaneous Lymphoma Group Study of 83 cases. *Blood*. 2008;111:838–845.

Witzig TE, Gordon LI, Cabanillas F, et al. Randomized controlled trial of yttrium-90-labeled ibritumomab tiuxetan radioimmunotherapy versus rituximab immunotherapy for patients with relapsed or refractory low-grade, follicular, or transformed B-cell non-Hodgkin lymphoma. *J Clin Oncol*. 2002;20:2453–2463.

Immunodeficiency-associated lymphoproliferative disorders

Boue F, Gabarre J, Gisselbrecht C, et al. Phase II trial of CHOP plus rituximab in patients with HIV-associated non-Hodgkin's lymphoma. *J Clin Oncol*. 2006;24:4123–4128.

Choquet S, Leblond V, Herbrecht R, et al. Efficacy and safety of rituximab in B-cell post-transplantation lymphoproliferative disorders: results of a prospective multicenter phase 2 study. *Blood*. 2006;107:3053–3057.

Ferreri AJ, Blay JY, Reni M, et al. Prognostic scoring system for primary CNS lymphomas: the International Extranodal Lymphoma Study Group experience. *J Clin Oncol*. 2003;21(2):266–272.

Heslop HE. Biology and treatment of Epstein-Barr virus–associated non-Hodgkin lymphomas. In: *Hematology: ASH Education Program Book*. Washington, DC: American Society of Hematology; 2005:260.

Kaplan LD, Lee JY, Ambinder RF, et al. Rituximab does not improve clinical outcome in a randomized phase 3 trial of CHOP with or without rituximab in patients with HIV-associated non-Hodgkin lymphoma: AIDS-Malignancies Consortium Trial 010. *Blood*. 2005;106:1538–1543.

Svoboda J, Kotloff R, Tsai DE. Management of patients with post-transplant lymphoproliferative disorder: the role of rituximab. *Transplant Int.* 2006;19:259-269.

Hodgkin lymphoma

Aleman BMP, Raemaekers JMM, Tirelli U, et al. Involved field radiotherapy for advanced Hodgkin lymphoma. *N Engl J Med.* 2003;348:2396–2406. *In a study of 421 patients with a CR to chemotherapy, the addition of involved-field radiation did not improve OS or disease-free survival. Patients with a PR to chemotherapy did appear to benefit from the addition of radiation therapy.*

Aleman BMP, van den Belt-Dusebout AW, Klokman WJ, Van't Veer MB, Bartelink H, van Leeuwen FE. Long-term cause-specific mortality of patients treated for Hodgkin's disease. *J Clin Oncol.* 2003;21:3431–3439.

Behringer K, Breuer K, Reineke T, et al. Secondary amenorrhea after Hodgkin's lymphoma is influenced by age at treatment, stage of disease, chemotherapy regimen, and the use of oral contraceptives during therapy: a report from the German Hodgkin's Lymphoma Study Group. *J Clin Oncol.* 2005;23:7555–7564.

Bhatia S, Robison LL, Oberlin O, et al. Breast cancer and other second neoplasms after childhood Hodgkin disease. *N Engl J Med.* 1996;334:745–751. *The risk of a second cancer was 7% 15 years after initial diagnosis and treatment of HD. Breast cancer was the most common and was associated with radiation therapy. The risk of breast cancer was 75 times higher than in the general population, with a probability approaching 35% by 40 years of age in these patients; the risk appeared highest in women treated with radiation therapy at ages 10 to 16 years.*

Bonadonna G, Bonfante V, Viviani S, Di Russo A, Villani F, Valagussa P. ABVD plus subtotal nodal versus involved-field radiotherapy in early-stage Hodgkin's disease: long-term results. *J Clin Oncol.* 2004;22:2835–2841.

Brune V, Tiacci E, Pfeil I, et al. Origin and pathogenesis of nodular lymphocyte-predominant Hodgkin lymphoma as revealed by global gene expression analysis. *J Exp Med.* 2008;205(10):2251–2268.

Campbell BA, Voss N, Pickles T, et al. Involved-nodal radiation therapy as a component of combination therapy for limited-stage Hodgkin's lymphoma: a question of field size. *J Clin Oncol.* 2008;26:5170–5174.

Canellos GP, Anderson JR, Propert KJ, et al. Chemotherapy of advanced Hodgkin disease with MOPP, ABVD, or MOPP alternating with ABVD. *N Engl J Med.* 1992;327:1478–1484. *Randomized trial comparing ABVD, MOPP/ABVD, and MOPP in advanced Hodgkin lymphoma.*

Connors JM, Noordijk EM, Horning SJ. Hodgkin lymphoma: basing the treatment on the evidence. In: *Hematology: ASH Education Program Book*. Washington, DC: American Society of Hematology; 2001:178–193. *The authors update the approach to early-stage disease, cooperative group trials in advanced-stage disease, and data related to the biology and treatment of lymphocyte-predominant HL.*

Diehl V, Franklin J, Pfreundschuh M, et al. Standard and increased-dose BEACOPP chemotherapy compared with COPP-ABVD for advanced Hodgkin disease [published correction appears in N Engl J Med. 2005;353:744]. *N Engl J Med.* 2003;348:2386–2395.

Diehl V, Sextro M, Franklin J, et al. Clinical presentation, course, and prognosis factors in lymphocyte-predominant Hodgkin's disease and lymphocyte-rich classic Hodgkin's disease. Report from the European Task Force Lymphoma Project on Lymphocyte-Predominant Hodgkin's Disease. *J Clin Oncol.* 1999;17:776–783.

Diehl V, Stein H, Hummel M, et al. Hodgkin lymphoma: biology and treatment strategies for primary, refractory, and relapsed disease. In: *Hematology: ASH Education Program Book*. Washington, DC: American Society of Hematology; 2003:225–247. *A summary of recent advances in the cell of origin and pathogenesis of HL, front-line treatment approaches for early- versus advanced-stage disease, and the management approach in patients with relapsed and refractory HL.*

Ekstrand BC, Horning SJ. Lymphocytic predominant Hodgkin disease. *Curr Oncol Rep.* 2002;4:424–433.

Ekstrand BC, Lucas JB, Horvitz SM, et al. Rituximab in lymphocyte-predominant Hodgkin disease. Results of a phase II trial. *Blood.* 2003;101:4285–4289.

Engert A, Pluetschow A, Eich HT, et al. Combined modality treatment of two or four cycles of ABVD followed by involved field radiotherapy in the treatment of patients with early stage Hodgkin lymphoma: update interim analysis of the Randomised HD10 Study of the German Hodgkin Study Group (GHSG) [abstract]. *Blood.* 2005;106:2673a.

Federico M, Bellei M, Brice P, et al. High-dose therapy and autologous stem-cell transplantation versus conventional therapy for patients with advanced Hodgkin lymphoma responding to front-line therapy. *J Clin Oncol.* 2003;21:2320–2325. *A study of 163 patients with unfavorable, advanced-stage HL who achieved a CR or PR to 4 initial courses of chemotherapy and were randomized to 4 additional courses of chemotherapy or HDT with ASCT. No significant differences were seen in 5-year OS or disease-free survival, indicating no benefit to HDT as initial therapy.*

Gallamini A, Hutchings M, Rigacci L, et al. Early interim 2-[18F] fluoro-2-deoxy-D-glucose positron emission tomography is prognostically superior to international prognostic score in advanced-stage Hodgkin's lymphoma: a report from a joint Italian-Danish study. *J Clin Oncol.* 2007;25:3746–3752.

Hasenclever D, Diehl V. A prognostic score for advanced Hodgkin disease. *N Engl J Med.* 1998;339:1506–1514. *An international panel evaluated prognostic factors and outcome in over 5000 patients with advanced HL. Seven factors were identified in multifactorial analyses that could be combined to establish an additive prognostic score.*

Horning SJ, Hoppe RT, Breslin S, Bartlett NL, Brown BW, Rosenberg SA. Stanford V and radiotherapy for locally extensive and advanced Hodgkin disease: mature results of a prospective clinical trial. *J Clin Oncol.* 2002;20:630–637. *An update of results of a combined chemotherapy plus irradiation approach for advanced HL employing a lower cumulative dose and shorter chemotherapy treatment schema.*

Meyer RM, Gospodarowicz MK, Connors JM, et al. Randomized comparison of ABVD chemotherapy with a strategy that includes radiation therapy in patients with limited-stage Hodgkin's lymphoma: National Cancer Institute of Canada Clinical Trials Group and the Eastern Cooperative Oncology Group. *J Clin Oncol.* 2005;23:4634–4642.

Ng AK, Bernardo MP, Weller E, et al. Long-term survival and competing causes of death in patients with early stage Hodgkin disease treated at age 50 or younger. *J Clin Oncol.* 2002;20:2101–2108.

Ramaswamy S, Golub TR. DNA microarrays in clinical oncology. *J Clin Oncol.* 2002;20(7):1932–1941.

Sieniawski M, Reineke T, Nogova L, et al. Fertility in male patients with advanced Hodgkin lymphoma treated with BEACOPP: a report of the German Hodgkin Study Group (GHSG). *Blood.* 2008;111:71–76.

CHAPTER 19

Chronic lymphocytic leukemia

Neil E. Kay and Vicki A. Morrison

Chronic lymphocytic leukemia, 555
Diagnosis, 557
Clinical and laboratory features, 559
Staging, 560
Prognostic factors, 560

Therapy, 564
Approach to newly diagnosed patients with high-risk disease, 569
Complications of CLL, 571
Quality-of-life issues, 572

Other indolent cell leukemias, 573
The future, 574
Bibliography, 574

Chronic lymphocytic leukemia

Incidence, epidemiology, and demographics

B-cell chronic lymphocytic leukemia (CLL) is a lymphoproliferative disorder manifested by a clonal expansion of mature, long-lived, B lymphocytes. The disease is identical to small lymphocytic leukemia (SLL); the clinical distinction is whether the leukemic (blood and marrow) or the nodal components of the disease predominate in a given patient. The 2001 World Health Organization classification scheme considers CLL and SLL in one category (CLL/SLL) because of shared clinicopathologic features. The mechanisms of why clonal B cells predominate in marrow or node are not clearly understood, but one possibility may be the ability of B lymphocytes to "home" to certain tissue sites, resulting in a clinical presentation that varies between predominant blood and marrow involvement versus involvement mostly in lymph node tissue. Although CLL is the most prevalent leukemia (~30% of all leukemia) in the Western hemisphere, its incidence is markedly different in various countries. In addition, ≥95% of the B-cell CLL cases in North America involve clonal B lymphocytes. In Asia, the incidence of CLL is much lower (5% of all leukemia), and the T-cell phenotype predominates. Individuals with CLL in the United States are more likely to be male, and the 2008 Surveillance, Epidemiology, and End Results (SEER) estimates predict that, of the 15,110 patients diagnosed with CLL, 8750 will be men and 6360 will be women. Using 2006 SEER data, the age-adjusted incidence rate is now estimated to be 4 per 100,000 men and women per year with approximately 0.46% of men and women born in 2008 anticipated to be diagnosed with CLL during their lifetime. Of note, recent surveys in Canada have shown a dramatic difference in incidence between cancer registry and centralized flow cytometry facilities with significantly more patients identified via flow methods. It may be necessary in the future to have adjustments of the incidence based on the more sensitive flow cytometry surveys of the population. The median age at diagnosis in the past was believed to be 60 to 65 years, with the incidence increasing steadily with age, reaching 40 per 100,000 per year in men in the eighth decade. During 2000 to 2005, according to the SEER database, the median age at diagnosis of CLL was found to be 72 years. CLL is virtually nonexistent in children and is rarely seen in adolescents. CLL is the only leukemia not typically associated with radiation exposure and has the strongest tendency for familial aggregation, currently estimated at approximately 10% of all CLL patients (see following section, Familial CLL). Historically, this disease has been described as a lymphoproliferative process, but several decades ago, Dameshek suggested that an additional defect in the leukemic cells' ability to undergo apoptosis would result in an accumulation of malignant B cells. This has been the dominant theory of the CLL B-cell accumulation process, but recent work using heavy-water (D_2O) cell labeling has definitely shown that there is a low but detectable proliferation level in B-cell CLL. Recently, significant insights into

---

Conflict-of-interest disclosure: *Dr. Kay*: consultancy: Cephalon; research funding: Celgene, Genentech, Polyphenon E International, Hospira; membership on board of directors or advisory committee: Genentech, Biogen Idec. *Dr. Morrison:* speakers' bureau: Merck, Pfizer, Genentech, Celgene, Amgen; membership on data safety monitoring board or scientific advisory committee: Merck, Celgene.
Off-label drug use: *Dr. Kay*: pentostatin and lenalidomide for CLL.

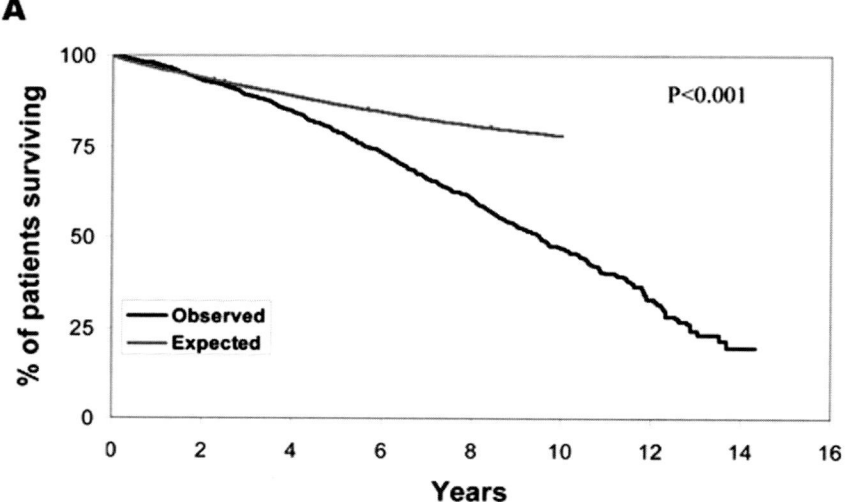

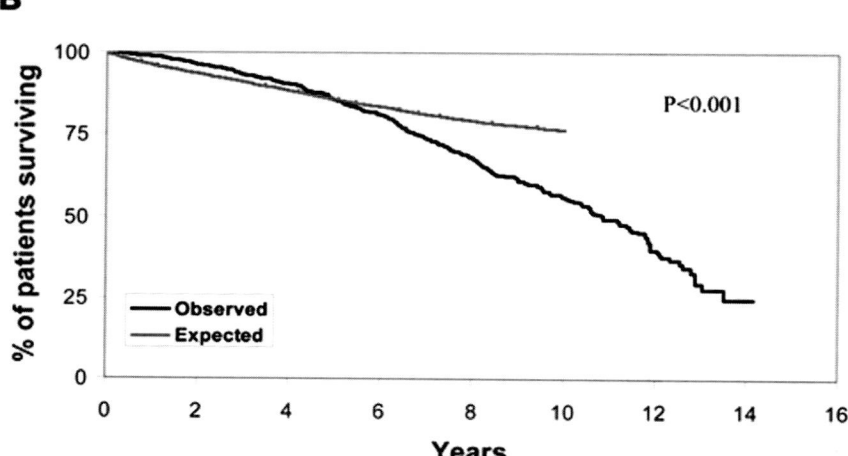

Figure 19-1 Overall survival of chronic lymphocytic leukemia (CLL) patients relative to age matched controls. Figure shows the survival from diagnosis of 2474 Mayo Clinic patients diagnosed with CLL since January 1995 as compared with the age-matched general Minnesota population. Shanafelt TD. Predicting clinical outcome in CLL: how and why. *Hematology: ASH Educ Book.* 2009: 421–429.

the pathogenesis of this disease have been uncovered including the remarkable "stereotypy" for B-cell receptors (BCRs), where fully 30% of CLL patients have B-cell clones that appear to be antigen driven. There is a second cohort of CLL where the B-cell clones are quite heterogenous in relation to the BCRs. The importance of the former group is that these BCRs seem close to those B cells that are a component of the innate immune system in contrast to the latter BCR group that may have been derived from the more mature B-cell population. Another significant biologic insight has been the detection of proliferation centers (focal aggregates of cells resembling prolymphocytes), primarily in lymph node and less so in bone marrow, that may be the sites that generate the progeny of circulating leukemic B cells.

The clinical course of this malignant disease is quite variable, and the complications that are associated with this entity are diverse, making management of any patient more complicated than might be thought by most hematologists. The more common clinical complications include autoimmune diseases, increased incidence of malignancies, immune deficits predisposing to infections, and transformation potential to more malignant lymphomas. Patients with CLL have been reported to have an increased incidence of nonhematologic neoplasms, particularly prostate, lung, or gastrointestinal cancer. However, skin cancer is the most commonly associated malignancy and can be a significant clinical problem even for early-stage and untreated patients.

Recent information suggests that CLL is a significant health problem affecting all ages of patients with this disease (Figure 19-1). Furthermore, it is important to know that women diagnosed with CLL have 5- and 10-year overall survival (OS) rates that exceed those of men. CLL is most common in whites and decreases in frequency in a descending order from blacks, Hispanics, American Indians and Native Alaskans, and Asians and Pacific Islanders. Importantly, the rarity of CLL among Asians and Pacific Islanders persists even in immigrants from these areas who have migrated to the Western hemisphere. This latter observation seems to indicate that there is a strong genetic component to the occurrence of CLL. Occupational or environmental exposure to radiation does not appear to predispose patients to a higher risk of developing CLL. Although acute myeloid leukemia, chronic myeloid leukemia, and acute lymphoblastic leukemia were increased among survivors of the atomic bomb at Hiroshima, to date, there has been no obvious increase in CLL. Studies for individuals at risk around the Chernobyl nuclear reactor accident again found increases in other types of leukemia but not CLL. There is no obvious relationship to toxic exposures with the possible exception of a relationship for men exposed to Agent Orange, the pesticide used in Vietnam. Finally, there is recent evidence that despite the fact that CLL is incurable, recent mortality trends for all CLL patients suggest that the newer treatment approaches have improved OS.

Familial CLL

Although B-cell CLL is known to be a heterogeneous disease, it is only recently that the familial component of CLL has been more thoroughly investigated. This entity is seen in approximately 5% to 10% of all CLL patients and has some distinct features that include earlier age at diagnosis; female prevalence; increased incidence of other lymphoproliferative disorders, such as non-Hodgkin lymphoma; and the more recently described, monoclonal B-cell lymphocytosis (MBL) (see later section, Monoclonal B-cell lymphocytosis) CLL in family members. Several case-control studies have shown that the relative risk ratio is high for first-degree relatives of CLL patients to develop CLL or other B-cell malignancies. Current information indicates that the prognostic parameters and clinical course of familial CLL is not clearly distinguishable from that of sporadic disease. In addition, it is not clear that the treatment responses for progressive disease have any discernible difference in familial versus sporadic CLL. The genetic etiology of CLL is unknown, and early work on familial CLL has not yet uncovered any obvious gene related to its pathogenesis; however, most recently, genome-wide analysis using single nucleotide polymorphisms does suggest that a small group of genes can be clearly related to the pathophysiology of CLL. These need to be validated and shown to play a clear role in the pathogenesis of familial CLL. For the practitioner, it is best to indicate to concerned CLL patients that their relatives are at relatively low risk of developing CLL or other lymphoproliferative disorders. Familial CLL is currently defined as a CLL case with at least one blood relative with CLL; however, this definition does not limit the type of familial relationships among the CLL cases. Kindred can show CLL in both closely related (eg, siblings) and in more distantly related (eg, cousins) relatives. Although this definition is clearly arbitrary, it is based on the fact that families with multiple individuals with CLL are rare. Indeed, it is common for most patients to have 1 or 2 first- or second-degree relatives with this diagnosis, but some of the familial clustering can be very dramatic; this latter observation strongly suggests a nonrandom chance finding. A limitation of this definition is the frequent lack of confirmation of the CLL diagnosis in the relative (ie, the self-reported family history). The CLL patient may not actually have familial CLL but rather a family history of another lymphoproliferative disorder (eg, follicular or mantle cell lymphoma) because the blood relatives of CLL patients are at increased risk of other B-cell malignancies. Thus, based on the presence or absence of blood relatives with CLL, it is feasible to consider 2 types of CLL: sporadic CLL patients who have no blood relatives having CLL and familial CLL patients who do have blood relatives with CLL. In addition, there is recent evidence that blood relatives of familial CLL patients have an increased incidence of circulating B cells with a phenotype that is identical to CLL leukemic B cells (so-called MBL; see later section on MBL), as well as increased risk of other B-cell lymphomas.

Key points

- Blood relatives of CLL patients have an increased risk of B-cell malignancies.
- CLL amongst all leukemias has the highest incidence of blood relatives also having CLL.
- Relatives are still at very low risk of acquiring or having CLL.
- MBL is present at an increased frequency in familial CLL.
- CLL is a common leukemia in North America with a higher incidence in males.
- The disease is more common in whites and does not change when nonwhites migrate to North America.
- CLL patients have a high incidence of other B-cell malignancies such as lymphoma.
- Common clinical complications include infections, autoimmune disease, and skin malignancies.
- No increase in B-cell CLL is seen in individuals exposed to ionizing radiation.
- CLL affects the health of all patients, regardless of the age of the patient with CLL.

Diagnosis

Differential diagnosis: cytogenetic, immunophenotypic, and molecular aspects

Cytogenetic abnormalities are present in approximately 80% of CLL cases when fluorescence in situ hybridization (FISH) techniques are used. The FISH approach is usually needed because CLL B cells do not divide readily on stimulation. The most common FISH-detected abnormality is a deletion in chromosome 13 at band q14 (55% of cases), followed by a deletion in chromosome 11 at q22-23 (18%). Less common abnormalities and their frequencies include trisomy 12

(16%) and deletions in chromosome arm del(17p13.1) (7%) and 6q (6%). A normal karyotype is seen in 18% of cases; however, the incidence of FISH-detectable defects increases with advancing stage. These abnormalities have been shown to be of prognostic importance, with the isolated finding of del13q associated with a favorable prognosis, whereas the presence of del(17p13.1) or del(11q22.3) confers a poor prognosis with regard to disease course and OS (see Prognostic factors section).

The immunophenotypic pattern of the CLL cells is important in distinguishing this entity from other low-grade lymphoproliferative disorders (Table 19-1). The B-cell CLL cells always express the pan-B-cell markers CD19 and CD20, as well as CD5, a T-cell marker. In addition, CD23 is generally positive and FMC7 is negative, distinguishing this disorder from mantle cell lymphoma, which is usually CD23 negative and FMC7 positive. These cells variably express CD38 and do not express CD10, CD103, and cyclin D1. Surface markers CD22 and CD79b are either negative or weakly expressed. Surface immunoglobulin (Ig), usually IgM or IgM and IgD, and either κ or λ, is dim or weakly expressed. The presence of a monoclonal paraprotein, usually IgM, in the serum occurs in <5% of cases, although with more sensitive techniques, this incidence increases.

Increasing data on the molecular aspects of CLL have been reported over the past decade. The tumor protein p53 resides on chromosome del(17p13.1), which is of prognostic importance and is associated with poor clinical outcome. In 85% of cases, high levels of the Bcl-2 protein are found with associated hypomethylation of the promoter region of the *Bcl-2* gene. This protein suppresses apoptosis, resulting in longevity of the malignant CLL clone. Ig variable heavy chain genes (IgV_H) may be mutated or unmutated. Patients with mutated genes (~50%) tend to have a more indolent disease course and a better prognosis than patients without mutations. CD38 expression has been found to have limited correlation with mutational status. However, ZAP-70 expression has better correlation with unmutated gene status. More information on this is discussed in the section on prognostic factors.

Is there a minimum level of blood B cells necessary for diagnosis of CLL?

The level of absolute blood lymphocytes (regardless of lineage) required for a diagnosis of B-cell CLL has declined significantly over the last several decades from approximately 25×10^9/L to 5×10^9/L. Recently, the International Workshop on Chronic Lymphocytic Leukemia (IWCLL) has stated, "The diagnosis of CLL requires the presence of at least 5×10^9 B lymphocytes/L (5000/L) in the peripheral blood. The clonality of the circulating B lymphocytes needs to be confirmed by flow cytometry" (Hallek et al, 2008). Although this may be a distinct improvement on the requirement of 5×10^9 lymphocytes/L for a diagnosis of CLL, it is unclear whether this new guideline will clearly designate those individuals who truly have CLL with potential for disease progression and the attendant clinical complications. With the suggestion that there is now a threshold for leukemic B cells to diagnose CLL, several issues arise including the uniform use of a standard approach to detect cells with a CLL B-cell phenotype and whether that approach will truly best define CLL disease. A recent study found that with this IWCLL-recommended B-cell threshold, many CLL patients with Rai stage 0 disease, using the old definition of CLL, would now be considered as having MBL (see following section). Further work substantiating the exact level of both absolute B-cell count and lymphocyte count will be needed to confirm what the best absolute level is for both.

Monoclonal B-cell lymphocytosis

Using sensitive multicolor flow cytometry, >3% of normal individuals can be found to contain blood lymphocytes that have the phenotype of CLL B cells. Thus, they will exhibit the presence of CD19, CD5, and CD23; weak expression of CD20 and CD79b; and either κ or λ immunoglobulin light chains. High-sensitivity flow cytometry allows for the detection of B cells with a CLL phenotype in numbers as low as 1 in 10,000 normal leukocytes. With this method, CLL-phenotype cells have been found in >3% of adults with otherwise normal blood counts. Initially, a lymphocytosis with <5000 CLL-phenotype

	sIg	CD20	CD5	CD23	CD10	CD103
Chronic lymphocytic leukemia	Weak	Weak	+	+	−	−
Lymphoplasmacytic lymphoma	Mod	+	−/+	+/−	−	−
Mantle cell lymphoma	Mod	+	+	− (partial)	−	−
Marginal zone: nodal/MALT lymphoma	+	+	−	−/+	−	−
Splenic marginal zone lymphoma	+	+	−/+	−/+	−	−/+
Follicular lymphoma	+	+	−	−/+	+/−	−
Hairy cell leukemia	+	+	−	−	−	+

Table 19-1 Chronic B-cell lymphoproliferative disorders defined based on immunophenotype.

− or −/+ = negative or weak; MALT = mucosa-associated lymphoid tissue; sIg = surface immunoglobulin.

B cells per liter and an absence of symptoms of CLL was defined as CLL-phenotype MBL. More recently, this has been clarified to classify someone as having MBL; the individual can have no other features of a lymphoproliferative disorder (ie, no lymphadenopathy, organomegaly, or cytopenia). It was not clear whether MBL could progress to CLL, but several recent studies have found that approximately 1% of MBLs will progress to CLL per year. In addition, for individuals with lymphocytosis and MBL, the CLL B cells will exhibit novel biomarkers that have been associated with both adverse and favorable outcomes. Thus, FISH defects such as chromosome 13q deletion or del(17p13.1), CD38-positive cells, and both mutated- and unmutated-type clones can be found in MBL blood B cells. Although the exact clinical or laboratory profiles that will best predict progression to overt CLL are not yet completely defined, recent reports indicate that the absolute B-cell level and the finding that CLL B cells are CD38 positive seem to be most strongly associated with time to progression. Currently, best estimates are that although the disease progression is slow for MBL compared with Rai stage 0 CLL, the Kaplan-Meir curves reveal a continuing slope indicating that MBL and CLL may have a relationship similar to that of monoclonal gammopathy of unknown significance and myeloma. However, the incidence of MBL appears to be approximately 100 times higher than the incidence of CLL; therefore, for most people with MBL, a "true" CLL will not be diagnosed in their lifetime. Other important features of MBL include the following: MBL can be found in individuals without lymphocytosis, increases in MBL incidence occur with age, and there is a marked increase in MBL in the family members of patients with a diagnosis of familial CLL (see earlier section on familial CLL).

Key points

- Cytogenetic abnormalities are common in CLL patients and are of prognostic importance.
- Deletions in chromosomes 17p or 11q are associated with a poorer prognosis.
- The malignant clonal lymphocytes in B-cell CLL are CD19, CD20, CD5, and CD23 positive.
- Mutated IgV_H gene rearrangements confer a more favorable prognosis compared with unmutated gene status.
- There is a typical surface immunophenotype that distinguishes CLL from other indolent B-cell disorders.
- FISH-detectable defects are common even in early-stage disease and can be associated with risk for disease progression.
- At diagnosis, in addition to the use of traditional prognostic factors (ie, β_2-microglobulin and Rai stage), it is important to know about other cellular features such as CD38, ZAP-70, and the IgV_H status for prognostic counseling (see section on prognostic factors).
- There is a new B-cell count level suggested to define CLL: an absolute level of greater than or equal to 5×10^9 B-cells per L.
- MBL can be a precursor state for progression to overt CLL.

Clinical and laboratory features

The diagnosis of CLL is often an incidental finding, noted when an absolute lymphocytosis ($>5 \times 10^9$/L) with mature-appearing lymphocytes is found on a complete blood cell (CBC) count often done for other medical purposes. Patients may commonly be asymptomatic at time of diagnosis. Alternatively, approximately 20% of patients will present with classical B-symptoms, including fever, night sweats, significant weakness, and weight loss. Patients may also present with symptoms referable to increasing lymphadenopathy or hepatosplenomegaly or related to marrow replacement or autoimmune complications, such as fatigue, dyspnea, or bleeding issues. Recurrent bacterial infections may also herald disease onset. Physical examination should specifically focus on the presence of peripheral lymphadenopathy, hepatomegaly (20% of cases), and/or splenomegaly (30%–40% of cases). The organomegaly may range from mild to massive.

Laboratory features are most remarkable for the presence of the previously noted mature lymphocytosis. Smudge cells are commonly present on the peripheral blood smear. These cells are also called basket cells and appear to be ruptured cells. Interestingly, there are recent reports that the level of smudge cells as measured in the peripheral smear is associated with OS. Approximately one-third of patients will have anemia or thrombocytopenia at diagnosis, although these are usually mild in degree. Autoimmune complications are a known complication in these patients (see Autoimmune complications section). At time of diagnosis, approximately 25% of patients will have a positive direct Coombs test. Over the disease course, autoimmune hemolytic anemia will occur in 10% to 25% of patients, with immune thrombocytopenia in 15% to 20%. Neutropenia may also be present as a reflection of marrow involvement by CLL. Hypogammaglobulinemia is a hallmark of this disorder, with increasing prevalence and severity with increasing disease duration and disease stage. The bone marrow differential generally has at least 30% lymphocytes, and the marrow may be normocellular or hypercellular. Marrow involvement may be in a nodular, interstitial, or diffuse pattern.

Key points

- At presentation, patients with CLL are often asymptomatic; likewise, some may present with increasing lymphadenopathy or hepatosplenomegaly or classical B-symptoms (eg, fever, night sweats, weight loss).
- On peripheral blood smear, a predominance of mature lymphocytes may be seen, in addition to smudge cells.
- The bone marrow will reveal >30% lymphocytes and may be normo- or hypercellular, with involvement by CLL in a nodular, interstitial, or diffuse pattern.
- Hypogammaglobulinemia is a hallmark of this disease.

Staging

Almost 35 years ago, Rai and colleagues devised and published a clinical staging system that predicted the OS of patients with CLL. This staging system was based on data derived and extracted from essentially a physical examination and a hemogram. The Rai system was modified shortly to be only 3 stages consisting of low, intermediate, and high risk (Table 19-2). This system was matched almost simultaneously by the system from Binet and colleagues, which is able to determine the prognostic predictions for survival of CLL patients. Since then, these systems continue to be used in the clinical investigation of CLL. For the first time, these staging systems enabled clinical investigators to compare patient features between clinical trials and are still used as routine templates for most research-based clinical investigations. However, both of these staging systems have limitations, the most prominent of which is the inability to predict which early-stage CLL patients are at higher risk to progress. In addition, neither the Rai nor Binet system permits a modification of prognosis as the disease progresses. Finally, the use of computed tomography scans of chest, abdomen, and pelvis remain controversial in routine usage for staging CLL patients. Only clinical trial evaluation will ultimately determine their usefulness in managing CLL patient care.

> **Key points**
> - The Rai staging system is still a valid system for prognostic counseling but does not meaningfully address early-stage patients who may progress.
> - Currently, computed tomography scans are not routinely incorporated into CLL staging.

Prognostic factors

The case for prognostic factors in CLL

CLL is one of the most common lymphoid malignancies, accounting for approximately 14% of all hematologic neoplasms, and given its cumulative aspect, there are estimated to be approximately 150,000 individuals in the United States living with CLL. We also know that CLL patients have a significantly shorter life expectancy than age-matched individuals from the general population. Compounding the latter fact is the knowledge that perhaps 70% to 80% of CLL patients are now diagnosed as Rai stage 0 at presentation. These early-stage patients have a marked heterogeneity in clinical course ranging from indolent disease for decades to very rapid progressive disease within a few years. Because CLL is an incurable disease and we have evidence that treatment of unselected early-stage patients at the time of diagnosis offers no survival advantage compared with treatment at the time of disease progression, many hematologists prefer a "watch and wait" strategy.

This current strategy is being challenged by 2 important clinical aspects: first, approximately 40% of early-stage patients with high risk will experience disease progression, and second, many CLL patients even with early-stage disease have significant and regular anxiety about their untreated CLL. The use of prognostic markers to assist in directing even early-stage patients to clinical trials that use modern and nontoxic therapy would seem to be reasonable. In addition, the ability to counsel patients about their disease mandates the use of prognostic markers and even prognostic models that incorporate the traditional and novel biomarkers of CLL disease process.

Traditional prognostic factors

The clinical course of patients with CLL may be quite variable, with some patients having an accelerated course,

Table 19-2 Chronic lymphocytic leukemia (CLL) clinical staging systems.

Binet classification			Rai classification				Median overall survival (years)
Stage	Definition	Patients (%)	Risk group	Stage	Definition	Patients (%)	
A	[lt]3 lymphoid areas	60	Low	0	Lymphocytosis only	30	[mt]10
B	[mt]3 lymphoid areas	30	Intermediate	I	Lymphadenopathy	25	5–7
				II	Hepatomegaly or splenomegaly ± lymphadenopathy	25	
C	Hemoglobin [lt]10 g/dL or platelets [lt]100 × 10³/dL	10	High	III	Hemoglobin [lt]11 g/dL	10	1–3
				VI	Platelets [lt]100 × 10³/dL	10	

Two systems have been widely used to classify stage of progression of CLL: Rai and Binet staging. These systems define early (Rai 0, Binet A), intermediate (Rai I/II, Binet B), and advanced (Rai III/IV, Binet C) stages of CLL based on the extent of lymphoid area involvement and the presence of anemia and thrombocytopenia.
From Kokhaei P, Palma M, Mellstedt H, Choudhury A. Biology and treatment of chronic lymphocytic leukemia. *Ann Oncol.* 2005;16 (Suppl 2):ii113–ii123.

whereas others have a more indolent process. Prior to the development of the newer molecular and genetic markers, a series of traditional prognostic factors were recognized. Median survival has been found to correlate with clinical stage, being >13 years with Rai stage 0 disease, 8 years for stage I disease, 6 years for stage II disease, 2 to 6 years for stage III disease, and 1.5 to 4 years for stage IV disease. A diffuse pattern of marrow involvement also portends a poorer prognosis than a nodular or interstitial pattern of involvement. A rapid lymphocyte doubling time (LDT) (<12 months) is also associated with a poorer prognosis than an LDT >1 year. Other poor prognostic factors (in some but not all series) include male sex, initial lymphocytosis of >50 × 10^9/L, elevated serum β_2-microglobulin, elevated serum lactate dehydrogenase, elevated serum thymidine kinase, and advanced age.

Novel biomarker prognostic factors in assessing high-risk subgroups of patients with CLL

Prognostic factors for determining CLL patients with high-risk disease are now clearly emerging as valuable tools for the patient and clinician. Even in early-stage CLL, approximately 50% of patients will exhibit high-risk prognostic biomarkers. The classical staging systems of Rai and Binet play a critical role in determining the natural course of the disease and the need for therapy but do not predict for the likelihood of disease progression among patients with early-stage disease (ie, Rai stage 0 or Binet stage A). Accurate prediction of disease outcome in early-stage disease is needed because >20% of patients eventually die of CLL-related causes, approximately 30% of patients with CLL are <65 years of age, and approximately 12% are <55 years of age. Even more concerning is that younger patients (for example, those <55 years old) appear to have a significantly higher risk of dying of CLL-related causes compared with older patients. Although the traditional prognostic parameters (reviewed later) are still helpful, novel biomarkers have provided significant insight into the biology of the disease and appear to be accurate predictors of disease progression and time to therapy even for early-stage disease. These biomarkers include the mutational status of the variable region of the Ig heavy chain (IgV_H), CD38, CD49d, ZAP-70, and genomic abnormalities most commonly detected by FISH (Table 19-3).

Table 19-3 Summary of potential outcomes associated with key prognostic markers* in patients with CLL.

Prognostic markers	Early-stage, previously untreated, or asymptomatic disease	Progressive disease requiring therapy	Advanced-stage or relapsed/refractory disease[†]
17p deletion[‡]	Disease progression, need for therapy, decreased OS	Decreased response to alkylators or F-based therapy; decreased PFS and OS to F-based therapy	Decreased TTP and OS with salvage FCR[d] or other chemotherapy
11q deletion	Disease progression, need for therapy, decreased OS	Decreased response to alkylators or F monotherapy; decreased PFS to F-based therapy	Decreased TTP and OS with salvage FCR therapy[§]
Unmutated IgV_H	Disease progression, need for therapy, decreased PFS and OS	Decreased response to alkylators; decreased response, PFS, and OS to F-based therapy; clinical relapse with auto-SCT	MRD-positive relapse and clinical relapse with auto-SCT
ZAP-70$^+$	Disease progression, need for therapy, decreased OS	Decreased response, PFS, and OS to F-based therapy	
CD38$^+$	Disease progression, need for therapy, decreased OS	Decreased response and PFS to F-based therapy	
Elevated β_2-microglobulin	Disease progression, decreased OS		Decreased TTP and OS with FCR therapy

*Outcomes associated with these prognostic markers are primarily based on univariate analysis and data from retrospective analyses outside of clinical trials.
[†]Patients with advanced-stage or fludarabine-refractory disease should be considered at high risk for disease progression and decreased survival regardless of other prognostic markers.
[‡]The presence of 17p− alone may be considered high risk for rapid disease progression and decreased survival in all clinical situations.
[§]In the study of salvage FCR therapy, genomic abnormalities were categorized only as unfavorable (ie, 17p−, 11q−, trisomy 12, or complex) versus favorable (normal or 13q− as the sole abnormality); unfavorable genomic abnormalities were an independent predictor of decreased TTP and OS in the multivariate analysis (Kay NE, O'Brien SM, Pettitt AR, Stilgenbauer S. The role of prognostic factors in assessing 'high-risk' subgroups of patients with chronic lymphocytic leukemia. *Leukemia*. 2007;21:1885–1891).
Auto-SCT = autologous stem cell transplantation; CLL = chronic lymphocytic leukemia; F = fludarabine; FCR = fludarabine, cyclophosphamide, and rituximab; MRD = minimal residual disease; OS = overall survival; PFS = progression-free survival; TTP = time to progression.

IgV_H mutation

IgV_H mutational status identifies 2 subgroups of CLL patients with different clinical outcomes and is predictive of survival in patients with CLL. In general, patients with mutated IgV_H constitute approximately 30% to 60% of CLL cases and have favorable outcomes, with a median survival of 10 to 20 years from time of diagnosis; however, patients with unmutated IgV_H have significantly poorer clinical courses, with a median survival of 5 to 10 years from diagnosis. This biomarker has a negative prognostic impact on survival even for patients with early-stage (ie, Binet stage A) CLL. Unmutated IgV_H has also been associated with decreased progression-free survival (PFS) among patients with early-stage, asymptomatic disease (from the CLL1 study of the German CLL Study Group). In addition, unmutated IgV_H has been associated with decreased PFS and OS in patients treated with upfront fludarabine-based combination regimens. The induction of durable minimal residual disease–negative remissions, even in patients with unmutated IgV_H status, have been shown for patients who do undergo allogeneic stem cell transplantation (SCT). This is likely due to the graft-versus-leukemia effect induced by allogeneic SCT. Determination of the mutational status is labor intensive and may not yet be practical in the routine clinical setting.

CD38, CD49d, and ZAP-70

It is likely that patients with an IgV_H status will be both CD38 and ZAP-70 positive, but this is not always true. CD38 is a cell surface antigen expressed on various hematopoietic and nonhematopoietic cells, including expression on B cells. Damle et al (1999) first showed that high levels of CD38 expression (CD38$^+$ in ≥30% of CLL cells) were found to significantly correlate with unmutated IgV_H, and this has been confirmed by subsequent studies. In several studies, CD38$^+$ predicted for both significantly shorter PFS (~3 years from diagnosis) and OS (~8–10 years from diagnosis). The use of CD38$^+$ status appears to also be useful for early-stage disease in that the association of decreased survival with CD38$^+$ has been found among patients with low- to intermediate-risk CLL, including those with previously untreated disease. Recent studies reported that CD38$^+$ was associated with decreased response and/or significantly shorter PFS in patients treated with first-line fludarabine-based therapy. The expression of CD38 is detectable by flow cytometry and therefore may be a more accessible alternative to determining IgV_H mutational status. Some confounding factors for CD38 as a surrogate marker for IgV_H status include that CD38 levels may change by >10% during the course of disease in a portion of patients but are only likely to alter the CD38 positivity status in very few patients; in addition, the relationship between CD38 and IgV_H status has been reported to be discordant in up to one third of CLL cases. Finally, CD38 expression is associated with other markers of cellular activation, including CD49d. CD49d is a cell surface antigen that functions at least as a cell adhesion molecule. Recent work has found that high expression of CD49d predicts for decreased survival outcomes in patients with CLL, and the cutoff value of 45% determined by flow cytometry can be used to best predict disease outcome for these patients.

ZAP-70 is an intracellular tyrosine kinase involved in normal T-cell signaling that was believed to be aberrantly expressed in CLL B cells. More recent work has found that ZAP-70 is expressed in normal activated tonsillar and splenic B cells. ZAP-70 was found to be highly predictive of IgV_H mutational status, with prognostic significance comparable to that of IgV_H status; patients with ZAP-70–positive CLL had a median survival of 8 to 9 years from the time of diagnosis compared with 24 years among patients with a ZAP-70–negative CLL. However, discordance in ZAP-70/IgV_H status has been found in >20% of CLL cases, which suggests that patients with ZAP-70 positivity may have worse outcomes regardless of IgV_H mutational status. The discordance may be explained by the more frequent occurrence of the del(11q22.3) and del(17p13.1) deletions (more high-risk FISH defects) among discordant cases with ZAP-70 negativity/unmutated IgV_H. The need for standardization of ZAP-70 assays makes this less available as a routine clinical assay, and until there is consensus on the methodology for measuring this parameter, the results for ZAP-70 in a particular patient needs to be viewed with caution.

Fluorescence in situ hybridization

Genomic abnormalities detected by interphase cytogenetic assays such as FISH are important prognostic indicators in CLL (Figure 19-2). In a landmark study, common recurring genetic abnormalities were placed in risk categories in a hierarchical model. Thus, from the worst clinical outcome to best outcome, the model proposed a progression of del(17p13.1), del(11q22.3), trisomy 12q, normal, and 13q– that differed significantly in terms of disease progression and OS. Notably, del(17p13.1) and del(11q22.3) were highly predictive of decreased survival, with patients with del(17p13.1) having the poorest outcomes with significantly shorter treatment-free interval (median, 9 months from diagnosis) and OS (median, 32 months from diagnosis) compared with other risk categories. FISH-detectable poor prognosis aberrations such as del(17p13.1) and del(11q22.3) have been found to be present in early-stage, untreated patients with CLL and have been associated with decreased PFS even among those with asymptomatic disease. The del(17p13.1) and del(11q22.3) abnormalities appear to be seen most often in patients with unmutated IgV_H status. Genomic aberrations detectable by FISH, including those known to be high-risk aberrations,

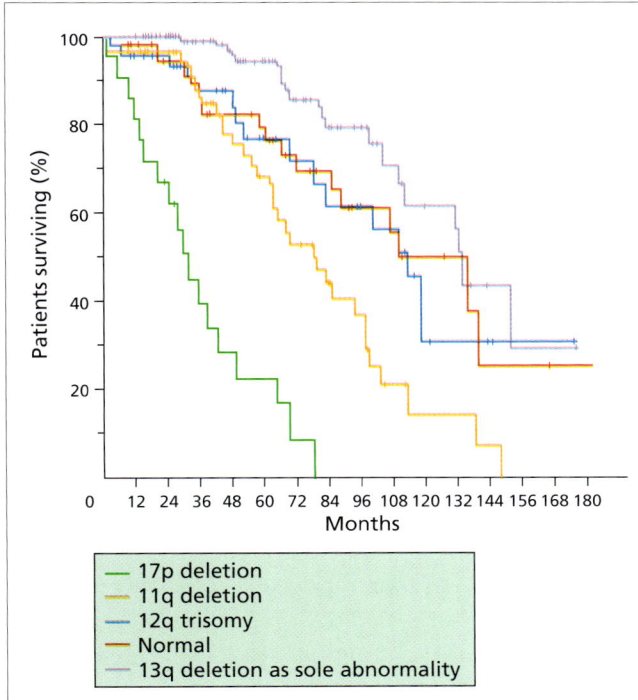

Figure 19-2 Probability of survival from the date of diagnosis among the patients in the 5 genetic categories. The median survival times for the groups with 17p deletion, 11q deletion, 12q trisomy, normal karyotype, and 13q deletion as the sole abnormality were 32, 79, 114, 111, and 133 months, respectively. Twenty-five patients with various other chromosomal abnormalities are not included in the analysis. From Dohner H, Stilgenbauer S, Benner A, et al. Genomic aberrations and survival in chronic lymphocytic leukemia. *N Engl J Med.* 2000;343:1910–1916.

may change over time during the course of disease in a given patient; one study, over a 5-year period, estimated that this may occur in 25% of patients with CLL.

Importantly, the presence of FISH-detected abnormalities has been shown to affect treatment outcomes in CLL. Recent information has demonstrated that del(17p13.1) and del(11q22.3) defects were significantly predictive of poorer response and shorter PFS and OS among patients with CLL treated with first-line fludarabine-based regimens. Treatment with single-agent alemtuzumab has been shown to be effective in patients with del(17p13.1) or *p53* mutations, even among patients with fludarabine-refractory CLL, suggesting that the use of FISH assays can help direct treatment choice.

Practical use of prognostic markers (traditional or novel) for newly diagnosed CLL versus previously treated or relapsed/refractory CLL

The ability of newer prognostic markers to predict outcomes is largely dependent on the clinical situation of each patient. A prognostic marker that may be useful in predicting disease progression in a patient with early-stage, previously untreated CLL may not be similarly predictive for this end point in a patient with previously treated, relapsed, and/or refractory disease. In addition, prognostic markers will likely predict for different end points, such as disease progression, OS, and/or resistance to therapy, and some markers may be predictive for several end points. To add to the complexity, prognostic markers may overlap in terms of ability to predict outcome, and the significance of a marker may not always be independent of the presence of other markers (hence, the absolute need to incorporate multivariate regression analysis in clinical studies). Moreover, it is plausible that different prognostic markers may be combined to provide a more refined approach to risk stratification. Currently, the novel prognostic markers, such as high-risk FISH defects [(del(17p13.1) and del(11q22.3)] and/or the presence of an unmutated IgV_H status, have clearly defined the likelihood of less effective responses to even the most aggressive of treatment approaches in CLL. However, it remains unclear whether individual patients are usefully served at diagnosis by the addition of newer prognostic variables such as CD38, IgV_H mutational status, or ZAP-70 to standard clinical measures such as LDT or Rai stage. As a result, it is important to continue to assess the helpfulness of these markers individually and collectively in the management of CLL patients. To this end, in the following sections, we review recent prognostic models that have been tested in CLL patients.

Prognostic models

Following are brief descriptions of models that use both traditional prognostic factors as well as more novel prognostic factors. The models are not completely definitive but are currently the best defined multivariate models for use in CLL.

Multivariate model using traditional prognostic factors

There has been a strong effort to develop a simple method of risk stratification in CLL where it would be feasible to use easily available parameters. Thus, an initial report in a large series of patients identified 6 factors (age, absolute lymphocyte count, sex, β_2-microglobulin, clinical stage, and number of nodal regions involved) and found that they were independently associated with patient survival. These factors were then combined in a prognostic index that was able to predict survival more accurately than clinical stage alone. This prognostic index was subsequently validated in an independent series of patients, further demonstrating that the index remained useful when applied exclusively to Rai stage 0 patients; in addition, it was able to predict time to treatment and OS.

Multivariate models using novel biomarkers

Recent studies using multivariate analyses have revealed the differential prognostic impacts of the newer prognostic markers depending on the covariates that were available for analysis. Both ZAP-70 and CD38 were significant independent prognostic factors for PFS in a multivariate regression model that included age, modified Rai stage, β_2-microglobulin, and soluble CD23; however, for analyses of survival, only ZAP-70 remained a significant prognostic indicator. In other studies, IgV_H mutational status, but not CD38, remained significantly predictive of decreased survival in a multivariate regression model that included, among other covariates, presence of genomic abnormalities. Various models consistently show that high-risk genomic alterations [ie, del(17p13.1), del(11q22.3)] and an unmutated IgV_H status are highly predictive of a poor clinical outcome. Multivariate analyses have also shown that 4 genetic subgroups based on risk models can be determined in order of poorer to better survival outcomes—presence of del(17p13.1) (regardless of IgV_H mutational status), presence of del(11q22.3) [no del(17p13.1) but regardless of IgV_H mutational status], unmutated IgV_H [no del(17p13.1) or del(11q22.3)], and mutated IgV_H [no del(17p13.1) or del(11q22.3)]. Importantly, the genetic risk categories used in this model were also applicable to patients with early-stage disease. For the most part, high-risk features have been assessed within the context of progressive disease requiring therapy, but increasingly, the novel biomarkers are showing high risk in early-stage CLL. Several studies in patients with early-stage, previously untreated CLL found that approximately 25% to 50% of patients will have high-risk features, including del(17p13.1) or del(11q22.3). It is generally found that the presence of del(17p13.1) alone can be considered a high-risk feature predictive of disease progression and/or potential resistance to alkylating agents and purine analog–based therapies. Data from ongoing phase III trials in patients with previously untreated CLL receiving fludarabine-based treatment have demonstrated the negative prognostic impact of several of the markers discussed earlier, including the presence of del(17p13.1) (decreased response, PFS, or OS), del(11q22.3) (decreased response or PFS), and unmutated IgV_H (decreased response or PFS). However, the frequency of del(17p13.1) is much lower in patients with early-stage or asymptomatic disease compared with patients with more advanced stages of CLL. In addition, the presence of del(17p13.1) in early-stage CLL does not always predict for a more aggressive disease course.

> **Key points**
>
> - Approximately 70% to 80% of CLL patients are now diagnosed as Rai stage 0 at presentation.
> - Early-stage CLL patients can progress more rapidly than predicted even if designated as stage 0.
> - Both novel and traditional prognostic markers can be a resource for more accurate predictions of early-stage CLL clinical outcome.
> - Unmutated-type clones more frequently also express high-risk features such as ZAP-70 and FISH defects such as del(17p13.1).
> - Genetic defects detected by FISH are the only novel biomarkers that may change dramatically as the disease progresses.
> - Certain high-risk, FISH-detectable defects, such as del(17p13.1) and del(11q22.3), are associated with poor outcome even to aggressive combination therapies.
> - Models using either traditional or novel biomarkers are now becoming available to help counsel patients.

Therapy

Initial therapy

Approaches to the initial therapy of the patient with CLL have undergone an evolution over the past several decades (Table 19-4). For 50 years, alkylating agents were the backbone of therapy for these disorders. With the introduction of the purine analogs in the 1990s, these agents came into general use for initial therapy. Over the past decade, combination chemoimmunotherapy approaches have been examined, adding agents such as rituximab and alkylators to the purine analog backbone of therapy. Alemtuzumab represented an alternative agent not only for initial therapy, but also for eradication of minimal residual disease. Most recently, bendamustine has been added to the therapeutic armamentarium for these patients.

Alkylator-based therapy

Alkylator-based therapy consisting of single-agent chlorambucil or, less commonly, cyclophosphamide has been used for many years. This therapy has been given alone or in combination with corticosteroids despite the lack of a survival advantage with the addition of this agent. Chlorambucil has been administered in a variety of schedules, including daily administration (0.1 mg/kg/d) and pulse intermittent dosing (0.4–1.0 mg/kg every 3 to 4 weeks). Although symptomatic improvement, including reduction in lymphadenopathy and organomegaly, is generally seen, with overall response rates ranging from 38% to 75%, there is only a 3% to 5% complete response (CR) rate, with recurrent disease after discontinuation of therapy and no survival advantage noted. Toxicities include myelosuppression and risk for therapy-related dysplasia with long-term use. This therapy is still used for many elderly patients due to its tolerability.

Table 19-4 Initial therapy of CLL: response results.

Schema	ORR	CR	nPR	PR
US-Canadian Intergroup Trial (CALGB 9011)*				
Fludarabine, 25 mg/m^2/d, Days 1–5	63%	20%	–	43%
Chlorambucil, 40 mg/m^2, Day 1	37%	4%	–	33%
Fludarabine + rituximab, concurrent/sequential (CALGB 9712)[†]				
Concurrent: fludarabine 25 mg/m^2/d, days 1–5, plus rituximab 375 mg/m^2/d, days 1+4 (cycle 1), then day 1 (cycles 2–6)	90%	47%	–	43%
Sequential: fludarabine, fludarabine + cyclophosphamide, followed by rituximab 375 mg/m^2/d, weekly × 4, repeated every 6 months	77%	28%	–	49%
Fludarabine + cyclophosphamide vs fludarabine (E2997)[‡]				
Fludarabine 20 mg/m^2/d, days 1–5 + cyclophosphamide 600 mg/m^2/d, day 1	74%	23%	–	50%
Fludarabine 25 mg/m^2/d, days 1–5	59%	5%	–	55%
Fludarabine + cyclophosphamide + rituximab (M.D. Anderson Cancer Center)[§]				
Fludarabine 25 mg/m^2/d, days 2–4 (cycle 1)/days 1–3 (cycles 2–6); cyclophosphamide 250 mg/m^2/d, days 2–4 (cycle 1)/days 1–3 (cycles 2–6); rituximab 375 mg/m^2/d, day 1 (cycle 1), 500 mg/m^2/d, day 1 (cycles 2–6)	95%	70%	10%	15%
Single-agent rituximab, first-line and maintenance therapy[‖]				
Rituximab 375 mg/m^2/d, days 1, 8, 15, and 22, followed by rituximab 375 mg/m^2/d, weekly × 4, every 6 months (for 2 years)	58%	9%	–	49%
Alemtuzumab vs chlorambucil[¶]				
Alemtuzumab 30 mg IV, thrice weekly for a maximum of 12 weeks	83%	24%	–	59%
Chlorambucil 40 mg/m^2/d, day 1	55%	2%	–	53%

*Rai KR, Peterson B, Appelbaum FR, et al. Fludarabine compared with chlorambucil as primary therapy for chronic lymphocytic leukemia. *N Engl J Med*. 2000;343:1750–1757.
[†]Byrd JC, Peterson BL, Morrison VA, et al. Randomized phase 2 study of fludarabine with concurrent versus sequential treatment with rituximab in symptomatic, untreated patients with B-cell chronic lymphocytic leukemia: results from Cancer and Leukemia Group B 9712 (CALGB 9712). *Blood*. 2003;101:6–14.
[‡]Flinn IW, Neuberg D, Grever MR, et al. Phase III trial of fludarabine plus cyclophosphamide compared with fludarabine for patients with previously untreated chronic lymphocytic leukemia: US Intergroup Trial E2997. *J Clin Oncol*. 2007;25:793–798.
[§]Keating MJ, O'Brien S, Albitar M, et al: Early results of a chemoimmunotherapy regimen of fludarabine, cyclophosphamide, and rituximab as initial therapy for chronic lymphocytic leukemia. *J Clin Oncol*. 2005;23:4079–4088.
[‖]Hainsworth JD, Litchy S, Barton JH, et al. Single-agent rituximab as first-line and maintenance treatment for patients with chronic lymphocytic leukemia or small lymphocytic lymphoma: a phase II trial of the Minnie Pearl Cancer Research Network. *J Clin Oncol*. 2003;21:1746–1751.
[¶]Hillmen P, Skotnicki A, Robak T, et al. Alemtuzumab compared with chlorambucil as first-line therapy for chronic lymphocytic leukemia. *J Clin Oncol*. 2007;25:5616–5623.
CALGB = Cancer and Leukemia Group B; CLL = chronic lymphocytic leukemia; CR = complete response; IV, intravenous; nPR = nodular partial response; ORR = overall response rate; PR = partial response.

Purine analogs

Although all 3 purine analogs (fludarabine, 2-chlorodeoxyadenosine, and pentostatin) have been studied in the treatment of CLL, fludarabine has gained the widest usage. Overall response rates range from 40% to 65%, with CR rates of 15% to 30% mostly based on nonrandomized phase II studies. The addition of prednisone to fludarabine therapy did not alter the response rate but resulted in an increased frequency of opportunistic infections. Several large prospective randomized trials compared the efficacy of fludarabine to alkylator-based regimens for the initial therapy of CLL patients. Fludarabine resulted in higher overall response and CR rates, as well as prolonged remission durations and PFS; however, no OS advantage has been seen with the use of this agent. The main toxicities of this agent are myelosuppression, fever, and infections, with the latter related to the drug's impact on cell-mediated immune function.

Rituximab

The anti-CD20 antibody rituximab has gained widespread use in the therapy of lymphoproliferative disorders including CLL. As a single agent, overall response rates are approximately 50% for previously untreated CLL, but for previously treated CLL, they are approximately 10% to 20% with <5% CRs. This may be related to the dim expression of CD20 on the surface of the malignant lymphocyte. This agent has also been studied in a dose-escalated manner with slightly higher response rates seen.

Combination purine analog–based chemotherapy and chemoimmunotherapy

With the impressive clinical results seen with the purine analogs, the next step has been to examine these agents as part of combination regimens. The combination of fludarabine plus cyclophosphamide (FC) had been compared with fludarabine alone in 3 large randomized phase III trials. In all of these trials, therapy with FC resulted in an improved overall response rate and CR rate and prolongation in PFS, although not in OS. However, this combination regimen is associated with more myelosuppression. In addition, only a small number of elderly patients were enrolled on these trials; thus, tolerability data in these patients are limited.

Fludarabine plus rituximab (FR) therapy has been studied in concurrent and sequential schedules. The CR rate was higher with concurrent versus sequential therapy (47% vs 33%, respectively), and despite more neutropenia with the concurrent regimen, no increase in infections was noted. When the FR regimen was compared with the single-agent fludarabine arm on the prior US Intergroup trial, FR was advantageous with regard to overall response rate (84% vs 63%), CR rate (38% vs 20%), 2-year PFS rate (67% vs 45%), and 2-year OS rate (93% vs 81%).

Lastly, the combination of fludarabine, cyclophosphamide, and rituximab (FCR) has been studied as initial CLL therapy. With a median follow-up of 6 years, overall response rate is 95%, with a 72% CR rate in the latest reports. Median time to progression is 80 months, with a 6-year failure-free survival rate of 51% and 6-year OS rate of 77%. In addition, molecular remissions were demonstrated in >40% of patients achieving a CR. In this single-institution setting, toxicities, including infectious complications, were manageable. At the present time, the FCR and FR regimens are being compared in the prospective phase III intergroup setting.

Although there has yet to be reported a randomized trial comparing FR to FCR, the recently completed German CLL Study Group CLL 8 trial suggests that FCR appears to be superior to FC combination therapy. The CR rate and time to disease progression were both significantly better for FCR-treated patients than FC-treated patients. However, it should be noted that the CR rate in the FCR arm of the CLL 8 trial was 44.5%, which is substantially lower than the 72% CR rate in the phase II experience of the M.D. Anderson Cancer Center. In this regard, the CR rate of the FCR arm of CLL 8 does not appear substantially different than the 47% CR rate in the multicenter, randomized, phase II trial of FR conducted by the Cancer and Leukemia Group B.

Other purine analogs

Two other purine analogs are pentostatin (deoxycoformycin) and cladribine. Pentostatin inhibits the enzyme adenosine deaminase, interfering with the cell's ability to process DNA. Cladribine, another purine analog (2-chlorodeoxyadenosine [2CDA]), is also postulated to work via inhibition of adenosine deaminase. Both of these drugs have been used for the treatment of hairy cell leukemia and CLL. The clinical activity of pentostatin in lymphoid malignancies was first noted in several case reports published in the early 1980s. Single-agent pentostatin was noted to be safe and active in advanced-stage and refractory patients in the initial phase I and II studies using a dose of 4 mg/m^2 given every 1 to 2 weeks. These responses were typically partial with few CRs. However, Kay and colleagues have used pentostatin with cyclophosphamide and rituximab (PCR) in the treatment of previously untreated CLL. This regimen generated a >90% overall response rate with a 41% CR rate, 22% nodular partial response rate, and 27% partial response rate. This regimen was equally effective in patients who were younger or older than 70 years of age. Patients who achieved a CR had a median duration of remission of 35.6 months. Despite treating a high-risk CLL cohort with advanced Rai stage, 71% were IgV_H, 34% were CD38 positive and ZAP-70 positive, and 36% had high-risk cytogenetics by FISH analysis. The regimen was also well tolerated with no evidence of excessive morbidity.

An initial study using combination pentostatin with cyclophosphamide (pentostatin at a dose of 4 mg/m^2 with cyclophosphamide at doses of 600 mg/m^2) was performed in patients with previously treated CLL. In this study, 23 patients with previously treated CLL achieved 17 responses (74%), including 4 CRs (17%), and toxicity appeared favorable. Building on this, a PCR combination was also tested for previously treated CLL. In 46 heavily pretreated patients, PCR was well tolerated with grade 3/4 toxicities limited to neutropenia, thrombocytopenia, and infection seen in 53%, 16%, and 28% of patients, respectively. This regimen was very active, with 75% of CLL patients achieving objective responses and 25% achieving a CR. The median response duration was 25 months, and OS was 44 months. Other combinations being tested with pentostatin include the addition of mitoxantrone to PCR regimens (PCRM). PCRM was administered to previously treated patients with CLL, and initial results suggest that it is very active, with an overall response rate of >90% observed, with approximately a quarter of the patients achieving a CR. With both PCR and PCRM, responses were achieved in patients who had previously been treated with fludarabine and/or were refractory to it. This suggests that the use of pentostatin-based regimens can be effective in some cases of relapsed/refractory CLL previously treated with fludarabine. Thus, pentostatin-based combination regimens have considerable activity for both previously untreated and relapsed/refractory CLL and can certainly be an option for previously treated CLL patients. Table 19-5 summarizes some recent pentostatin-based trials for upfront and salvage treatment options for CLL patients.

Cladribine has received less attention in CLL, but there are several recent reports that suggest that it has activity in combinations for this disease. Phase II and III studies of cladribine monotherapy achieved similar clinical responses as alkylating agent–based treatments, but cladribine was associated with more cytopenias and immune suppression. Thus, in one study, there was a retrospective comparison of the efficacy and toxicity of 2CDA plus cyclophosphamide (CC regimen) in 20 patients with previously untreated B-cell CLL who all had a del(17p13.1) deletion. This trial of the CC regimen consisted of 2CDA at a dose of 0.12 mg/kg and cyclophosphamide at a dose of 250 mg/m^2 given intravenously for 3 consecutive days, and cycles were repeated at 28-day intervals for up to 6 cycles; 16 (80%) of 20 patients responded to CC, 10 patients (50%) obtained a CR and 6 patients (30%) obtained a PR. Treatment toxicity was believed to be acceptable, with infection, the most common grade 3/4 complication, seen in 6 patients. Ongoing phase III trials are comparing cladribine to fludarabine-containing regimens, and these data will be of interest given the recent clinical information from the CC regimen.

Alemtuzumab

Alemtuzumab, an anti-CD52 monoclonal antibody, is now approved for initial therapy of CLL, based on a trial in which it demonstrated superior outcome results compared with chlorambucil. Alemtuzumab has also been incorporated into a variety of combination therapy regimens, in some as part of

Table 19-5 Recent pentostatin-based trials for upfront and salvage treatment options for CLL patients.

Schema	ORR, No. (%)	CR, No. (%)	nPR, No. (%)	PR, No. (%)
Pentostatin 4 mg/m^2, cyclophosphamide 600 mg/m^2, and rituximab 375 mg/m^2 every 21 days for 6 cycles*†	24 (75)	8 (25)	1 (3)	15 (47)
Pentostatin 4 mg/m^2, cyclophosphamide 600 mg/m^2, rituximab 375 mg/m^2 (omitted from cycle 1), mitoxantrone (dose escalated in phase I portion starting at 6, 8, and 10 mg/m^2) all administered on day 1 of 28-day cycles for a total of 6 treatments*‡	15 (94)	4 (25)	0	11 (69)
Pentostatin 2 mg/m^2, cyclophosphamide 600 mg/m^2, and rituximab 375 mg/m^2 for 6 cycles§‖	58 (91)	26 (41)	14 (22)	18 (28)
Pentostatin 4 mg/m^2 and rituximab given every 21 days; rituximab was given at 100 mg/m^2 IV at day 1, then 375 mg/m^2 IV on days 3 and 5 of the first treatment cycle; during cycles 2 to 6, rituximab was given at 375 mg/m^2 as a single IV infusion on day 1 of weeks 4, 7, 10, 13 and 16; total of 6 cycles§¶	26 (79)	9 (30)	0	19 (49)
Pentostatin 4 mg/m^2, cyclophosphamide 600 mg/m^2, and rituximab 375 mg/m^2 (PCR) every 21 d for 6 cycles followed by Campath (CA). Campath is either short-term CA (4 weeks) or longer-term CA (18 weeks) depending upon PCR response[b,#]	17 (46%)	0	0	17 (46%)

*Previously treated.

†Lamanna N, Kalaycio M, Maslak P, et al. Pentostatin, cyclophosphamide, and rituximab is an active, well-tolerated regimen for patients with previously treated chronic lymphocytic leukemia. *J Clin Oncol.* 2006;24:1575–1581.

‡Lamanna N, Heaney ML, Brentjens RJ, Jurcic JG, Weiss MA. Pentostatin, cyclophosphamide, rituximab, and mitoxantrone (PCRM): a new highly active regimen for patients with chronic lymphocytic leukemia (CLL) previously treated with PCR or FCR. *Blood.* 2007;110(11):3115.

§Previously untreated.

‖Kay NE, Geyer SM, Call TG, et al. Combination chemoimmunotherapy with pentostatin, cyclophosphamide, and rituximab shows significant clinical activity with low accompanying toxicity in previously untreated B chronic lymphocytic leukemia. *Blood.* 2007;109:405–411.

¶Kay N, Wu W, Byrd JC, et al. Cyclophosphamide remains an important component of treatment in CLL patients receiving pentostatin and rituximab based chemoimmunotherapy. *Blood.* 2008;12(11):43.

#Kay NE, Kim HT, Kempin S, et al. Predictors of clinical outcome to pentostatin, cyclophosphamide and rituximab (PCR) followed by Campath for relapsed/refractory CLL: a study of the Eastern Cooperative Oncology Group, E2903. *Blood.* 2008;112(Abstract):387.

Data from Lamanna N, Kay NE. Pentostatin treatment combinations in chronic lymphocytic leukemia. *Clin Adv Hematol Oncol.* 2009;7:386–392.

CLL = chronic lymphocytic leukemia; CR = complete response; IV, intravenous; nPR = nodular partial response; ORR = overall response rate; PCR = pentostatin, cyclophosphamide, and rituximab; PR = partial response.

consolidation therapy after fludarabine-based induction therapy. This agent appears to be more effective in eradicating peripheral blood and marrow disease than in clearing bulky nodal disease. In addition, achievement of minimal residual disease may be achieved with alemtuzumab. It may be administered by either a subcutaneous or intravenous route, with the latter associated with risk of infusion reactions. The most significant toxicity of alemtuzumab is associated infectious complications, especially with regard to cytomegalovirus (CMV) reactivation, which is estimated to occur in 15% to 25% of patients. Routine antiviral, antifungal, and *Pneumocystis* prophylaxis is generally used. In addition, Epstein-Barr virus–positive lymphoproliferative disorders have been reported in alemtuzumab-treated patients. In preliminary studies, this agent appears to have activity in CLL patients with deletions in chromosome arm del(17p13.1).

Bendamustine

Bendamustine is a bifunctional agent, with both an alkylating group and a purine-like benzamidazole ring. In a randomized phase II trial, bendamustine was compared with chlorambucil for initial CLL therapy. Not only were the overall response and CR rates higher with bendamustine (59% vs 26% and 27% vs 2%, respectively), but median PFS was also prolonged with this agent (18 vs 6 months, respectively). This agent was well tolerated, with myelosuppression being the most common adverse effect. Infusion reactions may also occur. Bendamustine was recently approved for use as initial therapy of CLL in the United States. Bendamustine is now being studied in clinical trials in combination with rituximab for previously untreated and relapsed/refractory CLL patients.

> **Key points**
>
> - There has been an evolution in the treatment approach to CLL over the past 5 decades, with initial therapy with alkylator-based therapy, such as chlorambucil, changing to purine analog–based therapy, especially fludarabine.
> - Building on the fludarabine backbone, other active agents, such as rituximab and cyclophosphamide, have been studied in combination regimens, resulting in improved therapeutic outcomes.
> - Alemtuzumab may be used as initial therapy or as an agent for consolidation in an attempt to achieve a state of minimal residual disease.
> - Bendamustine is the newest approved agent for the therapy of CLL.
> - The purine analogs, as well as alemtuzumab, have unique effects on cell-mediated immunity, resulting in opportunistic infectious complications, with implications for prophylactic antimicrobial therapy.
> - Hematopoietic SCT is an option for therapy of CLL patients, although it has limitations.

Relapsed/refractory CLL: workup and treatment options

The dilemma for CLL patients who have relapsed or are refractory to prior treatments is the significant drug resistance of the residual leukemic B cells. In addition, the patients are often suffering from residual marrow toxicity and immune suppression, which result in increased rates of infections that can often be opportunistic in nature (see later section, Infectious complications). Nevertheless, there are treatment options for these patients, including combination agents and novel single-agent approaches. These will be briefly reviewed here, and we will begin with some general considerations when treating relapsed CLL patients.

The approach to reinitiating therapy for CLL patients who have relapsed after initial therapy is similar to that applied for initial therapy assessment. Patients should have an indication for treatment with the indications discussed earlier for previously untreated CLL because previously treated CLL patients may acquire additional cytogenetic abnormalities, in particular del(17p13.1) or other FISH-detectable defects including complex abnormalities (ie, 2 defects rather than 1). It has been estimated that the incidence of del(17p13.1) may increase to approximately 50% in heavily treated patients. Unfortunately, when del(17p13.1) is found, there are significant limitations on treatment efficacy. The other prognostic parameters (CD38, ZAP-70, and IgV_H mutational status) probably do not need to be reassessed because these parameters do not change with time. Prior to initiation of therapy, a bone marrow analysis should be performed if cytopenias are present to confirm that CLL is the cause and to exclude other potential causes including autoimmune-induced cytopenias, transformed lymphoma, marrow toxicity from prior therapy, or development of treatment-related myelodysplasia. In general, CLL patients who have relapsed should be treated according to the indications outlined in National Cancer Institute-96 Working Group guidelines. For the patient under the age of 70 who has experienced a good clinical response (usually at least a partial response) with initial therapy for $\geq$12 months, the use of the original treatment, particularly if it was a combination regimen such as FCR, FR, or PCR, is recommended. If the patient has a high-risk FISH defect, then it may be necessary to consider adding an investigational agent or placing the patient on a clinical trial. If a CR is obtained in the absence of high-risk FISH, a reasonable approach is to observe the patient on an every 3- to 4-month basis. For patients who are younger and have a high-risk FISH defect such as del(17p13.1) or who did not achieve a CR to therapy, it may be prudent to discuss with the patient whether he or she would be interested in nonmyeloablative SCT. For relapsed patients who are 70 years or older and are considered in excellent physiologic status, retreatment with the same therapy or investigational agents in clinical trials can also be considered.

Approach to newly diagnosed patients with high-risk disease

In the past decade, it has been found that the IgV_H gene mutational status is of significant prognostic importance. The median time to initial therapy in one large study was 3.5 years in patients with unmutated IgV_H, compared with 9.2 years in patients with mutated IgV_H. Because of these differing natural histories, several groups have opted to examine the impact of early treatment intervention in newly diagnosed patients at high risk. In a German CLL Study Group trial, patients with at least 2 of 4 high-risk features (high-risk cytogenetic abnormalities, elevated thymidine kinase level, predicted LDT >12 months, and unmutated IgV_H status) will be randomized to FCR therapy or observation. Likewise, in a US Intergroup trial, newly diagnosed patients with unmutated IgV_H status will be randomized to FR therapy or observation with later treatment. Results of these 2 large trials will be of great interest to ascertain whether the natural history of these high-risk CLL patients can be altered with early therapeutic intervention.

> **Key points**
> - CLL is a heterogeneous disease with different clinical courses.
> - Ongoing clinical trials are assessing the impact of early therapeutic intervention in patients with disease at high risk of early clinical progression.

Options for the relapsed/refractory CLL patient

There are a large variety of unique biologic agents with non-overlapping mechanisms of action that are in phase I and II studies. However, a few are in a more mature state of study and/or are close to US Food and Drug Administration approval and will be briefly mentioned here. These agents are currently only given for CLL therapy as part of clinical trial investigations.

Lenalidomide

Lenalidomide is an immunomodulatory drug that is a more potent analog of thalidomide. Its chemical structure is a 3-(4-amino-1,3-dihydro-1-oxo-2H-isoindol-2-yl)-2,6-piperidinedione. The mechanism of action is not known, but this drug can have pleiotropic effects that modulate the tumor microenvironment. There are now 2 published trials for relapsed/refractory CLL in which patients were given either lenalidomide 25 mg orally for 21 days every 28 days for up to 12 months or lenalidomide 10 mg daily with a dose escalation by 5 mg daily every 28 days (median dose, 10 mg/d). In both trials, responses were seen in <50% of patients, and most were partial responses. However, the higher dose trial did find a few CRs with negative minimal residual disease. Importantly, in both trials, responses were seen in high-risk CLL patients (ie, bulky disease, high-risk FISH). Some notable toxicities included a flare reaction and hematologic problems. A flare reaction was observed in approximately 50% of patients, with 8% having a grade 3 or 4 flare in the high-dose trial, and several patients needed to discontinue therapy. The flare reaction can be characterized as sudden onset of tender enlargement of lymph nodes associated with fever and even a rash. Marked leukocytosis and lymphocytosis can be a component of this toxicity, and careful management is advised, along with considering the possibility of this being a transformed lymphoma. To manage these flares, it is recommended to use low-dose prednisone (10–20 mg/d), but sometimes a methylprednisolone pack may be needed to alleviate the flare reaction with anti-inflammatory medication. Hematologic toxicity can be considerable, with grade 3 or 4 neutropenia and thrombocytopenia occurring in >50% of patients. It is rare to see serious infections with this drug. There is currently a large, multicenter trial randomizing patients to low-dose (10 mg) or high-dose (25 mg) lenalidomide for patients with relapsed and refractory CLL. It is important to use this drug only in well-designed and monitored clinical trials given the potential for severe flares and the hematologic toxicities.

Flavopiridol

Flavopiridol (alvocidib) is a unique agent that has been characterized as being capable of inducing caspase-3-independent apoptosis of CLL B cells. It is an N-methylpiperidinyl chlorophenyl flavone that is known to be a p53-independent agent for inducing CLL B-cell apoptosis. The study of this agent is an excellent lesson concerning the need to perform pharmacokinetic analyses of newer drugs. This agent was first tested in phase I clinical studies and was given by 72-hour continuous intravenous infusion. However, despite achieving reasonable plasma concentrations, there was no important clinical activity noted in phase II studies. Ultimately, the lack of efficacy found via the continuous intravenous dosing schedules was found to be related to the increased binding of flavopiridol to human serum proteins, resulting in less effective plasma dose levels. Subsequent investigation by Grever et al found that a bolus dosing achieves the necessary plasma dose levels, and a phase II study administering flavopiridol 50 mg/m^2 by 1-hour intravenous bolus for 3 consecutive days to 36 heavily pretreated relapsed patients found an 11% response rate (mostly partial responses), and one patient experienced a tumor lysis syndrome. Then, additional pharmacokinetic modeling determined that a novel dosing schedule of a 30-minute intravenous bolus followed by 4-hour continuous infusion would achieve a proper plasma level and induce apoptosis of CLL cells in vivo. Subsequent phase I studies of flavopiridol in patients with relapsed CLL used a planned dose escalation, for both the bolus and continuous infusions, which resulted in determination of safe bolus and continuous-infusion schedules for this drug. However, it is still prudent to use aggressive safety monitoring and carefully monitor serum potassium levels with prompt intervention for hyperkalemia to maximize the safe administration of flavopiridol. Tumor lysis syndrome requiring hemodialysis can occur typically with the first treatment dose and is most frequently seen in patients with total white blood cell counts of $\geq 200 \times 10^9$/L. It is currently recommended that patients with extremely high peripheral lymphocyte counts undergo cytoreduction before receiving flavopiridol. The initial work on the phase I study found a 45% response rate (all partial responses), with many patients having high-risk FISH and patients with bulky nodes achieving response. The median duration of PFS was 12 months. The more recent updates with the phase II studies in CLL continue to confirm the high level of activity in high-risk and bulky node disease.

HuMax-CD20 (ofatumumab)

HuMax-CD20 (ofatumumab) is a fully humanized, high-affinity monoclonal antibody that targets an epitope on CD20 molecules that is not the same as rituximab. HuMax-CD20 is able to induce complement-dependent cytotoxicity at higher levels than rituximab probably related to the former antibody's higher affinity binding to CD20. This latter result suggests that HuMax-CD20 may have more effective antitumor activity. Results of a phase I/II trial demonstrated an overall response rate of 46%, and one patient had a nodular partial response, with the remainder of responses being all partial responses. The median time to treatment progression was 161 days in responders, and the median time to next treatment was approximately 1 year. Toxicity was predominately grade 1 or 2 infectious events in 48% of patients. A phase III registration study of HuMax-CD20 in patients with CLL characterized as bulky resistant or double refractory to fludarabine and alemtuzumab was recently completed and reported. The results show surprisingly high levels of responses for both categories with response rates of 51% and 44% for double-refractory and bulky-refractory cohorts, respectively.

Stem cell transplantation

There are currently 3 options for hematopoietic SCT in CLL: autologous, allogeneic myeloablative, and allogeneic nonmyeloablative SCT.

Autologous SCT for patients with CLL may have limited applicability. This process is complicated by the presence of clonal cells in the stem cell product, as well as preexistent myelosuppression from prior CLL therapies, especially the purine analogs, which limit stem cell mobilization. Finally, therapy-related myelodysplastic syndrome or acute myeloid leukemia is a concern in these patients, occurring in up to 10% of patients in several large autologous transplantation series. A pattern of continuing relapse is found in patients undergoing autologous SCT, with no plateau in survival seen. Outcome is more favorable in patients who undergo this process while in CR or with minimal residual disease.

The use of allogeneic SCT is primarily limited by the advanced age of the majority of patients with this disorder. However, in contrast to autologous procedures, stem cell mobilization and contamination are not issues, and the favorable immunologic graft-versus-leukemia effect is seen. Although data are limited for myeloablative procedures, preparative regimens with total body irradiation appear to result in better outcomes than chemotherapy-only regimens. The 3-year disease-free survival of approximately 50% after myeloablative allogeneic SCT is clearly better than that seen with autologous procedures. However, 100-day transplantation-related mortality has approached 30% to 40% in several large series.

More recently, the utility of nonmyeloablative allogeneic SCT has been examined in patients with CLL. Although transplantation-related mortality is lower than with myeloablative procedures, significant graft-versus-host disease, both acute and chronic, may occur in these patients. Chronic graft-versus-host disease may be seen in up to 75% of patients, although data are limited. Successful engraftment generally occurs, and as with autologous procedures, patients with resistant disease have a poorer outcome. At the present time, these procedures are best considered for patients as part of a clinical trial.

Key points

- As with patients with previously untreated CLL, patients with relapsed CLL should also meet standard indications for therapy.
- Patients with relapsed CLL often have additional FISH-detectable defects.
- Patients with del(17p13.1) often respond incompletely to renewed therapy.
- CLL patients with favorable prognostics and who have >1 year of response to their initial chemoimmunotherapy may be retreated successfully with the same regimen.
- A variety of new agents with novel mechanisms of action can be offered to the relapsed patient.
- Autologous SCT is limited by issues of contamination of the stem cell product by the malignant clone, therapy-related myelodysplasia, and a continuing pattern of relapses.
- Allogeneic SCT is limited most often by the advanced age of CLL patients.
- Myeloablative allogeneic SCT is early in clinical trial evaluation.

Complications of CLL

Autoimmune complications

The autoimmune cytopenias are clinically very important and can be a serious complication of CLL. The most common presentations of autoimmune cytopenias are autoimmune hemolytic anemia and immune thrombocytopenia, with a lower frequency of pure red blood cell aplasia and only rare patients who have autoimmune granulocytopenia. The earlier diagnosis of CLL and improvements in treatment have altered the presentation and prevalence of autoimmune cytopenia in patients with CLL. The current published data indicate a cumulative risk of approximately 5% to 10%. An important point is that autoimmune cytopenias can occur as a complication of all clinical stages of CLL at any time in the disease course, and although somewhat controversial, they are believed to be precipitated by treatment with the use of either single-agent purine analogs or alkylating agents. One recent study found that the presence of autoimmune cytopenias does not confer a worse outcome for CLL patients, but appropriate and timely diagnosis and management of these complications are critical.

The Rai and Binet clinical staging systems for CLL do not mandate detection of the etiology of cytopenias—that is, whether the cytopenia is an autoimmune disorder versus bone marrow failure. It is clear that this distinction is important for appropriate management of CLL patients. Thus, to know which patients have cytopenias due to autoimmune disease, bone marrow failure, or a combination of these pathologies, the workup requires at least a bone marrow examination. This requirement for CLL patients who are to begin treatment, because of the presence of cytopenia, is encouraged by the 2008 IWCLL update of the National Cancer Institute-96 Working Group guidelines.

Autoimmune cytopenias are a discrete complication of CLL requiring specific evaluation and management. These complications can appear at any time in the disease course as well. There is no standard treatment for autoimmune-induced cytopenias in CLL. Typically, patients without progressive CLL respond well to immunosuppressives including prednisone, cyclosporine, azathioprine, or rituximab. Patients with autoimmune hemolytic anemia or autoimmune thrombocytopenia are initially started on prednisone (eg, 1 mg/kg/d) until the laboratory parameters indicate that the hemolytic or thrombolytic process is controlled. At that time, the prednisone can be gradually tapered with close monitoring of the autoimmune features. In patients who fail to respond to high-dose prednisone or are unable to tolerate this agent, cyclosporine or other immunosuppressive agents, including the use of rituximab, may be helpful and steroid-sparing. In selected refractory patients, splenectomy can be a helpful option for the ultimate control of either red blood cell or platelet destruction. If patients are to receive chemotherapy for the underlying CLL, it is important to stabilize the autoimmune process before starting such therapy. Patients who receive a rituximab-based approach might also experience respiratory distress and a cytokine release syndrome following the rapid administration of rituximab. Therefore, a cautious approach to administration of the initial dose of this monoclonal antibody is required, which can include slow infusion rates or an initial thrice-weekly approach. It is not unusual to prepare the patient with diphenhydramine, acetaminophen, and possibly even steroid infusions such as dexamethasone for the initial course of therapy.

Although most patients will respond to these approaches, initial response duration can often be short lived, and most patients require intermittent or long-term maintenance therapy. In patients who require treatment for both progressive CLL and autoimmune cytopenia, purine analog–containing regimens are usually avoided because of the concern about exacerbating the autoimmunity. These patients, however, can be treated with combinations of corticosteroids, alkylating agents, and rituximab. In addition, patients who are refractory to the usual single-agent immunomodulating or immunosuppressive approaches can be managed with combination approaches. In a small series of patients using a combination of rituximab, corticosteroids, and an alkylator, this combination approach showed durable responses in most patients with a good level of tolerance. This regimen requires further testing but does offer an option for refractory autoimmune disease in CLL.

Infectious complications

Infections remain a major cause of morbidity and mortality in CLL patients, despite advances in the treatment of this disorder. The pathogenesis of infection is multifactorial, including inherent immune defects related to the primary disease process, such as hypogammaglobulinemia, as well as therapy-related immunosuppression. A spectrum of infectious complications is characteristic for specific therapeutic agents in CLL. With alkylator-based therapy, most infections are bacterial, caused by common Gram-positive and -negative organisms, with the respiratory tract being the most common site of infection. The purine analogs cause quantitative and qualitative T-cell abnormalities. As a result, patients receiving fludarabine have more major infections and herpes virus infections than those receiving chlorambucil. However, *Pneumocystis*, *Aspergillus*, and CMV infections are uncommon. Risk factors for infection in fludarabine-treated patients include advanced-stage disease, prior CLL therapy, response to therapy, elevated serum creatinine, hemoglobin <12 g/dL, and decreased serum IgG. Treatment with alemtuzumab is complicated by frequent opportunistic infections, with CMV reactivation being especially problematic, occurring in 10% to 25% of patients. For prevention of infection in CLL patients, the use of vaccinations and immunoglobulin replacement has been examined but is still somewhat controversial. Recommendations for prophylactic antimicrobial therapy are based on results from CLL treatment trials and anecdotal reports and are specific for a given therapeutic agent.

Transformation to prolymphocytic leukemia or Richter transformation

Up to 10% to 15% of patients with CLL will develop a Richter transformation to a high-grade lymphoproliferative disorder—most commonly, although not exclusively, diffuse large B-cell lymphoma. By immunophenotypic and cytogenetic studies, it remains controversial as to whether this transformation arises more commonly from clonal evolution of the CLL or from the appearance of a new clonal B-cell process. In limited series, this has been estimated to occur at a median of 2 years after diagnosis. Presentation is often with fever, rapidly increasing lymphadenopathy or hepatosplenomegaly, and markedly elevated lactate dehydrogenase. Diagnosis is most commonly made by a lymph node or bone marrow biopsy. Treatment is based on the diagnostic histology and often includes anthracycline-based combination chemotherapy. Prognosis tends to be poor, with refractory disease being common and survival generally being <6 months.

In 2% to 5% of CLL patients, transformation to prolymphocytic leukemia (PLL), with at least 55% of peripheral blood lymphocytes being prolymphocytes, may occur. Progressive cytopenias and splenomegaly may also be seen. As with Richter's transformation, therapy is often ineffective, and the prognosis is poor. Alemtuzumab is commonly used in the treatment of these patients, with purine analogs less commonly used.

Other second malignancies

Second malignancies occur at an increased incidence in CLL patients, as compared with the general population. It has been estimated that they may be seen in up to 25% of patients. The majority are common malignancies, such as lung, gastrointestinal, skin, and other epithelial cancers. The cause of death is related to these second malignancies in 7% to 10% of patients. In addition, therapy-related myelodysplasia or acute myeloid leukemia may be seen in these patients. In a large intergroup trial, these latter disorders more commonly occurred in patients receiving initial therapy with concurrent chlorambucil plus fludarabine compared with patients receiving either chlorambucil or fludarabine as a single agent.

> **Key points**
> - Even early-stage CLL patients may have clinical complications, including autoimmune disease.
> - Autoimmune hemolytic anemia and thrombocytopenias are common complications of CLL; autoimmune neutropenia and pure red blood cell aplasia are less frequent.
> - If CLL patients have cytopenias, the cause should be determined to be autoimmune-induced or bone marrow failure-induced or both.
> - Usually, the autoimmune complications can be managed by immunosuppressive therapies and/or splenectomy in the case of autoimmune hemolytic anemia or immune thrombocytopenia.
> - The spectrum of infections seen in CLL patients is definitely influenced by the specific therapy rendered.
> - Both purine analogs and alemtuzumab result in significant defects in cell-mediated immunity.
> - CMV reactivation is a significant issue in patients receiving alemtuzumab therapy, occurring in 10% to 25% of patients.
> - Ten percent to 15% of CLL patients will develop transformation to a high-grade non-Hodgkin lymphoma (Richter transformation), manifested by rapidly increasing lymphadenopathy/hepatosplenomegaly, fever, and elevated lactate dehydrogenase.
> - Transformation to PLL occurs in a minority of CLL patients (2% to 5%).
> - Prognosis for patients with either transformation to a high-grade non-Hodgkin lymphoma or PLL is poor.
> - Second malignancies, including lung, colon, and skin cancers, are more common in patients with CLL than in the general population.

Quality-of-life issues

CLL is a common disease, with many patients diagnosed at an early stage and often not placed on therapy. This is a reasonable approach considering randomized phase III trials demonstrating no increase in survival for treatment of early-stage disease and considering the fact that there is no cure for this disease. Although this approach is based on clinical trial data, it can be psychologically difficult for patient who recognizes that he or she has a significant health problem but whose physician is not going to administer any therapy for some time. For CLL patients, there is also uncertainty about what their diagnosis of CLL means to family members, their own livelihood, and their functional status, which may be an issue depending on their professional demands. Finally, patients usually have little understanding of CLL and thus are heavily reliant on their physician to provide information about the illness and support them as they adjust to the implications of the diagnosis. In sum, there are significant emotional issues for the CLL patient that can impact on their quality of life (QOL). Recent studies have examined the influence of physician and patient factors on both emotional distress and QOL in CLL patients.

One study was an international Web-based survey of CLL patients that used standardized instruments to evaluate fatigue and QOL. When CLL patients were evaluated at the time of diagnosis, most patients had physical, functional, and overall QOL scores similar to or better than both published population norms and samples of patients with other types of malignancy. In distinct contrast, the emotional QOL scores of CLL patients were significantly lower than both the general population and individuals with other malignancies. In this study, more than half the patients thought about their diagnosis daily. In addition, although the overwhelming majority of patients felt that their doctor understood how their disease was progressing, approximately 70% did not appreciate that their doctor understood how CLL affected their QOL, which included both their anxiety and/or worry. There was also a significant association in terms of satisfaction with their physician based on the patients' measured emotional and overall QOL. Importantly, in this study, the use of specific euphemistic phrases by the doctor to characterize the patient's CLL such as "Do not worry, you have a good leukemia" was also associated with lower emotional QOL among patients. These studies demonstrate that the physician's role in helping the patient adjust to the physical, intellectual, and emotional challenges of CLL appears to significantly impact the patient's QOL.

> **Key points**
>
> • Even patients with early-stage, untreated CLL have significant anxiety about their diagnosis.
> • Physicians can play a key role in allaying patients' anxiety by inquiring about their concerns and by not using certain phrases that downplay the diagnosis of CLL.

Other indolent cell leukemias

Within the B-cell lymphoproliferative disorders, PLL, hairy cell leukemia, marginal zone lymphoma, and lymphoplasmacytic lymphoma must be considered when patients with a lymphocytosis are believed to have a diagnosis of CLL. The correlation of morphologic, immunophenotypic, and clinical information usually allows differentiation of CLL from these other disorders. However, when the morphology is confusing, the use of immunophenotype analysis is critically important in understanding the specific chronic lymphoid leukemia existing in a given patient. Although discussed earlier, it is important to remember that CLL B cells have a characteristic immunophenotype that can differentiate CLL from other low-grade or indolent B-cell leukemias (Table 19-1). Thus, leukemic CLL cells express a variety of B-cell markers, including dim surface Ig (sIg), CD19, dim CD20 and CD23, and the pan-T-cell marker CD5. Kappa or lambda restriction is always present, establishing the presence of a clonal B-cell population. Some key features that may suggest other low-grade B-cell leukemias in the patient include the presence of CD10, FMC7, or CD79b (usually absent on CLL cells) or bright expression of CD11c, CD20, or CD25 (found to be usually dim on CLL cells).

Prolymphocytic leukemia

PLL is a distinct clinical entity, with a de novo PLL having a more aggressive clinical course than CLL, usually in patients over the age of 70, and with a high peripheral lymphocyte count with a predominance of prolymphocytes. The morphologic appearance in the blood can be distinct, with cells having a large nucleolus, and can be found in >55% of the circulating lymphocytes. Patients with PLL frequently have enlarged spleens, even massive splenomegaly, without impressive lymphadenopathy. Many patients with massive splenomegaly will have an associated abdominal discomfort and early satiety, whereas lymphadenopathy is often minimal. The immunophenotypic profile is different than that of CLL or the prolymphocytic transformation that can be seen with CLL. Unlike CLL cells, PLL cells express dense surface IgM positivity and are FMC7 positive/CD23 negative, but only approximately a third of PLL cases are CD5 positive. Some cases carry the t(11;14) abnormality. Given similarities in immunophenotype, the distinction from mantle cell lymphoma with lymphocytosis may be difficult. Accurate recognition of PLL is important because the response to treatments used for CLL is suboptimal in these patients. Standard therapies for this rare lymphoproliferative disease are not clear, but there are anecdotal reports of responses to purine nucleoside analogs. Both fludarabine and cladribine (2CDA) have generated clinical responses in PLL but less frequently when PLL occurs in the setting of CLL. Alemtuzumab may also be an option for these patients. Splenectomy may be useful for symptomatic splenomegaly or cytopenias due to splenic sequestration.

Hairy cell leukemia

Bouroncle and colleagues have described the clinical features of hairy cell leukemia (HCL), which is a rare disease described over 50 years ago. The usual patient is a male age 50 to 60 years who presents with pancytopenia, splenomegaly, and infections. The marrow aspirate can be a dry tap and can initially look like myelofibrosis because there can also be increased reticulin fibrosis in the marrow biopsy. The specific diagnosis is based on the morphology of hairy cell projections and a positive tartrate-resistant acid phosphatase (TRAP) stain. The immunophenotype is sIg, CD19, CD20, CD22, CD11c, cd25, and CD103 positive. The usual choice of therapy is pentostatin or cladribine because they both are highly effective. Thus, it is typical to see high response rates and very durable responses with these agents. The short course and durability of cladribine has resulted in this agent being used more frequently for HCL. The high level of CD20 on the HCL leukemic cells has encouraged treatment with rituximab. HCL is also discussed in Chapter 18.

Marginal zone lymphoma

Marginal zone lymphoma can present with circulating lymphoid clonal B cells; thus, it is in the differential diagnosis of CLL-like disorders. However, this disease process may be indolent, and diagnostically and prognostically, it is different from CLL. Patients with marginal zone lymphoma have been reported to respond to either splenectomy or rituximab, depending on the extent of bone marrow involvement and cytopenias.

Lymphoplasmacytic lymphoma

Lymphoplasmacytic lymphoma is also an indolent B-cell leukemia but frequently presents with hybrid features that resemble both CLL and Waldenström macroglobulinemia. The neoplastic cells most often have a morphology of the bone marrow cells that features a plasmacytic lymphocyte and can be distinguished from CLL by flow-based immunophenotyping.

T-cell CLL and other chronic T-cell leukemias

In North America, <5% of CLL is of the T-cell subtype. T-cell CLL is much more common in Asia. T-cell CLL disease can have a PLL morphology and an immunophenotype that is CD4, CD8, or CD16 positive. Commonly, patients with T-cell PLL present with very high lymphocyte blood levels, splenomegaly, progressive lymphadenopathy, and pancytopenia due to marrow failure. These patients are older and less responsive to standard chemotherapy. Alemtuzumab has been reported to provide some therapeutic response, but there is a clear need for experimental approaches to improve on the therapy of this disease. More recently, the use of alemtuzumab (anti-CD52) has been helpful in the treatment of these patients. Patients with cutaneous T-cell lymphoma frequently have circulating morphologically abnormal lymphoid cells where immunophenotype can be used to detect the T-cell nature of the malignant cell. It is not infrequent to find that the T-cell leukemia patients have a history of recurrent infiltrative skin lesions. Cutaneous T-cell lymphoma patients will eventually progress to exhibit obvious lymphadenopathy, and unfortunately, these patients have a deficient immune system that is associated with increasing infectious complications.

Mantle cell lymphoma

Mantle cell lymphoma may present with a circulating neoplastic cell that morphologically can be confused with the leukemic CLL B cell. However, the distinctive immunophenotypic profile, the characteristic cytogenetics [t(11:14)] demonstrable by FISH, and the expression of cyclin D1 will enable mantle cell lymphoma to be recognized. Because mantle cell lymphoma can have a more aggressive clinical course and require different chemotherapy than CLL, this diagnostic distinction is critically important. Thus, the recommendation for mantle cell lymphoma is that, in the differential of a malignant lymphocytosis, FISH and immunophenotypic analysis should be done promptly. For a more complete description of mantle cell lymphoma, see Chapter 18.

> **Key points**
>
> - There are several other indolent leukemias or lymphomas to be considered in patients with a clonal blood lymphocytosis.
> - For patients who had a diagnosis of CLL made several years ago, it is prudent to redo the flow cytometry to confirm that the leukemic cells carry the signature phenotype of CLL.
> - Immunophenotype and FISH probes are usually very helpful in distinguishing the various diseases associated with lymphocytosis.

The future

The remarkable advances in the understanding of this common incurable and complicated disease have been due in part to the high-level science done in this very accessible leukemic disease. The application of these advances can be best seen by the following: a more accurate diagnosis, dissection of prognostic cohorts even in early-stage disease, outlining important progression events, specific determination of residual disease, and most important, determination of agents that can undermine the resistance to cell death and drug resistance that is such a prominent feature of the leukemic CLL B cell. The next time this chapter is rewritten, it is hoped that we will be much closer to the real goal—more frequent and durable responses in the vast majority of CLL patients and even cures in some.

Bibliography

Chronic lymphocytic leukemia

Abrisqueta P, Pereira A, Rozman C, et al. Improving survival in patients with chronic lymphocytic leukemia (1980–2008): the Hospital Clinic of Barcelona experience. *Blood*. 2009;114:2044–2050.

Boice JD, Cohen SS, Mumma MT, et al. Mortality among radiation workers at Rocketdyne (Atomics International), 1948–1999. *Radiat Res.* 2006;166:98–115.

Brenner H, Gondos A, Pulte D. Trends in long-term survival of patients with chronic lymphocytic leukemia from the 1980s to the early 21st century. *Blood.* 2008;111:4916–4921.

Crowther-Swanepoel D, Wild R, Sellick G, et al. Insight into the pathogenesis of chronic lymphocytic leukemia (CLL) through analysis of IgVH gene usage and mutation status in familial CLL. *Blood.* 2008;111:5691–5693.

Cuttner J. Increased incidence of hematologic malignancies in first-degree relatives of patients with chronic lymphocytic leukemia. *Cancer Invest.* 1992;10:103–109.

Di Bernardo MC, Crowther-Swanepoel D, Broderick P, et al. A genome-wide association study identifies six susceptibility loci for chronic lymphocytic leukemia. *Nat Genet.* 2008;40:1204–1210.

Flynn JM, Byrd JC, Diehl LF. The causes of death and the impact of age on the survival of patients with chronic lymphocytic leukemia. *Blood.* 1999;84(Abstract):298b.

Federico Caligaris-Cappio F, Ghia P. Novel insights in chronic lymphocytic leukemia: are we getting closer to understanding the pathogenesis of the disease? *J Clin Oncol.* 2008;26:4497–4503.

Gluzman D, Imamura N, Sklyarenko L, Nadgornaya V, Zavelevich M, Machilo V. Patterns of hematological malignancies in Chernobyl clean-up workers (1996–2005). *Exp Oncol.* 2006;28:60–63.

Goldgar DE, Easton DF, Cannon-Albright LA, Skolnick MH. Systematic population-based assessment of cancer risk in first-degree relatives of cancer probands. *J Natl Cancer Inst.* 1994;86:1600–1608.

Goldin LR, Pfeiffer RM, Li X, Hemminki K. Familial risk of lymphoproliferative tumors in families of patients with chronic lymphocytic leukemia: results from the Swedish Family-Cancer Database. *Blood.* 2004;104:1850–1854.

Ishibe N, Albitar M, Jilani IB, Goldin LR, Marti GE, Caporaso NE. CXCR4 expression is associated with survival in familial chronic lymphocytic leukemia, but CD38 expression is not. *Blood.* 2002;100:1100–1101.

Ishibe N, Sgambati MT, Fontaine L, et al. Clinical characteristics of familial B-CLL in the National Cancer Institute Familial Registry. *Leuk Lymphoma.* 2001;42:99–108.

Marwick C. Link found between Agent Orange and chronic lymphocytic leukaemia. *BMJ.* 2003;326:242.

Matasar MJ, Ritchie EK, Consedine N, Magai C, Neugut AI. Incidence rates of the major leukemia subtypes among US Hispanics, blacks, and non-Hispanic whites. *Leuk Lymphoma.* 2006;47:2365–2370.

Mauro FR, Giammartini E, Gentile M, et al. Clinical features and outcome of familial chronic lymphocytic leukemia. *Haematologica.* 2006;91:1117–1120.

Preston DL, Kusumi S, Tomonaga M, et al. Cancer incidence in atomic bomb survivors. Part III: leukemia, lymphoma and multiple myeloma, 1950–1987. *Radiat Res.* 1994;137:S68–S97.

Ries Lag MD, Krapcho M, Mariotto A, et al, eds. National Cancer Institute. SEER Cancer Statistics Review. SEER Data submission 1975–2004. Vol. 2007. Bethesda, MD: National Cancer Institute; 2007.

Xie Y, Davies SM, Xiang Y, Robison LL, Ross JA. Trends in leukemia incidence and survival in the United States (1973–1998). *Cancer.* 2003;97:2229–2235.

Seftel MD, Demers AA, Banerji V, et al. High incidence of chronic lymphocytic leukemia (CLL) diagnosed by immunophenotyping: a population-based Canadian cohort. *Leuk Res.* 2009;33:1463–1468.

Diagnosis

Crespo M, Bosch F, Villamor N, et al. ZAP-70 expression as a surrogate for immunoglobulin-variable-region mutations in chronic lymphocytic leukemia. *N Engl J Med.* 2003;348:1764–1775.

Crowther-Swanepoel D, Wild R, Sellick G, et al. Insight into the pathogenesis of chronic lymphocytic leukemia (CLL) through analysis of IgVH gene usage and mutation status in familial CLL. *Blood.* 2008;111:5691–5693.

Cuttner J. Increased incidence of hematologic malignancies in first-degree relatives of patients with chronic lymphocytic leukemia. *Cancer Invest.* 1992;10:103–109.

Di Bernardo MC, Crowther-Swanepoel D, Broderick P, et al. A genome-wide association study identifies six susceptibility loci for chronic lymphocytic leukemia. *Nat Genet.* 2008;40:1204–1210.

Dohner H, Stilgenbauer S, Benner A, et al. Genomic aberrations and survival in chronic lymphocytic leukemia. *N Engl J Med.* 2000;343:1910–1916.

Goldgar DE, Easton DF, Cannon-Albright LA, Skolnick MH. Systematic population-based assessment of cancer risk in first-degree relatives of cancer probands. *J Natl Cancer Inst.* 1994;86:1600–1608.

Goldin LR, Pfeiffer RM, Li X, Hemminki K. Familial risk of lymphoproliferative tumors in families of patients with chronic lymphocytic leukemia: results from the Swedish Family-Cancer Database. *Blood.* 2004;104:1850–1854.

Hallek M, Cheson BD, Catovsky D, et al. Guidelines for the diagnosis and treatment of chronic lymphocytic leukemia: a report from the International Workshop on Chronic Lymphocytic Leukemia updating the National Cancer Institute-Working Group 1996 guidelines. *Blood.* 2008;111:5446–5456.

Hamblin TJ. Prognostic makers in chronic lymphocytic leukaemia. *Best Pract Res Clin Haematol.* 2007;20:455–468.

Ishibe N, Albitar M, Jilani IB, Goldin LR, Marti GE, Caporaso NE. CXCR4 expression is associated with survival in familial chronic lymphocytic leukemia, but CD38 expression is not. *Blood.* 2002;100:1100–1101.

Ishibe N, Sgambati MT, Fontaine L, et al. Clinical characteristics of familial B-CLL in the National Cancer Institute Familial Registry. *Leuk Lymphoma.* 2001;42:99–108.

Wiestner A, Rosenwald A, Barry TS, et al. ZAP-70 expression identifies a chronic lymphocytic leukemia subtype with unmutated immunoglobulin genes, inferior clinical outcome, and distinct gene expression profile. *Blood.* 2003;101:4944–4951.

Clinical and laboratory features

Nowakowski GS, Hoyer JD, Shanafelt TD, et al. Using smudge cells on routine blood smears to predict clinical outcome in chronic lymphocytic leukemia: a universally available prognostic test. *Mayo Clin Proc.* 2007;82(4):449–453.

Nowakowski GS, Hoyer JD, Shanafelt TD, et al. Percentage of smudge cells on routine blood smear predicts survival in chronic lymphocytic leukemia. *J Clin Oncol.* 2009;27(11): 1844–1849.

Staging

Binet JL, Leoprier M, Dighiero G, et al. A clinical staging system for chronic lymphocytic leukemia: prognostic significance. *Cancer.* 1977;40:855–864.

Rai KR, Sawitsky A, Cronkite EP, Chanana AD, Levy RN, Pasternack BS. Clinical staging of chronic lymphocytic leukemia. *Blood.* 1975;46:219–234.

Prognostic factors

Byrd JC, Gribben JG, Peterson BL, et al. Select high-risk genetic features predict earlier progression following chemoimmunotherapy with fludarabine and rituximab in chronic lymphocytic leukemia: justification for risk-adapted therapy. *J Clin Oncol.* 2006;24:437–443.

Crespo M, Bosch F, Villamor N, et al. ZAP-70 expression as a surrogate for immunoglobulin-variable-region mutations in chronic lymphocytic leukemia. *N Engl J Med.* 2003;348: 1764–1775.

Damle RN, Wasil T, Fais F, et al. Ig V gene mutation status and CD38 expression as novel prognostic indicators in chronic lymphocytic leukemia. *Blood.* 1999;94:1840–1847.

Del Principe MI, Del Poeta G, Buccisano F, et al. Clinical significance of ZAP-70 protein expression in B-cell chronic lymphocytic leukemia. *Blood.* 2006;108:853–861.

Dewald GW, Brockman SR, Paternoster SF, et al. Chromosome anomalies detected by interphase fluorescence in situ hybridization: correlation with significant biological features of B-cell chronic lymphocytic leukaemia. *Br J Haematol.* 2003;121:287–295.

Kay NE, O'Brien SM, Pettitt AR, Stilgenbauer S. The role of prognostic factors in assessing 'high-risk' subgroups of patients with chronic lymphocytic leukemia. *Leukemia.* 2007;21: 1885–1891.

Krober A, Bloehdorn J, Hafner S, et al. Additional genetic high-risk features such as 11q deletion, 17p deletion, and V3–21 usage characterize discordance of ZAP-70 and VH mutation status in chronic lymphocytic leukemia. *J Clin Oncol.* 2006;24:969–975.

Krober A, Seiler T, Benner A, et al. V(H) mutation status, CD38 expression level, genomic aberrations, and survival in chronic lymphocytic leukemia. *Blood.* 2002;100:1410–1416.

Lin KI, Tam CS, Keating MJ, et al. Relevance of the immunoglobulin VH somatic mutation status in patients with chronic lymphocytic leukemia treated with fludarabine, cyclophosphamide, and rituximab (FCR) or related chemoimmunotherapy regimens. *Blood.* 2009;113: 3168–3171.

Nolz JC, Tschumper RC, Pittner BT, Darce JR, Kay NE, Jelinek DF. ZAP-70 is expressed by a subset of normal human B-lymphocytes displaying an activated phenotype. *Leukemia.* 2005;19:1018–1024.

Orchard JA, Ibbotson RE, Davis Z, et al. ZAP-70 expression and prognosis in chronic lymphocytic leukaemia. *Lancet.* 2004;363:105–111.

Oscier DG, Gardiner AC, Mould SJ, et al. Multivariate analysis of prognostic factors in CLL: clinical stage, IGVH gene mutational status, and loss or mutation of the p53 gene are independent prognostic factors. *Blood.* 2002;100:1177–1184.

Shanafelt TD, Jenkins G, Call TG, et al. Validation of a new prognostic index for patients with chronic lymphocytic leukemia. *Cancer.* 2009;115:363–372.

Shanafelt TD, Witzig TE, Fink SR, et al. Prospective evaluation of clonal evolution during long-term follow-up of patients with untreated early-stage chronic lymphocytic leukemia. *J Clin Oncol.* 2006;24:4634–4641.

Stilgenbauer S, Dohner H. Genotypic prognostic markers. *Curr Top Microbiol Immunol.* 2005;294:147–164.

Tam CS, Shanafelt TD, Wierda WG, et al. De novo deletion 17p13.1 chronic lymphocytic leukemia shows significant clinical heterogeneity: the M.D. Anderson and Mayo Clinic experience. *Blood.* 2009;114:957–964.

Wierda WG, O'Brien S, Wang X, et al. Prognostic nomogram and index for overall survival in previously untreated patients with chronic lymphocytic leukemia. *Blood.* 2007;109:4679–4685.

Wiestner A, Rosenwald A, Barry TS, et al. ZAP-70 expression identifies a chronic lymphocytic leukemia subtype with unmutated immunoglobulin genes, inferior clinical outcome, and distinct gene expression profile. *Blood.* 2003;101:4944–4951.

Zent CS, Call TG, Hogan WJ, Shanafelt TD, Kay NE. Update on risk-stratified management for chronic lymphocytic leukemia. *Leuk Lymphoma.* 2006;47:1738–1746.

Therapy

Kay NE, Geyer SM, Call TG, et al. Combination chemoimmunotherapy with pentostatin, cyclophosphamide, and rituximab shows significant clinical activity with low accompanying toxicity in previously untreated B chronic lymphocytic leukemia. *Blood.* 2007;15;109(2):405–411.

Approach to newly diagnosed patients with high-risk disease

Grever MR, Leiby JM, Kraut EH, et al. Low-dose deoxycoformycin in lymphoid malignancy. *J Clin Oncol.* 1985;3(9):1196–1201.

Grever MB, Lucas DM, Dewald GW, et al. Comprehensive assessment of genetic and molecular features predicting outcome in patients with chronic lymphocytic leukemia: results from the US intergroup phase III trial E2997. *J Clin Oncol.* 2007;25:799–804.

Hamblin TJ, Davis Z, Gardiner A, et al. Unmutated Ig V(H) genes are associated with a more aggressive form of chronic lymphocytic leukemia. *Blood*. 1999;94:1848–1854.

Treatment options for newly diagnosed and relapsed/refractory CLL patients

Aivado M, Schulte K, Henze L, Burger J, Finke J, Haas R. Bendamustine in the treatment of chronic lymphocytic leukemia: results and future perspectives. *Semin Oncol*. 2002;29:19–22.

Byrd JC, Gribben JG, Bercedis LP, et al. Select high-risk genetic features predict earlier progression following chemoimmunotherapy with fludarabine and rituximab in CLL: justification for risk-adapted therapy. *J Clin Oncol*. 2006;24:437–443.

Byrd JC, Murphy T, Howard RS, et al. Rituximab using a thrice weekly dosing schedule in B-cell chronic lymphocytic leukemia and small lymphocytic lymphoma demonstrates clinical activity and acceptable toxicity. *J Clin Oncol*. 2001;19:2153–2164.

Byrd JC, Peterson BL, Morrison VA, et al. Randomized phase 2 study of fludarabine with concurrent versus sequential treatment with rituximab in symptomatic, untreated patients with B-cell chronic lymphocytic leukemia: results from Cancer and Leukemia Group B 9712 (CALGB 9712). *Blood*. 2003;101:6–14.

Chanan-Khan A, Miller KC, Musial L, et al. Clinical efficacy of lenalidomide in patients with relapsed or refractory chronic lymphocytic leukemia: results of a phase II study. *J Clin Oncol*. 2006;24:5343–5349.

Cheson BD, Rummel MJ. Bendamustine: rebirth of an old drug. *J Clin Oncol*. 2009;27:1492–1501.

Coiffier B, Lepretre S, Pedersen LM, et al. Safety and efficacy of ofatumumab, a fully human monoclonal anti-CD20 antibody, in patients with relapsed or refractory B-cell chronic lymphocytic leukemia: a phase 1–2 study. *Blood*. 2008;111:1094–1100.

Dighiero G, Maloum K, Desablens B, et al. Chlorambucil in indolent chronic lymphocytic leukemia. *N Engl J Med*. 1998;338:1506–1511.

Dreger P, Brand R, Michallet M. Autologous stem cell transplantation for chronic lymphocytic leukemia. *Semin Hematol*. 2007;44:246–251.

Dreger P, Corradini P, Kimby E, et al. Chronic Leukemia Working Party of the EMBT. Indications for allogeneic stem cell transplantation in chronic lymphocytic leukemia: the EBMT transplant consensus. *Leukemia*. 2007;21:12–17.

Eichhorst BF, Busch R, Hopfinger G, et al. Fludarabine plus cyclophosphamide versus fludarabine alone in first-line therapy of younger patients with chronic lymphocytic leukemia. *Blood*. 2006;107:885–891.

Ferrajoli A, Lee BN, Schlette EJ, et al. Lenalidomide induces complete and partial remissions in patients with relapsed and refractory chronic lymphocytic leukemia. *Blood*. 2008;111:5291–5297.

Flinn IW, Neuberg D, Grever MR, et al. Phase III trial of fludarabine plus cyclophosphamide compared with fludarabine for patients with previously untreated chronic lymphocytic leukemia: US Intergroup Trial E2997. *J Clin Oncol*. 2007;25:793–798.

Gribben JG. Role of allogeneic hematopoietic stem-cell transplantation in chronic lymphocytic leukemia. *J Clin Oncol*. 2008;26:4864–4865.

Gribben JG. Stem cell transplantation in chronic lymphocytic leukemia. *Biol Blood Marrow Transplant*. 2009;15:53–58.

Hainsworth JD, Litchy S, Barton JH, et al. Single-agent rituximab as first-line and maintenance treatment for patients with chronic lymphocytic leukemia or small lymphocytic lymphoma: a phase II trial of the Minnie Pearl Cancer Research Network. *J Clin Oncol*. 2003;21:1746–1751.

Hillmen P, Skotnicki A, Robak T, et al. Alemtuzumab compared with chlorambucil as first-line therapy for chronic lymphocytic leukemia. *J Clin Oncol*. 2007;25:5616–5623.

Huhn D, von Schilling C, Wilhelm M, et al. Rituximab therapy for patients with B-cell chronic lymphocytic leukemia. *Blood*. 2001;98:1326–1331.

Keating MJ, Flinn I, Jain V, et al. Therapeutic role of alemtuzumab (Campath-1H) in patients who have failed fludarabine: results of a large international study. *Blood*. 2002;99:3554–3561.

Keating MJ, O'Brien S, Albitar M, et al. Early results of a chemoimmunotherapy regimen of fludarabine, cyclophosphamide, and rituximab as initial therapy for chronic lymphocytic leukemia. *J Clin Oncol*. 2005;23:4079–4088.

Keating MJ, O'Brien SO, Lerner S, et al. Long-term follow-up of patients with chronic lymphocytic leukemia (CLL) receiving fludarabine regimens as initial therapy. *Blood*. 1998;92:1165–1171.

Kharfan-Dabaja MA, Anasetti C, Santos ES. Hematopoietic cell transplantation for chronic lymphocytic leukemia: an evolving concept. *Biol Blood Marrow Transplant*. 2007;13:373–385.

Kharfan-Dabaja MA, Kumar A, Behera M, et al. Systematic review of high dose chemotherapy and autologous haematopoietic stem cell transplantation for chronic lymphocytic leukemia: what is the published evidence? *Br J Haematol*. 2007;139:224–242.

Kluin-Nelemans HC, Coenen JL, Boers JE, et al. EBV-positive immunodeficiency lymphoma after alemtuzumab-CHOP therapy for peripheral T-cell lymphoma. *Blood*. 2008;112:1039–1041.

Leporrier M, Chevret S, Cazin B, et al. Randomized comparison of fludarabine, CAP, and ChOP in 938 previously untreated stage B and C chronic lymphocytic leukemia patients. *Blood*. 2001;98:2319–2325.

Lissitchkov T, Arnaudov G, Peytchev D, Merkle K. Phase I/II study to evaluate dose limiting toxicity, maximum tolerated dose, and tolerability of bendamustine HCl in pre-treated patients with B-chronic lymphocytic leukaemia (Binet stages B and C) requiring therapy. *J Cancer Res Clin Oncol*. 2006;132:99–104.

Lundin J, Kimby E, Bjorkholm M, et al. Phase II trial of subcutaneous anti-CD52 monoclonal antibody alemtuzumab (Campath-1H) as first-line treatment for patients with B-cell chronic lymphocytic leukemia (B-CLL). *Blood*. 2002;100:768–773.

Lundin J, Porwit-MacDonald A, Rossmann ED, et al. Cellular immune reconstitution after subcutaneous alemtuzumab (anti-CD52 monoclonal antibody, CAMPATH-1H) treatment as first-line therapy for B-cell chronic lymphocytic leukaemia. *Leukemia*. 2004;18:484–490.

Montserrat E. Further progress in CLL therapy. *Blood*. 2008;1123:924–925.

O'Brien S, Kantarjian H, Beran M, et al. Results of fludarabine and prednisone therapy in 264 patients with chronic lymphocytic leukemia with multivariate analysis-derived prognostic model for response to treatment. *Blood*. 1993;2:1695–1700.

O'Brien SM, Kantarjian HM, Thomas DA, et al. Alemtuzumab as treatment for residual disease after chemotherapy in patients with chronic lymphocytic leukemia. *Cancer*. 2003;98:2657–2663.

O'Brien S, Moore JO, Boyd TE, et al. Randomized phase III trial of fludarabine plus cyclophosphamide with or without oblimersen sodium (Bcl-2 antisense) in patients with relapsed or refractory chronic lymphocytic leukemia. *J Clin Oncol*. 2007;25:1145–1120.

Osterborg A, Kipps TJ, Mayer J, et al. Ofatumumab (HuMax-CD20), a novel CD20 monoclonal antibody, is an active treatment for patients with CLL refractory to both fludarabine and alemtuzumab or bulky fludarabine-refractory disease: results from the planned interim analysis of an international pivotal trial. *Blood*. 2008;112(Abstract):328.

Rai KR, Byrd JC, Peterson BL, Larson RA. A phase II trial of fludarabine followed by alemtuzumab in previously untreated chronic lymphocytic leukemia (CLL) patients with active disease: Cancer and Leukemia Group B (CALGB) study 19901. *Blood*. 2002;100:205a–206a.

Rai KR, Byrd JC, Peterson BL, et al. Subcutaneous alemtuzumab following fludarabine for previously untreated patients with chronic lymphocytic leukemia (CLL): CALGB study 19901. *Blood*. 2003;102:676a–677.

Rai KR, Peterson B, Appelbaum FR, et al. Fludarabine compared with chlorambucil as primary therapy for chronic lymphocytic leukemia. *N Engl J Med*. 2000;343:1750–1757.

Robak T. The place of cladribine in the treatment of chronic lymphocytic leukemia: a 10-year experience in Poland. *Ann Hematol*. 2005;84:63–70.

Sorror ML, Storer BE, Maloney DG, et al. Outcomes after allogeneic stem cell transplantation with nonmyeloablative or myeloablative conditioning regimens for treatment of lymphoma and chronic lymphocytic leukemia. *Blood*. 2008;111:446–452.

Tam CS, O'Brien S, Wierda W, et al. Long-term results of the fludarabine, cyclophosphamide, and rituximab regimen as initial therapy of chronic lymphocytic leukemia. *Blood*. 2008;112:975–980.

Wendtner CM, Ritgen M, Schweighofer CD, et al. Consolidation with alemtuzumab in patients with chronic lymphocytic leukemia (CLL) in first remission: experience on safety and efficacy within a randomized multicenter phase III trial of the German CLL Study Group (GCLLSG). *Leukemia*. 2004;18:1093–1101.

Wierda W, O'Brien S, Wen S, et al. Chemoimmunotherapy with fludarabine, cyclophosphamide, and rituximab for relapsed and refractory chronic lymphocytic leukemia. *J Clin Oncol*. 2005;23:4070–4078.

Complications of CLL

Anaissie EJ, Kontoyiannis DP, O'Brien S, et al. Infections in patients with chronic lymphocytic leukemia treated with fludarabine. *Ann Intern Med*. 1998;129:559–566.

Cooperative Group for the Study of Immunoglobulin in Chronic Lymphocytic Leukemia. Intravenous immunoglobulin for the prevention of infection in chronic lymphocytic leukemia. *N Engl J Med*. 1988;319:902–907.

Eichhorst BF, Busch R, Schweighofer C, et al. Due to low infection rates no routine anti-infective prophylaxis is required in younger patients with chronic lymphocytic leukaemia during fludarabine-based first line therapy. *Br J Haematol*. 2006;136:63–72.

Francis S, Karanth M, Pratt G, et al. The status on immunoglobulin V_H gene mutation status and other prognostic factors on the incidence of major infections in patients with chronic lymphocytic leukemia. *Cancer*. 2006;107:1023–1033.

Hamblin TJ. Autoimmune disease and its management in chronic lymphocytic leukemia. In: Cheson B, ed. Chronic Lymphocytic Leukemias. 2nd ed. New York, NY: Marcel Dekker; 2001:435–458.

Hensel M, Kornaker M, Yammeni S, et al. Disease activity and pretreatment, rather than hypogammaglobulinemia, are major risk factors for infectious complications in patients with chronic lymphocytic leukemia. *Br J Haematol*. 2003;122:600–606.

Hisada M, Biggar RJ, Greene MH, et al. Solid tumors after chronic lymphocytic leukemia. *Blood*. 2001;98:1979–1981.

Landgren O, Pfeiffer RM, Stewart L, et al. Risk of second malignant neoplasms among lymphoma patients with a family history of cancer. *Int J Cancer*. 2007;120:1099–1102.

Mauro FR, Foa R, Cerretti R, et al. Autoimmune hemolytic anemia in chronic lymphocytic leukemia: clinical, therapeutic, and prognostic features. *Blood*. 2000;95:2786–2792.

Morrison VA, Byrd JC, Peterson BL, et al. Adding rituximab to fludarabine therapy for patients with untreated chronic lymphocytic leukemia (CLL) does not increase the risk of infection: Cancer and Leukemia Group B (CALGB) study. *Blood*. 2003;102:440a.

Morrison VA, Rai KR, Peterson B, et al. Impact of therapy with chlorambucil, fludarabine, or fludarabine plus chlorambucil on infections in patients with chronic lymphocytic leukemia: Intergroup Study Cancer and Leukemia Group B 9011. *J Clin Oncol*. 2001;19:3611–3621.

Morrison VA, Rai KR, Peterson B, et al. Therapy-related myeloid leukemias are observed in patients with chronic lymphocytic leukemia after treatment with fludarabine and chlorambucil: results of an intergroup study (CALGB 9011). *J Clin Oncol*. 2002;20:3878–3884.

Robertson LE, Pugh W, O'Brien S, et al. Richter's syndrome: a report on 39 patients. *J Clin Oncol*. 1993;11:1985–1989.

Sinisalo M, Aittoniemi J, Kayhty H, et al. Vaccination against infections in chronic lymphocytic leukemia. *Leuk Lymphoma*. 2003;44:649–652.

Wadhwa P, Morrison VA. Infectious complications of chronic lymphocytic leukemia. *Semin Oncol*. 2006;33:240–249.

Yee KW, O'Brien SM, Giles FJ. Richter's syndrome: biology and therapy. *Cancer J*. 2005;11:161–174.

Zent CS, Ding W, Schwager SM, et al. The prognostic significance of cytopenia in chronic lymphocytic leukaemia/small lymphocytic lymphoma. *Br J Haematol*. 2008;141:615–621.

Quality-of-life issues

Cella D, Zagari MJ, Vandoros C, Gagnon DD, Hurtz HJ, Nortier JW. Epoetin alfa treatment results in clinically significant improvements in quality of life in anemic cancer patients when referenced to the general population. *J Clin Oncol*. 2003;21:366–373.

Charlson ME, Pompei P, Ales KL, MacKenzie CR. A new method of classifying prognostic comorbidity in longitudinal studies: development and validation. *J Chronic Dis*. 1987;40:373–383.

Levy V, Porcher R, Delabarre F, Leporrier M, Cazin B, Chevret S. Evaluating treatment strategies in chronic lymphocytic leukemia: use of quality-adjusted survival analysis. *J Clin Epidemiol*. 2001;54:747–754.

Shanafelt TD, Bowen D, Venkat C, et al. Quality of life in chronic lymphocytic leukemia: an international survey of 1482 patients. *Br J Haematol*. 2007;139:255–264.

Shanafelt TD, Bowen DA, Venkat C, et al. The physician-patient relationship and quality of life: lessons from chronic lymphocytic leukemia. *Leuk Res*. 2009;33:263–270.

Other indolent cell leukemias

Arcaini L, Paulli M, Burcheri S, et al. Primary nodal marginal zone B-cell lymphoma: clinical features and prognostic assessment of a rare disease. *Br J Haematol*. 2007;136:301–304.

Dearden CE. T-cell prolymphocytic leukemia. *Med Oncol*. 2006;23:17–22.

Dearden CE, Matutes E, Cazin B, et al. High remission rate in T-cell prolymphocytic leukemia with CAMPATH-1H. *Blood*. 2001;98:1721–1726.

Oh SY, Ryoo BY, Kim WS, et al. Nodal marginal zone B-cell lymphoma: analysis of 36 cases. Clinical presentation and treatment outcomes of nodal marginal zone B-cell lymphoma. *Ann Hematol*. 2006;85:781–786.

Papadaki T, Stamatopoulos K, Belessi C, et al. Splenic marginal-zone lymphoma: one or more entities? A histologic, immunohistochemical, and molecular study of 42 cases. *Am J Surg Pathol*. 2007;31:438–446.

CHAPTER 20

Plasma cell dyscrasias

Irene M. Ghobrial, Jacob P. Laubach, and Paul G. Richardson

Plasma cell development, 581
Etiology and incidence, 582
Molecular pathogenesis, 583

Plasmacytoma, 597
Other plasma cell disorders, 597
Acknowledgment, 599

Bibliography, 599

Plasma cell dyscrasias include monoclonal gammopathy of undermined significance (MGUS), multiple myeloma (MM), plasmacytoma, Waldenström macroglobulinemia (WM), amyloidosis (AL), and POEMS syndrome (polyneuropathy, organomegaly, endocrinopathy monoclonal gammopathy, and skin changes). MGUS, smoldering MM, and symptomatic MM represent a spectrum of the same disease. MGUS is characterized by a serum monoclonal protein <30 g/L, <10% plasma cells in the bone marrow, and absence of end-organ damage (Kyle and Rajkumar, 2009). Smoldering (asymptomatic) MM is characterized by having a serum immunoglobulin (Ig) G or IgA monoclonal protein of 30 g/L or higher and/or 10% or more plasma cells in the bone marrow but no evidence of end-organ damage. Symptomatic or active MM is characterized by any level of monoclonal protein and the presence of end-organ damage that consists of the CRAB criteria (hypercalcemia, renal insufficiency, anemia, or bone lesions) (Kyle and Rajkumar, 2009). Table 20-1 summarizes the diagnostic criteria of monoclonal gammopathies.

MM is a plasma cell malignancy that characteristically involves extensive infiltration of bone marrow (BM), with the formation of plasmacytomas, as clusters of malignant plasma cells inside or outside of the BM milieu (Kyle and Rajkumar, 2004, 2008). Consequences of this disease are numerous and involve multiple organ systems. Disruption of BM and normal plasma cell function leads to anemia, leukopenia, hypogammaglobulinemia, and thrombocytopenia, which variously result in fatigue, increased susceptibility to infection, and, less commonly, increased tendency to bleed. Disease involvement in bone creates osteolytic lesions, produces bone pain, and may be associated with hypercalcemia (Kyle and Rajkumar, 2004, 2008). Plasmacytomas extending into soft tissue may also cause symptoms specific to the tissue involved, such as spinal cord compression. A hallmark of the disease is expression of abnormal monoclonal (M) protein, classically attributed to switch mutations in the Ig genes. M protein is secreted into the blood by malignant plasma cells in the majority of patients with MM and can contribute further to complications, including renal dysfunction, hyperviscosity syndrome, and peripheral neuropathy. Binding of M protein to plasma proteins may also lead to metabolic disturbance and contribute to clotting deficiencies. MM is characteristically diagnosed by the detection of elevated levels of M protein in the serum and/or urine and the presence of plasma cells in the BM. The most common presenting symptoms are bone pain and fatigue (Kyle and Rajkumar, 2008).

Plasma cell development

B-cell maturation consists of early (antigen-independent) and late (antigen-dependent) stages, ultimately terminating in the development of the plasma cell (Katogi and Kudo, 2005; Hagman and Lukin, 2006; Fairfax et al, 2008). Early development is initiated by the rearrangement of genes for

Conflict-of-interest disclosure: Dr. Ghobrial: research funding: Millennium; honoraria: Millennium, Celgene; speakers' bureau: Millennium, Celgene, Novartis; membership on board of directors or advisory committee: Millenium; advisory board: Celgene, Novartis. Dr. Laubach: membership on board of directors or advisory committee: Novartis; advisory board: Novartis. Dr. Richardson: speakers' bureau: Celgene, Millennium, Johnson & Johnson; membership on board of directors or advisory committee: Celgene, Millennium, Johnson & Johnson; advisory board: Celgene, Millenium.
Off-label drug use: Dr. Ghobrial: bortezomib use in Waldenström macroglobulinemia, use of lenalidomide in upfront therapy for myeloma. Dr. Richardson: upfront use of lenalidomide.

Table 20-1 Diagnostic criteria for monoclonal gammopathies.*

Disorder	Disease definition
MGUS	Serum monoclonal protein level <3 g/dL, bone marrow plasma cells <10%, and absence of end-organ damage, such as lytic bone lesions, anemia, hypercalcemia, or renal failure, that can be attributed to a plasma cell proliferative disorder
SMM (also referred to as asymptomatic multiple myeloma)	Serum monoclonal protein (IgG or IgA) level ≥3 g/dL and/or bone marrow plasma cells ≥10%, absence of end-organ damage, such as lytic bone lesions, anemia, hypercalcemia, or renal failure, that can be attributed to a plasma cell proliferative disorder
Multiple myeloma	Bone marrow plasma cells ≥10%, presence of serum and/or urinary monoclonal protein (except in patients with true nonsecretory multiple myeloma), plus evidence of lytic bone lesions, anemia, hypercalcemia, or renal failure that can be attributed to the underlying plasma cell proliferative disorder
Solitary plasmacytoma	Biopsy-proven solitary lesion of bone or soft tissue with evidence of clonal plasma cells, normal skeletal survey, and MRI of spine and pelvis, and absence of end-organ damage, such as anemia, hypercalcemia, renal failure, or additional lytic bone lesions, that can be attributed to a plasma cell proliferative disorder

*Adapted from Rajkumar V, et al. Multiple myeloma: diagnosis and treatment. *Mayo Clin Proc.* 2005;80:1371-1382, with permissions.
Ig = immunoglobulin; MGUS = monoclonal gammopathy of undetermined significance; MRI = magnetic resonance imaging; SMM = smoldering multiple myeloma.

the heavy and light chains of antibodies, a process referred to as V/(D)/J recombination. The earliest B-precursor cell shows rearrangement of the Ig heavy chain, which is then followed by light chain rearrangement. The κ-light chain genes rearrange first; if neither κ locus is productively rearranged, then the λ gene loci undergo rearrangement. Once a successful light chain rearrangement occurs, the cell will express the complete Ig molecule on its surface, which identifies it as a mature B cell. Mature B cells will typically express either IgM or IgD on their surfaces, and this surface expression is critical to cell survival and maturation because they then become plasma cells of memory B cells (Hagman and Lukin, 2006; Fairfax et al, 2008).

CD10 (CALLA, the common acute lymphoblastic leukemia antigen) and CD19 are expressed on immature B cells (pro-B and B precursor) that have begun heavy chain rearrangement. Terminal deoxynucleotidyl transferase (TdT), a DNA polymerase important for nucleotide chain elongation during gene rearrangement, is also expressed at this stage. CD20 is then expressed as cells rearrange light chains and express surface Ig, and the expression of CD10 and TdT is lost. The mature but antigen-naive B cell leaves the BM to circulate and populate lymphoid organs such as lymph nodes, spleen, and mucosa-associated lymphoid tissue (MALT) (Fairfax et al, 2008).

The late, or antigen-dependent, stages of B-lymphocyte development begin when a naive B cell recognizes an antigen with its membrane-bound antibody. These B cells collect in germinal centers of the various lymphoid organs and begin to divide and undergo several types of genetic modification (Clark MR et al, 2005). Somatic hypermutation is a process by which cells introduce mutations into the variable region genes. These mutations result in antibodies that may have a higher or lower affinity for the antigen. Those that produce a higher affinity antibody will persist and become either plasma cells or memory B cells, whereas those that fail to produce functional antibody at this stage will undergo apoptosis. Class switching involves changing the heavy chain that is expressed to produce other antibody classes—IgG, IgA, or IgE. Although this switch does not alter antibody affinity, the change in class of antibody will alter its effector function and thereby affect the immune response (Fairfax et al, 2008).

Etiology and incidence

The etiology of myeloma and other plasma cell dyscrasias is not known. Risk factors other than race and sex include environmental agents such as radiation and certain chemicals, as well as presence in first-degree relatives, indicating familial predisposition in some patients (Kyle and Rajkumar, 2007; Vachon et al, 2009). Several studies indicate that myeloma risk increases with cumulative exposure to ionizing radiation (Brown et al, 2008). Chemicals such as dioxin and other herbicides and pesticides have also been shown to increase the risk of myeloma as much as 3- to 4-fold (Kyle and Rajkumar, 2007). In a recent study, the prevalence of MGUS among pesticide applicators was twice that in a population-based sample of men from Minnesota, adding support to the hypothesis that specific pesticides are causatively linked to myelomagenesis (Landgren, Kyle, Hoppin, et al, 2009).

Recent studies suggest that an asymptomatic MGUS stage consistently precedes MM (Landgren, Kyle, Pfeiffer, et al, 2009). MGUS is present in 3% of persons >50 years old and in 5% of persons >70 years old. The risk of progression to MM or a related disorder is 1% per year (Kyle and Rajkumar, 2005). Patients with risk factors consisting of an abnormal serum free light chain ratio, non-IgG MGUS, and an elevated serum M protein ≥15 g/L had a risk of progression at 20 years of 58%, compared with 37% with 2 risk factors present, 21% with 1 risk factor present, and 5% when none of the risk factors were present (Rajkumar et al, 2004). The cumulative probability of progression to active MM or AL was 51% at 5 years, 66% at 10 years, and 73% at 15 years; the median time to progression (TTP) was 4.8 years (Rajkumar et al, 2007). A study of the natural history of smoldering MM (SMM) suggests that there are 2 different types: evolving SMM and nonevolving SMM (Dimopoulos, Spencer, et al, 2009). Evolving SMM is characterized by a progressive increase in M protein and a shorter median TTP of 1.3 years. Nonevolving SMM has a stable M protein that changes more abruptly at the time of progressive disease, with a median TTP of 3.9 years (Dimopoulos, Spencer, et al, 2009).

The incidence of MM increases with age, with an average age at diagnosis of 65 years; is more common in people of West African heritage; and is the second most common hematologic malignancy after non-Hodgkin lymphoma (Jemal et al, 2009). The incidence in the United States is 20,580 cases, and the estimated number of deaths is 10,580 according to the 2009 estimates (Jemal et al, 2009).

Molecular pathogenesis

Genetic and epigenetic regulation of MM

A number of chromosomal translocations have been identified in plasma cell dyscrasias (Fonseca et al, 2004). The most common primary translocations involve the Ig heavy chain locus in association with many partner genes, including cyclin D1, cyclin D3, and *FGFR3/MMSET* (Bergsagel et al, 2005; Fonseca et al, 2003; Hideshima et al, 2004). These appear to occur during Ig heavy chain class switch recombination, suggesting that the final transforming event arose in a postgerminal center B cell. A common secondary event appears to involve c-*myc* and is associated with tumor progression (Hideshima et al, 2004).

The rearranged Ig genes are somatically hypermutated in a manner compatible with antigen selection. By conventional analyses, karyotypic abnormalities are detected in MM at a frequency of 30% to 50% in large studies of MM tumors. The frequency and extent of karyotypic abnormalities correlate with the stage, prognosis, and response to therapy. For example, approximately 20% are abnormal in stage I disease, 60% are abnormal in stage III disease, and >80% are abnormal in extramedullary tumor. By interphase fluorescence in situ hybridization (FISH) analysis, 2 studies reported that at least 1 chromosome is trisomic in 96% or 89% of MM tumor samples, respectively. Although conventional karyotypes are not routinely reported for MGUS, it appears that a substantial fraction of MGUS plasma cells are aneuploid as well. By FISH analysis, the incidence of trisomy for at least 1 chromosome was 43% and 53% in 2 studies of MGUS cells; in the former, 61% of the cells had an aneuploid DNA content by image analysis. The characteristic numerical abnormalities are monosomy 13 and trisomies of chromosomes 3, 5, 7, 9, 11, 15, and 19. Nonrandom structural abnormalities most frequently involve chromosome 1 with no apparent locus specificity; 14q32 (IgH) locus occurs in 20% to 40%; 11q13 (bcl-1) locus occurs in approximately 20% but mostly translocated to 14q32; 13q14 interstitial deletion occurs in 15%; and 8q24 occurs in approximately 10%, with approximately half of these involved in a translocation. Importantly, similar translocations occur in MGUS and MM, including t(4;14)(p16.3;q32) and t(14;16)(q32;q23), without any obvious clinical or biologic correlation. Table 20-2 summarizes chromosomal alternations of myeloma.

The hallmark genetic lesion in many B-lymphocyte tumors involves dysregulation of an oncogene as a consequence of a translocation involving the IgH locus (14q32.3) occurring in approximately 20% to 40% of MM with an abnormal karyotype; less frequently, variant translocations involve 1 of the IgL loci, (2p12) or λ(22q11) (Hideshima et al, 2004). The incidence of these translocations is significantly higher in the extramedullary phase of the disease and in cell lines, perhaps due to a higher number of metaphase spreads that are examined.

Table 20-2 Myeloma chromosomal alterations.

Chromosome anomalies: incidence
 Conventional banding: 30%-50% of patients
 Interphase FISH: >90% of patients
 SKY: ? ~100%

Specific chromosome changes
 14q32: majority of cases
 11q13: most common (bcl-1 locus, 30%)
 4p16 (FGFR3, MMSET, 25%)
 8 q24 (c-*myc*, 5%)
 16q23 (c-*maf*, 1%)
 6p25 (*Irf4*, rare)
 13 deletion (Rb)

Sources: Bergsagel L et al. Promiscuous translocations into immunoglobulin heavy chain switch regions in multiple myeloma. *Proc Natl Acad Sci USA*. 1996;93:13931–13936.
Facon T, Avet-Loiseau H, Guillerm G, et al. Chromosome 13 abnormalities identified by FISH analysis and serum β$_2$-microglobulin produce a powerful myeloma staging system for patients receiving high-dose therapy. *Blood*. 2001;97:1566.
Fonseca R, Bailey RJ, Ahmann GJ, et al. Genomic abnormalities in monoclonal gammopathy of undetermined significance. *Blood*. 2002;100:1417.
Kuehl WM, Bergsagel PL. Multiple myeloma: evolving genetic events and host interactions. *Nat Rev Cancer*. 2002;2:175.
Tricot G. *Br J Hematol* 2002;116:211.

In approximately 30% of these translocations, the partner chromosomal locus is 11q13 (bcl-1, cyclin D1), but in most cases, the partner is not identified (14q32+). The expression level of *cyclin D1, cyclin D2,* or *cyclin D3* messenger RNA (mRNA) in MM and MGUS is distinctly higher than in normal plasma cells, comparable to the levels of cyclin D2 mRNA expressed in normal proliferating peripheral blood (Bergsagel et al, 2005). Normal hematopoietic cells, including normal B lymphocytes, plasma cells, and peripheral blood cells, express cyclin D2 and/or D3, but little or no cyclin D1. Almost all MM tumors dysregulate at least 1 of the cyclin D genes. Ig translocations that dysregulate cyclin D1 or cyclin D3 occur in approximately 20% of MM tumors. Cyclin D1 is expressed in nearly 40% of tumors without t(11;14) translocations, whereas levels of cyclin D2 are seen in the remaining tumors (Bergsagel et al, 2005).

Other recurrent partner loci have been identified infrequently, including 8q24 (c-*myc*) in <5%, 18q21 (*bcl-2*), 11q23 (*MLL-1*), and 6p21.1 (Hideshima et al, 2004). By combining conventional karyotypic analysis with a comprehensive Southern blot assay, which detects translocations involving IgH switch regions, it has become apparent that most MM cell lines and 1 primary tumor fully examined have IgH translocations that mainly involve IgH switch regions. FISH studies have also shown that IgH gene rearrangements are present in 73% of MM patients. The apparent oncogene dysregulated by the t(4;14) is the fibroblast growth factor receptor 3 (*FGFR3*) gene, and it is possible that dysregulated expression of *FGFR3*, as a result of t(4;14), receives an *FGFR3*-mediated signal from fibroblast growth factor (FGF) produced by stromal cells in the BM microenvironment (Keats et al, 2003). The t(4;14) in MM regulates both *FGFR3* and a novel gene, *MMSET*, resulting in *IgH/MMSET* hybrid transcripts. Ectopic expression of *FGFR3* promotes MM cell proliferation and prevents apoptosis, and its oncogenic potential has been tested in a murine model confirming its capacity to transform hemopoietic cells (Chen et al, 2005). There is evidence that elevated expression of c-*myc* and selective expression of 1 c-*myc* allele may occur frequently in MM, even though structural genetic changes near c-*myc* have been identified in only 10% to 20% of tumor cells.

Ras mutations occur in approximately 39% of newly diagnosed MM patients, and the frequency of *ras* mutations increases with disease progression (Fonesca et al, 2004). Mutations of N- and K-*ras* are rarely detected in solitary plasmacytoma and MGUS but occur more frequently in MM (9%-30%) and in the majority of terminal disease or plasma cell leukemia (PCL) patients (63%-70%). Activating mutations of the *ras* oncogenes may also result in growth factor independence and suppression of apoptosis in MM.

p53 mutations are not frequent in MM and are a late event in the disease; *p53* mutations occur in 5% of inactive MM and in 20% to 40% of acute PCL. Thus, *p53* mutations may cause a block of plasmablastic apoptosis and differentiation at the final stages of plasma cell maturation (Alvino et al, 1999).

As mentioned previously, chromosome 13 deletions are present in >50% of MM patients and considered to be associated with poor prognosis. However, these deletions are also associated with MGUS, and their role in transformation of MGUS to MM is thus at present undefined (Bernasconi et al, 2002; Fonesca et al, 2002). Furthermore, the presence of chromosome 13 deletion by FISH does not significantly affect survival of chromosomal hyperdiploidy MM patients. Interestingly, chromosome 13 deletions are not predictive of poor outcome with bortezomib, in contrast to other agents, including high-dose dexamethasone (Richardson, Barlogie, et al, 2005).

Gene expression profiling, array comparative genomic hybridization, and spectral karyotyping and multiplex FISH have confirmed and extended results from conventional cytogenetics and FISH (Carrasco et al, 2006). These techniques have allowed prognostic classification and insights into the pathogenesis of MM based on genetic abnormalities (Carrasco et al, 2006).

Figure 20-1 summarizes the critical role of cyclin D dysregulation in the pathogenesis of MM.

Epigenetics in MM

Classic genetics alone cannot explain the diversity of phenotypes within a population or the different susceptibilities to disease in twins (Esteller, 2008). Epigenetics is defined as heritable changes in gene expression that do not involve a change in DNA sequence. Epigenetics have now been widely accepted as major regulators of tumor suppressors and oncogenes and in the development of many tumor types (Esteller, 2006, 2007). The main epigenetic changes include DNA methylation and histone modification (Esteller, 2007, 2008). MicroRNAs (miRNAs) are a recently discovered group of small RNA molecules involved in the regulation of gene expression (Cowland et al, 2007).

A study examined the aberrant promoter methylation profile of 14 known or suspected tumor suppressor genes in leukemias (n = 48), lymphomas (n = 42), MMs (n = 40), and MGUS (n = 20) (Takahashi et al, 2004). Ten of the genes studied were methylated at frequencies of 29% to 68% in one or more tumor types. In general, the methylation pattern of MGUS was similar to that of MM, although the methylation frequencies were lower (the methylation index of MGUS was 0.15, and the index of MM was 0.3) (Takahashi et al, 2004). Another study with

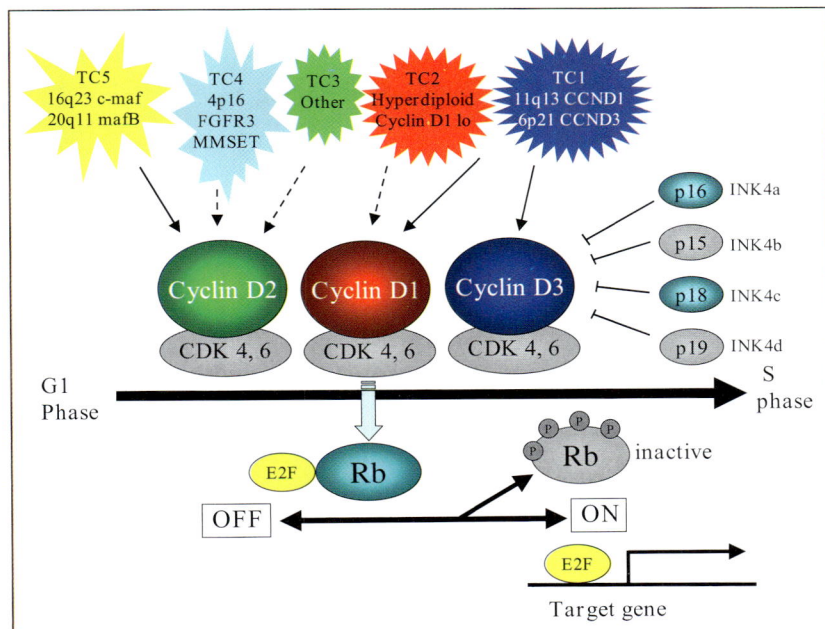

Figure 20-1 The critical role of cyclin D dysregulation in the pathogenesis of multiple myeloma (MM) highlights the importance of the cyclin D/Rb pathway and suggests that there may be a therapeutic window in targeting this pathway for all molecular subtypes of MM.

32 cases of MM and 19 cases of MGUS found significantly increased methylation of $p16$ ($P = .001$), $SHP1$ ($P \leq .001$), and E-$cadherin$ ($P \leq .001$) genes in the MM cases compared with the MGUS cases. Methylation of DAP kinase and estrogen receptor genes was comparable in MM and MGUS (Chim et al, 2007). However, a different study using plasma cells from 33 patients with MGUS and 33 patients with MM were isolated and analyzed for p15(INK4b) and p16(INK4a) methylation by methylation-specific polymerase chain reaction. Selective methylation was found in 19% for p16(INK4a), 36% for p15(INK4b), and 6.5% for both genes in MGUS, and frequencies were similar in MM, suggesting that methylation of these genes is an early event not associated with transition from MGUS to MM (Guillerm et al, 2001). These studies indicate that methylation of some tumor suppressor genes may be related to tumor progression from MGUS to MM and highlight the role of epigenetics in this disease.

Several recent studies have examined the role of miRNA in MM (Lionetti et al, 2009; Pichiorri et al, 2008; Roccaro et al, 2009; Ronchetti et al, 2008). A recent study examined the role of miRNA in the malignant transformation of plasma cells (Pichiorri et al, 2008). This study identified overexpression of miR-21, miR-106b approximately 25 cluster, and miR-181a and miR-181b in MM and MGUS samples with respect to healthy plasma cells. Selective up-regulation of miR-32 and miR-17 approximately 92 cluster was identified in MM patients and cell lines but not in MGUS patients or healthy plasma cells. Furthermore, 2 miRNAs, miR-19a and miR-19b, that are part of the miR-17 approximately 92 cluster, were shown to down-regulate expression of $SOCS$-1, a gene frequently silenced in MM that plays a critical role as inhibitor of interleukin (IL)-6 growth signaling. They also identified p300-CBP–associated factor, a gene involved in p53 regulation, as a bona fide target of the miR-106b approximately 25 cluster, miR-181a and miR-181b, and miR-32. Xenograft studies using human MM cell lines treated with miR-19a, miR-19b, miR-181a, and miR-181b antagonists resulted in significant suppression of tumor growth in nude mice (Pichiorri et al, 2008). Another recent study showed an MM-specific miRNA signature characterized by underexpression of miRNA-15a/-16 and overexpression of miRNA-222/-221/-382/-181a/-181b ($P < .01$) (Roccaro et al, 2009). miRNA-15a and miRNA-16-1 are both located on chromosome 13. The functional role of miRNA-15a and miRNA-16 was further investigated and showed that they regulate proliferation and growth of MM cells in vitro and in vivo (Roccaro et al, 2009). These data indicate that miRNAs play a pivotal role in the biology of MM and represent important targets for novel therapies in MM.

Role of the BM microenvironment in MM pathogenesis

Despite limits to our understanding of the molecular events of neoplastic transformation in MM, advances have been made in understanding the biology of the disease. The BM microenvironment appears to be fundamental for the proliferation, survival, and resistance of myeloma (Roodman, 2002). Cytokines, such as IL-6, play important roles in the pathogenesis and progression of the disease and its pathophysiologic manifestations (Hideshima et al, 2001). BM stromal cells (BMSCs) are a major source of IL-6, which acts to promote myeloma cell survival by inhibiting apoptosis. IL-6 also contributes to bone loss in myeloma by stimulating osteoclast formation and inhibiting bone formation (Hideshima et al, 2001). It has been demonstrated that malignant plasma cells interact with extracellular matrix (ECM) proteins and that these interactions protect the cells from chemotherapy- and radiation therapy–induced cell death.

MM cells home to the BM and adhere to ECM proteins and to BMSCs, a process that not only localizes tumor cells in the BM milieu but also has important functional sequelae. Specifically, adhesion of MM cells to ECM proteins confers cell adhesion–mediated drug resistance (CAM-DR), and binding of MM cells to BMSCs triggers transcription and secretion of cytokines (ie, IL-6, insulin-like growth factor-1 [IGF-1], or vascular endothelial growth factor [VEGF]) from BMSCs, which not only promotes growth, survival, and migration of MM cells, but also further confers resistance to conventional chemotherapy (Damiano et al, 1999; Damiano and Dalton, 2000; Damiano, 2002). Therefore, delineation of mechanisms mediating MM cell growth, survival, and drug resistance in the BM milieu provides the framework to develop and validate novel therapeutic agents to improve the outcomes of patients with MM.

Role of adhesion molecules

Adhesion molecules mediate both homotypic and heterotypic adhesion of MM cells to either ECM proteins or BMSCs (Uchiyama et al, 1992; Podar et al, 2007). Adhesion molecules CD44, very late antigen 4 (VLA-4, CD49d), VLA-5 (CD49e), leukocyte function-associated antigen 1 (LFA-1, CD11a), neuronal adhesion molecule (NCAM, CD56), intercellular adhesion molecule (ICAM-1, CD54), syndecan-1 (CD138), and MPC-1 mediate homing of MM cells to the BM. Subsequently, tumor cells bind to type I collagen and fibronectin (ECM proteins) via syndecan-1 and VLA-4 on MM cells, respectively, and to BMSCs (ie, via VLA-4) on MM cells to VCAM-1 (CD106) on BMSCs (Uchiyama et al, 1992). This MM cell adherence to BMSCs not only localizes tumor cells in the BM microenvironment, but also has important functional and clinical sequelae (Uchiyama et al, 1992). Elevated level of serum syndecan-1 correlates with increased tumor cell mass, decreased metalloproteinase-9 activity, and poor prognosis. Furthermore, adhesion of MM cells via syndecan-1 to collagen induces matrix metalloproteinase-1, thereby promoting bone resorption and tumor invasion. Moreover, binding via VLA-4 on MM cells to the fibronectin up-regulates *p27Kip1* and other genetic changes, which confer CAM-DR (Chauhan et al, 1996; Shain et al, 2009). Importantly, serum IL-6 and IL-6 receptors are prognostic factors in MM and reflect the proliferative fraction of MM cells within patients. C-reactive protein (CRP), an acute-phase reactant synthesized in the liver in response to IL-6, can serve as a surrogate prognostic factor. IL-6 or CRP, either alone or coupled with β_2-microglobulin (β2M) as a measure of MM cell mass, provides the framework for a biologically based staging system in MM.

Because adhesion molecules play a crucial role in the pathogenesis of MM, targeting these molecules could be potential novel therapeutic strategies (Schmidmaier and Baumann, 2008).

Role of cytokines in MM
Interleukin-6

Although some MM cells secrete IL-6 and grow in an autocrine fashion, IL-6 is primarily produced in BMSCs and mediates paracrine MM cell growth (Hideshima et al, 2001, 2005). IL-6 secretion from BMSCs is up-regulated by many molecules/cytokines (ie, CD40, tumor necrosis factor-α [TNF-α], VEGF, IL-1β, transforming growth factor-β [TGF-β]) and MM cell adherence. Importantly, nuclear factor (NF)-κB plays a central role in cytokine- and adhesion-mediated IL-6 up-regulation and specific inhibition of NF-αB blocks IL-6 secretion (Chauhan et al, 1997). Many MM cell lines and patient tumor cells respond to IL-6. Interestingly, CD45$^+$ MM cells have recently been identified as those MM cells responsive to IL-6.

Clinically, serum IL-6 and IL-6 receptors are prognostic factors in MM and reflect the proliferative fraction of MM cells within patients. CRP, an acute-phase reactant synthesized in the liver in response to IL-6, can serve as a surrogate prognostic factor (Guo and Chen, 2006). IL-6 or CRP, either alone or coupled with β2M as a measure of MM cell mass, provides the framework for a biologically based staging system in MM. Treatment strategies targeting IL-6, including antibodies to IL-6 and IL-6 receptor as well as IL-6 superantagonists, that block IL-6 binding to its receptor mediate signaling for IL-6R binding but do not activate downstream signaling. To date, however, only transient responses have been observed (Richardson, Mitsiades, et al, 2007).

Insulin-like growth factor-1

IGF-1 is a multifunctional peptide that regulates cell proliferation, differentiation, and apoptosis (Pene et al, 2002). In the circulation, IGF-I binds primarily to the main IGF binding protein, IGFBP-3. Several studies of risk in malignancies including lung, breast, prostate, and colorectal cancer suggest that high concentrations of circulating IGF-1 are associated with an increased risk of cancer, whereas high IGFBP-3 concentrations are associated with a decreased risk. However, the direct relationship of serum IGF-1 level and prognosis in MM has not yet been clarified. Indeed, mean IGF-1 level does not differ between myeloma patients and controls. However, IGF-1 was a strong indicator of prognosis (Guo and Chen, 2006). Therapies targeting IGF-1, such as inhibitors of IGF-1 receptor, have already shown preclinical anti-MM activity and will undergo clinical evaluation (Mitsiades et al, 2004)

Vascular endothelial growth factor

VEGF is a known angiogenic factor in both solid tumor and hematologic malignancies (Podar and Anderson, 2005). In MM, it is produced both by MM cells and BMSCs and may account, at least in part, for the increased angiogenesis observed in MM patients' BM (Le Gouill et al, 2004). It has been shown that increased microvessel density (MVD) in MM patients' BM specimens is associated with poor prognosis, and BM MVD at diagnosis is an important prognostic factor for survival of patients who undergo autologous transplantation as frontline therapy (Kumar, Gertz, et al, 2004; Guo and Chen, 2006).

Figure 20-2 shows cytokine-mediated signaling cascades in MM. Figure 20-3 shows the interaction of MM cells with the BM microenvironment including cytokine secretion and interaction with osteoclasts, osteoblasts, and BM endothelial cells.

Role of angiogenesis in MM

BM endothelial cells (BMECs) are also involved in the initial homing of myeloma cells to the BM stromal compartment, and medullary angiogenesis in active MM is driven by the paracrine activation of BMEC by angiogenic cytokines and proteases secreted by myeloma cells, fibroblasts, and osteoclasts. The adhesion between MM cells and BMSCs up-regulates many cytokines with angiogenic activity, most notably VEGF and basic fibroblast growth factor (bFGF) (Podar and Anderson, 2005). In myeloma cells, these angiogenic factors may also be produced constitutively as a result of oncogene activation and/or genetic mutations (Rajkumar and Witzig, 2000).

Evidence for the importance of angiogenesis in the pathogenesis of MM was obtained from BM samples from MM patients (Kumar, Gertz, et al, 2004). The level of BM angiogenesis, as assessed by grading and/or MVD, is consistently increased in patients with active MM compared with patients with inactive disease or MGUS, a less advanced plasma cell disorder (Kumar, Gertz, et al, 2004). Among patients with active MM, MVD has been directly correlated with the degree of plasma cell proliferation and infiltration, revealing MVD to be an adverse prognostic marker (Rajkumar and Kyle, 2001).

BMSCs from MM patients were found to express VEGF and bFGF in addition to several other proangiogenic

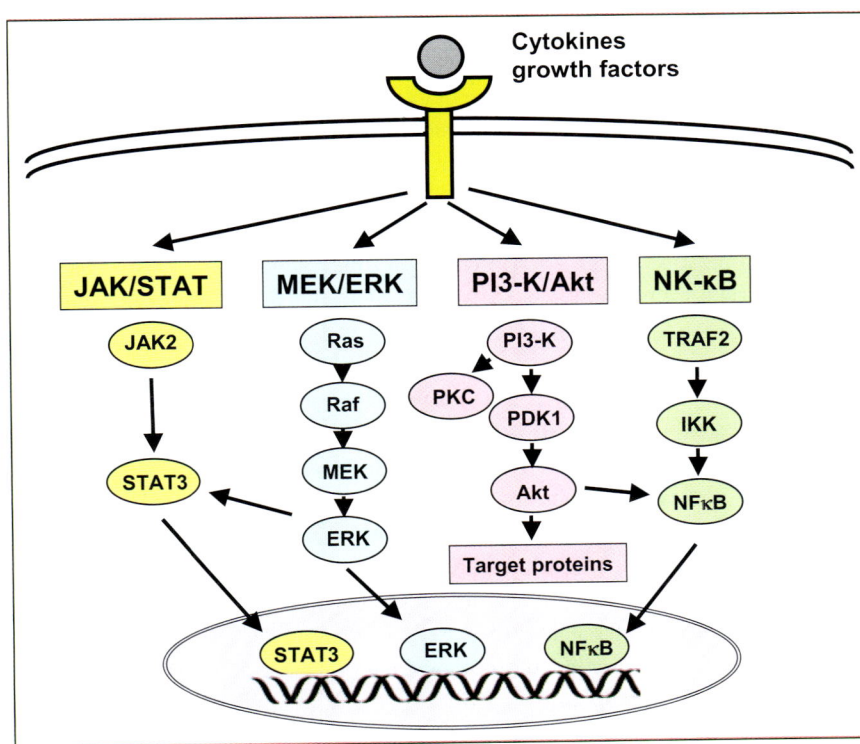

Figure 20-2 Cytokine-mediated signaling cascades in MM. IL-6 triggers Ras/Raf/MEK/ERK-mediated proliferation; induces JAK2/STAT3 signaling promoting MM cell survival and activates PI3K/Akt signaling, thereby mediating antiapoptosis and drug resistance in MM cells. IGF-1, VEGF, and SDF-1α activate ERK and PI3K/Akt signaling cascades. TNFα triggers NFκB activation, thereby enhancing MM cell-BMSC adherence and cytokine secretion.

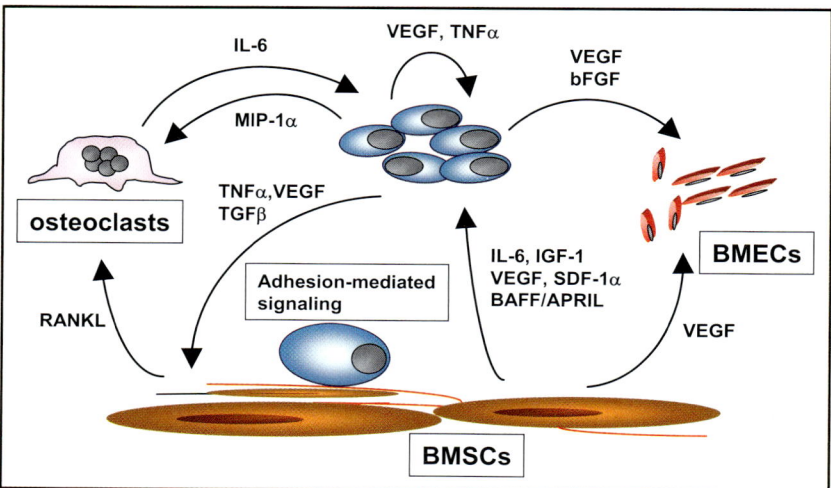

Figure 20-3 Growth factors for MM cells in the BM microenvironment. MM cells secrete VEGF, bFGF, TNFα, TGFβ, and MIP-1α. BMSCs secrete IL-6, VEGF, SDF-1α, and RANKL. Cytokines secreted from either MM cells or BMSCs further augment these cytokine secretions. TNFα, VEGF and TGFβ from MM cells enhance IL-6 secretion from BMSCs. VEGF and bFGF trigger angiogenesis in BM endothelial cells. MIP-1α and RANKL trigger osteoclast formation, thereby inducing bone destruction in MM. Osteoclasts also produce IL-6, promoting MM cell growth and antiapoptosis.

molecules, including angiopoietin-1 (Ang-1), TGF-β, platelet-derived growth factor (PDGF), hepatocyte growth factor (HGF), IL-1, and others (Alexandrakis et al, 2004). An analysis in newly diagnosed MM found a correlation between MVD, syndecan-1 (in blood and BM), and level of serum HGF (Scudla et al, 2006).

Role of chemokines and cell trafficking in MM

MM is characterized by the presence of multiple lytic lesions in most patients, indicating continuous spread of MM cells into and out of the BM (Kyle and Rajkumar, 2004). Indeed, studies have demonstrated the presence of a small number of circulating plasma cells in >70% of patients with MM (Nowakowski et al, 2005), indicating that progression of MM occurs through the continuous trafficking of malignant cells to new sites of the BM. Therefore, adhesion of MM cells to the BM niches is not a static process, but an active dynamic process that involves migration of the malignant cells to the specific BM niches, adhesion to the microenvironment, and egress or mobilization of some of these cells into the peripheral circulation to home to other new sites in the BM.

Migration of cells through the blood to the BM niches requires active navigation, a process termed *homing*. Homing is thought to be a coordinated, multistep process that involves signaling by stromal derived factor-1 (SDF-1) and its chemokine receptor CXCR4; activation of adhesion receptors such as lymphocyte function–associated antigen 1 (LFA-1) and VLA-4/5; cytoskeleton rearrangement; and activation of metalloproteases MMP2/9 (Kollet et al, 2003; Avecilla et al, 2004; Lapidot et al, 2005). Other cytokines that also regulate migration of MM cells include VEGF and IGF-1. Studies of chemokine receptors in MM have demonstrated that MM cell lines express high levels of CXCR3, CXCR4, CCR1, and CCR6. The ligands of these receptors are MIP-1α, MIP-1β, SDF-1, CXC, and RANTES. Of these, the CXCR4/SDF-1 axis plays a critical role in regulating migration and adhesion of MM cells. Studies to identify expression of chemokine receptors in MM have shown large variations in CXCR4 expression ranging from 10% to 100% (Moller et al, 2003). SDF-1 induces migration of MM cells in vitro and homing into the BM in vivo. In addition, SDF-1 induces modest proliferation of MM cells, as well phosphorylation of MEK1/2, p42/44 MAPK, and AKT in a time-dependent fashion in MM cell lines and primary MM cells (Hideshima et al, 2002). CXCR4 is essential for the migration of MM cells in vitro and their homing in vivo (Alsayed et al, 2007). CXCR4 knockdown led to significant inhibition of migration to SDF-1 in MM cell lines and primary CD138+ cells (Alsayed et al, 2007).

Mobilization or egress of cells out of the BM could be enhanced by disrupting the SDF-1/CXCR4 axis. This may occur by decreasing the concentration of endogenous SDF-1 (eg, after infusion of granulocyte colony-stimulating factor [G-CSF] or cyclophosphamide) in BM as performed for stem cell transplantation (SCT) in MM (Petit et al, 2002); by the cleavage and inactivation of SDF-1 by proteases in the BM (Lapidot, 2001); or by up-regulation of CXCR4 expression by hypoxia. Mobilization of stem cells from the BM may also occur if CXCR4 is inhibited (Flomenberg et al, 2005). Inhibitors of CXCR4 such as AMD3100 (Genzyme, Cambridge, MA) have been shown to induce mobilization of stem cells (Broxmeyer et al, 2005; Grignani et al, 2005). AMD3100 is a bicyclam molecule that reversibly blocks the binding of CXCR4 with SDF-1 (De Clercq, 2005). A recent report showed that the CXCR4 inhibitor AMD3100 induced disruption of the interaction of MM cells with the BM reflected by mobilization of MM cells into the circulation in vivo, with kinetics that differed from that of hematopoietic stem cells (Azab et al, 2009). AMD3100 enhanced sensitivity to bortezomib in vitro by disrupting adhesion of MM cells to stromal cells. The combination of AMD3100 and bortezomib induced significant tumor reduction (Azab et al, 2009).

Osteoclasts in MM

Osteolytic bone lesions develop in >70% to 80% of patients throughout the axial skeleton and are one of the major sources of morbidity and mortality for patients with MM (Callander and Roodman, 2001). These lesions are frequently associated with severe and debilitating bone pain and pathologic fractures (Melton et al, 2005). There is a balance between bone destruction and new bone formation; however, in more advanced disease, this balance is lost, resulting in bone destruction and the development of osteolytic lesions (Bataille et al, 1989). Bone destruction develops adjacent to MM cells, yet not in areas of normal BM. Furthermore, new bone formation, which would normally develop at sites of prior bone destruction, is absent with evidence of apoptotic osteoblasts (Taube et al, 1992). The lack of osteoblasts explains why nuclear medicine bone scans underestimate the degree of bone destruction in patients with MM. The bone lesions that develop rarely heal, even when patients are in a complete remission. As a consequence of increased bone destruction, nearly 15% of patients develop hypercalcemia. The combination of hypercalcemia, pathologic fractures, nerve compression, and severe bone pain leads to significant morbidity and mortality for patients with MM (Roodman, 2004).

There are several factors implicated in osteoclast activation, including receptor activator of NF-κB ligand (RANKL), macrophage inflammatory protein-1α (MIP-1α), IL-3, and IL-6 (Roodman, 2009). RANKL is a member of the TNF family and serves a major role in the increased osteoclastogenesis implicated in MM bone disease (Roodman, 2004). MM cell binding to neighboring stromal cells within the BM of patients with MM results in increased RANKL expression. This leads to an increase in osteoclast activity through the binding of RANKL to its receptor on osteoclast precursor cells, which further promotes their differentiation (Ehrlich and Roodman, 2005). RANKL is also involved in inhibition of osteoclast apoptosis.

Osteoblasts in MM

Several factors are felt to be responsible for the suppressed osteoblast activity observed in MM; however, their precise role is just beginning to be identified. Some of these markers include IL-3, dickkopf 1 (DKK1), secreted frizzled-related protein-2 (sFRP-2), and IL-7 (Tian et al, 2003; Ehrlich et al, 2005; Giuliani et al, 2005; Oshima et al, 2005). Certain factors (DKK1 and sFRP-2) appear to affect the Wnt signaling pathway, critical for osteoblast differentiation (Canalis et al, 2005), whereas others (IL-3 and IL-7) do not appear to directly affect this signaling pathway. These are soluble inhibitors of signaling pathways that affect osteoblast differentiation and not osteoblast survival, suggesting that their inhibitory effects should be reversible when MM cells are no longer present (Huston and Roodman, 2006). A soluble inhibitor of the Wnt signaling pathway, DKK1, is produced by osteoblasts and plays a critical role in osteoblast differentiation (Tian et al, 2003; Oshima et al, 2005). DKK1 is important in osteoblast suppression in myeloma (Tian et al, 2003). DKK1 is secreted by MM cells and inhibits osteoblast differentiation. A high correlation of *DKK1* gene expression levels with the extent of bone disease was demonstrated in MM patients. In contrast, other investigators have found *DKK1* not to be expressed by MM cells (Tian et al, 2003; Oshima et al, 2005), no evidence of up-regulation after MM cell binding to preosteoblasts, and an absence of blockade on the inhibitory effects of MM cell lines on human osteoblast differentiation when treated with antibody to DKK1. A more recent study showed that levels of DKK1 were elevated in patients with MM as compared with either patients with MGUS or normal controls. A sustained decrease in levels after autologous SCT correlated with a normalization of markers of bone turnover, suggesting a return of osteoblast activity (Politou et al, 2006). Another study demonstrated that treating severe combined immunodeficiency (SCID) mice implanted with rabbit bone rudiments containing primary myeloma cells with an antibody to DKK1 decreased bone destruction, increased bone formation, and decreased tumor growth (Yaccoby et al, 2007).

Diagnostic evaluation

Although some patients with MM are asymptomatic at the time of presentation, most patients present with symptoms. The most common presenting complaint is bone pain from lytic lesions or compression fractures, but patients may also be symptomatic from anemia, hypercalcemia, or renal insufficiency. Recurrent infections are frequent as a result of impaired cellular immunity and the reduced levels of normal Ig.

The initial evaluation of a suspected monoclonal gammopathy should include both serum and urine protein electrophoresis with immunofixation to identify and quantify the M protein (Table 20-3). The majority of patients will have a detectable M protein, but approximately 1% to 3% can present with a nonsecretory myeloma that does not produce light or heavy chains (Kyle and Rajkumar, 2008, 2009). True nonsecreting myeloma is rare because, with the availability of serum free light chain testing, it is recognized that M protein is present. The most common M protein is IgG, followed by IgA and light chain only disease. IgD and IgE are

Table 20-3 Monoclonal gammopathy: staging studies.

Complete blood count, including differential to assess for circulatory plasma cells
Chemistry with BUN, creatinine
Serum protein electrophoresis with immunofixation
Quantitative immunoglobulins
24-hour urine immunoelectrophoresis
Skeletal survey (plain films)
Serum β_2-microglobulin, albumin
Bone marrow aspirate and biopsy
Cytogenetics/FISH
Serum free light chain
MRI
PET scan

BUN 5 blood urea nitrogen; FISH = fluorescent in situ hybridization; MRI = magnetic resonance imaging; PET = positron emission tomography.

relatively uncommon and can be more difficult to diagnose because their M spikes are often small (Kyle and Rajkumar, 2008). Up to 20% of patients will produce only light chains, which may not be detectable in the serum because they pass through the glomeruli and are excreted in the urine. The standard evaluation of a documented monoclonal gammopathy includes a complete blood count with differential, calcium, serum urea nitrogen, and creatinine. As mentioned previously, serum free light chain testing is also a useful diagnostic test (Piehler et al, 2008). Bone disease is best assessed by skeletal survey. Bone scans are not a sensitive measure of myelomatous bone lesions because the radioisotope is poorly taken up by the lytic lesions. Magnetic resonance imaging (MRI) is useful for the evaluation of solitary plasmacytoma of bone, for more sensitive detection of marrow and lytic lesions (positron emission tomography [PET]) than skeletal survey, and for the evaluation of paraspinal and epidural components (Mulligan, 2005; Dimopoulos, Spencer, et al, 2009). A BM aspiration and biopsy are important to quantify the plasma cell infiltrate and add important prognostic information with cytogenetic evaluation, including FISH. Additional prognostic information can be obtained with serum β2M and CRP.

Staging/prognostic factors

The criteria for the diagnosis of MM, SMM, and MGUS are detailed in Table 20-1. Distinction among these entities is important for making treatment decisions and prognostic recommendations.

Several staging systems exist. The most widely used myeloma staging system since 1975 has been the Durie–Salmon, in which the clinical stage of disease is based on several measurements including levels of M protein, serum hemoglobin value, serum calcium level, and the number of bone lesions. The International Staging System (ISS), developed by the International Myeloma Working Group, is now more widely used (Greipp et al, 2005). Both are outlined in Table 20-4. This validated system is based on 2 prognostic factors, serum levels of β2M and albumin, and is comprised of 3 stages: β2M ≤3.5 mg/L and albumin ≥3.5 g/dL (median survival, 62 months; stage I); β2M <3.5 mg/L and albumin <3.5 g/dL or β2M ≥3.5 to <5.5 mg/L (median survival, 44 months; stage II); and β2M ≥5.5 mg/L (median survival, 29 months; stage III) (Greipp et al, 2005). With an increased understanding of the biology of myeloma, other factors have been shown to correlate well with clinical outcome and are now commonly used. These factors are also listed in Table 20-4. Cytogenetic abnormalities as detected by FISH techniques have been shown to identify patient populations with very different outcomes. Loss of the long arm of chromosome 13 is found in up to 50% of patients and is associated

Table 20-4 Staging systems for multiple myeloma: Durie–Salmon staging system and International Staging System (ISS).

Stage	Durie–Salmon system	ISS staging system
I	Hemoglobin value >10 g/dL	β2M ≤3.5 and albumin ≥3.5 g/dL
	Calcium normal or ≤12 mg/dL	C-reactive protein ≤4.0 mg/dL
	Normal skeletal survey or solitary plasmacytoma	Plasma cell labeling index <1%
	Low M protein with an IgG <5 g/dL or IgA <3 g/dL	Absence of chromosome 13 deletion
	Bence Jones protein >4 g/24 hours	Low serum IL-6 receptor levels
		Long duration of initial plateau phase
		Chemotherapy/glucocorticoid-sensitive disease
		Median survival of 62 months
II	Neither stage I nor stage III	β2M <3.5 g/dL Albumin <3.5 g/dL OR β2M 3.5 to <5.5 mg/dL Median survival of 44 months
III	One of the following: Hemoglobin value <8.5 g/dL Calcium >12 mg/dL Multiple lytic lesions High M component with an IgG >7 g/dL or IgA >5 g/dL Bence Jones protein >12 g/24 hours	β2M ≥5.5 Median survival of 29 months

*Durie–Salmon subclassification of A or B with A having normal renal function (creatinine < 2.0 mg/dL) and B having abnormal renal function (creatinine > 2.0 mg/dL).
β2M = β$_2$-microglobulin; Ig = immunoglobulin; IL = interleukin.

with poor prognosis, as is a hypodiploid karyotype (Paul et al, 2009). Specifically t(4;14) and −17p13.1 are typically associated with poor outcome; in contrast, t(11;14) and hypodiploidy are associated with improved survival (Kyrtsonis et al, 2009).

Survival

The survival of myeloma patients has increased in the last decade. A recent study examined the outcome of 2 groups of patients seen at Mayo Clinic, one from the time of diagnosis and the other from the time of relapse, to examine the survival trends over time (Kumar et al, 2008). Among 387 patients relapsing after SCT, a clear improvement in overall survival (OS) from the time of relapse was seen, with those relapsing after year 2000 having a median OS of 23.9 months versus 11.8 months ($P < .001$) for those who relapsed prior to this date. Patients treated with one or more of the newer drugs (eg, thalidomide, lenalidomide, bortezomib) had longer survival from relapse (30.9 vs 14.8 months, respectively; $P < .001$). In a larger group of 2981 patients with newly diagnosed myeloma, patients diagnosed in the last decade had a 50% improvement in OS (44.8 vs 29.9 months, respectively; $P < .001$) (Kyle and Rajkumar, 2009).

Another study estimated trends in age-specific 5- and 10-year relative survival of patients with MM in the United States from 1990-1992 to 2002-2004 from the 1973 to 2004 database of the Surveillance, Epidemiology, and End Results (SEER) Program. Techniques of period analysis were used to show most recent developments. Overall, 5-year relative survival increased from 28.8% to 34.7% ($P < .001$), and 10-year relative survival increased from 11.1% to 17.4% ($P < .001$) between 1990-1992 and 2002-2004. Much stronger increases were seen in the age group younger than 50 years, leading to 5- and 10-year relative survival rates of 56.7% and 41.3%, respectively, in 2002-2004, and in the age group 50 to 59 years, leading to 5- and 10-year relative survival rates of 48.2% and 28.6%, respectively, in 200-2004. By contrast, only moderate improvement was seen in the age group 60 to 69 years, and essentially no improvement was achieved among older patients (Kyle and Rajkumar, 2004, 2008).

Treatment

Patients with MGUS should have repeat protein studies approximately every 6 months for 2 to 3 years to assess possible progression and annually thereafter. Patients with SMM should be followed approximately every 3 months with serum protein electrophoresis, blood counts, and creatinine, and with skeletal survey every 12 months or sooner if new symptoms develop. Individuals with progressive disease should be considered for treatment. Evidence of progressive disease includes increasing M protein, declining hemoglobin, increased creatinine, lytic lesions, or recurrent infections related to depressed levels of normal Ig.

Patients should not receive treatment unless they have symptomatic MM. The criteria used to determine initiation of therapy are the CRAB criteria defined as calcium elevation (>11.5 g/dL), renal insufficiency (creatinine >2 mg/dL), anemia (hemoglobin <10 g/dL or 2 g $<$ normal), and bone disease (lytic or osteopenic). Other examples of active disease include repeated infections, secondary AL, hyperviscosity, or hypogammaglobulinemia.

Frontline therapy for symptomatic MM includes either conventional chemotherapy or high-dose chemotherapy (HDT) supported by autologous or allogeneic SCT, depending on patient characteristics such as performance status, age, availability of a sibling donor, comorbidities, and, in some cases, patient and physician preferences. Response to therapy is commonly measured by a reduction in M protein levels in serum and/or urine and the reduction in size or disappearance of plasmacytomas. The international uniform response criteria for MM have expanded upon the European Group for Blood and Marrow Transplantation criteria to provide a more comprehensive evaluation system (Durie et al, 2006). Despite high response rates to frontline therapy, virtually all patients eventually relapse. Thus, research efforts are concentrated on improving frontline therapy to enhance and prolong response, reduce the rate of relapse, and improve the efficacy of treatment at relapse. Importantly, achievement of response has been associated with improved survival in SCT trials with high-dose therapy. Similarly, TTP has been shown to be an important surrogate for improved survival. Table 20-5 shows the international uniform response criteria for MM.

Initial therapy for patients eligible for SCT

Patients with newly diagnosed myeloma who are considered eligible for HDT and SCT should avoid alkylators such as melphalan, which can interfere with adequate stem cell mobilization, regardless of whether an early or delayed transplantation is contemplated. Several new combinations have improved the response and survival of patients with MM. The introduction of targeted therapeutic agents such as thalidomide, bortezomib, and lenalidomide has revolutionized options of treatment in patients with MM. These novel agents, in combination with dexamethasone or cytotoxic therapies, have shown better responses compared with traditional agents such as single-agent dexamethasone or conventional chemotherapy, such as high-dose dexamethasone or doxorubicin, vincristine, and intermittent high-dose dexamethasone (VAD).

Table 20-5 Definitions.

Response category

CR	Negative immunofixation on the serum and urine and disappearance of any soft tissue plasmacytomas and ≤ 5% plasma cells in bone marrow
sCR	CR as described above, plus: normal free light chain (FLC) ratio and absence of clonal cells in bone marrow by immunohistochemistry or immunofluorescence
VGPR	Serum and urine M protein detectable by immunofluorescence but not on electrophoresis or 90% or greater reduction in serum M protein plus urine M protein level <100 mg per 24 hours
PR	≥ 50% reduction of serum M protein and reduction in 24-hour urinary M protein by ≥ 90% or to < 200 mg per 24 hours
	If the serum and urine M protein are unmeasurable, a ≥ 50% decrease in the difference between involved and uninvolved FLC levels is required in place of the M protein criteria
	If serum and urine M protein are unmeasurable, and serum free light assay is also unmeasurable, ≥ 50% reduction in plasma cells is required in place of M protein, provided baseline bone marrow plasma cell percentage was ≥ 30%
	In addition to the above listed criteria, if present at baseline, a ≥ 50% reduction in the size of soft tissue plasmacytomas is also required
SD	Not meeting criteria for CR, VGPR, PR, or progressive disease

Relapse subcategory

Progressive disease   any one or more of the following:

  Increase of ≥ 25% from baseline in:

  – Serum M component and/or (the absolute increase must be ≥0.5 g/dL)

  – Urine M component and/or (the absolute increase must be ≥200 mg/24 h)

  – Only in patients without measurable serum and urine M protein levels: the difference between involved and uninvolved FLC levels. The absolute increase must be ≥10 mg/dL

  – Bone marrow plasma cell percentage: the absolute % must be ≥10%

  – Definite development of new bone lesions or soft tissue plasmacytomas or definite increase in the size of existing bone lesions or soft tissue plasmacytomas

  – Development of hypercalcemia (corrected serum calcium >11.5 mg/dL or 2.65 mmol/L) that can be attributed solely to the plasma cell proliferative disorder

Clinical relapse   one or more of the following:

  – Development of new soft tissue plasmacytomas or bone lesions.

  – Definite increase in the size of existing plasmacytomas or bone lesions. A definite increase is defined as a 50% (and at least 1 cm) increase as measured serially by the sum of the products of the cross-diameters of the measurable lesion

  – Hypercalcemia (>11.5 mg/dL) [2.65 mmol/L]

  – Rise in serum creatinine by 2 mg/dL or more [177 mmol/L or more]

Relapse from CR   one or more of the following:

  – Reappearance of serum or urine M protein by immunofixation or electrophoresis

  – Development of ≥ 5% plasma cells in the bone marrow

  – Appearance of any other sign of progression (ie, new plasmacytoma, lytic bone lesion, or hypercalcemia)

Durie BG, Harousseau JL, Miguel JS, et al. International uniform response criteria for multiple myeloma. *Leukemia.* 2006;20:1467–1473.
CR = Complete response; PR = partial response; SCR = stringent complete response; SD = stable disease; VGPR = very good partial response.

Thalidomide in newly diagnosed transplantation-eligible patients

Several phase III clinical trials have shown that the combination of thalidomide and dexamethasone (TD) is superior to dexamethasone alone in induction therapy in transplantation-eligible patients with newly diagnosed MM. Rajkumar et al (2006) randomized 207 individuals with newly diagnosed MM to either TD or dexamethasone; TD included thalidomide 200 mg daily and dexamethasone 40 mg on days 1 to 4, 9 to 12, and 17 to 20. The combination of TD showed a superior overall response rate (ORR; 63% vs 41%) and complete response (CR) rate (4% vs 0%) compared with the dexamethasone arm. In a second phase III trial of TD versus dexamethasone in 470 transplantation-eligible MM patients, the combination of TD showed an ORR of 64%, whereas dexamethasone alone produced an ORR of 46% (Rajkumar, Rosinol, et al, 2008). TTP was significantly longer in patients who received the combination (22.6 vs 6.5 months). Another study by Macro et al (2006) randomized 203 patients with previously untreated MM to either 4 cycles of TD or 3 cycles of VAD induction, followed by high-dose melphalan 200 mg/m^2 and autologous SCT (ASCT). The rate of very good partial response (VGPR) or better was higher in the TD group prior to stem cell collection (24.7% vs 7.3%) compared with the group receiving VAD chemotherapy. The most common adverse effects of thalidomide include deep vein thrombosis, rash, neuropathy, and bradycardia.

Bortezomib in newly diagnosed transplantation-eligible patients

Harousseau et al (2008) randomized 480 newly diagnosed MM patients to induction therapy with either VAD or bortezomib plus dexamethasone (VD). A second randomization was then performed to either receive or not receive 2 cycles of dexamethasone, cyclophosphamide, etoposide, and cisplatin (DCEP) consolidation prior to ASCT. VD was superior to VAD induction with respect to rates of VGPR or better (46.7% vs 18.6%) and CR/near CR (nCR; 21.3 vs 8.3%). Clinical benefit associated with VD persisted after ASCT with respect to rates of VGPR or better (40.8% vs 28.8%) and CR/nCR (71.8% vs 51%). Response rates were not improved in either treatment group by DCEP consolidation. Another ongoing phase III study randomized 883 transplantation-eligible patients to either VAD or bortezomib plus doxorubicin and dexamethasone (PAD) followed by stem cell mobilization and either single or tandem ASCT (Sonneveld et al, 2008). Patients in the VAD group then received maintenance therapy with thalidomide 50 mg daily, whereas patients in the PAD arm received bortezomib 1.3 mg/m^2 every other week as maintenance. In a preliminary analysis, PAD induction was superior to VAD with respect ORR (80% vs 64%), rate of VGPR orbetter (41% vs 17%), and CR rate (5% vs 0%). The benefit of PAD was also observed after ASCT, with superior ORR (92% vs 77%) and CR rate (15% vs 4%). In the PAD arm, bortezomib maintenance deepened responses further, with an increase in the CR/nCR rate from 23% to 35%. The main adverse effects of bortezomib are peripheral neuropathy, thrombocytopenia, and gastrointestinal symptoms and herpes zoster reactivation. The incidence of bortezomib-associated neuropathy appears to be cumulative and is reversible in most cases with interruption of therapy or dose modification (Richardson et al, 2006; Badros et al, 2007).

Lenalidomide in newly diagnosed transplantation-eligible patients

A phase II trial of lenalidomide 25 mg on days 1 to 21 and dexamethasone 40 mg on days 1 to 4, 9 to 12, and 17 to 20 of each 28-day cycle showed an ORR rate of 91%, with partial response (PR), VGPR, and CR rates of 35%, 38%, and 18%, respectively (Lacy et al, 2007). In the phase III Eastern Cooperative Oncology Group (ECOG) E4A03 trial, 445 patients with newly diagnosed MM were randomized to receive lenalidomide 25 mg on days 1 to 21 and either high-dose dexamethasone (RD; 40 mg daily on days 1-4, 9-12, and 17-20) or low-dose dexamethasone (Rd; 40 mg on days 1, 8, 15, and 22) (Rajkumar, Jacobus, et al, 2008). There was a higher degree of grade $\geq$3 toxicity that occurred in 50% of RD-treated patients as opposed to 30% of patients who received Rd. Rd yielded superior OS rates compared with RD (96% vs 88% at 1 year and 87% vs 75% at 2 years, respectively). However, RD was superior to Rd in the ORR (82% vs 70%, respectively). This study led to a significant change in the dosing of dexamethasone in all subsequent trials and in clinical care.

Another phase III trial of lenalidomide and dexamethasone compared with placebo/dexamethasone was conducted in 198 patients (Southwest Oncology Group [SWOG] trial S0232) (Zonder et al, 2007). In arm A, lenalidomide was given at 25 mg/d (28 of 35 days for 3 induction cycles, then 21 of 28 days as maintenance thereafter) plus high-dose dexamethasone (HD; 40 mg on days 1-4, 9-12, and 17-20 induction, then days 1-4 and 15-18 maintenance); in arm B, HD (same induction and maintenance schedules) was given plus placebo. Estimated 1-year progression-free survival (PFS) was 77% (arm A) versus 55% (arm B) ($P = .002$). The ORR was 85.3% (minor response [MR], 79.4%; CR, 22.1%) versus 51.3% (MR, 26.2%; CR, 3.8%) on arms A and B, respectively ($P = .001$). Myelosuppression and vascular thrombotic events are the most common toxicities observed with lenalidomide. It is not associated with neuropathy. Concern has been raised regarding the impact of lenalidomide on stem cell collection prior to ASCT. A decrease in the total number of CD34$^+$ stem cells collected has been observed in patients mobilized with G-CSF after induction with lenalidomide plus dexamethasone as compared with induction with VAD, TD, or dexamethasone alone (Kumar et al, 2007).

Combination of these agents in newly diagnosed transplantation-eligible patients

A phase III study randomized 480 transplantation-eligible patients with newly diagnosed MM to bortezomib, thalidomide, and dexamethasone (VTD) or TD (Cavo et al, 2008). Preliminary analysis has demonstrated the superiority of VTD compared with TD with respect to ORR (92% vs 78.5%), CR/nCR rate (33% vs 12%), and rate of VGPR or better

(61% vs 30%). Although the use of bortezomib and thalidomide in combination prompted concern for peripheral neuropathy, the toxicity profile associated with this regimen has been manageable. Bortezomib in combination with lenalidomide and dexamethasone (RVD) has also proven to be effective in the treatment of newly diagnosed and relapsed MM (Richardson, Jagannath, et al, 2007). A phase II trial of 66 patients showed a response rate (>PR) to date of 98%, including 52% CR/nCR/VGPR (Richardson, Jagannath, et al, 2007).

Induction therapy for non–transplantation-eligible patients
Thalidomide

Several phase III trials have shown that thalidomide in combination with melphalan and prednisone (MPT) is an effective regimen for patients with newly diagnosed MM who are ineligible for ASCT. In one randomized phase III trial by Palumbo, Bringhen, et al (2006), MPT was compared with melphalan and prednisone (MP) in 255 previously untreated individuals 60 years of age or older. The ORR and nCR/CR rate among patients who received MPT were 76% and 27.9%, respectively, compared with 47.6% and 7.2%, respectively, in the MP group. In another phase III trial by Facon et al (2007), 447 individuals between the age of 65 and 75 years with previously untreated MM were randomly assigned to receive MP, MPT, or 2 courses of VAD followed by reduced-intensity ASCT using melphalan 100 mg/m^2. A PR or better was achieved in 35% of patients treated with MP, 76% of those treated with MPT, and 65% of those who received VAD followed by melphalan-ASCT. CR rates were 2%, 13%, and 18% in the MP, MPT, and VAD followed by melphalan-ASCT arms, respectively. Although response rates in the MPT and melphalan-ASCT arms were similar, MPT produced superior PFS (27.5 vs 19.4 months) and median OS (51.6 vs 38.3 months).

Bortezomib

In a phase III trial, 682 ASCT-ineligible patients with previously untreated MM were randomized to either bortezomib plus melphalan and prednisone (VMP) or MP alone (San Miguel et al, 2008). All patients received melphalan 9 mg/m^2 and prednisone 60 mg/m^2 on days 1 through 4 of each 6-week cycle, whereas bortezomib was administered in the combination arm at 1.3 mg/m^2 on days 1, 4, 8, 11, 22, 25, 29, and 32 during cycles 1 to 4 and on days 1, 8, 22, and 29 during cycles 5 to 9. VMP was superior to MP in terms of the study's primary end point of TTP (24 vs 16.6 months), as well as secondary end points of CR rate (30% vs 4%) and duration of response (19.9 vs 13.1 months).

Lenalidomide

A phase I/II trial of 54 patients with newly diagnosed MM and age ≥65 years was performed using lenalidomide 5 to 10 mg on days 1 to 21, for 9 monthly cycles; melphalan 0.18 to 0.25 mg/kg orally on days 1 to 4; and prednisone 2 mg/kg on days 1 to 4 (R-MP) (Palumbo, Falco, et al, 2006). After 3 cycles, CR was observed in 10% of patients, PR was observed in 60%, and response <50% was observed in 30%; no progressive disease occurred. Major grade 3 and 4 adverse events were hematologic toxicities: neutropenia (58%) and thrombocytopenia (21%). R-MP was well tolerated with manageable toxicity. Significant response rate was observed.

Intensification therapy

Although not curative, HDT/SCT improves CR rates and prolongs median OS in myeloma by approximately 12 months, with a low treatment-related mortality (reported as <5%, and in most institutions, now ≤1%) (Harousseau, 2005). Melphalan 200 mg/m^2 is the most widely used preparative regimen (Harousseau, 2005). The first phase III trial in >200 patients was reported by Attal et al (1996) and demonstrated a survival benefit for HDT/SCT compared with standard chemotherapy, with an event-free survival (EFS) rate at 5 years of 28% versus 10% in the high-dose versus conventional-dose groups, respectively. Several phase II studies have demonstrated the activity of HDT/SCT in patients with MM (Kumar, Lacy, et al, 2004). Another randomized trial (the Program for the Study and Treatment of Hematological Malignancies, Spanish Society of Hematology [PETHEMA] study) of intensified therapy plus autologous transplantation compared with intensified therapy alone did not demonstrate a survival benefit with the transplantation arm, suggesting that more intense induction therapy may be helpful without myeloablative therapy (Blade et al, 1998). Randomization in this study was limited to patients with responding disease, and the trial included 164 patients.

Although HDT/SCT prolongs survival in younger patients with myeloma, its timing (early vs delayed) is an area of debate (Bensinger et al, 2009; Rotta et al, 2009). Early transplantation is more typical than delayed. Given effective new agents to treat myeloma, some patients and physicians may choose to delay transplantation. Clinical trials are being performed to examine this question further as novel therapies are integrated into initial therapy and as maintenance.

With tandem HDT/SCT, patients receive a second planned HDT/SCT after recovery from the first procedure. The French Myeloma Intergroup (IFM) 94 randomized trial found significantly better EFS and OS in recipients of double versus single HDT/SCT, but in only a subset of patients

(Harousseau, 2005). Survival advantage from the tandem approach was primarily limited to patients achieving PR or less with the first SCT and with good prognostic factors. Conversely, patients achieving CR with the first SCT and patients with poorer prognostic factors (eg, chromosome 13 deletion and high β2M at presentation) did not appear to benefit from the second intensification (Paul et al, 2009). A similar benefit was also demonstrated in a randomized trial conducted in Italy; 2 other randomized trials are yet to show significant improvement in OS with tandem ASCT, but they have shorter follow-up (Harousseau, 2005). In both the French and Italian trials, the benefit of a second HDT/SCT was restricted to patients who failed to achieve a CR or VGPR (>90% reduction in M protein level) with the first procedure (Harousseau, 2005). Quality of life studies will be required to determine whether EFS is a valid end point in these comparisons.

A recent phase III trial has shown that the addition of thalidomide to tandem SCT, compared with tandem SCT and no thalidomide, led to better CR (62% vs 43%, $P < .001$) and improved 5-year EFS (56% vs 44%, $P = .01$) (Barlogie et al, 2008). However, OS after relapse did not improve.

The advantages of allogeneic HDT/SCT include lack of graft contamination with tumor cells and presence of a graft-versus-myeloma effect. However, only 5% to 10% of patients are candidates because of age, availability of an human leukocyte antigen (HLA)-matched sibling donor, and adequate organ function (Harousseau, 2005; Bensinger et al, 2009). Furthermore, the high treatment-related mortality, mainly related to graft-versus-host disease (GVHD), has made conventional allogeneic transplantations unacceptable for most patients with myeloma. Despite this, a small number of patients achieve prolonged disease-free survival, and thus, this approach remains an option. Fully myeloablative allogeneic transplantation is controversial. Treatment-related mortalities have approached 50%, which prompted closure of the North American allogeneic SCT arm of S9321, although European studies suggest that a subgroup of patients (approximately 20%) achieve long-term disease-free survival with an allogeneic approach (Bruno et al, 2009). Nonmyeloablative allogeneic SCT has also demonstrated activity in myeloma, with evidence of a graft-versus-myeloma effect in small numbers of patients, although such "mini transplants" with donor lymphocyte infusions remain investigational (Bensinger et al, 2009). Several recent trials have been conducted using nonmyeloablative conditioning regimens. The best results have been reported in newly diagnosed patients with a tandem approach of ASCT (to reduce tumor burden to minimal levels) followed by an HLA-identical sibling donor mini-allogeneic transplantation, with a treatment-related mortality of approximately 10% to 15% and a high risk of acute and chronic GVHD (Bruno et al, 2009). At this time, allogeneic transplantation remains investigational and should be considered only in the context of clinical trials (Stewart, 2009).

Maintenance therapy

Maintenance therapy remains controversial in MM, and further studies are needed. One of the most significant studies tested thalidomide in a randomized phase III trial from the IFM; the IFM-99 02 trial assessed the impact of thalidomide maintenance on duration of response after SCT in 780 patients (Attal et al, 2006). At 29 months of median follow-up from randomization (2 months after the second transplantation), patients randomized to thalidomide had improvement in EFS compared with patients randomized to no treatment or to pamidronate alone (arm 3 vs arm 1 vs arm 2, 52% vs 36% vs 37%; $P = .002$). Another study published by Barlogie et al (2006) using thalidomide as maintenance in combination with dexamethasone and interferon after tandem transplantations showed no survival advantage with the addition of thalidomide. This was because the OS after relapse or progression was significantly lower in the thalidomide-treated patients ($P = .001$). Therefore, the role of thalidomide as maintenance therapy remains to be defined. Bortezomib has been used in maintenance therapy after SCT in the HOVON-65/GMMG-HD4 study (Sonneveld et al, 2008). The response rates were significantly higher on the PAD arm, even at the time of maintenance therapy, indicating that bortezomib maintenance may be efficacious in MM. Similarly, lenalidomide is being tested in multiple clinical trials including a large randomized study of low-dose lenalidomide or placebo after SCT that is being conducted by the Cancer and Leukemia Group B (CALGB) cooperative group.

Treatment of relapsed and refractory MM
Thalidomide

The activity of thalidomide was first demonstrated in a phase II trial by Singhal et al (1999) in which 84 individuals with relapsed and refractory MM received thalidomide monotherapy at doses ranging from 200 to 800 mg/d. The ORR in this heavily pretreated population was 32%. The 2-year EFS and OS rates of 169 patients who ultimately enrolled onto this trial were 20% and 48%, respectively (Barlogie et al, 2001), with 10-year EFS and OS rates of 6% and 10%, respectively (van Rhee et al, 2008). These results were confirmed by other clinical trials involving thalidomide. A systematic review of 42 phase II trials involving 1674 patients with relapsed and refractory MM showed that thalidomide monotherapy produces an ORR of 29% and a median OS of 14 months (Glasmacher et al, 2006).

Bortezomib

Phase I and II studies involving individuals with relapsed MM demonstrated manageable treatment-associated toxicity and significant activity in this setting (Orlowski et al, 2002; Richardson et al, 2003; Jagannath et al, 2004). These studies were followed by a phase III study in which 669 patients with relapsed MM were randomized to receive either bortezomib 1.3 mg/m^2 on days 1, 4, 8, and 11 of each 21-day cycle for eight 3-week cycles followed by treatment on days 1, 8, 15, and 22 for 5-week cycles or dexamethasone 40 mg on days 1 through 4, 9 through 12, and 17 through 20 for four 5-week cycles followed by treatment on days 1 through 4 for five 4-week cycles (Richardson, Sonneveld, et al, 2005). Bortezomib was superior to high-dose dexamethasone with respect to ORR (38 vs 18%), CR rate (6% vs 1%), median TTP (6.22 vs 3.49 months), and 1-year OS rate (80% vs 66%). With extended follow-up of study participants, the ORR and CR rates among bortezomib-treated patients increased to 43% and 95%, respectively (Richardson, Sonneveld, et al, 2007). The median OS was 29.8 months in the bortezomib arm versus 23.7 months in the dexamethasone arm.

The addition of anthracyclines to bortezomib has also shown high efficacy in MM. In a phase III trial of 646 patients with relapsed MM, patients received either bortezomib 1.3 mg/m^2 on days 1, 4, 8, and 11 of each 21-day cycle or the same regimen of bortezomib in combination with pegylated liposomal doxorubicin 30 mg/m^2 on day 4 (Orlowski et al, 2007). The combination was more superior to bortezomib alone in terms of median TTP (9.3 vs 6.5 months) and 15-month OS (76% vs 65%). Although grade 3 and 4 toxicities such as anorexia, vomiting, thrombocytopenia, neutropenia, and hand-foot syndrome occurred more frequently with the doublet, cardiac toxicity was only minimally increased with the combination, and rates of neuropathy were nearly equivalent.

Lenalidomide

Two large, randomized, phase III clinical trials in relapsed MM—the MM-009 North American study and the MM-010 European/Israeli/Australian study—have been published (Dimopoulos et al, 2007; Weber et al, 2007). Study participants were randomized to either placebo or lenalidomide 25 mg on days 1 to 21 of each 28-day cycle. Dexamethasone 40 mg was administered to both treatment groups on days 1 to 4, 9 to 12, and 17 to 20 during the first 4 cycles and on days 1 to 4 only thereafter. Lenalidomide and dexamethasone produced superior ORRs in both MM-009 (61% vs 19.9%) and MM-010 (60% vs 24%). Median TTP, the primary end point of the trial, was significantly longer in both the MM-009 (11.1 vs 4.7 months) and MM-010 (11.3 vs 4.7 months) studies. Subgroup analysis of MM-009 and MM-010 demonstrated that, as compared with dexamethasone alone, lenalidomide plus dexamethasone conferred a benefit in ORR, TTP, and PFS regardless of prior thalidomide exposure (Wang et al, 2008).

The list of novel agents is rapidly increasing as new targets are identified, and further investigation of these novel strategies, both alone and in combination, for the treatment of MM is warranted as part of a continued effort to improve patient outcome. Thus, participation in clinical trials is critical and a cornerstone of patient management in the relapsed or relapsed/refractory setting. Until recently, management strategies for patients with MM have been limited. With the introduction of novel targeted therapies and combinations with these and other agents, the opportunity to improve responses in this patient population has dramatically increased. Understanding of the gene expression profiling, multiple cellular signaling pathways, and microenvironmental events involved both in the pathogenesis of MM and in mechanisms underlying relapse has already improved and should aid further in the design of future treatment strategies to combat this otherwise fatal disease.

Supportive care

Several agents and treatments are important components of the supportive care for patients with MM. Bisphosphonates, such as pamidronate or zoledronic acid, reduce skeletal events in patients with lytic bony lesions, and monthly infusions of one of these agents are part of the standard care of patients with lytic lesions (Kyle and Rajkumar, 2008; Roodman, 2009). Complications include osteonecrosis of the jaw, which, although rare, can be challenging (Kyle and Rajkumar, 2008). Avoidance of invasive dentistry and prolonged use of inhibitors in cases where infiltration occurs during bisphosphonate therapy are important considerations. Albuminemia secondary to pamidronate can be seen, as well as glomerulonephropathy with zoledronic acid. Treatment involves cessation of bisphosphonate, and the nephropathy is usually reversible.

The role of plasma exchange in patients with acute renal failure at the onset of MM was assessed in a randomized study of 104 patients (Clark WF et al, 2005). Study participants were randomly assigned to conventional therapy plus 5 to 7 plasma exchanges of 50 mL/kg of body weight of 5% human serum albumin for 10 days or conventional therapy alone. There was no conclusive evidence that plasma exchanges substantially reduced a composite outcome of death, dialysis dependence, or glomerular filtration rate at 6 months (Clark et al, 2005).

Anemia is common in myeloma, due to direct marrow effects of the myeloma, renal insufficiency, or chemotherapy. Recombinant human erythropoietin (rhEPO) can improve both the hemoglobin level and quality of life in patients with MM (Kyle and Rajkumar, 2008).

Other elements of supportive care in MM relate to the specific complications of the disease. Radiation therapy can be useful for painful lytic lesions or spinal compression fractures[3]. Orthopedic consultation is important for impending fractures in weight-bearing bones. Kyphoplasty is also as a useful modality in managing significant myelomatous involvement of the spinal column. Hypercalcemia is treated primarily with intravenous fluids and bisphosphonates. The risk of renal dysfunction is reduced by maintaining hydration and by avoiding nephrotoxins such as intravenous contrast dye or aminoglycoside antibiotics and by judicious use of nonsteroidal anti-inflammatory drugs. Because of the hypogammaglobulinemia associated with the disease, patients are also at considerable risk of infection, particularly at later stages of the disease. Therefore, antibiotics are an important part of the supportive care of patients with advanced myeloma (Kyle and Rajkumar, 2008).

Plasmacytoma

Patients who present with an apparent solitary bone lesion should be staged carefully to eliminate the possibility of more generalized disease. The most common site is the vertebral column, followed by the pelvis, femur, and humerus (Kyle and Rajkumar, 2004). All patients with solitary plasmacytoma of bone have either no or low levels of M protein in serum or urine, and serum levels of normal Ig are usually preserved, but patients may have elevated serum free light chains (Dingli et al, 2006). Marrow biopsies are negative for increased plasma cells. MRI of the spine is an important tool and may reveal abnormalities not previously detected by skeletal survey and thus may upstage up to a quarter of patients to MM (Dimopoulos, Spencer, et al, 2009). Local therapy for solitary plasmacytoma of bone consists of radiotherapy of 40 to 50 Gy. PET–computed tomography scan may be a useful staging modality in such patients (Dimopoulos, Spencer, et al, 2009). Patients with subsequent disappearance of any detectable M protein by immunofixation and no evidence of active disease have the longest stability and a chance of cure. Otherwise, the majority of patients progress to myeloma within a median of 2 years; only 20% remain free of disease at 10 years (Kyle and Rajkumar, 2008).

A solitary extramedullary soft tissue plasmacytoma is more likely to be truly localized than a plasmacytoma of bone (Kyle and Rajkumar, 2008). The most common sites are in the upper respiratory tract (nasal cavity, sinuses, or pharyngeal lynx), but they can also occur in the gastrointestinal tract, central nervous system, urinary bladder, thyroid, breast, testes, parathyroid gland, or lymph nodes. Careful staging is necessary to rule out systemic disease. Because they are more likely to remain localized, there is a relatively high chance of cure with localized radiotherapy of 40 to 50 Gy; approximately 70% of patients will be alive and disease free at 10 years.

Other plasma cell disorders

Amyloidosis

Table 20-6 summarizes the characteristics of the next 3 types of plasma cell disorders. AL is an uncommon disorder in which proteins change conformation, aggregate, and form fibrils that infiltrate tissues leading to organ failure and death (Comenzo, 2009). The most frequent types are light chain (AL) derived from monoclonal B-cell disorders producing amyloidogenic Ig light chains and the hereditary and "senile systemic" (ATTR) variants from mutant and wild-type transthyretin (*TTR*). Diagnosis requires tissue biopsy. AL is more frequent and causes more organ disease than ATTR. Although both can cause cardiomyopathy and heart failure, AL progresses more quickly, so survival depends on timely diagnosis. Typing is usually based on clinical and laboratory findings with monoclonal gammopathy evaluation and, if indicated, *TTR* gene testing (Comenzo, 2009). Direct tissue typing is required when a patient has 2 potential amyloid-forming proteins. In coming years, widespread use of definitive proteomics will improve typing. Amyloid is an infiltrative fibrillar protein with light chain sequences for each patient identical to those of the light chains produced by the monoclonal plasma cells. Of patients with MM, 10% have evidence of concurrent AL. Serum and urine immunofixation studies reveal an M protein in 80% of patients, with λ-light chains more frequent than κ-light chains. AL should be suspected in patients with myeloma or a monoclonal gammopathy who show evidence of unexplained fatigue or weight loss, cardiomyopathy, orthostatic hypotension, macroglossia, nephrotic syndrome, carpal tunnel syndrome, peripheral or autonomic neuropathy, periorbital purpura, or hepatomegaly. Diagnosis is confirmed by the presence of apple-green birefringence on polarized light examination of a tissue biopsy stained with Congo red. Survival is usually poor but is shortest in those patients with cardiomyopathy, orthostatic hypotension, renal failure, hepatomegaly, cachexia, or overt MM. Treatment of AL is similar to that for myeloma, although the amyloid deposits are generally irreversible, and an aim of therapy is to retard further amyloid deposition (Comenzo, 2009). Options of therapy include melphalan and dexamethasone, ASCT, and novel therapies including thalidomide, bortezomib, and

Table 20-6 Other plasma cell disorders.

Waldenström macroglobulinemia	IgM monoclonal gammopathy (regardless of the size of the M protein) with >10% bone marrow lymphoplasmacytic infiltration (usually intertrabecular) by small lymphocyes that exhibit plasmacytoid or plasma cell differentiation and a typical immunophenotype (eg, surface IgM$^+$, CD5$^\pm$, CD10$^-$, CD19$^+$, CD20$^+$, CD23$^-$) that satisfactorily excludes other lymphoproliferative disorders, including chronic lymphocytic leukemia and mantle cell lymphoma
	IgM MGUS is defined as serum IgM monoclonal protein level <3 g/dL, bone marrow lymphoplasmacytic infiltration <10%, and no evidence of anemia, constitutional symptoms, hyperviscosity, lymphadenopathy, or hepatosplenomegaly
	Smoldering Waldenström macroglobulinemia (also referred to as indolent or asymptomatic) is defined as serum IgM monoclonal protein level ≥3 g/dL and/or bone marrow lymphoplasmacytic infiltration ≥10% with no evidence of end-organ damage, such as anemia, constitutional symptoms, hyperviscosity, lymphadenopathy, or hepatosplenomegaly
Amyloidosis (AL)	Presence of an amyloid-related systemic syndrome (such as renal, liver, heart, gastrointestinal tract, or peripheral nerve involvement) with positive amyloid staining by Congo red in any tissue (eg, fat aspirate, bone marrow, or organ biopsy); plus evidence that amyloid is light chain-related, established by direct examination of the amyloid (immunoperoxidase staining, direct sequencing); plus evidence of a monoclonal plasma cell proliferative disorder (serum or urine M protein, abnormal free light chain ratio, or clonal plasma cells in the bone marrow)
	Approximately 2%-3% of patients with amyloidosis will not meet the requirement for evidence of a monoclonal plasma cell disorder and the diagnosis must be made with caution in these patients
POEMS syndrome	Presence of a monoclonal plasma cell disorder, peripheral neuropathy, and at least 1 of the following 7 features: osteosclerotic myeloma, Castleman disease, organomegaly, endocrinopathy (excluding diabetes mellitus or hypothyroidism), edema, typical skin changes, and papilledema
	The absence of either osteosclerotic myeloma or Castleman disease should make the diagnosis suspect
	Elevations in plasma or serum levels of vascular endothelial growth factor and thrombocytosis are common features of the syndrome and are helpful when the diagnosis is difficult

Adapted with permission, from Rajkumar V, et al. Multiple myeloma: diagnosis and treatment. *Mayo Clin Proc.* 2005;80:1371–1382.
Ig = immunoglobulin; MGUS = monoclonal gammopathy of undetermined significance.

lenalidomide Patients with impaired renal function often experience increased toxicity with melphalan at 200 mg/m^2; therefore, the dose should be attenuated to 140 mg/m^2 to minimize occurrence of renal failure requiring dialysis, the risk of which is 5% (Dispenzieri et al, 2008). Participation in clinical trials for patients with these rare diseases is critical to improve the outcome and survival.

POEMS syndrome

POEMS (polyneuropathy, organomegaly, endocrinopathy monoclonal gammopathy, and skin changes) syndrome is a plasma cell dyscrasia that typically presents with a sensorimotor peripheral neuropathy (Dispenzieri, 2005). Other features include hyperpigmentation, hypertrichosis, thickened skin, papilledema, lymphadenopathy, peripheral edema, hepatomegaly, splenomegaly, and hypothyroidism. Patients with POEMS syndrome are younger (median age, 51 years) and have longer average survivals (median, 8 years) than patients with symptomatic myeloma (Dispenzieri et al, 2003). The clinical course is commonly one of progressive neuropathy, and in almost all cases, the Ig light chain type is λ. Bone lesions are characteristically osteosclerotic. Therapy for POEMS syndrome includes radiation therapy if sclerotic disease is localized and is similar to clinical myeloma if diffuse. Treatment approaches include autoSCT, steroid-based therapy, and lenalidomide, which, with less neurotoxicity than thalidomide, is seen as a promising new agent in this setting (Dispenzieri et al, 2004; Dispenzieri, 2005).

Lymphoplasmacytic lymphoma (WM)

WM, termed lymphoplasmacytic lymphoma in the World Health Organization classification, is an indolent lymphoid malignancy composed of mature plasmacytoid lymphocytes that produce monoclonal IgM (Ghobrial et al, 2003; Leleu et al, 2008; Treon, 2009). The disease affects predominantly older patients, who present with anemia, lymphadenopathy, purpura, splenomegaly, elevated serum viscosity, neurologic signs and symptoms, or combinations of these findings. Lytic bone lesions are typically absent. The lymphoma cells may express a variety of markers, including CD5, CD19, CD20, CD38, and surface or cytoplasmic Ig. Symptoms may be due to tumor infiltration (marrow, spleen, or lymph nodes), circulating IgM macroglobulin (hyperviscosity, cryoglobulinemia, or cold agglutinin hemolytic anemia), and tissue deposition of IgM or other proteins (neuropathy, glomerular disease, and/or amyloid).

Asymptomatic patients should be observed. Patients with a disease-related hemoglobin level <10 g/L, platelet count <100 × 10^9/L, bulky adenopathy or organomegaly, symptomatic hyperviscosity, peripheral neuropathy, AL, cryoglobulinemia, cold agglutinin disease, or evidence of disease transformation should be considered for therapy (Morel et al, 2009). Plasmapheresis should be considered for symptomatic hyperviscosity. Options of therapy for newly diagnosed patients with WM include the use of rituximab as monotherapy or in combination with cyclophosphamide, nucleoside analog, bortezomib, or thalidomide (Chen et al, 2007; Vijay and Gertz, 2008). Similar options can be used in the salvage setting (Dimopoulos, Gertz, et al, 2009). Newer agents such as everolimus can also be considered in the treatment of WM (Ghobrial et al, 2008; Treon, 2009). Time to response after rituximab usually exceeds 3 months on average. In a significant proportion of patients, a transient increase of serum IgM may occur immediately after initiation of rituximab. The combination of bortezomib and rituximab with or without dexamethasone has shown significant activity in the upfront or relapsed setting in WM (Treon et al, 2009). There is a high rate of peripheral neuropathy with the use bortezomib at the usual dosing schedule of twice a week (Treon et al, 2009). Therefore, current clinical trials are using once-a-week regimens and showing promising activity.

Key points

- MGUS is present in approximately 3% of individuals >70 years of age.
- MM may be treated with a variety of therapeutic regimens, including SCT. Thalidomide and derivatives, including lenalidomide, as well as other novel agents, such as bortezomib, which is a first-in-class proteasome inhibitor, are promising new approaches that now offer a significantly more positive outlook for patients with this otherwise incurable malignancy.
- Bisphosphonates are an important component of supportive care to decrease skeletal complications in myeloma.
- AL may be suspected in myeloma patients with cardiomyopathy, peripheral neuropathy, nephrotic syndrome, and macroglossia.
- WM presents clinically as an indolent B-cell lymphoma and may respond to nucleoside analogs, combination chemotherapy, or rituximab; promising investigational advances are also being made using combinations with novel agents.

Acknowledgment

The authors gratefully acknowledge the assistance of Jennifer Stedman in the preparation of this chapter.

Bibliography

Alexandrakis MG, Passam FJ, Ganotakis E, et al. Bone marrow microvascular density and angiogenic growth factors in multiple myeloma. *Clin Chem Lab Med*. 2004;42:1122–1126.

Alsayed Y, Ngo H, Runnels J, et al. Mechanisms of regulation of CXCR4/SDF-1 (CXCL12)-dependent migration and homing in multiple myeloma. *Blood*. 2007;109:2708–2717.

Alvino S, Marcucci M, Canzoniere D, et al. IL-6, p53 and proto-oncogene c-myc play different roles as biological markers of plasma cell dyscrasias. *Clin Ter*. 1999;150:197–202.

Attal M, Harousseau JL, Leyvraz S, et al. Maintenance therapy with thalidomide improves survival in patients with multiple myeloma. *Blood*. 2006;108:3289–3294.

Attal M, Harousseau JL, Stoppa AM, et al. A prospective, randomized trial of autologous bone marrow transplantation and chemotherapy in multiple myeloma. Intergroupe Francais du Myelome. *N Engl J Med*. 1996;335:91–97.

Avecilla ST, Hattori K, Heissig B, et al. Chemokine-mediated interaction of hematopoietic progenitors with the bone marrow vascular niche is required for thrombopoiesis. *Nat Med*. 2004;10:64–71.

Azab AK, Runnels JM, Pitsillides C, et al. The CXCR4 inhibitor AMD3100 disrupts the interaction of multiple myeloma cells with the bone marrow microenvironment and enhances their sensitivity to therapy. *Blood*. 2009;113:4341–4351.

Badros A, Goloubeva O, Dalal JS, et al. Neurotoxicity of bortezomib therapy in multiple myeloma: a single-center experience and review of the literature. *Cancer*. 2007;110:1042–1049.

Barlogie B, Desikan R, Eddlemon P, et al. Extended survival in advanced and refractory multiple myeloma after single-agent thalidomide: identification of prognostic factors in a phase 2 study of 169 patients. *Blood*. 2001;98:492–494.

Barlogie B, Pineda-Roman M, van Rhee F, et al. Thalidomide arm of Total Therapy 2 improves complete remission duration and survival in myeloma patients with metaphase cytogenetic abnormalities. *Blood*. 2008;112:3115–3121.

Barlogie B, Tricot G, Anaissie E, et al. Thalidomide and hematopoietic-cell transplantation for multiple myeloma. *N Engl J Med*. 2006;354:1021–1030.

Bataille R, Chappard D, Marcelli C, et al. Mechanisms of bone destruction in multiple myeloma: the importance of an unbalanced process in determining the severity of lytic bone disease. *J Clin Oncol*. 1989;7:1909–1914.

Bensinger WI. Role of autologous and allogeneic stem cell transplantation in myeloma. *Leukemia*. 2009;23:442–448.

Bergsagel PL, Kuehl WM, Zhan F, Sawyer J, Barlogie B, Shaughnessy J Jr. Cyclin D dysregulation: an early and unifying pathogenic event in multiple myeloma. *Blood*. 2005;106:296–303.

Bernasconi P, Cavigliano PM, Boni M, et al. Long-term follow up with conventional cytogenetics and band 13q14 interphase/metaphase in situ hybridization monitoring in monoclonal gammopathies of undetermined significance. *Br J Haematol*. 2002;118:545–549.

Blade J, San Miguel JF, Escudero ML, et al. Maintenance treatment with interferon alpha-2b in multiple myeloma: a prospective randomized study from PETHEMA (Program for the Study and Treatment of Hematological Malignancies, Spanish Society of Hematology). *Leukemia*. 1998;12:1144–1148.

Brown LM, Gridley G, Check D, Landgren O. Risk of multiple myeloma and monoclonal gammopathy of undetermined significance among white and black male United States veterans with prior autoimmune, infectious, inflammatory, and allergic disorders. *Blood*. 2008;111:3388–3394.

Broxmeyer HE, Orschell CM, Clapp DW, et al. Rapid mobilization of murine and human hematopoietic stem and progenitor cells with AMD3100, a CXCR4 antagonist. *J Exp Med*. 2005;201:1307–1318.

Bruno B, Giaccone L, Sorasio R, Boccadoro M. Role of allogeneic stem cell transplantation in multiple myeloma. *Semin Hematol*. 2009;46:158–165.

Callander NS, Roodman GD. Myeloma bone disease. *Semin Hematol*. 2001;38:276–285.

Canalis E, Deregowski V, Pereira RC, Gazzerro E. Signals that determine the fate of osteoblastic cells. *J Endocrinol Invest*. 2005;28:3-7.

Carrasco DR, Tonon G, Huang Y, et al. High-resolution genomic profiles define distinct clinico-pathogenetic subgroups of multiple myeloma patients. *Cancer Cell*. 2006;9:313–325.

Cavo M, Tacchetti P, Patriarca F, et al. Superior complete response rate and progression-free survival after autologous transplantation with up-front velcade-thalidomide-dexamethasone compared with thalidomide-dexamethasone in newly diagnosed multiple myeloma. *Blood*. 2008;111:Abstract 158.

Chauhan D, Kharbanda S, Ogata A, et al. Interleukin-6 inhibits Fas-induced apoptosis and stress-activated protein kinase activation in multiple myeloma cells. *Blood*. 1997;89:227–234.

Chauhan D, Uchiyama H, Akbarali Y, et al. Multiple myeloma cell adhesion-induced interleukin-6 expression in bone marrow stromal cells involves activation of NF-kappa B. *Blood*. 1996;87:1104–1112.

Chen CI, Kouroukis CT, White D, et al. Bortezomib is active in patients with untreated or relapsed Waldenstrom's macroglobulinemia: a phase II study of the National Cancer Institute of Canada Clinical Trials Group. *J Clin Oncol*. 2007;25:1570–1575.

Chen J, Lee BH, Williams IR, et al. FGFR3 as a therapeutic target of the small molecule inhibitor PKC412 in hematopoietic malignancies. *Oncogene*. 2005;24:8259–8267.

Chim CS, Liang R, Leung MH, Kwong YL. Aberrant gene methylation implicated in the progression of monoclonal gammopathy of undetermined significance to multiple myeloma. *J Clin Pathol*. 2007;60:104–106.

Clark MR, Cooper AB, Wang LD, Aifantis I. The pre-B cell receptor in B cell development: recent advances, persistent questions and conserved mechanisms. *Curr Top Microbiol Immunol*. 2005;290:87–103.

Clark WF, Stewart AK, Rock GA, et al. Plasma exchange when myeloma presents as acute renal failure: a randomized, controlled trial. *Ann Intern Med*. 2005;143:777–784.

Comenzo RL. How I treat amyloidosis. *Blood*. 2009;114:3147–3157.

Cowland JB, Hother C, Gronbaek K. MicroRNAs and cancer. *APMIS*. 2007;115:1090–1106.

Damiano JS. Integrins as novel drug targets for overcoming innate drug resistance. *Curr Cancer Drug Targets*. 2002;2:37–43.

Damiano JS, Cress AE, Hazlehurst LA, Shtil AA, Dalton WS. Cell adhesion mediated drug resistance (CAM-DR): Role of integrins and resistance to apoptosis in human myeloma cell lines. *Blood*. 1999;93:1658–1667.

Damiano JS, Dalton WS. Integrin-mediated drug resistance in multiple myeloma. *Leuk Lymphoma*. 2000;38:71–81.

De Clercq E. Potential clinical applications of the CXCR4 antagonist bicyclam AMD3100. *Mini Rev Med Chem*. 2005;5:805–824.

Dimopoulos MA, Gertz MA, Kastritis E, et al. Update on treatment recommendations from the Fourth International Workshop on Waldenstrom's Macroglobulinemia. *J Clin Oncol*. 2009;27:120–126.

Dimopoulos M, Spencer A, Attal M, et al. Lenalidomide plus dexamethasone for relapsed or refractory multiple myeloma. *N Engl J Med*. 2007;357:2123–2132.

Dimopoulos M, Terpos E, Comenzo RL, et al. International myeloma working group consensus statement and guidelines regarding the current role of imaging techniques in the diagnosis and monitoring of multiple Myeloma. *Leukemia*. 2009;23:1545–1556.

Dingli D, Kyle RA, Rajkumar SV, et al. Immunoglobulin free light chains and solitary plasmacytoma of bone. *Blood*. 2006;108:1979–1983.

Dispenzieri A. POEMS syndrome. *Hematology Am Soc Hematol Educ Program*. 2005:360–367.

Dispenzieri A, Kyle RA, Lacy MQ, et al. POEMS syndrome: definitions and long-term outcome. *Blood*. 2003;101:2496–2506.

Dispenzieri A, Merlini G, Comenzo RL. Amyloidosis: 2008 BMT Tandem Meetings (February 13–17, San Diego). *Biol Blood Marrow Transplant*. 2008;14:6-11.

Dispenzieri A, Moreno-Aspitia A, Suarez GA, et al. Peripheral blood stem cell transplantation in 16 patients with POEMS syndrome, and a review of the literature. *Blood*. 2004;104:3400–3407.

Durie BG, Harousseau JL, Miguel JS, et al. International uniform response criteria for multiple myeloma. *Leukemia*. 2006;20:1467–1473.

Ehrlich LA, Chung HY, Ghobrial I, et al. IL-3 is a potential inhibitor of osteoblast differentiation in multiple myeloma. *Blood*. 2005;106:1407–1414.

Ehrlich LA, Roodman GD. The role of immune cells and inflammatory cytokines in Paget's disease and multiple myeloma. *Immunol Rev*. 2005;208:252–266.

Esteller M. Epigenetics in cancer. *N Engl J Med.* 2008;358:1148–1159.

Esteller M. Epigenetics provides a new generation of oncogenes and tumour-suppressor genes. *Br J Cancer.* 2006;94:179–183.

Esteller M. Epigenetics provides a new generation of oncogenes and tumour-suppressor genes. *Br J Cancer.* 2007;96(Suppl):R26-R30.

Facon T, Mary JY, Hulin C, et al. Melphalan and prednisone plus thalidomide versus melphalan and prednisone alone or reduced-intensity autologous stem cell transplantation in elderly patients with multiple myeloma (IFM 99–06): a randomised trial. *Lancet.* 2007;370:1209–1218.

Fairfax KA, Kallies A, Nutt SL, Tarlinton DM. Plasma cell development: from B-cell subsets to long-term survival niches. *Semin Immunol.* 2008;20:49–58.

Flomenberg N, Devine SM, Dipersio JF, et al. The use of AMD3100 plus G-CSF for autologous hematopoietic progenitor cell mobilization is superior to G-CSF alone. *Blood.* 2005;106:1867–1874.

Fonseca R, Bailey RJ, Ahmann GJ, et al. Genomic abnormalities in monoclonal gammopathy of undetermined significance. *Blood.* 2002;100:1417–1424.

Fonseca R, Barlogie B, Bataille R, et al. Genetics and cytogenetics of multiple myeloma: a workshop report. *Cancer Res.* 2004;64:1546–1558.

Fonseca R, Debes-Marun CS, Picken EB, et al. The recurrent IgH translocations are highly associated with nonhyperdiploid variant multiple myeloma. *Blood.* 2003;102:2562–2567.

Ghobrial IM, Chuma S, Sam A, et al. Phase II trial of the mTOR inhibitor RAD001 in relapsed and/or refractory Waldenstrom macroglobulinemia: the Dana Farber Cancer Institute Experience. *Blood.* 2008;112:Abstract 1011.

Ghobrial IM, Gertz MA, Fonseca R. Waldenstrom macroglobulinaemia. Lancet Oncol. 2003;4:679–85.

Giuliani N, Colla S, Morandi F, et al. Myeloma cells block RUNX2/CBFA1 activity in human bone marrow osteoblast progenitors and inhibit osteoblast formation and differentiation. *Blood.* 2005;106:2472–2483.

Glasmacher A, Hahn C, Hoffmann F, et al. A systematic review of phase II trials of thalidomide monotherapy in patients with relapsed or refractory multiple myeloma. *Br J Haematol.* 2006;132:584–593.

Greipp PR, San Miguel J, Durie BG, et al. International staging system for multiple myeloma. *J Clin Oncol.* 2005;23:3412–3420.

Grignani G, Perissinotto E, Cavalloni G, Carnevale Schianca F, Aglietta M. Clinical use of AMD3100 to mobilize CD34+ cells in patients affected by non-Hodgkin's lymphoma or multiple myeloma. *J Clin Oncol.* 2005;23:3871–3872.

Guillerm G, Gyan E, Wolowiec D, et al. p16(INK4a) and p15(INK4b) gene methylations in plasma cells from monoclonal gammopathy of undetermined significance. *Blood.* 2001;98:244–246.

Guo YQ, Chen SL. The significance of IGF-1, VEGF, IL-6 in multiple myeloma progression. *Zhonghua Xue Ye Xue Za Zhi.* 2006;27:231–234.

Hagman J, Lukin K. Transcription factors drive B cell development. *Curr Opin Immunol.* 2006;18:127–134.

Harousseau JL. Stem cell transplantation in multiple myeloma (0, 1, or 2). *Curr Opin Oncol.* 2005;17:93–98.

Harousseau JL, Mathiot C, Attal M, et al. Bortezomib/dexamethasone versus VAD as induction prior to autologous stem cell transplantation (ASCT) in previously untreated multiple myeloma (MM): updated data from IFM2005/01 trial. *J Clin Oncol.* 2008;26:Abstract 8505.

Hideshima T, Bergsagel PL, Kuehl WM, Anderson KC. Advances in biology of multiple myeloma: clinical applications. *Blood.* 2004;104:607–618.

Hideshima T, Chauhan D, Hayashi T, et al. The biological sequelae of stromal cell-derived factor-1alpha in multiple myeloma. *Mol Cancer Ther.* 2002;1:539–544.

Hideshima T, Nakamura N, Chauhan D, Anderson KC. Biologic sequelae of interleukin-6 induced PI3-K/Akt signaling in multiple myeloma. *Oncogene.* 2001;20:5991–6000.

Hideshima T, Podar K, Chauhan D, Anderson KC. Cytokines and signal transduction. *Best Pract Res Clin Haematol.* 2005;18:509–524.

Huston A, Roodman GD. Role of the microenvironment in multiple myeloma bone disease. *Future Oncol.* 2006;2:371–378.

Jagannath S, Barlogie B, Berenson J, et al. A phase 2 study of two doses of bortezomib in relapsed or refractory myeloma. *Br J Haematol.* 2004;127:165–172.

Jemal A, Siegel R, Ward E, Hao Y, Xu J, Thun MJ. Cancer statistics, 2009. *CA Cancer J Clin.* 2009;59:225–249.

Katogi R, Kudo A. B cell development and Ig gene rearrangement. *Nippon Rinsho.* 2005;63(Suppl 4):243–247.

Keats JJ, Reiman T, Maxwell CA, et al. In multiple myeloma, t(4;14)(p16;q32) is an adverse prognostic factor irrespective of FGFR3 expression. *Blood.* 2003;101:1520–1529.

Kollet O, Shivtiel S, Chen YQ, et al. HGF, SDF-1, and MMP-9 are involved in stress-induced human CD34+ stem cell recruitment to the liver. *J Clin Invest.* 2003;112:160–169.

Kumar S, Dispenzieri A, Lacy MQ, et al. Impact of lenalidomide therapy on stem cell mobilization and engraftment post-peripheral blood stem cell transplantation in patients with newly diagnosed myeloma. *Leukemia.* 2007;21:2035–2042.

Kumar S, Gertz MA, Dispenzieri A, et al. Prognostic value of bone marrow angiogenesis in patients with multiple myeloma undergoing high-dose therapy. *Bone Marrow Transplant.* 2004;34:235–239.

Kumar S, Lacy MQ, Dispenzieri A, et al. High-dose therapy and autologous stem cell transplantation for multiple myeloma poorly responsive to initial therapy. *Bone Marrow Transplant.* 2004;34:161–167.

Kumar SK, Rajkumar SV, Dispenzieri A, et al. Improved survival in multiple myeloma and the impact of novel therapies. *Blood.* 2008;111:2516–2520.

Kyle RA, Rajkumar SV. Epidemiology of the plasma-cell disorders. *Best Pract Res Clin Haematol.* 2007;20:637–664.

Kyle RA, Rajkumar SV. Criteria for diagnosis, staging, risk stratification and response assessment of multiple myeloma. *Leukemia.* 2009;23:3-9.

Kyle RA, Rajkumar SV. Monoclonal gammopathy of undetermined significance. *Clin Lymphoma Myeloma*. 2005;6:102–114.

Kyle RA, Rajkumar SV. Multiple myeloma. *N Engl J Med*. 2004;351:1860–1873.

Kyle RA, Rajkumar SV. Multiple myeloma. *Blood*. 2008;111:2962–2972.

Kyrtsonis MC, Maltezas D, Tzenou T, Koulieris E, Bradwell AR. Staging systems and prognostic factors as a guide to therapeutic decisions in multiple myeloma. *Semin Hematol*. 2009;46:110–117.

Lacy MQ, Gertz MA, Dispenzieri A, et al. Long-term results of response to therapy, time to progression, and survival with lenalidomide plus dexamethasone in newly diagnosed myeloma. *Mayo Clin Proc*. 2007;82:1179–1184.

Landgren O, Kyle RA, Hoppin JA, et al. Pesticide exposure and risk of monoclonal gammopathy of undetermined significance (MGUS) in the Agricultural Health Study. *Blood*. 2009;113:6386–6391.

Landgren O, Kyle RA, Pfeiffer RM, et al. Monoclonal gammopathy of undetermined significance (MGUS) consistently precedes multiple myeloma: a prospective study. *Blood*. 2009;113:5412–5417.

Lapidot T. Mechanism of human stem cell migration and repopulation of NOD/SCID and B2mnull NOD/SCID mice. The role of SDF-1/CXCR4 interactions. *Ann N Y Acad Sci*. 2001;938:83–95.

Lapidot T, Dar A, Kollet O. How do stem cells find their way home? *Blood*. 2005;106:1901–1910.

Le Gouill S, Podar K, Amiot M, et al. VEGF induces Mcl-1 up-regulation and protects multiple myeloma cells against apoptosis. *Blood*. 2004;104:2886–2892.

Leleu X, Roccaro AM, Moreau AS, et al. Waldenstrom macroglobulinemia. *Cancer Lett*. 2008;270:95–107.

Lionetti M, Agnelli L, Mosca L, et al. Integrative high-resolution microarray analysis of human myeloma cell lines reveals deregulated miRNA expression associated with allelic imbalances and gene expression profiles. *Genes Chromosomes Cancer*. 2009;48:521–531.

Macro M, Divine M, YUzunhan Y, et al. Dexamethasone+thalidomide (dex/thal) compared to VAD as a pre-transplant treatment in newly diagnosed multiple myeloma (MM): a randomized trial. *Blood*. 2006;108:57a.

Melton LJ 3rd, Kyle RA, Achenbach SJ, Oberg AL, Rajkumar SV. Fracture risk with multiple myeloma: a population-based study. *J Bone Miner Res*. 2005;20:487–493.

Mitsiades CS, Mitsiades NS, McMullan CJ, et al. Inhibition of the insulin-like growth factor receptor-1 tyrosine kinase activity as a therapeutic strategy for multiple myeloma, other hematologic malignancies, and solid tumors. *Cancer Cell*. 2004;5:221–230.

Moller C, Stromberg T, Juremalm M, Nilsson K, Nilsson G. Expression and function of chemokine receptors in human multiple myeloma. *Leukemia*. 2003;17:203–210.

Morel P, Duhamel A, Gobbi P, et al. International prognostic scoring system for Waldenstrom's macroglobulinemia. *Blood*. 2009;114:2375–2385.

Mulligan ME. Imaging techniques used in the diagnosis, staging, and follow-up of patients with myeloma. *Acta Radiol*. 2005;46:716–724.

Nowakowski GS, Witzig TE, Dingli D, et al. Circulating plasma cells detected by flow cytometry as a predictor of survival in 302 patients with newly diagnosed multiple myeloma. *Blood*. 2005;106:2276–2279.

Orlowski RZ, Nagler A, Sonneveld P, et al. Randomized phase III study of pegylated liposomal doxorubicin plus bortezomib compared with bortezomib alone in relapsed or refractory multiple myeloma: combination therapy improves time to progression. *J Clin Oncol*. 2007;25:3892–3901.

Orlowski RZ, Stinchcombe TE, Mitchell BS, et al. Phase I trial of the proteasome inhibitor PS-341 in patients with refractory hematologic malignancies. *J Clin Oncol*. 2002;20:4420–4427.

Oshima T, Abe M, Asano J, et al. Myeloma cells suppress bone formation by secreting a soluble Wnt inhibitor, sFRP-2. *Blood*. 2005;106:3160–3165.

Palumbo A, Bringhen S, Caravita T, et al. Oral melphalan and prednisone chemotherapy plus thalidomide compared with melphalan and prednisone alone in elderly patients with multiple myeloma: randomised controlled trial. *Lancet*. 2006;367:825–831.

Palumbo A, Falco P, Falcone A, et al. Oral revlimid plus melphalan and prednisone (R-MP) for newly diagnosed multiple myeloma: results of a multicenter phase I/II study. *Blood*. 2006;108:Abstract 800.

Paul E, Sutlu T, Deneberg S, et al. Impact of chromosome 13 deletion and plasma cell load on long-term survival of patients with multiple myeloma undergoing autologous transplantation. *Oncol Rep*. 2009;22:137–142.

Pene F, Claessens YE, Muller O, et al. Role of the phosphatidylinositol 3-kinase/Akt and mTOR/P70S6-kinase pathways in the proliferation and apoptosis in multiple myeloma. *Oncogene*. 2002;21:6587–6597.

Petit I, Szyper-Kravitz M, Nagler A, et al. G-CSF induces stem cell mobilization by decreasing bone marrow SDF-1 and up-regulating CXCR4. *Nat Immunol*. 2002;3:687–694.

Pichiorri F, Suh SS, Ladetto M, et al. MicroRNAs regulate critical genes associated with multiple myeloma pathogenesis. *Proc Natl Acad Sci U S A*. 2008;105:12885–12890.

Piehler AP, Gulbrandsen N, Kierulf P, Urdal P. Quantitation of serum free light chains in combination with protein electrophoresis and clinical information for diagnosing multiple myeloma in a general hospital population. *Clin Chem*. 2008;54:1823–1830.

Podar K, Anderson KC. The pathophysiologic role of VEGF in hematologic malignancies: therapeutic implications. *Blood*. 2005;105:1383–1395.

Podar K, Richardson PG, Hideshima T, Chauhan D, Anderson KC. The malignant clone and the bone-marrow environment. *Best Pract Res Clin Haematol*. 2007;20:597–612.

Politou MC, Heath DJ, Rahemtulla A, et al. Serum concentrations of Dickkopf-1 protein are increased in patients with multiple myeloma and reduced after autologous stem cell transplantation. *Int J Cancer*. 2006;119:1728–1731.

Rajkumar SV, Jacobus S, Callander N, Fonseca R, Vesole D, Greipp P. A randomized phase III trial of lenalidomide plus high-dose dexamethasone versus lenalidomide plus low-dose dexamethasone in newly diagnosed multiple myeloma (E4A03): a trial coordinated by the Eastern Cooperative Oncology Group. *Blood*. 2006;108:239a.

Rajkumar SV, Kyle RA. Angiogenesis in multiple myeloma. *Semin Oncol*. 2001;28:560–564.

Rajkumar SV, Kyle RA, Therneau TM, et al. Presence of monoclonal free light chains in the serum predicts risk of progression in monoclonal gammopathy of undetermined significance. *Br J Haematol*. 2004;127:308–310.

Rajkumar SV, Lacy MQ, Kyle RA. Monoclonal gammopathy of undetermined significance and smoldering multiple myeloma. *Blood Rev*. 2007;21:255–265.

Rajkumar S, Jacobus N, Callander R, et al. Randomized trial of lenalidomide plus high-dose dexamethasone versus lenalidomide plus low-dose dexamethasone in newly diagnosed myeloma (E4A03), a trial coordinated by the Eastern Cooperative Oncology Group: analysis of response, survival, and outcome. *J Clin Oncol*. 2008;26:Abstract 8504.

Rajkumar SV, Rosinol L, Hussein M, et al. Multicenter, randomized, double-blind, placebo-controlled study of thalidomide plus dexamethasone compared with dexamethasone as initial therapy for newly diagnosed multiple myeloma. *J Clin Oncol*. 2008;26:2171–2177.

Rajkumar SV, Witzig TE. A review of angiogenesis and antiangiogenic therapy with thalidomide in multiple myeloma. *Cancer Treat Rev*. 2000;26:351–362.

Richardson PG, Barlogie B, Berenson J, et al. A phase 2 study of bortezomib in relapsed, refractory myeloma. *N Engl J Med*. 2003;348:2609–2617.

Richardson PG, Barlogie B, Berenson J, et al. Clinical factors predictive of outcome with bortezomib in patients with relapsed, refractory multiple myeloma. *Blood*. 2005;106:2977–2981.

Richardson PG, Briemberg H, Jagannath S, et al. Frequency, characteristics, and reversibility of peripheral neuropathy during treatment of advanced multiple myeloma with bortezomib. *J Clin Oncol*. 2006;24:3113–3120.

Richardson P, Jagannath, S, Raje, N, et al. Lenalidomide, bortezomib, and dexamethasone (Rev/Vel/Dex) as front-line therapy for patients with multiple myeloma (MM): preliminary results of a phase 1/2 study. *Blood*. 2007;110:Abstract 187.

Richardson P, Mitsiades C, Schlossman R, et al. The treatment of relapsed and refractory multiple myeloma. *Hematology Am Soc Hematol Educ Program*. 2007:317–323.

Richardson PG, Sonneveld P, Schuster MW, et al. Bortezomib or high-dose dexamethasone for relapsed multiple myeloma. *N Engl J Med*. 2005;352:2487–2498.

Richardson PG, Sonneveld P, Schuster M, et al. Extended follow-up of a phase 3 trial in relapsed multiple myeloma: final time-to-event results of the APEX trial. *Blood*. 2007;110:3557–3560.

Roccaro AM, Sacco A, Thompson B, et al. microRNAs 15a and 16 regulate tumor proliferation in multiple myeloma. *Blood*. 2009;113:6669–6680.

Ronchetti D, Lionetti M, Mosca L, et al. An integrative genomic approach reveals coordinated expression of intronic miR-335, miR-342, and miR-561 with deregulated host genes in multiple myeloma. *BMC Med Genomics*. 2008;1:37.

Roodman GD. Pathogenesis of myeloma bone disease. *Blood Cells Mol Dis*. 2004;32:290–292.

Roodman GD. Pathogenesis of myeloma bone disease. *Leukemia*. 2009;23:435–441.

Roodman GD. Role of the bone marrow microenvironment in multiple myeloma. *J Bone Miner Res*. 2002;17:1921–1925.

Rotta M, Storer BE, Sahebi F, et al. Long-term outcome of patients with multiple myeloma after autologous hematopoietic cell transplantation and nonmyeloablative allografting. *Blood*. 2009;113:3383–3391.

San Miguel JF, Schlag R, Khuageva NK, et al. Bortezomib plus melphalan and prednisone for initial treatment of multiple myeloma. *N Engl J Med*. 2008;359:906–917.

Schmidmaier R, Baumann P. Anti-adhesion evolves to a promising therapeutic concept in oncology. *Curr Med Chem*. 2008;15:978–990.

Scudla V, Budikova M, Pika T, et al. Comparison of serum levels of selected biological parameters in monoclonal gammopathy of undetermined significance and multiple myeloma. *Vnitr Lek*. 2006;52:232–240.

Shain KH, Yarde DN, Meads MB, et al. Beta1 integrin adhesion enhances IL-6-mediated STAT3 signaling in myeloma cells: implications for microenvironment influence on tumor survival and proliferation. *Cancer Res*. 2009;69:1009–1015.

Singhal S, Mehta J, Desikan R, et al. Antitumor activity of thalidomide in refractory multiple myeloma. *N Engl J Med*. 1999;341:1565–1571.

Sonneveld P, Van der Holt B, Schmidt-Wolf I, et al. First analysis of HOVON-65/GMMG-HD4 randomized phase III trial comparing bortezomib, adriamycin, dexamethasone (PAD) vs VAD as induction treatment prior to high dose melphalan (HDM) in patients with newly diagnosed multiple myeloma (MM). *Blood*. 2008;112:Abstract 653.

Stewart AK. Reduced-intensity allogeneic transplantation for myeloma: reality bites. *Blood*. 2009;113:3135–3136.

Takahashi T, Shivapurkar N, Reddy J, et al. DNA methylation profiles of lymphoid and hematopoietic malignancies. *Clin Cancer Res*. 2004;10:2928–2935.

Taube T, Beneton MN, McCloskey EV, Rogers S, Greaves M, Kanis JA. Abnormal bone remodelling in patients with myelomatosis and normal biochemical indices of bone resorption. *Eur J Haematol*. 1992;49:192–198.

Tian E, Zhan F, Walker R, et al. The role of the Wnt-signaling antagonist DKK1 in the development of osteolytic lesions in multiple myeloma. *N Engl J Med*. 2003;349:2483–2494.

Treon SP. How I treat Waldenstrom's macroglobulinemia. *Blood*. 2009.

Treon SP, Ioakimidis L, Soumerai JD, et al. Primary therapy of Waldenstrom macroglobulinemia with bortezomib, dexamethasone, and rituximab: WMCTG Clinical Trial 05–180. *J Clin Oncol*. 2009;27:3830–3835.

Uchiyama H, Barut BA, Chauhan D, Cannistra SA, Anderson KC. Characterization of adhesion molecules on human myeloma cell lines. *Blood*. 1992;80:2306–2314.

Uchiyama H, Barut BA, Mohrbacher AF, Chauhan D, Anderson KC. Adhesion of human myeloma-derived cell lines to bone marrow stromal cells stimulates interleukin-6 secretion. *Blood*. 1993;82:3712–3720.

Vachon CM, Kyle RA, Therneau TM, et al. Increased risk of monoclonal gammopathy in first-degree relatives of patients with multiple myeloma or monoclonal gammopathy of undetermined significance. *Blood*. 2009;114:785–790.

van Rhee F, Dhodapkar M, Shaughnessy JD Jr, et al. First thalidomide clinical trial in multiple myeloma: a decade. *Blood*. 2008;112:1035–1038.

Vijay A, Gertz MA. Current treatment options for Waldenstrom macroglobulinemia. *Clin Lymphoma Myeloma*. 2008;8:219–229.

Wang M, Dimopoulos MA, Chen C, et al. Lenalidomide plus dexamethasone is more effective than dexamethasone alone in patients with relapsed or refractory multiple myeloma regardless of prior thalidomide exposure. *Blood*. 2008;112:4445–4451.

Weber DM, Chen C, Niesvizky R, et al. Lenalidomide plus dexamethasone for relapsed multiple myeloma in North America. *N Engl J Med*. 2007;357:2133–2142.

Yaccoby S, Ling W, Zhan F, Walker R, Barlogie B, Shaughnessy JD Jr. Antibody-based inhibition of DKK1 suppresses tumor-induced bone resorption and multiple myeloma growth in-vivo. *Blood*. 2007;109:2106–2111.

Zonder J, Crowley, J, Hussein, M, et al. Superiority of lenalidomide (Len) plus high-dose dexamethasone (HD) compared to HD alone as treatment of newly-diagnosed multiple myeloma (NDMM): results of the randomized, double-blinded, placebo-controlled SWOG trial S0232. *Blood*. 2007;110:Abstract 77.

Index

Note:
Page numbers followed by "f" refer to figures; those followed by "t" refer to tables.

A

AA/PNH syndrome, 459, 459f
Abciximab, 196
ABO incompatible HSCTs, transfusion therapy, 313–315, 314t
ABO/Rh(D) typing, transfusion therapy, pretransfusion testing, 306–307, 306t
ABO system, transfusion therapy, 291–292, 293t
Acanthocytosis, 155, 155f
Accuracy, defined, 263
Acid(s), nucleic, digestion and separation of, 6, 7f
Acquired bone marrow failure syndromes, 450–472. *See also specific syndromes and* Bone marrow failure syndromes
Acquired coagulation factor deficiencies, conditions associated with, 183, 183t
Acquired immunodeficiency syndrome (AIDS)–related retroviruses, transfusion therapy and, 324
Acquired underproduction anemias, 109–132. *See also specific anemias and* Underproduction anemias, acquired
Activated partial thromboplastin time (aPTT)
 in laboratory hematology, 277–279, 278f
 PT and, combined abnormalities of, in laboratory hematology, 279, 279f
Acute chest syndrome, sickle cell disease and, 146
Acute hemolytic reactions, transfusion therapy and, 321–322
Acute intermittent porphyria (AIP), 103
Acute leukemia
 ET transformation to, 430
 platelet function–related, 258t, 259
Acute lung injury, transfusion-related, 323
Acute lymphoblastic leukemia (ALL), 489–503
 in adolescents, treatment of, 501
 classification of, 489
 cytogenetics of, 490–491, 491t
 described, 489
 diagnosis of, 489
 G-CSF and GM-CSF in, 77
 HSCT for, 359–360
 immunophenotyping in, 489–490
 minimal residual disease detection in, 493
 molecular genetics of, 491–492

 pediatric, cryptic translocation identification of, 15
 Ph$^+$, 500–501
 precursor B-cell/T-cell
  in adults, treatment of, 498–503. *See also* Precursor B-cell/T-cell ALL, in adults, treatment of
  in children, treatment of, 494–498. *See also* Precursor B-cell/T-cell ALL, in children, treatment of
 prognosis of, 489
 prognostic factors in, 492–493, 492t
 subgroups of, in children, 497–498
 treatment of, 493–503
  pharmacogenomics and, 17
  supportive care in, 493–494
 in young adults, treatment of, 501
Acute myelogenous leukemia
 G-CSF and GM-CSF in, 77
 HSCT for, 358–359
 secondary, in PV, treatment of, 424
Acute myeloid leukemia (AML), 475–487
 causes of, 475
 classification of, 476, 476t, 477t
 clinical manifestations of, 475
 defined, 475
 epidemiology of, 475
 FAB classification of, 476, 476t
 incidence of, 475
 nucleophosmin mutations in, 15
 in older patients, 481
 pediatric, 483
 prognostic factors in, 477–479, 478t
 relapse of, 480–481
 residual, monitoring of, 480–481
 treatment of, 479–480
 WHO classification of, subtypes, 476, 476t, 477t
Acute promyelocytic leukemia (APL), 481–482, 482f
ADAMTS13, 250, 251f
 assays for, in acquired thrombocytopenia testing, 286
Adenosine deaminase (ADA) excess, 159
Adenosine diphosphate (ADP) receptor antagonists, 196
Adhesion molecules, in molecular pathogenesis of MM, 586
Adolescent(s), ALL in, treatment of, 501
ADP receptor antagonists. *See* Adenosine diphosphate (ADP) receptor antagonists
Adsorption, differential, defined, 318
Adult erythropoiesis, 335
Adult T-cell leukemia/lymphoma, 536

Aggressive lymphomas
 described, 516
 indolent lymphoma transformation to, 528
Aggressive NK-cell leukemia, 536–537
AGM region. *See* Aorto-gonadal-mesonephros (AGM) region
AHA. *See* Autoimmune hemolytic anemia (AHA)
AIDS. *See* Acquired immunodeficiency syndrome (AIDS)
AIP. *See* Acute intermittent porphyria (AIP)
AITL. *See* Angioimmunoblastic T-cell lymphoma (AITL)
ALA dehydratase deficiency, 103
ALCL. *See* Anaplastic large-cell lymphoma (ALCL)
Alemtuzumab, for CLL, 567–568
ALK-negative ALCL, 538
ALK-positive ALCL, 537–538
Alkylator-based therapy, for CLL, 564, 565t
ALL. *See* Acute lymphoblastic leukemia (ALL)
Allele(s), 6
 defined, 20
Allele-specific oligonucleotide, 17
 defined, 20–21
Allergic reactions, transfusion therapy and, 322–323
Allogeneic HSCT, 337–352
 benign hematologic disorders–related, conditioning for, 343
 class I antigens in, 337, 337f
 class II antigens in, 337, 337f
 clinical case, 339, 341
 complications of, 343–352, 344t, 346t–347t. *See also specific types, e.g.,* Graft-versus-host disease (GVHD), allogeneic HSCT and
  bleeding, 351
  cardiac/pulmonary toxicity, 350–351
  DAH, 351
  graft failure, 347–348
  GVHD, 343–347, 344t, 346t–347t
  infections, 348–349
  IPS, 351
  iron overload, 351–352
  obstructive airway disease, 351
  TMA, 351
  VOD/SOS, 349–350
 conditioning regimens, 342–343, 342t
 donor leukocyte infusions in, 339–340
 donor types in, 340–342
 genomic variation in, 343

| 605

graft-versus-tumor effects of, 339–340
GVHD and, 338–342
histocompatibility and HLA typing in, 337–339, 337f–339f
in MDS management, 471–472
myeloablative regimens, 342
nonmyeloablative/reduced-intensity conditioning in, 342t, 343
stem cell sources for, 337
Allogeneic stem cell transplantation (allo-SCT)
for adult ALL in CR1, 501–502
beyond CR1, 502–503
for CML, 403–405
high-dose chemotherapy and, for follicular lymphoma, 525
mobilization of peripheral blood stem cells from normal donors for, G-CSF and GM-CSF in, 78
Alloimmune complications, consultative hematology for, 41–42
Alloimmunization, to HLA antigens, prevention of, 302–303
Allo-SCT. *See* Allogeneic stem cell transplantation (allo-SCT)
Alphanate, for von Willebrand disease, 226
α thalassemia, 138–140, 139f
Alternative splicing, 3–4
defined, 21
Amegakaryocytic thrombocytopenia, congenital, 444t, 450
American College of Chest Physicians (ACCP) guidelines, in genetic thrombophilias testing, 193–194
American Society of Clinical Oncology (ASCO), guidelines for myeloid growth factors uses, 76–77, 76t
AML. *See* Acute myeloid leukemia (AML)
Amyloidosis, 597–598, 598t
Anaplastic large-cell lymphoma (ALCL), 537
ALK-negative, 538
ALK-positive, 537–538
primary cutaneous, 536
Ancestin. *See* Stem cell factor
Anemia(s). *See also specific types*
aplastic, 450–457. *See also* Aplastic anemia
of cancer, 129–130
chemotherapy-induced, darbepoetin alfa for, 84
in children, consultative hematology for, 62–63
of chronic disease/inflammation, 114–115
complex/multifactorial, 128–130, 129t
congenital dyserythropoietic, 444t, 448–449, 448f
Diamond-Blackfan, 444t, 447–448
of the elderly, 128–129, 129t
Fanconi, 443–447, 444t, 445f. *See also* Fanconi anemia
hemolytic, 133–177. *See also specific types and* Hemolytic anemias
HIV infection–related, 130
erythropoietin for, 81–82
in ICU, consultative hematology in, 35–36

iron deficiency, 110–114, 111t, 112f, 113t
megaloblastic, 115–121. *See also* Megaloblastic anemias
myelophthisic, 127–128, 128f
in newborns, consultative hematology for, 57–59, 57f, 58t
nonmyelodysplastic sideroblastic, 120, 120f
in patients receiving cancer-related chemotherapy/radiation therapy, erythropoietin for, 82
PMF-related, treatment of, 435–436
during pregnancy, consultative hematology for, 42–43
pregnancy-related, 128
in preterm infants, erythropoietin for, 81
underproduction, acquired, 109–132. *See also specific anemias and* Underproduction anemias, acquired
Anemia of prematurity, 81
Angiogenesis, in molecular pathogenesis of MM, 587–588
Angioimmunoblastic T-cell lymphoma (AITL), 537
Ann Arbor staging system, 518, 518t
for Hodgkin lymphoma, 543, 543t
Anneal, defined, 21
Anorexia nervosa, anemia associated with, 121, 121f
Anthracycline, for advanced-stage DLBCL, 529–530
Antibody(ies)
antiphospholipid. *See* Antiphospholipid antibody(ies); Antiphospholipid antibody (APLA) syndrome
antiplatelet, platelet function related to, 258t, 259
platelet, assays for, in acquired thrombocytopenia testing, 285
Antibody screening, transfusion therapy, pretransfusion testing, 307–308
Anticoagulant(s), 197–202. *See also specific drugs*
fondaparinux, 199
heparins, 197–199
lupus, in children, consultative hematology for, 63–64
thrombin inhibitors, 199
VKAs, 200–201, 200f, 201t, 202t
for VTE, 205, 205t
Anticoagulation, bridging, management of patients receiving, 29, 29t
Antifibrinolytic agents, for von Willebrand disease, 226
Antigen(s)
CD10, development of, 582
CD19, development of, 582
CD38, in assessing high-risk subgroups of patients with CLL, 561t, 562
CD49d, in assessing high-risk subgroups of patients with CLL, 562
class I, in allogeneic HSCT, 337, 337f
class II, in allogeneic HSCT, 337, 337f
human platelet, platelet transfusion therapy, 298

Antiphospholipid antibody(ies), thrombophilia due to, 184t, 187–188, 187f. *See also* Antiphospholipid antibody (APLA) syndrome
Antiphospholipid antibody (APLA) syndrome
consultative hematology in, 39
general information, 187
management of, 188
pediatric considerations, 188
prevalence of, 187
risk for thrombosis, 188
testing for, 187–188, 187f
thrombophilia due to, 184t, 187–188, 187f
Antiplatelet agents, 195–197
ADP receptor antagonists, 196
aspirin, 195
GPIIb/IIIa receptor antagonists, 196–197
pediatric considerations, 197
phosphodiesterase inhibitors, 196
Antiplatelet antibodies, platelet function related to, 258t, 259
Antisense, RNA interference therapy and, DNA technology applications to, 18–19
Antisense oligonucleotides, 18
defined, 21
Antithrombin deficiency
assays for, in acquired thrombocytopenia testing, 287
thrombophilia due to, 184t, 186–187
Antithrombotic drugs, 195–202. *See also specific drugs*
anticoagulants, 197–202
antiplatelet agents, 195–197
thrombolytic agents, 202
Aorto-gonadal-mesonephros (AGM) region, 335
Aperture impedance counters, in laboratory hematology, 264
Apheresis, transfusion therapy, 308–312, 309t
exchange transfusion, 310
PBSC harvesting, 310–312
plasma exchange/plasmapheresis, 308–310, 309t
APL. *See* Acute promyelocytic leukemia (APL)
Aplasia(s), pure red cell, 125–127, 125f, 125t, 126f
Aplastic anemia, 450–457
classification of, 451t, 452t
clinical case, 451, 457
clinical presentation of, 453
defined, 450–451
differential diagnosis of, 454–455, 454f
epidemiology, causes, and pathogenesis of, 451–453, 452t, 453f
HSCT for, 361–362
idiopathic, differential diagnosis of, 452t
transfusion therapy, 312, 321
treatment of, 455–457
bone marrow transplantation in, 456
described, 455

immunosuppressive therapy in, 456–457
vs. bone marrow transplantation, 457
late clonal complications with, 457
supportive care, transfusions, and hematopoietic growth factors in, 455–456
APLA syndrome. *See* Antiphospholipid antibody (APLA) syndrome
aPTT. *See* Activated partial thromboplastin time (aPTT)
Argatroban, 199
Arterial clots, thrombosis and, 180
Arterial thromboembolism, 210–212, 210t
in absence of arteriosclerosis, 210–211, 210t
atrial fibrillation and, prevention of, 211
childhood stroke due to, 211–212
neonatal stroke due to, 211
peripheral arterial disease due to, 211
stroke and, prevention of, 211
Arterial thrombosis, in absence of arteriosclerosis, 210–211, 210t
Arteriosclerosis, arterial thrombosis in absence of, 210–211, 210t
Arthritis, rheumatoid, neutropenia and, 378t, 382
Arthropathy(ies), hemophilic, 228
Artificial heart valves, during pregnancy, consultative hematology for, 49–50
ASCO. *See* American Society of Clinical Oncology (ASCO)
ASCO/American Society of Hematology, erythropoietin guidelines of, 83
Aspirin, 195
Asymptomatic MM, defined, 582t
Atrial fibrillation, prevention of, 211
Autoimmune cytopenias
after HSCT, transfusion therapy, 315
CLL and, 571
Autoimmune diseases, HSCT for, 361–362
Autoimmune hemolytic anemia (AHA), 160–171, 161t
clinical manifestations of, 163–164
cold, 160–161, 161t
described, 28
laboratory findings in, 163–164, 163f, 164t
mixed, 161, 161t
pathophysiology of, 160–161, 161t
transfusion therapy, 318–319
treatment of, 164–165
warm, 160, 161t
Autoimmune thrombocytopenia, transfusion therapy, 319
Autoinflammatory diseases, neutrophil-related, 386–387
Autologous HSCT, 352–354, 354t
complications of, 354, 354t
conditioning regimens, 354
HSC collection and manipulation in, 352–354
infections due to, 354, 354t

Automated blood cell counting, in laboratory hematology, 263–266, 264f
Azacitidine, in MDS management, 470

B
Babesiosis, hemolytic anemias due to, 174, 174f
Bacteria, RBC membrane injury caused by, hemolytic anemias due to, 172–173
Bacterial infections, transfusion-related, 323–324
Bartonellosis, hemolytic anemias due to, 174
Basophil(s), in myeloid disorders, 375
B cell(s)
in CLL, minimum level of, 558
development of, 511–512
B-cell CLL. *See* Chronic lymphocytic leukemia (CLL)
B-cell lymphocytosis, monoclonal, 558–559
B-cell lymphomas
aggressive, 528–535
Burkitt lymphoma, 532–533
DLBCL, 529–532. *See also* Diffuse large B-cell lymphoma (DLBCL)
MCL, 532–533
PMBCL, 532
diffuse large, 529–532. *See also* Diffuse large B-cell lymphoma (DLBCL)
indolent, 521–526. *See also* Follicular lymphoma
primary mediastinal (thymic) large, 532
B-cell mutations, DNA technology applications to, 15
B-cell neoplasms, WHO classification of, 514, 515t
BCR-ABL1 positive gene, CML, 398–406
Bendamustine
for CLL, 568
for relapsed and refractory follicular lymphoma, 524–525
Benign hematologic disorders, conditioning for, in allogeneic HSCT, 343
Bernard-Soulier syndrome, 255, 255t
ß thalassemia, 136–138, 136f
BFU-E. *See* Burst-forming units–erythroid (BFU-E)
Biomarker(s)
in assessing high-risk subgroups of patients with CLL, 561–563, 561t, 563f
in CLL, multivariate models using, 564
Bite(s), spider, hemolytic anemias due to, 171–172
Bleeding. *See also* Bleeding disorders; Hemorrhage; Hemostasis
allogeneic HSCT and, 351
excessive, approach to patient with, 219–220
management of
heparins in, 197
VKAs in, 201, 201t

postoperative, consultative risk assessment for, 32
risk of, consultative preoperative assessment of, 27–30, 28t, 29t
Bleeding disorders, 217–240. *See also* Bleeding; Hemostasis
fibrinolysis, 236–238
hemophilias, 227–233
hemostatic process in, 217–219, 218f
with normal screening hemostasis tests, in laboratory hematology, 282–283
platelet function disorders, 220–223
von Willebrand disease, 223–227
Blood cell counting, automated, in laboratory hematology, 263–266, 264f
Blood clots, arterial, thrombosis and, 180
"Bloodless" medicine, 326–327
Blood smears, peripheral examination of, in laboratory hematology, 266–267, 266t
Blood substitutes, transfusion therapy, 326–327
BMECs. *See* Bone marrow endothelial cells (BMECs)
BMT. *See* Bone marrow transplantation (BMT)
Bone marrow
aspirate and biopsy of, in laboratory hematology, 267–268, 267t
samples for ancillary studies, preparation of in laboratory hematology, 268
Bone marrow culture, long-term, stem cell–related, 331–332
Bone marrow endothelial cells (BMECs), in molecular pathogenesis of MM, 587–588
Bone marrow engraftment, analysis of, 18
Bone marrow failure
causes of, 443
described, 443
PNH evolution and, 459
Bone marrow failure syndromes, 443–474. *See also specific types*
acquired, 450–472
CAMT, 444t, 450
CDAs, 444t, 448–449, 448f
congenital, 443–450
Diamond-Blackfan anemia, 444t, 447–448
dyskeratosis congenita, 444t, 449–450
Fanconi anemia, 443–447, 444t, 445f
MDSs, 462–472
PNH, 458–461
Bone marrow microenvironment, in molecular pathogenesis of MM, 585–586
Bone marrow transplantation (BMT). *See also* Hematopoietic stem cell transplantation (HSCT)
for aplastic anemia, 456
immunosuppressive therapy vs., for aplastic anemia, 457
improvement of neutrophil production in patients with delayed

engraftment or graft failure after, G-CSF and GM-CSF in, 78
neutrophil recovery after, acceleration of, G-CSF and GM-CSF in, 78
Bortezomib, for MM
  in newly diagnosed transplantation-eligible patients, 593
  in non-transplantation-eligible patients, 594
  relapsed or refractory, 596
Branch retinal vein occlusion (BRVO), 209
British Columbia Cancer Agency, 528
BRVO. See Branch retinal vein occlusion (BRVO)
Budd-Chiari syndrome, 207–208
Burkitt-like lymphoma, 533
Burkitt lymphoma, 532–533
  in children and adults, treatment of, 494
Burst-forming units–erythroid (BFU-E), erythropoiesis and, 109
Bypassing agents, 231

C
C4b-binding protein (C4b-BP), 184–185
CAMT. See Congenital amegakaryocytic thrombocytopenia (CAMT)
Cancer(s)
  anemia of, 129–130
  germ cell, HSCT for, 364
  VTE due to, 192
Capping, defined, 21
Carbohydrate antigen systems, transfusion therapy, 293t, 295
Carboxyhemoglobinemia, 149–150
Cardiac toxicity, allogeneic HSCT and, 350–351
Cardiac valve hemolysis, fragmentation hemolysis due to, 169–170
Cardiopulmonary surgery, transfusion therapy during, 321
Castleman disease, consultative hematology for, 55–56
Catastrophic APLA syndrome, in ICU, consultative hematology in, 39
Catheter-related thrombosis, 207
CCI. See Corrected count increment (CCI)
CD markers, clinically useful, 271t
CD10 antigen, development of, 582
CD19 antigen, development of, 582
CD38 antigen, in assessing high-risk subgroups of patients with CLL, 561t, 562
CD49d antigen, in assessing high-risk subgroups of patients with CLL, 562
CDAs. See Congenital dyserythropoietic anemias (CDAs)
cDNA. See Complementary DNA (cDNA)
Cell(s), iPS, 13
  defined, 22
Cell biology, of MDSs, 468
Cell trafficking, in molecular pathogenesis of MM, 588–589
CEL not otherwise specified. See Chronic eosinophilic leukemia (CEL) not otherwise specified

Central nervous system (CNS), precursor B-cell/T-cell ALL effects on
  in children, treatment of, 496
  prevention of, 499–500
Central nervous system (CNS) disease, sickle cell disease effects on, 146
Central retinal vein occlusion (CRVO), 209
Cerebral and sinus vein thrombosis, 209
Cerebral sinovenous thrombosis, 209
CFU-E. See Colony-forming units–erythroid (CFU-E)
CFU-GEMM. See Colony-forming unit–granulocyte erythroid-monocyte macrophage (CFU-GEMM)
CFU-S assay. See Spleen colony-forming unit (CFU-S) assay
CGD. See Chronic granulomatous disease (CGD)
CGH. See Comparative genomic hybridization (CGH)
Chédiak-Higashi syndrome (CHS), 378t, 379t, 381–382
Chemical agents, hemolytic anemias due to, 171–172
Chemoimmunotherapy, purine analogs with, for CLL, 566
Chemokine(s), in molecular pathogenesis of MM, 588–589
Chemotherapy
  for advanced-stage follicular lymphoma, 522–524, 523t
  anemia due to, darbepoetin alfa for, 84
  febrile neutropenia due to, prevention of, G-CSF and GM-CSF in, 75–76
  high-dose, allogeneic SCT and, for follicular lymphoma, 525
  for Hodgkin lymphoma, 543–547, 545t
  neutropenia due to, 378t, 384–385
  for NHLs, combination therapy, 522–523, 523t
  thrombocytopenia due to
    prevention of, IL-11 in, 86
    TPO for, 86
Childhood stroke, 211–212
Children
  ALL in
    cryptic translocation identification of, 15
    subgroups of, 497–498
  AML in, 483
  antiplatelet agents in, 197
  APLA syndrome in, 188
  Burkitt lymphoma in, treatment of, 494
  cobalamin (vitamin B$_{12}$) deficiency in, 119
  consultative hematology in
    anemia, 62–63
    ITP, 63
    lupus anticoagulants, 63–64
  FVL in, 182
  Hodgkin lymphoma in, treatment of, 546–547
  NHLs in, 540–541
  precursor B-cell/T-cell ALL in, treatment of, 494–498. See also Precursor B-cell/T-cell ALL, in children, treatment of

primary ITP in, management of, 245
protein C deficiency in, 184
protein S deficiency in, 185–186
solid tumors in, HSCT for, 364–365
transfusion therapy in, 315–319. See also Transfusion therapy, pediatric issues related to
VKAs in, 201
Chimeric, defined, 13, 21
CHL. See Classical Hodgkin lymphoma (CHL)
Chlorambucil, for CLL, 564, 565t
Chromatic, 2
  defined, 21
Chromosomal alterations, in MM, 583, 583t
Chromosomal translocations, in NHLs, 513, 513t
Chromosome(s), defined, 2, 21
Chronic disease, anemia of, 114–115
Chronic eosinophilic leukemia (CEL) not otherwise specified, 413–414
  clinical features of, 413–414
  course/prognosis of, 414
  described, 413
  diagnostic criteria for, 414
  epidemiology of, 413
  treatment of, 414
Chronic granulomatous disease (CGD), 386, 387f
Chronic lymphocytic leukemia (CLL), 555–579
  B-cell, 555–579
    minimum level of, 558
  clinical and laboratory features of, 559
  clinical course of, 556
  complications of, 571–572
  cytogenetic abnormalities in, 557–559, 558t
  demographics of, 555–557, 556f
  described, 555
  diagnosis of, 557–559, 558t
  epidemiology of, 555–556, 556f
  familial, 557
  future research on, 574
  high-risk, newly diagnosed patients with, treatment of, 569–570
  high-risk subgroups with, assessment of, novel biomarkers prognostic factors in, 561–563, 561t, 563f
  HSCT for, 361
  immunophenotypic pattern of, 558
  incidence of, 555–556
  molecular aspects of, 558
  monoclonal B-cell lymphocytosis, 558–559
  newly diagnosed vs. previously treated or relapsed/refractory, prognostic factors for, 563
  prognostic factors in, 560–564
    biomarkers, 561–563, 561t, 563f
    multivariate models using, 564
    case for, 560
    for newly diagnosed CLL vs. previously treated or relapsed/refractory CLL, 563
    outcomes associated with, 561, 561t
    traditional, 560–561
      multivariate model using, 563–564

prognostic models in, 563–564
quality-of-life issues related to, 572–573
relapsed or refractory
  treatment of, 569–570
  workup and treatment options for, 568
second malignancies related to, 572
staging of, 560, 560t
survival of, 556, 556f
T-cell, 574
transformation to prolymphocytic leukemia or Richter transformation, 572
treatment of, 564–570
  alemtuzumab in, 567–568
  alkylator-based therapy in, 564, 565t
  bendamustine in, 568
  cladribine in, 566–567
  combination purine analog-based chemotherapy and chemoimmunotherapy in, 566
  flavopiridol in, 569–570
  HuMax-CD20, 570
  initial, 564–568, 565t
  lenalidomide in, 569
  pentostatin in, 566–567, 567t
  purine analogs in, 565–567, 565t, 567t
  for relapsed or refractory CLL, 568
  rituximab in, 565–566, 565t
  SCT in, 570
Chronic myelogenous leukemia (CML), 398–406
  clinical features of, 400
  course/prognosis of, 405–406, 405t
  described, 398
  diagnostic criteria for, 400–402, 401t
  epidemiology of, 398
  HSCT for, 360–361
  pathobiology of, 398–400, 399f
  treatment of, 402–405
    for advanced disease, 404
    allogeneic transplantation, 403–404
    graft-versus-leukemia effect and reduced-intensity conditioning regimens in, 404
    imatinib mesylate in, 402, 404
    SCT in, 403–404
    second-generation TK inhibitors in, 402–403
Chronic myeloid leukemia
  clinical features of, 401t
  minimal residual disease in, monitoring of, 17
  neutrophilia in, 377
Chronic neutrophilic leukemia (CNL), 406–407
  clinical features of, 406
  course/prognosis of, 407
  described, 406
  diagnostic criteria for, 406
  epidemiology of, 406
  neutrophilia in, 377
  pathobiology of, 406
  treatment of, 406–407
Chronic renal failure
  darbepoetin alfa for, 84
  erythropoietin in, 80–81

Chronic T-cell leukemias, 574
Chronic thromboembolic pulmonary hypertension, 206
CHS. See Chédiak-Higashi syndrome (CHS)
Cilostazol, 196
cis-acting regulatory elements, 4
  defined, 21
Cladribine, for CLL, 566–567
Class I antigens, in allogeneic HSCT, 337, 337f
Class II antigens, in allogeneic HSCT, 337, 337f
Classical Hodgkin lymphoma (CHL), 541–542
  lymphocyte-depleted, 542
  lymphocyte-rich, 542
  mixed cellularity, 542
  nodular sclerosis, 542
  prevalence of, 541
CLL. See Chronic lymphocytic leukemia (CLL)
Clonal, defined, 21
Clonal abnormalities, 8
Clopidogrel, 196
Clostridial sepsis, hemolytic anemias due to, 172
CML. See Chronic myelogenous leukemia (CML)
CMV. See Cytomegalovirus (CMV)
CNL. See Chronic neutrophilic leukemia (CNL)
CNS. See Central nervous system (CNS)
CNV. See Copy number variant (CNV)
Coagulation, phases of, 217–219, 218f
Coagulation factor activity assays, in laboratory hematology, 276
Coagulation factor deficiency, acquired, conditions associated with, 183, 183t
Coagulopathy, in newborns, consultative hematology for, 61
Cobalamin (vitamin B_{12}) deficiency
  anemia associated with, 116–119, 116f, 117t, 118t
  causes of, 116–117, 117t
  complications of, 117–118
  described, 116
  diagnosis of, 118, 118t
  in infants and children, 119
  prevalence of, 117
  treatment of, 118–119
Coding sequence, 1
Codon(s), 4
  defined, 21
  termination, 4
    defined, 23
Colony-forming assays, stem cell–related, 331–332, 333f
Colony-forming unit(s)–erythroid (CFU-E), erythropoiesis and, 109
Colony-forming unit–granulocyte erythroid-monocyte macrophage (CFU-GEMM), erythropoiesis and, 109
Communication, interphysician, effective principles of, 27, 28t

Comparative genomic hybridization (CGH)
  defined, 21
  molecular studies–related, 9
Complementary, defined, 21
Complementary DNA (cDNA), 11
  defined, 21
  structure of, 1
Complex/multifactorial anemias, 128–130, 129t
Conditioning regimens
  in allogeneic HSCT, 342–343, 342t
  in autologous HSCT, 354
Congenital amegakaryocytic thrombocytopenia (CAMT), 444t, 450
Congenital bone marrow failure syndromes, 443–450. See also specific syndromes and Bone marrow failure syndromes
Congenital dyserythropoietic anemias (CDAs), 444t, 448–449, 448f
Congenital erythropoietic porphyria, 106–107
Congenital heart surgery, ECMO and, in neonates, 316–317
Constitutive promoter, 12
  defined, 21
Consultative hematology, 27–73
  for alloimmune complications, 41–42
  for atypical lymphoproliferative processes, 55–56, 55t
  for Castleman disease, 55–56
  consultant's role and effectiveness in, 27
  for drug-related abnormalities, 41
  effective, principles of, 27, 28t
  in excessive warfarin dosing risk assessment, 34, 35t
  for hematologic complications of solid organ transplantation, 40–42, 41t
  in hemostatic agents risk assessment, 30–31
  ICU-related, 35–39. See also Intensive care unit (ICU), consultative hematology in
  in intraoperative risk assessment, 30
  for leukocytosis, 53, 54t
  for leukopenia, 53–55, 54t
  for lymphadenopathy, 55, 55t
  for mild thrombocytopenia, 52–53
  in pediatric patients, 57–64. See also Children, consultative hematology in; Newborn(s), consultative hematology in
  for persistent polyclonal lymphocytosis, 55
  in postoperative bleeding risk assessment, 32
  in postoperative thrombosis prophylaxis, 32–34, 33t, 35t
  in posttransplantation erythrocytosis, 40
  during pregnancy, 42–52. See also Pregnancy, consultative hematology during
  in preoperative assessment of bleeding risk, 27–30, 28t, 29t
  for PTLDs, 40–41, 41t

for splenomegaly, 56–57, 56t
for surgery and invasive procedures, 27–34
in thromboprophylaxis, 32–34, 33t, 35t
in transfusion risk assessment, 31–32
transfusion-related, 40
Consumptive thrombocytopenia, transfusion therapy, 319
Contraceptive(s), estrogen, VTE due to, 192–193
Conventional cytogenetics, 8
Coping sequence, defined, 21
Copper, hemolytic anemias due to, 171
Coproporphyria, hereditary, 103
Copy number variant (CNV), 6
 defined, 21
Cord blood donors, in allogeneic HSCT, 340–341
Corrected count increment (CCI), 301
CR1, adult ALL in, treatment of, allo-SCT in, 501–502
CREGs. See Cross-reactive groups (CREGs)
Critically ill patients, thrombocytopenia in, 253–254
Crossmatching, transfusion therapy, pretransfusion testing, 308
Cross-reactive groups (CREGs), 298t
CRVO. See Central retinal vein occlusion (CRVO)
Cryoprecipitate, transfusion therapy, 305
Cryptic translocation, in pediatric ALL identification, 15
Culture-initiating cells, long-term, stem cell–related, 332
Cutaneous porphyrias, 105–107, 105f
Cyclic neutropenia, 378t, 379t, 380–381
Cyclophosphamide, for CLL, 564, 565t
Cytochemical stains, in laboratory hematology, 267–268, 267t
Cytogenetics
 in ALL, 490–491, 491t
 in CLL, 557–559, 558t
 conventional, 8
 defined, 21
 in laboratory hematology, 270
 in lymphoproliferative disorders, 513–514, 513t
 in MDSs, 466–468, 467t
 techniques in, molecular studies–related, 8–10
Cytokine(s), in molecular pathogenesis of MM, 586–587, 587f, 588f
Cytomegalovirus (CMV), transfusion therapy and, 325
Cytometry, flow, in laboratory hematology, 268–269, 269t
Cytopenia(s)
 autoimmune
  after HSCT, transfusion therapy, 315
  CLL and, 571
 idiopathic, of undetermined significance, 469
Cytoreductive therapy(ies)
 for CML, 404
 for ET, 429–430, 429t
 for PV, 423–424
Cytosine-phosphate-guanine (CpG) islands, 470

D
Dabigatran, 202
DAH. See Diffuse alveolar hemorrhage (DAH)
Dapsone, hemolytic anemias due to, 171
Darbepoetin alfa, 84–85, 84f
 adverse effects of, 85
 for chemotherapy-induced anemia, 84
 for chronic renal failure, 84
Decitabine, in MDS management, 470–471
Deep vein thrombosis (DVT)
 diagnosis of, 204
 postoperative, treatment of, consultative risk assessment for, 33–34
 postthrombotic syndrome, 205–206, 206f
 prevention of, 203, 203t
 symptoms of, 203–204
 treatment of, acute, 204–205
 upper extremity, 207
Deferasirox, in hereditary hemochromatosis management, 101
Deferoxamine, in hereditary hemochromatosis management, 100–101
Definitive erythropoiesis, 335
Degenerate, 4
 defined, 21
Delayed hemolytic reactions, transfusion therapy and, 322
Dendritic cells, in myeloid disorders, 376
Diabetes mellitus, G-CSF in, 79
Diamond-Blackfan anemia, 444t, 447–448
DIC. See Disseminated intravascular coagulation (DIC)
Dicer, 5
 defined, 21
Differential adsorption, defined, 318
Diffuse alveolar hemorrhage (DAH), allogeneic HSCT and, 351
Diffuse large B-cell lymphoma (DLBCL), 529–532
 advanced-stage, treatment of, 529–530
 clinical case, 529
 composition of, 529
 features of, 529
 localized, treatment of, 531
 relapsed and refractory, treatment of, 532
 treatment of, response to, assessment of, 531–532
Dipyridamole, 196
Disequilibrium, linkage, 6
Disomy, uniparental, 3
 defined, 23
Disseminated intravascular coagulation (DIC)
 fragmentation hemolysis due to, 170
 thrombocytopenia in ICU due to, consultative hematology in, 37–38
DITP. See Drug-induced thrombocytopenia (DITP)
DLBCL. See Diffuse large B-cell lymphoma (DLBCL)

DNA
 complementary, 11
 structure of, 1
DNA methylation, 2–3
DNA probe, 6
DNA technology
 clinical applications of, 13–20
  expression profiling, diagnostic- and treatment-related, 17
  germline mutations–related, 13–15, 14f
  novel therapies and, 18–20, 19t
  somatic mutations–related, 15–17, 16f
  stem cell transplantation–related, 18
 microarray, expression arrays, 11–12
Döhle bodies, 376, 377f
 in May-Hegglin syndrome, 253, 253f
Donor(s), in allogeneic HSCT
 cord blood donors, 340–341
 haploidentical-related donors, 341–342
 related donors, 340
 types of, 340–342
 unrelated donors, 340
Donor leukocyte infusions, in allogeneic HSCT, 339–340
Down syndrome, AML with, 483
Drosha, 5
 defined, 21
Drug(s)
 abnormalities related to, consultative hematology for, 41
 immune hemolytic anemia due to, 161–162, 162t
 neutropenia due to, 378t, 383–384, 384t
 platelet function inhibition by, 258t, 259–260
Drug-induced thrombocytopenia (DITP), 246–248
 described, 246–247
 diagnosis of, 247
 in ICU, consultative hematology in, 37
 mechanism of, 247
Duffy antigen system, transfusion therapy, 293–294, 293t
Durie-Salmon staging system, for MM, 590, 590t
DVT. See Deep vein thrombosis (DVT)
Dyscrasia(s), plasma cell, 581–604. See also Plasma cell dyscrasias
Dyskeratosis congenita, 444t, 449–450
Dysproteinemia(s), platelet function–related, 258t, 259

E
ECMO. See Extracorporeal membrane oxygenation (ECMO)
Elderly
 AML in, 481
 anemia of, 128–129, 129t
Elliptocytosis, hereditary, 153f, 154–156
Eltrombopag, in MDS management, 470
Embolism, pulmonary. See Pulmonary embolism (PE)
Endocrine system
 abnormalities of, underproduction anemias due to, 123–124
 HSCT effects on, 365

Endonuclease(s), restriction, 6, 7f
  defined, 22
Endothelial cells, bone marrow, in molecular pathogenesis of MM, 587–588
Enhancer(s), 4
  defined, 21
Enteropathy-associated T-cell lymphoma, 538–539
Enzyme(s), RBC, abnormalities of, 156–159
Eosinophil(s), in myeloid disorders, 375
Eosinophilia, myeloid (and lymphoic) neoplasms associated with, 410–413
Epigenetic(s), 2–3
  defined, 21
  in molecular pathogenesis of MM, 584–585
Epoetin alfa. See Erythropoietin (epoetin alfa)
Eptifibatide, 196–197
Erythrocyte analysis, in laboratory hematology, 264–265
Erythrocyte production, requirements for, 109
Erythrocyte sedimentation rate (ESR), in laboratory hematology, 272
Erythrocytosis, posttransplantation, consultative hematology for, 40
Erythroid growth factors, 80–85. See also specific factors
  darbepoetin alfa, 84–85, 84f
  erythropoietin, 80–85
Erythropoiesis
  adult, 335
  BFU-E and, 109
  CFU-E and, 109
  CFU-GEMM and, 109
  definitive, 335
  primitive, 335
  progression of, 109
Erythropoietic protoporphyria, 106
Erythropoietin (epoetin alfa), 80–84
  adverse effects of, 84
  for anemia
    HIV infection–related, 81–82
    in patients receiving cancer-related chemotherapy/radiation therapy, 82
    in preterm infants, 81
  ASCO/American Society of Hematology guidelines for, 83
  in chronic renal failure, 80–81
  FDA regulations for, 82
  FDA-approved indications for, 80t
ESR. See Erythrocyte sedimentation rate (ESR)
Essential thrombocytopenia (ET), 425–430
  biologic features of, 426
  bone marrow/cytogenetic findings in, 428
  clinical features of, 426, 426t
  clonality of, 425
  course/prognosis of, 428
  diagnostic criteria for, 427, 427t
  differential diagnosis of, 427
  incidence of, 425
  JAK2/MPL mutations in, 425–426
  laboratory features of, 427–428, 427f
  pathobiology of, 425–426
  during pregnancy, 430
  thrombohemorrhagic risk associated with, 428–429
    prevention/management of, 430
  transformation to acute leukemia, 430
  treatment of, 429–430, 429t
Essential thrombocytosis, 190
Estrogen contraceptives, VTE due to, 192–193
ET. See Essential thrombocytopenia (ET)
Ewing sarcoma, in children, HSCT for, 365
Exchange transfusion, 310
Exome, defined, 21
Exon(s), 1
  defined, 21
Expression arrays, 11–12
Expression profiling, DNA technology applications to, diagnostic- and treatment-related, 17
Extracorporeal membrane oxygenation (ECMO), congenital heart surgery and, in neonates, 316–317
Extranodal NK/T-cell lymphoma, nasal type, 538

F
FAB classification, of AML, 476, 476t
Factor V Leiden (FVL)
  general information, 180–181, 181f
  management of, 182
  pediatric considerations, 182
  prevalence of, 181
  risk for thrombosis, 181–182
  testing for, 181, 184t
  thrombophilia due to, 180–182, 181f, 184t
Factor VIII, elevated levels of, thrombophilia due to, 188–189
Factor VIII deficiency (hemophilia A), 227–233. See also Hemophilia(s)
Factor IX deficiency (hemophilia B), 227–233. See also Hemophilia(s)
Factor deficiencies
  acquired, 234
  multiple, 234
  rare, 233–236
    causes of, 233–234
    clinical presentation of, 234, 235t
    diagnosis of, 234–235
    gaps in knowledge, 236
    outcomes of, 236
    pathophysiology of, 17
    prognosis of, 236
    treatment of, 235–236
Faggot cell, 482, 482f
Familial CLL, 557
Familial Mediterranean fever (FMF), 386
Familial polycythemic states, in PV, 418–419
Familial thrombocytopenia, 252–253, 253f
Fanconi anemia, 443–447, 444t, 445f
  clinical case, 443
  clinical features of, 446–447
  diagnosis of, 446–447
  epidemiology of, 443, 445
  pathobiology of, 445–446, 445f
  treatment of, 447
Febrile neutropenia
  chemotherapy-induced, prevention of, G-CSF and GM-CSF in, 75–76
  described, 77
  prevention of
    G-CSF and GM-CSF in, 75t, 76
    perfilgrastim in, 76
  risk factors for, 77, 77t
Febrile reactions, transfusion therapy and, 322
Ferroportin disease, 100
FFP. See Fresh frozen plasma (FFP)
FGFR1 abnormalities, myeloid (and lymphoid) neoplasms associated with, 413
Fibrin, formation and degradation of, in hemostatic process, 217, 218f
Fibrinogen assays, in laboratory hematology, 280
Fibrinolysis
  abnormalities in, thrombophilia due to, 191–192, 191f
  disorders of, 236–238
    causes of, 236–237
    clinical presentation of, 237
    gaps in knowledge, 237–238
    outcomes of, 237
    pathophysiology of, 236
    prognosis of, 237
    treatment of, 237
Filgrastim, 74–80
  FDA-approved indications for, 74, 74t
  in MDS management, 470
FISH. See Fluorescence in situ hybridization (FISH)
Flanking sequences, 1–2
  defined, 21
Flavopiridol, for relapsed or refractory CLL, 569–570
FLIPI. See Follicular Lymphoma International Prognostic Index (FLIPI)
Flow cytometry, in laboratory hematology, 268–269, 269t
Fludarabine, for CLL, 565, 565t
Fluorescence in situ hybridization (FISH)
  in assessing high-risk subgroups of patients with CLL, 562–563, 563f
  defined, 21
  molecular studies–related, 8–9
FMF. See Familial Mediterranean fever (FMF)
Folic acid deficiency, anemia associated with, 119–120
Follicular lymphoma, 521–526
  advanced-stage, treatment of, 522–524, 523t
  clinical case, 522
  described, 521
  FLIPI in, 519, 519t

localized, management of, 521–522
relapsed and refractory, treatment of, 524–525
treatment of
high-dose chemotherapy and ASCT in, 525
tumor vaccine in, 525–526
variants of, 521
Follicular Lymphoma International Prognostic Index (FLIPI), IPI and, comparison between, in follicular lymphoma, 519, 519t
Fondaparinux, 199
Foot strike hemolysis, fragmentation hemolysis due to, 171
Fragmentation hemolysis, 169–171
causes of, 169–171
clinical case, 169, 170
described, 169, 169f
pathophysiology of, 169
Frameshift mutation, 4
defined, 21
French-American-British (FAB) classification, of AML, 476, 476t
Fresh frozen plasma (FFP), transfusion therapy, 304–306
FVL. See Factor V Leiden

G
Gammopathy(ies), monoclonal, diagnostic criteria for, 581, 582t
Gastrointestinal abnormalities, underproduction anemias due to, 124
Gaucher disease, 392–393, 392f
G-CSF. See Granulocyte colony-stimulating factor (G-CSF)
Gene(s)
anatomy of, 1–3, 2f
BCR-ABL1 positive, CML, 398–406
defined, 1, 21
structural, 4
defined, 23
structure of, 1–2
Gene expression, control of, 4–5, 5f
Gene expression profile, 11
defined, 21
Gene rearrangement studies, in lymphoproliferative diseases, 15
Gene regulation, 4
defined, 21
Gene signatures, in lymphoma, 517–518
Gene therapy, DNA technology applications to, 19–20, 19t
Gene transfer, methods of, 19, 19t
Genetic(s)
mendelian, described, 3
molecular. See Molecular genetics
in molecular pathogenesis of MM, 583–584, 583t, 585f
Genetic code, 4
defined, 21
Genetic information, flow of, 2f, 3–5, 5f
Genetic Information Nondiscrimination Act (GINA), 193

Genomics
in allogeneic HSCT, 343
defined, 21
described, 5–6
Genotype(s), *HFE*, in HFE hemochromatosis, prevalence of, 97, 97t
German Hodgkin Study Group (GHSG), 544
German Low Grade Lymphoma Study Group (GLSG), 534
Germ cell cancer, HSCT for, 364
Germline (inherited) mutations, DNA technology applications to, 13–15, 14f
GHSG. See German Hodgkin Study Group (GHSG)
GINA. See Genetic Information Nondiscrimination Act (GINA)
Glanzmann thrombasthenia, 255–256, 255t
Global hemostasis tests, in laboratory hematology, 280–281
Global primary hemostasis screening tests, 285
GLSG. See German Low Grade Lymphoma Study Group (GLSG)
Glucose-6-phosphate dehydrogenase (G6PD) deficiency
hemolytic anemias and, 157–159, 158t, 159f
testing for, in laboratory hematology, 274
Glycolytic pathway, abnormalities of, 157, 157f
GM-CSF. See Granulocyte-macrophage colony-stimulating factor (GM-CSF)
GPIIb/IIIa antagonists, oral, 197
GPIIb/IIIa receptor antagonists, 196–197
Graft-versus-host disease (GVHD)
allogeneic HSCT and, 338–347, 344t, 346t–347t
acute, 344–345, 344t
chronic, 345–347, 346t–347t
syngeneic autologous, 352
transfusion-associated, 325–326
Graft-versus-leukemia (GVL) effect, of allograft, in CML management, 404
Graft-versus-tumor effects, of allogeneic HSCT, 339–340
Granule deficiency, neutrophil-specific, 386
Granulocyte(s)
collection and storage of, 303–304
described, 373
in myeloid disorders, 373–375, 374t, 375f
procedure, 304
transfusion therapy, 303–304
Granulocyte antigen systems, 303
Granulocyte colony-stimulating factor (G-CSF), 74–80
in acceleration of neutrophil recovery after bone marrow transplantation, 78
adverse effects of, 79
in ALL, 77

in AML, 77
clinical uses of, 75–79, 76t, 77t
described, 74
in diabetes mellitus, 79
in febrile neutropenia prevention, 75t, 76, 77
in HIV infection, 79
in leukapheresis, 79
leukemia risk with, 80
in MI, 79
in mobilization of autologous peripheral blood stem cells and enhancement of neutrophil recovery after transplantation, 77–78
in mobilization of peripheral blood stem cells from normal donors for allogeneic transplantation, 78
in myelodysplasia, 79
new versions of, 80
pegylated methionyl, 74–75, 75t
in pneumonia, 79
potential clinical uses of, 79
in prevention of severe chronic neutropenia, 78
Granulocyte-macrophage colony-stimulating factor (GM-CSF), 75–80
in acceleration of neutrophil recovery after bone marrow transplantation, 78
adverse effects of, 80
clinical uses of, 75–79, 76t, 77t
described, 75
in febrile neutropenia prevention, 75t, 76, 77
leukemia risk with, 80
in mobilization of autologous peripheral blood stem cells and enhancement of neutrophil recovery after transplantation, 77–78
in myelodysplasia, 79
new versions of, 80
in prevention of severe chronic neutropenia, 78
Granulopoiesis, 373–374
Growth factor(s)
hematopoietic, in MDS management, 469–470
in MDS management, 469–470
Growth factors, erythroid, 80–85. See also *specific factors*
Gunther disease, 106–107
GVHD. See Graft-versus-host disease (GVHD)

H
Hairy cell leukemia (HCL), 528, 573–574
Haploidentical-related donors, in allogeneic HSCT, 341–342
HCL. See Hairy cell leukemia (HCL)
HDAC inhibitors. See Histone deacetylase (HDAC) inhibitors
Heart valves, artificial, during pregnancy, consultative hematology for, 49–50

Helicobacter pylori, MALT lymphoma and, 511, 516–517, 526
HELLP syndrome
  fragmentation hemolysis due to, 170–171
  during pregnancy, consultative hematology for, 43t, 44–45
Hemaphagocytic lymphohistiocytosis (HLH), 388–390, 389f, 390t
Hematologic disorders, benign, conditioning for, in allogeneic HSCT, 343
Hematologic malignancies, during pregnancy, consultative hematology for, 50–52
Hematologic values, for newborns, 58t
Hematology
  consultative, 27–73. *See also* Consultative hematology
  laboratory, 263–290. *See also* Laboratory hematology
  molecular basis of, 1–26. *See also* Molecular studies, in hematology
Hematopoiesis
  cellular basis of, 331–371
  normal, in laboratory hematology, 269–270
  optogeny of, 334–335
Hematopoietic growth factors (HGFs), 74–91
  for aplastic anemia, 455–456
  darbepoetin alfa, 84–85, 84f
  erythroid growth factors, 80–85
  G-CSF, 74–80. *See also* Granulocyte colony-stimulating factor (G-CSF)
  in MDS management, 469–470
  myeloid growth factors, 74–80
  platelet growth factors, 85–87
  stem cell factor, 87
Hematopoietic stem cell(s) (HSCs)
  assays, 331–332, 333f
  biologic properties of, 335
  circulation of, 333
  collection and manipulation of, in autologous HSCT, 352–354
  concepts related to, 331–334, 333f, 334f
  enrichment strategies, 335–354
  ex vivo expansion of, 336
  hierarchal differentiation of, 333, 334f
  historical perspective of, 331
  homing of, 333
  immunophenotype in, 335–336
  mobilization of, 333
  niche for, 332–333
  number of, 332
    required for engraftment, 336–337
  physical properties of, 335
  properties of, 331
Hematopoietic stem cell transplantation (HSCT). *See also* Stem cell transplantation (SCT)
  ABO incompatible, transfusion therapy, 313–315, 314t
  for ALL, 359–360
  allogeneic, 337–352. *See also* Allogeneic HSCT

for AML, 358–359
for anaplastic anemia, 361–362
autoimmune cytopenia after, 315
for autoimmune diseases, 361–362
autologous, 352–354, 354t. *See also* Autologous HSCT
candidates for, 312–315, 314t
  infusion procedure, 312–313
for CLL, 361
for CML, 360–361
described, 336–337
endocrine effects of, 365
for germ cell cancer, 364
for hemoglobinopathies, 362–364
for Hodgkin lymphoma, 356–357, 546
for immune deficiency disorders, 363–364
indications for, 354–365. *See also specific disorders*
for inherited metabolic disorders, 364
late effects of, 365–366
long-term follow-up, 365–366
lymphoproliferative disorders due to, 366
musculoskeletal effects of, 366
for NHL, 354–356
for plasma cell dyscrasias, 357–358
psychosocial effects of, 366
for PV, 424
second malignancies and, 366
for sickle cell disease, 363
for solid tumors, 364–365
  in children, 364–365
syngeneic, 352
for thalassemia major, 362–363
Hemochromatosis
  causes of, 97t
  defined, 96
  hereditary, 96–101. *See also* Hereditary hemochromatosis
  natural history of, 98, 98f
Hemoglobin
  abnormalities of, 134–151
  disorders of, 135–151
    classification of, 135
    sickle cell disease, 140–147
    thalassemia, 136–140
  function of, 135
  production of, 134–135, 134f
  in RBCs, level of, 296
  structure of, 135
Hemoglobinopathy(ies)
  Hemoglobin S, solubility testing for, 273–274, 274f
  HSCT for, 362–364
  screening and diagnosis of, 273–274, 274f
Hemoglobinuria
  march, fragmentation hemolysis due to, 171
  paroxysmal cold, 295
  paroxysmal nocturnal, 166–168, 458–461. *See also* Paroxysmal nocturnal hemoglobinuria (PNH)
Hemoglobulin, unstable, 148–149
Hemoglobulin C disease, 148

Hemoglobulin D disease, 148
Hemoglobulin E disease, 147–148
Hemoglobulin H disease, 150–151
Hemoglobulinopathy(ies), acquired, 149–151
Hemolysis
  abnormalities of RBCs and, 134–159
  cardiac valve, 169–170
  described, 133
  foot strike, 171
  fragmentation, 169–171. *See also* Fragmentation hemolysis
  immune, hemolytic anemias due to, 163f, 173
  in PNH, 459
Hemolytic anemias, 133–177. *See also specific types and* Hemoglobin
  acanthocytosis, 155, 155f
  acquired hemoglobinopathies, 149–151
  AHA, 160–161, 161t
  α thalassemia, 138–140, 139f
  autoimmune. *See* Autoimmune hemolytic anemia (AHA)
  ß thalassemia, 136–138, 136f
  carboxyhemoglobulinemia, 149–150
  chemical or physical agents and, 171–172
  classification of, methods of, 133, 133t
  described, 133–134
  extrinsic abnormalities of RBCs and, 160–175. *See also specific types*
  fragmentation hemolysis, 169–171
  G6PD deficiency, 157–159, 158t, 159f
  glycolytic pathway abnormalities, 157, 157f
  gram-positive/gram-negative organisms causing, 172–173
  hemoglobulin C disease, 148
  hemoglobulin D disease, 148
  hemoglobulin E disease, 147–148
  hemoglobulin H disease, 150–151
  hexose-monophosphate shunt abnormalities, 157–159, 158t, 159f
  immune, drug-induced, 161–162, 162t
  infections and, 172–175
  methemoglobinemia, 150, 150t
  in newborns, 59
  nucleotide metabolism abnormalities, 159
  overview of, 133
  oxygen affinity mutants, 149
  PNH, 166–168, 458–461
  RBC enzyme abnormalities, 156–159
  RBC membrane abnormalities, 151–156
  Rh deficiency (null) syndrome, 156
  sickle cell disease, 140–147
  stomatocytosis, 156, 156f
  sufhemoglobinemia, 150
  thalassemia, 136–140
  unstable hemoglobin, 148–149
Hemolytic reactions
  acute, transfusion therapy and, 321–322
  delayed, transfusion therapy and, 322
Hemolytic uremic syndrome (HUS), 250–252
  clinical features of, 250
  diagnosis of, 251–252

management of, 252
pathogenesis of, 250–251
TTP and, thrombocytopenia in ICU due to, consultative hematology in, 38–39
Hemolytic uremic syndrome–thrombotic thrombocytopenic purpura (HUS-TTP). *See* Thrombotic thrombocytopenic purpura–hemolytic uremic syndrome (TTP-HUS)
Hemophagocytic syndrome, 253
Hemophilia(s), 227–233
　acquired, 228
　clinical presentation of, 227–228
　diagnosis of, 228–229, 228f
　gaps in knowledge, 233
　mild, 228
　moderate, 228
　outcomes of, 232–233
　pathophysiology of, 227
　prognosis of, 232–233
　severe, 228
　treatment of, 229–232, 229t, 230t, 232t
Hemophilic arthropathy, 228
Hemorrhage. *See also* Bleeding
　diffuse alveolar, allogeneic HSCT and, 351
　intraoperative, consultative risk assessment for, 30
Hemostasis
　described, 274–275
　disorders of, 241–262. *See also specific types*
　　DITP, 246–248
　　HIT, 248–250, 248t, 249f
　　ITP, 243–250
　　platelet function–related, 254–260. *See also* Platelet function disorders
　laboratory hematology for, 274–285
　overview of, 217–219, 218f
　platelet function in, 242–243, 242f
　primary, disorders of, 220–227. *See also specific disorders, e.g.,* Platelet function disorders
　　platelet function–related, 220–227
　　von Willebrand disease, 223–227
　screening coagulation testing in, 275–282, 276f–279f, 282t, 283f, 284f
　　coagulation factor activity assays, 276
　　mixing studies, 275–276
　　preanalytical variables, 275
　secondary, disorders of, 227–236
　　hemophilias
　　　A, 227–233
　　　B, 227–233
　　rare factor deficiencies, 233–236. *See also* Factor deficiencies, rare
Hemostatic agents, consultative risk assessment for, 30–31
Hemostatic process, phases of, 217–219, 218f
Heparin(s), 197–199
　in bleeding management, 197
　low molecular weight, 199
　mechanism of action of, 197

resistance to, 198
thrombocytopenia due to, 197–198, 248–250, 248t, 249f
unfractionated, 198
Heparin-induced thrombocytopenia (HIT), 197–198, 248–250, 248t, 249f
　assays for, in acquired thrombocytopenia testing, 285–286
　clinical features of, 248, 248t
　described, 248
　diagnostic tests for, 249, 249f
　treatment of, 249–250
Heparin resistance, 198
Hepatic vein thrombosis, 207–208
Hepatitis, transfusion-related, 324
Hepatitis/AA syndrome, 451
Hepatosplenic T-cell lymphoma, 538
Hereditary coproporphyria, 103
Hereditary elliptocytosis, 153f, 154–156
Hereditary hemochromatosis, 96–101
　clinical case, 96, 101
　described, 96–97
　ferroportin disease, 100
　HFE
　　clinical presentation of, 98–99
　　diagnosis of, 98, 98f
　　epidemiology of, 97–98, 97t
　　pathophysiology of, 97–98, 97t
　　prevalence of, 97, 97t
　　screening for, 99
　　treatment of, 99
　juvenile form of, 100
　treatment of, 100–101
Hereditary hemochromatosis *HFE* protein, 94–95
Hereditary spherocytosis, 152–154, 152t, 153f
　clinical manifestations of, 152–153
　laboratory evaluation of, 153, 153f
　pathophysiology of, 152, 152t
　treatment of, 153–154
Hexose-monophosphate shunt, abnormalities of, 157–159, 158t, 159f
HFE. See Hereditary hemochromatosis
HFE genotypes, in HFE hemochromatosis, prevalence of, 97, 97t
HFE protein, 94–95
HGFs. *See* Hematopoietic growth factors (HGFs)
Hirudin(s), 199
Histiocyte(s)
　disorders of, 388–392, 389f, 390t, 391f
　　HLH, 388–390, 389f, 390t
　tissue, in myeloid disorders, 375–376
Histiocytosis(es)
　HLH, 388–390, 389f, 390t
　Langerhans cell, 390–392, 391f
　non–Langerhans cell, 392
Histocompatibility, in allogeneic HSCT, 337–339, 337f–339f
Histone deacetylase (HDAC) inhibitors, in MDS management, 471
HIT. *See* Heparin-induced thrombocytopenia (HIT)
HIV infection

anemia associated with, 130
erythropoietin for, 81–82
G-CSF in, 79
HLA. *See* Human leukocyte antigen (HLA)
HLH. *See* Hemaphagocytic lymphohisticytosis (HLH)
Hodgkin lymphoma, 541–547
　advanced-stage, treatment of, 544–546
　Ann Arbor staging system for, 543, 543t
　in children, treatment of, 546–547
　classical, 541–542. *See also* Classical Hodgkin lymphoma (CHL)
　disease types in, 514t, 541
　early-stage, treatment of, 543–544
　HRS cell in, 541
　HSCT for, 356–357
　incidence of, 541
　nodular lymphocyte-predominant, 542–543
　pathology of, 541
　prognostic scoring system for, 543, 543t
　relapsed or refractory, treatment of, 546–547
　staging and prognostic factors in, 543, 543t
　subtypes of, 514, 514t, 541
　treatment of, 543–547, 545t
　　for advanced-stage disease, 544–546
　　chemotherapy in, 543–547, 545t
　　for children, 546–547
　　for early-stage disease, 543–544
　　HSCT in, 546
　　long-term complications of, 547
　　for relapsed or refractory disease, 546–547
Hodgkin Reed-Sternberg (HRS) cell, in Hodgkin lymphoma, 541
Homeostasis, iron
　proteins in, 93–95, 95t
　regulation of, 93–96, 94f, 95t, 96f
Homocysteine pathway, 189, 190f
Homocystinuria, thrombophilia due to, 189, 190f
Homologous recombination, 13
　defined, 21
HPAs. *See* Human platelet antigens (HPAs)
HRS cell, in Hodgkin lymphoma, 541
HSCs. *See* Hematopoietic stem cell(s)
HSCT. *See* Hematopoietic stem cell transplantation (HSCT)
HTLVs. *See* Human T-cell lymphoprotrophic viruses (HTLVs)
Human immunodeficiency virus (HIV) infection. *See* HIV infection
Human leukocyte antigen(s) (HLAs)
　alloimmunization to, prevention of, 302–303
　platelet transfusion therapy, 297–298, 298t
Human leukocyte antigen (HLA) typing, in allogeneic HSCT, 337–339, 337f–339f
Human platelet antigens (HPAs), platelet transfusion therapy, 298
Human T-cell lymphoprotrophic viruses (HTLVs), transfusion therapy and, 324

Humate-P, for von Willebrand disease, 226
HuMax-CD20 (ofatumumab), for relapsed or refractory CLL, 570
HUS. *See* Hemolytic uremic syndrome (HUS)
Hybridization techniques, molecular studies–related, 6–8, 7f
Hyper-IgD syndrome, 386–387
Hyperimmunoglobulin E syndrome, 385–386
Hypertension, pulmonary
   chronic thromboembolic, 206
   VTE and, 206
Hypocellular MDS, 468–469
Hypomethylating agents, in MDS management, 470–471

I
ICU. *See* Intensive care unit (ICU)
Idiopathic aplastic anemia, differential diagnosis of, 452t
Idiopathic cytopenias of undetermined significance, 469
Idiopathic pneumonia syndrome (IPS), allogeneic HSCT and, 351
Idiopathic thrombocytopenic purpura. *See* Immune thrombocytopenia (ITP)
Idraparinux, 202
IGF-1. *See* Insulin-like growth factor-1 (IGF-1)
IgV_H mutation, in assessing high-risk subgroups of patients with CLL, 562
IL-6. *See* Interleukin(s), IL-6
IL-11. *See* Interleukin(s), IL-11
Imatinib mesylate, for CML, 402, 404
Immune complex mechanism, 160
Immune deficiency disorders
   HSCT for, 363–364
   lymphoproliferative disorders associated with, 539–541
   pediatric, transfusion therapy for, 317–318
Immune hemolysis, hemolytic anemias due to, 163f, 173
Immune hemolytic anemia, drug-induced, 161–162, 162t
Immune thrombocytopenia (ITP), 243–246
   described, 243–244
   differential diagnosis of, 244t
   primary
      in adults, management of, 245–246
      in children
         consultative hematology for, 63
         management of, 245
      clinical features of, 244
      described, 243–244
      diagnosis of, 244–245
      pathophysiology of, 244
      persistent, after splenectomy, 246
   secondary, described, 243
   treatment of, emergency, 246
Immune tolerance induction (ITI), 231

Immunoglobulin(s), transfusion therapy, 305–306
Immunohistochemical stains, in laboratory hematology, 267t, 268
Immunomodulatory drugs, in MDS management, 471
Immunophenotyping
   in CLL, 558
   of HSCs, 335–336
   in lymphoproliferative disorders, 512–513, 513t
Immunosuppressive therapy
   for aplastic anemia, 456–457
   bone marrow transplantation vs., for aplastic anemia, 457
Immunotherapy, in MDS management, 471
Imprinting, 3
   defined, 21
Indolent cell leukemias, 573–574
Indolent lymphomas, described, 516
Induced pluripotent stem (iPS) cells, 13
   defined, 22
Induction therapy, for non-transplantation-eligible patients with MM, 594
Infant(s)
   cobalamin (vitamin B_{12}) deficiency in, 119
   preterm, anemia in, erythropoietin for, 81
Infection(s)
   allogeneic HSCT and, 348–349
   autologous HSCT and, 354, 354t
   CLL and, 571–572
   hemolytic anemias due to, 172–173
      babesiosis, 174, 174f
      bartonellosis, 174
      clinical case, 172, 175
      clostridial sepsis, 172
      immune hemolysis associated with, 163f, 173
      malaria, 173–174, 173f
      parasitic infestations of RBCs, 173–174, 173f, 174f
      RBC membrane injury caused by bacteria, 172–173
   thrombocytopenia and, 253
   in ICU, consultative hematology in, 37–38
   transfusion-related, 323–325. *See also specific types*
   viral, NHLs and, 517
Inferior vena cava filters, VTE and, 206–207
Inflammation, anemia of, 114–115
Inherited metabolic disorders, HSCT for, 364
Inherited platelet function defects, treatment of, 257–258
Inherited platelet function disorders, 254–258, 255t. *See also* Platelet function disorders, inherited
INRs, elevated, management of, VKAs in, 201, 201t
Insulin-like growth factor-1 (IGF-1), in molecular pathogenesis of MM, 586–587

Intensification therapy, for MM, 594–595
Intensive care unit (ICU), consultative hematology in, 35–39
   for anemia, 35–36
   catastrophic antiphospholipid antibody syndrome, 39
   thrombocytopenia, 36–39. *See also* Thrombocytopenia, in ICU, consultative hematology in
Interleukin(s)
   IL-6, in molecular pathogenesis of MM, 586
   IL-11, 86–87
      adverse effects of, 86–87
      in prevention of chemotherapy-induced thrombocytopenia, 86
International Bone Marrow Transplant Registry, 525
International Prognostic Index (IPI)
   FLIPI and, comparison between, in follicular lymphoma, 519, 519t
   in NHLs, 518–519, 519t
International Prognostic Scoring System (IPSS; 1997), 466, 466t
International Staging System (ISS), for MM, 590, 590t
Interphysician communication, effective, principles of, 27, 28t
Intraoperative hemorrhage, consultative risk assessment for, 30
Intron, defined, 22
In utero transfusion, 315
IPS. *See* Idiopathic pneumonia syndrome (IPS)
iPS cells. *See* Induced pluripotent stem (iPS) cells
IPSS. *See* International Prognostic Scoring System (IPSS)
Iron
   absorption of, 94
   balance of, regulators of, 93–96, 94f, 95t, 96f
   described, 93
   dysregulation of, 114–115
   toxicity of, 93
   transferrin-bound, 95
Iron chelation therapy, 100–101
   in MDS management, 469
Iron deficiency anemia, 110–114, 111t, 112f, 113t
   causes of, 110–112, 111t
   described, 110
   diagnosis of, 112–113, 112f, 113t
   symptoms of, 112
   treatment of, 113–114
Iron homeostasis
   proteins in, 93–95, 95t
   regulation of, 93–96, 94f, 95t, 96f
Iron overload
   allogeneic HSCT and, 351–352
   causes of, 93, 100–101
Iron overload syndromes, 93–107
   hereditary hemochromatosis, 96–101
ITI. *See* Immune tolerance induction (ITI)
ITP. *See* Immune thrombocytopenia (ITP)

J

JAK2/MPL mutation, in ET, 425–426
JAK2 mutations, in PV, 415
JAK2 V617F mutation, thrombophilia due to, 190

K

Kasabach-Merritt syndrome, fragmentation hemolysis due to, 171
Kell antigen system, transfusion therapy, 293–294, 293t
Kidd antigen system, transfusion therapy, 293–294, 293t
Kidney disease, underproduction anemias due to, 121–123, 122f
Knockout mice
  defined, 22
  molecular studies-related, 12–13
Kostmann syndrome, 378–380, 378t, 379t
Kozak sequence, 4
Kx protein, 294

L

Laboratory hematology, 263–290
  for acquired thrombocytopenia, 285–288. *See also* Thrombocytopenia, acquired, specialized testing for
  ancillary testing, 268–272, 269t, 271t–274t
  aPTT, 277–279, 278f
  automated blood cell counting, 263–266, 264f
  bleeding disorders with normal screening hemostasis tests, 282–283
  bone marrow aspirate and biopsy, 267–268, 267t
  cytogenetics, 270
  ESR, 272
  fibrinogen assays, 280
  flow cytometry, 268–269, 269t
  in G6PD, 274
  general concepts, 263
  global hemostasis tests, 280–281, 285
  hematopoiesis, 269–270
  for hemoglobinopathies, 273–274, 274f
  for hemostasis, 274–282, 285. *See also* Hemostasis, screening coagulation testing in
  immunohistochemical stains, 267t, 268
  molecular diagnostics, 270, 272
  PCR, 270, 272
  peripheral blood smear examination, 266–267, 266t
  platelet function tests, 283–285, 284f
  PT, 277, 277f
  for PT and aPTT combined abnormalities, 279, 279f
  reptilase time, 280
  terminology related to, 263
  for thromboses, 274–275
  TT, 280
  vWF assays, 281–282, 282t, 283f, 284f

LAD. *See* Leukocyte adhesion deficiency (LAD)
Langerhans cell histiocytosis (LCH), 390–392, 391f
Large granular lymphocyte leukemia, 378t, 382–383
LCH. *See* Langerhans cell histiocytosis (LCH)
Lenalidomide
  for MDS, 471
  for MM
    in newly diagnosed transplantation-eligible patients, 593
    in non-transplantation-eligible patients, 594
    relapsed or refractory, 596
  for relapsed or refractory CLL, 569
Lenograstim, 74–80
  indications for, 74
Leucine zipper(s), 4–5
  defined, 22
Leukapheresis, G-CSF in, 79
Leukemia(s). *See also specific types, e.g.,* Chronic myelogenous leukemia (CML)
  acute
    ET transformation to, 430
    platelet function–related, 258t, 259
  acute lymphoblastic, 489–503. *See also* Acute lymphoblastic leukemia (ALL)
  acute myelogenous. *See* Acute myelogenous leukemia
  acute myeloid, 475–487. *See* Acute myeloid leukemia (AML)
  acute promyelocytic, 481–482, 482f
  aggressive NK-cell, 536–537
  chronic eosinophilic, not otherwise specified, 413–414. *See also* Chronic eosinophilic leukemia (CEL) not otherwise specified
  chronic lymphocytic, 555–579. *See also* Chronic lymphocytic leukemia (CLL)
  chronic myelogenous, 398–406. *See also* Chronic myelogenous leukemia (CML)
  chronic myeloid. *See* Chronic myeloid leukemia
  chronic neutrophilic, 377, 406–407. *See also* Chronic neutrophilic leukemia (CNL)
  G-CSF and GM-CSF and, 80
  hairy cell, 528, 573–574
  indolent cell, 573–574
  large granular lymphocyte, 378t, 382–383
  lymphocytic, T-cell large granular, 536
  myeloid, specimen allocation for, 269t
  prolymphocytic, 573
    CLL transformation to, 572
  T-cell, chronic, 574
Leukocyte(s)
  analysis of, in laboratory hematology, 265
  passenger, 297
Leukocyte adhesion deficiency (LAD), 385

Leukocytosis, consultative hematology for, 53, 54t
Leukoerythroblastic peripheral smear, 127, 128f
Leukopenia
  acquired, causes of, 54, 54t
  consultative hematology for, 53–55, 54t
Linkage analysis, defined, 22
Linkage disequilibrium, 6, 338
  defined, 22
Lipoprotein(a), thrombosis due to, 192
Liver disease, underproduction anemias due to, 124, 124f
LMWH. *See* Low molecular weight heparin (LMWH)
Long-term culture-initiating cells (LTC-ICs), stem cell–related, 332
Low molecular weight heparin (LMWH), 199
LTC-ICs. *See* Long-term culture-initiating cells (LTC-ICs)
Lung injury, acute, transfusion-related, 323
Lupus anticoagulants, in children, consultative hematology for, 63–64
Lymphadenopathy, consultative hematology for, 55, 55t
Lymphoblastic lymphomas, 503–504
  incidence of, 503
  prevalence of, 503
  treatment of, 504
    late complications of, 504
Lymphocyte(s), development of
  B-cells, 511–512
  overview of, 511–512, 512t
  T cells, 512
Lymphocyte-depleted CHL, 542
Lymphocyte-rich CHL, 542
Lymphocytic leukemias, chronic, 555–579. *See also* Chronic lymphocytic leukemia (CLL)
Lymphocytosis
  B-cell, monoclonal, 558–559
  persistent polyclonal, consultative hematology for, 55
Lymphohistiocytosis, hemaphagocytic, 388–390, 389f, 390t
Lymphoid neoplasms, 410–413. *See also* Myeloid (and lymphoid) neoplasms
Lymphoma(s), 511–554. *See also specific types and* Lymphoproliferative disorders
  aggressive
    described, 516
    indolent lymphoma transformation to, 528
  anaplastic large cell, 537
    primary cutaneous, 536
  B-cell. *See* B-cell lymphomas
  biology of, 512, 512t
  Burkitt, 532–533
    in children and adults, treatment of, 494
  Burkitt-like, 533
  classification of, 514, 514t, 515t

follicular, 521–526. See also Follicular lymphoma
gene signatures in, 517–518
Hodgkin, 541–547. See also Hodgkin lymphoma
indolent, described, 516
lymphoblastic, 503–504. See also Lymphoblastic lymphoma
lymphoplasmacytic, 527, 574, 598–599, 598t
MALT, 511, 526
causative organisms, 516–517
Helicobacter pylori and, 516–517
mantle cell, 533–535, 574
HSCT for, 355–356
marginal zone, 526–527, 574. See also Marginal zone lymphomas (MZLs)
minimal residual disease detection in, 17
non-Hodgkin. See Non-Hodgkin lymphomas (NHLs)
primary CNS, 540
T-cell. See T-cell lymphomas
treatment of, assessment of, PET in, 520, 520t
Lymphoplasmacytic lymphomas, 527, 574, 598–599, 598t
Lymphoproliferative disorders. See also Lymphoma(s)
diagnostic testing in, 512–514, 513t
gene rearrangement studies in, 15
immunodeficiency-associated, 539–541
immunophenotyping in, 512–513, 513t
molecular genetics/cytogenetics in, 513–514, 513t
morphology of, 512
posttransplantation. See Posttransplantation lymphoproliferative disorders (PTLDs)
specimen allocation for, 269t
Lymphoproliferative processes, atypical, consultative hematology for, 55–56, 55t
Lysosomal storage diseases, 392–393, 392f

M
Macroglobulinemia, Waldenström, 527–528, 598–599, 598t
Major histocompatibility complex (MHC), described, 337
Malaria, hemolytic anemias due to, 173–174, 173f
Malignancy(ies)
hematologic, during pregnancy, consultative hematology for, 50–52
second
after HSCT, 366
CLL and, 572
Malnutrition, anemia associated with, 120–121, 121f
MALT lymphomas, 511, 526
causative organisms, 516–517
Helicobacter pylori infection and, 511, 516–517, 526

Mantle cell lymphoma (MCL), 533–535, 574
HSCT for, 355–356
March hemoglobinuria, fragmentation hemolysis due to, 171
Marginal zone lymphomas (MZLs), 526–527, 574
hairy cell leukemia, 528, 573–574
lymphoplasmacytic lymphomas, 527
nodal, 526–527
splenic, 527
Waldenström macroglobulinemia, 527–528, 598–599, 598t
Marrow failure states, underproduction anemias due to, 125–127, 125f, 125t, 126f
Massive transfusion, procedures and indications for, 320–321
Mastocytosis, systemic, 407–410. See also Systemic mastocytosis
May-Hegglin syndrome, Döhle bodies in, 253, 253f
May-Thurner syndrome, 205
MCL. See Mantle cell lymphoma (MCL)
MDSs. See Myelodysplastic syndromes (MDSs)
Megaloblastic anemias, 115–121. See also *specific types*
causes of, 120
cobalamin (vitamin B_{12}) deficiency, 116–119, 116f, 117t, 118f
described, 115–116
folic acid deficiency, 119–120
malnutrition and, 120–121, 121f
nonmyelodysplastic sideroblastic anemias, 120, 120f
trace element deficiencies and, 120–121, 121f
Mendelian genetics, described, 3
Mesenteric vein thrombosis, 208
Metabolic disorders, inherited, HSCT for, 364
Methemoglobinemia, 150, 150t
Methylation, 2
defined, 22
DNA, 2–3
Methylenetetrahydrofolate reductase (MTHFR), thrombophilia due to, 189, 190f
MGUS. See Monoclonal gammopathy of undetermined significance (MGUS)
MHC. See Major histocompatibility complex (MHC)
MI. See Myocardial infarction (MI)
Microangiopathy(ies), thrombotic, 250–252, 251f, 252f. See also Thrombotic microangiopathy(ies) (TMAs)
Microarray, defined, 22
microRNAs, 5
defined, 22
Minimal residual disease
in CML, monitoring of, 17
in lymphomas, detection of, 17
Mixed cellularity CHL, 542
MM. See Multiple myeloma (MM)

MNSs antigen systems, transfusion therapy, 293–294, 293t
Molecular biology, of MDSs, 466–468, 467t
Molecular diagnostics, in laboratory hematology, 270, 272
Molecular genetics
of ALL, 491–492
in lymphoproliferative disorders, 513–514, 513t
Molecular studies
DNA technology in, 13–20. See also DNA technology, clinical applications of
gene therapy–related, 19–20, 19t
in hematology, 1–26
analytic techniques, 6–11
basic concepts, 1–6, 2f, 5f
CGH, 9
cytogenetic techniques, 8–10
DNA microarray technology, 11–12
FISH, 8–9
hybridization techniques, 6–8, 7f
PCR, 10–11, 10f
proteomics, 12
sequence-based studies, 10
SNP chips, 9
transgenic and knockout mice models, 12–13
Molecule(s), adhesion, in molecular pathogenesis of MM, 586
Molgramostim, 75
Monoclonal B-cell lymphocytosis, 558–559
Monoclonal gammopathies, diagnostic criteria for, 581, 582t
Monoclonal gammopathy of undetermined significance (MGUS)
defined, 582t
staging and prognostic factors in, 590–591, 590t
treatment of, 591–597, 592t
Monocyte(s), in myeloid disorders, 375–376
Monocytopenia, 388
Monocytosis, 388
MPDs. See Myeloproliferative disorders (MPDs)
MPNs. See Myeloproliferative neoplasms (MPNs)
MPN-U. See Myeloproliferative neoplasm-unclassified (MPN-U)
mRNA splicing, 3
MTHFR. See Methylenetetrahydrofolate reductase (MTHFR)
Mucosa-associated lymphoid tissue (MALT) lymphomas. See MALT lymphomas
Multiple-factor deficiencies, 234
Multiple myeloma (MM)
asymptomatic, defined, 582t
causes of, 582–583
defined, 582t
described, 581
diagnostic evaluation, 589–590, 590t
incidence of, 583
molecular pathogenesis of, 583–589, 583t, 585f, 587f, 588f
adhesion molecules in, 586

angiogenesis in, 587–588
BMECs in, 587–588
cell trafficking in, 588–589
chemokines in, 588–589
chromosomal alterations in, 583, 583t
cytokines in, 586–587, 587f, 588f
epigenetics in, 584–585
genetic and epigenetic regulation in, 583–584, 583t, 585f
IGF-1 in, 586–587
IL-6 in, 586
osteoblasts in, 589
osteoclasts in, 589
VEGF in, 587, 587f, 588f
pathogenesis of, bone marrow microenvironment in, 585–586
relapsed or refractory, treatment of, 595–596
smoldering. See Smoldering multiple myeloma (SMM)
staging and prognostic factors in, 590–591, 590t
staging systems for, 590, 590t
survival rates, 591
treatment of, 591–597, 592t
initial therapy for patients eligible for SCT, 591–592
intensification therapy in, 594–595
maintenance therapy in, 595
in newly diagnosed transplantation-eligible patients
bortezomib in, 593
combination therapy, 593–594
lenalidomide in, 593
thalidomide in, 592–593
for non-transplantation-eligible patients, induction therapy in, 594
supportive care in, 596–597
Musculoskeletal system, HSCT effects on, 366
Mutation(s)
B-cell, DNA technology applications to, 15
frameshift, 4
defined, 21
germline, DNA technology applications to, 13–15, 14f
IgV_H, in assessing high-risk subgroups of patients with CLL, 562
JAK2, in PV, 415
JAK2 V617F, thrombophilia due to, 190
JAK2/MPL, in ET, 425–426
nucleophosmin, in AML, 15
prothrombin 20210, thrombophilia due to, 182–183, 184t
somatic, DNA technology applications to, 15–17, 16f
T-cell, DNA technology applications to, 15
Mycosis fungoides, 535–536
Myeloablative regimens, in allogeneic HSCT, 342
Myelodysplasia, G-CSF and GM-CSF in, 79
Myelodysplastic syndromes (MDSs), 462–472
causes of, 462, 464

cell biology of, 468
classification of, 462, 464t
cytogenetics of, 466–468, 467t
described, 462, 463f
diagnosis of, 465
epidemiology of, 462, 464
hypocellular, 468–469
idiopathic cytopenias of undetermined significance, 469
molecular biology of, 466–468, 467t
platelet function–related, 258t, 259
prognosis of, 466, 466t
treatment of, 469–472
allogeneic HSCT in, 471–472
goals of, 469
growth factors in, 469–470
HDAC inhibitors in, 471
hypomethylating agents in, 470–471
immunomodulatory drugs in, 471
immunotherapy in, 471
iron chelation in, 469
transfusions in, 469
Myelofibrosis(es), primary, 431–437. See also Primary myelofibrosis (PMF)
Myeloid disorders, 373–396
basophils in, 375
dendritic cells in, 376
eosinophils in, 375
Gaucher disease, 392–393, 392f
granulocytes in, 373–375, 374t, 375f. See also Granulocyte(s); Neutrophil(s)
granulopoiesis in, 373–374
histiocyte disorders, 388–392, 389f, 390t, 391f
lysosomal storage diseases, 392–393, 392f
monocytes in, 375–376
monocytopenia, 388
monocytosis, 388
neutropenia in, 378–385. See also Neutropenia
neutrophil clearance in, 374
neutrophil extravasation in, 374–375, 375f
neutrophil function disorders, 385–387, 387f. See also Neutrophil function disorders
neutrophil release in, 374
neutrophilia in, 376–378, 377f, 377t. See also Neutrophilia
Niemann-Pick disease, 393
tissue histiocytes in, 375–376
Myeloid growth factors, 74–80
clinical uses of, guidelines for, 76–77, 76t
G-CSF, 74–80. See also Granulocyte colony-stimulating factor (G-CSF)
Myeloid leukemia, specimen allocation for, 269t
Myeloid (and lymphoid) neoplasms
eosinophilia-related, 410–413
FGFR1 abnormalities and, 413
PDGFRA rearrangement and, 411–412
PDGFRB rearrangement and, 412

Myeloma(s), multiple. See Multiple myeloma (MM)
Myeloperoxidase deficiency, 385
Myelophthisic anemia, 127–128, 128f
Myeloproliferative disorders (MPDs)
neutrophilia in, 377–378
platelet function–related, 258–260, 258t
specimen allocation for, 269t
thrombophilia due to, 190
Myeloproliferative neoplasms (MPNs), 397–441. See also specific disorders
CEL not otherwise specified, 413–414
classification of, 397–398, 398t
CML, 398–406
CNL, 406–407
described, 397–398
epidemiology of, 398
ET, 425–430
MPN-U, 437
myeloid (and lymphoid) neoplasms, 410–413. See also Myeloid (and lymphoid) neoplasms
PMF, 431–437
PV, 414–425
systemic mastocytosis, 407–410
Myeloproliferative neoplasm-unclassified (MPN-U), 437
Myocardial infarction (MI), G-CSF in, 79
MZLs. See Marginal zone lymphomas (MZLs)

N
NAIT. See Neonatal alloimmune thrombocytopenia (NAIT)
National Comprehensive Cancer Network (NCCN), guidelines for myeloid growth factors uses, 76–77, 76t
National Health and Nutrition Examination Study (NHANES III), 128
NCCN. See National Comprehensive Cancer Network (NCCN)
Neonatal alloimmune neutropenia, 378t, 379t, 382
Neonatal alloimmune thrombocytopenia (NAIT), 298
Neonatal exchange transfusion, 315
Neonatal stroke, defined, 211
Neonatal transfusion, 315–317
Neonate(s). See Newborn(s)
Neoplasm(s)
B- and T-cell, WHO classification of, 514, 515t
lymphoid, 410–413. See also Myeloid (and lymphoid) neoplasms
myeloproliferative, 397–441. See also Myeloproliferative neoplasms (MPNs)
Neuroblastoma, in children, HSCT for, 364–365
Neutropenia
causes of, 378, 378t
chemotherapy-induced, 378t, 384–385
chronic, severe, prevention of, G-CSF and GM-CSF in, 78–79

classification of, 378, 378t
clinical case, 378–380, 382–385
cyclic, 378t, 379t, 380–381
defined, 378
differential diagnosis of, 378, 379t
drug-induced, 378t, 383–384, 384t
febrile. *See* Febrile neutropenia
idiosyncratic drug reactions and, 378t, 383–384, 384t
in myeloid disorders, 378–385. *See also specific disorders, e.g.,* Kostmann syndrome
  chemotherapy-induced neutropenia, 378t, 384–385
  CHS, 378t, 379t, 381–382
  cyclic neutropenia, 378t, 379t, 380–381
  drug-induced neutropenia, 378t, 383–384, 384t
  large granular lymphocyte leukemia, 378t, 382–383
  neonatal alloimmune neutropenia, 378t, 379t, 382
  NI-CINA, 378t, 383
  primary autoimmune neutropenia, 378t, 379t, 382
  RA, 378t, 382
  SDS, 378t, 379t, 381
  secondary autoimmune neutropenia, 378t, 382
  severe congenital neutropenia, 378–380, 378t, 379t
  Sjögren syndrome, 378t, 382
  SLE, 378t, 382
  WHIM syndrome, 378t, 379t, 381
neonatal alloimmune, 378t, 379t, 382
in newborns, consultative hematology for, 59–60
nonimmune chronic idiopathic, 378t, 383
primary autoimmune, 378t, 379t, 382
secondary autoimmune, 378t, 382
severe congenital, 378–380, 378t, 379t
Neutrophil(s)
  described, 373
  hemeostasis of, 374, 375f
  in myeloid disorders, 373–375, 374t, 375f
    clearance of, 374
    extravasation of, 374–375, 375f
    release of, 374
Neutrophil function disorders, 385–387, 387f
  autoinflammatory diseases, 386–387
  CGD, 386, 387f
  clinical case, 385
  described, 385
  FMF, 386
  hyper-IgD syndrome, 386–387
  hyperimmunoglobulin E syndrome, 385–386
  LAD, 385
  MPD deficiency, 385
  neutrophil-specific granule deficiency, 386
Neutrophilia
  causes of, 376, 377t

in CML, 377
in CNL, 377
defined, 376
in myeloid disorders, 376–378, 377f, 377t
in myeloproliferative disorders, 377–378
Neutrophil-specific granule deficiency, 386
Newborn(s)
  component therapy in, 316
  consultative hematology in, 57–62, 57f, 58t
    anemia, 57–69, 57f, 58t
    coagulopathy, 61
    neutropenia, 59–60
    thrombocytopenia, 60–61
    thrombosis, 61–62
  ECMO and congenital heart surgery in, 316–317
  hematologic values for, 58t
Next-Gen sequencing, 10
  defined, 22
NHANES III. *See* National Health and Nutrition Examination Study (NHANES III)
NHLs. *See* Non-Hodgkin lymphomas (NHLs)
NI-CINA. *See* Nonimmune chronic idiopathic neutropenia (NI-CINA)
Niemann-Pick disease, 393
NLPHL. *See* Nodular lymphocyte-predominant Hodgkin lymphoma (NLPHL)
NMD. *See* Nonsense-mediated decay (NMD)
Nodal MZL, 526–527
Nodular lymphocyte-predominant Hodgkin lymphoma (NLPHL), 542–543
Nodular sclerosis CHL, 542
"No-LASH," 519
Noncoding sequences, 1
  defined, 22
Non-Hodgkin lymphomas (NHLs), 516–539
  aggressive-type, HSCT for, 354–355
  Ann Arbor staging system in, 518, 518t
  B-cell lymphomas, aggressive, 528–535. *See also* B-cell lymphomas, aggressive
  categories of, 515t, 516
  in children, 540–541
  classification of, 516
  described, 516
  development of, risk factors for, 512, 512t
  epidemiology of, 516
  FLIPI in, 519, 519t
  gene signatures in, 517–518
  HSCT for, 354–356
  indolent
    HSCT for, 356
    transformation to aggressive lymphoma, 528
  indolent B-cell, 521–526. *See also* Follicular lymphoma
  indolent vs. aggressive, 516

IPI in, 518–519, 519t
MCL, 533–535, 574
  HSCT for, 335–336
molecular characterization of, 517
MZLs, 526–527
pathogenesis of, 516–517
phenotypic markers and chromosomal translocations in, 513, 513t
PTCLs, 535–539. *See also* Peripheral T-cell lymphomas (PTCLs)
REAL classification of, 516
staging and prognostic factors in, 518–520, 518t–520t
treatment of
  assessment of, PET in, 520, 520t
  chemotherapy combinations in, 522–523, 523t
  follow-up care, 520–521
viral infections associated with, 517
Nonimmune chronic idiopathic neutropenia (NI-CINA), 378t, 383
Non-Langerhan cell histiocytoses, 392
Nonmyeloablative/reduced-intensity conditioning, in allogeneic HSCT, 342t, 343
Nonmyelodysplastic sideroblastic anemias, 120, 120f
Nonsense-mediated decay (NMD), 4
  defined, 22
Northern blotting
  defined, 22
  described, 8
Nucleated RBCs, in laboratory hematology, 265
Nucleic acid(s), digestion and separation of, 6, 7f
Nucleic acid hybridization, 6
  defined, 22
Nucleophosmin mutations, in AML, 15
Nucleotide(s)
  defined, 1, 22
  metabolism of, abnormalities of, 159
Null syndrome, 156
Nutritional deficiencies, underproduction anemias due to, 110–115, 111t, 112f, 113t. *See also specific anemias, e.g.,* Iron deficiency anemia

O
Obstructive airway disease, transplantation-related, allogeneic HSCT and, 351
Ofatumumab, for relapsed or refractory CLL, 570
Older adults, AML in, 481
Oligonucleotide(s)
  allele-specific, 17
    defined, 20–21
  antisense, 18
    defined, 21
  defined, 22
  described, 18
  in germline mutations screening, 14–15, 14f

Oncogene(s), 15
  defined, 22
1000 Genomes Project, 6
Oprelvekin. See Interleukin(s), IL-11
Optical counters, in laboratory hematology, 264
Organ dysfunction, underproduction anemias due to, 121–125, 122f, 124f. See also specific types, e.g., Kidney disease
  endocrine abnormalities, 123–124
  gastrointestinal abnormalities, 124
  kidney disease, 121–123, 122f
  liver disease, 124, 124f
Osteoblast(s), in molecular pathogenesis of MM, 589
Osteoclast(s), in molecular pathogenesis of MM, 589
Oxygen affinity hemoglobulin mutants, 149

P
PAI-1. See Plasminogen activator inhibitor-1 (PAI-1)
"Paired-end reads," 10
Panagglutinating, defined, 318
Pancytopenia
  differential diagnosis of, 452t
  specimen allocation for, 269t
P antigen system, transfusion therapy, 293t, 295
Parasitic infestation of RBCs, hemolytic anemias due to, 173–174, 173f, 174f
Paroxysmal cold hemoglobinuria (PCH), 295
Paroxysmal nocturnal hemoglobinuria (PNH), 166–168, 458–461
  clinical case, 166, 168, 458, 461
  clinical manifestations of, 167, 460
  defined, 458
  diagnosis of, 459–460
  evolution of, bone marrow failure and, 459
  hemolysis in, 459
  laboratory diagnosis of, 167
  laboratory findings in, 166–167, 459–460
  pathophysiology of, 166, 168, 458–459, 459f
  prognosis of, 168, 461
  thrombophilia due to, 190–191
  thrombosis in, 459
  treatment of, 167–168, 460–461
Parvovirus B19, transfusion therapy and, 325
Passenger leukocyte(s), 297
PBSCs. See Peripheral blood stem cell(s) (PBSCs)
PCH. See Paroxysmal cold hemoglobinuria (PCH)
PCNSL. See Primary CNS lymphoma (PCNSL)
PCR. See Polymerase chain reaction (PCR)
PDGFRA rearrangement, myeloid (and lymphoid) neoplasms associated with, 411–412

PDGFRB rearrangement, myeloid (and lymphoid) neoplasms associated with, 412
PE. See Pulmonary embolism (PE)
Pegfilgrastim, 74–75, 75t
Pegylated methionyl G-CSF, 74–75, 75t
Pentostatin, for CLL, 566–567, 567t
Pentoxifylline, 196
Periodic fever syndromes, 386–387
Peripheral arterial disease, arterial thromboembolism and, 211
Peripheral blood smears, examination of, in laboratory hematology, 266–267, 266t
Peripheral blood stem cell(s) (PBSCs), harvesting of, transfusion therapy, 310–312
Peripheral T-cell lymphomas (PTCLs), 535–539
  adult T-cell leukemia/lymphoma, 536
  aggressive, 536–537
  aggressive NK-cell leukemia, 536–537
  AITL, 537
  ALCL, 537
  ALK-negative ALCL, 538
  ALK-positive ALCL, 537–538
  described, 535
  enteropathy-associated, 538–539
  extranodal NK/T-cell lymphoma, nasal type, 538
  hepatosplenic, 538
  indolent, 535–536
  mycosis fungoides, 535–536
  not otherwise specified, 537
  prevalence of, 535
  primary cutaneous, 539
  primary cutaneous aggressive epidermotropic CD8$^+$ T-cell lymphoma, 539
  primary cutaneous ALCL, 536
  primary cutaneous CD4$^+$ small/medium T-cell lymphoma, 536
  rare subtypes, 538
  SCPTCL, 538
  Sézary syndrome, 535–536
  T-cell large granular lymphocytic leukemia, 536
Persistent polyclonal lymphocytosis, consultative hematology for, 55
PET. See Positron emission tomography (PET)
PFA. See Platelet function analyzer (PFA)
Ph$^+$ ALL, treatment of, 500–501
Pharmacogenomics, ALL treatment and, 17
Phenazopyridine, hemolytic anemias due to, 171
Phenotypic markers, in NHLs, 513, 513t
Phlebotomy, for PV, 421–422, 422f, 422t
Phosphodiesterase inhibitors, 196
Physical agents, hemolytic anemias due to, 171–172
PIDs. See Primary immune deficiencies (PIDs)
Plasma cell(s), development of, 581–582
Plasma cell dyscrasias, 581–604. See also specific types, e.g., Multiple myeloma (MM)

  amyloidosis, 597–598, 598t
  causes of, 582–583
  described, 581
  diagnostic evaluation, 589–590, 590t
  HSCT for, 357–358
  incidence of, 583
  molecular pathogenesis of, 583–589, 583t, 585f, 587f, 588f
  plasmacytomas, 597
  POEMS syndrome, 598, 598t
  staging and prognostic factors in, 590–591, 590t
  survival rates, 591
  treatment of, 591–597, 592t
    initial therapy for patients eligible for SCT, 591–592
Plasmacytoma(s), 597
  solitary, defined, 582t
Plasma exchange, transfusion therapy, pretransfusion testing, 308–310, 309t
Plasmapheresis, transfusion therapy, pretransfusion testing, 308–310, 309t
Plasma products, transfusion therapy, 304–306
Plasmaproliferative disorders, specimen allocation for, 269t
Plasminogen activator inhibitor-1 (PAI-1), thrombosis due to, 192
Plasminogen deficiency, thrombosis due to, 191
Platelet(s)
  analysis of, in laboratory hematology, 265–266
  biology of, 241–243, 242f
  collection and storage of, 298–299
    clinical case, 299
  disorders of, number and function-related, 241–262. See also Platelet function disorders
  function of, in hemostasis, 242–243, 242f
  production of, normal, 243
  single-donor, 298
  structure of, 241
  transfusion therapy, 297–303. See also Platelet transfusion
Platelet activation, in hemostatic process, 217, 218f
Platelet adhesion disorders, 255, 255t
Platelet aggregation disorders, 255, 255t
Platelet antibodies, assays for, in acquired thrombocytopenia testing, 285
Platelet function
  defects of, inherited, treatment of, 257–258
  drugs inhibiting, 258t, 259–260
Platelet function analyzer (PFA)
  in excessive bleeding evaluation, 219
  in platelet function disorders evaluation, 221
Platelet function disorders, 220–223, 254–260
  acquired, 258–260, 258t
  causes of, 4–5
  clinical case, 254

clinical presentation of, 221
described, 254
diagnosis of, 221–222
gaps in knowledge, 223
inherited, 254–258, 255t
    Bernard-Soulier syndrome, 255, 255t
    Glanzmann thrombasthenia, 255–256, 255t
    platelet adhesion disorders, 255, 255t
    platelet aggregation disorders, 255, 255t
    platelet procoagulant activities disorders, 255t, 257
    platelet secretion disorders, 255t, 256–257
    signal transduction disorders, 255t, 256–257
    SPD, 255t, 256–257
myeloproliferative disorders, 258–260, 258t
outcomes of, 223
pathophysiology of, 220
prognosis of, 223
treatment of, 222–223
Platelet function tests, 283–285, 284f
Platelet growth factors, 85–87
    IL-11, 86–87
    TPO, 85–86
Platelet number, regulation of, 243
Platelet procoagulant activities, disorders of, 255t, 257
Platelet products, characteristics and indications for, 296t
Platelet secretion, disorders of, 255t, 256–257
Platelet transfusion, 297–303
    dose, 301
    HLA system, 297–298, 298t
    HPAs, 298
    infectious complications of, 300, 301t
    procedure, 300–303, 301t
    product selection, 300–301, 301t
    prophylactic, 300
    refractoriness of, diagnosis and management of, 301
Platelet transfusion therapy, 303
PLL. *See* Prolymphocytic leukemia (PLL)
PMBCL. *See* Primary mediastinal (thymic) large B-cell lymphoma (PMBCL)
PMF. *See* Primary myelofibrosis (PMF)
Pneumonia(s), G-CSF in, 79
PNH. *See* Paroxysmal nocturnal hemoglobinuria (PNH)
POEMS (polyneuropathy, organomegaly, endocrinopathy monoclonal gammopathy, and skin changes) syndrome, 598, 598t
Polyadenylation, 3
    defined, 22
Polycythemia vera (PV), 190, 414–425
    absolute vs. relative, 416–417, 417t
    ambiguous cases, 419
    AML in, treatment of, 424
    biologic abnormalities of, 415–416
    clinical case, 414
    clinical features of, 416, 416t
    clonality of, 415

course/prognosis of, 420–421
described, 415
diagnostic criteria for, 419
differential diagnosis of, 416–419, 417t, 418t
familial polycythemic states, 418–419
histopathologic features of, 419–420, 420f
JAK2 mutations, 415
laboratory features of, 419–420, 420f
leukemic transformation in, 420–421
molecular testing for, 419
pathobiology of, 415–416
pregnancy with, 424
primary vs. secondary, 417–418, 418t
thrombohemorrhagic risk associated with, 421, 421t
treatment of, 421–424
    acute thrombosis–related, 423
    cytoreductive therapy in, 423–424
    HSCT in, 424
    phlebotomy in, 421–422, 422f, 422t
    symptomatic therapy in, 422–423
    thromboprophylaxis in, 422–423
Polymerase chain reaction (PCR)
    in germline mutations screening, 14–15, 14f
    in laboratory hematology, 270, 272
    molecular studies–related, 10–11, 10f
    quantitative, 11
        defined, 22
    real-time, 11
        defined, 22
    reverse transcriptase, 11
Polymorphism, defined, 22
Porphyria(s), 101–107
    acute, 103–105, 104f
        AIP, 103
        ALA dehydratase deficiency, 103
        clinical features of, 103–104
        diagnostic algorithm for, 104–105, 104f
        hereditary coproporphyria, 103
        metabolic effects in, 103
        treatment of, 105
        variegate porphyria, 103
    acute intermittent, 103
    clinical case, 101, 107
    cutaneous, 105–107, 105f
    described, 101–102
    erythropoietic, congenital, 106–107
    genetic, clinical, and biochemical features of, 102t
    nonacute, 105–107, 105f
    variegate, 103
Porphyria cutanea tarda, 105–106, 105f
Porphyric syndromes, 101–102, 102f
Portal vein thrombosis, 208
Positron emission tomography (PET), in lymphoma therapy assessment, 520, 520t
Postoperative bleeding, consultative risk assessment for, 32
Postoperative thrombosis, consultative risk assessment for, 32–34, 33t, 35t
Postthrombotic syndrome, 205–206, 206f
Posttransfusion purpura (PTP), 298

Posttransplantation erythrocytosis, consultative hematology for, 40
Posttransplantation lymphoproliferative disorders (PTLDs)
    consultative hematology for, 40–41, 41t
    HSCT and, 366
    WHO classification of, 41, 41t
Prader-Willi syndrome
    mechanisms of, 3
    uniparental disomy in, 3
Prasugrel, 196
Precision, defined, 263
Precursor B-cell/T-cell ALL
    in adults
        beyond CR1, treatment of, allo-SCT in, 502–503
        treatment of
            allo-SCT in, 501–502
            CNS prophylaxis–related, 499–500
            induction phase, 498
            intensification (consolidation) therapy in, 499
            maintenance therapy in, 500
            novel therapies in, 503
            relapse-related, 502
            risk-directed, 500
    in children, treatment of, 494–498
        CNS-directed, 496
        intensification (consolidation) therapy in, 495
        maintenance therapy in, 495–496
        relapse-related, 496–497
        remission induction in, 494–495
        SCT in, 496
        targeted therapies in, 497
Predictive value, defined, 263
Pregnancy
    consultative hematology during, 42–52
        anemia, 42–43
        artificial heart valves, 49–50
        clinical case, 42
        hematologic malignancies, 50–52
        thrombocytopenia, 43–45, 43t
        thromboembolism, 46–49, 47t–48t, 50t, 51t
        thrombophilia, 46–49, 47t–48t, 50t, 51t
        von Willebrand disease, 45–46
    ET during, 430
    PV and, 424
    sickle cell disease in, 146–147
Prematurity, anemia of, 81
Premessenger RNA (premRNA), 3
    defined, 22
premRNA. *See* Premessenger RNA (premRNA)
Preterm infants, anemia in, erythropoietin for, 81
Pretransfusion testing, 306–308, 306t
    ABO/Rh(D) typing, 306–307, 306t
    antibody screen and specificity identification, 307–308
    crossmatching, 308
Primaquine, hemolytic anemias due to, 171
Primary autoimmune neutropenia, 378t, 379t, 382
Primary CNS lymphoma (PCNSL), 540

Primary cutaneous aggressive epidermotropic CD8+ T-cell lymphoma, 539
Primary cutaneous ALCL, 536
Primary cutaneous CD4+ small/medium T-cell lymphoma, 536
Primary cutaneous PTCL, 539
Primary immune deficiencies (PIDs), lymphoproliferative disorders associated with, 539
Primary mediastinal (thymic) large B-cell lymphoma (PMBCL), 532
Primary myelofibrosis (PMF), 431–437
   clinical case, 431
   clinical features of, 432, 432t, 434, 434f
   course/prognosis of, 434–435, 435t
   diagnosis of, 432–433, 433t
   differential diagnosis of, 433, 433t
   histopathologic features of, 434, 434f
   incidence of, 431
   laboratory features of, 433, 433t
   morphologic features of, 434, 434f
   pathobiology of, 431
   treatment of, 435–437
     anemia-related, 435–436
     general considerations in, 435
     newer agents in, 436
     SCT in, 436–437
     splenomegaly-related, 436
Primary Rituximab and Maintenance (PRIMA) study, 524
Primitive erythropoiesis, 335
Probe(s), defined, 6, 22
Prognostic scoring system, for Hodgkin lymphoma, 543, 543t
Prolymphocytic leukemia (PLL), 573
   CLL transformation to, 572
Promoter, defined, 22
Promoter region, 4
Protein(s). *See also* Protein C deficiency; Protein S deficiency
   C, described, 183
   HFE, 94–95
   in iron homeostasis, 93–95, 95t
   Kx, 294
Protein C deficiency
   assays for, in acquired thrombocytopenia testing, 287
   general information, 183
   management of, 184
   pediatric considerations, 184
   prevalence of, 183
   risk for thrombosis, 183–184
   testing for, 183, 183t, 184t
   thrombophilia due to, 183–184, 183t, 184t
Protein S deficiency
   assays for, in acquired thrombocytopenia testing, 287–288
   general information, 184–185
   management of, 185
   pediatric considerations, 185–186
   prevalence of, 185
   risk for thrombosis, 185
   testing for, 183t, 184t, 185
   thrombophilia due to, 183t, 184–186, 184t

Proteomics, molecular studies–related, 12
Prothrombin 20210 mutation, thrombophilia due to, 182–183, 184t
Prothrombin time (PT)
   aPTT and, combined abnormalities of, in laboratory hematology, 279, 279f
   in laboratory hematology, 277, 277f
Protoporphyria, erythropoietic, 106
Protozoal infections, transfusion-related, 323–324
Psychosocial factors, HSCT effects on, 366
PT. *See* Prothrombin time (PT)
PTCLs. *See* Peripheral T-cell lymphomas (PTCLs)
PTLDs. *See* Posttransplantation lymphoproliferative disorders (PTLDs)
PTP. *See* Posttransfusion purpura (PTP)
Pulmonary embolism (PE)
   diagnosis of, 204
   postthrombotic syndrome, 205–206, 206f
   prevention of, 203, 203t
   symptoms of, 203–204
   treatment of, acute, 204–205
Pulmonary hypertension
   chronic thromboembolic, 206
   VTE and, 206
Pulmonary toxicity, allogeneic HSCT and, 350–351
Pure red cell aplasia, underproduction anemias due to, 125–127, 125f, 125t, 126f
Purine, defined, 1, 22
Purine analogs, for CLL, 565–567, 565t, 567t
   chemoimmunotherapy with, 566
PV. *See* Polycythemia vera (PV)
Pyrimidine, defined, 1, 22
Pyrimidine-5'-nucleotide deficiency, 159
Pyropoikilocytosis, hereditary, 153f, 154–156
Pyruvate kinase deficiency, 157, 157f

Q
Quality of life, CLL effects on, 572–573
Quantitative PCR, 11
   defined, 22
Quebec platelet disorder, 255t, 257

R
RA. *See* Rheumatoid arthritis (RA)
Radioimmunotherapy, for follicular lymphoma
   advanced-stage, 524
   relapsed and refractory, 524
RBCs. *See* Red blood cell(s) (RBCs)
Real-time PCR, 11
   defined, 22
Reanneal, defined, 22
Recombinant FVIIa (rFVIIa), for platelet function disorders, 222–223
Red blood cell(s) (RBCs)

   abnormalities of
     extrinsic, hemolysis due to, 160–175
     in laboratory hematology, 266–267, 266t
   ABO system, 291–292, 293t
   carbohydrate antigen systems, 293t, 295
   characteristics of, 296t
   clinical case, 297
   collection and storage in, 295
   Duffy antigen system, transfusion therapy, 293–294, 293t
   hemoglobin level in, 296
   immune injury to, hemolytic anemia due to, 160–165, 161t
   indications for, 296t
   intrinsic abnormalities of, hemolysis due to, 134–159
   Kell antigen system, 293–294, 293t
   Kidd antigen system, transfusion therapy, 293–294, 293t
   maturation of, factors in, 109
   MNSs antigen systems, 293–294, 293t
   nucleated, in laboratory hematology, 265
   P antigen system, 293t, 295
   parasitic infestation of, hemolytic anemias due to, 173–174, 173f, 174f
   Rh system, 292–293, 293t
   transfusion therapy, 291–297, 293t
   procedure, 295–297, 296t
   for sickle cell disease, 145–146
Red blood cell (RBC) enzymes, abnormalities of, 156–159
Red blood cell (RBC) mass, 109
Red blood cell (RBC) membrane
   abnormalities of, 151–156
     hereditary elliptocytosis, 153f, 154–156
     hereditary pyropoikilocytosis, 153f, 154–156
     hereditary spherocytosis, 152–154, 152t, 153f
     types of, 151
   injuries of, bacterial-related, hemolytic anemias due to, 172–173
   protein composition and assembly in, 151–152, 151f
Reduced-intensity conditioning regimens, in CML management, 404
Reference ranges, predictive, 263
Refractory cytopenia of childhood, 462
Renal failure, chronic
   darbepoetin alfa for, 84
   erythropoietin in, 80–81
Renal vein thrombosis, 209
Reptilase time, in laboratory hematology, 280
Restriction endonucleases, 6, 7f
   defined, 22
Restriction fragment length polymorphism (RFLP), 7–8
   defined, 22
Reticulocyte counts, in laboratory hematology, 265
Retinal vein thrombosis, 209–210
Retrovirus(es), 15

AIDS-related, transfusion therapy and, 324
  defined, 23
Reverse transcriptase, defined, 23
Reverse transcriptase polymerase chain reaction (RT-PCR), 11
  defined, 23
Reverse transcriptase reaction, 17
Revised European-American Lymphoma (REAL) classification, of NHLs, 516
RFLP. See Restriction fragment length polymorphism (RFLP)
rFVIIa. See Recombinant FVIIa (rFVIIa)
Rheumatoid arthritis (RA), neutropenia and, 378t, 382
Rh deficiency (null) syndrome, 156
Rh system, transfusion therapy, 292–293, 293t
Ribavirin, hemolytic anemias due to, 171
Ribosome(s), 4
  defined, 23
Richter transformation, CLL transformation to, 572
RISC (RNA-induced silencing complex), 5, 5f
  defined, 23
Rituximab
  for advanced-stage DLBCL, 529–530
  for CLL, 565–566, 565t
  for follicular lymphoma
    advanced-stage, 523–524
    relapsed and refractory, 524
Rivaroxaban, 202
RNA
  premessenger, defined, 22
  transfer, 4
RNA interference therapy, antisense and, DNA technology applications to, 18–19
RNA polymerase II, 3
  defined, 23
Romiplostim, in MDS management, 470
RT-PCR. See Reverse transcriptase polymerase chain reaction (RT-PCR)

S
Sarcoma(s), Ewing, in children, HSCT for, 365
Sargramostim
  FDA-approved indications for, 75, 75t
  in MDS management, 470
Schistocyte(s), 169, 169f
Schwachman-Diamond syndrome (SDS), 378t, 379t, 381
SCPTCL. See Subcutaneous panniculitis-like T-cell lymphoma (SCPTCL)
Screening coagulation testing, in laboratory hematology, 275–282, 276f–279f, 282t, 283f, 284f
SCT. See Stem cell transplantation (SCT)
SDPs. See Single-donor platelets (SDPs)
SDS. See Schwachman-Diamond syndrome (SDS)
Secondary autoimmune neutropenia, 378t, 382

SEER. See Surveillance, Epidemiology, and End Results (SEER; 2008)
Sensitivity, defined, 263
Sepsis(es), clostridial, hemolytic anemias due to, 172
Sequence-based studies, molecular studies–related(s), 10
Serum monoclonal protein, defined, 582t
Severe chronic neutropenia, prevention of, G-CSF and GM-CSF in, 78–79
Severe Chronic Neutropenia International Registry, 79
Severe congenital neutropenia, 378–380, 378t, 379t
Sézary syndrome, 535–536
Shunt(s), hexose-monophosphate, abnormalities of, 157–159, 158t, 159f
Shwachman-Bodian-Diamond syndrome, 378t, 379t, 381
Sickle cell disease, 140–147
  acute chest syndrome and, 146
  anemia in, acute exacerbations of, causes of, 143, 143f
  clinical case, 140, 147
  clinical manifestations of, 142–144, 143t, 144f
  CNS disease and, 146
  course of, 147
  described, 140–141, 141f
  HSCT for, 363
  laboratory features of, 141t, 142
  pathophysiology of, 141–142, 141t
  pregnancy and, 146–147
  randomized clinical trials in, 144t
  transfusion therapy, 319–320
  treatment of, 144–146, 144t
    for painful episodes, 145
    preventive interventions in, 144–145
    RBC transfusion in, 145–146
Sickle cell syndromes, described, 140
Sickle-hemoglobin C disease, 144, 144f
Signal transduction, disorders of, 255t, 256–257
Silencer(s), 4
  defined, 23
Single-donor platelets (SDPs), 298
Single nucleotide polymorphism(s) (SNPs), 5
  defined, 23
  tag, 6
  defined, 23
Single nucleotide polymorphism (SNP) chips, molecular studies–related, 9
siRNAs. See Small interfering RNAs (siRNAs)
  defined, 23
Sjögren syndrome, neutropenia and, 378t, 382
SLE. See Systemic lupus erythematosus (SLE)
Small interfering RNAs (siRNAs), 5
SMM. See Smoldering multiple myeloma (SMM)
Smoldering multiple myeloma (SMM). See also Multiple myeloma (MM)

defined, 582t
staging and prognostic factors in, 590–591, 590t
treatment of, 591–597, 592t
SNPs. See Single nucleotide polymorphism(s) (SNPs)
Solid organ transplantation, hematologic complications of, consultation for, 40–42, 41t
Solid tumors
  in children, HSCT for, 364–365
  HSCT for, 364–365
Solitary plasmacytoma, defined, 582t
Somatic (acquired) mutations, DNA technology applications to, 15–17, 16f
Southern blot analysis, 6, 15, 16f
  defined, 23
  in laboratory hematology, 270
Southwest Oncology Group (SWOG), 523–524
SPD. See Storage pool deficiency (SPD)
Specificity, defined, 263
Specificity identification, transfusion therapy in, pretransfusion testing, 307–308
Spherocytosis, hereditary, 152–154, 152t, 153f. See also Hereditary spherocytosis
Spider bites, hemolytic anemias due to, 171–172
Splanchnic vein thrombosis, 190
Spleen colony-forming unit (CFU-S) assay, 331, 332f
Splenectomy, persistent primary ITP after, 246
Splenic MZLs, 527
Splenic sequestration, 252
Splenic vein thrombosis, 209
Splenomegaly
  causes of, 56, 56t
  consultative hematology for, 56–57, 56t
  PMF-related, 436
Splicing
  alternative, 3–4
    defined, 21
  defined, 23
Stain(s)
  cytochemical, in laboratory hematology, 267–268, 267t
  immunohistochemical, in laboratory hematology, 267t, 268
Stem cell factor, 87
  adverse effects of, 87
  in peripheral blood stem cells mobilization, 87
Stem cell transplantation (SCT), 331–371. See also Hematopoietic stem cell transplantation (HSCT)
  allogeneic. See Allogeneic stem cell transplantation (allo-SCT)
  for CML, 403–404
  DNA technology applications to, 18
  hematopoietic. See Hematopoietic stem cell transplantation (HSCT)
  for MM, initial therapy for patients eligible for, 591–592

for PMF, 436–437
for precursor B-cell/T-cell ALL, 496
for relapsed or refractory CLL, 570
Stent(s), venous, VTE and, 207
Stomatocytosis, 156, 156f
Storage pool deficiency (SPD), 255t, 256–257
acquired, 259
Stroke
childhood, 211–212
neonatal, defined, 211
prevention of, 211
Structural gene, 4
defined, 23
Subcutaneous panniculitis-like T-cell lymphoma (SCPTCL), 538
Sulfhemoglobinemia, 150
Superficial thrombophlebitis, 202–203
Surveillance, Epidemiology, and End Results (SEER; 2008), on CLL, 555
SWOG. See Southwest Oncology Group (SWOG)
Syngeneic autologous GVHD, 352
Syngeneic transplantation, 352
Systemic lupus erythematosus (SLE), neutropenia and, 378t, 382
Systemic mastocytosis, 407–410
classification of, 407, 408f, 409t
clinical features of, 407–408
course/prognosis of, 410
described, 407
diagnostic criteria for, 408, 409t
epidemiology of, 407
pathobiology of, 407
treatment of, 410

T
TAFI. See Thrombin-activatable fibrinolysis inhibitors (TAFI)
tag SNPs, 6
defined, 23
T cell(s), development of, 512
T-cell CLL, 574
T-cell large granular lymphocytic leukemia, 536
T-cell leukemias
adult, 536
chronic, 574
T-cell lymphomas
adult, 536
angioimmunoblastic, 537
enteropathy-associated, 538–539
hepatosplenic, 538
peripheral, 535–539
primary cutaneous aggressive epidermotropic CD8$^+$, 539
primary cutaneous CD4$^+$ small/medium, 536
subcutaneous panniculitis-like, 538
T-cell mutations, DNA technology applications to, 15
T-cell neoplasms, WHO classification of, 514, 515t
Termination codon, 4
defined, 23

Ternary complex mechanisms, 160–161, 161t
Thalassemia(s), 136–140
α, 138–140, 139f
ß, 136–138, 136f
in children, consultative hematology for, 63
clinical case, 136, 140
Thalassemia major, HSCT for, 362–363
Thalidomide
for MDS, 471
for MM
in newly diagnosed transplantation-eligible patients, 592–593
in non-transplantation-eligible patients, 594
relapsed or refractory, 595
Thrombasthenia, Glanzmann, 255–256, 255t
Thrombin-activatable fibrinolysis inhibitors (TAFI), thrombosis due to, 192
Thrombin inhibitors, 199
Thrombin time (TT), in laboratory hematology, 280
Thrombocytopenia
acquired, specialized testing for, 285–288
assays for platelet antibodies, 285
assays for thrombophilia, 286–288
assays for TTP and vWF cleaving protease, 286
for HIT, 285–286
amegakaryocytic, congenital, 444t, 450
autoimmune, transfusion therapy, 319
chemotherapy-induced
prevention of, IL-11 in, 86
TPO for, 86
consumptive, transfusion therapy, 319
in critically ill patients, 253–254
drug-induced, 246–248. See also Drug-induced thrombocytopenia (DITP)
essential, 425–430. See also Essential thrombocytopenia (ET)
familial, 252–253, 253f
heparin-induced, 197–198, 248–250, 248t, 249f. See also Heparin-induced thrombocytopenia (HIT)
in ICU
consultative hematology in, 36–39
DIC-related, 37–38
drug-related, 37
infection-related, 37–38
diagnosis of, 36–37, 36t
prevalence of, 36
immune, 243–246. See also Immune thrombocytopenia (ITP)
immune causes of, 243–250
with infection, 253
massive transfusion-induced, in ICU, consultative hematology in, 38
mild, consultative hematology for, 52–53
in newborns, consultative hematology for, 60–61
nonimmune causes of, 250–254, 251f–253f

during pregnancy, consultative hematology for, 43–45, 43t
Thrombocytosis, essential, 190
Thromboembolism
arterial, 210–212, 210t. See also Arterial thromboembolism
during pregnancy, consultative hematology for, 46–49, 47t–48t, 50t, 51t
prophylaxis for, consultative risk assessment for, 32–33, 33t, 34t
venous, unproked, causes of, 179, 180, 180f
Thrombolytic agents, 202
Thrombophilia(s), 179–215. See also specific types, e.g., Factor V Leiden
antithrombin deficiency, 184t, 186–187
APLA syndrome, 184t, 187–188, 187f
assays for, in acquired thrombocytopenia testing, 286–288
factor VIII elevation, 188–189
fibrinolysis abnormalities and, 191–192, 191f
FVL, 180–182, 181f, 184t
homocystinuria, 189, 190f
JAK2 V617F mutation, 190
MPDs, 190
MTHFR, 189, 190f
during pregnancy, consultative hematology for, 46–49, 47t–48t, 50t, 51t
protein C deficiency, 183–184, 183t, 184t
protein S deficiency, 183t, 184–186, 184t
prothrombin 20210 mutation, 182–183, 184t
splanchnic vein thrombosis, 190
testing for, 193–195, 193t–195t
adult hematologist's approach to, 194, 194t, 195t
author's approach to, 194–195, 194t, 195t
candidates for, 193–194, 193t
consensus guidelines, 193
pediatric hematologist's approach to, 194–195
reasons for or against, 193–194, 193t
results of
acute thrombosis, heparin, and vitamin K antagonists effects on, 183, 184t
interpretation of, 195
patient education related to, 195
types of, 180–195
Thrombophlebitis, superficial, 202–203
Thrombopoietin (TPO), 85–86
for chemotherapy-induced thrombocytopenia, 86
thrombopoietin receptor c-Mpl and, 243
Thrombopoietin (TPO) receptor c-Mpl, thrombopoietin and, 243
Thrombosis(es), 179–215
acute, PV-related, treatment of, 423–424
antithrombin deficiency and, 186
antithrombotic drugs for, 195–202. See also Antithrombotic drugs
APLA syndrome and, 188

arterial, in absence of arteriosclerosis, 210–211, 210t
catheter-related, 207
causes of, 179–180, 180f
cerebral and sinus vein, 209
cerebral sinovenous, 209
deep vein. *See* Deep vein thrombosis (DVT)
defined, 179
drugs for, 195–202. *See also specific drugs and* Antithrombotic drugs
FVL and, 181–182
hepatic vein, 207–208
laboratory hematology for, 274–285
lipoprotein(a) and, 192
mesenteric vein, 208
in newborns, consultative hematology for, 61–62
PAI-1 and, 192
pathophysiology of, 179–180, 180f
plasminogen deficiency and, 191
in PNH, 459
portal vein, 208
postoperative, consultative risk assessment for, 32–34, 33t, 35t
protein C deficiency and, 183–184
protein S deficiency and, 185
prothrombin 20210 mutation and, 182
renal vein, 209
retinal vein, 209–210
risk factors for, threshold model of, 179, 180f
TAFI and, 192
tPA and, 191–192
venous. *See* Venous thrombosis(es)
Thrombotic microangiopathy(ies) (TMAs), 250–252, 251f, 252f
allogeneic HSCT and, 351
clinical features of, 250
diagnosis of, 251–252, 252f
management of, 252
pathogenesis of, 250–251, 251f
Thrombotic thrombocytopenic purpura (TTP), 250–252, 251f, 252f
assays for, in acquired thrombocytopenia testing, 286
clinical features of, 250
diagnosis of, 251–252, 252f
management of, 252
pathogenesis of, 250–251, 251f
Thrombotic thrombocytopenic purpura–hemolytic uremic syndrome (TTP-HUS)
fragmentation hemolysis due to, 170
during pregnancy, consultative hematology for, 43t, 45
thrombocytopenia in ICU due to, consultative hematology in, 38–39
Ticlopidine, 196
Tirofiban, 197
Tissue histiocytes, in myeloid disorders, 375–376
Tissue plasminogen activator (tPA), thrombosis due to, 191–192
TK inhibitors, second-generation, for CML, 402–403

TMAs. *See* Thrombotic microangiopathy(ies) (TMAs)
tPA. *See* Tissue plasminogen activator (tPA)
TPO. *See* Thrombopoietin (TPO)
Trace element deficiencies, anemia associated with, 120–121, 121f
TRALI. *See* Transfusion-related acute lung injury (TRALI)
trans-acting factor, 4–5
defined, 23
Transcription
defined, 23
genetic information flow and, 2f, 3–4
Transcription factors, 4–5
defined, 23
Transferrin-bound iron, 95
Transfer RNAs (tRNAs), 4
defined, 23
Transfusion(s), 291–329. *See also* Transfusion therapy; *specific types, e.g.,* Red blood cell(s) (RBCs)
AHA, 318–319
apheresis, 308–312, 309t
aplastic anemia, 312, 321, 455–456
autoimmune thrombocytopenia, 319
blood substitutes, 326–327
during cardiopulmonary surgery, 321
consumptive thrombocytopenia, 319
exchange, 310
granulocyte, 303–304
in HSCT candidates, 312–315, 314t
massive, 320–321
procedures and indications for, 320–321
platelet, 297–303. *See also* Platelet transfusion
RBC, 291–297, 293t
thrombocytopenia in ICU due to, consultative hematology in, 38
Transfusion-related acute lung injury (TRALI), 323
Transfusion therapy. *See also* Transfusion(s)
consultative hematology in, 40
consultative risk assessment for, 31–32
in MDS management, 469
pediatric issues related to, 315–319
congenital heart surgery and, 316–317
ECMO and, 316–317
immune disorders, 317–318
in utero transfusion, 315
neonatal component therapy, 316
neonatal exchange transfusion, 315
neonatal transfusion, 316–317
pretransfusion testing, 306–308, 306t
risks associated with, 321–327
AIDS-related retrovirus, 324
allergic reactions, 322–323
bacterial/protozoal transmission, 323–324
CMV, 325
febrile reactions, 322
GVHD, 325–326
hemolytic reactions
acute, 321–322
delayed, 322

hepatitis, 324
HTLVs, 324
infectious complications, 323–325
parvovirus B19, 325
reduction strategies, 326–327
TRALI, 323
West Nile virus, 325
sickle cell disease, 319–320
in special clinical settings, 312–321
Transgenic mice
defined, 23
molecular studies–related, 12–13
Translation
defined, 23
genetic information flow and, 2f, 4
Translocation(s)
chromosomoal, in NHLs, 513, 513t
cryptic, in pediatric ALL identification, 15
Translocation breakpoint, 9
defined, 23
Transplantation(s)
allogeneic
for CML, 403–405
mobilization of peripheral blood stem cells from normal donors for, G-CSF and GM-CSF in, 78
bone marrow. *See* Bone marrow transplantation; Hematopoietic stem cell transplantation (HSCT)
hematopoietic stem cell. *See* Hematopoietic stem cell transplantation (HSCT)
neutrophil recovery after, mobilization of autologous peripheral blood stem cells and enhancement in, G-CSF and GM-CSF in, 77–78
solid organ, hematologic complications of, consultation for, 40–42, 41t
stem cell. *See* Stem cell transplantation (SCT)
syngeneic, 352
Transplantation assays, stem cell–related, 332
tRNAs. *See* Transfer RNAs
Trousseau syndrome, 203
TT. *See* Thrombin time (TT)
TTP. *See* Thrombotic thrombocytopenic purpura (TTP)
TTP-HUS. *See* Thrombotic thrombocytopenic purpura–hemolytic uremic syndrome (TTP-HUS)
Tumor(s), solid
in children, HSCT for, 364–365
HSCT for, 364–365

U
Underproduction anemias
acquired, 109–132. *See also* Megaloblastic anemias; *specific anemias, e.g.,* Cobalamin (vitamin B_{12} deficiency
anemia of chronic disease/inflammation, 114–115
causes of, 109–110, 110t

iron deficiency anemia, 110–114, 111t, 112f, 113t
megaloblastic anemias, 115–121
nutritional deficiencies and, 110–115, 111t, 112f, 113t
organ dysfunction and, 121–125, 122f, 124f
complex/multifactorial, 128–130, 129t
marrow failure states leading to, 125–127, 125f, 125t, 126f
secondary to marrow infiltration or abnormalities in marrow microenvironment, 127–128, 128f
Unfractionated heparin, 198
Uniparental disomy, 3
defined, 23
Unstable hemoglobulin, 148–149
Upper extremity(ies), DVT of, 207
Uremia, platelet function–related, 258t, 259

V
Vaccine(s), tumor, for follicular lymphoma, 525–526
Value(s)
hematologic, for newborns, 58t
predictive, defined, 263
Variegate porphyria, 103
Vascular endothelial growth factor (VEGF), in molecular pathogenesis of MM, 587, 587f, 588f
VEGF. See Vascular endothelial growth factor (VEGF)
Venoocclusive disease/sinusoidal obstruction syndrome (VOD/SOS), allogeneic HSCT and, 349–350
Venous stents, VTE and, 207
Venous thromboembolism (VTE), 202–210
cancer and, 192
described, 202
diagnosis of, 204
estrogen contraceptives and, 192–193
family history of, 192
inferior vena cava filters in, 206–207
prevalence of, 202
prevention of, 203, 203t
pulmonary hypertension due to, 206
recurrence of, risk factors for, 205–206, 206f
superficial thrombophlebitis, 202–203
symptoms of, 203–204
treatment of
acute, 204–205
anticoagulants in, 205, 205t
unprovoked, causes of, 179, 180, 180f
venous stents in, 207
Venous thrombosis(es)
causes of, 179, 180, 180f
hepatic, 207–208
mesenteric, 208
portal, 208
renal, 209
retinal, 209–210
splanchnic, 190
splenic, 209
unusual, 207–210
Vitamin K antagonists (VKAs), 200–201, 200f, 201t, 202t
classes of, 200–201
for elevated INRs and bleeding, 201, 201t
mechanism of action of, 200, 200f
monitoring and dose requirement, 200
new agents in development, 201–202
pediatric considerations, 201
periprocedural interruption of, 201, 202t
VKAs. See Vitamin K antagonists (VKAs)
VOD/SOS. See Venoocclusive disease/sinusoidal obstruction syndrome (VOD/SOS)
von Willebrand disease, 223–227, 255t
causes of, 224, 224t
classification of, 224, 224t
clinical presentation of, 224–225
diagnosis of, 224t, 225, 226f
gaps in knowledge, 226–227
pathophysiology of, 223–224
during pregnancy, consultative hematology for, 45–46
treatment of, 225–226
von Willebrand factor (vWF) assays, in laboratory hematology, 281–282, 282t, 283f, 284f
von Willebrand factor (vWF) cleaving protease, assays for, in acquired thrombocytopenia testing, 286
VTE. See Venous thromboembolism (VTE)
vWF assays. See von Willebrand factor (vWF) assays

W
Waldenström macroglobulinemia, 527–528, 598–599, 598t
Warfarin, 200–201
excessive dosing of, consultative risk assessment for, 34, 35t
Watson–Crick base pairing, 1, 5
Western blotting
defined, 23
described, 8
West Nile virus, transfusion therapy and, 325
WHIM (warts, hypogammaglobulinemia, infections, and myelokathexis) syndrome, 378t, 379t, 381
WHO. See World Health Organization (WHO)
WHO Classification of Tumors of Hematopoietic and Lymphoid Tissues, 514
World Health Organization (WHO) classification
AML subtypes, 476, 476t, 477t
B- and T-cell neoplasms, 514, 515t
NHLs, 516
PTLDs, 41, 41t

X
Ximelagatran, 202

Y
Young adults, ALL in, treatment of, 501

Z
ZAP-70, in assessing high-risk subgroups of patients with CLL, 561t, 562
Zinc-finger, 4–5
defined, 23